BREASTFEEDING KINETICS

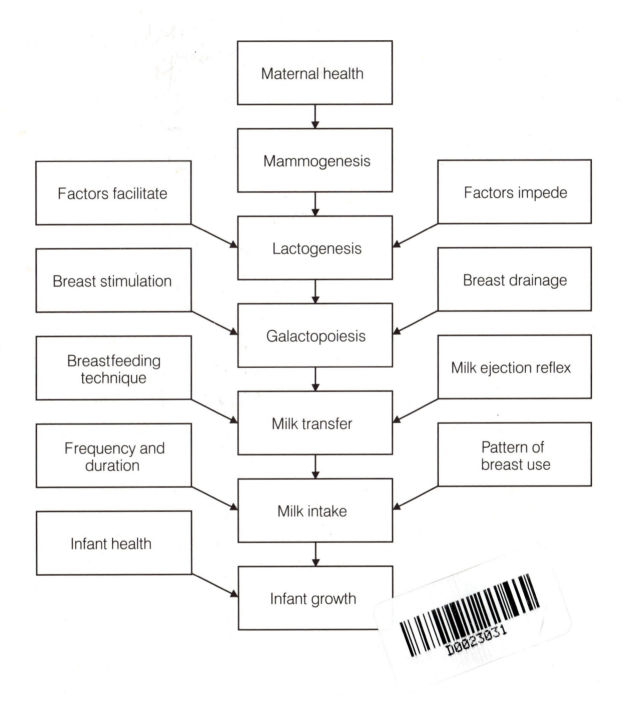

Source: Livingstone, V.: Problem-Solving Formula for Failure to Thrive in Breast-fed Infants, *Canadian Family Physician* 36:1542, 1990.

Breastfeeding and Human Lactation

The Jones and Bartlett Series in Nursing

Adult Emergency Nursing Procedures, Proehl

Basic Steps in Planning Nursing Research, Third Edition, Brink/Wood

Bone Marrow Transplantation, Whedon

Cancer Chemotherapy: A Nursing Process Approach, Barton Burke et al.

Cancer Nursing: Principles and Practice, Second Edition, Groenwald et al.

Chemotherapy Care Plans, Barton Burke

A Clinical Manual for Nursing Assistants, McClelland/Kaspar

Children's Nutrition, Lifshitz/Finch/Lifshitz

Chronic Illness: Impact and Intervention, Second Edition, Lubkin

Clinical Nursing Procedures, Belland/Wells

A Comprehensive Curriculum for Trauma Nursing, Bayley/Turcke

Comprehensive Maternity Nursing, Second Edition, Auvenshine/Enriquez

Concepts in Oxygenation, Ahrens/Rutherford

Critical Care Review, Wright/Shelton

Emergency Care of Children, Thompson

Essential Medical Terminology, Stanfield

Family Life: Process and Practice, Janosik/Green

Fundamentals of Nursing with Clinical Procedures, Second Edition, Sundberg

1991-1992 Handbook of Intravenous Medications, Nentwich

Handbook of Oncology Nursing, Johnson/Gross

Health Assessment in Nursing Practice, Third Edition, Grimes/Burns

Health and Wellness, Fourth Edition, Edlin/Golanty

Healthy People 2000, U.S. Department of Health & Human Services

Human Development: A Life-Span Approach, Fourth Edition, Freiberg

Instruments for Clinical Nursing Research, Oncology Nursing Society

Intravenous Therapy, Nentwich

Introduction to the Health Professions, Stanfield

Introduction to Human Disease, Third Edition, Crowley

Journal of Perinatal Education, ASPO

Management and Leadership for Nurse Managers, Swansburg

Management of Spinal Cord Injury, Second Edition, Zejdlik

Math for Health Professionals, Third Edition, Whisler

Medical Terminology, Stanfield

Memory Bank for Chemotherapy, Preston

Memory Bank for IVs, Second Edition, Weinstein

Memory Bank for Medications, Second Edition, Kostin/Evans

Mental Health and Psychiatric Nursing: A Caring Approach, Davies/Janosik

The Nation's Health, Third Edition, Lee/Estes

Nursing and the Disabled: Across the Lifespan, Fraley

Nursing Assessment: A Multidimensional Approach, Third Edition, Bellack/Edlund

Nursing Diagnosis Care Plans for Diagnosis-Related Groups, Neal/Paquette/Mirch

Nursing Management of Children, Servonsky/Opas

Nursing Pharmacology, Second Edition, Wallace/Wardell

Nursing Research: A Quantitative and Qualitative Approach, Roberts/Burke

Nutrition and Diet Therapy: Self-Instructional Modules, Second Edition, Stanfield

Pediatric Emergency Nursing Procedures, Bernardo/Bove

Perioperative Nursing Care, Fairchild

Perioperative Patient Care, Second Edition, Kneedler/Dodge

A Practical Guide to Breastfeeding, Riordan

Psychiatric Mental Health Nursing, Second Edition, Janosik/Davies

Ready Reference of Common Emergency and Prehospital Drugs, Cummings

Ready Reference for Critical Care, Strawn

The Research Process in Nursing, Third Edition, Dempsey/Dempsey

Understanding/Responding, Second Edition, Long/Prophit

Writing a Succesful Grant Application, Second Edition, Reif-Lehrer

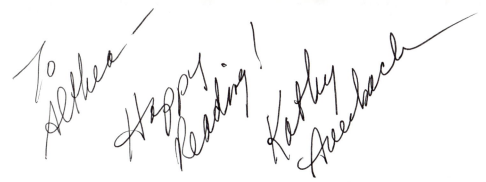

Breastfeeding and Human Lactation

Jan Riordan, EdD, RN, IBCLC

Professor of Nursing, Kansas Newman College
Nurse Researcher, St. Joseph Medical Center
Wichita, Kansas

Kathleen G. Auerbach, PhD, IBCLC

Complemental Faculty Member
Department of Maternal-Child Nursing
Rush-Presbyterian-St Luke's Medical Center
Chicago, Illinois
Lactation Consultant and Researcher (Private Practice)
Homewood, Illinois

JONES AND BARTLETT PUBLISHERS
BOSTON   LONDON

Editorial, Sales, and Customer Service Offices

Jones and Bartlett Publishers
One Exeter Plaza
Boston, MA 02116
1-617-859-3900
1-800-832-0034

Jones and Bartlett Publishers International
P O Box 1498
London W6 7RS
England

Library of Congress Cataloging-in-Publication Data

Breastfeeding and human lactation / edited by Jan Riordan and Kathleen
  G. Auerbach.
    p.   cm.
   Includes bibliographical references and index.
   ISBN 0–86720–343–9
   1. Breast feeding. I. Riordan, Jan. II. Auerbach, Kathleen G.
   [DNLM: 1. Breast Feeding. 2. Infant Nutrition. 3. Lactation.
4. Milk, Human.   WS 125 B8293]
RJ216.B775   1993
649′.33—dc20
DNLM/DLC
for Library of Congress   92–49067
                                                        CIP

Section Cover Photo Credits:
p. 1. Sergei Vasiliev; p. 79. WHO/PAHO (19834); p. 179. Sergei Vasiliev;
p. 347. WHO (20532); p. 541. St. Joseph Medical Center.

Cover art: *Dakota Mother and Child* by Ioyan Mani. Courtesy of *Canadian Art Prints, Inc.*

Printed in the United States of America
97 96 95 94   10 9 8 7 6 5 4 3

We dedicate this book to the thousands
of breastfeeding women and their babies
around the globe who have taught us
and who continue to allow us to learn from them.

Contents

Preface

Since *A Practical Guide to Breastfeeding* was published in 1983, almost a decade ago, much has happened that affects breastfeeding. Not all of these events were positive. In 1983, U.S. breastfeeding rates were still climbing; now in 1992, fewer mothers in the U.S. are breastfeeding, despite the U.S. Surgeon General's goal that breastfeeding rates reach 75% by 1990. Formula sales, on the other hand, have tripled over the past 10 years and represent a major drain on government economies around the world. Fear of the spread of AIDS through breastfeeding has reduced the use of pooled, banked human milk; many milk banks have closed or expanded their services into other areas in order to survive. Governmental support for breastfeeding continues to be less than it should be, given its enormous importance.

Breastfeeding is health promotion in its purest form. Only a decade ago, the primary health benefit of breastfeeding was immunologic protection from gastrointestinal infection and disease. Indeed, some alternatives to breastfeeding have proven disastrous for babies. We now know that breastmilk reduces many other infections in the baby, as well as certain chronic diseases later in life and recognize that lactation also benefits mothers in both short- and long-term ways. For example, 10 years ago, we did not know that the lactating mother is at less risk for calcium depletion than the nonlactating, postpartum woman.

Other changes have occurred. The National Center for Health Statistics reported that there were 4.1 million live births in the United States during 1990, a jump of four percent from the previous year. The percentage of women employed outside the home was 33% in 1950. By 1990, this figure rose to 70% and 53% of women who are employed, either full- or part-time, have preschoolers. Because the traditional stay-at-home mother and her at-work husband make up only seven percent of the U.S. population, health care should develop care delivery systems for widely differing family patterns.

The length of a hospital stay after normal delivery has dropped from five days to two days or less in the United States. While such short stays mean that breastfeeding mothers and babies return home less likely to be exposed to hospital infections and to supplementary feedings, this brief time allows almost no opportunity for teaching. Mothers, still needing care themselves, return home to assume full-time child care before they feel physically able to do so.

A new profession—lactation consulting—has emerged. Since 1985, more than 2,000 health-care workers from 15 countries have been certified by the International Board of Lactation Consultants Examiners, Inc. Hundreds of hospitals now employ lactation consultants, an idea almost unheard of only a few years ago. The *Journal of Human Lactation,* edited by one of the authors of this textbook, is now a widely read and respected publication.

This book represents more than 50 years of the authors' combined clinical experiences. Why did we choose to write a large reference book on breastfeeding? It was time for a new book that brings together in a single resource both clinical techniques and research findings. The relationship between daily clinical practice and concepts is reciprocal—just as clinical practice improves as a result of research outcomes, so clinical observations point the way to research studies. This book identifies more than 2,000 research studies to support our clinical recommendations. Readers will note that many of the research studies discussed in this book give credence to information that observant clinicians have known for years.

Nearly every chapter in this book contains a section that focuses on the clinical implications of the information provided. And every chapter contains references deemed by the authors to be the most important from the vastly expanded basic research and clinical literature—with particular emphasis on those articles that have appeared since the mid-1980s. The color photographs on the end pages give readers visualizations of phenomena that are difficult to describe in words, but which must be recognized in clients.

The chapters in *Part One* set the stage on which the information in later chapters can be placed. This section focuses on "the big picture," placing lactation and breastfeeding in a historical and sociocultural context and identifying different ways in which the breastfeeding family functions within that context.

Part Two focuses on another kind of "big picture": basic anatomic and biologic imperatives. Appropriate clinical application of particular techniques must be based on a clear understanding of the physical underpinnings of a particular behavior. Thus this section, too, provides the background against which to assess other aspects of the lactation course and breastfeeding behavior.

Part Three concerns itself with the breastfeeding baby. Not every baby is born at term or healthy at birth. Pre-term babies' special needs and how to support their mothers as they express milk and later feed directly is addressed; in addition, we critically evaluate breastfeeding devices and recommend how and when they are most appropriately used. In spite of evidence to the contrary, jaundice continues to be a diagnosis that results in clinical decisions that interfere with breastfeeding.

We discuss the lactating mother in *Part Four,* noting that breastfeeding skills are not instinctive in the human. Thus, teaching the basics of *what* to do, *when* to do it, and *how* is a primary care-giving goal when assisting the new lactating mother. Ideally, the mother learns about breastfeeding before her baby's birth; her learning continues when she puts her baby to breast during the early postpartum period. We then take a look at maternal problems that can occur during the breastfeeding course, and the effect of the mother's employment on lactation. We conclude with a discussion of maternal sexuality and fertility, their relationship to one another and to lactation.

In *Part Five* we examine newer aspects of the field of lactation, including lactation consulting, and review the development and current activities of human milk banking. We take a careful look at research—how it is conducted, why ongoing research is needed, how research findings can be applied in clinical settings, and how clinical experiences can lead to new research endeavors.

An extensive glossary of key terms relating to lactation can be found in this book and in the accompanying *Study Guide.* The *Study Guide* provides suggestions for instructors in college-level courses in lactation and for individuals preparing to seek certification as lactation consultants. To avoid confusion between the word *nursing*—meaning the profession—and nursing, meaning breastfeeding, *nursing* (italicized) in the book refers to the profession. The masculine pronoun has been used to denote the infant or child throughout the book as a matter of convenience in distinguishing the child from the breastfeeding mother. Nurses, lactation consultants, and other health-care workers are referred to in the feminine gender, recognizing that males serve in various health-care professions.

As this book goes to press we are entering a new millennium as witnesses to an historic shift in the dominant social paradigm that is redefining the roles of women in society. Women activists campaigning for birthing and breastfeeding rights have been at the forefront of the consumer movement of the last quarter century. Women have the right to be fully, not partially, informed—to take fully active, not institutionally constrained, roles in childbearing and childrearing. We view this book as our contribution to the continuing effort to truly inform women of their right to nourish their babies in the only way that has proven its worth over thousands of years.

Contributors

Lois Arnold, MPH, IBCLC
Executive Director
Human Milk Banking Association of North America, Inc.
West Hartford, Connecticut

Debi Leslie Bocar, RN, MS, MEd, IBCLC
Lactation Consultant
Mercy Health Center
Oklahoma City, Oklahoma

Mary-Margaret Coates, MS, IBCLC
Certified Lactation Consultants of Colorado
Wheat Ridge, Colorado

Betty Ann Countryman, RN, MN
Assistant Professor, Maternal-Child Nursing
Indiana University School of Nursing (Retired)
Indianapolis, Indiana

Richard A. Guthrie, MD
Professor, Department of Pediatrics
University of Kansas School of Medicine at Wichita
Director, Diabetes Center
St. Joseph Medical Center
Wichita, Kansas

Roberta Hewat, RN, MSN, IBCLC
Assistant Professor, School of Nursing
University of British Columbia
Vancouver, British Columbia, Canada

Kathy I. Kennedy, MA
Senior Research Associate
Family Health International
Research Triangle Park, North Carolina

Henry H. Mangurten, MD
Director of Neonatology
Lutheran General Hospital
Chicago, Illinois

Paula P. Meier, RN, DNSc
Assistant Professor of Maternal/Child Nursing
Coordinator of Perinatal Graduate Program
Department of Maternal Child Health
University of Illinois
Chicago, Illinois

Linda Shrago, RN, MS, IBCLC
Lactation Consultant
Mercy Health Center
Oklahoma City, Oklahoma

Marsha Walker, RN, IBCLC
Director, Breastfeeding Support Program
Harvard Community Health Plan
Wellesley, Massachusetts

Acknowledgments

We gratefully acknowledge the people who helped and supported us during the writing of this book, in particular: Gail Ausdenmoore (Leewood, KS); Jan Barger and Jill Barger (Wheaton, IL); Virginia Brackett (Evanston, IL); Roger Clark (Wichita, KS); Donna Corrieri (Boca Raton, FL); Barbara Hardin (Cicero, IL); Angela Jacobi (Chicago, IL); Linda Kutner (Mooresville, NC); Kathleen Lindstrom (Abbotsford, BC); Margaret Marquardt (Long Beach, CA); Chris Mulford (Swarthmore, PA); Ellen Petok (Woodland Hills, CA); Faith Ploude (Miami, FL); Jeanne Rago (Morristown, NJ); Ros Escott (Hobart, Tasmania); Calayne Stanton (Spring Hill, KS); Peggy Toman (Oshkosh, WI); Lorna Weixelman (Wichita, KS); Ruth Wester (San Diego, CA); Gina Woodley (Wichita, KS); and Linda Zielinski (Boise, ID).

The seemingly tireless reviewers who improved the text include:

Helen Armstrong, UNICEF Baby Friendly Project, Tuft University (Boston, MA)

Jan Barger, International Lactation Consultant Association (Wheaton, IL)

Fred Chang, University of Kansas School of Medicine (Wichita, KS)

Mary Margaret Coates, Colorado La Leche League and Breastfeeding Coalition (Denver, CO)

Sarah Danner, Private midwifery practice (Ashburnham, MA)

Ann Flores, St. Joseph Medical Center (Wichita, KS)

Vergie Hughes, Georgetown University Community Milk Bank (Washington, DC)

Miriam Labbok, Georgetown University (Washington, DC)

Verity Livingstone, University of British Columbia (Vancouver, BC)

Chele Marmet, Lactation Institute and Breastfeeding Clinic (Los Angeles, CA)

Joan Melzer, Kansas Newman College (Wichita, KS)

Maureen Minchin, Nursing Mothers Association of Australia (Armadale, Victoria, Australia)

Gerald Nelson, University of Kansas School of Medicine (Wichita, KS)

Rosanne Orlando, Brookhaven Memorial Medical Center (Bohemia, NY)

Virginia Phillips, Nursing Mothers Association of Australia (Brisbane, Adelaide, Australia)

Ellen Shell, Lactation Institute and Breastfeeding Clinic (Los Angeles, CA)

JoAnne Scott, International Board of Lactation Consultant Examiners (Annandale, VA)

Arnold Tanis, Private pediatric practice (Hollywood, FL)

We extend thanks to La Leche League International for providing the foundation for our breastfeeding education as La Leche League leaders and to institutions who welcomed us to their libraries to explore their treasures: St. Joseph Medical Center and the University of Kansas School of Medicine (Wichita, KS); Crerar Library, University of Chicago, and Rush-Presbyterian-St. Luke's Medical Center (Chicago, IL).

We lovingly acknowledge our families; Hugh, Michael, Neil, Shirley, Brian, and Quinn Riordan, Teresa and Richard Chenoweth, Renee and Kevin Garty, and Doug Auerbach who encourage and nurture us.

Breastfeeding and Human Lactation

Breastfeeding and Human Lactation

SECTION

ONE

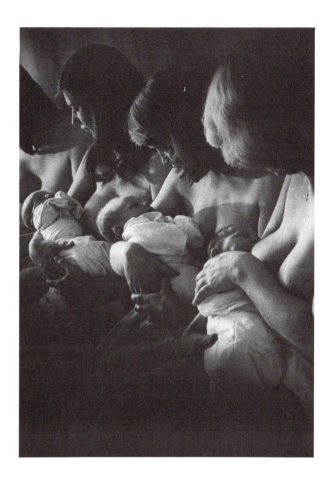

Historical and Sociocultural Context of Infant Feeding

Lactation and breastfeeding exist within the constraints of each culture in which the physical function and the behavior are practiced. Just as the breastfeeding course flows and ebbs in a mother's life, so also has it experienced flows and ebbs in different cultures through the years. While clearly playing an important beneficial role in the health of women and infants, the importance of breastfeeding *as a human behavior* is reflected in society over time by how it is practiced—when, where, for how long—and under what circumstances it is not allowed.

The theoretical constructs that allow us to examine the family—identifying its individual members and their unique roles, as well as their relationships and how each contributes to a sum greater than its parts—also enable us to identify issues specific to the breastfeeding family, be it affluent, nonwhite, low income, or headed by teen-age parents.

1

Tides in Breastfeeding Practice

INTRODUCTION

Throughout the world today, an infant is apt to receive less breast milk than at any time in the past. Until the 1940s, the prevalence of breastfeeding was high in nearly all societies. Although the feeding of manufactured milks and baby milks had begun before the turn of the century in parts of Europe and North America, the practice spread slowly during the next decades. It was still generally limited to portions of population elites, and it involved only a small percentage of the world's population. During the post-World War II era, however, the way most mothers fed their infants in industrialized regions began to change, and the export of these new practices to developing nations was underway.

EVIDENCE ABOUT BREASTFEEDING PRACTICES

LARGE-SCALE SURVEYS

How do we know what we "know" about the prevalence of breastfeeding? (Prevalence is used here to mean the combined effect of breastfeeding initiation rates and breastfeeding continuance rates.) Before attempting to trace trends in infant feeding practices, it is helpful to consider the nature of the evidence. National surveys which produced the kind of representative data that allow statistical evaluation are available only for the last 35 years. These consist primarily of national fertility or natality surveys, as well as marketing surveys conducted by manufacturers of artificial baby milks. In the United States, the National Fertility Studies of 1965 and 1970, sponsored by the National Institute of Child Health and

MARY-MARGARET COATES

Human Development, and the National Surveys of Family Growth of 1973 and 1976, sponsored by the National Center for Health Statistics, included questions on breastfeeding along with questions on other aspects of fertility (Hendershot, 1980; Hirschman & Butler, 1981). National Natality Surveys, which collected data in 1969 and 1980 on how newborns were fed, were also conducted by the National Center for Health Statistics (Forman et al., 1985). Results of several market surveys made between 1955 and 1989 have also been published (Martinez & Nalezienski, 1979; Ryan et al., 1991).

Outside the United States, representative data for countries in Latin America, Asia, Africa, and the Middle East are derived from three sources. World Fertility Surveys conducted from 1972 to 1984 were sponsored by the Office of Population within the United States Agency for International Development (USAID), the United Nations Fund for Population Activities, and the United Kingdom Office of Development Assistance (Lightbourne & Singh, 1982). The World Health Organization began ongoing surveys on infant feeding in the mid-1970s. Finally, demographic and health surveys were initiated in 1984; these ongoing surveys are sponsored jointly by the USAID and governments of host countries in which the surveys are made.

SMALL SURVEYS

Local or special-purpose studies document the variety of practices within smaller regions or population segments. Before 1955 such studies provided the only quantitative information available on breast-

3

feeding. Bain's (1948) compilation of the incidence of breastfeeding in U.S. hospitals was the first such published study of practices in that country.

OTHER EVIDENCE

Until the last few decades, breastfeeding was the unremarkable norm. Thus, what we "know" about breastfeeding from much earlier times often must be inferred from evidence of other methods of feeding infants. Most historical material available in English-language literature derives from a rather limited geographic area: Western Europe, Asia Minor, the Middle East, and North Africa. Written materials, which include verses, legal statutes, religious tracts, personal correspondence, inscriptions, and medical literature, extend back to before 2000 B.C.

Some of the earliest existing medical literature deals at least in passing with infant feeding. An Egyptian medical encyclopedia, the Papyrus Ebers (c. 1500 B.C.), contains recommendations for increasing a mother's milk supply (Fildes, 1986). The first writings to discuss infant feeding in detail are those of the physician Soranus, who practiced in Rome around A.D. 100; his views were widely repeated by other writers up through the mid-1700s. It is not immediately apparent to what degree these early exhortations either reflected or influenced actual practices. Many writings before A.D. 1800 deal primarily with wet nurses or how to hand-feed infants. Both were practices of only a small, socially privileged, portion of the population.

Archeological evidence provides our information on infant feeding prior to 2000 B.C. Some of the earliest artifacts are pottery figurines from the Middle East which depict lactating goddesses, such as Ishtar of Babylon and Isis of Egypt. Their abundance suggests that lactation was held in high regard (Fildes, 1986). These first appear in sites c. 3000 B.C., when pottery-making first became widespread in that region. Information about infant feeding may also be derived from paintings, inscriptions, and infant feeding implements.

Modern ethnography has a place of special importance. By documenting the infant feeding practices of present-day non-technological, hunter-gatherer, herding, and farming societies, ethnographers expand our knowledge of the range of "normal" breastfeeding practices. At the same time, they provide a richer appreciation of cultural practices which enhance the prevalence of breastfeeding. Such studies are also our best window onto breastfeeding

practices of 10,000 years ago, which may in fact be the biological norm for *Homo sapiens sapiens.*

In summary, the historical aspect of this chapter deals with a limited social stratum in a limited geographic region. However, the common threads provide a useful context within which we may better understand modern breastfeeding practices, especially in Western cultures.

THE BIOLOGICAL NORM IN INFANT FEEDING

EARLY HUMAN EVOLUTION

The class *Mammalia* is characterized principally by the presence of breasts (*mammae*) which secrete and release a fluid that for a time is the sole nourishment of the young. This manner of sustaining newborns is extremely ancient; it dates back to the late Mesozoic era, some 100 million years ago. (See Fig. 1–1.) Hominid precursors first appeared about four million years ago; the genus *Homo* has existed about two million years. The currently dominant human species, *Homo sapiens sapiens,* has existed for only 40, 000 years. How breastfeeding was practiced by our earliest ancestors is not known, but certain other information about Paleolithic societies which existed 10,000 years ago sheds light on this question.

EARLY BREASTFEEDING PRACTICES

Diets reconstructed by archeological methods reveal that the Late Paleolithic era was populated by pre-agricultural peoples who ate a wide variety of fruits, nuts, vegetables, meat (commonly small game), fish, and shellfish. This diet closely resembles that of twentieth-century, hunter-gatherer societies (Eaton & Konner, 1985). Therefore, the infant feeding practices of societies today may reflect breastfeeding practices of much earlier prehistoric times. Consider the breastfeeding practices of the ¡Kung of the Kalahari Desert in southern Africa (Konner & Worthman, 1980) as well as hunter-gatherer societies of Papua New Guinea and elsewhere (Short, 1984). Breastfeeding among these people is frequent (averaging four feeds per hour) and short (about two minutes per feed). It is equally distributed over a 24-hour period and continues for two to four years. These breastfeeding patterns are considered by some to be a direct inheritance of practices which prevailed at the end of a long, and dietetically stable,

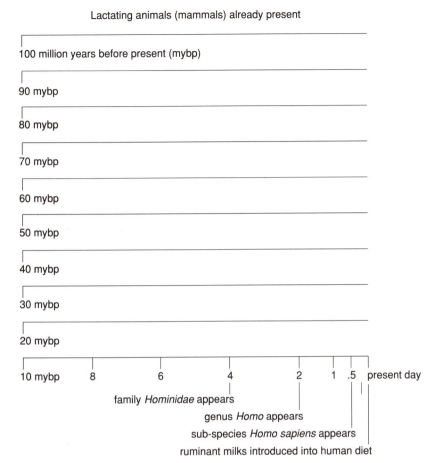

Lactating animals (mammals) already present

100 million years before present (mybp)

90 mybp

80 mybp

70 mybp

60 mybp

50 mybp

40 mybp

30 mybp

20 mybp

10 mybp   8   6   4   2   1 .5 present day

family *Hominidae* appears

genus *Homo* appears

sub-species *Homo sapiens* appears

ruminant milks introduced into human diet

FIGURE 1–1. The antiquity of lactation. Arrows mark approximate times of first appearance of lactating precursors of modern humans, and of regular use of non-human animal milk by humans.

evolutionary period which ended about 10,000 B.C. This assumption is supported by observations of the human's closest primate relative, the chimpanzee, which secretes a milk quite similar to that of humans, suckles several times an hour, and sleeps with and nurses its young at night (Short, 1984).

THE REPLACEMENT OF MATERNAL BREASTFEEDING

However, the practice of giving foods other than maternal breast milk is deeply rooted. Both written and archeological records show that by 2000 B.C. some babies were being wet-nursed or fed animal milks. Considering the biological impetus for mothers to breastfeed infants, why have some mothers sought other foods for their own infants? At one end of the spectrum are women or infants with debilities or deformities that prevent lactation or suckling. At the other end are the women about whom one Euro-

pean writer of the 1300s remarked, "Women nowadays are too delicate or too haughty, or they do not like the inconvenience" (Bernard of Gordon, 1309). In between these two extremes there are many economic, social, familial and personal factors which can affect the mother. These factors may interact with the mother/infant dyad to reduce a milk supply below the infant's needs, or to produce the perception that this has happened, or to convince a mother that she cannot or should not breastfeed.

When women choose other foods for their infants, two conditions are met: (1) alternative foods are available and (2) the use of these alternative foods is socially acceptable. Alternatives become acceptable when maternal breastfeeding is impossible, or when it appears to give no social or health advantage to the mother or to the infant, while the alternative food or method of feeding does appear to offer such advantages. Mothers acclimate to the idea of feeding their infants foods other than their own breast milk under many different circumstances. During the past century the increasing availability of manufactured baby milks for infants has made the replacement of breast milk easier. These two factors—the desire to feed other foods and the availability of acceptable foods—closely intertwine.

WET-NURSING

Wet-nursing may not have been the earliest alternative to maternal breastfeeding, but it was the only one likely to enable the infant to survive. Wet-nursing is common, although not universal, in traditional societies of today and by inference among ancient human societies. A woman who is already lactating may have been the most obvious choice for a wet nurse; but women who stimulate lactation without a recent pregnancy have been described in many traditional societies (Slome, 1976; Wieschhoff, 1940).

Wet-nursing for hire is mentioned in some of the oldest surviving texts, which implies that the practice was well established, even in ancient times. The Babylonian Code of Hammurabi (c. 1700 B.C.) forbade a wet nurse to substitute a new infant for one who had died. The Book of Exodus in the Old Testament (c. 1250 B.C.) records the hiring of a wet nurse for the foundling Moses; the fact that the "wet nurse" was Moses's own mother is incidental. The epic poems of Homer, written down around 900 B.C., contain references to wet nurses. A treatise on pediatric care from India, written during the second century A.D., contains instructions on how to qualify a wet nurse when the mother could not provide milk. The Koran, written about A.D. 500, also permits parents to "give your children out to nurse."

Although wet-nursing has had an almost unbroken history from the earliest times to the present, the popularity of the practice among the elite classes who most used it has waxed and waned, and wet nurses have played a mixed role. Although wet nurses were slaves in ancient Greece and Rome, they were respected members of the household. They lived in the infant's home and often remained a servant in the family long after infants were weaned. The custom of boarding the wet nurse continued among the aristocracy in medieval Europe.

In England during the 1600s and 1700s, as well as elsewhere in Europe, the middle classes began to employ wet nurses. The use of less attentive nurses and the sending of infants greater distances from home allowed less maternal supervision of either nurse or infant. Often an infant was not seen by his parents from the time he was given to the nurse until he was returned home after weaning (if he lived). But by the latter part of the 1700s the use of wet nurses, except in foundling hospitals, was on the decline in North America and England, as public concern increased over the moral character of wet nurses and the quality of care they provided.

Throughout this long period wet nurses were used sometimes because of maternal debility, but more often because it was the social expectation of the class of women who could afford to hire them. Thus the use of wet nurses by social elites foreshadows the demographic pattern later seen in the use of manufactured baby milks.

HAND-FED FOODS

The agricultural revolution. The idea that animal milks are suitable foods for human infants is reflected in myths—such as that of Romulus and Remus, the mythical founders of Rome, who are usually depicted as being suckled by a wolf. It may then come as a surprise to realize that the current most popular hand-fed infant foods, animal milks and cereals, did not become part of the human diet until well along in the evolutionary history of *Homo sapiens sapiens.* Cereal grains first appeared only about 10,000 years ago, and animal milks somewhat later (McCracken, 1971). The widespread adoption of these foods was made possible by the development of agriculture and, later, animal husbandry. Because of the availability of new weaning foods, periods of lactation, which normally lasted for three to four years, were shortened to about two years in farming and herding societies (Schaefer, 1986).

Gruels. In much of the world the soft foods most commonly added to the infant diet have been gruels containing a liquid, a cereal, and other substances added for variety or nutrition. The cereal might be rice, wheat, or corn. The grain might be boiled and mashed; ground and boiled; or, as in the case of bread crumbs, ground, baked, crushed, and heated. The liquid might be animal milk, meat broth, or water; eggs or butter might also be added. Where grains are not commonly eaten, similar soft foods for infants are based on starchy plants such as taros, cassavas, or plantains.

Animal milks. Animal milks are a relatively recent addition to the human diet. This is implied genetically by the common lack of lactase, an enzyme necessary for the digestion of the milk sugar, lactose, in children. In cultures which do not use animal milks, such as those in Bangladesh or Thailand, some children may be lactose intolerant before one year of age; in those which do use animal milks, the onset of lactose intolerance occurs considerably later—after 10 years of age in Finland (Simoons, 1980). Adult lactose tolerance is common only in cultures in which animal milks have traditionally been an important part of the diet, such as those of northern Europe and western Asia (McCracken, 1971).

Feeding vessels. The earliest "vessel" used to hand feed an infant was undoubtedly the human hand, and the foods so fed were probably soft or mashed, rather than liquid. The earliest crafted vessels used for feeding liquids were probably animal horns pierced by holes in the tips; such horns continued to be used into the 1900s in parts of Europe. The oldest pottery vessel thought to have been used for infant feeding, a small spouted bowl found in an infant's grave in France, is dated c. 2000–1500 B.C. (Lacaille, 1950). Small spouted or football-shaped bowls have been found in infant burial sites in Germany (c. 900 B.C.) and in the Sudan in North Africa (c. 400 B.C.) (Lacaille, 1950). They attest to the fact that hand feeding of infants has been attempted for more than three millenia. (See Fig. 1–2.)

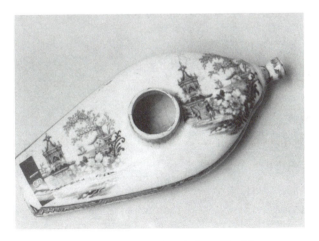

FIGURE 1–2.   Photograph of English Staffordshire Spode nursing bottle c. 1825. (Courtesy V. H. Brackett.)

TIMING OF THE INTRODUCTION OF HAND-FEEDING

What archeological evidence cannot tell us is why these infants were hand-fed. Neonates may temporarily be offered other foods (prelacteal feeds); young infants may be offered occasional tastes of other foods, and they will be offered increasing amounts of soft foods as they transfer to the adult diet (mixed feeds). Finally, infants may be reared from birth on other foods (artificial feeding).

Prelacteal feeds. Many of the world's infants, even those who later will be fully breastfed, receive other foods as newborns. Of 120 traditional societies (and by inference in many ancient preliterate societies) whose neonatal feeding practices have been described, 50 delay the initial breastfeeding more than two days, and some 50 more delay it from one to two days. The reason: to avoid the feeding of colostrum, which is described as being dirty, contaminated, bad, bitter, constipating, insufficient, or stale (Morse, Jehle & Gamble, 1990).

Early medical writers in the eastern Mediterranean region (Greece, Rome, Asia Minor, and Arabia) and later in Europe—from Soranus through those of the 1600s—also discouraged the feeding of colostrum. Medical writers recommend avoiding breastfeeding for periods as short as one day (Avicenna, c. A.D. 1000) to as long as three weeks (Soranus, c. A.D. 100). Commonly, the newborn was first given a "cleansing" food designed to promote passage of meconium: honey, sweet oils such as almond, or sweetened water or wine were most often used.

In Europe, the fear of feeding colostrum may have contributed to the undermining of maternal breastfeeding—at least among the upper classes—and spread the practice of wet-nursing (Deruisseau, 1940). A similar charge has been leveled at prelacteal bottle feeds. These are commonly given in Western (or Western-style) hospital nurseries; they seem to undermine breastfeeding and to increase the use of manufactured baby milk (Verronen et al., 1980; Winikoff et al., 1986). One can only wonder if routine Western hospital practices, which include delayed first breastfeeding and prelacteal feeds of water or artificial baby milk, are technological vestiges of this widespread traditional "taboo."

Not all published work supports the idea that prelacteal feeds and a delay in initiating breastfeeding reduce the likelihood of successful lactation (Richards, 1986). Ensuing successful breastfeeding may be associated with the maternal perception that prelacteal feeds are appropriate, and in positive maternal behavior following the commencement of breastfeeding: nearly constant contact with or close proximity to the infant; breastfeeding *ad lib* day and night; and no further use of feeding bottles (Woolridge, Greasley & Silpisornkosol, 1985; Nga & Weissner, 1986).

Mixed feeds. Based on current practices of many traditional societies, early mixed feedings may be the most common infant feeding regimen (Dimond & Ashworth, 1987; Kusin, Kardjati & van Steenbergen, 1985; Latham et al., 1986; Wieschhoff, 1940).

Mixed feeding occurs even during the time when breastmilk forms the foundation of the infant diet and in societies where breastfeeding continues into the second or third year of life. In non-Western cultures hand-fed foods include tea infusions, mashed fruits, and/or a variety of starchy gruels or pastes. Where the use of a particular food dominates a culture, e.g., rice in many parts of Asia, that food is usually the principal supplemental infant food (Jelliffe, 1962). These foods may form any portion of the infant diet. In some non-Western cultures they are offered in such a way that they supplement, rather than replace, breastmilk (Whitehead, 1985) and thus do not appreciably hasten complete weaning. The use of feeding bottles, however, can shorten the weaning interval—that period between full sustenance by breastmilk and full sustenance by table foods (Winikoff & Laukaran, 1989).

Hand-feeding from birth. In a few regions of northern Europe (such as Switzerland and Finland) a cool, dry climate and a tradition of dairy farming permit the survival of infants on cow milk that is hand-fed from birth. From at least the 1400s, in these regions, breastfeeding was actively discouraged (Fildes, 1986). In France some foundlings, as well as infants with syphilis, were fed directly from goats; this practice was first described in writings in the 1500s, and it persisted until the early 1800s (Wickes, 1953a). Out of necessity, foundling hospitals of the 1700s and 1800s in Europe and the United States hand-fed infants, but with appalling mortality rates: up to 100% died. (See Fig. 1–3.) However, by the mid-1900s in industrialized countries, hand-

feeding from birth had become the norm and hand-fed infants did survive and grow.

TECHNOLOGICAL INNOVATIONS IN INFANT FEEDING

THE SOCIAL CONTEXT

During the late 1800s and the early 1900s, high infant mortality—even among infants cared for at home—was a major public concern. Physicians and parents as well recognized that poorly nourished children were more susceptible to illness. Between 1910 and 1915 the then newly created United States Children's Bureau sponsored several studies of infant mortality in major cities. Each shows that babies fed artificial milks were three to five times as likely to die as those who were breastfed. The studies also docu-

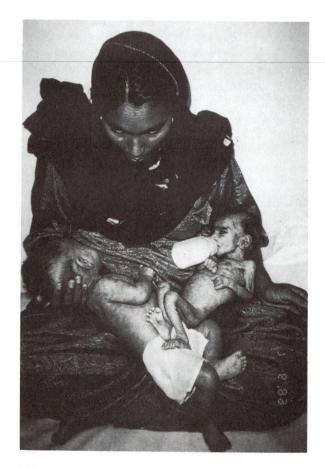

FIGURE 1–3. UNICEF photograph of thriving breastfed twin and his dying bottle-fed sister. (Courtesy of Children's Hospital, Islamabad, Pakistan.)

mented that both the rate of breastfeeding and the rate of infant mortality were linked: each increased steadily as family income decreased. In summarizing these results Williamson (1915) commented:

> . . . the disadvantages of a low income were sufficient to offset the greater prevalence of breast feeding among the babies of the poorer families.

During this same period a similar observation was made in England, where high infant mortality prevailed among poor, working-class mothers, 80% of whom breastfed their infants (Levenstein, 1983).

At the same time that women's aspirations for community service and commercial involvement were rising, Victorian beliefs about modesty discouraged breastfeeding in public. Advertising, which promoted bodily cleanliness, may have led to associating breast milk with body fluids that were unclean or noxious—a notion that persists to this day, at least in North America (Morse, 1989). Advances in the prevention of disease, largely through public health measures related to sanitation, extended an expanding faith in "modern science" to the field of "modern medicine." Women's magazines developed a wide audience of readers interested in female accomplishments outside the home, modern attitudes, and technological innovations; these same magazines reinforced concerns abut infant health. An 1880 issue of *The Ladies' Home Journal* contained this statement:

> If fed from your breast, be sure that the quantity and quality supply his demands. If you are weak or worn out, your milk cannot contain the nourishment a babe needs . . . (Apple, 1986).

THE TECHNOLOGICAL CONTEXT

Between about 1860 and 1910, scientific advances and technological innovations created many new options in infant feeding that appeared to enhance infant survival. The upright feeding bottle and rubber nipple, each of which could be cleaned thoroughly, made artificial feeding easier and safer. New foods to be used with this equipment appeared. Large-scale dairy farming produced abundant supplies of cow milk, which was marketed first as canned evaporated milk and later in condensed (i.e., highly sweetened to retard spoilage) or dried forms. This technological ferment, fueled both by need for improved infant health-care and a popular belief in the ability of science and technology to provide answers, attracted analytical chemists. Around 1850 chemists had

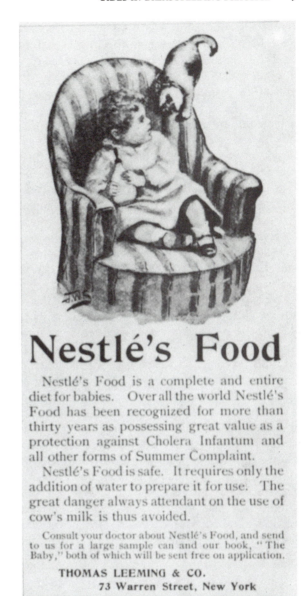

FIGURE 1–4. 1895 advertisement for artificial infant milk. (*The Ladies' Home Journal* 12:26, 1895).

begun to turn their attention to food products. Early investigations, now viewed as rudimentary, into the composition of human and cow milk convinced them that ". . . the combined efforts of the cow and the ingenuity of man" could construct a food the equal of human milk (Gerrard, 1974). Patented foods, such as Liebig's Food and Nestlé's Milk Food, were first marketed in Europe and the United States in the 1860s. The Nestlé's product was a mixture of flour, cow milk, and sugar, which was to be dissolved in milk or water before feeding. Milk modifiers, such as Mellin's Food, and milk foods, such as Horlick's Malted Milk, were popular in the United States by the 1880s. Both mothers and members of the newly emerging medical specialty of pediatrics were courted by manufacturers of these baby foods. Extravagant claims for these foods (Liebig's Food was called "the most perfect substitute for mother's milk") were combined with artful advertising which played on fears for the health of the infant and faith in modern science (Apple, 1986). (See Fig. 1–4.)

In the 1890s a physician, Thomas Rotch, developed a complex system of modifying cow milk so that it more closely resembled human milk. Rotch observed that the composition of human milk varies and that the digestive capacities of infants do so as well. He devised mathematical formulae to denote the proportions of fat, sugar, and protein in cow milk which particular infants required at a particular age (Rotch, 1907). The result was an exceedingly complex system of feeding which required constant intervention by the physician, who often changed the "formula" weekly. Supervising infant feeding then became a principal focus of the newly emerging specialty of pediatrics.

Commercial advertising promoted the use of manufactured infant milks to both mothers and physicians. The basic themes—a mother's concern for her infant's health, the perfection of the manufactured product, and the difficulty of breastfeeding—have persisted over the years (Apple, 1986). By 1910, whether the maternal ability to lactate was disappearing from the species was a question meriting discussion at child welfare conferences (Levenstein, 1983).

THE ROLE OF THE MEDICAL COMMUNITY

Regulation of childbirth. During the early part of this century, childbirth moved from home or midwife-attended births to hospitals, where a birthing woman was separated from her family and attended by a physician. During the middle part of this century, hospital routines and the use of general anesthesia during labor and delivery separated mother and infant much of the time in the early postpartum period. Bottle-feedings by nursery staff became increasingly common. Normal postpartum hospital stays in the United States lengthened; during the 1930s and 1940s they were sometimes as long as two weeks. This period, intended to permit the mother

to recuperate from childbirth, often resulted instead in a return home with an impaired breastmilk supply and a baby who was accustomed to bottle-feeds. Bain (1948) notes that babies who were older than eight days at discharge were less apt to be breastfed than were younger ones.

Regulation of Breastfeeding

Underlying many changes in the feeding of infants was a "regulatory" frame of mind, the seeds of which had been sown in Europe as early as the 1500s. The advent of book printing about this time permitted a much wider dissemination of works on infant care. Their authors shared a concern for the high incidence of gastrointestinal illness in infants and for high infant mortality rates. Overfeeding was deemed a central factor in both. Writers on child care responded by advocating the regulation of feeding in order to prevent presumed overfeeding.

M. Ettmüller (1703), writing in the mid-1600s, was not the first to recommend infrequent feedings:

> Nothing is more apt to disorder the child than suckling it too often, since large quantities of milk stagnating in the stomach, must needs corrupt . . . especially if fresh milk be pour'd in before the preceeding be digested.

Some 250 years later in 1900, Pierre Budin (1907), a French obstetrician famous for his early interest in premature infants and for his advocacy of breastfeeding, was nonetheless typical of many others in recommending small feedings:

> . . . it is better at first to give too little than too much, (for an underfed infant failed to gain weight but it was free from digestive troubles). . . .

Even medical writers who strongly recommended breastfeeding also recommended highly regulated times for feedings—a fixed number of feedings at fixed times. William Cadogan (1749), whose firm endorsement of breastfeeding and largely sound advice prompted many privileged English women to breastfeed, advocated only four feeds per day at equal intervals, and no night feeds! A prototype mothercraft manual by Hugh Smith (1774) contains excellent advice: to feed colostrum and to allow the newborn to suckle frequently to stimulate lactation. However, it then instructs mothers to limit feeds, beginning at one month, to five per day timed at 7:00 and 10:00 A.M. and 1:00, 6:00, and 11:00 P.M. About 50 years later, Thomas Bull (1849), after recommending *ad lib* feeds for the first 10 days, instructed mothers to feed the rest of the first month at regular four-hour intervals day and night, because he also believed that irregular feeding harmed the infant. After one month the night feed was to be eliminated.

These influential publications began the process of removing the management of infant feeding from the mother, or from the realm of women in general, and placing it in the hands of usually male "authorities." Cadogan (1749) commended this change which put "men of sense rather than foolish unlearned women" in charge, and Rotch (1907) deplored that "mothers and nurses . . . dominated the physicians."

Regulation and industrialization. This "regulatory" frame of mind fit nicely with the needs of the growing industrial sector of the economy, which relied on efficiency and schedules governed by the clock. Societal perceptions of infants' innate characteristics and needs were interpreted in this light (Millard, 1990). Early in the twentieth century, infants were seen as needing order imposed onto their characters from the outside:

> . . . an infant two days old may be forming either a good or a bad habit. A child that is taken up whenever it cries is trained into a bad habit; the same principle is true in reference to nursing a baby to stop its crying. Both these habits cultivate self-indulgence and a lack of self-control . . . (Rossiter, 1908).

"Good" mothering thus drifted towards meeting the letter of schedules often imposed by the medical profession rather than meeting the mutual needs of mother and infant as expressed by and interpreted within the dyad.

Although the approval of rigid external schedules diminished after the 1960s, it is still assumed in medical literature that lactation functions better when both mother and baby develop feeding schedules. The lack of a schedule is usually perceived as abnormal by both mother and physician (Millard, 1990). Neither externally imposed schedules nor supposedly innate ones are guaranteed to meet the mutual needs of a given dyad. Unfortunately, certain employment skills, such as an awareness of time and responsiveness within a hierarchial authority structure, are those least apt to

enable a person to accommodate the irregularities of early breastfeeding.

Regulation of contraception. During the late 1950s and early 1960s, the widespread acceptance of oral contraceptives may have reinforced the decline in breastfeeding (Meyer, 1968). Contraceptives containing estrogen and progesterone reduce breast milk volume and thus contribute to lactation insufficiency. Moreover, women who planned to use oral contraceptives were discouraged from breastfeeding in order to avoid passing those hormones to the infant. During this period several million women per year in the United States alone were thereby removed from the pool of potential breastfeeders. Currently marketed low-progesterone contraceptives pose fewer hazards to the maternal milk supply and the baby, and often they are routinely recommended to mothers nursing young infants.

The accommodation between physicians and infant milk manufacturers. The relationship between physicians and infant food manufacturers has in general promoted mothers' dependency on either the manufacturer or the physician for information on infant feeding. In the late 1800s as proprietary infant foods were being developed, manufacturers advertised to both groups. By the 1920s, some preparations were advertised to mothers but could be purchased only by prescription or used only after consulting a physician: the package contained no instructions for use. By 1932 the American Medical Association essentially required baby-milk manufacturers to advertise only to the medical profession (Greer & Apple, 1991). Manufacturers and physicians recognized the mutual economic benefits of this policy, which were clearly spelled out in many advertisements placed by formula manufacturers such as Mead Johnson (1930) in medical journals in the 1930s:

> When mothers in America feed their babies by lay advice, the control of your pediatric cases passes out of your hands, Doctor. Our interest in this important phase of medical economics springs, not from any motives of altruism, philanthropy or paternalism, but rather from a spirit of enlightened self-interest and co-operation because (our) infant diet materials are advertised only to you, never to the public.

Despite several early studies that showed breast-fed infants to be healthier than bottle-fed ones

(Grulee, Sanford & Herron, 1934; Howarth, 1950; Woodbury, 1922), many physicians acted for years as if there were little advantage to breastfeeding. This persistent view was expressed up through the 1960s. For instance, Aitken and Hytten (1960) reported:

> . . . with modern standards of hygiene artificial feeding on simple mixtures of cow's milk, water and sugar is a satisfactory substitute for breast feeding. . . .

Likewise, Hill (1968) noted:

> . . . formula feeding has become so simple, safe, and uniformly successful that breast-feeding no longer seems worth the bother.

It was not until the 1970s that medical research began to identify the complex immunological properties of breast milk (Gerrard, 1974). These discoveries led to a wider recognition that immunological factors, rather than the avoidance of contamination in other infant foods, were a chief cause of the better health documented in breastfed infants. Some authorities contend that breastmilk does benefit infants living in impoverished conditions, but deny that it confers any advantage to well nourished infants living in hygienic surroundings. As newer research on the lifelong health consequences of having consumed breastmilk versus artificial baby milks becomes better known, even this argument becomes increasingly difficult to defend (Cunningham, Jelliffe & Jelliffe, 1991).

In 1988 two infant food manufacturers began mass marketing their products directly to consumers. Whether advertising to the public will further undermine breastfeeding, and whether it will increase the cost of the products advertised, have yet to be determined.

PREVALENCE OF BREASTFEEDING

UNITED STATES, ENGLAND, EUROPE

The recent past. The net result of these shifts in technology and attitudes has been a rapid decline in the prevalence of breastfeeding in Western nations since the 1940s. In the United States the proportion of newborns receiving any breastmilk at one week postpartum declined steadily to a low of 25% in 1970 (Martinez & Krieger, 1985). The proportion of newborns exclusively breastfed at hospital discharge

was even lower: it declined from 38% in 1946 (Bain, 1948) to 21% in 1956 and only 18% by 1966 (Meyer, 1968). The period of most dramatic decline of breastfeeding coincided with economic factors in the United States (and perhaps in other countries) that encouraged major migrations from rural to urban areas. As one example, between 1945 and 1970 approximately five million African-Americans moved from the rural South to the urban North. The association between internal migration from rural to urban areas and a decline in breastfeeding also has been noted in developing countries (Jelliffe & Jelliffe, 1978, p. 223).

During the 1970s the trend to artificial feeding reversed. (See Fig. 1–5.) The reasons are not clear (Eckhardt & Hendershot, 1984) but seem to have been part of a widespread desire of many to include simpler, more natural practices in their lives. Voluntary groups which offer information and support to women interested in breastfeeding, such as La Leche League International in the United States, Nursing Mothers' Association of Australia, and Amningshjalpen of Sweden, were formed in the 1950s and 1960s. Such groups both assisted individual women and focused attention on the benefits of breastfeed-

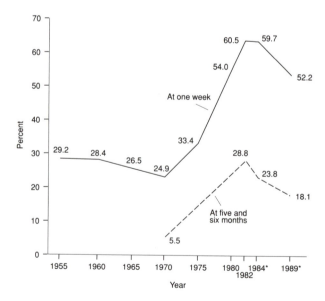

FIGURE 1–5. Percentage of infants in the United States receiving any breastmilk at birth (upper curve) and at five and six months (lower curve), 1955–1989. (* 1984 and 1989 data, in hospital and at six months.) Based on data from Martinez and Krieger (1985) and Ryan et al. (1991).

ing. Women of higher socioeconomic status were among the first to return to breastfeeding. In Western nations women who breastfeed are more likely to possess some characteristics of this group (Grossman et al., 1990). This increase leveled off in the early 1980s and has fallen steadily since then.

Current breastfeeding practices.   One marketing study made in the United States in 1989 showed that only 52% of hospital-born infants received any breastmilk in the hospital; only 18% were still receiving any breastmilk by six months of age. These figures compare with those of 63% and 24% for 1984, respectively (Ryan et al., 1991). Whether a given mother breastfeeds is influenced by many interrelated factors which include but are not restricted to race or ethnic group, age, education, affluence, and where she lives. In general, breastfeeding initiation is more common among older Caucasian women of higher socioeconomic status; in the United States, breastfeeding rates are higher in the West and lower in the East and Southeast. In England the percentage of first babies breastfed dropped from 74% in 1980 to 69% in 1985/86. Between 1985 and 1986, 64% of all babies surveyed were breastfed, and 22% were still breastfed at six months. Class differences were also marked: the initiation rate of the highest socioeconomic class (87%) was twice that of the lowest (43%) (Lancet, 1988). In 1988, about 60% of all mothers delivering in Sheffield, United Kingdom, intended to breastfeed. At one month, only 32% were doing so. These figures are 10 and seven percentage points lower respectively than in 1981 (Emery, Scholey & Taylor, 1990).

The World Health Organization (WHO) reports (1989a) that breastfeeding initiation rates are increasing in Europe and are as high as 90% or more in Scandinavia, Switzerland, Austria, Bulgaria, Germany, and Hungary. Scandinavia is notable because breastfeeding initiation is high in all social classes. Portugal, Poland, and Hungary are notable because of their high continuation rate: nearly 90% of infants who are initially breastfed are still breastfed during the fourth month of life.

DEVELOPING REGIONS

The role of colonial empires.   Patterns of declines in the prevalence of breastfeeding have been noted in non-Western regions somewhat later than in the West. Between World Wars I and II, British,

French, and German colonial empires controlled fully a quarter of the inhabited globe and a quarter of the world's population. These empires served as vehicles for the expansion of markets for artificial baby milks.

Colonial ruling elites, through the accepted practices of their social class in their country of origin, and as a way of placing social distance between themselves and the nationals of the country in which they lived, were much more likely to feed their infants artificial milks than to breastfeed. That most of these infants survived is due in large part to the higher levels of sanitation and medical care that their position in life afforded them. Thus colonial elites served as unwitting role models for indigenous peoples.

Concern for the health of colonial peoples led many health-care workers to transmit Western attitudes towards infant feeding to the populations they served—by example, by direct recommendations, and by the training provided to indigenous health-care providers.

> Westerners have traditionally assumed that foods good for them must be good for all people and have passed these prejudices on to foreign nationals trained in Western schools (McCracken, 1971).

Perhaps because Western medical personnel were successful at treating many other health problems, local populations were prepared to accept attitudes which encouraged the use of artificial baby milks. Health-care personnel in hospitals helped to introduce the use of manufactured baby milks and contributed to undermining breastfeeding (Winikoff & Laukaran, 1989).

Colonial transportation and communication networks, as well as health-care clinics and hospitals aided the advertisement and sale of artificial baby milks to this huge population. The decline in breastfeeding accelerated after World War II, in part because of greater contact between Western health-care personnel and populations in developing countries, and in part because relief projects shipped surpluses of skim milk, produced in abundance by the large dairy industry in the United States, to war-torn countries (Wade, 1974). Between 1976 and 1977, 42 transnational companies manufactured, distributed and/or marketed infant milk products in four countries surveyed: Ethiopia, Nigeria, India, and the Philippines (WHO, 1981).

Infant feeding and infant mortality. The relation between infant feeding and infant mortality is complex. Although widespread artificial feeding has been associated with markedly poorer infant survival—both in Western nations early in this century and in developing nations in the mid- and late-1900s—the reverse is not always the case. High breastfeeding rates do not necessarily mean low mortality rates. Infant mortality has tended to be highest among populations in which breastfeeding was most common: the poor. Rural mothers in Ethiopia and Zaire reported that at least 30% of their infants died, although 97% of mothers were breastfeeding at 18 months postpartum, as were 80% of a similar group of mothers in rural Zaire (WHO, 1981).

Although artificial feeding has been associated with poorer infant health—both in Western nations early in this century and in developing nations in the mid-1900s—a decrease in infant mortality does not necessarily reflect a return to breastfeeding. The advent of primary health care for a large portion of a population may explain decreases in infant mortality in the face of declines in breastfeeding. In Nicaragua, the proportion of infants breastfed at six months declined 25 percentage points (from 58% to 33%) between 1977 and 1988. During this same period, infant mortality declined from about 10% to about 6.5% (Sandiford et al., 1991). It seems clear that the pervasive problems of poverty, in both Western and non-Western locales, were at the root of the appalling infant mortality in impoverished populations.

During the 1970s, when breastfeeding rates were generally increasing in Western nations, they continued to decline in the more populous developing regions. Between the late 1970s and the mid- to late-1980s, however, trends in developing nations varied. During this period breastfeeding initiation rates stayed about the same or increased slightly in 15 Asian, African, and Latin American countries: Indonesia, Sri Lanka, Thailand; Kenya, Ghana, Senegal, Tunisia, Morocco; Colombia, Dominican Republic, Ecuador, Mexico, Peru, and Trinidad/Tobago. However, the median duration of any breastfeeding decreased in twice as many (10) countries as it increased (five); and the greatest decline (5-1/2 months in Thailand) was twice the greatest increase

(2-1/2 months in Ghana and Trinidad/Tobago) (Dr R. F. Sharma, personal communication, 1991).

Characteristics of breastfeeding women. Generalizations about demographic characteristics most likely to predict who will breastfeed have many exceptions. In general, rural women are more likely to begin breastfeeding, and to breastfeed longer, than urban ones; poorer mothers are more likely to breastfeed than more affluent ones. The urban poor, often recent immigrants from more rural areas, are the mothers among whom breastfeeding rates are declining most rapidly. However, in Kenya and Trinidad/Tobago, increases in median duration during the 1980s occurred in a broad range of socioeconomic and educational levels. During this same period in the Dominican Republic the median duration of breastfeeding rose among urban and among employed mothers, although the overall median duration dropped 15% (Dr R. K. Sharma, personal communication, 1991).

The regions discussed below are those defined by the World Health Organization in its compilations of breastfeeding practices.

REGIONAL BREASTFEEDING PRACTICES

Eastern Mediterranean. Breastfeeding initiation rates exceed 90%, but many infants begin receiving supplements at four weeks, and most are supplemented by three months. (See Fig. 1–6.) In Tunisia this three-month figure represents a decline in the median duration of full breastfeeding of two months (Sharma et al., 1992); only 10% of urban Yemeni infants were fully breastfed at three months. Although more than 50% of infants in this region are still breastfeeding at one year of age, the range is quite wide, depending on the country and the mother's social position. High-status mothers wean earlier in Pakistan (none are breastfeeding at one year) and Egypt (where the average duration is six months). Almost 60% of low-income mothers in Pakistan are still breastfeeding at one year; similar mothers in Egypt breastfeed on the average nearly 19 months (WHO, 1989b).

Africa. During the mid-1980s in Africa, more than 95% of infants began life breastfeeding. Water or other foods were added by one month in most countries; supplemented breastfeeding was nearly

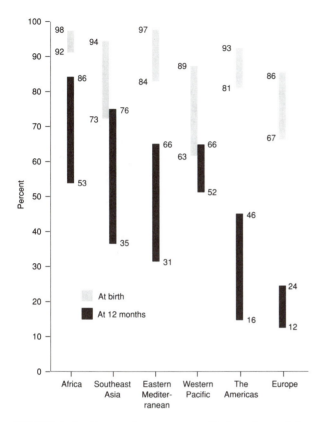

FIGURE 1–6. Range of percentages of infants breastfed during the 1980s at birth (upper bar) and at 12 months (lower bar), in six regions of the world. Based on data from World Health Organization (1989a).

universal by three months. During the 1980s the median duration of full breastfeeding declined in several countries, including Kenya and Senegal. Earlier complete weaning is becoming more common, although total duration remains high by Western standards: the median duration of any breastfeeding ranges up to 21 months, as is true in Ghana (WHO, 1989a; Sharma et al., 1992).

Southeast Asia. Initiation rates remain high, from about 75% to 95%, in Southeast Asia and in the Western Pacific, although mixed feeding is common after the first month. The duration of breastfeeding is highly variable; it may be as low as four months in urban areas or as long as 20 or more months in rural ones. During the 1980s, median duration declined

from 20 to 15 months in Thailand, reflecting changes in rural breastfeeding practices (WHO, 1989a; Sharma et al., 1992).

Western Pacific. This region has the lowest average initiation rate, about 75%, outside of Europe or North America. Rural and low-income women in less developed countries tend to have noticeably higher initiation and continuance rates than do their urban or high-income counterparts. The trend is reversed in industrialized countries of this region (Japan, Australia, New Zealand), and there the demographic pattern is similar to that of the United States (Hitchcock, 1990; WHO, 1989b). In these countries, breastfeeding increased during the 1980s; one study shows an 88% initiation rate in Australia, and that 55% of mothers were breastfeeding at three months. In Japan in 1985, 92% of infants were fully or partially breastfed during their first month (Manami Hasegawa, Tohori College of Medical Care Technology, Yonango, Japan, 1991).

Latin America. In most Latin American countries close to 90% of infants begin breastfeeding, although mixed feeding is widespread by one month. Moreover, urban/rural differences are pronounced. Urban mothers initiate breastfeeding slightly less frequently than do rural ones, and they wean much more quickly. Many urban infants are weaned by six months, and most are weaned by one year (WHO 1989b); their rural counterparts may still be breastfeeding at 18 months or longer (Sharma et al., 1992).

THE COST OF NOT BREASTFEEDING

To see a world in a grain of sand and a heaven in a wild flower, Hold infinity in the palm of your hand and eternity in an hour. —William Blake, "Auguries of Innocence," c. 1803

Although isolated voices championed breastfeeding throughout its years of steady decline, not until the 1970s did more organized efforts to reverse the trend begin. What prompted this change? Basic, clinical, and demographic research increasingly demonstrated the benefits of breastmilk and breastfeeding to the infant, and of lactation and breastfeeding to the mother. Later still, it has come to be recognized that there is a cost to not breastfeeding.

HEALTH RISKS OF MANUFACTURED INFANT MILKS

To the infant. It has been recognized since the advent of manufactured infant milks that infants fed these products suffered more illness (Howarth, 1905; Woodbury, 1922; Grulee, Sanford & Herron, 1934). This observation is confirmed by more recent studies (Fallot, Boyd & Oski, 1980; Chen, Yu & Li, 1988; Cunningham, 1991). At the time of the earlier studies, the immunological role of breastmilk was unclear; most deleterious effects of such milks were attributed to contamination. In more recent decades it has become established that artificial baby milks increase the risk of ill health because they lack immunological and other health-promoting factors present in human milk. In addition they contain nutrients that are foreign or in non-physiologic proportions (Minchin, 1987). Furthermore, the *act* of bottle-feeding differs from that of breastfeeding in ways that may contribute to health problems in some infants (Mathew & Bhatia, 1989). Artificially fed infants are denied the benefits of "autoimmunization," whereby the breast produces antibodies to organisms to which the infant has been exposed (Fishaut et al., 1981). Immunization may be less effective in artificially fed infants, because manufactured milks do not enhance the immune response to vaccination (Pabst & Spady, 1990).

Recent research shows that artificially fed infants are more susceptible to gastrointestinal infections caused by *Campylobacter* (Ruiz-Palacios et al., 1990), cholera (Glass et al., 1983), and shigella (Cleary et al., 1989), as well as to urinary tract infections (Marild, Jodal & Hanson, 1990; Piscane, Graziano & Zona, 1990). Artificial infant milks may help respiratory pathogens become established (Andersson et al., 1986), and infants so fed are more likely to develop ear infections (Forman et al., 1984; Kero & Piekkala, 1987). Grulee, Sanford and Herron (1934) noted that infants fed cow milk were more likely to have eczema; infants fed manufactured infant milks are also more likely to manifest allergic signs (Chandra, Pusi & Hamed, 1989; Working Group on Cow's Milk Protein Allergy, 1988). One of these signs may be disturbed sleep (Kahn et al., 1987). In premature infants, artificial feeds are a significant risk factor for the serious condition of necrotizing enterocolitis (Lucas & Cole, 1990). Bottle-feeds are associated with poorer oxygenation during feedings in both premature infants (Meier & Anderson, 1987) and term neonates (Mathew & Bhatia, 1989).

To the child and adult. The effects of artificial feeding may extend well beyond infancy. Artificial feeding is implicated in some disease entities which develop in childhood, such as celiac disease (Greco et al., 1988; Kelly et al., 1989), diabetes (Mayer, Hamman & Gay, 1988; Scott, 1990), and lymphoma (Davis, Savitz & Graubard, 1988). Adults with inflammatory bowel disease (Calkins & Mendeloff, 1986) or Crohn's disease (Bergstrand & Hellers, 1983) are more likely to have been fed artificially. Bottle-feeding is also associated with oral malocclusion (Labbok & Hendershot, 1987).

To the mother. Artificial feeding also affects maternal health. In the absence of lactational amenorrhea, additional pregnancies may strain her health. Mothers who bottle-feed their infants are more likely than breastfeeding mothers to develop osteoporosis (Cummings, Kelsey & Nevitt, 1985), premenopausal breast cancer (McTiernan & Thomas, 1986), and ovarian cancer (Schneider, 1987).

ECONOMIC COSTS OF FEEDING MANUFACTURED INFANT MILKS

The presence or absence of breastfeeding affects the economics of the family, the community, and the nation. Some of these effects are more pronounced in less developed regions, but to a degree they affect both elite and poor populations in technologically advanced regions.

To the family. Although lactation imposes some demands on the mother to follow a more substantial diet, these needs are moderated by gastric changes which allow women to metabolize foods more efficiently while lactating (Illingworth et al., 1986; Uvnas-Moberg et al., 1987) and by the water conservation effect of prolactin (Dearlove & Dearlove, 1981). Moreover, the contraceptive effect of full, unrestricted breastfeeding reduces a woman's physical and economic costs of childbearing (Jackson, 1988; Kennedy et al., 1989).

The direct monetary costs of rearing a breastfeeding infant are markedly lower than those of rearing an artificially fed one. In industrial nations, the cost of manufactured baby milks may exceed the cost of additional food for the lactating mother by two or three times; in developing nations the ratio is many times more. In regions where one-third to one-half of those in large urban areas live in poverty, the cost of manufactured products required to provide adequate nutrition (and implements with which to feed them) is a significant portion of the family income (Serva, Karim & Ebrahim, 1986). Other members of the family may eat more poorly because the baby is artificially fed.

Equally important is the reduced need for medical care by breastfed infants (particularly those who are exclusively breastfed). The frequency and severity of illnesses in a young infant is often inversely related to the proportion of his diet which comes from breastmilk (Chen, Yu & Li, 1988). More breastfeeding increases an infant's intake of high quality protein and a variety of other needed nutrients, and it decreases exposure of the infant to potential pathogens in other foodstuffs (Habicht, DaVanzo & Butz, 1988).

Because full breastfeeding, which includes frequent feeds throughout a 24-hour period, tends to delay resumption of ovulation (Lewis et al., 1991), spacing between births tends to increase. Especially in a family living at the subsistence level, the older a child is when displaced from the breast, and the fewer the children in a family, the more likely each is to be healthy. Briend, Wojtyniak and Rowland (1988) state that in malnourished communities, breastfeeding may substantially increase child survival up to three years of age. On the other hand, the time expended in breastfeeding may to some degree reduce maternal time available for other family activities, including the production of food or other items of economic necessity, meal preparation, and caring for other family members. Traditional cultures usually allow a period, up to a few weeks, during which the mother is relieved of many of her normal duties, is provided extra (or special) foods, and is allowed to devote the majority of her time to her new infant. This postpartum "settling in" period is markedly attenuated in most Western societies.

Thus the breastfed infant stands a significantly greater likelihood of surviving. The maternal investment in pregnancy and lactation, and the familial investment in time and money, is repaid by the survival of a child; it is lost to the family when that child dies.

To the community and state. Community or national units that provide health care must respond to the local epidemiology of infant illness, in which

feeding may play a major role. Morbidity is more prevalent in artificially fed infants (Jason, Nieburg & Marks, 1984; Kovar et al., 1984) regardless of location. The increase of the infant population, resulting from the loss of the contraceptive effect of breastfeeding, also serves to increase the need for pediatric health care.

A little-discussed aspect of the decline of breastfeeding is that certain sectors of an economy can become dependent on the payrolls met and taxes paid by infant milk manufacturers, especially if capital funds are obtained from outside the country. Once they become a financial presence in a country, those manufacturers may be politically and economically difficult to dislodge, despite increases in health costs elsewhere in the economy.

Nonetheless, manufactured milk products which are widely used for infant feeding are subsidized by the diversion of resources—land, dairy cattle, and people to manage both—as well as manufacturing capacity pulled from other possible uses. Or such products must be purchased on the international market, and such purchases may markedly affect a nation's balance of trade. Jelliffe and Jelliffe (1978, p. 270) estimate that 150 cans of ready-to-feed manufactured baby milk are used during the first six months of artificial feeding. When one considers that more than 20 million babies are born annually in Africa alone, it becomes apparent that providing adequate volumes of manufactured milks represent a staggering burden and a largely unnecessary diversion of human and monetary resources from other more beneficial programs. At a time when environmental issues have become paramount, these unnecessary uses of power and raw material, not to mention the handling of discarded packaging, is an increasing concern.

PROMOTION OF BREASTFEEDING

Many studies in North America and Europe, especially in Britain and Sweden, have attempted to define the relative characteristics of women who do and who do not breastfeed. This information then gives direction to efforts for promoting breastfeeding. A flaw of many studies is the lack of a clear definition of what behavior was termed "breastfeeding." Breastfeeding behaviors of interest include: (1) initiation of any breastfeeding with the newborn; (2) initiation of exclusive breastfeeding; (3) duration of exclusive breastfeeding; and (4) duration of any breastfeeding. The adoption of a consistent terminology by researchers, such as that proposed by Labbok and Krasovec (1990), will aid interpretation and comparison of study results.

CHARACTERISTICS OF WOMEN WHO BREASTFEED

Initiation of lactation. Consistently since the 1970s, breastfeeding in North America and Western Europe has been more likely to be initiated by older Caucasian women of higher social class: they are more affluent, have more years of formal education, are non-smokers, have attended childbirth classes, have more social support, and intend to breastfeed. By contrast, the exclusive feeding of manufactured infant milks occurs among lower income, non-Caucasian women who smoke and have fewer years of formal education. The conclusion of Grossman and colleagues (1990) that low-income women who chose to breastfeed were more likely to be similar in several respects (such as age, education, and most sources of support) to high-income women who breastfeed is important. Regional differences impinge on women in both the United States and Canada: in general, the incidence of breastfeeding increases from east to west in both countries; in the United States it increases also from south to north. Breastfeeding is little practiced among indigenous peoples of both countries.

Infants who are larger at birth are more likely to be breastfed at one week (Forman et al., 1985; Ryan et al., 1990). Houston and Field (1988) note that smaller babies are more apt to be fed on a routine schedule, which perhaps increases the difficulty of establishing breastfeeding.

Role of the health care system. The role of the health-care system in both undermining and enhancing the initiation of breastfeeding is widely debated. The usual division of care of the breastfeeding dyad—between a gynecologist/obstetrician and a pediatrician—makes the identification and resolution of breastfeeding problems more difficult. Many studies show that few physicians discuss breastfeeding with their patients (although pediatricians are more likely to do so). In any case, few mothers rely on a physician's advice when deciding whether to breastfeed (Mansbach et al., 1984).

Many hospital practices have been implicated in undermining breastfeeding. In an attempt to increase breastfeeding initiation rates, the following changes have been recommended:

- minimize obstetric medication
- breastfeed immediately after birth
- keep mother and infant together during the hospital stay
- place no restrictions on the frequency or duration of breastfeeds
- avoid routine bottle supplements of water or manufactured infant milks, especially before the baby is established at the breast
- withhold complementary samples of artificial baby milk or booklets produced by infant food manufacturers in "gift packs" and given to mothers upon discharge from the hospital
- and enhance among all staff a positive attitude toward, and consistent, correct information about, breastfeeding.

Continuance of lactation. The duration, as opposed to initiation, of lactation is strongly affected by the mother's determination to continue breastfeeding in a predominantly bottle-feeding society (Bottorff, 1990; Coreil & Murphy, 1988). It also may be adversely affected by additional factors, including admission of the neonate into a special-care nursery, even if the reason for admission was minor and transient (Kemper, Forsyth & McCarthy, 1989; Persson, 1985). Early supplementation of breastfeeding with manufactured infant milks is strongly implicated in shortening the duration of breastfeeding both in the United States (Kurinij, Shiono & Rhoads, 1988) and in developing nations (Winikoff & Laukaran, 1989).

Mothers who are physically able to lactate and nurse healthy infants may seek other foods when they perceive that their baby requires more than they are able to provide. Such a perception may be "real," in that the infant's health would indeed benefit from increased breastmilk intake. The volume of breast milk made available to the infant may reflect any one, or a combination, of three factors: (1) intrinsic maternal lactational capacity; (2) the effectiveness of infant suckling; and (3) the mother's "socially determined" capacity, i.e., the amount of milk she produces as a function of cultural attitudes towards breastfeeding and cultural constraints on breastfeeding behavior (see end leaves).

A mother's attentiveness to her infant also has a strong socially determined component. A mother also may seek other foods when she perceives that her breastfed infant needs more maternal attention than she feels she can, or should have to, provide. Infant nursing patterns, general contentedness, and/or sleeping behavior that differ markedly from maternal expectations may prompt the feeding of supplements. Although the relative role which each factor plays may vary among individuals, cultural constraints on breastfeeding behavior are always important determinants of breastmilk transfer.

PROMOTION EFFORTS

The many ways of encouraging mothers to breastfeed their own infants, "breastfeeding promotion," may be considered to lie on a continuum. At one end, in societies where breastfeeding is the cultural norm, "promotion" consists of assuming that mother and infant will breastfeed. This is combined with social arrangements, such as special foods for the mother or lightened duties, especially within the first few weeks after birth, which help to ensure that breastfeeding becomes well established. At the other end, in societies in which artificial feeding is the norm, "promotion" often consists of people—sometimes government officials, often health-care professionals or members of population elites—encouraging others to breastfeed, without at the same time removing cultural barriers to breastfeeding. An index of the status of breastfeeding in a culture positions that culture on this continuum.

Exhortation. Perhaps the commonest form of "breastfeeding promotion" has been exhortation. Caesar (in 48 B.C.) ridiculed, and Tacitus (c. A.D. 100) deplored, Roman mothers who left their children in the care of wet nurses (Hymanson, 1934). During the 1500s in Europe, when breastfeeding was infrequently practiced among the aristocracy, long poems addressed to this class attempted to convince mothers of the cruelty of not breastfeeding (Davidson, 1953). Stricter Protestant sects of this era considered breastfeeding a religious duty, and women belonging to these sects were more likely to breastfeed. By the early 1600s women who did not breastfeed were condemned by Puritan clergy, both from the pulpit and in religious tracts. Elizabeth, Countess of Lincoln, the only woman from the aristocracy who condemned wet-nursing in print during this period, was from a Puritan family (Fildes, 1986, p. 99).

Statements by Health Organizations. In 1978 the American Academy of Pediatrics (Committee on Nutrition, 1978) and the Canadian Paediatric Society jointly issued a statement endorsing breastfeeding—as part of the World Health Organization's program to identify 1979 as the International Year of the Child. Similar public endorsements by other professional organizations of physicians, nurses, and nutritionists began to appear several years later (Coates, 1990).

Governmental Support: the United States. In 1978, the United States Public Health Service defined National Health Objectives for 1990. Among these was that 75% of women should breastfeed at hospital discharge and 35% at six months, as opposed to the actual 1978 figures of 45% and 21% (United States Department of Health and Human Services, 1980). Since these goals were not met by 1990, they were reasserted as goals for the year 2000. To help find ways to work towards these goals, the Surgeon General convened a Workshop on Breastfeeding and Human Lactation in 1984.

The Special Supplemental Food Program for Women, Infants, Children (WIC). Although other government agencies in the United States also work to improve infant nutrition, the WIC program probably directly affects the most people. This program, established in 1972, provides free nutrition counseling and food supplements, including manufactured baby milks, to low-income mothers and their infants. This clientele comes from the population segment in the United States least likely to breastfeed (MacGowan et al., 1991).

The WIC program follows in the footsteps of infant welfare programs in France, England, and the United States of the 1890s and early 1900s in which centers were provided where infants could be weighed and examined weekly. These centers also provided cow milk ("fresh and clean" in some, sterilized in others) to non-breastfeeding mothers in an effort to reduce infant illness and death caused by the use of contaminated milks. By 1903 such milk dispensaries were already being accused of discouraging breastfeeding because they seemed to endorse the use of other infant milks (Wickes, 1953b). Even today, government-sponsored distribution of free milk in Nicaragua, which has occurred since 1970, has been seen as one reason for the decline of breastfeeding there (Sandiford et al., 1991).

WIC has become the largest purchaser of manufactured infant milk—fully 40% of all formula sold—in the United States. For years WIC paid the full retail price; by 1991, when by law WIC was required to purchase manufactured infant milks from the lowest bidder (usually in the form of a rebate from the manufacturer), bids typically came in less than a penny apart in unit price. It has been estimated that in 1988 the purchase of artificial milks for WIC infants' first month of life amounted to more than $30 million (Lazarov, 1989).

Formula manufacturers traditionally have maintained close ties with this important customer in additional ways. A large U.S. manufacturer of artificial baby milk, which bids on WIC contracts, publishes WIC's house newsletter, *WIC Currents.* Formula manufacturers have provided clinics with informational pamphlets on breastfeeding and posters of breastfeeding women; the company logo is prominently displayed on both.

However, in the latter half of the 1980s, the promotion of breastfeeding became an important goal within WIC. Compared with non-breastfeeding mothers, breastfeeding women now have a higher priority for enrollment in WIC programs: they are provided more, and more varied, foods; plus, their benefits persist longer—one year, as opposed to six months for non-breastfeeders.

During the 1980s WIC obtained funds which allowed improved training of WIC nutritionists with respect to breastfeeding, permitted research on how to encourage low-income women to breastfeed, and enabled demonstration projects through which breastfeeding rates have in fact been increased. Reinforcing this commitment is a 1991 directive which bans formula advertising on any item used or displayed in WIC clinics and requires that the formula itself be stored out of sight of clients.

The World Health Organization.   In the 1970s, the deleterious effects of manufactured baby milks on infant health and survival became better appreciated, and the role of advertising in spreading the use of these milks became increasingly suspect. In 1981 the World Health Organization approved, by a vote

of 118 to one (the United States was the dissenting country which voted not to support ratification of the Code), the International Code of Marketing of Breast-milk Substitutes. The Code provides a model of marketing practices which permits the availability of manufactured baby milks, but forbids their advertisement directly to consumers. (See boxed list of provisions on p. 21.) It also seeks to balance the information provided by infant milk manufacturers, in both written "educational" material and in the text or pictures on containers of the product (Armstrong, 1988; IBFAN/IOCU, 1985). An individual country may adopt the International Code in the manner that best fits the needs of that country. In some, as in the United States, no action has been taken, and formula manufacturers are bound only by voluntary adherence to the industry-written "codes of ethics." A few other countries have adopted and do enforce various aspects of the Code.

The Code focuses attention on ways in which the infant formula industry influences both consumers and professionals to support the use of their products. Direct advertising to consumers may be the most obvious, but what Jelliffe and Jelliffe (1978) have called "manipulation by assistance" is also effective. For example, formula manufacturers not only provide free formula to hospital nurseries, but assist in the design of those nurseries (to promote separation of mother and infant), donate equipment to hospitals (gowns for premature infants, for example) and to individual physicians, and support conferences (including some dealing with breastfeeding). They even entertain hospital staff at company-sponsored events; in 1990 in one midwestern U.S. city hospital staff was taken on an outing to the dog races. These "gifts" are treated by the companies as marketing expenses.

As individuals and institutions become financially dependent on such gifts and enmeshed in social relationships with company salespersons, it becomes more difficult to avoid promotion by tacit endorsement of artificial baby milks. By highlighting such practices, the Code may make health-care professionals more aware of the intent behind them, and thus perhaps more resistant to their allure.

In 1990 the World Health Organization and UNICEF were instrumental in the development of the Innocenti Declaration, which restated the importance of breastfeeding for maternal and child health. It set forth four goals to be met by 1995: (1) the establish-

---

WHO/UNICEF CODE FOR MARKETING BREAST-MILK SUBSTITUTES

- No advertising of these products to the public.
- No free samples to mothers.
- No promotion of products in health-care facilities.
- No company mothercraft nurses to advise mothers.
- No gifts or personal samples to health workers.
- No words or pictures idealizing artificial feeding, including pictures of infants, on the products.

- Information to health workers should be scientific and factual.
- All information on artificial feeding, including the labels, should explain the benefits of breastfeeding, and the costs and hazards associated with artificial feeding.
- Unsuitable products, such as condensed milk, should not be promoted for babies.
- All products should be of a high quality and take into account the climatic and storage conditions of the country where they are used.

---

ment of national breastfeeding coordinators; (2) the practice of Ten Steps to Successful Breastfeeding by maternity services (see boxed checklist on this page); (3) the implementation of the WHO Code; and (4) enactment of enforceable laws for protecting the breastfeeding rights of employed women (UNICEF, 1990). The World Alliance for Breastfeeding Action, a multinational coalition of individuals and private organizations involved in research and

promotion of breastfeeding, works to ensure that the goals of the Innocenti Declaration are met.

Legislation. Legislation intended to increase the prevalence of breastfeeding may mandate actions which encourage breastfeeding or which discourage feeding of artificial baby milks (or use of wet nurses) or both. Lycurgus, who was King of Sparta about 350 B.C., set an early example: he required not only that

---

TEN STEPS TO SUCCESSFUL BREASTFEEDING*

Every facility providing maternity services and care for newborn infants should:

1. Have a written breastfeeding policy that is routinely communicated to all health-care staff.
2. Train all health-care staff in skills necessary to implement this policy.
3. Inform all pregnant women about the benefits and management of breastfeeding.
4. Help mothers initiate breastfeeding within 30 minutes after birth.
5. Show mothers how to breastfeed, and how to maintain lactation even if they should be separated from their infants.

6. Give newborn infants no food or drink other than breast milk, unless *medically* indicated.
7. Practice rooming-in—allow mothers and infants to remain together—24 hours a day.
8. Encourage breastfeeding on demand.
9. Give no artificial teats or pacifiers (also called dummies or soothers) to breastfeeding infants.
10. Foster the establishment of breastfeeding support groups and refer mothers to them on discharge from the hospital or clinic.

From: Protecting, Promoting and Supporting Breastfeeding: The Special Role of Maternity Services. A joint WHO/UNICEF statement, Geneva, 1989, World Health Organization.
*These steps form the basis for the "Baby Friendly Hospital Initiative."

mothers nurse their own infants, but that nursing mothers be shown kindness and respect (Hymanson, 1934).

A more modern example is legislation following the model of the World Health Organization Code of Marketing of Breast-Milk Substitutes. The advertising of infant feeding bottles and artificial infant milks was forbidden by law in the mid-1970s in Papua New Guinea; both are still available, but only by prescription. The benefits of breastfeeding were publicized to the general population and to health workers. This dual approach increased the prevalence of breastfeeding among children who were less than two years of age by 23%—from 65% in 1976 to 88% in 1979 (Biddulph, 1981). In 1986, the government of the Philippines banned the distribution of free and subsidized artificial infant milks to hospitals, and it imposed fines or prison sentences on violators of the ban. The distribution of such milks intended for young infants declined by 95% between 1986 and 1988. Although it remains to be seen whether this policy will result in an increase in breastfeeding, the policy now makes it less convenient and more expensive for mothers to use artificial infant milks in the hospital (Popkin, Fernandez & Avila, 1990).

Private support movements. In the 1950s and 1960s, at the same time that breastfeeding was becoming less prevalent, individuals interested in breastfeeding and sharing information about breastfeeding found each other and formed mutual-support groups. La Leche League was founded in the United States in 1956; Nursing Mothers' Association of Australia started up in 1965, and Ammenhjelpen of Sweden opened in 1968. La Leche League now has over 3,500 groups in 46 countries around the world. Its manual is translated into eight languages, and it provides some information in 28 others. Members of groups such as these, by their demonstration that even "modern" mothers can breastfeed, and by their requests to medical personnel for information about medical practices that enhance the ease of breastfeeding, have been a major force behind the dissemination of technical information concerning lactation, human milk, and breastfeeding that began in the late 1970s. To better reach low-income women, who are not commonly La Leche League members, the organization has begun training peer counselors. These counselors, low-income women who have breastfed and have completed a training

program, offer breastfeeding advice and support in clinics which serve low-income populations. Such counselors can be very effective: a Chicago WIC clinic reported an eight-fold increase in breastfeeding during a six-month period in which peer counselors were available (Heiser, 1990). La Leche League is officially recognized as a "Non-Governmental Organization" qualified to consult on breastfeeding to organizations such as the United Nations and the United States Agency for International Development.

Public/private coalitions. The Healthy Mothers/Healthy Babies coalition in the United States informally brings together representatives of the United States Department of Agriculture, the Department of Health and Human Services, and some 60 other public agencies and private organizations for the purpose of promoting prenatal and infant care—including breastfeeding. Market research conducted by the Public Health Service provides a better focus on efforts to promote breastfeeding to low-income women (Wittenberg, 1983).

ELEMENTS OF BREASTFEEDING PROMOTION PROGRAMS

Between the mid-1970s and mid-1980s, the prevalence of breastfeeding generally increased in North America, Europe, and some British Commonwealth countries. During this period, the "promotion" of breastfeeding tended to take one of three forms: (1) encouragement and information provided by other breastfeeding mothers; (2) efforts by individuals and policy statements of professional organizations which supported hospital maternity-unit policies favorable to breastfeeding; and (3) popular articles, usually in women's magazines, which discussed the benefits of breastfeeding. These efforts are all important, but they are not solely responsible for creating the favorable climate necessary for a greater prevalence of breastfeeding. Two other components of a comprehensive promotion program for encouraging breastfeeding have been noted by Jelliffe and Jelliffe (1989). They are: (4) services and legislation which protect a woman's right to breastfeed when she is employed outside of the home; and (5) regulation of marketing practices of the infant-formula industry.

The first three components generally involve individual efforts—those of breastfeeding mothers, hospital personnel, and writers. The fourth and fifth components require legislative sanctions. A sixth component is also necessary, but is even more difficult to obtain, because it requires changes in attitudes of society at large: acceptance of the need for mother/child togetherness and the right of the breastfeeding dyad to participate in social, civic, and commercial activities outside the home. For many women, the ultimate barrier to breastfeeding is not sore nipples, night-time nursing, or employment outside the home. It is the disapproval they encounter from men, as well as from other women—either for "wasting" education and career skills by staying home with their breastfeeding infants; or for taking their breastfeeding infant with them to work, church, school, or perhaps to a city council or parent-teacher meeting. A goal for all mothers, whether they are breastfeeding or not, should be to empower women so that they are able to attend to all their duties, maternal as well as civic, religious, and professional, and to do so concurrently if need be.

CONCLUSION

Humans evolved within the mammalian lineage, which has provided a species-specific milk for the nourishment and protection of the young of each species. For millennia the staple of the human infant's diet has been human milk obtained directly from the human breast, commonly in situations where no other food was suitable. Within the last century or so, as breastfeeding became associated with more restrictive aspects of women's lives, as breastmilk was thought by some to be inferior to increasingly available manufactured infant milks, and as use of manufactured milks became a hallmark of privileged segments of society, large portions of both lay and health-care populations came to believe that there was little reason to persist in traditional breastfeeding practices.

In the 1990s, however, it has become increasingly clear that breastfeeding confers health and psychological advantages on the breastfeeding infant—and to the child and adult into which that infant will grow. Breastfeeding enhances aspects of maternal health as well. Breastfeeding is economically frugal and ecologically sound. Breastfeeding is important. Most mothers and most health-care providers now recognize this.

Those who do breastfeed, or who promote the re-establishment of breastfeeding as the norm in infant feeding, do so not because there are no alternatives but because the alternatives are inferior. Unfortunately, the belief that breastfeeding is the optimal way to nourish an infant may not be enough to empower a woman to breastfeed. Knowledge of beneficial breastfeeding practices and the social acceptance of those practices is also required. Currently, the prevalence of breastfeeding reflects the importance which society places on it, as measured by the degree to which breastfeeding mothers and infants are accepted in the life of the community at large. Returning breastfeeding wisdom to the public domain, and reintegrating it into the social fabric so that women who wish to breastfeed may do so without hindrance, is the challenge that awaits.

REFERENCES

Aitken, FC, and Hytten, FE: Infant feeding: comparison of breast and artificial feeding, *Nutr Abstr and Rev* 30:341–71, 1960.

American Academy of Pediatrics Committee on Nutrition, and the Nutrition Committee of the Canadian Paediatric Society: Breast-feeding; a commentary in celebration of the International Year of the Child, *Pediatrics* 62:591–601, 1978.

Andersson, B, et al.: Inhibition of attachment of Streptococcus pneumoniae and Haemophilus influenzae by human milk and receptor oligosaccharides, *J Infec Dis* 153:232–37, 1986.

Apple, RD: "Advertised by our loving friends": the infant formula industry and the creation of new pharmaceutical markets, 1870–1910, *J Hist Med Allied Sci* 41:3–23, 1986.

Armstrong, H: The International Code of Marketing of Breast-Milk Substitutes, Part Two of a Series, *J Hum Lact* 4:194–99, 1988.

Bain, K: The incidence of breast feeding in hospitals in the United States, *Pediatrics* 2:313–20, 1948.

Bergstrand, O, and Hellers, G: Breast-feeding during infancy in patients who later develop Crohn's disease, *Scand J Gastroenterol* 18:903–6, 1983.

Bernard of Gordon (Bernardus Gordonius): *Regimen sanitas*, Vatican Palatine Latin manuscript 1174, 1309. Cited in Fildes, op. cit., p. 47.

Biddulph J: Promotion of breast-feeding: Experience in Papua New Guinea. In Jelliffe, DB, and Jelliffe, EF, eds., *Advances in international maternal and child health, vol. 1*, Oxford, 1981, Oxford Press. Cited in Huffman, S, 1984, op. cit.

Blake, W: Auguries of Innocence. In Spencer, H, Houghton, WE, and Barrows, H, eds., *British literature from Blake to the present day*, Boston, 1952, D.C. Heath & Co., pp. 22–23.

Bottorf, JL: Persistence in breastfeeding: a phenomenological investigation, *J Adv Nurs* 15:201–09, 1990.

Briend, A, Wojtyniak, B, and Rowland, MGM: Breast feeding, nutritional state, and child survival in rural Bangladesh, *Br Med J* 296:879–82, 1988.

Budin, P: *The nursling* (WJ Maloney, trans.), London, 1907. Cited in Wickes, 1953b, op. cit.

Bull, T: *Hints to mothers,* 6th ed., London, 1849. Cited in Wickes, 1953a, op. cit.

Cadogan, W: *An essay on nursing and the management of children from their birth to three years of age,* London; J Roberts, 1749 (3rd ed. 1769). Cited in Kessen, 1965; pp. 10–30 op. cit.

Calkins, BM, and Mendeloff, AI: Epidemiology of inflammatory bowel disease, *Epidemiol Rev* 8:60–91, 1986.

Chandra, RK, Pusi, S, and Hamed, A: Influence of maternal diet during lactation and use of formula feeds on development of atopic eczema in high-risk infants, *Br Med J* 299:228–30, 1989.

Chen, Y, Yu, S, and Li, W: Artificial feeding and hospitalization in the first 18 months of life, *Pediatrics* 81:58–62, 1988.

Cleary, TG, et al.: Human milk immunoglobulin A antibodies to Shigella virulence determinants, *Infec Immunol* 57:1675–79, 1989.

Coates, MM, ed.: Policy statements. In *The lactation consultant's topical review and bibliography of the literature on breastfeeding,* Franklin Park, 1990, La Leche League International, 188 pp.

Coreil, J, and Murphy, JE: Maternal commitment, lactation practices, and breastfeeding duration, *JOGNN* July/Aug: 273–78, 1988.

Cummings, SR, Kelsey, JL, and Nevitt, MC: Epidemiology of osteoporosis and osteoporotic fractures, *Epidemiol Rev* 7:178–208, 1985.

Cunningham, AS, Jelliffe, DB, and Jelliffe, EFP: Breast-feeding and health in the 1980s: a global epidemiologic review, *J Pediatr* 118:659–66, 1991.

Davidson, WD: A brief history of infant feeding, *J Pediatr* 43:74–87, 1953.

Davis, MK, Savitz, DA, and Graubard, BI: Infant feeding and childhood cancer, *Lancet* 2(8607):365–68, 1988.

Dearlove, JC, and Dearlove, BM: Prolactin, fluid balance, and lactation, *Br J Obstet Gynaecol* 88:652–54, 1981.

Deruisseau, LG: Infant hygiene in the older medical literature, *Ciba Symposia* 2:530–60, 1940.

Dimond, HJ, and Ashworth, A: Infant feeding practices in Kenya, Mexico and Malaysia: the rarity of the exclusively breastfed infant, *Human Nutr, Appl Nutr* 41A:51–64, 1987.

Eaton, SB, and Konner, M: Paleolithic nutrition: a consideration of its nature and current implications, *N Engl J Med* 312:283–89, 1985.

Eckhardt, KW, and Hendershot, GE: Analysis of the reversal in breast feeding trends in the early 1970s, *Public Health Rep* 99:410–15, 1984.

Emery, JL, Scholey, S, and Taylor, EM: Decline in breast feeding, *Arch Dis Child* 65:369–72, 1990.

Ettmuller, M: *Etmullerus Abrig'd,* 2nd ed., London, 1703. Cited in Wickes, 1953a, op cit.

Fallot, ME, Boyd, JL III, and Oski, FA: Breastfeeding reduces incidence of hospital admissions for infection in infants, *Pediatrics* 65:1121–24, 1980.

Fildes, VA: *Breasts, bottles, and babies: A history of infant feeding,* Edinburgh, 1986, Edinburgh University Press, 462 pp.

Fishaut, M, et al.: Bronchomammary axis in the immune response to respiratory syncytial virus, *J Pediatr* 99: 186–89, 1981.

Forman, MR, et al.: The PIMA infant feeding study: breast feeding and respiratory infections during the first year of life, *Int J Epidemiol* 13:447–53, 1984.

Forman, MR, et al.: Exclusive breast-feeding of newborns among married women in the United States: the National Natality Surveys of 1969 and 1980, *Am J Clin Nutr* 42:864–69, 1985.

Gerrard, JW: Breast-feeding: second thoughts, *Pediatrics* 54:757–64, 1974.

Glass, RI, et al.: Protection against cholera in breast-fed children by antibodies in breast milk, *N Engl J Med* 308:1389–92, 1983.

Greco, L, et al.: Case control study on nutritional risk factors in celiac disease, *J Pediatr Gastroenterol Nutr* 7:395–99, 1988.

Greer, FR, and Apple, RD: Physicians, formula companies, and advertising: a historical perspective, *Am J Dis Child* 145:282–86, 1991.

Grossman, LK, et al.: The infant feeding decision in low and upper income women, *Clin Pediatr* 29:30–37, 1990.

Grulee, CG, Sanford, HN, and Herron, PH: Breast and artificial feeding: influence on morbidity and mortality of twenty thousand infants, *JAMA* 103:735–39, 1934.

Habicht, J-P, DaVanzo, J, and Butz, WP: Mother's milk and sewage: their interactive effect on infant mortality, *Pediatrics* 88:456–61, 1988.

Heiser, B: Reaching out to all, *Breastfeeding Abstr* 9:19–20, 1990.

Hendershot, GE: *Trends in breast feeding,* United States Dept. of Health and Human Services, No. 80–1250, Hyattsville, Maryland, 1980, National Center for Health Statistics.

Hill, LF: A salute to La Leche League International, *J Pediatr* 73:161–62, 1968.

Hirschman, C, and Butler, M: Trends and differentials in breast feeding: an update, *Demography* 18:39–54, 1981.

Hitchcock, NE: Infant feeding in Australia: an historical perspective, *Breastfeed Rev* 2:71–77, 1990.

Houston, MJR, and Field, PA: Practices and policies in the initiation of breastfeeding, *JOGNN* Nov/Dec:418–24, 1988.

Howarth, WJ: The influence of feeding on the mortality of infants, *Lancet* 2:210–13, 1905.

Huffman, SL: Determinants of breastfeeding in developing countries: overview and policy implications, *Stud Fam PLANN* 15:170–83, 1984.

Hymanson, A: A short review of the history of infant feeding, *Arch Pediatr* 51:1–10, 1934.

Illingworth, PJ, et al.: Diminution in energy expenditure during lactation, *Br Med J* 292:437–41, 1986.

IBFAN/IOCU: *Protecting infant health: a health worker's*

guide to the International Code of Marketing of Breast-milk Substitutes, Penang, Malasia, 1985, IBFAN/IOCU.

Jackson, RI: Ecological breastfeeding and child spacing, *Clin Pediatr* 27:373–77, 1988.

Jason, JM, Nieburg, P, and Marks, JS: Mortality and disease associated with infant-feeding practices in developing countries, *Pediatrics* 74:702–727, 1984.

Jelliffe, DB: Culture, social change and infant feeding: current trends in tropical regions, *Am J Clin Nutr* 10:19–45, 1962.

Jelliffe, DB, and Jelliffe, EFP: *Human milk in the modern world,* Oxford, 1978, Oxford University Press, 500 pp.

———: World-wide breast feeding programmes—consideration of key components, *J Trop Pediatr* 35:144–46, 1989.

Kahn, A, et al.: Difficulty in initiating and maintaining sleep associated with cow's milk allergy in infants, *Sleep* 19: 116–21, 1987.

Kelly, DW, et al.: Rise and fall of coeliac disease, 1960–1985, *Arch Dis Child* 64:1157–60, 1989.

Kemper, K, Forsyth, B, and McCarthy, P: Jaundice, terminating breast-feeding, and the vulnerable child, *Pediatrics* 84:773–78, 1989.

Kennedy, K, et al.: Consensus statement on the use of breastfeeding as a family planning method, *Contraception* 39:477–96, 1989.

Kero, P, and Piekkala, P: Factors affecting the occurrence of acute otitis media during the first year of life, *Acta Paediatr Scand* 76:618–23, 1987.

Kessen, W: *The child.* New York: John Wiley & Sons, 1965.

Konner, M, and Worthman, C: Nursing frequency, gonadal function, and birth spacing among iKung hunter-gatherers, *Science* 207:788–91, 1980.

Kovar, MG, et al.: Review of the epidemiologic evidence for an association between infant feeding and infant health, *Pediatrics* 74:615–638, 1984.

Kurinij, N, Shiono, PH, and Rhoads, GG: Breast-feeding incidence and duration in black and white women, *Pediatrics* 81:365–71, 1988.

Kusin, JA, Kardjati, S, and van Steenbergen, W: Traditional infant feeding practices: right or wrong? *Soc Sci Med* 21:283–86, 1985.

Labbok, M, and Hendershot,GE: Does breast-feeding protect against malocclusion? An analysis of the 1981 Child Health Supplement to the National Health Interview survey, *Am J Prev Med* 3:227–32, 1987.

Labbok, M, and Krasovec, K: Toward consistency in breastfeeding definitions, *Stud Fam Plann* 21:226–30, 1990.

Lacaille, AD: Infant feeding-bottles in prehistoric times, *Proc Roy Soc Med* 43:565–68, 1950.

Lancet: Present day practice in infant feeding (editorial), *Lancet* 1:975–76, 1988.

Latham, MC, et al.: Infant feeding in urban Kenya: a pattern of early triple nipple feeding, *J Trop Pediatr* 32:276–80, 1986.

Lazarov, M.: Testimony of Minda Lazarov, Director, Tennessee Breastfeeding Promotion Project, before the Subcommittee on Nutrition and Investigations of the Senate Committee on Agriculture, Nutrition and Forestry, June 15, 1989. Available from the Tennessee Department of Health and Environment.

Levenstein, H: "Best for babies" or "Preventable infanticide"? The controversy over artificial feeding of infants in America, 1880–1920, *J Am Hist* 70:75–94, 1983.

Lewis, PR, et al.: The resumption of ovulation and menstruation in a well-nourished population of women breastfeeding for an extended period of time, *Fertil Steril* 55:529–36, 1991.

Lightbourne, R, and Singh S, with Green, CP: The World Fertility Survey: charting global childbearing, *Pop Bull* 37:7–55, 1982.

Livingstone, V: Problem-solving formula for failure to thrive in breast-fed infants, *Can Fam Phys* 36:1541–45, 1990.

Lucas, A, and Cole, TJ: Breast milk and neonatal necrotising enterocolitis, *Lancet* 336(8730):1519–23, 1990.

MacGowan, RJ, et al.: Breast-feeding among women attending Women, Infants, and Children clinics in Georgia, 1987, *Pediatrics* 87:361–66, 1991.

Mansbach, IL, et al.: Advice from the obstetrician and other sources: do they affect women's breastfeeding practices? A study among different Jewish groups in Jerusalem, *Soc Sci Med* 19:157–62, 1984.

Marild, S, Jodal, U, and Hanson, LA: Breastfeeding and urinary-tract infection, *Lancet* 336(8720):942, 1990.

Martinez, GA, and Krieger, FW: 1984 milk-feeding patterns in the United States, *Pediatrics* 76:1004–8, 1985.

Martinez, GA, and Nalezienski, JP: The recent trend in breast-feeding, *Pediatrics* 64:686–92, 1979.

Mathew, OP, and Bhatia, J: Sucking and breathing patterns during breast- and bottle-feeding in term neonates: effects of nutrient delivery and composition, *Am J Dis Child* 143:588–92, 1989.

Mayer, EJ, Hamman, RF, and Gay, EC: Reduced risk of IDDM among breast-fed children: The Colorado IDDM Registry, *Diabetes* 37:1625–32, 1988.

McCracken, RD: Lactase deficiency: an example of dietary evolution, *Curr Anthrop* 12:479–517, 1971.

McTiernan, A, and Thomas, DB: Evidence for a protective effect of lactation on risk of breast cancer in young women: results from a case-control study, *Am J Epidemiol* 124:353–58, 1986.

Mead Johnson (advertisement):*JAMA* 95:22, 1930.

Meier, P, and Anderson, GC: Responses of small preterm infants to bottle- and breast-feeding, *MCN* 12:97–105, 1987.

Meyer, HF: Breast feeding in the United States. Report of a 1966 national survey with comparable 1946 and 1956 data, *Clin Pediatr* 7:708–15, 1968.

Millard, AV: The place of the clock in pediatric advice: rationales, cultural themes, and impediments to breastfeeding, *Soc Sci Med* 31:211–21, 1990.

Minchin, M: Infant formula: a mass, uncontrolled trial in perinatal care, *Birth* 14:25–35, 1987.

Morse, JM: "Euch, those are for your husband!" Examination of cultural values and assumptions associated with breast-feeding, *Health Care Women Int* 11:223–232, 1989.

Morse, JM, Jehle, C, and Gamble, D: Initiating breastfeeding: a world survey of the timing of postpartum breastfeeding, *Int J Nurs Stud* 27:303–13, 1990.

Nestlé's Food (advertisement): *The Ladies' Home Journal* 9:26, 1892.

Nga, NT, and Weissner, P: Breast-feeding and young child nutrition in Uong Bi, Quang Ninh province, Vietnam, *J Trop Pediatr* 32:137–39, 1986.

Pabst, HF, and Spady, DW: Effect of breast-feeding on antibody response to conjugate vaccine, *Lancet* 336(8710): 269–70, 1990.

Persson, LA: Multivariate approaches to the analysis of breast-feeding habits, *Bull WHO* 63:1129–36, 1985.

Piscane, A, Graziano, L, and Zona, G: Breastfeeding and urinary tract infection, *Lancet* 336(8706):50, 1990.

Popkin, BM, Fernandez, ME, and Avila, JL: Infant formula promotion and the health sector in the Philippines, *Am J Public Health* 80:74–75, 1990.

Richards B: Early suckling and prolonged breast-feeding (letter), *Am J Dis Child* 141:741, 1986. Reply: Taylor, PM, Maloni, JA, and Brown, DR: *Am J Dis Child* 141:741, 1986.

Rossiter, FM: *The practical guide to health, a popular treatise on anatomy, physiology, and hygiene, with a scientific description of diseases, their causes and treatment, designed for nurses and home use*, 1908, Pacific Press Publishing Association. Reprinted in part (pp. 462–63, pp. 500–506) in *J Hum Lact* 7:89–91, 1991.

Rotch, TM: An historical sketch of the development of percentage feeding, *NY Med J* 85:532–37, 1907.

Ruiz-Palacios, GM, et al.: Protection of breast-fed infants against Campylobacter bacteria by antibodies in human milk, *J Pediatr* 116:707–13, 1990.

Ryan, AS, et al.: Duration of breast-feeding patterns established in hospital: influencing factors. Results from a national survey, *Clin Pediatr* 29:99–107, 1990.

Ryan, AS, et al.: Recent declines in breast-feeding in the United States, 1984–1989, *Pediatrics*, 88:719–27, 1991.

Sandiford, P, et al.: Why do child mortality rates fall? An analysis of the Nicaraguan experience, *Am J Public Health* 81:30–37, 1991.

Schaefer, O: The impact of culture on breastfeeding patterns, *J Perinatol* 6:62–65, 1986.

Schneider, AP III: Risk factor for ovarian cancer, *N Engl J Med* 317:508–9, 1987.

Scott, FW: Cow milk and insulin-dependent diabetes mellitus: is there a relationship? *Am J Clin Nutr* 51:489–91, 1990.

Serva, V, Karim, H, and Ebrahim, GJ: Breast-feeding and the urban poor in developing countries, *J Trop Pediatr* 32:127–29, 1986.

Short, RV: Breast feeding, *Scient Am*, 250:35–41, 1984.

Simoons, FJ: Age of onset of lactose malabsorption, *Pediatrics* 66:646–48, 1980.

Slome, C: Nonpuerperal lactation in grandmothers, *J Pediatr* 49:550–52, 1976.

Smith, H: *Letters to married women on nursing and the management of children*. The 3rd edition, revised and considerably enlarged, London, 1774. Cited in Fildes, 1986, op. cit.

United Nations Children's Fund: Innocenti Declaration on the Protection, Promotion and Support of Breastfeeding, Florence, Italy, 1 August 1990. UNICEF, Nutrition Cluster (H-8F), 3 United Nations Plaza, New York, New York 10017.

United States Department of Health and Human Services, Public Health Service: *Promoting health/preventing disease: objectives for the nation*, Washington, 1980, US Government Printing Office.

Uvnas-Moberg, K, et al.: Release of GI hormones in mother and infant by sensory stimulation, *Acta Paediatr Scand* 76:851–60, 1987.

Verronen, P, et al.: Promotion of breastfeeding: effect on neonates of change of feeding routine at a maternity unit, *Acta Paediatr Scand* 69:279–82, 1980.

Wade, N: Bottle-feeding: Adverse effects of a Western technology, *Science* 184:45–48, 1974.

Whitehead, RG: The human weaning process, *Pediatrics* 75(suppl. 1):189–93, 1985.

Wickes, IG: A history of infant feeding. Part III. Eighteenth and nineteenth century writers, *Arch Dis Child* 28:332–40, 1953a.

Wickes, IG: A history of infant feeding. Part V. Nineteenth century concluded and twentieth century, *Arch Dis Child* 28:495–502, 1953b.

Wieschhoff, HA: Artificial stimulation of lactation in primitive cultures, *Bull Hist Med* 8:1403–15, 1940.

Williamson, MA: *Infant mortality: Montclair, NJ: A study of infant mortality in a suburban community*, Washington, 1915, United States Department of Labor, Children's Bureau.

Winikoff, B, et al.: Dynamics of infant feeding: mothers, professionals, and the institutional context in a large urban hospital, *Pediatrics* 77:357–65, 1986.

Winikoff, B, and Laukaran, VH: Breast feeding and bottle feeding controversies in the developing world: evidence from a study in four countries, *Soc Sci Med* 29:859–868, 1989.

Wittenberg, CK: Summary of market research for "Healthy Mothers, Healthy Babies" campaign, *Public Health Rep* 98:356–59, 1983.

Woodbury, RM: The relation between breast and artificial feeding and infant mortality, *Am J Hyg* 2:668–87, 1922.

Woolridge, MW, Greasley, V, and Silpisornkosol, S: The initiation of lactation: the effect of early versus delayed contact for suckling on milk intake in the first week postpartum. A study in Chiang Mai, northern Thailand, *Early Hum Dev* 12:269–78, 1985.

Working Group on Cow's Milk Protein Allergy. Cow's milk allergy in the first year of life, *Acta Paediatr Scand* Suppl. 348:2–14, 1988.

World Health Organization: *Contemporary patterns of breast-feeding*, Geneva, 1981, World Health Organization.

———: The prevalence and duration of breast-feeding: Updated information, 1980–1989. Part I. *Wkly Epidem Rec* 42:321–23, 1989a.

———: The prevalence and duration of breast-feeding: Updated information, 1980–1989. Part II. *Wkly Epidem Rec* 43:331–34, 1989b.

2

The Cultural Context
of Breastfeeding

DEFINITIONS AND CHARACTERISTICS

Culture exerts a major influence on a mother's attitude towards breastfeeding and how she decides to feed her baby. Attitudes and patterns of infant feeding cannot be understood without placing them in their specific cultural context. The purpose of this chapter is to look at breastfeeding as a human behavior that is sensitive to cultural influence and social change.

Culture is defined as the values, beliefs, norms, and practices of a particular group which are learned, shared and guide thinking, decisions and actions in a patterned way (Leininger, 1985). Culture provides implicit and explicit codes of behavior. Culture is:

- *Learned* both through language and socialization
- *Shared,* often unconsciously, by all members of a cultural group who are then bound together under one identity
- An *adaptation* to specific conditions related to environmental and technical factors and to the availability of natural resources
- A *dynamic,* ever-changing process.

From a practical standpoint, a society's culture consists of whatever one has to know or believe in order to operate in a manner acceptable to its members (van Esterik, 1988). It is a blueprint for human behavior that helps us to gain a clearer understanding of individual behaviors. Women and their families have a right to expect that their cultural needs will be met as they are helped with breastfeeding and lactation. Without understanding the mother's cultural practices, our care and intervention could do more harm than good.

JAN RIORDAN

THE DOMINANT CULTURE

Every society has a dominant culture, the values of which are shared by the majority of its members as a result of early common experiences. Although there are approximately 100 ethnic groups in the United States (Spector, 1985), the dominant cultural group is that of white, middle-class Protestants—descendants of northern Europeans who immigrated to the United States several generations ago. Characteristic norms of this group are a high school education; a conservative value system; family orientation; commitment to higher education for one's children; a work ethic which dictates that individuals should work and are failures if they are unemployed; materialism; a personal faith in God; the quest for physical beauty; cleanliness; high technology; punctuality; independence; and free enterprise. The dominant health culture in the United States views birth as dangerous for the mother and neonate. Breastfeeding is seen as the optimal method of infant feeding, but difficult to accomplish and an intimate private act not to be practiced in public.

In the United States, Western allopathic medicine is viewed as "professional" health care; any medical tradition outside this system is considered traditional folk medicine with its accompanying connotations of primitive, "useless," "lay," and "outdated" (Boyle & Andrews, 1989). The dominant U.S. health system marketplace is comprised of the hospital, the health worker's office, and community health departments. The folk belief system marketplace cen-

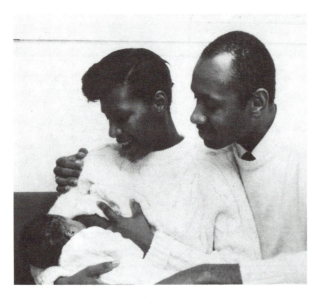

FIGURE 2–1. Each family has its own expectations about breastfeeding that are partially based on culture.

ters around the home of the client or the homes of their extended kin (Scott & Stern, 1985).

According to Scott and Stern (1985), there are three types of consumers of health care:

1. the corporate buyer, who buys the dominant health care system completely
2. the careful shopper, who balances between the folk health system and the dominant health system
3. the cultural buyer, who buys only the folk health system.

Folk health beliefs may be combined with health care beliefs of the dominant culture. For instance, Scott and Stern (1985) found that black women in northern Louisiana selected bicultural elements from the influences of folk treatments offered by older women in their culture as well as scientific Western-style remedies.

Ethnocentrism may be defined as being centered in one's own ethnic or cultural system, i.e., judging the world by one's own standards, or believing that "my group is best." When caring for culturally diverse groups, nurses and health-care workers at first tend to ethnocentric, believing that their own professional, scientifically based practices are superior. Most of the health-care workers reading this book have been socialized into their profession within the framework of a Western health-care system which emphasizes the biomedical model and is based on the white, working- and middle-class value system. If this system is the *only* model that is used to evaluate and implement care, the nurse or lactation consultant is ethnocentric. Fortunately, once health-care workers are exposed to other cultures, they begin to appreciate why certain behavior and values have been effective in that culture and move beyond ethnocentric behaviors (Tripp-Reimer, Brink & Saunders, 1984).

The opposite of ethnocentrism is *cultural relativism,* in which the care provider recognizes and appreciates cultural differences and treats each client with deference to her cultural background. She builds on and uses cultural variations instead of seeing them as obstacles.

In order to be able to provide for optimal care, the caregiver must first understand her *own* reaction to cultural differences and then appreciate how these cultural values affect the lives of her clients. By discovering areas of commonality between herself and the mother, the nurse or care provider will then be better able to recognize and deal with cultural similarities and variations between the client and herself (Orque, Bloch & Monrroy, 1983). This process is illustrated in Fig. 2–2.

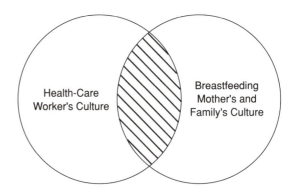

FIGURE 2–2. Shared values and beliefs. Orque MS, Block B, & Monrroy, LS: *Ethnic nursing care: A multicultural approach,* St. Louis, 1983, The C.V. Mosby Co., p. 19.

"Cultural relativism likewise recognizes variation within cultures, such as the diverse ethnic groups in the United States. At one time people expected and hoped that these ethnic and cultural groups would blend into one common whole. It has not worked out that way; many third and fourth generation Americans proudly claim and identify with their ethnic heritage. Brownlee (1978) describes a clinic worker in Boston who was annoyed at the way local residents generalized about the city's many cultural groups: "Haitian is like this, Hispanic is like that, you know those Italians all lie . . . and oh, those Puerto Ricans, they never ever. . . ." Brownlee felt these stereotypes blinded people to the diversity *within* each of these many groups.

ASSESSING CULTURE

To provide culturally appropriate care, nurses and other care providers must first systematically gather information about a culture. Ethnographic fieldwork is vital to obtain data about the components of a given culture. For example, in the early 1980s infant feeding practices in four developing countries were studied by collecting data on mother-child pairs using large-scale sample surveys. The researchers collected other information from government documents and extensive personal interviews (van Esterik & Elliott, 1986; see also Winikoff, 1988).

Cultural elements that are important to assess include language, foodways, dress, patterns of social behavior, religious customs, rituals, use of time and space, nonverbal communication, health-illness belief systems, and economic-political systems. Collecting cultural data is a skill that must be studied, learned and practiced to know the right questions to ask and the right way to ask those questions. The health-care worker should collect sufficient data to compile as complete a picture as possible without becoming overwhelmed with too much raw data and information.

The most useful methods of gathering cultural information are by conducting focus groups, interviewing key informants, and reviewing current literature (Labbok, personal communication, 1991). Focus groups are group interviews in which information is collected from a group discussion among four to

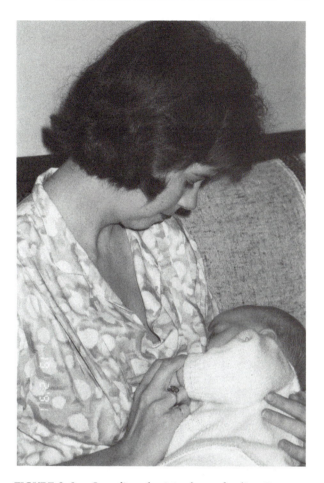

FIGURE 2–3.   Canadian physician breastfeeding. Recognizing one's own cultural values is the basis of appreciating cultural diversity. (Courtesy G. Arsenault.)

ten participants who discuss their thoughts and experiences about breastfeeding or other selected topics. In a focus group women are more likely to share ideas with other group members; this triggers additional thought and in-depth discussion not possible in a one-to-one interview. The following techniques can provide other rich sources of cultural data:

- find a close confidant and other good informants to help you "bridge the gap" between cultures
- talk with "ordinary" family members (mothers, fathers, grandmothers, older children) who can alert the care provider to divergent cultural beliefs among the family

- talk with people who serve as a social support to mothers in early infant care matters (female relatives, grandmothers, fathers)
- visit hospitals and clinics and talk with nurses and physicians
- get to know local leaders and residents of the community who are widely respected
- learn through formal, in-depth interviews and informal conversations
- learn through both participating in and observing behaviors
- gather clues from overheard conversations and unsolicited comments.

Surveys are not considered useful because people tend to say what they think the investigator wants them to say, regardless of their real feelings and attitudes. Existing cultural assessment tools (Brownlee, 1978; Giger & Davidhizar, 1991; Orque, Bloch & Monrroy, 1983) may be easily adapted to gather information on childbearing and infant feeding practices within a given culture. Such a guide is given in the boxed chart on this page.

It is essential to assess and understand infant feeding practices and styles when choosing culturally appropriate policy and breastfeeding promotion strategies. For example, people living in Kenya consider formula a "superfood" and consider breastfeeding an activity or *process* rather than the means of obtaining a *product* (like formula). These beliefs will likely influence any infant feeding programs or policies developed in that country (van Esterik & Elliott, 1986). Also helpful is demographic data which show breastfeeding trends within a certain area. For example, data that shows traditional rural women are more likely to breastfeed and to do so longer than urban mothers (Ebrahim, 1976; Guthrie et al., 1983) may influence how one might plan a breastfeeding promotion program designed to reach the urban mothers as well as the rural ones. Rural people are also more likely to continue traditional rituals than are urban families who may not have even heard of these practices.

A simple but effective method for evaluating the value of a cultural practice (Williams & Jelliffe, 1972) is to consider whether the practice is beneficial, harmless, harmful, or uncertain to a particular outcome:

- *Is it beneficial?* Several cultures prohibit the lactating mother from having intercourse because

---

Guide for Assessing Culture

General
- History, origins of the cultural group
- Custom, values
- Behaviors and attitudes

Communication
- Language patterns (verbal and nonverbal)
- Language barriers
- Use of time and space
- Art and literature

Family
- Childbearing and childrearing practices
- Family organization, roles, decision-making
- Kinship patterns
- Housing
- Food habits

Health Practices
- Healing systems (folk or cultural healers vs. bio-medical)
- Health beliefs
- Effect of illness on family
- Biological variations

Religion
- Tenets and practices
- Rituals and restrictions

Social/political systems
- Type of political system governing health and welfare
- Educational system
- Income levels per capita
- Degree of technology in use

Infant care and feeding practices
- Input from family and support persons
- Level of knowledge
- Traditions, rituals and taboos
- Values concerning breastmilk and other infant foods
- Attitude toward breastfeeding (process vs. product)

it is believed that that semen poisons her breast-milk (Counts, 1984). A side benefit of this practice is enhanced fertility control. Such beliefs assure that infants continue to be breastfed and are well nourished and nurtured, since many cultures pro-scribe breastfeeding when a woman becomes pregnant again. Cultural practices such as carrying a baby close, breastfeeding on demand, and spac-ing children by long-term breastfeeding are like-wise considered beneficial (Jimenez & Newton, 1979; Konner & Shostak, 1987).

- *Is it harmless?* Placing an amulet or charm of gar-lic around the baby's neck to protect him from "the evil eye," or pinning a belly band around his abdomen to prevent an umbilical hernia are harmless practices. If the mother eats garlic to prevent illness, the practice is harmless to her baby even though her milk will smell like garlic (Mennela & Beauchamp, 1991).

- *Is it harmful?* Routine supplementation of the breastfeeding baby and separation of the mother and infant after birth are common practices in the United States and are clearly harmful. There are many cultures in which colostrum is consid-ered poisonous and unfit for the infant (Baums-lag, 1987; Counts, 1984; Fernandez & Popkin, 1988). The newborn is fed by a lactating relative or is given gruel until the "true" milk comes in, thereby depriving the baby of the concentrated immune properties of colostrum. Another harm-ful belief is that breastmilk causes diarrhea and that breastfeeding must be stopped when diar-rhea occurs (Guthrie et al., 1983).

- *Is it uncertain?* Some practices fall into this "gray" area. Until more information is gathered, they cannot be evaluated. For example, while working as a part of a nursing team in the Domini-can Republic, I noted that women avoided eating fresh fruits for two weeks after delivery. This is a common cultural restriction in Hispanic cultures. Although our current knowledge does not permit judgments about food taboos, they merit further study (Eaton-Evans & Dugdale, 1986).

LANGUAGE BARRIERS

When working with families who speak a different language, ideally the care provider is able to under-stand and speak that language. If she cannot, the care provider should study the language spoken by the breastfeeding families she frequently serves. Rapport is difficult when language differences are a barrier.

When it is necessary to have a translator, a trained interpreter is able to rephrase words so they are more understandable and acceptable to the culture. When using a translator, talk slowly, avoid using slang and subjectives (e.g., "would" and "if") and speak in a normal voice. It also may be wise to tape record the discussion with the mother, so that the taped discussion may be used again.

Even with a translator, there may be problems, since there are different dialects within some coun-tries. Vietnamese, for example, is a language which has many regional dialects. Or a word may have dif-ferent shades of meaning in different regions of the country. In preparing a flip chart and audiocassette for encouraging breastfeeding among mothers in the Dominican Republic, I used the word "amamantar" to mean breastfeeding, as it does in many Spanish-speaking countries. However, much to the amuse-ment of the Dominican mothers, it meant "milk the cow" to them.

Most people who are new to a culture are shy. Out of respect for the people they are dealing with, they may nod their head and say "yes" even though they may disagree or not understand what is being said. An example of this is described by Bowles (1987). On a postpartum unit a student nurse cared for an East Indian woman who spoke very little English. Whenever the doctor or nurse asked if she was going to breastfeed or bottle-feed, she would say, "bottle"; consequently she was given a lactation supressant. After the woman was discharged, the student and her instructor made a home visit to find the mother and baby happily breastfeeding under the safe su-pervision of the child's grandmother. Failure to rec-ognize that the mother's "bottle-feeding" reply was a cultural masquerade in response to being in a "bot-tle-culture" resulted in giving her a medication that could have ended her ability to breastfeed.

Whenever possible, provide printed materials on breastfeeding in the family's language. Information sheets on breastfeeding in many different languages may be ordered from La Leche League Interna-tional.*

---

*La Leche League International, P.O. Box 1209, Franklin Park IL 60131–8209. To order by telephone with VISA or MasterCard, call 708–455–7730.

THE EFFECTS OF CULTURE ON BREASTFEEDING

In the United States, care providers work increasingly with Indochinese families who have immigrated there in search of a new life and opportunities. Immigrants tend to adopt cultural practices of the new country; for these newcomers, adaptation has meant bottle-feeding instead of breastfeeding. For many of them, breastfeeding becomes a choice, neither a cultural norm nor an economic necessity. The women may be wrongly told that it is the custom in the United States to bottle-feed babies. A local community health nurse asked a Vietnamese mother, "But, didn't your mother breastfeed you?" The woman replied, "Yes, but that's the old way. We're in a new land now."

Very few Vietnamese and IndoChinese women who live in the United States breastfeed. In a survey (Serdula et al., 1991) of Southeast Asian infants living in a low-income area of St. Paul, Minnesota, 93% of those born in their native land had been breastfed compared with 10% of those born in the United States. Their mothers, in their eagerness to acculturate, turn away from their cultural heritage of breastfeeding. The father of the baby is likely to agree with his wife, especially if their baby is a boy, in the belief that their son will grow to be physically larger (and more like American males) and to have "harder bones" if he is fed formula.

Consider the influences of a new culture when a mother receives a formula discharge pack from the hospital and free formula through the WIC program in the land "where babies don't die." Consider, too, the messages she receives when she sees the stacks of formula in the supermarket and the magazine pictures of attractive mothers bottle-feeding their babies. (See Table 2–1.)

The overwhelming influence of environment on breastfeeding is not limited to Southeast Asian immigrants to the United States. Chinese who immigrated the Glasgow, U.K., likewise gave up breastfeeding after arriving in that country. Only 2% of the Chinese babies born in Glasgow were breastfed, while 81% of those born in Hong Kong of the same mother had been breastfed (Koh, 1981).

Well-meaning efforts to acculturate recent immigrants can also disrupt breastfeeding by separating mothers from their babies. For example, new Vietnamese-Americans are encouraged, and sometimes even paid, to attend government-sponsored English classes. Because there classes are important, and breast pumping is unacceptable to many Indochinese mothers (La Du, 1985), formula is given instead. These breastfeeding mothers should be allowed to keep their babies with them in class.

TABLE 2–1   POSSIBLE CULTURAL BELIEFS AND PRACTICES

	Asian	**American Black**	**Hispanic/Chicano**
Beliefs about health	Seen as a balance of energy—yin vs. yang	Able to be productive, a state of harmony with the universe	Health is state of equilibrium; disease due to an imbalance
Support/resource person for a new mother	Mother, mother-in-law	Older woman with experience; peers	Mother often is cared for by her own mother
Infant feeding	Mother prefers to formula-feed; sees formula as "superfood" that will make baby grow larger; may bottle-feed in hospital, and both breastfeed and bottle-feed at home; does not use breast pump	Most mothers in low socioeconomic group, choose formula-feeding; breastfeeding may be embarrassing; early introduction of solids	Mother likely to breastfeed; may wait three days if she considers colostrum to be "dirty"; gives baby small amounts of family foods
Family and parenting	Male babies are preferred; father is head of household	Fear "spoiling" baby; grandmother (mother of mother) helps parent	Mother is homemaker, father is provider
Infant care	Hot-cold foods to treat illnesses; feel responsible for baby's behavior; bring baby to social events, church	May put excess clothing on baby to keep him warm; abundant use of oil on baby's scalp and skin	Infant must be protected from the "evil eye" (mal ojo); various remedies are used to treat fallen (depressed) fontanel; female ears pierced; male may not be circumcised

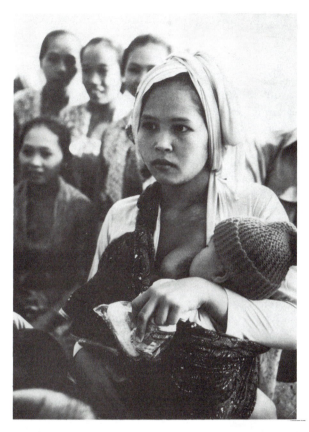

FIGURE 2–4.   Well-nourished woman and breastfeeding infant in Searo, where breastfeeding is a basic part of the life process. (Courtesy WHO.)

Breastfeeding in a public place or in the presence of friends is an activity that is extremely sensitive to cultural norms. For instance, in Saudi Arabia it is not uncommon to see a totally veiled woman baring her breast to feed her infant in public with no one taking notice—except, perhaps, a foreigner. In France, a woman in a topless swimming suit on certain beaches is perfectly acceptable. However, a French woman would hesitate, or at least cover herself carefully, while breastfeeding in public—even in a restaurant near the "topless" beach. Modesty is important for the Mexican-American mother and may be viewed as inconsistent with breastfeeding in public (Wright et al., 1988).

Cultural attitudes towards modesty and breastfeeding may be compared to attitudes about the degree of difficulty of breastfeeding. In Kenya, breastfeeding is not considered a particularly difficult or problematic activity, although it is thought to

be time consuming. Women do not worry or complain about breastfeeding; in a survey by van Esterik and Elliot (1986), most women had no problems associated with it. Because breastfeeding is viewed as a natural process, medical personnel in that country are not aware that mothers might need help with breastfeeding; as a result, there are few instructions or rules for successfully managing breastfeeding problems.

RITUALS

Rituals associated with infant feeding are critical elements in assessing the culture's infant feeding practices. Unfortunately the word "ritual" has come to connote a meaningless ceremonial act. Actually, rituals can have a significant effect if the individual believes in them. Eating a special food or praying to a patron saint to increase the milk supply are cultural rituals that work for some people, just as taking a pill on the advice of a Western-trained doctor may have a positive effect—even if the medicine is a sugar pill. Researchers call this the placebo effect, which is based on the observation that if one "believes" that a particular action will have a desired effect, it will.

In the Philippines the ritual of *lihi* assures a good flow of rich milk. The ceremony involves stroking the mother's breasts with broken papaya leaves and stalks of sugar cane. The white sap of the papaya ensures that the mother's milk will be copious, thick and white, while the cane guarantees that it will be sweet (Guthrie et al., 1983). In certain rural areas of Japan, figurines and paintings depicting a woman with a bounteous milk supply are displayed in the belief that they increase the mother's milk. (See Fig. 2–5.) A picture of a breastfeeding mother seated in front of a waterfall has been used in the United States for similar effect. One of the authors of this book, Kathleen Auerbach, kept a notice that states, "This is a positive thinking area," in her office where mothers sat during lactation consultations. Its message was not lost on the clients, many of whom commented that they needed such a reminder while working through breastfeeding difficulties. Commonly practiced rituals in the United States which are harmful to breastfeeding include separation of mother and baby after birth and routine glucose water feeds.

A purgative made from the maskreti plant is fed to Haitian babies soon after birth to "clean his insides"

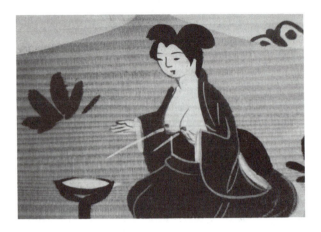

FIGURE 2–5.   Votive picture (*ema* in Japanese). This wooden plaque is given to the breastfeeding mother by the temple. She, in turn, prays to the plaque for sufficient milk. If her wish is fulfilled, she writes her name and age on the plaque and dedicates it to the temple. (Courtesy K. Sawada.)

(Harris, 1987). The prenatal preparation of nipples that is still popular in some Western countries could be considered a ritual that psychologically prepares the mother for the breastfeeding experience, even if it is not necessary from a physiological point of view.

COLOSTRUM

In many cultures throughout the world, colostrum is accepted and encouraged as the first food for infants. Others, believing that colostrum is "old" milk that has been in the breasts for months and is unfit for the newborn, express it and throw it away until the "true" milk appears on the second or third day (Conton, 1985; Fishman, Evans & Jenks, 1988). In the first chapter of this book, Mary-Margaret Coates points out that the fear of feeding colostrum helped spread the practice of wet-nursing in years past. Baumslag (1987) points out that in many developing countries mothers do not give their babies this first milk because they fear it to be "pus" or "poison." This belief exists among people in countries thousands of miles apart, including the Indians of Guatemala and Africans in Sierra Leone and Lesotho. On Vanatinai Island in the Coral Sea, the mother feeds her baby about one hour after birth, but she must first drink *mwaoli* tea and then express the contents of her breasts in the belief that she must rid them of the residue of fats, coconut, fish, wild game or pig

which she ate during her pregnancy (Lepowsky, 1985).

RESUMING SEXUAL RELATIONS

A vestige of medieval European thought, the notion that semen contaminates breastmilk, is widespread in many developing countries (Conton, 1985; Counts, 1984). It assumes that (1) there is a physiological connection between the uterus and the breast and (2) the mother's milk may become contaminated by sexual contact and make a baby sick. The Lusi people in New Britain, Papua New Guinea, believe that new parents should refrain from sexual activity lest the semen enter and contaminate the breastmilk through "cords" that are thought to link the uterus and breast. This is especially true if the semen is from a man other than the baby's father. Restraint from sexual relations should:

> continue until the child has achieved a certain independence, variously expressed as when it is old enough to tell its parents of its dreams or when it is old enough to gather shell fish or try to spear small fish in the shallows: about three years of age. When a child has reached this stage, people anticipate no problems should a mother have another baby. In fact many women opined that this was the ideal spacing of children (Counts, 1984).

Labbok (1981) points out that sexual abstinence in the postpartum period serves two functions: it enhances the mother's physical recovery from the trauma of the birth and it prevents subsequent pregnancy.

WET-NURSING

Wet-nursing is a long-established practice in many developing countries. Traditionally, a child whose mother has died or who was otherwise unable to breastfeed is either passed around among breastfeeding women or adopted by a lactating mother whose child has recently died (Counts, 1984). Among Japanese and Thai mothers of Chinese ancestry, breastmilk can be shared between infants of the same sex, but not those of the opposite sex. In cultures in which breastmilk is viewed as a conduit for ancestral power, it is not unusual for wet nurses to be restricted to women from the mother or father's clan or lineage (Lepowsky, 1985; van Esterik, 1988).

In the United States, where cross-nursing (Krantz & Kupper, 1981) is rarely discussed but often practiced, it is more likely for sisters to nurse one another's babies, rather than for an unrelated acquaintance to do so.

CHILDBIRTH PRACTICES

Childbirth, like breastfeeding, is heavily influenced by culture. Mercer and Stainton (1984) clarify the role of culture in childbirth as providing norms that influence attitudes, values, and interpretations of personal and interpersonal experience. The "fire rest" is a ritual carried out after childbirth in Southeast Asian and Caribbean cultures (Fishman, Evans & Jenks, 1988). Traditional Filipino childbirth practices, for example, expect the new mother to sit in a special slotted chair over hot coals for one hour each day for nine days after giving birth to restore her reproductive organs. This procedure is called "drying" or "roasting" and also involves restricting the mother's diet according to "hot" and "cold" foods. The mother is not allowed to bathe for two weeks after delivery until the "fresh uterus" returns to its normal shape with the help of massages administered by a midwife. A special bath is given at this time to remove unclean substances from the body through perspiration (McKenzie & Chrisman, 1977).

In Melanesia and Polynesia the mother lies beside a coconut fire while her women friends massage her with oil (Kitzinger, 1990). To involute the uterus and to prevent vaginal discharge later, a Vietnamese woman may squat over a small coal fire or a cauldron of steaming water filled with alcohol, lemon grass or Chinese medicine (Mathews & Manderson, 1981). The Haitian version of this postpartum warming is known as the "three baths"—two baths in water boiled with special leaves and later a cold bath followed by a cleansing purge (Harris, 1987).

A seclusion period of about 40 days is common in many cultures. The purpose of this time of seclusion for the mother and baby varies according to the culture. However, Jimenez and Newton (1979) report that it permits a mother to:

- become acquainted with her baby
- establish her milk supply

- reduce her own and her infant's exposure to infectious diseases
- protect others from her "unclean" state following childbirth.

At the same time, these new mothers rarely stay completely secluded and pampered as there is work to be done and the mother becomes bored.

In Korea, the mother's mother-in-law traditionally takes care of her after birth and serves as her "doula." During her pregnancy Korean women undergo *Thae Kyo* or education-teaching of the fetus. In this ancient tradition a mother-in-law trains her daughter-in-law to be a mother (Pope, M: personal communication, Seoul, Korea, 1989). *Thae Kyo* instructs the expectant mother that to avoid bad luck in having her baby she should not see fires or fights, she must think pure thoughts and eat "pretty" foods, and she must always walk in a straight line.

INFANT CARE

Swaddling or bundling is an ancient practice still used today for maintaining the infant's body temperature and soothing him. Both swaddling and carrying the baby also free the mother's hands for other tasks. In many parts of rural Nigeria, an infant is wrapped on his mother's back all day and sleeps with her at night. During the first 40 days, the baby is snugly wrapped, a practice that ensures that the infant stays warm and reduces his energy requirements (Omuloulu, 1982).

In Bogota, Colombia, and other parts of world which do not have intensive care nurseries, premature infants who are clinically stable go directly to the mother as early as two to three hours after birth. By being held in an upright position, skin-to-skin between their mother's beasts, they are kept warm (Anderson, Marks & Wahlberg, 1986).

In any culture, swaddling the baby and carrying him close typifies mothers who practice unrestricted breastfeeding. The Zambian infant is secured to his mother's body as early as 24 hours after delivery with a *dashica,* or long piece of cloth. The baby rides on the mother's hip in the *dashica,* and his head is not supported. As a result, the Zambian infant maintains a strong shoulder girdle to keep his head steady and develops early head control. A specially woven strong cotton cloth folded in a special way, the

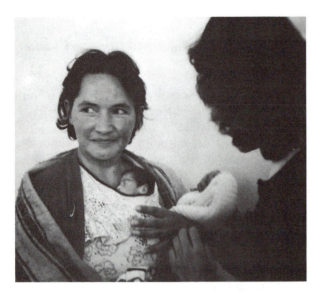

FIGURE 2–6. A premature infant in Bogota goes home 12 hours after birth, cradled skin-to-skin with his mother. (Courtesy G. C. Anderson.)

aquawo, is the infant carrier in Bolivia. The *aquawo* can be turned around to several positions to facilitate breastfeeding. In Mexico, a woman uses a long, wide shawl called a *rebozo* for carrying her infant while she goes about her daily activities. Many different types of baby carriers are seen everywhere in the United States. Their use suggests that mothers and fathers, regardless of their cultural backgrounds, recognize and enjoy the convenience these carriers afford. Women who work in the fields use a cradleboard device that functions much like swaddling. Carrying the infant swaddled to his mother's body develops muscle tone and seems to encourage alertness. Being carried about during normal daily activities offers many opportunities for tactile, visual, and social stimulation. Have you ever found yourself peering into a pair of curious eyes that belong to a baby in a back carrier? You may find yourself irresistibly carrying on animated "baby" conversation with this little creature who responds to every clever thing you say.

Babies in the Dominican Republic are not secured to their mother in any fashion but are carried in their arms in a horizontal position until they are old enough to sit up by themselves. Because it is believed that a baby can break his neck easily if his head is not held, a mother will become visibly anxious when the nurse assesses his head control. While in the Dominican Republic, I learned to be very cau-

tious when doing this—always reassuring the mother that I would not harm her baby. This experience points out the necessity of incorporating cultural beliefs into nursing practice.

An infant may be affected by diseases recognized only in that culture. In Spanish-speaking cultures, the most common is *mollera caída* (fallen fontanel). The health professional interprets a depressed fontanel in the baby as a symptom of dehydration, whereas a Chicana mother may see it as curable illness caused by removing her nipple while the baby is still suckling—or by the baby falling. One mother explained that her baby's fontanel had fallen in church after she was accidently knocked over in her baby seat: "My mother-in-law diagnosed her right away as having *mollera caída.* She could tell because when the baby sucked, there was a different sound to it and there was no grip to it. She was then taken to the curandera (healer) who cured her by applying pressure on the infant's palate with her thumbs." (Ehling, 1981).

Another Chicano and Puerto Rican folk disease is *mal de ojo* (or evil eye), which is presumably caused by someone who admired the baby but did not touch him. It is also thought to be caused by people with very strong glances. Symptoms of *mal de ojo* are sometimes vague, but the baby is usually very unhappy, cries continuously, cannot sleep, and may even die (Lacay, 1981). The cure is effected by finding the person who is thought to have given the infant the evil eye and having her touch the baby. Lactation consultants (LCs) working with such clients should take care to touch the baby when admiring him to avoid being thought of as the cause of a later case of *mal de ojo.*

Babies often are outfitted with special ornaments or bands which have a specific purpose. Chicano grandmothers often worry a great deal about the infant's umbilicus and may insist that the baby wear a belly band (*fajita*) to prevent an umbilical hernia. Haitian babies may have a band of cloth around their abdomen to develop a strong body and a sense of balance (Harris, 1987). A traditional necklace protects the Laotian newborn (La Du, 1985). Babies in Papua New Guinea are protected from disease by special rituals, such as blackening the top of the baby's head with burnt coconut husk (Lepowsky, 1985). In the Philippines, applying charred chicken gizzard to the baby's lips is believed to prevent diarrhea (Guthrie, 1983).

In most cultures the infant sleeps with or close to his mother. The Chinese infant frequently sleeps in his parent's bed or in the same room with them at night. The first year is characterized by warmth and security, and he is lavished with attention by everyone in the family. Extended family members who live nearby are close to the infant. Traditionally, Chinese infants are not allowed to cry, but are immediately picked up and rocked or carried by a member of the family in a back sling (Char, 1981).

MATERNAL FOODS

Whether she lives on a mountaintop in remote Tibet, in a dusty Mexican village, or in an American suburb or urban high-rise apartment, the lactating woman produces milk that is amazingly homogeneous in composition—despite the wide diversity of foods she consumes. Only the milk of a woman who is severely malnourished will be measurably diminished in its nutrient content and volume since body nutrients are depleted before the milk suffers.

Part of understanding a culture involves becoming acquainted with its "foodways"—the way in which a distinct group selects, prepares, consumes, and otherwise uses portions of the available food supply (Suitor & Hunter, 1980). "Food behavior" denotes and describes the foodways of an individual. The list of various ethnic foods in Table 2–2 gives an overview of the wide variety of food patterns followed by lactating women.

For more than half the inhabitants of this planet, including lactating women, beans, rice, and grains are daily fare. Fruits and vegetables appear seasonally, and meat is found in the family cooking pot only on special occasions. When it does appear, it is poultry, goat, horse, or dog, instead of beef. In most cultures meat plays a minor part in flavoring rice, beans, and vegetables, not the major role it has served in affluent Western industrialized countries.

The daily food pattern of a breastfeeding mother in Mexico who eats very little meat might concern us if we did not have a basic knowledge of amino acids and complementary proteins. Beans, a staple item in Mexican foodways, provides an incomplete protein when served alone because they are low in methionine, an essential amino acid. This deficiency, however, is completely corrected when beans are served with a food high in methionine,

such as whole grain breads or cereals. Complementary proteins can be achieved by numerous combinations. For example, eggs or a milk product will balance the protein and amino acids of a meal consisting primarily of plant proteins. However, two protein foods cannot complement each other if they have similar amino acids in their composition. For this reason, nuts and black-eyed peas are not complementary proteins, because both legumes lack the same amino acids. Some examples for using complementary proteins are given in Table 2–3.

FOODS THAT INCREASE BREASTMILK

Almost all cultures abound with an array of prescriptive foods for lactating women. In the United States, beer and brewer's yeast have been touted as galactogogues—i.e., foods that are thought to increase milk secretion and improve letdown. Parturient mothers in a number of countries gratefully accept the chicken soup given to them. In addition to its fluid value, chicken soup, a perennially favorite medicinal food, contains calcium, as well as sodium to maintain electrolyte balance. Village mothers in Kaliai, Papua New Guinea, do not worry about the production of adequate milk, for it can be readily increased by drinking lots of fluids, especially fish soup and green coconut liquid (Counts, 1984).

In Mexico, the use of a wide variety of galactagogues was a common practice until recent times. The herbalist's "bible" in Mexico recommends anise and cotton seeds to increase breastmilk (Vargas, 1979). In traditional Japan a low-calorie diet (rice, gruel, soup, vegetables) for mothers during the immediate postpartum period was believed to help the secretion of milk. Lactating women in Japan were also encouraged to eat lotus roots. Since the root has many holes, it was thought to prevent plugged milk ducts. Another Japanese tradition was to wrap rice or red beans in a cotton cloth made to look like a small breast. A woman who wished to have enough milk for her coming baby offered one of these breast models to Buddha as she prayed. Later, she cooked and ate the rice or beans (Sawada, 1981).

Ethnographic records of North American Indians show that the Navajo woman's milk supply was believed to increase if she drank broth made from blue corn meal (Moore, 1969). The Ojibwa Indians encouraged the intake of wild rice, lake trout, and white fish. In the Philippines, soups containing

TABLE 2–2   BRIEF DESCRIPTIONS OF AN ASSORTMENT OF ETHNIC AND REGIONAL FOODS

Grain group

Anadama: Cornmeal-molasses yeast bread (New England)

Bagels: Bread dough shaped like a donut, cooked in water, then baked; chewy (Jewish-American

Bulgur: Granular wheat product with nutlike flavor, served like rice (Middle Eastern)

Brioche: Type of egg-rich French roll, often served at breakfast

Challah: Braided eggbread

Chapatis: Unleavened bread used by Indians

Croissants: Flaky crescent shaped rolls (French)

Crumpets: Muffinlike product cooked on griddle; often served toasted (British)

Grits: Coarsely ground hominy (corn product) (Southern USA)

Johnnycake: Cornbread (New England)

Kasha: Coarsely ground grain toasted before cooking in liquid

Latkes: Pancakes

Limpa: Rye bread (Swedish)

Mush: Cooked cereal (often cornmeal)

Pasta: Macaroni, spaghetti, noodles in variety of forms (Italian)

Polenta: Cornmeal (Italian)

Scones: Round, flat, unleavened, sweetened bread product (British)

Sopapillas: Fried bread (rich dough) (Mexican)

Tortillas: Thin rounds of leathery dough made from lime-treated corn or from wheat flour, often fried until crisp (Mexican)

Fruit and vegetable group

Bok choy: Green leafy, stalklike vegetable (Oriental)

Chayote: Green or white squashlike vegetable eaten raw, cooked, or pickled (Mexican)

Dandelion greens: Young leaves from wild dandelion plants, eaten raw or cooked

Greens in "pot liquor" ("likor"): Green leafy vegetables such as kale or turnip, mustard or collard greens, cooked with salt pork, served with cooking liquid (Southern USA)

Jalapeños: Hot peppers

Kelp: Seaweed

Papaya: Large, yellow, melon-like tropical fruit

Prickly pear: Fruit of a cactus

Viandas: Starchy tropical vegetables such as sweet potato, cassava, plantain (banana-like in appearance) (Puerto Rican

Meat group

Adobo: Meat, soy sauce (Filipino)

Chitterlings: Pork intestine, tripe (soul food)

Chorizo: Sausage (Mexican)

Escargots: Snails (French)

Falafel: Mashed chick peas mixed with other ingredients and fried (Israeli)

Feijoada: Blackbeans, meat (Brazilian)

Finnan haddie: Smoked haddock

Frijoles refritas: Refried pinto or calico beans (Mexican)

Gefilte fish: Ground or flaked fish seasoned and shaped into balls (Jewish-American)

Hog maw: Stomach of pig (Southern USA)

Jerky: Dried meat strips

Kibee: Fresh raw lamb, ground, seasoned; eaten uncooked (Middle Eastern)

Kielbasa: Polish sausage

Miso: Soybean paste

Pepperoni: Italian hot sausage

Sauerbrauten: Pot roast marinated in acidic sauce (German)

Sashimi: Raw fish (Japanese)

Teriyaki: Broiled beef marinated in sweet soy sauce (Hawaiian)

Mixed dishes

Couscous: Semolina, meat stew (North African)

Goulash: Stew usually seasoned with paprika (Hungarian)

Gumbo: Okra and meat stew, thickened with filé (pulverized sassafras leaves) (Louisiana Creole)

Hoppin John: Blackeyed peas and rice (Southern USA)

Jambalaya: Rice, ham, and seafood (Louisiana Creole)

Moussaka: Eggplant casserole (Greek)

Scrapple: Pork and cornmeal (Pennsylvania Dutch)

Tacos: Fried tortillas filled with meat or beans, vegetables, hot sauce, (Mexican)

Wonton: Stuffed dough, fried or cooked in broth (Chinese)

Others

Baklavah: A layered pastry rich in honey (Greek)

Butterhorns: Sweet pastry

Cracklins: Crispy pieces left after pork fat is rendered (Southern)

Fatback: Fat from belly of pig

Kuchen: Cake

Lard: Pork fat rendered to be used like shortening

Salt pork: Salted pork fat, sometimes with bit of meat

Sofrito: Specially seasoned tomato sauce used by Puerto Ricans

Spumoni: Fruit ice cream (Italian)

Strickle sheets: Coffee cake (Pennsylvania Dutch)

Strudel: Paper-thin pastry with fruit filling or cheese (German)

Tzimmes: Carrot-prune dessert (Jewish-American)

From Suitor, CW, and Hunter, MF: *Nutrition: principles and application in health promotion,* Philadelphia, 1980, J.B. Lippincott Co.

TABLE 2–3 COMPLEMENTING PROTEINS—COMBINING PROTEINS SO THAT THEIR AMINO ACID STRENGTHS AND WEAKNESSES BALANCE OUT, RESULTING IN A MIXTURE OF FOODS WITH GOOD BIOLOGICAL VALUE

			Relative amino acid content	
Food category	**Examples**		**Lysine**	**Methionine**
Legumes	Peanut butter	Chili beans	+ to ++	—
Grains	Whole wheat bread	Corn bread	—	+
	Combination		Adequate	
Grains	Rye bread	Puffed rice	—	+
Milk	Cheese	Milk	+ +	+
	Combination		Good	Very good

From Suitor, CW, and Hunter, MF: *Nutrition: principles and application in health promotion,* Philadelphia, 1980, J.B. Lippincott Co.
+The protein contains more of the amino acid than does a high-quality protein.
+ +The protein is very high in the amino acid in comparison to a high-quality protein.
—The protein is low in the amino acid in comparison to a high-quality protein.

marungay leaves and papayas are supposed to make the milk flow; sour foods, however, are believed to decrease milk and to increase lochia (Affonso, 1978). Pakistani galactogogues include cumin, cotton seeds and goat's stomach; in India fried ginger and black pepper are recommended (Baumslag, 1987).

FOOD RESTRICTIONS
Food restrictions or taboos regarding the postpartum diet are common; many restrictions result in diets that are similar to those for sick people. Over a long period, such limited nutrition would seriously deplete the mother's nutritional reserves, making her more susceptible to infection, exhaustion, and other effects of malnutrition. Currently, we have no good evidence that the common maternal food restrictions found in many cultures help the infant; neither can we say that they harm the mother. Many people in the United States still believe that hot spicy foods have a deleterious effect on milk supply. If this were true, however, the Spanish, East Indians, and Italians would have died out long ago.

Restricting fruit in the postpartum diet is a com-

TABLE 2–4 EXAMPLES OF CULTURAL PRACTICES THAT PROMOTE ADEQUATE NUTRIENT INTAKE

Culture	**Nutritious foods that are rarely eaten**	**Cultural corrections**
Chinese	Milk	Cooking bones in acid solution to make soup provides an excellent source of calcium.
		Soybean products such as tofu and many Chinese greens are good sources of calcium.
Mexican	Milk	*Corn* tortillas are prepared with lime-soaked* corn and therefore contribute significant amounts of calcium to the diet.
Italian	Milk	Calcium-rich cheeses are popular.
Southern black	Milk	Buttermilk may be used occasionally.
		Calcium-rich greens are popular vegetables.
Puerto Rican	Bread	Viandas such as plantains are similar to bread in nutritive value.
		Rice is popular and is a good substitute if whole grain or enriched.

From Suitor, CW, and Hunter, MF: *Nutrition: principles and application in health promotion,* Philadelphia, 1980, J.B. Lippincott Co.
*Lime is a calcium salt.

mon practice in many Spanish-speaking cultures, including some Mexican-Americans. Haitian women avoid foods that are white after the baby is born because they are thought to increase vaginal discharge. One way to get around this is to add another food (for instance, coffee to milk) to color it. (Harris, 1987). (See Table 2–4.)

Severe restrictions that cause nutritional deprivation seem unnecessarily harsh and are difficult to understand. The custom of *pautang* in Malaya includes six weeks of restricted food intake by the postpartum mother (Mead & Newton, 1967). To the Hmong, boiled chicken rice and hot water is the only appropriate nourishment for the first month after delivery, and family members often bring food to the hospital in portable stacking food carriers typical of their homeland (Nelson & Hewitt 1983).

For many cultural groups, foodways involve a balance that must be maintained to sustain health or be restored when illness occurs. Balance between opposing energy forces is based on the Greek theory of body humors. After centuries of dissemination throughout the world, this theory now appears as the hot (caliente)-cold (frio or fresco) system in Hispanic cultures. Other people such as the Vietnamese, Chinese, East Indians, and Arabs also use a hot-cold system to some extent. Classifying foods as "hot" or "cold" in a given culture has little to do with their form, color, texture, or temperature, although "hot" foods are believed to be more easily digested than cold foods. Instead, the classification is based on the food's effect on an illness or condition, which is itself categorized as "hot" or "cold." During the last trimester of pregnancy, the unborn child is believed to be "hot"; therefore the mother is in a hot state. Once the child is born, accompanied by a loss of blood, a "cold" condition exists for both. To correct this imbalance, women believe that they need humorally warming foods; to replace heat and energy, they may lie near or over smouldering coals. Failure to observe these puerperal prescriptions is thought to have serious long-term medical implications (Fishman, Evans & Jenks, 1988; Mathews & Manderson, 1981).

Traditional Chinese consider chicken, squash, and broccoli to be hot. Cold foods include melon, fruits, soybean sprouts, and bamboo shoots. In India, milk may be hot or cold depending on where a person lives. In Hispanic cultures, cold foods include most fresh vegetables, tropical fruits, dairy products, beans, squash, and some meats. Hot foods—cereal grains, chili peppers, temperate-zone fruits, goat's milk, oils, and beef—serve to balance the cold foods. Since the potential listing of hot and cold foods in any particular culture is almost endless, we must do our own ethnographic homework regarding the belief system of the cultures with whose members we are working.

Among Vietnamese women who delivered infants in Australia in the early 1980s, foods restricted after childbirth included raw vegetables and all fruit. Among Vietnamese-Chinese mothers, bananas, cabbage, soy-milk soft drinks and unboiled water were also prohibited (Mathews & Manderson, 1981).

Another belief system concerning food balance is the Chinese, yin-yang theory. In America, the system is practiced by people who use macrobiotics. Like the hot-cold theory, the basis of the yin-yang belief rests on a proper balance between opposing energy forces. On one side yin represents "female," a negative force (cold, emptiness, darkness); on the other side yang represents "male," a positive force (warmth, fullness, light). Too much of either yin or yang food is considered threatening to health. Whether a food is considered yin or yang depends on the effect it is thought to have on the body and is not associated with color, texture, or other obvious characteristics. Without an extensive orientation for things Chinese, it is difficult to understand the yin-ness or yang-ness of food.

Traditional cultures have used medicinal herbs extensively. For instance, Cambodian mothers who have immigrated to the United States still use tiger balm and ginger root for treating their children's illnesses (Rosenberg, 1986). Northern Mexicans make special teas from so-called "hot" plants such as sesame and absinthe, and in some parts of Latin America herb teas are drunk in the evening to stimulate milk for the morning (Baumslag, 1987). Herbs taken by the breastfeeding mother may have pharmacologic effects on her baby, including irritation of the mucosal lining of the intestine and an increase in the release of flatus. As a result, some breastfed infants of mothers who regularly consume herbs have increased gas and loose stools. Unless it becomes troublesome and an allergic response occurs, it is more important for the mother to continue enjoying her favorite herbs than to stop using them because of her baby's minor stool changes.

VEGETARIANS

For reasons of health, religion, ethnic values, or economy, many people worldwide are vegetarians. Two general classifications are recognized: (1) lacto-ovo-vegetarians, who use eggs and dairy products in addition to plant foods and (2) vegans, who use only plant foods. A lactating vegetarian who eats a wide variety of grains, legumes, nuts, fruits, vegetables and dairy products has a nutritionally sound diet. Frequently, families in industrial nations who practice vegetarianism by choice are quite knowledgeable about nutrition. They are rarely obese and have superior diet patterns because they conscientiously avoid processed, empty-calorie foods. Concerns about breastfeeding usually center on whether the mother is consuming adequate protein and vitamin B_{12} since this vitamin is not found in vegetable protein. Even a strict vegan diet can be carefully planned and supplemented if need be. Supplemental vitamins, fortified soy milk and fortified yeast are all good sources of B_{12}.

Women who consume large amounts of green vegetables sometimes produce milk that has a greenish tint. This also can occur among women taking advantage of large quantities of certain foods when they are in season. "Green" milk, although not at all harmful to the infant, can be rather unnerving at first to the unwary until they understand the cause.

BREASTFEEDING IN SPECIFIC COUNTRIES

Russia

In economically troubled Russia, increasing numbers of Russian women, influenced by the advertising of German formula companies, are formula-feeding their babies. Russian physicians are attempting to reverse this trend by warning women about infant health problems, especially allergies, that are caused by not breastfeeding. New mothers remain in the hospital for 7–14 days, have paid maternity leave for 18 months, and are assured of returning to their same job. Children are considered a "privileged class"; maternity care, education and health care are all free. Additionally, Russian families are financially rewarded by the government for having children; yet Russian women are reluctant to have children, they limit their families to one or two. Like their U.S. counterparts, Russian mothers are exhausted from their dual role ("you work all day, then you shop, then cook—our men watch TV and don't do their fair share") and depressed about their bleak conditions and lack of living space (Riordan: personal communication with Russian women in Leningrad, summer, 1989).

Japan

Almost all women now deliver their infants in a hospital or clinic. Even though Japanese mothers may have been breastfed four or five years themselves, they accept formula for their babies. At three months almost one-half of the mothers are still breastfeeding; by six months it drops to one-third. Breastfeeding rates have risen since the 1970's probably because the Ministry of Health in Japan actively promotes breastfeeding. Japanese mothers are inclined to follow "doctor's orders" and are reluctant to challenge their physician's (mostly male) opinion. Many young Japanese women experience a dissonance between their culture's old-world values (staying home, raising children, breastfeeding) and values of today (working, career, bottle-feeding). (Riordan, personal communication, M. Hasegawa, 1991; J. Ohuchi, 1987.)

Korea

Korean mothers are taken care of by their mothers-in-law postpartum and look to them for advice about feeding and caring for their babies; therefore breastfeeding promotion efforts must include mothers-in-law. About half of Korean babies are formula-fed with formulas imported from the West and advertised as "the second kind of mother's milk" (Riordan, personal communication, M. Pope, 1988.)

A basic diet guide for balanced vegetarian meals includes:

- Grains, legumes, nuts, and seeds: Six or more servings including several slices of whole grain bread, beans, and some nuts or seeds
- Vegetables: Three servings or more, including one or more servings of dark leafy greens
- Fruit: One to four pieces including citrus fruits for a raw source of vitamin C
- Milk and eggs: Dairy products (if the baby does not show an allergic response) and eggs to meet basic protein requirements.

RELIGIOUS INFLUENCES

Religion also influences the diet of the breastfeeding woman. If she is a Seventh-Day Adventist or a member of certain Eastern religious sects, she practices vegetarianism. Orthodox Muslim and Black Muslim women are expected to breastfeed their babies according to religious teachings, and Islamic dietary regulations prohibit pork, animal shortening, products containing gelatin, and alcoholic beverages. No animal meat can be eaten unless it has been slaughtered in a prescribed manner. During the month-long Ramadan fast, Muslims are not allowed to eat or drink anything between sunrise and sunset. If they are not exempt, this practice imposes a hardship on pregnant and lactating women who require a regular intake of fluid and calories (Prentice et al., 1983).

An orthodox Jewish mother will closely observe dietary laws that prohibit pork products and shellfish. According to these laws, meat and milk cannot be eaten at the same meal. After meat is eaten, she must wait before consuming milk products. Dietary counseling must include planning her daily meals so that she takes in adequate calcium and phosphorus from milk products or substitute foods.

THE "DOULA"

Much has been written about the importance of social support of the breastfeeding woman. Raphael (1973), who coined the word "doula," explains the characteristics of such a person as one who is knowledgeable in the breastfeeding process and who "mothers the mother." To undertake this important task, different cultures designate a specific person or persons to this role. Usually, but not always, this is an older female, often the mother's mother, mother-in-law or aunt who has breastfeeding experience and who passes her knowledge on to the mother. At the same time, she assists the mother with her household work and protects her from the stresses of the outside world.

WEANING

Weaning, a time when childhood illness and death is more likely in developing countries, is a key issue in studies of cross-cultural child-care practices. Cultural assessment includes the timing and types of foods given to infants as well as weaning practices. While they are breastfed, infants typically thrive and grow. When a substantial proportion of their dietary intake is from food other than breastmilk, growth rates falter and the effects of morbidity come into play. Woolridge (1991) suggests, as a rule of thumb, that when 25 to 50% of a baby's kilocalories come from breastmilk, the milk will protect the baby from environmental pathogens. At the same time, every breastfed infant reaches a point when breastmilk alone can no longer meet its nutritional needs, and solid foods are necessary.

Early solid and semisolid infant foods given by mothers vary widely across cultures (Table 2–5) as does the timing of their introduction. Worldwide there is a high rate of both the initiation of breastfeeding and the too early supplementation with other foods. Although infants in Papua New Guinea are not introduced to supplemental foods until six months of age (Lepowsky, 1985), which is optimal, this is not the usual pattern. In a comparison study of how mothers feed their infants in four diverse countries, Winikoff and colleagues (1988) noted that early infant supplements were common. The majority of Kenyan babies are given food supplements before they are four months old (van Esterik & Elliott, 1986; Dimond & Ashworth, 1987); in East Java, force feeding by hand is a common practice from as early as few days after birth (van Steenbergen et al., 1991).

What implications can we derive from these diverse practices in infant feedings? Van Esterik (1988) suggests looking at a culture's breastfeeding "style," i.e., the cultural assumptions underlying infant feeding practices, to distinguish between breastfeeding as a process and breastmilk as product. According

TABLE 2–5 EXAMPLES OF INFANT SOLID FOODS ACROSS CULTURES

Culture	Foods	Reference
Brazil	Grain products, beans, bean broth, herb teas	Wright & Oliveria, 1989
Egypt	Biscuit, bread, yolk	Raphael, 1984
India	Rice	Raphael, 1984
Solomon Islands	Premasticated taro (sweet potato)	Akin, 1985
Papua New Guinea	Yam, taro, banana, pumpkin, papaya	Lepowsky, 1985 Marshall, 1983
Fiji Islands	Broth of cooked starch or leafy vegetables, mashed papaya	Katz, 1984
Kenya	Maize, millet and sorghum porridges	van Esterik & Elliott, 1986
Korea	Boiled rice, beans, barley, dried fish	M. Pope, Personal communication, Seoul, Korea 1989
United States	Mashed banana, chicken pieces, uncooked fruit	La Leche League, 1991
Turkey	Yogurt, cereals, eggs	Koctürk & Zetterström, 1986

From van Esterik, P, and Elliott T: Infant feeding style in urban Kenya. *Ecol Food Nutr* 18:183–95, 1986.

to this model, a given culture will tend to emphasize breastfeeding style either as a process or a means to obtain a product. When breastfeeding is considered a process, supplements are small in amount and are not given to replace breastfeeding. For example, mothers in Kenya perceive breastfeeding as a process—something that mothers and infants do and not solely as food for the infant. As such, finger-feeding the baby small amounts of food from the family cooking pot is part of the socialization of the infant, and meals consist of several foods. Since breastmilk is not considered a product, it is not thought to be either superior or inferior to other foods.

When breastmilk is thought of as a product, the emphasis changes to the characteristics of the milk:

> It is produced from food but is not easily affected by the particulars of a mother's diet. Breastmilk is considered sweet and light (not heavy) and is warm in quality and temperature. Cold milks are harmful for the infant. There is only one product produced from the breast and that is breastmilk (van Esterik & Elliott, 1986).

In the United States, breastfeeding is primarily thought of as a product that can be closely approximated, although not completely replaced, by formula. The emphasis is on its nutritional and immu-

nologic properties as opposed to nonproduct issues such as fertility, maternal satisfaction and feelings of closeness to her baby. If breastfeeding is primarily seen as a product in a given culture, it is seldom considered as an integral part of the maternal experience.

Weaning from the breast is a process during which mothers gradually introduce their babies to culturally assigned foods as they continue to breastfeed. According to Raphael (1984), mothers worry as much about the availability of additional foods as they do about the amount of milk they produce. Weaning begins with the introduction of sources of food other than breastmilk and ends with the last breastfeeding. Three types of weaning have been described:

1. *Gradual weaning* takes place over several weeks or months.
2. *Deliberate weaning* is a conscious effort initiated by the mother in order to end breastfeeding at a particular point in time.
3. *Abrupt weaning* is an immediate cessation of breastfeeding, which may be forced on the baby by the mother or on mother and baby by others.

Weaning practice can affect infant health, particularly in developing countries or inner-city areas where weaning diarrhea is prevalent. In cultures in which food is available sporadically or is meager, *kwashiorkor,* a severe form of protein deficiency, appears during the transition from breastmilk to other foods. In the Ga language of Accra, Ghana, the term *kwashiorkor* means "the disease of the deposed baby" (Dr. Cicely Williams, lecture, Tulane University, 1975). Identifying the reasons women wean early sheds considerable light on the beliefs and attitudes that influence the continuation of breastfeeding.

Reasons for early weaning are similar in many cultures. For example the following six reasons which poor Philippine mothers report for early termination of breastfeeding are similar to those of women living in North America (Guthrie et al., 1983):

1. *Infant Diarrhea:* The test of whether a baby tolerates her breastmilk or any other food is whether it causes diarrhea.
2. *Insufficient milk:* The baby is not satisfied after breastfeeding.
3. *Mother returns to work:* Selling foods on the street requires that the mother be exposed to the hot sun; since milk would lie in the breast for many hours, it is not fit for the baby.
4. *Mother becomes sick:* The mother may stop breastfeeding because she has an infectious disease such as diphtheria or tuberculosis or *Bughat.* This is a culture-bound syndrome, a vague illness that only women who have borne children can develop. If the healer is not successful, the mother terminates breastfeeding.
5. *Baby refuses breast:* The mother is uncertain why her baby refuses to continue nursing but suspects that her milk is no longer good. The mother tastes it to see if it is thin, watery, or salty.
6. *Milk is salty or not good:* The mother almost always stops breastfeeding if she decides that her milk is salty. One mother raised six children on one breast because she decided that the milk of the other was salty at her first pregnancy.

Examples of gradual, deliberate, or abrupt weaning may be found in any culture. Specially prepared rice, the major infant food in East Java, is hand-fed in small amounts to almost all infants, and all babies breastfeed (van Steenbergen et al., 1991). Rice, finger-fed in small amounts, initiates the Thai baby to a rice culture and helps to stave off spiritual parents who might come to take the baby away (Woolridge,

1991). It is gradual weaning, however, that is the least traumatic both to the infant and the mother. Breastfed infants in a poor community on the periphery of Lima, Peru, for example, are given nondairy complementary foods beginning around five to six months of age (de Kanashiro et al., 1990). La Leche League mothers around the world typically wean their babies from the breast "gradually with love" over many months or even years (La Leche League Int., 1991).

Various stages in infant development are sometimes used as cues to begin *deliberate* weaning. A common belief among African cultures is that the child should be walking before weaning is attempted. Some kind of independence is implicit in the concept of weaning, so it seems reasonable that the child be self-sufficient in locomotion before leaving the dependency of its mother's breast. In many Western cultures, teething is a developmental reference point thought to signal readiness to wean. In others, subsequent pregnancy signals the time to wean. Usually a toddler or child will spontaneously wean with a new pregnancy. The reasons include a diminished milk supply, changes in the milk composition and a less desirable taste.

Rage, withdrawal and depression are typical behaviors of a baby or child forcibly weaned from breastfeeding. Martinez (1978) reports that this rejection is so important that it is considered the foundation of the hot-cold syndrome used in Spanish-speaking cultures:

> In the process of weaning, the Mexican child is subjected to a prolonged period of acute rejection. As a result of this experience, he forms strong subconscious associations between warmth and acceptance (or intimacy), on the one hand, and between cold and rejection (or withdrawal), on the other. In adult life, these associations appear in those beliefs initially concerned with the problem of personal security; theories about nourishment and about the prevention and cure of disease and injury. On the conscious level, the hot-cold syndrome is a basic principle of human physiology, and it functions as a logical system for dealing with the problem of disorder and disease. On a subconscious level, however, the hot-cold syndrome is a model of social relations.

Some rather harsh techniques have been used to bring about *abrupt* weaning. One time-honored method calls for pepper, garlic, ginger or onion to be applied to the mother's breasts to discourage the baby from breastfeeding (Aquino, 1981). In the Fiji Islands weaning of *kali* (to separate) is a four-day period of abrupt weaning during which the breast is denied to the infant and the baby's food is cooked specially in a separate pot. The infant is not allowed to sleep with the mother until after weaning and is sometimes cared for by one of the mother's female relatives in another household for this period of time (Katz, 1984).

In cultures in which early weaning from both bottle and breast is a common practice, long-term breastfeeding is accepted by a minority within the cultural context. The sight of a walking child calmly sliding into his mother's lap for milk and deftly opening her buttons to gain access to her breasts is shocking and subject to ridicule in some cultures. The term *closet nursing* describes a practice that has evolved in the United States in response to criticism of breastfeeding that extends beyond the dominant culture's expectations (Avery, 1977; Morse & Harrison, 1987). With *closet nursing,* breastfeeding continues by mutual consent of mother and child, but only in secret. The mother and baby usually have a "code" word for breastfeeding that can be used in public (Wrigley & Hutchinson, 1990).

IMPLICATIONS FOR PRACTICE

Every culture has its visible elements (housing, clothing, food) and its invisible elements (attitudes, tradition, values); an understanding of both of these attributes contributes significantly to communication between the breastfeeding client and the health-care provider (Brownlee, 1978).

Here are a few specific folkways about infants and ways to handle them:

- Touching the baby of a Spanish-speaking family while admiring him helps avoid giving the baby *mal de ojo.*
- If an anemic breastfeeding mother is not vegetarian and if she believes anemia is a yin condition, she will more readily accept the suggestion of consuming more meat, a yang food, to improve her iron status (Suitor & Hunter, 1980).
- If the baby burps during the feeding, according

to some Hispanic mothers, the air goes to the breast and stops the flow of milk so that her milk duct becomes plugged. To validate her belief, it can be suggested that if this happens, she should switch to the other breast and then back to the first breast to release the "air."
- Another Mexican-American belief is that the milk in the breast will sour if a woman is upset or angry. Sour milk, of course, should never be fed to the baby. If the mother's husband or partner is angry with her, she can avoid an argument by pleading that her milk will become sour, thereby avoiding the problem (Frantz, personal communication, 1981).
- To deal with the cultural belief that colostrum is "bad," suggest to mothers that the first few drops of "impure" milk may be expressed and discarded before the mother breastfeeds and that "the sooner you breastfeed, the better the milk:" van Esterik, 1988; Skeel & Good, 1988).
- Immigrant mothers may be served foods which traditionally are forbidden to postpartum women, such as raw vegetables and fruit for Vietnamese mothers. If the dietary department of an institution is aware of this, it can provide alternate foods to these women.
- Many Indochinese women living in the United States formula-feed their infant, at least while in the hospital, and then both breastfeed and bottle-feed after leaving the hospital; therefore, lactation suppressants and formula discharge packs are not appropriate.
- If mothers in any culture believe that certain foods can promote lactation, encouraging these women to bring these foods to the postpartum unit will enhance breastfeeding and provide a clear signal that the health-care system supports breastfeeding (Chan-Yip & Kramer, 1983).

When sufficient food is available, additional calories (20 to 25%) needed during lactation are easily supplied by nutrients in a variety of foods compatible with the mother's cultural and personal preference. Given that food is plentiful, the most reliable guide for the amount of foods and fluids a lactating mother needs is her appetite and thirst. Nutrition education is needed when it appears that her diet is insufficient and there are clinical signs such as anemia, excessive weight loss, or possibly a lessened supply of breastmilk.

Regardless of the culture, weaning is ideally a collaborative effort in which both the mother and baby reach a state of readiness to begin weaning around the same time. In a culture in which unrestricted breastfeeding is practiced, with the child breastfeeding for a prolonged period, the mother has very little ambivalence when she decides to wean saying, "You, child, have had enough milk!" (Mead & Newton, 1967). Unfortunately this is not always the case.

While weaning practices vary from culture to culture weaning is thought to be least traumatic when it is slow, gradual and related to the needs of the child. It is essential to identify factors which influence continuation or early termination of breastfeeding in order to develop appropriate programs to assist the mother in maintaining breastfeeding. Women involved in long-term breastfeeding develop a special bond with their baby. A mother's choice of how long she wishes to breastfeed is an individual right that may not mesh within the context of her culture. All breastfeeding families have the right to be treated in a non-judgmental manner which accepts the cultural diversity that they represent.

A practical question has been raised regarding breastfeeding promotion programs: Should these programs establish goals for exclusive breastfeeding which might be difficult to achieve? Or is it preferable to promote partial breastfeeding rather to set impractical goals? A wise philosopher once said that the answer is the question—both may be found within the culture, if we only look for them.

SUMMARY

The study of childrearing patterns of a culture is crucial to all health-care professionals who work with new and growing families. It is through the patterns of childrearing that the seeds of a culture are planted, grow and thrive. Cultural awareness is liberation from egocentric views in which one looks at the universe and sees oneself and one's beliefs in the center. The study of any culture begins with the awareness that there is a significant difference between one's own cultural values and those of other people; this also applies to the breastfeeding woman and her family.

Analysis of the breastfeeding style within the cultural context is critically linked to social action and policy decisions regarding breastfeeding promotion and teaching. For those who look carefully, so-called cultural "obstacles" to solving problems usually include the solutions too. It is within the cultural context underlying infant feeding problems that solutions must ultimately emerge. Changes, if they are to last, must originate from within a culture, not be imposed from without.

REFERENCES

Affonso, DO: The Filipino American. In Clark, A, ed: *Culture, childbearing, health professionals,* Philadelphia, 1978, F. A. Davis Co., pp. 128–53.

Akin, KG: Women's work and infant feeding practices: traditional and transitional practices on Malita, Solomon Islands. *Ecol Food Nutr* 16:55–73, 1985.

Anderson, GC, Marks, EA, and Wahlberg, V: Kangaroo care for premature infants, *AJN* 86:807–9, 1986.

Aquino, CJ: The Filipino in America. In Clark A, ed.: *Culture and childrearing,* Philadelphia, 1981, F.A. Davis Co., pp. 166–90.

Avery, JL: Closet nursing: A symptom of intolerance and a forerunner of social change? *Keep Abreast J* 2:212–26, 1977.

Baumslag, N: Breastfeeding: cultural practices and variations, *Adv International Mat and Child Hlth* 7:36–50, 1987.

Bowles, BC: Cultural masquerade (letter), *J Hum Lact* 3:157, 1987.

Boyle, JS, and Andrews, MM: *Transcultural concepts in nursing care,* Glenview, Illinois, 1989, Scott, Foresman & Co. Little, Brown & Co.

Brownlee, AT: *Community, culture and care: A cross-cultural guide for health workers,* St. Louis, 1978, The C.V. Mosby Co.

Chan-Yip, AM, and Kramer, MS: Promotion of breastfeeding in a Chinese community in Montreal, *CMAJ* 129:955–58, 1983.

Char, EL: The Chinese American. In Clark, A, ed.: *Culture and childrearing,* Philadelphia, 1981, F.A. Davis Co., pp. 141–164.

Conton, L: Social, economic and ecological parameters of infant feeding in Usino, Papua New Guinea, *Ecol Food Nutr* 16:39–54, 1985.

Counts, DA: Infant care and feeding in Kaliai, West New Britain, Papua New Guinea, *Ecol Food Nutr* 15:49–59, 1984.

de Kanashiro, C, et al.: Consumption of food and nutrients by infants in Huascar (Lima) Peru, *Am J Clin Nutr* 52:995–1004, 1990.

Dimond, HJ, and Ashworth, A: Infant feeding practices in Kenya, Mexico and Malaysia: The rarity of the exclusively breast-fed infant, *Hum Nutr, Appl Nutr* 41A:51–64, 1987.

Eaton-Evans, J, and Dugdale, AE: Food avoidance by breastfeeding mothers in South East Queensland, *Ecol Food Nutr* 19:123–29, 1986.

Ebrahim, GJ: Cross-cultural aspects of breastfeeding. In *Breastfeeding and the mother, Ciba Foundation Symposium 45,* Amsterdam, 1976, Elsevier Scientific Publishing Co.

Ehling, MB: The Mexican American (El Chicano). In Clark, A, ed.: *Culture and childrearing,* Philadelphia, 1981, F.A. Davis Co., pp. 193–209.

Fernandez, MA, and Popkin, BM: Prelacteal feeding patterns in the Philippines, *Ecol Food Nutr* 21:303–14, 1988.

Fishman, C, Evans, R, and Jenks, E: Warm bodies, cool milk: conflicts in post partum food choice for Indochinese women in California, *Soc Sci Med* 26:1125–32, 1988.

Giger, JN, and Davidhizar, RE: *Transcultural nursing,* St. Louis, 1991, Mosby Year Book, p. 5.

Guthrie, GM, et al.: Early termination of breastfeeding among Philippine urban poor, *Ecol Food Nutr* 12:195–202, 1983.

Harris, K: Beliefs and practices among Haitian American women in relation to childbearing, *J Nurs-Midwif* 32:150–55, 1987.

Jimenez, MH, and Newton, N: Activity and work during pregnancy and the postpartum period: a cross-cultural study of 202 societies, *Am J Obstet Gynecol* 135:171–76, 1979.

Katz, MM: Infant care in a group of outer Fiji Islands, *Ecol Food Nutr* 15:323–39, 1984.

Kitzinger, S: *The crying baby,* London, 1990, Penguin Group.

Koctürk, TA, and Zeterström, R: Breastfeeding among Turkish mothers living in suburbs of Istanbul and Stockholm—a comparison, *Acta Paediatr Scand* 75:216–21, 1986.

Koh, THHG: Breastfeeding among the Chinese in four countries, *J Trop Pediatr* 27:88–91, 1981.

Konner, M, and Shostak, M: Timing and management of birth among the iKung: Biocultural interaction in reproductive adaptation, *Cult Anthrop* 2(1):11–27, 1987.

Krantz, JZ, and Kupper, NS: Cross-nursing: wet-nursing in a contemporary culture, *Pediatrics* 67:715–17, 1981.

Labbok, M: Pregnancy in traditional societies. In Ahmed, P: *Pregnancy, childbirth and parenthood,* New York, 1981, Elsevier Scientific Publishing Co.

Lacay, GI: The Puerto Rican in mainland America. In Clark, A ed.: *Culture and childrearing,* Philadelphia, 1981, F.A. Davis Co., pp. 211–27.

La Du EB: Childbirth care for Hmong families, *MCN* 10:382–85, 1985.

La Leche League International, *The womanly art of breastfeeding,* 5th ed., Franklin Park, Illinois, 1991, The League.

Leininger, M: *Qualitative research methods in nursing,* Orlando, Florida, 1985, Grune & Stratton, Inc.

Lepowsky, MA: Food taboos, malaria and dietary change: Infant feeding and cultural adaptation of a Papua New Guinea Island, *Ecol Food Nutr* 16:105–26, 1985.

Marshall, LB: Infant feeding practices among clinical nursing staff in urban Papua New Guinea, *Int J Nurs Stud* 20:63–74, 1983.

Martinez, RA: *Hispanic, culture and health care: fact, fiction, folklore,* St. Louis, 1978, The C.V. Mosby Co.

Mathews, M, and Manderson, L: Vietnamese behavioral and dietary precautions during confinement, *Ecol Food Nutr* 11:9–16, 1981.

McKenzie, JL, and Chrisman, NJ: Healing, herbs, gods and magic: Folk health beliefs among Filipino-Americans, *Nurs Outlook* 25:326–29, 1977.

Mead, M, and Newton, N: Cultural patterning of perinatal behavior. In Richardson, SA, and Buttmacher, AF, eds.: *Childbearing: its social and psychological aspects,* Baltimore, 1967, The Williams & Wilkins Co., p. 142–243.

Mennella, JS, and Beauchamp, GK: Maternal diet alters the sensory qualities of human milk and the nursling's behavior, *Pediatrics* 88:737–44, 1991.

Mercer, RT, and Stainton, MC: Perceptions of the birth experience: A cross-cultural comparison, *Health Care Women Int* 5:29–47, 1984.

Moore, WH, ed.: Nutrition, growth and development of North American Indian children, Department of Health, Education, and Welfare, Publ. No. 72–76, Washington, D.C., 1969, National Institutes of Health.

Morse, JM, and Harrison, MJ: Social coercion for weaning, *J Nurs-Midwif* 32:205–10, 1987.

Nelson, CN, and Hewitt, MA: An Indochinese refugee population in a nurse-midwife service, *N Nurs-Midwif* 28:9–14, 1983.

Omuloulu, A: Breastfeeding practice and breastmilk intake in rural Nigeria, *Hum Nutr, Appl Nutr* 36A:445–51, 1982.

Orque, MS, Bloch, B, and Monrroy, LSA: *Ethnic nursing care: A multicultural approach,* St. Louis, 1983, The C.V. Mosby Co.

Prentice, AM, et al.: Metabolic consequences of fasting during Ramadan in pregnant and lactating women, *Hum Nutr Clin Nutr* 37C:283–94, 1983.

Raphael, D: *The tender gift: breastfeeding,* Englewood Cliffs, New Jersey, 1973, Prentice-Hall, Inc.

Raphael, D: Weaning is always: The anthropology of breast feeding behavior, *Ecol Food Nutr,* 15:203–13, 1984.

Rosenberg, JA: Health care for Cambodian children: Integrating treatment plans, *Pediatr Nurs* 12:118–25, 1986.

Sawada, K: Breastfeeding customs in Japan, Proceedings of Eighth International Conference of La Leche League, International, Chicago, 1981.

Scott, MDS, and Stern PN: The ethno-market theory: factors influencing childbearing health practices of northern Louisiana Black women, *Health Care Women Int* 6:45–61, 1985.

Serdula, MK, et al.: Correlates of breast-feeding in a low-income population of whites, blacks, and Southeast Asians, *J Am Diet Assoc* 91:41–45, 1991.

Skeel, LS, and Good, ME: Mexican cultural beliefs and breastfeeding: a model for assessment and intervention, *J Hum Lact* 4:160–63, 1988.

Spector, RE: *Cultural diversity in health and illness,* 2nd ed. New York, 1985, Appleton–Century–Crofts, p. 3.

Suitor, CW, and Hunter, MF: *Nutrition: principles and application in health promotion,* Philadelphia, 1980, J.B. Lippincott Co., pp. 53–64.

Tripp-Reimer, T, Brink, P, and Saunders, JM: Cultural assessment: content and process, *Nurs Outlook* 32:78–82, 1984.

van Esterik, P: The cultural context of infant feeding. In Winikoff, B, Castle, MA, and Laukaran, VH: *Feeding infants in four societies: Causes and consequences of mothers' choices,* New York, 1988, Greenwood Press, pp. 187–201.

van Esterik, P, and Elliott, T: Infant feeding style in urban Kenya, *Ecol Food Nutr* 18:183–95, 1986.

van Steenbergen, WM, et al.: Nutritional transition during infancy in East Java, Indonesia: 1. A longitudinal study of feeding pattern, breast milk intake and the consumption of additional foods, *Eur J Clin Nutr* 45:67–75, 1991.

Vargas, LA: Traditional breastfeeding methods in Mexico. In Rapheal, D, ed. : *Breastfeeding and food policy in a hungry world,* New York, 1979, Academic Press, Inc.

Williams, C, and Jelliffe, D: *Mother and child health: Delivering the services,* Oxford, 1972, Oxford University Press.

Winikoff, B: Summary. In Winikoff, B, Castle, MA, and Laukaran, VH: *Feeding infants in four societies: Causes and consequences of mothers' choices,* New York, 1988, Greenwood Press.

Woolridge, M: Breastfeeding in the US and Thailand, International Lactation Consultant Association, Miami, July 16–19, 1991.

Wright, AL, et al.: Infant feeding practices among middle-class Anglos and Hispanics, *Pediatrics* 82:496–503, 1988.

Wright, MG, and Oliveira, JE: Infant feeding in a low-income Brazilian community, *Ecol Food Nutr* 23:1–12, 1989.

Wrigley, EA, and Hutchinson: S: Long-term breastfeeding: the secret bond, *J Nurs-Midwif* 35:35–41, 1990.

SUGGESTED READINGS

Erlinda, MA, Fernandez, L, and Popkin, BM: Prelacteal feeding patterns in the Philippines, *Ecol Food Nutr* 21:303–14, 1988.

Jelliffe, DB, and Jelliffe, EFP: Education of the public for successful lactation *Ecol Food Nutr* 2:127–32.

Kokinos, M, and Dewey, K: Infant feeding practices of migrant Mexican-American families in northern California, *Ecol Food Nutr* 18:209–20, 1986.

Lee, PA: Health beliefs of pregnancy and postpartum Hmong women, *West J Nurs Res* 8:83–93, 1986.

Rorabaugh, ML: The pediatric nurse practitioner in South East Asia: A personal account, *Pediatr Nurs* 9:263–66, 1983.

Scrimshaw, SC, et al.: Factors affecting breastfeeding among women of Mexican origin or descent in Los Angeles, *Am J Public Health* 77:467–70, 1987.

3

Families

KATHLEEN G. AUERBACH

INTRODUCTION

The care provider working with the breastfeeding mother must always be cognizant of the family from which that mother comes and into which her child will be born and reared. To a very real degree, when we help a breastfeeding mother and baby, we are helping a family. In order to place the breastfeeding family in a social context, the care provider must first recognize that "family" is a term which is variously defined and experienced. A variety of theories have been proposed to explain how families work. While every family is expected to perform similar functions, how those functions are recognized and accomplished will vary.

Certain families need special attention. A case in point is the single pregnant adolescent, who may not have others on whom she can depend, and who has greater needs than if she were married or part of a well-established support network. The family living in poverty may need to breastfeed to provide the baby with protections that are only available in human milk; however, in most settings in the developed world, the poorest mothers are least likely to breastfeed. Care providers need to be cognizant of the breastfeeding promotion programs that have been developed with such families in mind.

This chapter, which examines the family from a developmental perspective, will enable the healthcare provider to gain insight into the ways in which this unique small group works and how it is influenced by others, including the social system surrounding it. The birth of a baby has rightly been described as a crisis insofar as it forces new ways of behavior on all family members. Issues pertaining to

the process of spousal and parent-child attachment are discussed. Particular attention is paid to the role of the father as a helpmate and supporter of his partner's dual role as mother and as breastfeeder. The special needs of the adolescent mother and of women living in poverty also are addressed in the discussion of breastfeeding promotion programs.

FAMILY FORMS AND FUNCTIONS

In the course of a lifetime, an individual experiences many family forms. Each meets different needs and serves different functions. Some include children; others do not. Some forms will be experienced only at certain times in the life cycle, while others may occur at several different times, although for different reasons. A traditional family is defined as one in which the mother is a full-time homemaker and primarily responsible for rearing the children, while her husband is a full-time worker outside the home. Although he is committed to seeing that the children are raised to adulthood, his role in their rearing is secondary to that of his wife. Although this form is often viewed as "ideal," it is experienced by only a small percentage of families, usually for a minority of the life of that family. A nuclear family is generally comprised of one or both parents and their children, who are either born to or adopted by them. An extended family usually contains lateral kin (such as aunts, uncles, and/or cousins) who occupy the same generational status as the parents and children in a nuclear family; or vertical kin, such as grandparents or grandchildren, who represent different generations than the parents and children in the nuclear family. In some cases, an extended family may include "fictive" kin—individuals who cannot trace lineage through blood or marriage ties to the nuclear family members, but who act, and are treated, as if they were related. An overt manifestation of such fictive kinship is calling an unrelated individual "aunt" or "uncle" or some other name implying relationship. The relationship between England's Prince Charles and the late Earl of Mountbatten is a case in point; Charles called the Earl his "honorary Grandfather," although they did not share such a blood relationship.

Examining how different family forms are likely to be experienced throughout an individual's lifetime can provide insight into the stresses that an individual is likely to encounter. It also reveals who people will lean on as they attempt to cope with those stresses. Take, for example, a hypothetical individual, whom we shall call Marsha. She begins life as part of her family of orientation (the family into which she was born or adopted). This family happens to be considered "traditional" because Marsha's mother has remained home since the birth of Marsha's older brother, and Marsha's father is the sole breadwinner. Marsha also has a younger sister and a younger brother, providing her with sibling relationships with both a same-sex and two opposite-sex siblings. If she marries, she will, with her husband, create her own family of procreation, the family unit into which her children will be born or adopted.

When Marsha goes away to college, she rooms with a series of other young single women. After she graduates and begins her first job as a commercial artist for a local public relations firm, she moves into her own apartment, reveling for the first time in her "very own space."

Four years after beginning her career, Marsha meets John, an architect who was a client of her firm. After a whirlwind courtship, and against the advice of their parents, the two marry and move into his apartment. Two years later, they buy a house in hopes of filling some of the upstairs bedrooms with children. Their wish is not long in coming. Just before their third wedding anniversary, Marsha gives birth to John, Jr. Three years later, Mary Jane is born. At the end of her pregnancy with John, Marsha quit her job. She was unwilling to allow her children to be "raised by someone else," although she had earlier vowed never to fall into what she thought of as the trap of full-time parenting that she had observed with her own mother. However, the closer she came to her own firstborn's birth, the less confident she was with what some of her friends described as "the modern way of babysitters, day care centers and being a full-time working wife." As a result, until Mary Jane was one year old, Marsha was a full-time homemaker while John was a full-time breadwinner; Marsha thus cared for their two children in a pattern much like that of both of their mothers.

Time away from work became increasingly difficult for Marsha. With Mary Jane a much more rambunctious toddler than her older quieter brother, Marsha decided to go back to work. "After all, MJ will only be one floor away from me. I called and there is space for her at the new daycare center in the same building as my old job, and Bernie said he'd take me back," she explained to John, who wasn't as keen as she about the idea. Unwilling to cause an argument, however, he agreed. For the next three years, both spouses worked fulltime.

As sometimes happens, neither spouse found their increasingly busy life conducive to maintaining communication. After 10 years of marriage, they experiment with a trial separation and then decide to divorce. Marsha maintains physical custody of the children insofar as they continue to live with her in the home that she and John had bought shortly after their marriage. John finds a small co-op apartment nearby so that the joint custody arrangement they worked out will enable him to see the children with minimal difficulty.

The two years that Marsha was single were difficult, but she felt that in many ways, she and the children had never been closer. Then she met Joe, a newly hired marketing specialist at her office. His ex-wife, who was very bitter about their divorce, had taken their three children, ages four to seven, to live out-of-state, although the divorce decree forbade it. However, Joe, in an attempt to remain cordial with his ex-wife so that he would be able to see his children, did not force her to return. Shortly after she married Joe, Marsha's children, ages 14 and 11, decided to live with John. This made Marsha a non-custodial parent, although she continued to see the children frequently. Six months after Marsha's children left her home, Joe's children returned to him for a visit; while there, Joe's wife was killed in a car accident. Joe then assumed full-time custody of the children, who remained with him and Marsha.

After a year with three small children at home, Marsha's own children did an about-face: they asked to come back to live with Joe and Marsha when John's job took him out-of-state. They continued to live there until they left for college.

A year after MJ left home for college, Joe was injured while working late on the evening of the San Francisco earthquake. He took early retirement. Marsha was secretly relieved that the work of caring for his teen-age children fell more heavily on Joe's shoulders once he became a full-time house-husband. This arrangement continued until Luci went into the Marines and Joe, Jr., received a scholarship to Harvard. Ten short months later, in the middle of a visit to a travel agent's office where he and Marsha were planning a special fifteenth anniversary cruise, Joe had a massive heart attack.

Marsha took the cruise alone and returned home to a house that was empty of people, but echoed with memories. She disliked staying in the house, which was so much larger than she needed, but she didn't have the psychic energy to move. A year after Joe's death, she was wakened in the middle of the night by a telephone call from a weeping MJ, who asked if she could come home. She and her husband Jason had had a terrible fight, and MJ was afraid he might become violent. Marsha put the front porch light on, set the tea kettle over a tiny flame, and made up the bed in MJ's old room.

For two years, MJ and her son, Jason, Jr., lived with grandma Marsha. Just before Marsha was getting ready to ask MJ to "get a grip" on her life and move out, Jason completed his drug-and-alcohol-rehabilitation program, rejoined a health and fitness club, won the intra-club weight-lifting championship, and appeared on Marsha's door to reclaim his family and "begin life anew." She kissed them all heartily and returned to enjoying the quiet of her "very own space." She contemplated taking early retirement at 62 and signing up for an around-the-world cruise.

Since leaving her own family of orientation, Marsha experienced ten different family configurations. If she moves in with her two sisters after selling her home, she may experience yet another form, that of a kin network that does not include different generations. Additionally, it is instructive to note that she has experienced what is often called a traditional nu-

clear family for only four of the ten years that she was married to John—and for less than one-tenth of her entire adult life since leaving her own family of orientation to go away to college. While this example is hypothetical, the life experiences that it represents are not atypical of those which are experienced by many people in developed nations today. (See boxed chart on p. 52.)

While the forms may vary, Spradley (1985) reports that each configuration of individuals who think of themselves as part of a family and call a particular group a family, are characterized by five universals:

1. It is a small social system.
2. It has its own culture and rules.
3. It has structure.
4. It has certain basic functions.
5. It moves through stages in its lifecycle.

The existence of these universals means that—regardless of its composition—a family provides certain elements to its members. These generally consist of affection, security, identity, affiliation, socialization, and controls (Spradley, 1985).

From the standpoint of a mother and infant, or a mother and young child, affection is important as an indication to the child that he is loved and appreciated for his own sake. Security comes from the establishment of physical and social restrictions that, along with other controls, set the boundaries by which appropriate behavior is identified and rewarded.

The family's identity is most often recognized by outsiders through a shared surname, which often places the members of that family within a larger social context, such as a neighborhood or community. Particularly in small towns, the members of a family may have a specific status that may have been established several generations earlier.

Affiliation is a recognition by its members that they relate to one another differently than they do with other individuals who are "non-family." The jokes that are made about meeting the parents and/or siblings of a future spouse for the first time are a recognition that not being a member of the family sets one apart—as different from—its members. Socialization refers to the means by which older family members teach younger members how to behave and what to value. A child who "minds his manners" when at a restaurant with grandparents has been socialized to behave in this manner by the members of his family

VARIOUS FAMILY FORMS AN INDIVIDUAL MAY EXPERIENCE IN A LIFETIME.

Age	Experience	Family Form
0–18	Living with family of orientation (two parents, three siblings)	Nuclear family (traditional)
19–25	College student; then working college graduate	Adult living with peers; alone
26–28	Newlywed	Nuclear dyad; two-career household
29–33	Two children born, three years apart	Nuclear family (traditional)
34–36	Marsha returns to work	Nuclear, two-career family
37–39	John and Marsha divorce	Marsha: single parent
		John: non-custodial parent
40–42	Marsha remarries; her children go to live with John	Marsha: non-custodial parent
		John: single parent
43–44	Joe's children come to live with Joe and Marsha	Marsha: stepparent
45–50	Marsha's children return to live with Marsha and Joe	"Blended" family
54–57	Joe's children leave home for military service and college	Nuclear dyad; non-traditional form
58	Joe dies	Adult living alone
59–61	MJ comes home with baby	Extended (three-generational) family
62	MJ moves back home with Jason	Aging adult living alone

Case study questions:

1. Identify in which developmental stage Marsha's family is at each juncture in her life when change dictates a different family form.
2. In what ways are these different family forms interfering with Marsha's progression through Duvall's developmental stages?
3. Using the tasks identified in Duvall's developmental stages, which tasks are most likely to be negatively affected as Marsha moves through different family forms? Which are likely to be achieved with the least effort?
4. When was Marsha's family expanding, remaining stable, contracting? In what ways were different needs required of the family at each of these developmental stages?

who have served as role models for correct behavior in public. Unacceptable behavior has been corrected in practice settings, including around the dinner table at home.

Finally, controls involve not only a recognition of appropriate behavior, but a mechanism for identifying and correcting inappropriate behavior. In cases where sex-role-specific behavior is expected, the boy who offers to wash dishes may be viewed as engaging in inappropriate behavior by some, although in his family, no such division of labor along gender lines is made. In many ways, identification of appropriate or inappropriate (or deviant) behavior is a recognition of subcultural norms or values. In a pluralistic society such as exists in the United States, where

many different subcultures and ethnic groups abound, the way in which behavior is structured and controlled may vary markedly from one family group to the next. Thus, breastfeeding in the living room in the presence of friends, male and female, may be viewed as completely acceptable in some families and as clearly incorrect behavior in others. For some mothers, breastfeeding requires draping a shawl around her shoulders and the baby's upper torso, while for others, no such restriction applies. The health-care worker assisting the breastfeeding mother is well-advised to ask for guidance about what the mother's family expects of her in order to provide advice that will be viewed as appropriate within that family setting.

Unlike the expectation that one lives in order to give birth to and raise children, today's families increasingly recognize that child-rearing will occupy only a portion of the entire life experience of a married couple (regardless of whether one or more marriages result). While a baby may be a culmination and reflection of the love its parents feel for one another, the presence of a baby is nearly always an added stress on the new family unit.

One way to identify how babies represent potential and on-going stress for the young couple is to recognize how family interaction patterns are affected by the addition of a new member.

The couple relationship is easy to understand. Each member of the couple relates to the other in a spousal relationship. Add one child and two new relationships are added: one linking the mother to the child and one linking the father to the child. In addition, the couple is now not only husband and wife but mother and father, and in assuming these roles each may view the other in new ways that are not always supportive of a continued spousal role (Majewski, 1986). When one adds another child, the relationships become even more complex. Both the mother and the father have new relationships with the new baby. In addition, as that baby begins to grow and develop, a sibling relationship will be added to the family that did not previously exist. Thus, in a two-person household, two relationships exist. In a three-person household, three

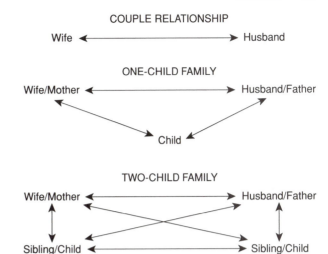

FIGURE 3–2. How family relationships change with the addition of a new member.

relationships exist; in a four-person household, while only four people live in the house, six relationships exist. (See Fig. 3–2.) With each additional person added to the family, more than one new relationship is also added, because each new person interacts with all other members of the family. It is not surprising to see how the addition of one new little person can represent a far different, potentially unstable, configuration than had existed before.

How families interact with health-care workers in a hospital or clinic setting often is related to the structure of the family in its own environment. If the husband/father makes all decisions relating to the family's role with the outside world, it may not be surprising that the woman, when asked when she will register at the hospital, looks to her husband and he answers! This may not reflect dependency on him so much as the couple's established way of organizing their life. However, if one were to ask the husband something that is the responsibility of the wife/mother, he would defer to her, for that is part of her role in their family.

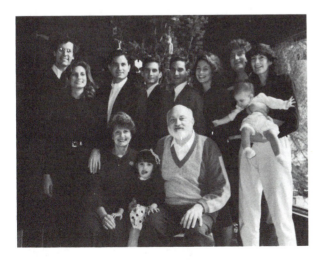

FIGURE 3–1. Three generations of family.

THE EFFECT OF A BABY ON A FAMILY

People have babies for many reasons. In addition to wanting to raise a family, other reasons for having a baby include:

- *Meeting a desire to nurture.* Sometimes it is the young wife who is the first to explicitly state her need to nurture; sometimes it is her husband. It is not that nurturing the spouse and the spousal relationship is not enough; rather, the spouse is seeking to nurture someone who is helpless, who "needs me more." Before agreeing to have a baby, some young couples will take on responsibility for a kitten or a puppy, which serves as a kind of surrogate baby. In some couples, the decision to become pregnant may be tinged with a good deal of concern about a pet's feelings of rejection after the baby comes. Will the pet be jealous and, if so, what can the couple do to help it accept the baby? Laughing at these concerns will be construed as insensitivity to real concerns relating to a set of established relationships between owner and pet.

- *Linking oneself to the future.* Especially for men, a child becomes their tangible link to immortality. In families practicing patrilineage, where a male heir is especially valued in order to pass on the family name, the desire for a son may be overwhelming. In an unpublished study that I conducted in the mid-1980s, nearly three-quarters of young adults in their early twenties preferred a firstborn male to a firstborn female child. For at least 40% of these young adults, the desire for a female child did not predominate until the fourth child.

- *Asserting adult status through parenthood.* In many cases, young teen-age parents often view the ability to impregnate or to become pregnant as an indication of their adulthood. The product of that ability is of lesser concern, particularly during the pregnancy, when a great deal of attention is often paid to the expectant mother.

- *Seeking acceptance by one's peer group.* Generally, if a couple has not had a baby by the time they have been married five years, often their peer group—unless they are the first to become parents—begins to question their motives for remaining child-free. According to one of the first studies of couples who did not have children (Nason & Poloma, 1976), the decision to remain child-free occurs in stages. At first there is a definite plan not to have children until a particular goal has been reached: they have purchased a home or found the "right" apartment; the husband or wife has reached a particular career level; they are earning a specific income; they

have been married at least three years. Less specific reasons follow; they simply aren't ready yet. Next they begin to realize the degree to which their lives will change if children are added, and they wonder if they really want to upset the apple cart. Finally, there's the realization that the biological clock has stopped ticking for them, and it's too late to have babies. If the peer group to which the couple belongs values a child-free lifestyle, and they wish to have children, they may find that a change of peer group is necessary if they want their decision to have children to be supported. Very often, "young marrieds" change from a mostly childfree cluster of recently married, two-career couples to a group of "young couples with children," as one after the other they begin raising children. The degree to which the peer group influences personal decision-making varies by group and by individual member. However, all individuals are swayed to one degree or another by the opinions and support offered by the group to which they look for social acceptance and support.

- *Fulfilling cultural expectations.* In some of her classic work, Margaret Mead describes cultures in which having a baby does not necessarily follow marriage; it may precede it. In many cases, in fact, having a baby as a result of casual sexual activity may enhance the young woman's "marriageability" (Mead, 1928). Certain cultural expectations, such as having a baby, are required if one is to establish a home apart from one's parents. In different subcultures in the United States, once one has been married a certain number of years, one is expected to have children.

- *Asserting one's sexuality.* In some cases, establishing oneself as an adult requires that one make clear one's adult sexual ability. Often this is linked to gaining adult status through parenthood, for one must become sexually active and prove one's sexual ability in order to impregnate or to become pregnant.

- *Seeking security for later life.* Although in most post-industrial societies, children are no longer viewed as a kind of social security for the aged, this view remains in other settings, especially among recent immigrant groups from developing countries where government old-age security programs are not part of their experience.

• *Serving as an outlet for personal creativity.* Having a baby is the ultimate expression of one's own creativity. The degree of satisfaction that new parents feel when others exclaim over the beauty of their baby and its "perfection" is verification of their success in producing such a winning creation.

• *Attaining or maintaining social status.* As with the appropriate timing of parenthood, having a baby may be a decision based on achieving or maintaining a certain social status. When couples say that they are having a baby because "it was time," or "it was the thing to do," they are reflecting pressure by their peer group; they also may be reflecting a sense that in order to reach a particular social plateau they must have children. In some businesses, young unmarried men were viewed as "less stable" than young married men. It was not lost on the social scientists studying these work settings that nearly all of the promotions were given to young married men "on the way up the corporate ladder." Among those same throngs of young professionals, young fathers received more promotions than young husbands without children. While appearing to have nothing to do with the business world the rationale behind such decision-making was that young husbands who become young fathers have responsibilities that are likely to make them want to get ahead, i.e., work harder for the company. When they do so, they are rewarded.

While the desire to nurture may seem, on the face of it, to be the most legitimate reason to have a baby, it is but one of many reasons that propel young couples and young single women into pregnancy and parenthood. The health-care worker who assists these clients needs to be aware that the reasons for the pregnancy may not be the same as she might have chosen herself. And, the value of the baby may differ from the value of the pregnancy in the mother's social scheme. All of these elements may play a role in whether the new mother chooses to breastfeed, and for how long.

FAMILY THEORIES

Numerous theories have been applied in an attempt to understand how families work, what influences them to work effectively, and how best to offer assis-

tance when they don't. One theory that seems particularly appropriate to health-care providers assisting young families was first proposed by Duvall (1971), who identifies eight separate stages in the family life cycle, each of which includes a variety of developmental tasks for its members. Duvall contends that failure to achieve certain developmental tasks will result in unhappiness among the family members and difficulty in meeting later developmental tasks. These stages and their tasks are elaborated in the extended outline on pp. 56–57.

Although Duvall was the first to propose a developmental-stages view of studying the family, she was not the only person to examine this theory. Aldous (1970) examined family interdependencies through the various positions and roles each member in the family assumes relative to the other. Using the notion of growth and change, she then traced the activities of different family members over time, dividing the family career into seven stages, as identified in the boxed listing on p. 57.

Note that Duvall and Aldous differ only in that the last two stages of Duvall's schema are collapsed into one by Aldous. Furthermore, while each new stage after Stage 1 and before the postparental or post-launching stages is keyed to the existence of children and where they are in the life cycle, no mention is made of later-born children and where their needs might place the family in its developmental progress. For example, a young mother marries in her late teens, perhaps precipitated by an unplanned pregnancy. In the Aldous scheme, she experiences a foreshortened establishment stage insofar as she begins marriage already pregnant! If her family is part of a research study 15 years later, however, where is her family placed? Perhaps she is now in a second marriage, the first having lasted but a short time. Now she is the mother of a teen-ager (Stage V for both Duvall and Aldous); however, she also is the mother of a six-month-old baby, who is the product of her second marriage. In many ways, she may be experiencing a very different life experience with this second baby than she did with her first. Not only is she older at the birth of her second child; her philosophy of childrearing, her evaluation of what is appropriate and inappropriate parenting behavior (including breastfeeding), as well as her spousal relationship, may be markedly different from her views and experiences in her first marriage. Should she also be viewed as occupying an earlier stage in the life cycle, one keyed to the age of her second baby?

DUVALL'S FAMILY DEVELOPMENTAL STAGES AND STAGE-SPECIFIC TASKS

Stage 1. Newly established couple (no children)

1. Establishing a home base in a place to call their own.
2. Establishing a mutually satisfactory system for getting and spending money.
3. Establishing mutually acceptable patterns of who does what and who is accountable to whom.
4. Establishing a continuity of mutually satisfactory sexual relationships.
5. Establishing systems of intellectual and emotional communication.
6. Establishing workable relationships with relatives.
7. Establishing ways of interacting with friends, associates, and community organizations.
8. Facing the possibility of children and planning for their arrival.
9. Establishing a workable philosophy of life as a couple.

Stage 2. Childbearing family (oldest child birth to 2-1/2 years)

1. Adapting housing arrangements for the life of the child (child-proofing).
2. Meeting the costs of family living.
3. Reworking patterns of responsibility and accountability.
4. Reestablishing mutually satisfying sexual relationships.
5. Refining intellectual and emotional communication systems for childbearing and childrearing.
6. Reestablishing working relationships with relatives.
7. Fitting into community life as a young family.
8. Planning for additional children in the family.
9. Reworking a suitable philosophy of life as a family.

Stage 3. Family with preschool children (oldest child 2–1/2 to 6 years)

1. Supplying adequate space, facilities, and equipment for the expanding family.
2. Meeting predictable and unexpected costs of family life with small children.
3. Sharing responsibilities within the expanded family and between members of the growing family.
4. Maintaining mutually satisfying sexual relationships and planning for future children.
5. Creating and maintaining effective communication systems within the family.
6. Cultivating the full potential of relationships with relatives within the extended family.
7. Tapping resources, serving needs, and enjoying contacts outside the family.
8. Facing dilemmas and reworking philosophies of life in the face of ever-changing challenges.

Stage 4. Family with school age children (oldest child 6 to 13 years)

1. Providing for children's activities and parents' privacy.
2. Staying financially solvent.
3. Cooperating to get things done.
4. Continuing to satisfy each other as marriage partners.
5. Effectively utilizing family communication systems.
6. Feeling close to relatives in the larger family.
7. Tying in with life outside the family.
8. Testing and retesting family philosophies of life.

Stage 5. Family with teen-agers (oldest child 13 to 20 years)

1. Providing facilities for widely differing needs.
2. Working out family money matters.
3. Sharing the tasks and responsibilities of family living.
4. Putting the marriage relationship into focus.
5. Keeping communications systems open.
6. Maintaining contact with the extended family.
7. Growing into the world as a family and as individuals.
8. Reworking and maintaining a philosophy of life.

Box continues

Stage 6. Family as launching center (oldest child gone to departure of youngest)

1. Rearranging physical facilities and resources.
2. Dealing with the costs that launching-center families encounter.
3. Reallocating responsibilities among grown and growing children.
4. Coming to terms as husband and wife.
5. Maintaining open systems of communication within the family and between the family and others.
6. Widening the family circle through release of young adult children and recruiting of new members by marriage.
7. Reconciling conflicting loyalties and philosophies of life.

Stage 7. Middle-aged family (empty nest to retirement)

1. Maintaining a pleasant and comfortable home.
2. Assuring security for the later years.
3. Carrying out household responsibilities.
4. Drawing closer together as a couple.

5. Maintaining contact with grown children's families.
6. Keeping in touch with brothers' and sisters' families and with aging parents.
7. Participating in community life beyond the family.
8. Reaffirming the values of life that have real meaning.

Stage 8. Aging family (retirement to death of spouse)

1. Finding a satisfying home for the later years.
2. Adjusting to retirement income.
3. Establishing comfortable household routines.
4. Nurturing each other as husband and wife.
5. Facing bereavement and widowhood.
6. Maintaining contact with children and grandchildren.
7. Caring for elderly relatives.
8. Keeping an interest in people outside the family.
9. Finding meaning in life.

From Duvall, EM: *Family Development,* 4th ed., Philadelphia, 1971, J. B. Lippincott Co.

One alternative view is to simply suggest that families expand and contract at different times. Thus, one might have the following set of stages:

- couple stage
- expansion stage
- stable stage
- contracting stage.

Such a scheme recognizes that most families begin as couples only. The expansion stage begins with the first pregnancy and continues until the birth of the last child. In some families, this stage may be very brief, the duration of one pregnancy only; in other families, it might last over two decades as new infants are continually added to the family. The stable stage involves that space of time when no members are being added or taken away. This stage is followed by the contracting stage, which begins when the oldest child leaves home to go to college, into the military, into a family of his or

---

ALDOUS'S DEVELOPMENTAL FAMILY STAGES

Stage 1. Establishment stage (engagement to marry up to first pregnancy)
Stage 2. Families with infants (begins with first pregnancy)
Stage 3. Families with preschool children
Stage 4. Families with school children
Stage 5. Families with adolescents
Stage 6. Families with young adults
Stage 7. Postparental families

her own creation or to some other setting where he no longer lives at home. This stage lasts until the only individuals remaining in the home are the original couple or their replacements in the family (if one or both of the original couple has remarried). However one views the family from a developmental perspective, the number of stages identified is not nearly so important as are the tasks expected of the family at different junctures in the life cycle.

The health-care worker assisting breastfeeding mothers is most likely to interact with members of families in Stage 2 or Stage 3 of Duvall's or Aldous's schema or the expansion phase of the family life cycle. It is important that they recognize the various tasks of these stages in order to identify how those tasks will influence decision-making and behavior related to infant feeding and other aspects of the early mother-child relationship.

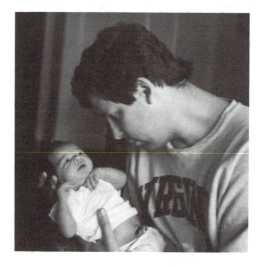

FIGURE 3–3.   A father attaches to his baby in much the same way as the mother.

FATHERS

ATTACHMENT TO THE BABY

Some investigators have emphasized the degree of similarity between mother-infant and father-infant behaviors in the attachment process in parents (Lamb, 1977). Classic among them is the work by Greenberg and Morris (1974), who observed that fathers present at the birth of the baby seemed to become more comfortable handling the baby sooner than those who were not present. Additionally, they described a sequence of touching that was remarkably similar to that engaged in by mothers. The fingertips are first used to make tentative contact with the extremities of the newborn; this is followed by a gradual movement of the hand until the entire palm is in contact with the baby's chest, face and/or head. Peterson, Mehl, and Leiderman (1979) also found that the father who participated at the birth by providing support to the mother was more likely to feel attached to his child than if he was not present at the birth. The authors recommend prenatal education and structuring of the birth environment to enhance the father's participation. Likewise, Bowen and Miller (1980) showed that presence of the father at delivery was important to paternal attachment behavior; those fathers who were present looked and talked to their infants more than fathers who did not attend the birth. A recent study found that fathers tend to progress from gazing to touching in the first fifteen minutes after birth and that enthusiastic reactions to the neonate were more likely when the father was not anxious about the mother's condition (Tomlinson, Ruthenberg & Carver, 1991). Jones (1981) reported that fathers who held their newborns within the first hour postpartum engaged in more nonverbal behavior with their infants one month later than those who did not hold the baby soon after birth. Additionally, they seemed less put off by infant irritability, often providing more care during such periods than was observed in other fathers. When fathers enter into caregiving roles from the first with their infants, they are more likely to feel that they are an important part of the baby's life (Fein, 1976; Lamb, 1976). Investigators who have examined the male parenting role have noted that the "emergent" role of the participative father has begun to be emphasized with greater frequency as an appropriate role in all social classes (Fein, 1978).

Recent examinations of the ways in which men evolve into fathers suggests that the role remains relatively invisible to others; it is a passive reflection of what is happening to the pregnant wife until after the baby's birth. When the baby begins to interact with the father directly, his role becomes more explicit—in his own mind as well as in the awarenesses of others (Jordan, 1990). In settings where men are heavily involved in child care, as when the father provides daily care of his children for many hours while the mother works away from home, or where the father assumes a "house-husband" role, boys and girls tend to grow up with more flexible views of what is "man's work" and "woman's work" (Robinson, 1979). The degree to which such flexibility is retained in the face of assumptions of stricter, more traditional sex-role behaviors as portrayed in children's literature, as well as the comments of others with whom the child interacts in school and elsewhere, remains to be seen. Levine (1977) notes that nurturing is a fundamentally human quality that need not be sex-specific. That it is viewed as "feminine" by many in more than one of the developed nations of the world must be seen as a cultural overlay rather than a reflection of inherent differences between males and females.

When the baby is born prematurely, the frequency of the father's visiting was found to be a predictor of later positive fathering behavior after the baby's discharge from the hospital (Levy-Shiff et al., 1990). These investigators found that when the fathers visited frequently, the baby's weight gain was more rapid, and the father's involvement with the baby at eight and 18 months after birth was more intensive, regardless of the mother's visiting patterns during the period when the baby was in the premature unit.

However, in one study of Australian fathers considered "highly participant" (Russell, 1982), it was found that fathers actually spent little time with their children. Kunst-Wilson and Cronenwett (1981) measured the amount of time fathers talked to their babies in the first three months and discovered that they did so less than three times per day, averaging only 37.5 seconds each time! Compared with the mothers, fathers spent very little time doing child-care tasks or in taking responsibility for them, nor were they simply "available" to their children in the same sense as the mothers. Ironically, these same fathers placed a high value on sharing in care-giving and reported deriving satisfaction from their interactions with their children.

BREASTFEEDING

The role of the father as a supporter of breastfeeding is frequently mentioned in the lay literature. Particularly when he has a "positive mind-set" relating to breastfeeding, it is thought that he can play an important role (Bishop & Bishop, 1978). However his negative feelings about breastfeeding also can have a major effect (Lerner, 1979). Although the "down" side of the father's role relative to breastfeeding is less recognized, Jordan (1986) and Jordan and Wall (1990) discuss the father's negative feelings. Breastfeeding is sometimes viewed as a means by which the mother denies him access to the baby by making exclusive the early infant feeding experience (Jordan, 1986).

Father identity is an expression of the nature of the marital relationship: the happier the marriage, the more positive the father's view of his parenting role (Soule, Standley & Copans, 1979). At the same time, the early days of fathering can be as stressful and disruptive to the father as mothering is to the mother; it is not at all unusual for a father to become disenchanted with his marriage after the first baby's birth (Wandersman, 1980). Jealousy of the mother's and infant's physical and emotional closeness, feelings of uselessness during breastfeeding, sexual frustration, and repulsion from the sight of full, dripping breasts are all realities for many fathers (Hangsleben, 1983). Some fathers feel ashamed of these emotions and tend not to talk about them; or they make joke about being jealous of the new baby.

The most comfortable place for fathers to express these socially unacceptable but very real feelings is with other new fathers, many of whom may harbor the same feelings. This is why childbirth education

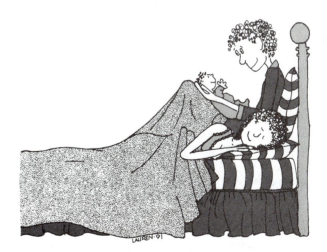

FIGURE 3–4. One of the many ways a dad helps with the care of his baby.

classes and La Leche League groups offer "fathers-only" classes where new fathers can openly share their feelings and perceptions about the realities of parenthood in an atmosphere of unconditional acceptance. The limitation of these get-togethers to new fathers is strictly enforced. Or experienced fathers can be invited to speak to parents at one session in a childbirth preparation series to talk about their needs and concerns. Fathers can help each other to realize that they are not alone in having ambivalent feelings about the closeness between their breastfeeding wives and babies and about giving up certain pleasures in exchange for new responsibilities. One reported:

> If I'd been more prepared that they would be this complete unit unto themselves, it would have been easier. For a while I felt left out, like I was around only to bring home the money and wasn't a part of it. I felt bad, then guilty about feeling bad. Before the baby came, my wife really spoiled me, you know, really adored and lavished attention on me. Then, whammo, she was pregnant three months after we were married and I wasn't getting that kind of treatment anymore. I resented it. Things really broke loose and we had a showdown; I finally had to open up and let her know how I really felt. After that, when it was all in the open, things got better. With the next baby, I don't think I'll go through those feelings again (Riordan, 1983, p. 101).

Support groups for new fathers validate a commitment to recognize the needs of new fathers—to help them develop coping strategies for optimal parenting of their breastfed baby. These father groups tend to attract fathers who are having more difficulty or who are more open in admitting to stress in adjusting. These are actions that can potentially strengthen family relationships in years ahead (Taubenheim & Silbernagel, 1988).

Implicit in the notion that breastfeeding prevents father-child closeness is acceptance of the assumption that the most (perhaps the *only*) significant way in which a father can interact with his child is by feeding him. Such an assumption is portrayed in advertisements of artificial feeding bottles that include statements like, "This is as close as some parents will ever get to breastfeeding." While detractors of the argument would suggest that such a view is inherently limiting, and therefore demeaning to the father, it is well to consider the thinking that underlies this view:

- feeding is something that should be shared if one is to be an "involved" parent
- feeding is a positive experience for the baby and the person feeding him
- breastfeeding is something only mothers can do; therefore, fathers should bottle-feed in order to have an opportunity to feed the baby, too
- without feeding the baby, the father cannot interact with the child.

The health-care worker first must recognize these concepts before she can encourage the father to consider the many other ways in which he can interact with the baby, particularly during the very early period when artificial feeding may pose a serious risk of breastfeeding failure. These options include:

- *Burping the baby after a feeding:* the necessity of burping is less an issue than the opportunity to frequently hold the baby when he is likely to be relaxed and somnolent; if a burp is obtained, the father also gains a sense of having accomplished something tangible that can be translated to mean "I am a good father"
- *Changing the baby's wet diapers:* a frequent occurrence
- *Changing the baby's soiled diapers:* a frequent occurrence, and one that is far less distasteful because the odor is less noxious than if the baby is artificially fed
- *Giving the baby a massage:* fathers who do so often find that they can put the baby to sleep with little effort; such activity often assists an overstimulated or colicky baby to relax sufficiently to fall asleep
- *Bathing the baby:* usually most happily accomplished after the baby begins to enjoy his bath
- *Rocking the baby:* while the mother is engaged in other activities
- *Singing or reading to the baby:* this activity can begin as soon after birth as the father wishes; often repeating the same songs which were played during the pregnancy will result in clear signals of recognition by the baby that are seen by the parents as an indication of their child's intelligence and receptivity to their ministrations

- *Playing with the baby:* although last in this list, it is usually the first thing that mothers will say fathers do best; often babies quickly identify fathers as "playthings" and mothers as "care-givers" because fathers spend proportionately more time tickling or playing with an infant and far less time with care-giving activity, such as changing, feeding, and cleansing; such expectations are most likely to occur in families where clearly different sex-role patterns are exhibited by mothers and fathers.

LEVELS OF FAMILY FUNCTIONING

In order to provide the most appropriate assistance for the young family, health-care workers must be able to determine how well the family is functioning. In so doing, help can be planned and provided in such a way that the family moves from a less effective to a more effective level of self-care. Tapia (1986) has identified different levels of functioning and the behaviors characteristic of each level. (See boxed outline below.)

While each family characterized by Tapia is labeled as if the group developed from infancy through adulthood, it is important to note that these families are not defined according to the age of the parent, but rather according to the maturity of their social action. A family in which the parents are adolescents, for example, may function at any one of the five levels identified by Tapia. In short, just as a family contains members of different ages and capabilities, each family functions at different levels. During stressful periods, a family that had functioned reasonably well previously may be so affected by stress

---

FOUR LEVELS OF FAMILY FUNCTIONING

Level 1: Infancy or Chaotic Family Functioning

1. Members live from day to day without an orientation to the future.
2. There is demonstrated distrust of outsiders and an inability to use community resources and services.
3. Members are hostile or show resistance to offers of help.
4. Parents are weak, showing immaturity and confusion in their roles within the family.
5. Family functions at a survival level.

Level 2: Childhood Family Functioning

1. Members have greater ability to trust, and thus have hope for a better way of life.
2. Parents, despite some confusion and role distortion, are willing to work together to benefit the family unit.
3. Members are able to meet basic survival needs.
4. Members are unable to change or to accept change.

Level 3: Adolescent Family Functioning

1. Family has more than the usual number of conflicts and problems.
2. Members are able to meet survival and physical needs, but emotional conflicts cause confusion for the children and others.
3. One parent is more adult in functioning than the other.
4. Parents are able to look for some solutions to problem; they are more future oriented.

Level 4: Adult Family Functioning

1. Families are normal, stable, healthy, happy and have fewer than the usual number of conflicts or problems.
2. Members are able to handle most problems as they arise.
3. Members are able to meet their physical and emotional needs.
4. Family may have problems related to growth and developmental tasks.
5. Members are willing and able to seek outside assistance to resolve problems.

From Tapia, JA: Fractionalization of the family unit. In Schuster, CS, and Asburn, SS, eds., *The process of human development.* Boston, 1986, Little, Brown & Co.

factors that its ability to function is seriously impaired; this results in its characterization as an adolescent rather than an adult family. In cases of extreme stress, some previously functioning families become chaotic, thereby failing to meet any of its members' needs and threatening its own ability to survive as a unit.

Tapia suggests that families at different levels of functioning require different levels of assistance from the health-care worker. A family in its *infancy*, whose organization is chaotic, will need to view the health-care provider as a partner as it moves through the health-care system. In some cases, this may mean that the nurse accompanies the pregnant mother through the corridors of a large hospital much like a mother who leads one of her offspring, in order to make sure that she finds her way through what must surely seem like an impenetrable maze. In other cases, it may mean sitting through her labor and assisting her each time she breastfeeds her newborn throughout her hospital stay. This role is like that of an older sibling who has been through the experience before and whose calmness and reassurance that all is well is highly valued. Honest answers to questions are most helpful as the new family attempts to understand their experience.

A family in its *childhood* needs somewhat less assistance than one in its infancy, but it is not yet ready for a helper simply to assist them. Instead, active teaching works better. If the baby needs to be diapered, the health-care provider may need to do this more than once while the new parents observe; she will then ask one of them to do so. When the new parent does so, assistance at each juncture in the procedure may be necessary.

The family that is moving through its own *adolescence* needs a helper who points out the family members' own abilities to cope. In this case, the health-care worker serves as an adult helper to the family and allows the new parents to take care of their own baby with freedom to seek help at their own pace. Something as simple as offering to teach the parents how to diaper their baby for the first time works well with this family.

The family that is functioning at an *adult* level views the health-care providers with whom they have contact as experts and "outside partners." These family members usually are adept at seeking information and are eager to engage in new activities on their own. They eagerly seek new information even as they are practicing new skills. The new breastfeeding mother who is operating at the adult level is ready to take in additional information related to what she is doing. For example, if she remarks that she feels sleepy shortly after she puts the baby to her breast, an explanation that this is one of the normal effects of the milk let-down response (Mulford, 1990) can help her to understand that she is not being worn out from breastfeeding, but is responding normally.

A *mature* family that is functioning at an optimal level only uses the health-care worker sporadically for assistance with breastfeeding. In such a setting, when questions arise, the family member will seek out the information; however, the mother will not lean on the nurse or the lactation consultant and expect her to make the decisions. Knowing where the family falls in this continuum of functioning assists the provider in determining how little or how much assistance the family needs. In situations where the needs of the family exceed the ability, time available, or skill level of the care provider, referral to other professionals may be the most appropriate action.

THE TEEN-AGE MOTHER

It is hard to identify a situation that is fraught with more difficulties than when a child has a child. The younger the mother when her first baby is born, the more likely she is to encounter problems that will impede her ability to care for herself or her baby. Wherever young women are expected to complete a high school education before they embark on adult roles, such as marriage and raising children, the teen-age mother is a visible reminder that society has failed to protect her from too early parenthood and that she has failed her society, which expects that parenthood comes after marriage and at least minimal schooling. Often for such young women schooling is interrupted (Mott & Maxwell, 1981) never to be resumed, while marriage—if it occurs—comes after, rather than before, the birth of her child. Subsequent pregnancies are likely to occur within two years of the first birth (Polit & Kahn, 1986).

When breastfeeding is brought into this picture, many care givers assume that the young mother is neither interested nor ready to "give" to another in this intimate way (Stotland & Peterson, 1985). As a result, the pregnant teen may not even be encouraged to plan how she will feed her baby. What her older sister or friends have done is what she assumes she will do. Too often, what they have done is to bottle-feed.

Yoos (1985) explored the infant feeding choices of 50 teen-age mothers. She found striking differences between those who chose bottle-feeding and those who chose breastfeeding. The bottle-feeders were more likely to live in an extended family setting (60%) rather than a nuclear family with two adults of the opposite sex, as did the breastfeeders (41%). Even more striking were the reasons given for their infant feeding choice. The bottle-feeders were much more likely to give reasons that the author described as "self-oriented" (79%), whereas the breastfeeding teens were much more likely to mention infant-oriented reasons (88%). Only among the bottle-feeders was breastfeeding equated with sex and therefore found to be inappropriate between mother and infant. Yoos suggests that adolescence is a period when self-centeredness is normal, making it difficult for the young woman to set aside concerns about herself in order to care for the needs of someone else. When parenthood impinges on adolescence, breastfeeding is a less likely choice because the mother has difficulty setting aside her own needs for her baby's.

The attitudes of teen-age boys and girls are telling, for they reflect the attitudes of their elders as well as their peers. Pascoe and Berger (1985) compared high school girls' attitudes about breastfeeding in the United States and Israel and found that Israeli girls were more likely to plan to breastfeed when they had children (68% vs. 42%) than were their counterparts in the United States. Most of the Israeli girls were themselves breastfed, compared with only one-third of the U.S. teens. Neither group, however, had discussed breastfeeding with their teen-age friends; in both groups, breastfeeding was considered less expensive than bottle-feeding, but it also was considered old-fashioned and thus not popular. These attitudes combined with the lack of understanding of the physiology of lactation may help to explain why teen-age girls need information about breastfeeding before they can be expected to make an informed choice, even in the face of another family member's experience with breastfeeding.

Another study of U.S. high school students' atti-

tudes about breastfeeding revealed that the greater their exposure to breastfeeding in the family or among friends, the more positive were their attitudes and the more knowledgeable they were about lactation. The age of the students at the time of the survey also influenced how knowledgeable they were; students in grades 11 and 12 were more likely than those in grades 9 and 10 to have read or heard about breastfeeding in a course. The authors concluded that early introduction of breastfeeding in a classroom setting can stimulate later discussion and increase the knowledge base from which later decisions will be made (Cusson, 1985).

An Australian study (Wolinski, 1989) looked at teens' attitudes about breastfeeding. Most of these students had seen a close relative or friend breastfeed, knew that they themselves had been breastfed and had seen a sibling at the breast (63–80%). Nevertheless, 31% of the students felt that women did not breastfeed because it was inconvenient to do so, because they had no milk (25%), because it was painful (24%) or embarrassing (18%). Almost all of the students, male and female, agreed that any infant, including their own future infants, should be breastfed at home alone, with only family or females present. More than 50% felt that it was inappropriate to breastfeed outside the home or when males were present. This suggests that even in a society in which a majority of infants are breastfed, privacy and modesty are concerns of teen-age girls and boys.

Another study of teens in Liverpool, U.K., revealed that while 75% of the students thought breastfeeding was healthier than bottle-feeding, 8% thought it was "rude" (Gregg, 1989). Both boys and girls felt that breastfeeding should be done in private, either alone or with just the baby's father or a female family member present. Almost none of these teens felt that breastfeeding should occur outside the mother's home. As with the Australian sample, students who had been breastfed themselves or who had seen a baby breastfed were more likely to say that they intended for their child to be breastfed. The investigator encouraged discussing breastfeeding as soon as possible to reduce the likelihood that it would be viewed as an embarrassing behavior and to "modify society's acceptance of the breast as a purely sexual organ," another factor very likely to have influenced the student's preference that breastfeeding occur only in the mother's home.

Teen mothers, when asked to identify their own needs following the birth of their baby, identified the infant's medical needs first, followed by daily physical care of the infant, psychosocial needs of mothers and babies, and lastly, the mother's own physical care (Howard & Sater, 1985). Mothers rated information about how to breastfeed and care for the breasts as important or very important. This high level of interest in meeting their baby's needs suggests that teen mothers are likely to be motivated to follow advice when it is offered.

In my experience working with teen mothers who just delivered a baby, I found that their questions were no different from older, more experienced women. All new mothers are concerned about how to help a baby grasp the breast, avoid sore nipples, and have sufficient milk. On the other hand, the kind of assistance offered to teens depends on their life situation. The teen mother living alone may need more assistance and referral to a breastfeeding support group in her local community. The teen mother living with her own mother—who may be caring for the baby while the teen is in school—may need to know about resources to draw on for additional information and support about breastfeeding. The teen mother living with the baby's father or another adult male needs to know how to balance her baby's needs and other people's plans for her. For example, if her friends want her to go to a school dance, she needs help recognizing that the baby is not a doll who can be propped on a shelf until the mother decides she wishes to play with it again. A happy breastfeeding experience—of whatever duration—helps the young mother to progress toward adulthood with a stronger and more positive sense of self and what she wants for her children in the future.

THE LOW-INCOME FAMILY

Families in an affluent society are expected to reflect the wealth of that society. When families in such a society are not affluent, they are confronted daily with reminders that they have failed to live up to the expectations of others. This is especially true in developed countries with a strong work ethic in which any degree of under- or unemployment is interpreted as personal failure and/or refusal to accept a basic tenet of that society. Comedians who have remarked that they didn't know they were poor until after they grew up and other people told them so

point out that children may not always know they are poor if the family does not act as if they are. Too often, however, particularly in urban neighborhoods located near affluent areas, the comparison of the "have's" and the "have not's" is overt and neverending. The family caught in such a situation often is well aware of their circumstances. In such families, daily concerns revolve around survival issues that rarely are of concern to their more affluent counterparts. Will I have enough money at the end of the day to buy some food? Will I be able to make that meatloaf stretch to the end of the week? How can I buy my kid some shoes so he can go to school? How can I afford the baby food the doctor says I should be feeding her? These and similar questions assail the parent attempting to preserve her or his family in a society in which it is expected that all parents will provide not only what is "best," but also that which is "more than or better than" what they experienced as children. Too often, that is an unattainable goal.

As with teen-age mothers, low-income mothers in the United States rarely choose to breastfeed. Poor women whose babies most need the benefits of human milk, which is far less costly to produce and far safer to use than artificial baby milks, are least likely to breastfeed.

OBSTACLES TO BREASTFEEDING AMONG LOW-INCOME FAMILIES

Background variables can predict whether a low-income woman will breastfeed. Grossman et al. (1989) found that if the woman were married, if she had at least a high-school education, if she began prenatal care in the first trimester, and if she were white or Hispanic, she was more likely to breastfeed than if she had less than a high-school education, if she began prenatal care in the second or third trimester, and if she were black. Additionally, the mother's expressed infant feeding choice during her pregnancy is likely to predict what she does after the baby's birth (Gabriel, Gabriel & Lawrence, 1986). Breastfeeding women were much more likely to do so if they declared their intention to breastfeed early in the pregnancy. Women who initially said they would bottle-feed were very likely to carry this through; women who were undecided about how to feed the baby were very likely to bottle-feed.

Ethnicity. Examining different beliefs that structure behaviors is one way to identify how best to work with women whose ethnicity differs from that of the helping professional (Fernandez & Guthrie, 1984). Skeel and Good (1988) point out that each culture or ethnic group has potentially harmful, harmless and helpful beliefs and practices that can influence breastfeeding initiation and duration. By attempting to work within the cultural constraints of the group to which the mother belongs, the lactation consultant can serve her client more completely and is more likely to be viewed as a helper rather than as one who "does not understand us." Rassin et al. (1984) have studied low-income women in three different ethnic groups. They suggest that the effect of ethnicity may be underestimated when attempting to identify background variables that influence breastfeeding initiation and/or duration rates. Trying to remove the effect of poverty from ethnicity is extremely difficult in a developed country where the likelihood of being poor and being black, for example, are both extremely high.

Lack of Support.   Barron et al. (1988) found that the availability of an outside source of support in the first six weeks postpartum nearly doubled the mean breastfeeding duration in a group of low-income women. In addition, the more breastfeeding friends the mother had, the longer was she likely to breastfeed (p<.05); furthermore, breastfeeding duration was positively related to her involvement in the WIC program of nutritional assistance. The involvement of WIC in promoting breastfeeding among their low-income clients has been discussed with increasing frequency since funds within the WIC allotment have been specifically earmarked for breastfeeding promotion. Kramer's recent discussion (1991) highlights the need for continuing work, particularly in the area of prenatal information and early postpartum support and assistance. He notes that too many WIC programs continue to accept and distribute materials from the infant formula companies. Training WIC personnel in how to assist breastfeeding women also may render this supplemental food program more effective in increasing the breastfeeding rate among the nation's low-income families.

Support from family members also makes a difference, according to Scrimshaw et al. (1987). In her study of more than 500 Mexican-American women in the Los Angeles area, she found that the influence of the mother's own mother, her husband, and other relatives or friends was much more important than that of doctors or nurses with whom they came in contact. In addition, rooming-in opportunities also influenced breastfeeding behavior, presumably through an increase in the number of hours per day in which mother and baby were housed together.

Confirmatory responses to the decision to breastfeed by important members of the mother's support system (Rassin, Richardson & Baranowski, 1986) may help to explain why ethnicity seems to exert such a strong influence on infant feeding choice. Additionally, the assumption by health workers that only certain women (e.g., white, middle-class, well-educated, first-time mothers) are interested in breastfeeding effectively shuts the door on future opportunities to reach women for whom breastfeeding could be a deliberate choice—if only they know it is an option for them (Manstead, Plevin & Smart, 1984).

Lack of Information.   Sometimes the reasons for not breastfeeding are related to lack of information. Kistin et al. (1990) studied low-income black women in the United States and found that prenatal education sessions which included far-ranging discussions about breastfeeding not only increased the likelihood that the women would choose to breastfeed, but also the likelihood that they would act on their choice when the baby was born, as well as for the duration of breastfeeding. The investigators concluded that "greater educational efforts in institutions and offices serving black, low-income, urban women might yield significant changes in breastfeeding rates" (Kistin et al., 1990). In Hill's study (1988), attendance at classes designed to inform low-income mothers about breastfeeding significantly increased the likelihood of their choosing breastfeeding *if* the women attended two or more classes. Among those who attended only one class, bottle-feeding was chosen *more* often than by those who did not attend any classes. This suggests that recognizing the benefits of breastfeeding and acknowledging a desire to breastfeed may come after being informed of the differences between artificial feeding and human milk feeding. Therefore, simply adding a session on infant feeding to childbirth preparation classes, or offering a one-time-only class on breastfeeding may not be sufficient to break down the barriers protecting the passive bottle-feeding choice (what everyone does)so that breastfeeding (I think I'll try that) can be considered and then implemented.

Hospital Practices.   Sometimes, the reasons for not breastfeeding are related to hospital factors. In Brazil, if the baby of a low-income mother received the breast first, that child was more likely to continue to breastfeed past six months. However, if something other than the breast was offered in the hospital, the mother was less likely to nurse as long. Often, the first feed in the hospital was followed later by supplementary water feedings, each of which reduced the duration of breastfeeding. It takes but a small leap of the imagination to understand why so many of the women who breastfed for short periods thought they had inadequate milk before their babies were four months old (Martines, Ashworth & Kirkwood, 1989).

Romero-Gwynn (1989) found that the only variable that predicted shortened duration of breastfeeding among her sample of Cambodian and Laotian immigrants was the use of formula giveaways in the hospital where the birth occurred. These women viewed such products as high-status items because of their extreme high cost and lack of availability in their home country. Their explanation of "insufficient milk" may simply have been a convenient hook, easily accepted without question by others, on which to hang their decision not to breastfeed, even though they had successfully breastfed older children prior to their immigration to the United States.

Hospital-based formula marketing.   The use of formula in the hospital also has been found to reduce the duration of breastfeeding (Samuels, Margen & Schoen, 1985). In this study, mothers in three different ethnic groups received care from a health maintenance organization (HMO). Formula use at that time was the single largest avoidable impediment and appeared to have both a direct effect on very early weaning in the first four weeks, as well as an increasingly cumulative effect through the first two months postpartum. Scrimshaw et al. (1987; see also Snell et al., 1992) found that the use of hospital formula negatively affected the duration of breastfeeding among Hispanic women in Los Angeles. Only one ounce of formula per day contributed to early weaning, even in the face of long duration of

breastfeeding in which the baby spent most of his time with the mother and she received both verbal and direct assistance to begin breastfeeding soon after birth. This finding may highlight the "valued" nature of formula feeding, particularly when it is introduced by authority figures in a hospital where the mother feels that she must emulate nurses' practices and follow doctors' recommendations.

Timing of solid food introduction.   In addition to formula use, the timing of solid foods also influences the duration of breastfeeding. In their low-income population, Hawkins, Nichols, and Tanner (1987) reported that the introduction of solid foods explained 32% of the variance in the duration of breastfeeding. Of interest in their sample were the additional findings that among short-term breastfeeders (four weeks or less) and moderate breastfeeders (5–24 weeks), inadequate milk supply or the baby's poor weight gain explained 50% and 37%, respectively, of the reasons for weaning the baby. Under problems experienced by these two groups, all of the short-term breastfeeders and nearly one-half of the moderate breastfeeders claimed inadequate milk supply to be a problem. What we do not know is how the timing of the introduction of solids related to an awareness of this problem and/or the decision to terminate breastfeeding. Might the problem have been secondary to early solid feedings and subsequent reduced breastfeeding frequency, or might the solids have been introduced in an effort to counter an inadequate milk supply that was reflected in poor infant weight gain?

Brogan and Fox (1984) also found that the introduction of solid foods influenced the duration of breastfeeding. In their comparison of low-income and middle-income women in one midwestern state, they found that weaning from the breast occurred earlier and that solid foods were introduced sooner in the low-income families than in the middle-income families. In a group of WIC recipients in New York City, similar results were obtained. Of additional interest from this study was the finding that receipt of information about breastfeeding from a physician or a nutritionist significantly delayed the time when solid foods were introduced. This suggests once again that information can be an important parameter for guiding infant feeding patterns (Bevan et al., 1984).

Comparison of high- and low-income breastfeeding and bottle-feeding women are closer when one compares them by feeding choice rather than by income status. Grossman et al. (1990a) found that breastfeeding women, whatever their income, were more like one another than the low-income breastfeeding women were to their bottle-feeding counterparts—particularly with regard to such variables as where they obtained support for their infant feeding choice, when they began prenatal care, when they decided to breastfeed, whether they had attempted to breastfeed a previous infant, and whether they viewed their previous breastfeeding experience as successful. This finding suggests that the same concerns are likely to affect all women, regardless of income; therefore, it is inappropriate to assume, simply on the basis of presumed maternal finances or social status, that a mother will not be interested in learning about, and later practicing, breastfeeding.

Sullivan and Jones (1986) present an innovation-decision process model to explain why some low-income women choose to breastfeed and why others do not. In this model, *knowledge* is an important first step to the innovative behavior. Before breastfeeding is likely to be chosen, the mother needs information on which to base her decision. Such knowledge is followed by *persuasion,* often in the form of discussions, video materials about breastfeeding that show other women doing so, and the experiences of other women, including friends and family members. *Making the decision* to breastfeed follows persuasion, and *implementation of the decision* occurs after the baby's birth. Postdelivery support of her decision to breastfeed leads to *confirmation* that hers was the right decision for her. When confirmation does not occur, or other factors interfere with her opportunity to have her decision confirmed, the mother is likely to stop nursing. In their study sample, maternal or infant complications that interfered with the opportunity to put breastfeeding into practice soon after delivery occurred in the confirmation process and contributed to a majority of those who later chose to bottle-feed. While this model was developed to explain why some low-income black women adopt breastfeeding, it could be applied to all women, regardless of income level; additional testing is needed to ascertain whether the model will hold up across income levels. (See following five-step checklist.)

INNOVATION DECISION-MAKING PROCESS

Step 1   Knowledge
Step 2   Persuasion
Step 3   Making the Decision
Step 4   Implementing the Decision
Step 5   Confirming the Decision

Confirming a mother's choice is another way of providing her with positive feedback. Low-income Hispanic women who were part of a WIC program responded positively to a hospital visit, phone call, letter, and/or group support at two weeks postpartum: they breastfed longer when compared with a group who received no such confirmation of breastfeeding (Saunders & Carroll, 1988). Differences in breastfeeding rates were most striking at four weeks postpartum: 95% of the women who had all three interventions were still breastfeeding, compared with 80% of those who received some but not all of the interventions, and 70% of those who received none. The decrement in weaning was slower in the group receiving all interventions, while the group receiving some or none of the interventions weaned at a faster rate. By 16 weeks, 67% of the total intervention group were still breastfeeding compared with 50% of the mothers in either of the other groups. The authors concluded that early and repeated postpartum breastfeeding support can be effective in increasing the duration of breastfeeding. The importance of repeated contact may help to explain why other studies involving only one contact—in the hospital (Lynch et al., 1986) or after the mother and baby go home (Grossman et al., 1990b)—have not shown similar positive results.

SOCIAL SUPPORT SYSTEMS

The role of supportive significant others cannot be underemphasized. Freedom of choice regarding infant feeding decisions is always couched within the social context in which it occurs. Thus, in a family in which extended breastfeeding is viewed as aberrant behavior, it is unlikely that the mother will choose to continue breastfeeding longer than when she receives a preponderance of positive, or at least neutral, reactions from her significant others. In another family in which breastfeeding is viewed as just another activity of two- or three-year-olds, extended breastfeeding is far more likely to occur. Insofar as the mother and her baby interact with significant others, their acceptance of such behavior must be taken into account when assessing how best to assist her. Woollett (1987) rightly notes that most women choose *to* breastfeed or *not to* breastfeed, rather than to bottle-feed, and that support systems, real or perceived, influence those choices.

Social support also influences the timing of weaning the baby from the breast. Usually pressure to wean, from family members and others, is more likely as the baby approaches or exceeds his twelfth month (Rogers, Morris & Taper, 1987). Morse and Harrison (1987) suggest that support moves gradually from active support for breastfeeding, often manifested in the first few months of the baby's life, to toleration of breastfeeding, to ignoring breastfeeding (sometimes interpreted as passive support for breastfeeding insofar as no negative statements are heard or negative action is taken), to active encouragement for weaning. This last stage usually is manifested sometime after the baby's sixth month and may grow markedly stronger after the baby's twelfth month in the developed world, when others view the baby as "too old" to breastfeed. Among Hong Kong families, bottle-feeders received support from their physicians, failed breastfeeders received no support for breastfeeding and were influenced by advertisements to use formula, and breastfeeders reported receiving a preponderance of support for breastfeeding. In addition, the successful breastfeeders were more aware of the risks of bottle-feeding than were the other groups (Hung, Ling & Ong, 1985).

Social support is especially important in the time period immediately following any life stress. One such stress, insofar as it necessitates changes in relationships and life patterns, is childbirth. Another is breastfeeding, particularly if the mother has not done so with an older child, or if she is the first in her family and/or group of friends to do so. Very often, mothers and others assume that the mode of feeding is the cause of other infant behaviors (Forsyth, Leventhal & McCarthy, 1985). If they receive advice that is inappropriate or that is based on faulty or incorrect assumptions (Anlar, Anlary & Tonyali, 1988;

Auerbach, 1990a), subsequent breastfeeding difficulty and even unnecessary weaning is more likely. Adaptation to change and the ability to cope with crises, small or large, is facilitated when support is offered by others (Cobb, 1976). Hart, Bax, and Jenkins (1980) found that home visits by a health visitor during the establishment of lactation improved the likelihood that the mother had a positive breastfeeding experience. In a group of working-class, first-time mothers, breastfeeding was more likely to occur— and to remain the only feeding method for the baby's first three months—when the mothers received support and information before, during, and after the baby's birth (Jenner, 1988). However, in a group of disadvantaged American mothers, McLorg and Bryant (1989) found that the advice of health-care workers was far less likely to be followed than was that of grandmothers, many of whom lived in the same house with the new mother. They recommended that health-care workers recognize the grandmother as a key informant and network person and involve her in health care and advice-giving.

It is unfortunate when health-care workers are not viewed as support resources. In one article, Auerbach (1979) reiterates how nurses in five different but related roles can assist the breastfeeding mother, providing her both information and specific assistance at a variety of points in her childbearing and childrearing career. Such assistance can enable the mother to feel that she is not "going it alone," but rather has a wealth of assistance on which she can call should the need arise.

The racial or ethnic group with which the mother identifies influences whom she seeks out for advice and assistance relating to childbearing and breastfeeding. Baranowski et al. (1983) found that those who are supportive of breastfeeding varies by ethnic group. For example, among their low-income Anglo-American sample, the male partner, the mother's own mother, the grandmother and the best friend all were supportive of breastfeeding. This pattern, with the exception of the best friend, was found among Mexican-Americans as well. However, among African-American respondents, less than half of these potential support individuals was found to be supportive of breastfeeding. Additionally, the percentage of individuals who were clearly not supportive was higher; this was particularly true of the best friend, who might have served as a role model for the mother if she were among the first in her group of friends to have a baby and to choose a method of infant feeding for the child. (See Table 3–1.)

In another study of WIC clients, Saunders and Carroll (1988) found that the more support the mother had for breastfeeding, the more likely she was to continue breastfeeding. They recommend that health-care workers make clear their support for breastfeeding and encourage other family members to support this choice as well. Pridham (1987) found that books, friends, and relatives were more likely to be cited as support resources than clinicians in the first three months of breastfeeding. Perhaps these mothers were looking to books as objective sources of information rather than advice, which they freely received from friends and relatives—often more frequently than through visits to the health-care worker.

I observed this following an emergency cesarean birth with a client who was a mental-health professional. Although breastfeeding proceeded uneventfully following the traumatic birth, it was several months later before the mother chose to talk about her fears for her own life and the life of her baby. This woman noted, with a good deal of bitterness, that—with one exception—her health-professional colleagues were least likely to provide support for her. Instead, she looked to her husband, other friends, and—in part—her parents (Albers, 1981). The lactation consultant served as her primary support for breastfeeding and, somewhat later, as an active listener regarding her continuing concerns relating to the emergency cesarean.

One factor that is important following early discharge from the hospital is the degree of support new mothers have at home. Lemmer (1987) found that women who chose early discharge also had more support at home than those who did not leave early. Since institutional economics rather than optimal health-care delivery governs the timing of many hospital discharges today, it is imperative that the health-care provider learn whether the new mother will have someone to whom she can turn at home. If she does not, steps need to be taken to provide follow-up support, or to arrange for home visitation by one of the many social-service organizations that provide such services. In addition, much of the teaching thought of as appropriate during the postpartum period may need to be shifted to a prenatal setting in order to free what little time is available for key planning issues at

TABLE 3–1 RACE/ETHNIC GROUP AND WHOSE ADVICE THE MOTHER CONSIDERS IMPORTANT

Ethnic group	Influential Person Regarding Breastfeeding
Anglo-American	Male partner/baby's father
	Grandmother (maternal and paternal)
	Mother's best friend
Mexican-American	Male partner/baby's father
	Grandmother (maternal and paternal)
Black-American	Peers
	Maternal grandmother

From Baranowski, T, et al.: Social support, social influence, ethnicity and the breastfeeding decision, *Soc Sci Med* 17:1599–1611, 1983; Cronenwett, LR, and Reinhardt, R: Support and breastfeeding: a review, *Birth* 14:199–203, 1987.

discharge. (See Chapter 9 for additional discussion of teaching elements to be brought up at discharge.)

How men support women varies. It has been found that reversion to traditional sex-roles is more likely shortly after the birth of a baby, when the baby's and mother's individual and related physical needs may require that she depend more on her husband than she has previously (Pleck, 1977). How the new family restructures its life to take into account previous patterns of behavior and newly recognized needs, some of which may be short-term and some of which may be long-term, will determine how readily the family—as a unit—continues to work.

BREASTFEEDING PROMOTION

Breastfeeding promotion can take several forms. For some people, it means the statements of support for breastfeeding by leaders in the health-care community: the American Academy of Pediatrics (Committee on Nutrition, 1980; AAP, 1982; Task Force Report, 1982); American Dietetic Association (ADA, 1986); Canadian Dietetic Association (CDA, 1989); International Pediatric Association (IPA, 1976); United States Public Health Service (Arango, 1984); and the International Lactation Consultant Association (ILCA, 1991). Words are cheap: only actions count. Breastfeeding promotion can be viewed as one leg of a three-legged stool; without the other two legs—support and protection—promotion cannot succeed (Auerbach, 1990b). The implications of this analogy are clear: breastfeeding promotion is a far more complex undertaking than simply putting up posters, or wearing buttons that identify the wearer as supporting breastfeeding, or eliminating advertising copy for artificial baby milks.

Advocacy requires knowledge of the goals of one's client(s) for whom one provides active support. Being an advocate, then, requires that the care-giving professional be willing to stick her neck out. Assuming the posture of an ostrich with its head in the sand to avoid the challenges that are going to be leveled at the advocate—particularly for behavior requiring change on the part of others—will not work. Being an advocate requires one to identify:

- the client for whom the advocacy is directed
- the purpose of the advocacy
- the resources of the advocate
- the persons in power who must be contacted and will be affected by the advocacy actions
- the receptivity of persons in power positions to the planned advocacy actions
- the actions that will need to be altered based on an evaluation of the advocacy action that is effected.

One important aspect of breastfeeding promotion is involving family and key community members, coupled with training and supervision of the primary health workers (Habicht, 1979). Chandler and Roush (1982), for example, have suggested that such individuals can serve as physician-extenders, reserving her or his time for crisis management rather than uneventful ongoing assistance. Clift (1989), noting how artificial formula is advertised over the radio in many developing countries, suggests that preventive health-behavior campaigns, of which breastfeeding promotion is an often overlooked example, can use the same media. If farm workers in China can be given messages extolling the appropriateness of family planning by electric megaphone from an all-terrain vehicle, why not a message about the importance of breastfeeding? One example of breastfeeding promotion that illustrates how the health-care worker incorporates her own skills and advocacy role with helping a mother reach her own personal breastfeeding goal is seen in Fig. 3–5.

The care provider should use a deliberative approach which requires direct interaction between herself and the mother and encourages two-way communication to assure that the information provided is not only understood but is relevant to the mother and her needs (Princeton, 1986). Such an approach is based on the assumption that the mother is able to identify what she needs and that she is an active player in the relationship between herself and the care provider. (See Table 3–2.) While phases 1 and 2 may occur in the hospital, they also may have to be dealt with if the mother is seen for the first time in her own home or at a community health center. Phase 3 is specific to a non-institutional setting and will, perhaps more than the previous phases, require recognition and acceptance of the legitimacy of cultural and social values and family concerns related to the baby as well.

Providing care that is meaningful to the mother and helpful to her as she cares for her baby must be a value of the health-care worker. If the worker sees high-tech care as the epitome of assistance but the mother is fearful of it, neither will be very happy with the other when the mother asks for, but does not necessarily receive, high-quality, low-tech care. Hanvey (1990) notes that unless the health-care worker in the community accepts as legitimate the notion that preventive care is as appropriate for her to provide as curative care, the most needed kind of maternal and newborn care will not be given.

While the WHO Code has stimulated some governments to design programs that promote breastfeeding (Koctürk & Zetterström, 1988; Rea & Berquó, 1990), the United States was the single developed country to vote against the WHO Code.

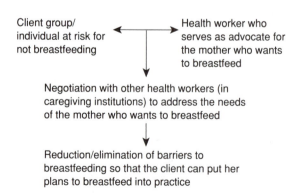

FIGURE 3–5.   The importance of assuming a partnership role with the client when promoting, supporting, and protecting the mother who wants to breastfeed.

**TABLE 3–2   THE DELIBERATIVE NURSING APPROACH TO ENSURE COMMUNICATION
AND UNDERSTANDING BY THE BREASTFEEDING MOTHER**

	Focus of Encounter	Elements of Encounter
Phase 1	The mother	Observation of nonverbal behavior
		Encourage mother to discuss her needs
Phase 2	The mother-infant dyad	Teach the art and science of breastfeeding, including specific skills relating to the mother's needs and the baby's behavior
Phase 3	The mother-infant dyad	Review issues that are still an issue for the mother, praise any evidence of her own and the baby's learning; relate her needs to community resources on which she can call

From Princeton, JC: Incorporating a deliberative nursing care approach with breastfeeding mothers, *Health Care Women Int* 7:277–93, 1986.

Members of the health-care community in the United States remain relatively uninformed about the existence of the WHO Code, or its significance for hospital routines and the activities of health workers relating to breastfeeding. Cadwallader and Olson (1986), as well as Burkhalter and Marin (1991), note that positive attitudes, knowledge and perceptions concerning breastfeeding are not enough. Training in how to assist the mother and on-going support of her efforts is also necessary if breastfeeding promotion is to result in a change in breastfeeding behavior. In a study by Cunningham and Segree (1990)—plus a report by Soysa, Fernando, and Abeywickrama (1988)—the health professionals who had contact with the women were found to impede rather than to positively reinforce their breastfeeding activities. The authors concluded that breastfeeding promotion requires that health-professional practices must be changed so that they support early initiation of breastfeeding. These practices should include opportunities for early breastfeeding, immediate postpartum contact, rooming-in, breastfeeding according to maternal or infant need, and eliminating formula feeding in the hospital—by the nurses as well as the mothers. Perhaps the most important change involves altering the attitudes of the health professionals who talk about breast being "best," but who foster maternal doubts by their actions, which impede breastfeeding practice.

A community-based breastfeeding promotion program included training of health-care providers, educational opportunities for the mothers, and mass-media efforts (Rodriguez-Garcia, Aumack & Ramos, 1990). The curriculum for health workers included recognition of the effect of cultural beliefs and myths on breastfeeding, as well as how to work with mothers for effective counseling. Continuing supervision and evaluation of the health workers' actions increased the likelihood that they offered consistent information. The active involvement of administrative personnel assured that the health workers felt their efforts were important and were supported by those in supervisory positions. The results were impressive: prior to the intervention program, breastfeeding initiation rates averaged 73%; after the intervention program was begun, nearly 90% of the women in the target communities began breastfeeding. Breastfeeding duration rates also increased.

Jelliffe (1975) is not the first, nor is she likely to be the last, to note that inclusion of instruction on the physiology of lactation, breast structure, *and* the practical application of that knowledge through instruction in breastfeeding management throughout the lactation course is essential if health-care workers are to be effective promoters of breastfeeding. The lack of such instruction in most medical and nursing schools makes it easy to understand why so few physicians and nurses feel adequately prepared to assist the mother who wants to breastfeed, or who is attempting to do so in spite of the impediments these same health providers (often unwittingly) have placed in her way.

We have already noted in this chapter that women in different ethnic groups, mothers of different ages, and women from different socioeconomic settings do not always respond in the same way to the opportunity to breastfeed. Koctürk and Zetterström (1989, p. 817) conclude that most promotional programs seem to be based on an assumption that mothers have the same needs regarding infant feeding, and that a single message such as "breast is best for baby" would be effective in motivating all mothers in the world, regardless of socioeconomical and cultural differences.

Getting beyond such assumptions is essential if specific groups of women are to be reached. One program which was successful used a structured approach that incorporated continuing training and motivation of the health-care workers who were in contact with the mothers. The authors found that motivation by the staff was not enough to change their behavior; specific implementation practices were needed (Palti et al., 1988).

Examples of breastfeeding promotion efforts in the United States include the activities of a prenatal clinic run by Santa Cruz County (California) Health Services Agency. It offered information about breastfeeding as part of the prenatal clinic beginning early in the third trimester, provided a group meeting once a month at the local WIC office, and made follow-up phone calls or home visits at 6, 12, and 24 weeks postpartum. This combination of activities increased breastfeeding rates substantially over the pre-project patterns (Skeel, McCarty & Pierce, 1986). In a migrant health clinic, mothers were given baby layettes if they attended a prenatal class session on breastfeeding. Of those Hispanic or black mothers who attended the class, 52% were breastfeeding at the time of hospital discharge compared with only 10% among those women of the same ethnic group who did not attend the prenatal class (Young & Kaufman, 1988).

In one study, both television commercials and print advertisements were run. The attitudes of teen-age girls toward breastfeeding were evaluated before and after the running of the print and video commercials. Only the television commercial was found to have influenced attitudes about breastfeeding. Sadly, knowledge scores about breastfeeding were unchanged by the commercial advertising campaign, suggesting that the visual medium may influence attitudes, but is unlikely to increase recall of specific facts about breastfeeding (Friel et al., 1989). Such social marketing has been found to have an impact on behavior, including infant feeding behavior.

The billboards that used to festoon the side of the roads in developing countries were there for a reason: since the adoption of the WHO Code, pictures of presumably healthy infants and formula tins are no longer seen. Instead, those advertisements have been replaced by those touting the wonders of infant foods, such as puréed solids and infant juices. The cost of such advertising would not be wasted if it were not effective (Clift, 1989).

Not all breastfeeding promotion programs work, however; Stokamer (1990) identified why one such program did not: administrators neither supervised nor supported the program, thereby reducing the likelihood that staff engaged in practices designed to assist, rather than interfere with, breastfeeding. Stokamer (1990) concludes: "If breastfeeding is important to the administration, it will be important to the staff." It is important to ask, however, how that "importance" is conveyed to the staff. Simply expecting them to "carry on," without providing them with the means to do so is not only self-defeating, but very likely to result in failure of the staff to share administration's sense that breastfeeding is important.

BREASTFEEDING PROGRAMS THAT WORK

Every cultural setting requires that a breastfeeding promotion program be geared to the specific needs of the target population, always keeping in mind those cultural elements that form the social boundaries. (See checklist of factors on p. 73.) In Honduras, one such breastfeeding promotion program that has met its objectives of increasing both breastfeeding initiation and duration is PROALMA. An evaluation and comparison of the first five years of the project has been reported recently (Popkin et al., 1991).

PROALMA is a multi-pronged program. It calls for changing:

- health professionals' knowledge about breastfeeding
- health professionals' attitudes about breastfeeding
- hospital policies—specifically, promoting breastfeeding within one hour after birth, rooming-in, and eliminating formula gift packs to mothers
- breastfeeding practices, including initiation and duration.

Between 1981 and 1987 rates of breastfeeding initiation increased from 80% to 93% in urban settings and from 95% to 98% in rural areas. Additionally, marked increases in the duration of breastfeeding occurred. In 1981, one-half of urban infants had been weaned by four months of age; in 1987, one-half of the urban infants were still breastfeeding at nine months of age. In 1981, one-half of the rural infants were still nursing at 15 months; in 1987, nearly two-thirds of the rural infants were still nursing at 15 months.

The attitudes and practices of health-care workers also changed. For example, in 1982, 35% of the physicians and 21% of the registered and auxiliary nurses recommended breastfeeding at birth; in 1986, 79% of the physicians and 88% of the nurses recommended breastfeeding at birth. Contraindications to breastfeeding were far less likely to be mentioned in 1986 than in 1982. For example, in 1982, 76% of the physicians and 81% of the nurses thought that a contagious disease was an appropriate reason for recommending against breastfeeding; in 1986, only 15% of the physicians and 20% of the nurses still believed this.

What made this program a success? Media coverage was part of the program when it began. Thus, the importance of training of health workers was given strong public support. In addition, the training of physicians and nurses enabled them to put into practice what they had learned: they were able to take a leadership role in the hospitals and clinics where they practiced. Such support assisted the mothers to get off to a good start with breastfeeding and helped

them to identify these healthworkers as obvious advocates for breastfeeding who could be called on to help them after they left the birth site.

Another program takes a different approach, and is based on the premise that how one's friendship network and support system feel about breastfeeding will strongly influence whether one chooses to breastfeed and how one does so (Bryant, 1982; McLorg & Bryant, 1989). Based on a series of focused interviews with low-income women in the southeastern United States, the "Best Start" program was developed. The program is aimed at reaching women who are least likely to breastfeed—low-income, often non-white, not always well educated. The training program includes four clearly identified objectives:

1. to identify the most common factors that deter low-income women from breastfeeding (this requires the trainee to know something about the women with whom she expects to be working)
2. to develop strategies for helping women overcome identified barriers to breastfeeding (these barriers may vary in different parts of the country and for different ethnic groups and subcultures)
3. to identify those factors that attract low-income women to breastfeeding (again, the trainee must know something about the population of women with whom she will be working)
4. to develop strategies for building on those appealing elements so that women will be encouraged to breastfeed (these attractive elements

---

CHECKLIST OF FACTORS CONTAINED IN AN OPTIMAL MULTI-FACETED BREASTFEEDING PROMOTION PROGRAM

- a clearly identified, measurable outcome variable
- media campaign that stimulates public support for the program
- ongoing active involvement of administrators and supervisory personnel at all levels of the health-care system
- training and on-going continuing education of health-care workers at all levels
- identification of specific hospital routines that are targeted for change

- specific techniques for informing women prenatally about breastfeeding
- specific techniques for assisting women immediately post-birth with breastfeeding
- specific techniques for assisting women throughout the lactation course with breastfeeding
- means of comparing the outcome variable prior to initiation of the program and at various time periods after implementation of the program

also will vary in different parts of the country and for different ethnic groups and subcultures).

Once these elements have been identified, information is provided that will assist the trainee to expand her or his understanding of appropriate and inappropriate ways of discussing breastfeeding. One typical example is the practice of asking pregnant women how they plan to feed their baby. If such a question is asked in advance of the mother having any information about breastfeeding other than what a neighbor, friend, or relative may have told her—and if she lives in an environment where bottle-feeding is highly visible—she is very likely to say "bottle-feeding" without giving it much thought. Such a response effectively shuts the door on any future discussion about breastfeeding that might have taken place had the original question not been asked. Alternatives to such an approach—with its self-defeating response—are discussed so that health workers will be in a better position to offer information that may encourage women to think about choosing breastfeeding when they may not have considered such a choice previously.

Specific barriers are then discussed and role-playing is used to assist those in the training program to practice how they might answer a prospective client's concerns. These barriers include:

- lack of confidence
- embarrassment
- loss of freedom
- the influence of family and friends
- dietary and health practices.

The last barrier can be a major stumbling block if a woman attending a WIC clinic understands that she has qualified for the supplemental food program because she is "nutritionally at risk." She may fear, but not voice her concerns, that if she hasn't been eating well enough to make a good baby without WIC food supplements, then she is very likely unable to make "good" milk either. Workers in such clinics may need to revise how they emphasize nutritional risk in order to assist mothers in understanding that milk production is far less dependent on food choices than is pregnancy.

Three counseling strategies are identified and examples are provided for each of the barriers identified earlier: eliciting the client's concerns, acknowl-

edging her feelings, and educating her by sharing information with her.

Finally, issues that attract women to breastfeeding—taking advantage of the unique health benefits to the baby that breastfeeding provides, enhancing the mother-infant bond, and providing a special time between mother and baby—are discussed, along with ways to use the "Best Start" program to cement these positive messages about breastfeeding. Originally designed for use in WIC offices, this program includes posters, informational pamphlets designed for a low-literacy audience, and video presentations that are designed to be used as public service announcements and to spark discussion in client focus groups. In some cases, WIC offices use selected segments of the video presentations to help mothers see that women like themselves—with similar concerns—think breastfeeding is best for them, not just for their babies. The pamphlets deal directly with the many concerns women have and then offer alternative views to help women see that such fears need not prevent them from breastfeeding. Such an honest approach legitimizes the concerns, but does not accept them as reasons for not breastfeeding; rather, they become the spur for serious consideration of ways to reduce their power as barriers. What remains to be done is a carefully controlled study in different settings to determine how effective these social marketing tools are in improving breastfeeding initiation and duration in low-income U.S. populations in which breastfeeding is least likely to occur.

SUMMARY

Different family forms reflect different needs of its members. Family developmental theories enable the health worker to identify specific family functions throughout the life cycle. The goal of the health-care provider should be to help the family to be able to meet its own needs without her assistance. Key issues related to family functioning are its placement within the support system and community of which it is a part. The early parenting period includes patterns of attachment behavior and how these reflect the growing competence of the parents as parents. In some cases, the father may be the mother's singular and most constant supporter; in other situations, he may be far less involved in the family and even less inclined to support breastfeeding.

Effective breastfeeding promotion goes beyond words and slogans. It requires tools for health providers, who will have contact with the breastfeeding father, as well as the mother. Promotion programs must be structured so that they take into consideration the cultural and social context within which the program and its participants function. Two such programs, one in a developing country, and one designed to reach low-income women in the United States, serve as examples of elements to consider.

Awareness of the social support system on which the mother can call, in addition to any health-care providers whom she might look to for assistance, is imperative for the care-giver attempting to provide ongoing information and help, particularly when that help is provided outside an institutional setting.

REFERENCES

Albers, RM: Emotional support for the breast-feeding mother, *Iss Compr Pediatr Nurs* 5:109–24, 1981.

Aldous, J: Strategies for developing family theory, *J Marr Fam* 33:250–57, 1970.

American Academy of Pediatrics: The promotion of breast-feeding, *Pediatrics* 69:654–61, 1982.

American Dietetic Association: Position of the American Dietetic Association: promotion of breast feeding, *J Am Diet Assoc* 86:1580, 1986.

Anlar, Y, Anlar, B, and Tonyali, A: Some factors influencing the time of lactation, *J Trop Pediatr* 34:198, 1988.

Arango, JO: Promoting breast feeding: a national perspective, *Public Health Rep* 99:559–65, 1984.

Auerbach, KG: The role of the nurse in support of breast feeding, *J Adv Nurs* 4:263–85, 1979.

Auerbach, KG: Breastfeeding fallacies: their relationship to understanding lactation, *Birth* 17:44–49, 1990a.

Auerbach KG: Breastfeeding promotion: why it doesn't work (editorial), *J Hum Lact* 6:45–46, 1990b.

Baranowski, T, et al.: Social support, social influence, ethnicity and the breastfeeding decision, *Soc Sci Med* 17:1599–1611, 1983.

Barron, SP, et al.: Factors influencing duration of breast feeding among low-income women, *J Am Diet Assoc* 88:1557–61, 1988.

Bee, DE, et al.: Breast-feeding initiation in a triethnic population, *Am J Dis Child* 145:306–9, 1991.

Bevan, ML, et al.: Factors influencing breast feeding in an urban WIC program, *J Am Diet Assoc* 84:563–67, 1984.

Bishop, WS, and Bishop, PA: Father-assisted breastfeeding, *Pediatr Nurs* 4:39–49, 1978.

Bowen, SM, and Miller, BC: Paternal attachment behavior as related to presence at delivery and preparenthood classes: a pilot study, *Nurs Res* 29:307–11, 1980.

Brodwick, M, Baranowski, T, and Rassin, DK: Patterns of infant feeding in a tri-ethnic population, *J Am Diet Assoc* 89:1129–32, 1989.

Brogan, BD, and Fox, HM: Infant feeding practices of low- and middle-income families in Nebraska, *J Am Diet Assoc* 84:560–63, 1984.

Bryant, CA: The impact of kin, friend and neighbor networks on infant feeding practices: Cuban, Puerto Rican and Anglo families in Florida, *Soc Sci Med* 16:1757–65, 1982.

Burkhalter, BR, and Marin, PS: A demonstration of increased exclusive breastfeeding in Chile, *Int J Gynaecol Obstet* 34:353–59, 1991.

Cadwallader, AA, and Olson, CM: Use of a breastfeeding intervention by nutrition paraprofessionals, *J Nutr Educ* 18:117–22, 1986.

Canadian Dietetic Association: Promoting breastfeeding: a role for the dietician/nutritionist: official position of the Canadian Dietetic Association, *J Can Diet Assoc* 50:211–14, 1989.

Chandler, CG, and Roush, RE: Training allied health professionals to deliver breast-feeding services to women in the pre- and postnatal periods, *J Allied Health* 11:124–30, 1982.

Clift, E: Social marketing and communication: changing health behavior in the Third World, *Am J Heath Prom* 3:17–24, 1989.

Cobb, S: Social support as a moderator of life stress, *Psychosom Med* 38:300–314, 1976.

Committee on Nutrition: Encouraging breast-feeding, *Pediatrics* 65:657–68, 1980.

Cronenwett, LR, and Reinhardt, R: Support and breastfeeding: a review, *Birth* 14:199–203, 1987.

Cunningham, WE, and Segree, W: Breast feeding promotion in an urban and a rural Jamaican hospital, *Soc Sci Med* 30:341–48, 1990.

Cusson, RM: Attitudes toward breast-feeding among female high-school students, *Pediatr Nurs* 10:189–91, 1985.

Duvall, EM: *Family development,* 4th ed., Philadelphia, 1971, J.B. Lippincott Co.

Fein, RA: The first weeks of fathering: the importance of choices and supports for new parents, *Birth Fam J* 3:53–58, 1976.

Fein, RA: Research on fathering: social policy and an emergent perspective, *J Soc Iss* 34:122–35, 1978.

Fernandez, EL, and Guthrie, GM: Belief systems and breastfeeding among Filipino urban poor, *Soc Sci Med* 19:991–95, 1984.

Forsyth, BW, Leventhal, JM, and McCarthy, PL: Mothers' perceptions of problems of feeding and crying behaviors, *Am J Dis Child* 139:269–72, 1985.

Friel, JK, et al.: The effect of a promotion campaign on attitudes of adolescent females towards breastfeeding, *Can J Public Health* 80:195–99, 1989.

Gabriel, A, Gabriel, KR, and Lawrence, RA: Cultural values and biomedical knowledge: choices in infant feeding, *Soc Sci Med* 23:501–9, 1986.

Greenberg, M, and Morris, N: Engrossment: the newborn's impact upon the father, *Am J Orthopsychiatry* 44:520–31, 1974.

Gregg, JEM: Attitudes of teenagers in Liverpool to breast feeding, *Br Med J* 299:147–48, 1989.

Grossman, LK, et al.: The infant feeding decision in low and upper income women, *Clin Pediatr* 29:30–37, 1990a.

Grossman, LK, et al.: The effect of postpartum lactation counseling on the duration of breast-feeding in low-income women, *Am J Dis Child* 144:471–74, 1990b.

Grossman, LK, et al.: Breastfeeding among low-income, high-risk women, *Clin Pediatr* 28:38–42, 1989.

Habicht, J-P: Assurance of quality of the provision of primary medical care by non-professionals, *Soc Sci Med* 13:67–75, 1979.

Hangsleben, KL: Transition to fatherhood: An exploratory study, *JOGN Nurs* 12:265–70, 1983.

Hanvey, L: Values in maternal and newborn care, *Can Nurse* 86:22–24, 1990.

Hart, H, Bax, M, and Jenkins, S: Community influences on breast feeding, *Child Care Health Dev* 6:175–87, 1980.

Hawkins, LM, Nichols, FH, and Tanner, JL: Predictors of the duration of breastfeeding in low-income women, *Birth* 14:204–9, 1987.

Hill, PD: Maternal attitudes and infant feeding among low-income mothers, *J Hum Lact* 4:7–11, 1988.

Howard, JS, and Sater, J: Adolescent mothers: self-perceived health education needs, *JOGN Nurs* 14:399–404, 1985.

Hung, BKM, Ling, L, and Ong, SG: Sources of influence on infant feeding practices in Hong Kong, *Soc Sci Med* 20:1143–50, 1985.

International Lactation Consultant Association: Position paper on infant feeding. Evanston, Illinois, 1991, ILCA.

International Pediatric Association Seminar: Recommendations for action programmes to encourage breast feeding, *Acta Paediatr Scand* 65:275–77, 1976.

Jelliffe, EFP: Introducing breast-feeding into modern health services, *J Trop Pediatr Env Health* 21:280–83, 1975.

Jenner, S: The influence of additional information, advice and support on the success of breast feeding in working class primiparas, *Child Care Health Dev* 14:319–28, 1988.

Jones, C: Father to infant attachment: effects of early contact and characteristics of the infant, *Res Nurs Health* 4:193–200, 1981.

Jordan, PL: Breastfeeding as a risk factor for fathers, *JOGNN* 15:94–97, 1986.

Jordan, PL: Laboring for relevance: expectant and new fatherhood, *Nurs Res* 39:11–16, 1990.

Jordan, PL, and Wall, VR: Breastfeeding and fathers: illuminating the darker side, *Birth* 17:210–13, 1990.

Kistin, N, et al.: Breast-feeding rates among black urban low-income women: effect of prenatal education, *Pediatrics* 86:741–46, 1990.

Klaus, MH, and Kennell, JH: *Maternal-Infant Bonding,* St. Louis, 1976, The C.V. Mosby Co., pp. 38–98.

Koctürk, T, and Zettestrom, R: Breast-feeding and its promotion, *Acta Paediatr Scand* 77:183–90, 1988.

Koctürk T, and Zetterström, R: The promotion of breast-feeding and maternal attitudes, *Acta Paediatr Scand* 78:817–23, 1989.

Kramer, MS: Poverty, WIC, and promotion of breast-feeding, *Pediatrics* 87:399–400, 1991.

Kunst-Wilson, W, and Cronenwett, L: Nursing care for the emerging family: promoting paternal behavior, *Res Nurs Health* 4:201–11, 1981.

Lamb, ME: Father-infant and mother-infant interaction in the first year of life, *Child Dev* 48:167–81, 1977.

Lamb, ME, ed.: *The role of the father in child development,* New York, 1976, John Wiley & Sons, Inc.

Lemmer, CM: Early discharge: outcomes of primiparas and their infants, *JOGNN* 16:230–36, 1987.

Lerner, HE: Effects of the nursing mother-infant dyad on the family, *Am J Orthopsychiatry* 49:339–48, 1979.

Levine, JA: Redefining the child care 'problem': men as child nurturers, *Child Educ* 54:55–61, 1977.

Levy-Shiff, R, et al.: Fathers' hospital visits to their preterm infants as a predictor of father-infant relationship and infant development, *Pediatrics* 86:289–93, 1990.

Lynch, SA, et al.: Evaluating effect of a breastfeeding consultant on the duration of breastfeeding, *Can J Public Health* 77:190–95, 1986.

McLorg, PA, and Bryant, CA: Influence of social network members and health care professionals on infant feeding practices of economically disadvantaged mothers, *Med Anthrop* 10:265–78, 1989.

Majewski, JL: Conflicts, satisfactions and attitudes during transition to the maternal role, *Nurs Res* 35:10–14, 1986.

Manstead, ASR, Plevin, CE, and Smart, JL: Predicting mothers' choice of infant feeding method, *Br J Soc Psychol* 23:223–31, 1984.

Martines, JC, Ashworth, A, and Kirkwood, B: Breast-feeding among the urban poor in southern Brazil: reasons for termination in the first 6 months of life, *Bull WHO* 67:151–61, 1989.

Mead, M: *Coming of Age in Samoa,* New York, 1928, Morrow Quill Paperbacks, pp. 147–57.

Morse, JM, and Harrison, MJ: Social coercion for weaning, *J Nurs Midwif* 32:205–10, 1987.

Mott, FL, and Maxwell, NL: School-age mothers: 1968 and 1979, *Fam Plann Perspect* 13:287–92, 1981.

Mulford, C: Subtle signs and symptoms of the milk ejection reflex, *J Hum Lact* 6:177–78, 1990.

Nason, EM, and Poloma, MM: *Voluntarily childless couples: the emergence of a variant life style.* Beverly Hills, 1976, Sage Publications.

Palti, H, et al.: Evaluation of the effectiveness of a structured breast-feeding promotion program integrated into a maternal and child health service in Jerusalem, *Isr J Med Sci* 24:342–48, 1988.

Pascoe, JM, and Berger, A: Attitudes of high school girls in Israel and the United States toward breast feeding, *J Adoles Health Care* 6:28–30, 1985.

Peterson, GH, Mehl, LE, and Leiderman, PH: The role of some birth-related variables in father attachment, *Am J Orthopsychiatry* 49:330–38, 1979.

Pleck, JH: The work-family role system, *Soc Prob* 24:417–27, 1977.

Polit, DF, and Kahn, JR: Early subsequent pregnancy among economically disadvantaged teenage mothers, *Am J Public Health* 76:167–71, 1986.

Popkin, BM, et al.: An evaluation of a national breast-feeding promotion programme in Honduras, *J Biosoc Sci* 23:5–21, 1991.

Pridham, KF: Meaning of infant feeding issues and mothers' use of help, *J Reprod Inf Psychol* 5:145–52, 1987.

Princeton, JC: Incorporating a deliberative nursing care approach with breastfeeding mothers, *Health Care Women Int* 7:277–93, 1986.

Rassin, DK, Richardson, CJ, and Baranowski, T: Ethnic determinants of lactation in a population of mothers in the United States. In Hamosh, M, and Goldman, AS, *Human Lactation 2*, New York, 1986, Plenum Publishing Corporation, pp. 69–81.

Rassin, DK, et al.: Incidence of breast-feeding in a low socioeconomic group of mothers in the United States: ethnic patterns, *Pediatrics* 73:132–37, 1984.

Riordan J: *A Practical Guide to Breastfeeding*, St. Louis: C. V. Mosby, 1983.

Rea, MF, and Berquó, ES: Impact of the Brazilian national breast-feeding programme on mothers in Greater São Paulo, *Bull WHO* 68:365–71, 1990.

Robinson, BE: Men caring for the young: an androgynous perspective, *Fam Coord* 28:553–59, 1979.

Rodriguez-Garcia, R, Aumack, KJ, and Ramos, A: A community-based approach to the promotion of breastfeeding in Mexico, *JOGNN* 19:431–38, 1990.

Rogers, CS, Morris, S, and Taper, LJ: Weaning from the breast: influences on maternal decisions, *Pediatr Nurs* 13:341–45, 1987.

Romero-Gwynn, E: Breast-feeding pattern among Indochinese immigrants in Northern California, *Am J Dis Child* 143:804–8, 1989.

Russell, G: High participant Australian fathers: some preliminary findings, *Merrill Palmer Q* 28:137–56, 1982.

Samuels, SE, Margen, S, and Schoen, EJ: Incidence and duration of breast-feeding in a health maintenance organization population, *Am J Clin Nutr* 42:504–10, 1985.

Saunders, SE, and Carroll, J: Post-partum breast feeding support:impact on duration, *J Am Diet Assoc* 88:213–15, 1988.

Scrimshaw, SCM, et al.: Factors affecting breastfeeding among women of Mexican origin or descent in Los Angeles, *Am J Public Health* 77:467–70, 1987.

Skeel, L, and Good, ME: Mexican cultural beliefs and breastfeeding: a model for assessment and intervention, *J Hum Lact* 4:160–63, 1988.

Skeel, L, McCarty, E, and Pierce, S: Promoting breast feeding among Hispanic women in Santa Cruz county, *Public Health Rep* 101:661–62, 1986.

Snell, BJ, et al.: The association of formula samples given at hospital discharge with the early duration of breastfeeding, *J Hum Lact* 8:67–72, 1992.

Soule, B, Standley, K, and Copans, SA: Father identity, *Psychiatry* 42:255–63, 1979.

Soysa, PE, Fernando, DN, and Abeywickrama, K: Role of health personnel in the promotion of breast feeding practices, *J Trop Pediatr* 34:75–78, 1988.

Spradley, BW: *Community Health Nursing: Concepts and Practice*, 2nd ed., Boston, 1985, Little, Brown & Co.

Stokamer, CL: Breastfeeding promotion efforts: why some do not work, *Int J Gynaecol Obstet* 31 (Suppl):61–65, 1990.

Stotland, NL, and Peterson, CH: A modest proposal: breastfeeding for the infants of adolescent mothers, *Adv Psychosom Med* 12:81–90, 1985.

Sullivan, J, and Jones, LC: Breastfeeding adoption by low-income black women, *Health Care Women Int* 7:295–309, 1986.

Tapia, JA: Fractionalization of the family unit. In Schuster, CS, and Ashburn, SS, eds., *The process of human development*, Boston, 1986, Little, Brown & Co.

Task Force Report: The promotion of breast-feeding, *Pediatrics* 69:654–61, 1982.

Taubenhein, AM, and Silbernagel, T: Meeting the needs of expectant fathers, *MCN* 13:110–13, 1988.

Tomlinson, PS, Rothenberg, MA, and Carver, LD: Behavioral interaction of fathers with infants and mothers in the immediate postpartum period, *J Nurs-Midwif* 36:232–39, 1991.

Wandersman, LP: The adjustment of father to their first baby: the roles of parenting groups and marital relationship, *Birth Fam J* 7:155–61, 1980.

Wolinski, M: Adolescent views on breastfeeding: a descriptive survey, *Breastfeeding Rev* 14:9–12, 1989.

Woollett, A: Who breastfeeds? The family and cultural context, *J Reprod Inf Psychol* 5:127–31, 1987.

Yoos, L: Developmental issues and the choice of feeding method of adolescent mothers, *JOGN Nurs* 14:68–72, 1985.

Young, SA, and Kaufman, M: Promoting breastfeeding at a migrant health center, *Am J Public Health* 78:523–25, 1988.

SECTION
TWO

Anatomic and Biologic Imperatives

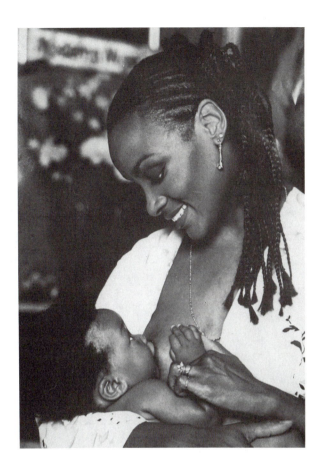

The female anatomy includes an organ whose physiology is designed to make milk at periodic intervals throughout the childbearing period. At the same time, the human breast produces a substance that meets most closely the needs of the infant for whom the milk was produced. No man-made substitute has yet been devised that nourishes the infant as well.

Viruses and bacteria stimulate particular protective reactions in the mother's body; when passed on through human milk these immunologic properties can provide important protections to the vulnerable infant. However, environmental contaminants and drugs can also be found in human milk. The question arises: if such contaminants and drugs can be found in the breast and in the milk it creates, to what degree do these elements represent acceptable or unacceptable risks when ingested by the breastfeeding infant?

4

Anatomy
and Psychophysiology
of Lactation

Breastfeeding is a symbiotic interchange between mother and child. While it is essential to understand the human female breast and the physiologic mechanisms of milk production, it is equally necessary to recognize the unique anatomy of the infant's oral structures and the physiologic mechanisms of suckling. Therefore, this chapter is divided into two parts: the first section focuses on the mother and the second section focuses on the infant. In lactation, as in all human biological systems, there is a working relationship between anatomy (form) and physiology (function). While function changes as form changes, the functional capacity of the human beast is not wholly dictated by form. Breast size, for instance, is a poor predictor of lactation success. The term psychophysiology used here reflects the sensitivity of breastfeeding to psychogenic influences. For example, for both the mother and the suckling infant, stress and fear can dramatically inhibit breastfeeding.

THE MOTHER

MAMMARY DEVELOPMENT

The mammary system is unlike other organ systems. From birth through puberty, pregnancy, and lactation, no other human organ displays such dramatic changes in size, shape, and function as does the breast. In humans, the female breasts serve more than one function: they first attract the sexual attentions of the male and then give nourishment and nurturing to the suckling infant. This first section, which focuses on the mother, describes breast development from embryo to adulthood, breast anatomy,

JAN RIORDAN

changes during pregnancy and lactation, and hormones which influence the course of lactogenesis.

In the embryo, breast development begins during the fourth week of gestation when a primitive milk streak develops from axilla to groin on the trunk of the embryo. This streak becomes the mammary ridge or milk line by the fifth week of embryonal life. The ridge or line is actually a thickening of epithelial cells in a localized ventrolateral area on the embryo. This thickening (the "milk hill" stage) continues through weeks seven and eight, accompanied by inward growth into the chest wall. Between 12 and 16 weeks, these specialized cells differentiate further into the smooth muscle of the nipple and areola. Also, during this period, epithelial cells continue to develop into mammary buds and then proliferate to form 15 to 25 epithelial branches that eventually become alveoli (Dawson, 1934; Vorherr, 1974).

Placental sex hormones enter fetal circulation and stimulate formation of channels (canalization) of the branched epithelial tissue. This process continues until the fetus reaches 32 weeks. From 32 to 40 weeks of gestation, lobular-alveolar structures containing colostrum develop. During this time, the fetal mammary gland mass increases four times over its original mass, and the nipple and areola develop further and become pigmented. After birth, mammary tissue of the neonate may secrete colostral milk ("witches" milk) that can be easily expressed.

Mammary gland development during childhood is limited to general growth. At puberty, estrogen becomes the major influence on breast growth. As pu-

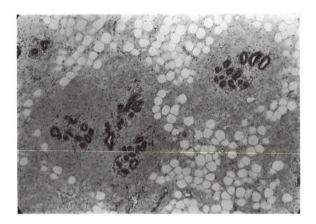

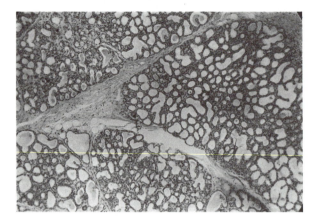

FIGURE 4–1 MAMMARY GLAND, INACTIVE

In the inactive mammary gland, connective tissue is abundant and glandular elements are minimal. Lobes and lobules are not well defined.

The grandular elements consist of groups of potential secretory tubules lined with cuboidal or low columnar epithelium. These are intralobular ducts with perhaps inactive alveoli at their terminal ends. Rarely is it possible to distinguish between ducts and alveoli. An occasional tubule lined with smaller cells may indicate a duct, or a tubule may be seen emerging from a lobule to join an interlobular duct. Tubules may be present in an indifferentiated form as solid cords of cells.

The tubules are surrounded by a loose, fine-fibered, vascular connective tissue with numerous fibroblasts, the intralobular connective tissue. Between the lobules are masses of dense collagenous fibers, the interlobular connective tissue in which adipose tissue is usually present. (*Source:* Victor B. Eichler, Kalamazoo, MI.)

FIGURE 4–2 MAMMARY GLAND DURING THE FIRST HALF OF PREGNANCY

Growth of secretory tubules with continued branchings of their terminal ends continues throughout the first half of pregnancy. Alveoli differentiate at the ends of the ducts but it is still difficult to distinguish intralobular ducts from alveoli. Most of the alveoli are empty but secretion is present in some.

The loose intralobular connective tissue enables the continued expansion of the ducts and alveoli. In addition to numerous fibroblasts, other cells appear in increasing numbers, mainly lymphocytes, plasma cells and eosinophils.

The lobules become more apparent and stand out distinctly in contrast to their indistinctness in the inactive gland. The dense interlobular connective tissue now appears as septa between the lobules of glandular tissue. Interlobular ducts, lined with columnar cells, course in these septa. These empty into large lactiferous ducts, lined usually with low pseudostratified columnar epithelium. Each lactiferous duct collects the secretions of a lobe. (*Source:* Victor B. Eichler, Kalamazoo, MI.)

berty begins (at 10 to 12 years of age), primary and secondary ducts grow and divide and form club-shaped terminal end buds that are associated with beginning function of the hypothalamus-pituitary-ovarian axis. The buds develop into new branches and small ductules of areolar buds, which later become the acini or alveoli in the mature breast. During each menstrual cycle, proliferation and active growth of duct tissue occurs during the follicular and ovulatory phases, reaching a maximum in the late luteal phase and then regressing. During each ovulatory cycle, peaks of ovarian steroids, primarily progesterone, foster further mammary development that never returns to its former state of the preceding cycle. Complete development of mammary function occurs only in pregnancy. At the same time, new budding of structures continues until about age 35 (Dabelow, 1957; Vorherr, 1974). In addition to es-

trogen and progesterone, prolactin and an epidermal growth factor or a specific mammary growth factor are other hormones thought to be required for mammary growth (Tonelli & Sorof, 1980).

STRUCTURE

The basic units of the mature glandular tissue are the *alveoli,* which are composed of secretory acinus units in which the ductules terminate. Each cluster of secretory cells of an alveolus is surrounded by a contractile unit of *myoepithelial cells* responsible for ejecting milk into the *ductules.* Each ductule then merges, without communicating with its neighbors, into a larger collecting *lactiferous* or *mammary duct.* Mammary ducts then widen into the *am-*

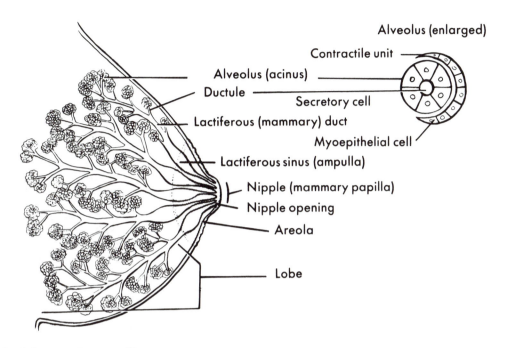

FIGURE 4–3   Schematic diagram of breast.

pullae or *lactiferous sinuses* located behind the nipple and the areola, the surrounding pigmented area of the breast. There are 15 to 20 subdivided *lobes* in each breast. (See Figs. 4–3 and 4–4.)

Between and around the uneven edges of the lobes is a thick layer of fat. As seen in Fig. 4–5, running vertically through the breast and attaching the deep layer of the subcutaneous tissue to the dermis of the skin are the *suspensory ligaments* or *Cooper's ligaments* named after a late 19th-century English surgeon (Clemente, 1985). The breast's structure is mainly given by the fibrous tissues that surround and course through it. Glandular tissue extends towards the axilla partly under the lateral border of the pectoralis majora; it is known as the *axillary tail.* (See Fig. 4–6.) Each breast of an adult woman weighs on the average 150 to 200 gm and increases to 400 to 500 gm (about one pound) during lactation.

The breast is highly vascularized. Blood is supplied to the breast mainly through the internal mammary (60%) and lateral thoracic (30%) arteries. The lymph vessels of the breast are numerous, and for the most part, join the lymph nodes of the axilla. The majority of lymph vessels follow the lactiferous ducts and thus converge towards the nipple, where they join a plexus situated beneath the areola (subareolar plexus).

The nerve supply of the breast is derived from the intercostal nerves of fourth, fifth, and sixth intercostal spaces. The fourth intercostal nerve penetrates the posterior aspect of the breast (left breast at 4 o'clock position, right breast at 8 o'clock position) and supplies the greatest amount of sensation to the nipple and to the areola. The breast has uneven patterns of sensation: the areola is the most sensitive part of the breast, the skin adjacent to the areola is less sensitive, and the nipple itself is the least sensitive. Larger breasts have less sensation than smaller breasts. Of women with small- or moderate-size breasts, those who have never been pregnant have greater sensation in their nipples and areolae (Courtiss & Goldwyn 1976). About midway to the nipple/areola the fourth intercostal nerve becomes more superficial. As it reaches the areola, it divides into five branches: one central, two upper and two lower. The lowermost branch consistently pierces the areola at the 5 o'clock position on the left side and at the 7 o'clock position on the right side. Any trauma to this nerve will cause some loss of sensation in the breast (Edgerton & McClary, 1958; Courtiss &

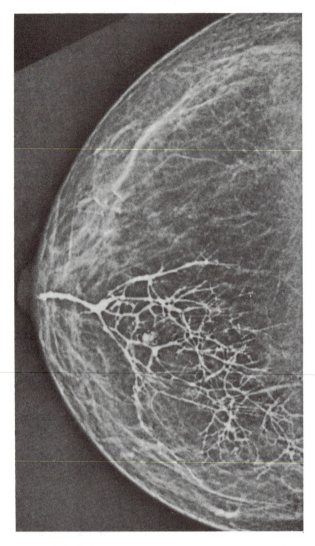

FIGURE 4–4 Contrast opacification of a single lactiferous duct demonstrates a branching network that defines a single lobe of the breast. From Kopans, DB: *Breast Imaging,* Philadelphia, 1989, J.B. Lippincott Co., p. 20.

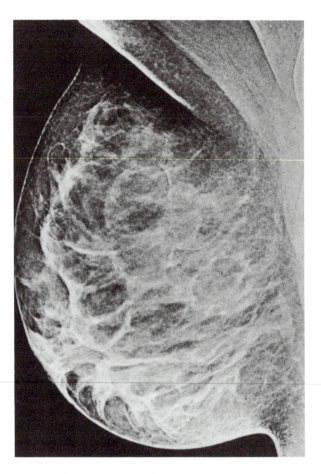

FIGURE 4–5 Curvlinear densities represent Cooper's ligaments. From Kopans, DB: *Breast Imaging,* Philadelphia, 1989, J.B. Lippincott Co., p. 20.

Goldwyn, 1976). If the lowermost nerve branch is severed, the mother loses sensation to the nipple and areola (Farina, Newby & Alani, 1980).

The covering smooth skin is modified at the center of each breast to form a *mammary papilla* or nipple into which the lactiferous sinuses open. There are 15 to 20 openings (pores) in the nipple. The nipple projects as a small cylindrical body with pigmented wrinkled skin slightly below the center of each breast at about the level of the fourth intercostal space. Surrounding the nipple is the *areola* within

which lie the tubercles of Montgomery, small sebaceous glands which enlarge during pregnancy. The tubercles of Montgomery range in number from approximately 4 to 28 on each breast. While it is widely stated that they provide nipple lubrication and antisepsis, there is neither evidence nor documentation of this function. The nipple and areola contain erectile smooth muscles. There are hair follicles around the nipple; most women have at least some nipple hair. In a lactating mother, the average diameter of the nipple areola is 6.4 cm; the average diameter of erectile portion of the nipple 1.6 cm and the length 0.7 cm (Ziemer, 1993).

VARIATIONS

From woman to woman, breasts vary in color, size, shape, function, and placement. Lobular size varies

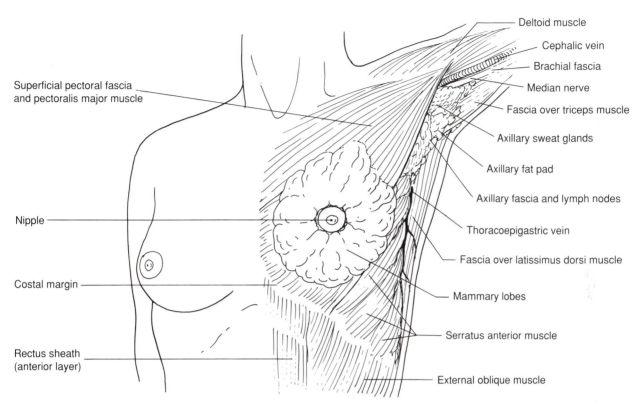

FIGURE 4–6   Anterior pectoral dissection showing the lobular nature of the mammary gland extending toward the axilla and its location anterior to the pectoralis major muscle. Includes the superficial axillary lymph and sweat glands. Adapted from Clemente, CD: *Anatomy: A regional atlas of the human body,* Philadelphia, 1978, Lea & Febiger.

within a single breast, from one breast to another, and from woman to woman. Moreover, asymmetry of breasts is very common—the left breast often larger than the right. The areola and nipple color vary according to complexion: pink in blonds, browner in brunettes, and black in black-skinned women (Love & Lindsey, 1990). *Supernumerary* nipple tissue or an *accessory* nipple may occur at any point along the milk line from the axilla to the groin (polymastia). Only rarely does a true or complete accessory mammary gland develop. The most common areas for an accessory breast to develop are in the axilla or on the thorax (see color plate).

Lack of full protraction of the nipple, when using the common pinch test (Figs. 4–11, *A* and *B*), is fairly common in primigravid women. The percentage of poor nipple protractility in women during their first pregnancy has been reported to range from 28 to 35 (Blaikeley et al., 1953; Hytten & Baird, 1958; Waller, 1946). The protractibility of the nipple gradually im-

proves during pregnancy and by puerperium most women have good nipple protraction. Generally, nipple protraction continues to improve with each subsequent pregnancy and lactation experience. Inch (1989) reviewed studies (Blaikeley et al., 1953; Hytten, 1954; Waller, 1946), on nipple protractility which were all conducted several decades ago, and found little relationship between protractility and subsequent breastfeeding difficulty. She concluded that because the infant makes a teat not from the nipple alone, but from the surrounding breast tissue, the actual shape of the nipple may be a secondary consideration.

While we know something about nipple protractility, there is little epidemiological data on nipple inversion. No published research study addresses the incidence of inverted nipples. Although true inversion appears to be a rare event it is difficult to treat. Usually the inversion is on one breast only, and the mother may breastfeed successfully from a single breast. When the inversion is bilateral, feedings at the breast may need to be supplemented.

PREGNANCY

During pregnancy the breasts grow larger, the skin appears thinner, and the veins become more prominent. The diameter of the areola increases from about 34 mm in early pregnancy to 50 mm postpartum (Hytten, 1954), although there is a wide range of areolar width in any population. As the nipples become more erect, pigmentation of the areola increases and the glands of Montgomery enlarge. Estrogen and progesterone exert their specific effect on the breast during pregnancy; the ductal system proliferates and differentiates under the influence of estrogen, while progesterone promotes an increase in size of the lobes, lobules, and alveoli.

Russo and Russo (1987) describe two distinct phases of pregnancy by which the breast attains its maximum development. The early stage is characterized by growth and proliferation of the ductal tree and further formation of lobules. During the second half of pregnancy, mammary changes involve continuation and accentuation of secretory activity. The acini or alveoli become distended by accumulation of colostrum. If the woman has an accessory breast, it may also swell. Just before and during childbirth, there is a new wave of mitotic activity which increases the total DNA of the gland (Vorherr, 1974; Salazar & Tobon, 1974). Following birth, milk is synthesized and released into the mammary acini and ductal system. As long as milk is removed regularly from the breast, the alveolar cells continue to secrete milk almost indefinitely (Vorherr, 1974).

HORMONAL INFLUENCES DURING PUERPERIUM

The hormonal trigger for milk production within the alveoli is the rapid decline of estrogen and progesterone following the expulsion of the placenta. After birth, a complex of several hormones coupled with stimulation of the let-down reflex direct the development of lactation. A great deal of information about these hormonal functions during lactation is now known through radioimmunoassay studies. The principal hormone in milk biosynthesis is prolactin.

Prolactin. During pregnancy, prolactin has an important role in increasing breast mass. The mammary ducts and alveoli mature and proliferate as prolactin levels steadily rise from the normal non-pregnancy level of 10–25 ng/mL to a peak of 200–400 ng/mL at term (Tyson et al., 1972). Lactation during pregnancy is inhibited by high levels of progesterone which interfere with prolactin action. As progesterone and estrogen levels abruptly drop after a woman gives birth, the anterior pituitary gland, no longer inhibited by these two hormones, releases very large amounts of prolactin. Fig. 4–7 describes the rise and fall of hormones during pregnancy and lactation.

Postpartum prolactin secretion is controlled by the hypothalamus. This control is largely inhibitory, in that whenever the pathway between the hypothalamus and the pituitary is disrupted, prolactin levels rise. When the nipple is stimulated, the hypothalamus inhibits the release of dopamine; this lower level of dopamine stimulates the release of prolactin and causes milk production (Chao, 1987). Stimulation of the nipple is reported to be sufficiently potent to cause the synthesis of breastmilk even in non-parturient individuals.

There are ample and well-documented reports that suckling stimulation alone can initiate lactation. Mead described the Mundugumore tribe in New Guinea, who customarily gave away one of each set of twins. The foster mother put the adopted baby constantly to her breast, and within a few weeks she had a good supply of milk. Similar examples have been reported from Asia, Africa, and Europe,

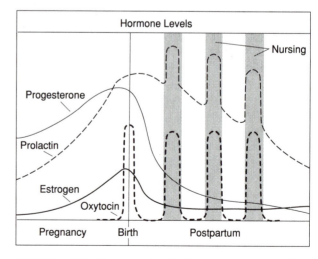

FIGURE 4–7 Hormone levels during pregnancy and lactation. Adapted from Love, S: *Dr. Susan Love's Breast Book,* Addison-Wesley, Boston, 1990, p. 34.

where women who have not been pregnant for years have adopted and suckled babies successfully. Even today in rural remote areas of the United States, this phenomenon is not unknown. Recently we received a well-documented report of a 60-year-old Mississippi grandmother who decided to adopt and nurse her grandchild when her daughter died. The milk appeared as expected, and the child was breastfed until he was able to walk.*

Plasma prolactin levels rise and fall proportionately to frequency, intensity, and duration of nipple stimulation. Prolactin levels usually double in response to suckling and peak somewhere between 15 minutes and 60 minutes after the initiation of suckling. During the first week after birth, prolactin levels in breastfeeding women fall about 50%. If a mother does not breastfeed, prolactin levels usually reach non-pregnant levels by seven days (Fig. 4–8) (Tyson et al., 1972; Speroff, Glass & Kase, 1989).

Battin et al. (1985) studied serum prolactin levels in eight breastfeeding women for 180 days postpartum. The infants of these mothers obtained almost all of their daily nutriment from breast milk. Mean baseline prolactin levels were 90 ng/mL at 10 days postpartum; afterwards they slowly declined but remained elevated at 180 days postpartum (44.3 ng/mL). At 10 days postpartum four women in the study who remained amenorrheic throughout the study had higher (about 110.0 ng/mL) baseline prolactin levels compared to the remaining four women

*From Newton, Michael, and Newton, Niles: The normal course and management of lactation, *Clinic Obstet Gyn* 5(1): 47, 1962.

(about 70.1 ng/mL) who spontaneously menstruated prior to 180 days. Other cross-sectional studies support the concept that serum prolactin levels remain elevated for as long as the mother nurses. Gross and Eastman (1979) found that nursing women in Australia had elevated prolactin levels at 66 weeks postpartum. An overview of prolactin serum levels during pregnancy and breastfeeding is seen in Fig. 4–8.

Prolactin is also present in the breastmilk itself. Yuen (1988) found milk prolactin content was highest in the early transition milk (about 43 ng/mL); afterwards it steadily declined but remained detectable in mature milk (about 11 ng/mL) until weaning up to 40 weeks postpartum. During suckling, the foremilk contained significantly more prolactin as compared with the hindmilk (about 29 vs. 21 ng/mL). Yuen concluded that (1) the release of prolactin into intra-alveolar secretions plays some role in the establishment and maintenance of lactation and (2) the early transmission of prolactin in the aqueous foremilk has an effect on intestinal fluid and electrolyte exchange in the newborn. Prolactin release is highest during suckling when a major portion of milk is secreted. When milk is removed by suckling, the alveoli partially collapse. Milk synthesis and secretion continue at this point, but to a smaller degree (Dabelow, 1957).

There is no relationship between the degree of postpartum breast engorgement and the level of circulating prolactin (West, 1979). A mother who smokes cigarettes will have lower prolactin levels (Baron et al., 1986); if she drinks beer, her prolactin levels will be higher (DeRosa et al., 1981).

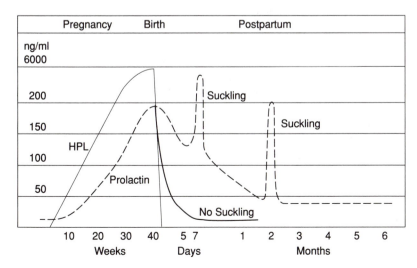

FIGURE 4–8 Fluctuation of HPL and prolactin serum levels in pregnancy and lactation. From Battin, DA, et al.: *Obstet Gynecol* 65:785–88, 1985; Tyson, JE, et al.: *Am J Obstet Gynecol* 113:14–20, 1972; Speroff, L, Glass, RH, and Kase, NG: *Clinical gynecology, endocrinology and infertility,* 4th ed. Baltimore, 1989, The Williams & Wilkins Co., p. 283.

The role of prolactin in the delay of fertility is well known. Prolactin delays the return of ovulation by inhibiting ovarian response to follicle-stimulating hormone (Bonnar et al., 1975). This topic is discussed extensively in Chapter 16 on fertility and sexuality. Prolactin reportedly has a relaxing effect, causing the breastfeeding woman to feel calm, even euphoric. As a result, higher prolactin levels may prevent or ameliorate postpartum blues in breastfeeding women.

The prolactin receptor theory. DeCarvalho et al. (1983) suggested that frequent feeding in early lactation stimulates a faster increase in milk output because suckling stimulates the development of receptors to prolactin in the mammary gland. According to DeCarvalho, the number of these receptors per cell increases in early lactation and remains constant thereafter. This theoretical framework is supported by animal studies (Lincoln & Renfrew, 1981; Sernia & Tyndale-Biscoe, 1979; Hinds & Tyndale-Biscoe, 1982) and by studies of breastfeeding mothers. There is evidence that when the mother breastfeeds early and often, milk production is greater, the infant gains more weight, and breastfeeding continues for a longer period than when early feedings are delayed and/or infrequent.

DeCarvalho (1983) demonstrated that infants gain more weight by their 15th day when they were breastfed an average of 9.9 times/day compared with infants in the control group who breastfed an average of 7.3 times/day. By the 35th day, however, postpartum milk intake and weight gain from birth were not significantly different between the two groups. This suggests that frequent feeding in early lactation stimulates a faster increase in milk output but that this output slows thereafter despite frequent breastfeedings. Humenick and Van Steenkiste (1983) found that women who had weaned their babies by eight weeks were much more likely than mothers who were still breastfeeding at that time to report longer time periods between each breastfeeding episode. They also were more likely to have used more supplements per day and to have perceived that feedings (in spite of their lesser frequency) occurred too often.

Zuppa et al. (1988) found that while serum prolactin levels were slightly lower in multiparous mothers compared with primiparous mothers in the first four postpartum days, the volume of milk obtained by the infants of the multiparous mothers was significantly higher. They concluded that multiparous women had a greater number of mammary gland receptors for prolactin. The implication here is that the controlling factor on breastmilk output is the number of prolactin receptors rather than the amount of prolactin in serum. More receptors may result in more than adequate milk production even in the presence of lower prolactin levels. This finding helps to explain why the infants of multiparous mothers begin gaining weight somewhat faster than those of primiparous mothers.

Human placental lactogen (HPL). Human placental lactogen is made by the placenta and is actively secreted into the maternal circulation starting in the second month of pregnancy. HPL reaches its maximum level (6,000 ng/mL) at term (Speroff, Glass & Kase, 1989). As yet, the role of HPL in lactogenesis is not clear (Neville & Berga, 1983); because it is produced in such large amounts, it may have a lactogenic effect.

Glucocorticoids. Glucocorticoids, hormones secreted by the adrenal glands, help to regulate water transport across the cell membranes during lactation. Cortisol, a main glucocorticoid, has little effect on the mammary system unless prolactin is present (Neville & Berga, 1983). The final differentiation of the alveolar epithelial cell in a mature milk cell takes place because prolactin is present but only after prior exposure to cortisol and insulin (Speroff, Glass & Kase, 1989).

Thyroid-stimulating hormone (TSH). Thyroid hormones promote mammary growth and lactation through a permissive rather than a regulatory role. Dawood et al. (1981) established a marked and significant increase in plasma TSH level on the third to fifth postpartum days. Thyroid hormones also play a general role in the health of the mother by regulating metabolic processes. Because the thyroid gland is an integral part of the complex endocrine system, a thyroid deficiency in the lactating mother can decrease the milk supply (Miyake, et al., 1989).

Prolactin inhibiting factor (PIF). PIF, a hypothalamic substance, either dopamine itself or mediated by dopamine, inhibits prolactin secretions (Diefenbach et al., 1976). Nipple stimulation suppresses PIF and dopamine, causing prolactin levels to rise and the breast to produce milk. Some drugs, such as phenothiazines and reserpine derivatives, increase breastmilk because they also inhibit PIF (Bohnet & Kato, 1985).

Thyrotropin-releasing hormone (TRH). TRH has been thought to increase TSH and prolactin levels. Therefore, TRH is thought to play a role in the control of prolactin secretion. Recently, however, Gehlbach, Bayliss, and Rosa (1989) were unable to conclude that TRH played any role in the release of prolactin when they measured plasma prolactin and TSH responses to breastfeeding during the first month postpartum.

LACTOGENESIS AND PSYCHOLOGICAL INFLUENCES
Through the mediation of the hypothalamus, the alveolar cells respond with milk secretion at the base of the alveolar cell, where small droplets are formed and migrate through to the cell membrane and then into the alveolar ducts for storage as shown by an ultrasound image in Fig. 4–9. The rate of milk synthesis after breastfeeding varies and ranged from 17 mL/hr to 33 mL/hr in one study (Arthur et al., 1989).

The highly vascularized secretory cells extract water, lactose, amino acids, fats, vitamins, minerals,

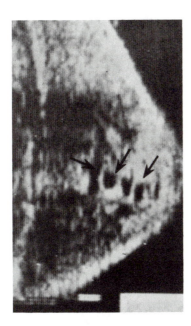

FIGURE 4–9 Ultrasound image showing milk-filled ducts. Mother lactating 10 months. From *Atlas of Breast Ultrasound*, Division of Ultrasound, Dept. of Radiology and Dept. of Pathology, Thomas Jefferson Univ. Medical College and Hospital, Philadelphia, 1980, p. 121.

and numerous other substances from the mother's blood, converting them to milk for her infant. Stores of adipose tissue laid down during pregnancy serve as stores that are drawn upon to provide substrate for milk synthesis (Agius & Williamson, 1980). It is thought that when the milk "comes in" or rapidly increases in volume with breast fullness 24 to 48 hours after birth, lactation shifts from endocrine control to autocrine control (Prentice et al., 1989).

The breast is not a passive container of milk but is an organ of active production that is infant, not hormone, driven. The removal of milk from the breasts facilitates continued milk production; conversely lack of adequate milk removal or stasis tends to limit breastmilk synthesis in the breasts. It is the quantity and quality of infant suckling or milk removal that governs breastmilk synthesis, not maternal hormones. This phenomenon, the supply-demand response, is a feedback control that regulates the production of milk to match the intake of the infant. A common adage that expresses this response is "The more the mother breastfeeds, the more milk there will be" (LLLI, 1991, p. 144). Akré (1989) observes that because lactation is an energy-intensive process, it makes evolutionary sense that there should be safeguards against wasteful overproduction as well as mechanisms for a prompt response to the infant's needs.

The supply-demand response is the somatic response to the infant's suckling that produces milk. Suckling stimulates afferent impulses in the sensory neurons of the areola which travel to the central nervous system. Responding to suckling, the posterior pituitary hormone, oxytocin, causes the milk ejection reflex or "let-down," a contraction of the myoepithelial cells surrounding the alveoli. The secreted milk is then ejected into the ductules and moved along to the lactiferous sinuses where it becomes readily available to the newborn through the nipple openings.

OXYTOCIN
Oxytocin levels in the blood rise within one minute of breast stimulation, remain elevated during the stimulation, and return to baseline levels within six minutes after stimulation of the nipple ends. This rise and fall of oxytocin levels continues at each feeding throughout the lactation course, even when the mother breastfeeds for an extensive period (Leake et al., 1983). The posterior pituitary contains a surpris-

ingly large store of oxytocin (3,000–9,000mU) when compared with the amount required to elicit the ejection reflex (50–100mU) (Lincoln & Paisley, 1982).

Oxytocin has another important function—to contract the mother's uterus. Uterine contractions help to control postpartum bleeding and to aid in uterine involution. The uterus not only contracts during breastfeeding but continues to contract rhythmically for as long as 20 minutes after the feeding. These cramps may be painful during the first few days postpartum. After involution is complete, however, these rhythmic pulsations may be a source of pleasure to the mother (Riordan & Rapp, 1980).

Through oxytocin mediation, these afferent pathways become so well established that let-down can occur even when the mother thinks of her baby. There are many anecdotal reports of spontaneous lactation in mothers who have weaned or who have never breastfed. On the other hand, stress or emotional upheaval can inhibit the let-down reflex and prolactin levels making less milk available to the infant (Newton & Newton, 1948). Chemically, stress and fear release adrenaline at the level of the mammary gland. Likewise, noradrenaline is released within the central nervous system. Both act to shut down the milk-ejection reflex (Lincoln & Paisley, 1982).

Whitworth's (1988) review of the importance of prolactin in milk production emphasizes that the hormone is essential for both initiating and maintaining milk production. While oxytocin appears to be keyed more closely to milk ejection, without prolactin, milk is not made. His discussion ends with the simple observation that "lactation . . . is controlled by the young, who in turn receive the benefits of milk secretion."

The influence of supplemental feedings on oxytocin and prolactin peaks was measured by Johnston and Amico (1986). They found that mothers who were not providing additional formula feedings to their infants had higher oxytocin levels over time than women who were giving their babies supplemental feedings. Not only did the non-supplementing women's oxytocin levels remain higher, they tended to climb over time, so that their oxytocin levels were higher at 15–24 weeks than they were at earlier periods (2–4 weeks and 5–14 weeks). In sharp contrast, the oxytocin levels of the mothers who were supplementing were lower at all time periods examined, and there was no rise in oxytocin peaks over time. In both of these groups of women, prolactin levels tended to decline over time. Among mothers who were not supplementing, however, prolactin levels were consistently higher at all time periods examined. These data suggest that over time prolactin levels can be expected to fall, but that oxytocin levels will continue to climb. However, when a mother supplements her baby with formula feedings, prolactin levels decline markedly and fall even further over time, while oxytocin levels remain depressed and do not climb. (See Fig. 4–10.)

The combination of these hormonal responses may contribute to reduced milk production and to the mother's perception—particular during periods of rapid infant growth and increased interest in breastfeeding—that she has insufficient milk to satisfy her infant. Prolactin and oxytocin levels that decline rapidly or remain depressed also may contrib-

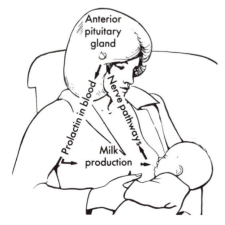

A

FIGURE 4–10 Release and effect of prolactin on milk ejection.

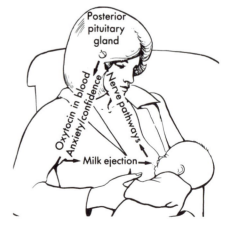

B

Release and effect of oxytocin.

ute to higher risk for early resumption of fertility during the lactation course.

GALACTORRHEA

Galactorrhea is the spontaneous secretion of milk from the breast under nonphysiological circumstances. Small amounts of milk or serous fluid are commonly expressed for weeks or months from women who have previously been pregnant and/or lactating. There are many anecdotal reports of spontaneous lactation that present an intriguing enigma. A case in point is that of a colleague, a pediatrician who suddenly began lactating after the death of her six-week-old infant whom she had not breastfed. Along with full breasts and dripping milk, she experienced uterine cramping. Abnormal milk secretion can be caused by several drugs, for example reserpine, methyldopa, and phenothiazines (see Chapter 6) or by the use of intrauterine devices containing copper (Horn & Scott, 1969).

Surprisingly, only 30% of women with galactorrhea have higher than normal prolactin levels (Frantz, Kleinberg & Noel, 1972); these women are otherwise healthy and have no history of menstrual irregularity or of infertility. It is suggested that these women may be excessively sensitive to normal circulating prolactin levels (Friesen & Cowden, 1989). For other women, galactorrhea is a symptom of a larger problem of hyperprolactinemia; in addition to a spontaneous milk secretion, they may also complain of amenorrhea, difficulty in becoming pregnant, and lack of libido. Any woman with persistent galactorrhea should be referred to a physician for a thorough physical exam and biochemical assessment.

CLINICAL IMPLICATIONS

BREAST ASSESSMENT

Usually little attention is given to prenatal assessment of the breast and nipples because of cultural inhibitions about the breast and physicians' lack of recognition of its importance. As a consequence, mothers may experience unnecessary feeding difficulties after delivery which could have been prevented. Nurses and lactation consultants practicing as primary care-givers are the ideal persons to do a prenatal breast assessment, particularly since physicians (especially male ones) often are reluctant to do so.

Ideal for teaching as well as for data gathering, physical assessment of the breast and nipples is done by both inspection and palpation. In inspecting the breasts, the following observations and questions are relevant.

Inspection. Size, symmetry, and shape of the breasts proper have minimal effect on lactation. The assessment provides the opportunity to reassure the woman with small breasts that she will be able to breastfeed and have a sufficient supply of milk. It should also be pointed out that having one breast larger or smaller than the other is usually normal. *Marked* asymmetry may be an indication of inadequate glandular tissue in a small minority of women. Inadequate glandular tissue may prevent the mother from being able to exclusively breastfeed; however, she can continue to enjoy the breastfeeding relationship if she provides the baby with additional nutrition while feeding from the breast (Neifert, Seacat & Jobe, 1985).

For the woman with large breasts, discussing the importance of a support bra and where it may be obtained is helpful. Holding and feeding her infant will not be the same for her as for mothers with average-sized breasts. Instead of simply holding the breast, the mother with large breasts may need to lift her breast and to hold or push part of the breast back for her infant to grasp the nipple and maintain an adequate airway. During this discussion, she may talk about some of her deeper feelings about having large breasts and her decision to breastfeed.

The skin of the breast should be inspected for any deviations. Skin turgor and elasticity can be assessed by gently pinching the skin, although the effect of elasticity on lactation is questionable. Women with previous pregnancies have more elastic skin, since it has been stretched from a previous pregnancy; women pregnant for the first time have firmer tissue.

A lateral incision in the vicinity of the cutaneous branch of the fourth intercostal nerve (left breast, 5 o'clock position; right breast, 7 o'clock position) from augmentation or reduction surgery may mean severed innervation of the nipple and areola (Farina, Newby & Alani, 1980). Surgery on the breast, especially if it involves an incision at the areola margin, is likely to interfere to some degree with milk production. However, even with such surgery, breastfeeding is possible for the majority of mothers. Breast reduction surgery, because of the greater likelihood of the movement and replacement of nipple tissue, is more likely than augmentation surgery to negatively influence later lactation performance (Neifert et al., 1990). Scar tissue from injury should be evaluated for its effect on skin elasticity and the degree to which nerve reactivity may have been affected.

Note should also be taken of any skin thickening and dimpling of the breast or nipple tissue. Although rare in a woman of childbearing age, such a change could be an early sign of a tumor.

Now is the time to ask, "Have your breasts grown during pregnancy?" Also inquire, "Have you had any tenderness and soreness?" An increase in breast size, swelling, and tenderness usually indicates adequately functioning breast tissue responsive to hormonal changes.

Next the nipple should be carefully inspected. (For the purpose of this discussion "nipple" includes the areola as well as the nipple shaft and pores.) If the nipples appear small, explain that the size of a woman's nipples is of secondary importance to their functional ability. Likewise, any nipple structural abnormality such as inversion should be assessed only in terms of its function. The look of the breast does not dictate its ability to function. A case in point may be seen in women who have sustained significant scarring from burns (see color plate). Second and third degree burns rarely extend so deeply into the parenchyma that they destroy the glandular tissue of the breast, even when the burns have occurred after adulthood. Significant scarring of the dermis and epidermis, however, may result in: (1) reduced sensation when the infant suckles; (2) minimal elasticity, thus requiring the mother to alter the baby's position at breast; and (3) reduced milk ejection if a nipple has been surgically reconstructed. Nevertheless, scar tissue on the breast or nipple does not, by itself, preclude breastfeeding.

Palpation.   After thorough hand washing, assess the nipple by compressing or palpating the areola between the forefinger and the thumb just behind the base of the nipple (the "pinch test"). This action simulates the compression that occurs when the infant is at breast. Because of possible nipple adhesions within the underlying connective tissue, a nipple that initially appears everted may retract inward on stimulation. Conversely, a nipple that appears flattened or inverted may, on palpation, evert; therefore a differentiation must be made between structure and function in assessing the nipples.

The classification of nipple function in Table 4–1

TABLE 4–1   CLASSIFICATION OF NIPPLE FUNCTION (SEE FIG. 4–11)

Protraction	Nipple moves forward; considered a normal functional response. No special interventions are needed.
Retraction	Instead of protracting, the nipple moves inward.
Minimal	An infant with a strong suck exerts sufficient pressure to pull the nipple forward. A weak or premature infant may have difficulties at first.
Moderate to severe	Retracts to a level even with or behind the surrounding areola. Intervention is helpful to stretch the nipple outward and improve protractility.
Inversion	On visual inspection all or part of the nipple is drawn inward within the folds of the areola.
Simple	The nipple moves outward to protraction with manual pressure or when cold (pseudoinversion).
Complete	The nipple does not respond to manual pressure because adhesions bind the nipple inward; very rarely there is congenital absence of the nipple.

is suggested as a standard terminology. It must be emphasized that although many primgravida women (Hytten, 1954; Waller, 1957) have nipples that tend to retract during pregnancy, most evert easily by the end of pregnancy and do not interfere with breastfeeding.

CLASSIFICATION OF NIPPLE FUNCTION
When the nipple is compressed using the pinch test, it responds in one of the ways identified in Fig. 4–11. This response may reflect degree of function.

Although flat or retracted nipples rarely cause breastfeeding problems because they may be treatable during pregnancy, we will discuss them. Dysfunction can be present in one nipple while the other is perfectly normal, or it can be present in both nipples. Retraction or inversion can prevent the infant from effectively milking the lactiferous sinuses that lie beneath the areola. Retraction or simple inversion identified in early pregnancy, however, does

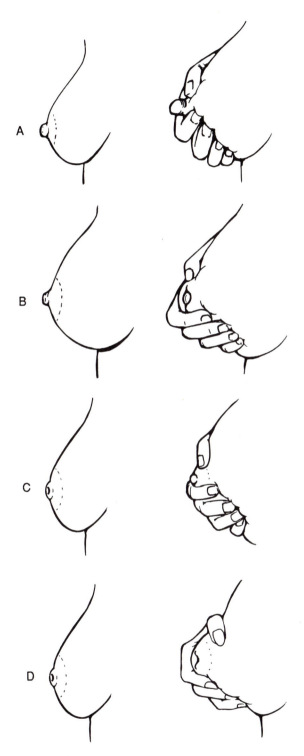

FIGURE 4–11 **A,** Protracting normal nipple. **B,** Moderate to severe retraction. **C,** Inverted-appearing nipple when compressed using pinch test will either invert farther inward or protract forward *(upper right)*. **D,** True inversion; nipple inverts further *(lower right)*.

not necessarily foretell later difficulty. The infant forms a "teat" not only from the nipple, but from surrounding breast tissue (Inch, 1989). When inversion is noted early in pregnancy, time is on the mother's side. As pregnancy progresses, hormonal changes increase the size and protractility of the nipples. She also has time to use interventions that help prevent subsequent feeding problems.

EARLY FREQUENT FEEDINGS

Encouraging early and frequent breastfeeding is a simple, low-cost recommendation contributing to a successful breastfeeding start (Johnson, 1976). If the infant is able to suckle effectively at the breast soon after birth, there is a direct relationship between the frequency and strength of suckling and subsequent availability of breastmilk. There appears to be an early "window of opportunity" for the infant's suckling to stimulate prolactin receptors (discussed earlier in this chapter) which, in turn, enhance milk production.

Salariya, Easton and Cater (1978) found that both early initiation of breastfeeding and frequent feedings thereafter contributed to longer breastfeeding duration. In their study, the group most likely to be breastfeeding at six weeks and at 12 weeks had begun breastfeeding within 10 minutes of delivery and continued to do so at two-hour intervals. The group least likely to be breastfeeding had a first breastfeed four to six hours after delivery and continued breastfeeding thereafter only every four hours. The authors concluded that early suckling had a stronger influence than did increased frequency of suckling, but that feeding every two hours helped to establish lactation sooner and to reduce the need for complementary feedings. They recommended putting the baby to breast as soon as possible after delivery—followed by two-hour feeds thereafter until lactation was well established, after which feeds on demand should continue.

Finally, a basic knowledge of anatomy and physiology is further put to valuable use when the lactation consultant or nurse translates basic concepts into easily understandable teaching materials for mothers and fathers such as those lesson plans covered in Chapter 8 on breastfeeding education and teaching. If a client understands that the reason for placing her baby as far back onto her areola as possible is because her milk is stored behind the nipple in "holding" containers (called lactiferous sinuses), then she will be more likely to do so. If a client realizes that a stressful environment may inhibit her milk supply, she can take action to reduce stressful situations over which she has control. Examples of the application of basic biologic principles of maternal lactation are legion and form the basis of many of the chapters that follow.

THE INFANT

The infant performs a series of complex oral movements to obtain sufficient nutriment from his mother's breast to meet daily nutritional requirements and to support his rapid growth, especially during the first few months of life. Suckling is a dynamic process, continually adjusting to a changing anatomy. The act of suckling involves far more than simply obtaining food. Bosma (1972) contends that "the infant's earliest autonomous functions are focused about his mouth and pharynx area, which is the principal site of interaction with his environment. The mouth is the cockpit of his awareness and of his most discriminate responses."

NEWBORN ORAL DEVELOPMENT

In the embryo, facial and pharyngeal regions develop from neural crest cells at about the time of neural tube closure. Further development is due to tissue differentiation from the endoderm, which later forms the digestive tract. During gestation, the fetus is able to swallow fluid as early as 11 weeks (Miller, 1982) and has a suck reflex at 24 weeks (Herbst, 1981). The rooting response and the linkage of sucking to swallowing is established by 32 weeks (Amiel-Tison, 1967; Bu'Lock, Woolridge & Baum, 1990). While these abilities are present relatively early in fetal development, the combination of sucking, swallowing, and breathing is not well coordinated until about 37 weeks (Bu'Lock, Woolridge & Baum, 1990).

At birth, the infant's mouth is vertically short in comparison with that of the adult. There is so little room that when the newborn's mouth is closed, the tongue is in lateral contact with the gums and with the roof of the mouth. There are other proportional differences in size and shape between the infant and the adult skull. (See Figs. 4–12 and 4–13.) The infant's lower jaw (mandible) is small and somewhat

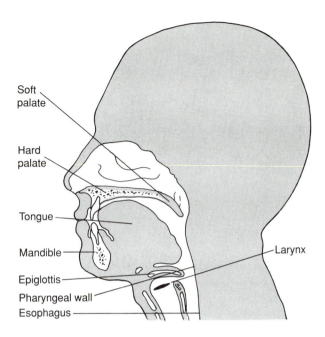

FIGURE 4–12 Midsagittal section of cranial and oral anatomy of an adult swallowing.

receded. Whereas the adult's hard palate is deeply arched and situated on a higher plane relative to the base of the skull, the infant's is short, wide and only slightly arched at birth. Corrugated transverse folds (rugae) on the hard palate assist the newborn in holding the breast during suckling.

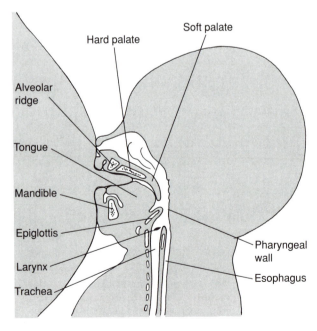

FIGURE 4–13 Midsagittal section of cranial and oral anatomy of an infant swallowing.

Because the infant's tongue fills his small oral cavity, the extent and the direction of tongue movement is limited. Taste buds on the tongue (mostly on tongue tip) are present at birth but the newborn has an increased suckling response only to sweet taste. The entire surface of the tongue is within the oral cavity. The infant's lips are well adapted to effect an airtight closure around the breast. The lips are partially everted so that the oral mucosa presents slightly externally; they have tiny swellings on the inner surface (eminences of the pars villosa) that facilitate holding the breast and areola in place (Bosma & Showacre, 1975; Ardran, Kemp & Lind, 1958).

During the first year after birth, the lower jaw grows downward creating a larger intraoral space. The tongue also gradually descends. By the fourth or fifth year of age, the tongue is attached directly to the epiglottis of the larynx. The frenulum is a fold of mucous membrane midline on the undersurface of the tongue that helps to anchor the tongue to the floor of the mouth. If the frenulum is too short for freedom of tongue movement, or placed too far forward for tongue extension upward or forward, it can interfere with the infant's ability to suckle (Notestine, 1990).

The infant's epiglottis lies just below the soft palate, unlike in the adult's, as seen in Fig. 4–13. This makes it possible for food to move laterally on the outside of the epiglottis and pass directly into the esophagus. The epiglottis plays an important role by closing off the pathway to the lungs when the infant swallows. This ensures that the milk will travel into the esophagus, rather than into the trachea. Relative to an adult larynx, the infant larynx is much higher in the oral cavity and occupies a larger space. It is short and funnel shaped (Crelin, 1973). As fluid passes through the mouth, the larynx elevates so that fluid can easily move into the pharynx. Because the larynx is high and elevated during swallowing, it is much less dependent upon the action of the epiglottis and upon closure of the vocal folds to protect the airway (Morris, 1982). The shape of the pharynx gradually changes as the child grows. At birth the pharynx curves very gradually downward to join the oral cavity. This curvature would prevent articulate speech even if the necessary central nervous system linkage were present. By puberty, the posterior walls of the nasal and oral segments join almost at a right angle.

The infant has pads of fat on both cheeks to assist with suckling. Each pad is a circumscribed layer of fat enclosed within its own capsule of fibrous connective tissue. It lies between the buccinator and masseter muscles. It is thought that buccal fat pads provide stability for suckling and reduce the likelihood of collapsing of the cheeks and buccinator muscles between the gums. When babies suck their own tongues, the degree of negative pressure is such that pulling in of the cheeks occurs, creating a characteristic dimpling. Collapsing of the cheeks is more likely in a premature baby who lacks the layer of fat (including that in the cheeks) that gives the full-term infant his characteristic plump facial appearance.

SUCKLING VS. SUCKING

The precise way in which an infant uses his oral/facial muscles to efficiently take in nourishment from his mother's breasts is vital information for health professionals, because some breastfeeding infants have initial difficulty getting on the breast, and a few continue to have suckling dysfunction. In a remarkable study of spontaneous feeding behavior (Widstrom et al., 1987) infants were placed in a prone position between their mother's breasts after an unmedicated delivery. The infants began sucking and rooting movements at an average of 15 minutes, hand-to-mouth movements at an average of 34 minutes, and spontaneously began to suckle after 55 minutes.

Does the infant suckle or suck at the breast? The words sucking and suckling are used interchangeably in much of the literature, although some individuals strongly prefer one term over the other. We use the two words interchangeably in this text.

> In the literature generally "sucking" and "suckling" are not distinguished, the terms being used indiscriminately and interchangeably to refer to "suckling." The baby is said to "suck" at its mother's nipple. The baby knows better than to do anything so foolish, for were he to "suck" the nipple all he would, for the most part, succeed in achieving would be to produce a partial vacuum in his mouth and fail to develop the ability to suckle properly. A baby sucks at the nozzle on the top of a bottle, but at the mother's breast a baby suckles.*

Traditionally, the baby "sucked," while the mother "suckled." When breastfeeding fell out of favor in the

*From Montagu, Ashley. In Raphael, D: *Breastingfeeding and Food Policy in a Hungry World,* New York, Academic Press, Inc., pp. 189–93.

United States, so did the word "suckle," because mothers were no longer suckling. Yet the word has not been out of use for so long that we have completely forgotten it. It hangs around the fringes of our collective memory, without our being quite sure of its meaning. Now that breastfeeding has made somewhat of a resurgence, and we have discovered that the mechanism by which babies extract milk from the breast differs considerably from the method they use on the bottle, we feel the need for separate words which differentiate the two acts. The word "suckle" would seem ideal to describe breastfeeding, and it has come to be used that way in modern American breastfeeding literature. The problem, however, is that it still retains its original meaning in the breastfeeding literature of many of the British Commonwealth countries.

Suck: (1) The action or an act of sucking milk from the breast; the milk or other fluid sucked at one time (p. 89).
      (2) To apply the lips to a teat, breast, the mother, nurse, or dam, for the purpose of extracting milk from, with the mouth (p. 90).
Suckle: (1) Transitive. To give suck to; to nurse (a child) at the the breast.
      (2) To cause to take milk from the breast or udder; to put to suck (p. 94).*

Physical therapy literature in the United States has adopted "suckling" to denote action to obtain breastmilk by an infant under four to six months and the word "sucking" to mean breastfeeding after that time. The shift in terminology, according to physical therapists, highlights the changes that occur in the infant's use of his mouth and tongue after the early months of life. Suckling describes the early stripping action on the areola and breast when tongue peristalsis moves from front to back. Morris (1982) calls it "a lick type of suck." As the first mid-year of life approaches, the oral space changes, both structurally and in the way an infant feeds. The oral cavity vertically elongates so that it is more spacious. The palate and epiglottis are no longer in apposition. The infant's tongue begins to elevate and to acquire a forward-backward movement; thus, it is possible for the infant to accept solid foods without choking. By six months, the baby's lips become more functional,

his neurological system matures, and he is able to make a variety of sounds (Morris, 1982).

Some experienced clinicians (Marmet, personal communication, 1990; Scott, personal communication, 1990) disagree, arguing that the infant's sucking pattern on the breast does not change over time at all. Instead, as infants develop, they become more versatile and develop a much wider repertoire of oral abilities, including the ability to carry a bolus of food from the front of the mouth to the back and swallow it. But they suck or suckle the same way they always have.

Babies suckle and swallow at a frequency of about once per second or faster when breastmilk is actively flowing. This rate is similar to that of other primates. If the milk flow lessens or stops, the infant will increase his rate to about two suckles per second (Wolff, 1968). In other words, when the milk flow increases, the rate of suckling decreases. Conversely, when milk flow is low, the rate of suckling is higher. Inch and Garforth (1989) describe the suckling rhythm as follows:

> When the baby first goes to the breast, short fast bursts of sucking can be observed. During this period no milk is flowing and unrelieved suction is applied to the surface of the nipple. Once the milk begins to flow it fills the oral cavity and relieves the negative pressure. As soon as this happens, the sucking pattern changes, and long, slow, continuous sucking supervenes. Very little milk transfer is necessary to cause the shift away from short, fast, continuous suckling.

Drewett and Woolridge (1979) observed that suckling rates fluctuate at different stages of the feeding and that the suckling rates are greater than that reported by Wolff (1968). The rate is 72.4 sucks/min during the first two minutes of feeding. It drops at two to four minutes to 70.8 sucks/min, and increases again to 73.3 and 74.9 sucks/minute at four to seven and seven to ten minutes.

Wolff (1968) originally defined two categories of suckling: nutritive (full and continuous milk flow) and non-nutritive (alternating suckling bursts and rests during minimal milk intake). Bowen-Jones, Thompson, and Drewett (1982). challenged the validity of these two categories. Their study showed that breastfeeding babies *always* suckle in bursts, with resting periods between bursts. If these resting

*From *The Oxford English Dictionary*, Volume X, "Sole/Sz," Oxford, 1961, The Clarendon Press.

periods are long, and only a small amount of milk is transferred, we call it "comfort nursing." The term "non-nutritive suckling" is now accepted to mean either (1) spontaneous suckling without anything being introduced into the infant's mouth (common during sleep), or (2) suckling prompted by something being introduced into the infant's mouth other than a liquid nutriment, e.g., a pacifier (McBride & Danner, 1987).

Non-nutritive suckling has important implications for development, especially under special circumstances such as prematurity. Measel and Anderson (1979) examined the effect of nonnutritive suckling in prematures and discovered that it increases peristalsis, enhances secretion of digestive fluids, and decreases crying in these infants. For more information about premature infant suckling patterns, see Chapter 10 on high-risk infants.

Several clinicians have examined the suckling process in great detail. With the advent of ultrasonography, it is now possible to accurately quantify suckling patterns, replacing earlier descriptions that only inferred what actually occurred. Detailed descriptions of infant suckling mechanics have been described by Morris (1982), Marmet and Shell (1984), Woolridge (1986), McBride and Danner (1987), and Smith et al. (1985). The following description of functional suckling at the breast is based on the work of these investigators. Figure 4–14 illustrates suckling movements.

1. The nipple and its surrounding areola and underlying breast tissue is drawn deeply into the infant's mouth; then the infant's lips and cheeks form a seal. The infant's lips are flanged outward around the mother's breast and are minimally involved.
2. The tip of the infant's tongue is maintained behind the lower lip and over the lower gum while the rest of the anterior tongue cups the areola of the breast.
3. During the feeding, the mother's nipple and areola elongates into a teat by suction created within the baby's mouth. The nipple extends back as far as the junction between the hard and soft palates. At its base, it is held between the upper gum and tongue, which covers the lower gum. The mother's nipple and areola tissue undergoes extensive changes during feeding.

Highly elastic, the nipple elongates about two to three times its resting length.

4. The jaw moves the tongue up, compressing the maternal areola against the infant's alveolar ridge which causes milk to be expressed from the lactiferous sinuses into the infant's mouth.
5. As the anterior portion of the tongue is raised, the posterior tongue is depressed and retracted in undulating or peristaltic motions, forming a groove that channels the milk to the back of the oral cavity where it stimulates receptors that initiate the swallowing reflex. This backward movement produces a negative pressure, similar to withdrawing a piston in an airtight syringe.
6. If the volume of milk taken is sufficient to trigger swallowing, the back of the tongue elevates and presses against the posterior pharyngeal wall. The soft palate rises and closes off the nasal passageways. The larynx then moves up and forward to close the trachea, propelling the milk into the esophagus. Afterwards the larynx returns to its previous position.
7. The infant lowers his jaw, the lactiferous sinuses refill and a new cycle begins. A rhythm is created by this sequence of vertical jaw movements and the depression and elevation of the posterior tongue. Each suck sequence is followed by a swallow. McBride and Danner (1987) describe the normal suck-swallow pattern:

As milk in the sinuses is depleted, several sucking sequences may occur before each swallow. The sucking-swallowing sequence is repeated approximately once per second in continuous fashion as long as milk is present and the infant is hungry. If the first one or two sucking sequences do not yield a palatable liquid, the normal infant will open and close his mouth in a tremorlike movement. The rapid jaw movement and the infant's tongue and lips stimulate tactile nerve endings in the mother's areola, initiating the release of oxytocin from her pituitary gland.

There are profound differences between bottle-feeding and breastfeeding as shown in Table 4–2. Generally, compared with bottle-feeding, breastfeeding infants suckle more times/day and maintain a higher level of oxygen pressure ($tcPO_2$) and skin temperature (Meier & Anderson, 1987; Mathew,

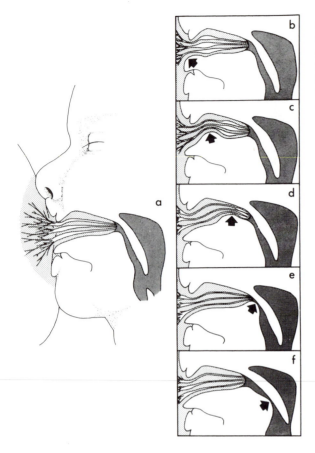

FIGURE 4–14   Shows a complete 'suck' cycle; the baby is shown in median section. The baby exhibits good feeding technique with the nipple drawn well into the mouth, extending back to the junction of the hard and soft palate (the lactiferous sinuses are depicted within the teat though these cannot be visualised on scans).

a. 'Teat' is formed from the nipple and much of the areola, with the lacteal sinuses, which lie behind the nipple, being drawn into the mouth with the breast tissue. The soft palate is relaxed and the nasopharynx is open for breathing. The shape of the tongue at the back represents its position at rest, cupped around the tip of the nipple.

b. The suck cycle is initiated by a welling up of the anterior tip of the tongue. At the same time, the lower jaw, which had been momentarily relaxed (not shown), is raised to constrict the base of the nipple, thereby 'pinching off' milk within the ducts of the teat (these movements are inferred as they lie outside the sector viewed in ultrasound scans).

c. The wave of compression by the tongue moves along the underside of the nipple in a posterior direction, pushing against the hard palate. This roller-like action squeezes milk from the nipple. The posterior portion of the tongue may be depressed as milk collects in the oropharynx.

d. & e. The wave of compression passes back past the tip of the nipple and pushes against the soft palate. As the tongue impinges on the soft palate the levator muscles of the palate contract raising it to seal off the nasal cavity. Milk is pushed into the oropharynx and is swallowed if sufficient has collected.

f. The cycle of compression continues and ends at the posterior base of the tongue. Depression of the back portion of the tongue creates negative pressure drawing the nipple and its milk contents once more into the mouth. This is accompanied by a lowering of the jaw which allows milk to flow back into the nipple.

In ultrasound scans it appears that compression by the tongue, and negative pressure within the mouth, maintain the tongue in close conformation to the nipple and palate. Events are portrayed here rather more loosely to aid clarity. From Woolridge, MW: The 'anatomy' of infant sucking, *Midwifery* 2:164–71, 1986.

TABLE 4–2   COMPARISONS BETWEEN BREASTFEEDING AND BOTTLE-FEEDING IN FULL-TERM INFANTS

Breastfeeding	Bottle-feeding	References
More frequent suckling/min Continuous suckling = 88 Intermittent suckling = 80	Less frequent suckling/min Continuous suckling = 63 Intermittent suckling = 58	Mathew, 1988
Breathing patterns Shortening of expiration Prolonging of inspiration	Breathing patterns Prolonged expiration Shortening of inspiration	Mathew, 1988
Oxygen saturation below 90% 2 out of 10 infants	Oxygen saturation below 90% 5 out of 10 infants	Mathew, 1988
Bradycardia 0 out of 10 infants	Bradycardia 2 out of 10 infants	Mathew, 1988
Extended opening of mouth to grasp mother's nipple	Less extension to grasp rubber teat	Maher, 1988
Infant's lips flanged outward, re-laxed and resting against the breast to make a seal	Lips closer together and pursed to maintain contact with rubber teat	McBride and Danner, 1987
Extensive mandibular (jaw) action	Minimal mandibular action	Maher, 1988
Tongue grooved around nipple; remains under nipple throughout feed; moves in peristaltic action from front to back	Tongue upward and thrust forward against end of teat, "piston-like," to control milk flow	Weber, Woolridge, and Baum, 1986 Woolridge, 1986 Marmet and Shell, 1984
Silent, except for soft swallow sounds, and (in older infants), coo-ing or "singing" sounds of pleasure	High-pitched squeak at end of intake of air prior to new suck	
Duration of feeding varies from short (few minutes) to long (30 minutes or longer)	Duration of feeding is usually 5–10 minutes	Ardan, Kemp, and Lind, 1958
Includes nutritive and non-nutri-tive suckling throughout the feed but less distinct differences	Involves nearly exclusively nutritive suckling	Woolridge, 1986

1988). The differences between bottle-feeding and breastfeeding premature infants are even greater. Meier and Pugh (1985) describe these differences from viewing videotapes of premature infants nurs-ing at the the breast and feeding from a bottle:

> For example, the infants had to open their mouths more widely to breast-feed than to bottle feed. Once they became accustomed to making this adjustment during breast-feeding, they attempted to do it while bottle-feeding. As a result, wide gaps could be seen between the commercial nipple and an infant's mouth during bottle-feedings, and "smacking" sounds could be heard while the infant was sucking.

Meier describes suckling patterns of premature in-fants in depth in Chapter 10, which deals with the high-risk infant.

BREATHING AND SUCKLING

In a normal, coordinated, nutritive suckling cycle, swallowing does not inhibit respiration, and breathing appears to continue throughout the suckling cycle (Morris, 1982), despite the assertion of Ardran, Kemp, and Lind (1958) that at the onset of the swallow, as the bulk of the bolus enters the pharynx, airflow is momen-tarily interrupted and then restored. Breathing move-ments appear related in a 1:1:1 sequence in a perfectly coordinated cycle of suckling, swallowing and breath-ing (Bu'Lock, Woolridge & Baum, 1990; Weber, Woolridge & Baum, 1986; Wolff, 1968). During unco-ordinated feedings, breathing is interrupted by swal-lowing and may be subordinate to it (Halverson, 1944; Logan & Bosma, 1976; Johnson & Salisbury, 1977).

Although suckling, swallowing, and breathing are generally well coordinated during a feeding, infant cyanosis is a relatively common event, especially in neonates. The neonate almost always recovers spontaneously (Mathew, 1988, p. 553) and often continues to suck and swallow despite cyanosis.

Unless hypoxic, the newborn is an obligate nose breather. This is due in part to the positioning of the soft palate, and to the lack of space in the mouth for air to be traveling in and out (Morris, 1982). While it is true that babies have ventilatory problems when the nasal passages are occluded, an infant is capable of breathing through the mouth when it is necessary (Rodenstein, Perlmutter & Stanescu, 1985).

CLINICAL IMPLICATIONS

The ability to suckle, even in many full-term infants, is not fully developed at birth and can be inhibited by drugs given to the mother during childbirth. Usually after several attempts, the infant latches on the breast and begins to suckle vigorously and effectively. These first feedings are critical because they imprint a suckling pattern that tends to be repeated in subsequent feedings.

SUCKLING ASSESSMENT
The infant's first few breastfeedings should be observed early in the neonatal period. Such observation enables the health-care worker to determine how well the infant roots, fixes, or latches on, and suckles the breast. Minor adjustments of maternal position or infant position can be made without interrupting or interfering with the mother and infant as they begin to learn how to breastfeed together.

If the infant cannot suckle the breast at all after several attempts, a visual evaluation and a digital examination may be appropriate. The roof of the mouth should be wide and gently domed. The tongue should be long enough to extend over the lower gum line, but not so long that it protrudes past the lips. The baby's response to a feather-light stroking of the center of the lower lip should be noted. In most cases, the infant who is alert will open his mouth wide and the tongue will come forward in response to such stimulation, as if seeking its source. The infant's frenulum (the small tissue tag under the tongue) should be far enough away from the tip of the tongue to prevent stricture during suckling. If it appears tight, a visual examination should be done to determine if the

frenulum prevents the tongue from elevating or extending sufficiently to produce the wave-like motion necessary for effective suckling (Marmet, Shell & Marmet, 1990).

When a finger is slid into the baby's mouth, the hard palate should feel intact. The tongue should groove around the finger. When the pad of the finger lightly touches the palate, the baby usually initiates a suck response that includes stroking by the tongue on the underside of the finger from knuckle to nail edge. In a healthy newborn, the strength of oral negative pressure is such that the examiner will feel as if the nailbed is being pulled deeper into the baby's mouth. The nature of the suckling action should be rhythmic, although some neonates quickly realize that the finger does not reward suckling and they cease doing so after several attempts.

Because the finger is not a breast with its soft areolar and nipple tissue, suckling at the breast should be the *first* experience of the infant if at all possible. Thereafter, a finger assessment may be attempted, although it is not necessary in most cases and should be used judiciously.

Even if the baby is found to have an anatomical variation, it may not interfere with effective suckling. However, any infant with a cleft palate, high palatal arch, or a short tongue may need interventions, most often provided by a team (physician, physical therapist, or speech therapist), in order to suckle. Marmet and Shell (1984) as well as McBride and Danner (1987) describe sequential steps to retrain dysfunctional suckling.

SUMMARY

Knowledge of maternal breast anatomy and the psychophysiology of lactation are necessary antecedents to clinical practice. The fundamental biologic principles of lactation discussed in this section are used, although not always consciously, in almost every clinical situation where lactation is involved. Knowledge of the structure and function of the normal breast and of infant suckling is necessary for appropriate assessment; knowing what is normal must precede recognizing the abnormal and recommending actions designed to support an optimal breastfeeding experience. Cooperation with the natural physiological mechanisms is more likely to lead to an uncomplicated breastfeeding experience; interference with these mechanisms can result in difficulty with breastfeeding for mother and/or infant.

At the same time, anatomy and physiology are but the building blocks in a larger picture of the breast-feeding/lactation experience. Physiologically most women are equipped to produce sufficient milk for their infant or infants. Yet the most commonly cited problem in breastfeeding in the United States, if not the world, is the mother's perception that she has an insufficient milk supply (Hill & Humenick, 1989). Social and cultural influences play a major role in the mother's perceptions of her ability to nourish her infant from her breasts. Succeeding chapters will explore the myriad of social, cultural, and psychologic aspects of breastfeeding.

REFERENCES

Agius, OL, and Williamson, DH: Lipogenesis in interscapular brown adipose tissue of virgin, pregnant, and lactating rats, *Biochem J* 190:447, 1980.

Akre, J: Infant feeding: The physiological basis, *World Health Organization Bulletin* (suppl.) vol. 67, Geneva, 1989.

Amiel-Tison, C: Neurological evaluation of the maturity of newborn infant, *Arch Dis Child* 43:89, 1967.

Ardran, GM, Kemp, MB, and Lind, J: A cineradiographic study of breast feeding, *Brit J Radiology* 31:156–62, 1958.

Arthur, PG, et al.: Measuring short-term rates of milk synthesis in breast-feeding mothers, *Quart J Exp Physiology* 74:419–28, 1989.

Baron, JA, et al.: Cigarette smoking and prolactin in women, *Br Med J* 293:482, 1986.

Battin, D, et al.: Effect of suckling on serum prolactin, luteinizing hormone, follicle-stimulating hormone, and estradiol during prolonged lactation, *Obstet Gynecol* 65:785–88, 1985.

Blaikeley, J, et al.: Breastfeeding—factors affecting success, *J Obstet Gynaec Brit Emp* 60:657–69, 1953.

Bohnet HG, and Kato, K: Prolactin secretion during pregnancy and puerperium: Response to metoclopramide and interactions with placental hormones, *Obstet Gynecol* 65:789–92, 1985.

Bonnar, J, et al.: Effect of breast-feeding on pituitary-ovarian function after childbirth, *Br Med J* 4:82–84, 1975.

Bosma, J: Form and function in the infant's mouth and pharynx. In Bosma, J, ed.: *Third symposium on oral sensation and perception*, Springfield, Ill., 1982, Charles C Thomas, Publisher, pp. 3–29.

Bosma, J, and Showacre, J: *Development of upper respiratory anatomy and function*, Rockville, Md., 1975, U.S. Dept. of Health, Education and Welfare, pp. 5–49.

Bowen-Jones, A, Thompson, C, and Drewett, RF: Milk flow and sucking rates during breast-feeding, *Dev Med Child Neurol* 24:626–33, 1982.

Bu'Lock, F, Woolridge, MW, and Baum, JD: Development of co-ordination of sucking, swallowing and breathing: Ultrasound study of term and preterm infants, *Dev Med Child Neurol* 32:669–78, 1990.

Chao, S: The effect of lactation on ovulation and fertility. In Lawrence, R, ed.: Breastfeeding, *Clin Perinatol* 14(1):39–49, 1987.

Clemente, CD: *Anatomy: A Regional Atlas of the Human Body*, Philadelphia, 1978, Lea and Febiger.

Clemente, CD: *Gray's anatomy* (30th ed.), Philadelphia, 1985, Lea & Febiger, pp. 1580–86.

Courtiss, EH, and Goldwyn, RM: Breast sensation before and after plastic surgery, *Plast Reconstr Surg* 58(1):1–12, 1976.

Crelin, ES: *Functional anatomy of the newborn*, New Haven, 1973, Yale University Press, pp. 27–33.

Dabelow, A: Die Milchdruse. In Bargmann, W, ed.: *Handbuch der Mikroskopischen Anatomic des Menschen*, vol. 3, part 3, Haut und sinnes organs, Berlin, 1957, Springer-Verlag, pp. 277–85.

Dawood, MY, et al.: Oxytocin release and plasma anterior pituitary and gonadal hormones in women during lactation, *J Clin Endocrinol Metab* 52:678–83, 1981.

Dawson, EK: A histological study of the normal mamma in relation to tumour growth. 1. Early development to maturity, *Edinb Med J* 41:653–82, 1934.

DeCarvalho, MD, et al.: Effect of frequent breast-feeding on early milk production and infant weight gain, *Pediatrics* 72:307–11, 1983.

DeRosa, G, et al.: Prolactin secretion after beer, *Lancet* 2:934, 1981.

Diefenbach, WP, et al.: Suppression of prolactin secretion by L-dopa in the stalk-sectioned rhesus monkey, *J Clin Endocrinol Metab* 43:638, 1976.

Division of Ultrasound, Dept of Radiology & Dept. of Pathology. *Atlas of Breast Ultrasound*, Philadelphia: Thomas Jefferson University Medical College & Hospital, 1980, p. 121.

Drewett, RF, and Woolridge, M: Sucking patterns of human babies on the breast, *Early Hum Dev* 315:315–21, 1979.

Edgerton, MT, and McClary, AR: Augmentation mammaplasty with special reference to use of polyvinyl alcohol sponge (Ivalon). Psychiatric implications and surgical indications, *Plast Reconstr Surg* 21:279, 1958.

Farina, MA, Newby, BG, and Alani, HM: Innervation to the nipple-areola complex, *Plast & Reconstruct Surg* 66(4):497–501, 1980.

Frantz, A, Kleinberg, DL, and Noel, G: Studies on prolactin in man, *Recent Prog Horm Res* 28:527–34, 1972.

Friesen, HG, and Cowden, EA: Lactation and galactorrhea. In DeGroot, LJ: *Endocrinology in Pregnancy*, Philadelphia, 1989, W.B. Saunders Co., pp. 2074–86.

Gehlbach, DL, Bayliss, P, and Rosa, C: Prolactin and thyrotropin responses to nursing during the early puerperium, *J Reprod Med* 34(4):295–98, 1989.

Gross, BA, and Eastman, DJ: Prolactin secretion during prolonged lactation amenorrhoea, *Aust NZ J Obstet Gynaecol* 19:95–99, 1979.

Halverson, HM: Mechanisms of early infant feeding, *J Genetic Psychol* 64:185–223, 1944.

Herbst, JJ: Development of suck and swallowing. In Lebenthal, E, ed.: *Textbook of gastroenterology and nutrition in infancy,* vol. 1, New York, 1981, Plenum Press, pp. 97–107.

Hill, PD, and Humenick, SS: Insufficient milk supply, *Image* 21:145–48, 1989.

Hinds, LA, and Tyndale-Biscoe, CH: Prolactin in the Marsupial *Macropus engenii* during the estrous cycle, pregnancy, and lactation, *Bio Reprod* 26:391–98, 1982.

Horn, HW, and Scott, JM: IUD insertion and galactorrhea, *Fertil Steril* 20:400–404, 1969.

Humenick, SS, and Van Steenkiste, S: Early indicators of breast-feeding progress, *Issues Comp Pediatr Nurs* 6:205–15, 1983.

Hytten, FE: Clinical and chemical studies in lactation IX: Breastfeeding in hospital, *Br Med J* 18:1447–52, 1954.

Hytten, FE, and Baird, D: The development of the nipple in pregnancy, *Lancet* 1:1201–4, 1958 (June 7).

Inch, S: Antenatal preparation for breastfeeding. In Enkin, M, and Keires, M, eds.: *Effective care in pregnancy and childbirth,* Oxford, 1989, Oxford University Press, pp. 335–42.

Inch, S, and Garforth, S: Establishing and maintaining breastfeeding. In Chalmers, I, Enkin, M, and Keirse, M, eds.: *Effective care in pregnancy and childbirth,* Oxford, 1989, Oxford University Press, pp. 1359–74.

Johnson, MW: Breastfeeding at one hour of age, *MCN* 1:12–16, 1976.

Johnson, P, and Salisbury, DM: Preliminary studies on feeding and breathing in the newborn. In Weiffenbach, JM, ed.: *Taste and Development: The genesis of sweet preference,* Department of Health, Education, and Welfare, Publ. No. (NIH)77–1068, Bethesda, Md., 1977, National Institutes of Health.

Johnstone, JM, and Amico, JA: A prospective longitudinal study of the release of oxytocin and prolactin in response to infant suckling in long term lactation, *J Clin Endocrinol Metab* 62:653–57, 1986.

Kopans, DB: *Breast imaging,* Philadelphia, 1989, J.B. Lippincott Co., p. 20.

La Leche League International: *The womanly art of breastfeeding* (5th ed.), Franklin Park, Ill., 1991, The League.

Leake, R, et al.: Oxytocin and prolactin responses in long-term breast-feeding, *Obstet Gynecol* 62:565–68, 1983.

Lincoln, DW, and Paisley, AC: Neuroendocrine control of milk ejection, *J Reprod Fertil* 65:571–86, 1982.

Lincoln, DW, and Renfrew, MB: Mammary gland growth and milk ejection in the Agile Wallaby, *Macropus afgilis,* displaying concurrent asynchronous lactation, *J Reprod Fertil* 63:193–96, 1981.

Logan, WJ, and Bosma, JF: Oral and pharyngeal dysphagia in infancy, *Pediatr Clin North Amer* 14:47–61, 1976.

Love, SM, and Lindsey, K: *Dr. Susan Love's breast book,* Reading, Mass., 1990, Addison-Wesley Publishing Co., Inc., pp. 3–20.

Maher, SM: An overview of solutions to breastfeeding and sucking problems. Franklin Park, Ill., La Leche League International, 1988, p. 4.

Marmet, C, and Shell, E: Training neonates to suck correctly, *MCN* 9:401–7, 1984.

Marmet, C, Shell, E, and Marmet, R: Neonatal frenotomy may be necessary to correct breastfeeding problems, *J Human Lact* 6:117–20, 1990.

Mathew, OP: Regulation of breathing patterns during feeding. In Mathew OP, and G. Sant Ambrogio, eds.: *Respiratory function of the upper airway,* New York, 1988, Marcel Dekker, Inc., pp. 535–60.

Mathew, OP, and Bhatia, J: Sucking and breathing patterns during breast- and bottle-feeding in term neonates, *Am J Dis Child* 143:588–92, 1989.

McBride, MC, and Danner, SC: Sucking disorders in neurologically impaired infants: Assessment and facilitation of breastfeeding, *Clin Perinatol* 14(1):109–30, 1987.

Measel, CP, and Anderson, GC: Nonnutritive suckling during tube feedings: Effect on clinical course in premature infants, *JOGNN* 8:265–72, 1979.

Meier, P, and Anderson, GC: Responses of small preterm infants to bottle- and breast-feeding, *MCN* 12:97–105, 1987.

Meier, P, and Pugh, EJ: Breast-feeding behavior in small preterm infants, *MCN* 10:396–401, 1985.

Miller, AJ: Deglutition, *Physiol Rev* 62:129–83, 1982.

Miyake, A, Tahara, M, and Tanizawa, O: *Eur J Obstet Gynecol Repro Bio* 33:49–53, 1989.

Montagu, A. In Raphael D, ed.: *Breastfeeding and Food Policy in a Hungry World,* New York: Academic Press Inc., 1979, pp. 189–193.

Morris, SE: *The normal acquisition of oral feeding skills: Implications for assessment and treatment,* New York, 1982, Therapeutic Media, pp. 19–29.

Neifert, M, et al.: The influence of breast surgery, breast appearance, and pregnancy-induced breast changes on lactation sufficiency as measured by infant weight gain, *Birth* 17:31–38, 1990.

Neifert, MR, Seacat, JM, and Jobe, WE: Lactation failure due to insufficient glandular development of the breast, *Pediatrics* 76(5):823–28, 1985.

Neville, MC, and Berga, SE: Cellular and molecular aspects of the hormonal control of mammary function: In Neville, MC, and Neifert, MR, eds.: *Lactation: Physiology, nutrition, and breast-feeding,* New York, 1983, Plenum Press, pp. 141–77.

Newton, M, and Newton, N: The let-down reflex in human lactation, *Pediatrics* 33:69–87, 1948.

Newton, M, and Newton, N: The normal course and management of lactation, *Clin Obstet Gynecol* 5:47, 1962.

Notestine, GE: The importance of the identification of ankyloglossia (short lingual frenulum) as a cause of breastfeeding problems, *J Hum Lact* 6:113–15, 1990.

Oxford English Dictionary, Volume X, "Sole/Sz." Oxford: Clarendon Press, 1961.

Prentice, A, et al.: Evidence for local feed-back control of human milk secretion, *Biochem Soc Trans* 17:489–92, 1989.

Riordan, J, and Rapp, E: Pleasure and purpose: the sensuousness of breastfeeding, *JOGNN* 9:109–12, 1980.

Rodenstein, DO, Perimutter, N, and Stanescu, DC: Infants are not obligatory nose breathers, *Am Rev Respir Dis* 131:343–47, 1985.

Russo, J, and Russo, IH: Development of the human mammary gland. In Neville, MD, and Daniel, CW, eds.: *The mammary gland: Development, regulation, and function,* New York, 1987, Plenum Press, pp. 67–93.

Salariya, EM, Easton, PM, and Cater, JI: Duration of breastfeeding after early initiation and frequent feeding, *Lancet* 2:1141–43, 1978.

Salazar, H, and Tobon, H: Morphologic changes of the mammary gland during development, pregnancy and lactation. In Josimovich, J, ed.: *Lactogenic hormones, fetal nutrition and lactation,* New York, 1974, Academic Press, Inc., pp. 1–18.

Sernia, C, and Tyndale–Biscoe, CH: Prolactin receptors in the mammary gland, corpus luteum and other tissues of the Tammar Wallaby, *Macropus engenii, J Endocrinol* 26:391–98, 1979.

Smith, WL, et al.: Physiology of sucking in the normal term infant using real-time ultrasound, *Radiology* 156:379–81, 1985.

Speroff, L, Glass, RH, and Kase, NG: *Clinical gynecologic endocrinology and infertility,* 4th ed., Baltimore, 1989, The Williams & Wilkins Co., pp. 283–311.

Tonelli, QJ, and Sorof, S: Epidermal growth factor requirement for development of cultured mammary gland, *Nature* 285:250–52, 1980.

Tyson, JE, et al.: Studies of prolactin in human pregnancy, *Am J Obstet Gynecol* 113:14–20, 1972.

Vorherr, H: Development of the female breast. In Vorrherr, H, ed.: *The Breast,* New York, 1974, Academic Press, Inc., pp. 1–18.

Waller, H: *The breasts and breastfeeding,* London, 1957, Heinemann, Medical Books.

Waller, H: The early failure of breastfeeding, *Arch Dis Child* 21:1–12, 1946.

Weber, F, Woolridge, MW, and Baum, JD: An ultrasonographic study of the organisation of sucking and swallowing by newborn infants, *Dev Med Child Neurology* 28:19–24, 1986.

West, CP: Hormonal profiles in lactating and non-lactating women immediately after delivery and their relationship to breast engorgement, *Am J Obstet Gynecol* 86:501–6, 1979.

Whitworth, NS: Lactation in humans, *Psychoneuroendocrinology* 13:171–88, 1988.

Widstrom, AM, et al.: Gastric suction in healthy newborn infants: Effects on circulation and developing feeding behaviour, *Acta Paediatr Scand.* 76:566–72, 1987.

Wolff, PH: The serial organization of sucking in the young infant, *Pediatrics* 42:943–956, 1968.

Woolridge, MW: The "anatomy" of infant sucking, *Midwifery* 2:164–71, 1986.

Yuen, BH: Prolactin in human milk: The influence of nursing and duration of postpartum lactation, *Am J Obstet Gynecol* 158:583–86, 1988.

Ziemer, M: Nipple skin changes during the first week of lactation. *JOGN Nurs* (in press, 1993).

Zuppa, AA, et al.: Relationship between maternal parity, basal prolactin levels and neonatal breast milk intake, *Biol Neonate* 53:144–47, 1988.

5

The Biologic Specificity
of Breastmilk

Breastmilk has been termed the perfect food for infants because it contains necessary nutrients in readily bioavailable forms while simultaneously providing many anti-infective components. Indeed, formula companies compete with one another by claiming that their product is "most like mother's milk." Moreover, breastmilk, like all other milks, is species-specific; it has been adapted throughout human existence to meet nutritional requirements of the human infant to ensure optimal growth, development, and survival.

Since the infant's birth weight normally requires about four to six months to double, the nutritional needs of the human baby must be substantially different from those of other mammals whose birth weight doubles much more rapidly. For example, a calf's birth weight is expected to double in six to seven weeks. Similar contrasts can be found across animal species.

Breastmilk has been referred to as "white blood" because it is considered similar to the placental blood of intrauterine life. Indeed, human milk is similar to unstructured living tissue such as blood, and it is capable of affecting biochemical systems, enhancing immunity, and even destroying pathogens. With the use of sophisticated laboratory techniques, many scientific investigators have substantiated the unique properties of human milk.

It is ironic that many of the complex properties of human milk described in this chapter have been identified through research funded by formula companies, which stand to make large sums of money if they can develop products for which they can claim a close resemblance to human milk.

JAN RIORDAN

MATURATIONAL CHANGES

Factors that influence milk composition are: stage of lactation, gestational age of the infant, age of the mother, the time frame (beginning or end) of the feed, and the baby's demand for milk. The stage of lactation is the most important factor affecting milk composition and volume. Lactogenesis is said to occur in two stages (Arthur, Smith & Hartmann, 1989). Stage one refers to the mammary gland developing the capacity to synthesize milk during late pregnancy. The second stage refers to the onset of copious milk secretion or the milk "coming in."

In the first stage colostrum predominates. The rate at which colostrum progressively changes to mature milk varies from mother to mother. The number of days postpartum has been shown to be an inadequate definition of colostrum. Humenick (1987) developed a Maturation Index of Colostrum and Milk (MICAM) to measure breastmilk maturation. (See Fig. 5–1.) She found that approximately 40% of women are producing late transitional milk at day 15, while others produce mature milk on day four. Mature milk is present in about one-half of women after approximately 10 days. She also showed that a faster milk maturation rate was associated with a greater infant weight gain at 28 days, and lower transcutaneous bilimeter readings.

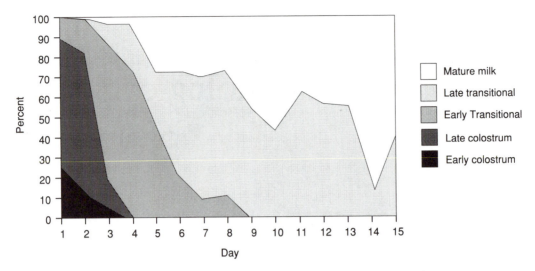

FIGURE 5–1   Milk type by day. (From Humenick, SS: The clinical significance of breast maturation rates, *Birth* 14(4):175, 1987.

Changes in concentrations of breastmilk lactose and citrate are markers of stage two of lactogenesis, or the onset of copious milk secretion which usually occurs between 24 and 48 hours after birth (Arthur, Smith & Hartmann, 1989).

Compared with mature milk, colostrum is more viscous, richer in protein and minerals, and poorer in carbohydrates, fat, and some vitamins. This high concentration of total protein and total ash (minerals) in colostrum gradually changes to reflect the infant's needs over the first few weeks as lactation becomes established. At the same time, it must be noted that the *total dose* of key components, such as immunoglobulins which the infant receives from breastmilk, *remains relatively constant throughout lactation* regardless of the amount of breastmilk provided by the mother. This happens because concentrations increase as total volume diminishes.

ENERGY, VOLUME AND GROWTH

Human milk is rich in nutrient proteins, nonprotein nitrogen compounds, lipids, oligosaccharides, vitamins, and certain minerals. In addition, it contains hormones, enzymes, growth factors, and many types of protective agents. Human milk contains about 10% solids for energy and growth; the rest is water, which is vital for maintaining hydration (Hamosh, 1985). Breastmilk is slightly acidic. The pH of colostrum is 7.45 and falls to a low of 7.0 during the second week of lactation. Thereafter the pH of milk remains at 7.0 and then rises gradually to 7.4 by 10 months. The significance of these changes during lactation is not known (Morriss et al., 1986).

CALORIC DENSITY

The caloric content or energy density of human milk is generally considered to be 65 kcal/100ml although published values differ. Garza et al. (1983) report 57.7/100 mL; Lepage et al. (1984) report 66.6; and Lemons et al. (1982) report 72.2. Using breastmilk as the "gold standard," the American Academy of Pediatrics (1976) recommends a calorie content of 67 kcal/100mL for commercial formulas.

Energy intakes of breastfed infants beyond the first month are *well below* the official Committee on Dietary Allowances (1980) and WHO/FAO (1980) recommendations. These state that infants should consume 115/kcal/kg/day up to six months, and 105 kcal/kg/day between six months and one year. Butte et al. (1984)—and Butte, Smith, and Garza (1990)—reported that during their first four months exclusively breastfed infants attained adequate growth with nutrient intakes substantially less than the current dietary recommendation. Likewise, Stuff and Nichols (1989) found that energy intake of infants fed human milk was about 20% below recommended levels. Caloric content did not increase after solid foods were added to the diet.

Wood et al. (1988) reported that breastmilk intake of 21 exclusively breastfed infants decreased significantly in terms of kcal/kg during the first five months of life for both sexes. Study infants were estimated to be receiving 128 kcal/kg at 14 days, but only 62.5 kcal/kg at five months. Garza, Stuff, and Butte (1986) found that energy intakes of breastfed infants remained approximately 70–75 kcal/kg from the third month on. Energy requirements have been overestimated for breastfed infants because they have been based on volumes of formula required by artificially fed infants.

The energy intakes of breastfed and formula-fed infants differ significantly. Total daily energy expenditure, minimal rates of energy expenditure, metabolic rates during sleep, rectal temperature, and heart rates are all found to be lower in breastfed infants. By eight months, breastfed infants have consumed about 30,000 kcal less than bottle-fed infants (Butte, Smith & Garza, 1990). Although this difference in energy intake should result in about a 2.7 kg mean difference of weight, such is not the case. To explain this discrepancy, Garza, Stuff, and Butte (1986) suggest that (1) differences in intake in the general population are not as great as those found in the babies studied; (2) energy expenditure differs substantially between breastfed and bottle-fed infants; or (3) composition of newly acquired tissue differs between these two groups. Another possibility is that the energy density of milk taken by a four-month-old is higher on the average than that taken by the same baby three months earlier. The four-month-old baby's suckle is more active, leading to a higher fat intake with lower volumes needed—i.e., breastmilk is more completely utilized with less wastage.

MILK VOLUME

The volume of milk must provide sufficient caloric energy to permit normal growth and development. Small amounts of colostrum, about 37 mL (range 7–123), are yielded in the first 24 hours postpartum (Hartmann & Prosser, 1984; Hartmann, 1987); the infant ingests approximately 7 to 14 mL at each feeding (Houston, Howie & McNeilly, 1983). This milk yield gradually increases for the first 36 hours, followed by a dramatic increase over the next 49 to 96 hours. By day five, volume is about 500 mL/day; it increases more slowly to about 750 mL/day during

months three to five of full breastfeeding, with a mean intake of about 800 mL/day at six months (Neville et al., 1988). These volumes are similar to others established by test weighing the infant (Dewey & Lonnerdal, 1983; Wood et al., 1988). By using pre- and post-feed weighings of infants, Dewey and Lonnerdahl (1983) found daily milk intake at one and six months to be 673 and 896 mL respectively, a difference of 223 mL per day. Likewise, Wood et al. (1988) found that the mean volume of milk intake of 21 study infants increased from 671 (day 15) to 789 mL during the first five months. As seen in Fig. 5–2, the volume of milk taken by thriving breastfed infants varies little over the first four months (Butte et al., 1984). Breastmilk intake slowly declines as other foods are added to the baby's diet.

There appear to be differences among women in the rate of milk synthesis. Arthur et al. (1989) measured the rate of milk synthesis in two women after breastfeeding and found that one synthesized milk at double the rate of the other. Studies indicate that the nutritional status of the mother does not affect milk volume unless the mother is severely malnourished (Neville & Oliva-Rasbach, 1987; Brown et al, 1986a; van Steenbergen et al., 1989; Forman et al., 1990). Even while fasting during Ramadan, Gambian women continued to supply their infants with sufficient milk by superhydrating themselves overnight (Prentice et al., 1984b).

Breastmilk volume varies widely from woman to woman and is limited only by the intake needs of the infant. For example, at five months infant intake of breastmilk can range from 200 (partial breastfeeding) to 3500 mL/day (wet nurse) (Neville & Oliva-Rasbach, 1987, p. 125). These differences can be culturally based. Australian women, for example, have more breastmilk than women in the United States. Hartmann (1987) found the average yield of well-nourished western Australian mothers to be in excess of 1100 mL in 24 hours during the first six months of lactation. Mothers breastfeeding twins produce in excess of 2100 mL/day in the early months. There are even seasonal differences in breastmilk volume that are influenced by a mother's need to work during harvest and her reluctance to introduce supplementary food for fear of diarrheal disease (Serdula, Seward & Marks, 1986; Whitehead et al., 1978).

In a healthy infant, breastmilk intake shows little or no correlation with maternal factors such as

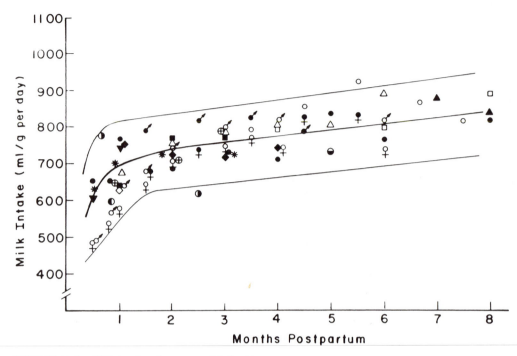

FIGURE 5-2   Milk intakes during established lactation. The lines show the smoothed mean from this study and ± 1 SD. Points are data from the literature obtained by test-weighing of fully breast-fed infants. From Neville, MC, et al: Studies in human lactation; milk volumes in lactating women during the onset of lactation and full lactation, *Am J Clin Nutr* 48:1381.

weight-for-height, weight gain, nursing frequency, maternal age, and parity (Dewey & Lonnerdal, 1983). Although birth weight is not a strong predictor of milk intake throughout lactation, infant weight at one month is. Thus, lactation performance during the first four weeks postpartum is a strong predictor of milk output during the subsequent period of full lactation (Neville & Oliva-Rasbach, 1987).

Two methodological problems must be addressed in lactation research. Inch and Renfrew (1989) point out the potential for error using pre- and postfeed test-weights to calculate breastmilk intake unless an integrated electronic balance is used. This type of balance calculates the mean value of a number of test-weighings over intervals of two to four seconds; readings are reproducible to within 2 g even if the baby moves vigorously. Another difficulty is the definition of "breastfed infants" as study subjects. Are all "breastfed" infants in the study receiving all of their

nutriment from breastfeeding? These issues are addressed more fully in Chapter 21 of this book.

INFANT GROWTH

Normal human growth is greatest during infancy. The infant gains about 10g/kg/day (about 5–7 oz per week) until about four weeks; then the gain drops to 1 g/kg/day (about 3 oz per week) by the end of the first year.

There are significant growth differences between breastfed and formula-fed infants. A review of international research (Butte et al., 1984; Jackson et al., 1964; Juex et al., 1983; Whitehead & Paul, 1981) shows breastfed infants gain weight more rapidly during the first three months and more slowly during the fourth, fifth, and sixth months of life. After the third month of life, weight gains of breastfeeding infants are consistently slower than those of formula-

TABLE 5–1 GENERAL GROWTH RATES BREAST VS. FORMULA

Type of Feeding	Growth Rate by Month		Body Size at 2 Years
	0–5	5–24	
Breast	Faster	Slower	Same
Bottle	Slower	Faster	Same

From Hui, VH: *Human nutrition and diet therapy,* Monterey, Calif., 1983, Wadsworth Publishing Co., p. 351.

fed infants; however head growth (both length and circumference) remains the same for both. Again, this suggests that formula-fed infants are being overfed. (See table 5–1.)

NUTRITIONAL VALUES

Breastmilk around the world is remarkably stable, varying only within a relatively narrow range. Constituents of colostrum and breastmilk are shown in Table 5–2. Yet, because breastfeeding is an interactive process, the infant helps determine the composition of the feed. During weaning, for example, the amounts of sodium and protein in breastmilk progressively increase; in contrast, concentrations of potassium, glucose, and lactose gradually decrease (Prosser, Saint & Hartmann, 1984). A profile of lactose, protein, and lipid concentrations in human milk for the first 30 days of lactation is seen in Fig. 5–3.

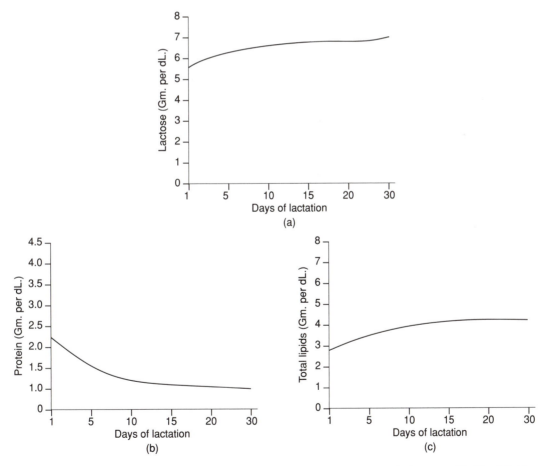

FIGURE 5–3   Lactose concentration in human milk. Protein concentration in human milk. Total lipid concentration in human milk.

TABLE 5–2   COMPOSITION OF HUMAN COLOSTRUM AND MATURE BREAST MILK

Constituent (per 100 mL)		Colostrum 1–5 days	Mature milk >30 days
Energy	kcal	58	70
Total solids	g	12.8	12.0
Lactose	g	5.3	7.3
Total nitrogen	mg	360	171
Protein nitrogen	mg	313	129
NPN	mg	47	42
Total protein	g	2.3	0.9
Casein	mg	140	187
α-Lactalbumin	mg	218	161
Lactoferrin	mg	330	167
IgA	mg	364	142
Amino acids (total)			
Alanine	mg	—	52
Arginine	mg	126	49
Aspartate	mg	—	110
Cystine	mg	—	25
Glutamate	mg	—	196
Glycine	mg	—	27
Histidine	mg	57	31
Isoleucine	mg	121	67
Leucine	mg	221	110
Lysine	mg	163	79
Methionine	mg	33	19
Phenylalanine	mg	105	44
Proline	mg	—	89
Serine	mg	—	54
Threonine	mg	148	58
Tryptophan	mg	52	25
Tyrosine	mg	—	38
Valine	mg	169	90
Taurine (free)	mg	—	8
Urea	mg	10	30
Creatine	mg	—	3.3
Total fat	g	2.9	4.2
Fatty acids (% total fat)			
12:0 lauric		1.8	5.8
14:0 myristic		3.8	8.6
16:0 palmitic		26.2	21.0
18:0 stearic		8.8	8.0
18:1 oleic		36.6	35.5
18:2, n-6 linoleic		6.8	7.2
18:3, n-3 linolenic		—	1.0
C_{20} and C_{22} polyunsaturated		10.2	2.9

TABLE 5–2   COMPOSITION OF HUMAN COLOSTRUM AND MATURE BREAST MILK *—cont'd*

Constituent (per 100 mL)		Colostrum 1–5 days	Mature milk >30 days
Cholesterol	mg	27	16
Vitamins			
Fat soluble			
Vitamin A (retinol equivalents)	μg	89	47
β-Carotene	μg	112	23
Vitamin D	μg	—	0.04
Vitamin E (total tocopherols)	μg	1280	315
Vitamin K_1	μg	0.23	0.21
Water soluble			
Thiamine	μg	15	16
Riboflavin	μg	25	35
Niacin	μg	75	200
Folic acid	μg	—	5.2
Vitamin B_6	μg	12	28
Biotin	μg	0.1	0.6
Pantothenic acid	μg	183	225
Vitamin B_{12}	ng	200	26
Ascorbic acid	mg	4.4	4.0
Minerals			
Calcium	mg	23	28
Magnesium	mg	3.4	3.0
Sodium	mg	48	15
Potassium	mg	74	58
Chlorine	mg	91	40
Phosphorus	mg	14	15
Sulphur	mg	22	14
Trace elements			
Chromium	ng	—	39
Cobalt	μg	—	1
Copper	μg	46	35
Fluorine	μg	—	7
Iodine	μg	12	7
Iron	μg	45	40
Manganese	μg	—	0.4,1.5
Nickel	μg	—	2
Selenium	μg	—	2.0
Zinc	μg	540	166

From Casey, CE, and Hambidge, KM: Nutritional aspects of human lactation. In *Lactation: physiology, nutrition and breastfeeding,* New York, 1983, Plenum Press.

FAT

The fat content of human milk, which provides about one-half of its calories, is its most variable component. The energy density of pre-term mother's milk is much greater than that of full-term mother's milk because of a 30% higher fat concentration (Atkinson, Anderson & Bryon, 1980). Triglycerides, the main constituents (98–99%) of milk fat, are readily broken down into free fatty acids and glycerol by the enzyme lipase, which is found not only in the infant's intestine but also in breastmilk itself. Thus an initial supply of energy from free fatty acids is available even before the milk reaches the intestines for digestion (Hamosh, 1985).

The lipid fraction of human milk provides essential acids and fat-soluble vitamins. Phospholipids and cholesterol compose about 0.5–0.8% of milk fat and are precursors for myelination and cell membrane synthesis (Hamosh, 1985). These two components are slightly more abundant in colostrum than in mature milk.

Breastfed and formula-fed infants have distinctly different plasma/fatty acid compositions: breastfeeders have higher levels of stearic, alpha-linolenic, and arachidonic acids, while formula-feeders have higher levels of oleic acid (Sanjurjo et al., 1988). Because formula is deficient in essential fatty acids, the body compensates by producing more oleic acid. The differences may have important consequences for the lipid structure of the infant's nervous system. Some free fatty acids and monoglycerides generated by milk lipases act against envelope viruses; they also have antibacterial and antifungal activities (Garza et al., 1987).

Although maternal dietary fat intake does not affect the total amount of fat in human milk, the types of fat in the diet do influence the composition of fatty acids in milk. For example black mothers in South Africa consuming a traditional maize diet have less monounsaturated fatty acid in their milk than their urban counterparts who eat more animal fats (van der Westhuyzen, Chetty & Atkinson, 1988). If the mother eats a high-carbohydrate, energy-replete diet, the proportion of triglycerides of medium-chain length fatty acids increases (Garza et al., 1987). Fatty acids of 18-carbon-chain length decrease almost proportionally. Studies are underway to determine if manipulating maternal diet can modify the fat content of human milk, in order to make it more digestible by low-birth-weight infants.

Since cholesterol levels (10–20 mg/dL) in human milk are considerably higher than those of formulas derived from bovine milk or vegetable products (Wagner & Stockhausen, 1988), cholesterol levels in adulthood might be expected to be higher in breastfed individuals. The reverse, however, may well be true: exposure to cholesterol in breastmilk may be an advantage later in life. At least one study (Osborn, 1968) reported that coronary artery disease in persons up to 20 years of age is seen less frequently in individuals who were breastfed. A "cholesterol-challenge" hypothesis proposes that exposure to cholesterol early in life may contribute to a more efficient cholesterol metabolism in adulthood and thus greater protection against heart disease. This hypothesis has been criticized on two counts. First, human milk is not high in cholesterol—10 to 15 mg/dL vs. none in formula. Second, the validity of a complex study which tries to measure the long-term effect of intake of different fats early in life is questionable (Jensen et al., 1988).

Fat content of milk varies diurnally; it is lowest about 6:00 A.M. and gradually increases to its highest point about 2:00 P.M. At any one feeding, the highest concentration of fat is at the end of the feeding in the "hindmilk." The rise of the fat content during a feeding has been interpreted as signalling the infant to stop (Hall, 1979; Cox, 1988).

LACTOSE

Lactose, a disaccharide, accounts for most of the carbohydrates in human milk, although small quantities of oligosaccharides, galactose, and fructose are also present. Although lactose concentration is relatively constant (7.0g/dL) in mature milk, it is affected by maternal diet. In a longitudinal study of breastfeeding Gambian women, Prentice (1980) found that the milk lactose concentration of these women was higher during the wet season (hungry period), when energy intakes were very low, than it was during the dry season when food was more plentiful.

Lactose enhances calcium absorption and metabolizes readily into galactose and glucose, which supply energy to the rapidly growing brain of the infant. Some oligosaccharides promote the growth of *Lactobacillus bifidus,* thus increasing intestinal acidity and stemming the growth of pathogens.

The enzyme lactase is necessary to convert lactose

into simple sugars that can be easily assimilated by the infant. The enzyme is present in the infant's intestinal mucosa from birth. Congenital or primary lactase deficiency is exceedingly rare; some authorities question its existence. Lactose intolerance, however, is common in many mammals as they grow older and is the result of diminishing activity of intestinal lactase after weaning. In humans, lactose intolerance is more prevalent among adults of Asian and African heritage.

PROTEIN

Protein content of mature human milk from well-nourished mothers is about 0.8 to 0.9% (Butte et al., 1984). Some of the protein in human milk is probably not nutritionally available to the infant; it serves immunological purposes instead. Although the protein content of human milk is less than one-half that of bovine milk, the high quality of protein in human milk compensates for its lower quantity and is sufficient for the energy needs of both term and pre-term infants (Gaull, 1985; Raiha, 1985).

Human milk contains casein and non-casein (whey) protein. Caseins account for 30% of the total protein in human milk, about one-half that in bovine milk. Non-casein or whey proteins, which predominate in milk, are acidified in the stomach forming soft flocculant curds. These quickly digest, supplying a continuous flow of nutrients to the baby. By contrast caseins, the primary protein in untreated bovine milk, form a tough, less digestible curd which requires high expenditure of energy for an incomplete digestive process.

Non-casein protein is comprised of five major components: alphalactalbumin, serum albumin, lactoferrin, immunoglobulins, and lysozyme. The latter three play important roles in immunological defense. The concentration of lactoferrin in milk is higher in iron-deficient women as compared with well-nourished mothers; therefore milk lactoferrin may also help protect the infant against iron deficiency (Raiha, 1985). A large number of other proteins (enzymes, growth modulators, and hormones) are present in low concentrations.

Nonprotein breastmilk nitrogen contains a number of free amino acids, including glutamic acid, glycine, alanine, valine, leucine, aspartic acid, serine, threonine, proline, and taurine. When amino acids exist singly or in free form they are known as free amino acids. Of these, leucine, valine, and threonine are essential amino acids; they must be consumed in the diet because the body does not manufacture them.

The percentage of protein in human colostrum is much greater than that in mature breastmilk. This high level is caused by the presence of several additional amino acids and antibody-rich proteins, especially secretory IgA and lactoferrin. All 10 essential amino acids are present in colostrum and account for approximately 45% of its total nitrogen content.

The importance to the baby of available nitrogen cannot be understated. Atkinson, Anderson and Bryan, (1980) have shown that the concentration of nitrogen in the milk of women who deliver pre-term infants is 20% greater than that in milk of women delivering at term. The higher levels of available protein and fat in pre-term mother's milk underscore the importance of using the milk of the pre-term infant's own mother rather than milk pooled from women in other stages of lactation. Donated milk, however, can be readily modified with components from other human milk to make a pre-term milk formula with none of the dangers of commercial, bovine-based, pre-term formulas.

VITAMINS

The amounts of vitamins in human milk vary markedly from one person to another because of diet and genetic differences. However it is generally true that human milk will satisfy the vitamin and trace mineral requirements of a full-term, healthy infant. Generally, as lactation progresses, the level of water-soluble vitamins in breastmilk increases and the level of fat-soluble vitamins declines. Fat-soluble vitamin (A,D,K,E) levels in human milk are minimally influenced by recent maternal diet as these vitamins can be drawn from storage in the body.

Fat soluble.   Human milk is a good source of vitamin A (200 IU/100mL) which is present mainly as retinol (40–53 ng/100mL). Its dietary precursor, β-carotene, is present in lower concentration than is retinol. Levels of vitamin A are highest in the first week after birth and gradually decline. Almost equal amounts of saturated and unsaturated fatty acids in human milk ensure excellent absorption of vitamin

A. West et al. (1986) reported that African children afflicted with xerophthalmia—a dry, thickened, lusterless condition of the eyeball resulting from a severe systemic deficiency of Vitamin A—were three times as likely as normal children to have stopped breastfeeding before age 24 months. Well-nourished mothers have sufficient levels of vitamin A; however, mothers with poor diet may be deficient. Milk from underprivileged Ethiopian mothers had less vitamin A and retinol than did that from European mothers (Gebre-Medhin et al., 1976).

Human milk has very little fat-soluble vitamin D. Concentrations in human milk range between 5 IU and 20 IU per liter. A water-soluble variant of vitamin D has been found (Lakdawala & Widdowson, 1977) but further study has not supported a major role for this compound (Reeve, Chesney & De Luca, 1982). Increased vitamin D intake results in increased levels in human milk (Specker et al., 1985). Ingestion of oral vitamin D supplements (60 ug/day) for two weeks raised the level of vitamin D in the milk of a lactating woman 40 times (Hollis, 1983).

Although rickets is rarely seen in breastfed children, especially if their mothers are well nourished, scattered reports of rickets have led the American Academy of Pediatrics to recommend vitamin D supplements (400 IU per day) for children subject to certain conditions (AAP, 1980). The risk of rickets is greatest for dark-skinned children living in inner-city areas, children whose clothing deters exposure of skin to the sun, and children of mothers eating vegetarian diets that exclude meat, fish, and dairy products.

The child who is adequately exposed to the sun (and thus to radiation-formed precursors of vitamin D) and whose mother consumes adequate nutrients may not need routine vitamin-D supplements (Greer & Marshall, 1989; Roberts et al., 1981). On the other hand, in light of a significant fall in vitamin levels in exclusively breastfed infants compared to partially breastfed infants (Markestad, 1983), and continued reports of rickets (Edidin et al., 1980; Hayward, Stein & Gibson, 1987), authors continue to recommend that breastfed babies receive supplemental vitamin D, an inexpensive and innocuous dietary supplement (Ala-Houhala, 1985; Worthington-Roberts & Williams, 1989).

Human colostrum is particularly rich in vitamin E (tocopherol). Milk of mothers with pre-term and term infants have similar levels of vitamin E (3 IU/100kcal), as well as β-carotene levels which are higher than in bovine milk levels (Ostrea et al., 1986; Jansson, Akesson & Holmberg, 1981). A deficiency of vitamin E in infancy can result in hemolytic anemia especially in the premature infant. As an antioxidant, vitamin E protects cell membranes in the retina and lungs against oxidant-induced injury. The requirement for vitamin E increases with intake of polyunsaturated fatty acids in breastmilk. Mothers who eat foods high in polyunsaturated fats and "fast foods" add to oxidant stress (Guthrie, Picciano & Sheehe, 1977).

Vitamin K, which is required for the synthesis of blood-clotting factors, is present in human milk in small amounts. Canfield and Hopkinson (1989) describe the problems in detecting how much vitamin K is actually present in human milk. Within a few days of birth, vitamin K is normally produced in sufficient quantities by enteric bacteria. However, neonates are susceptible to vitamin-K deficiency until ingestion of copious amounts of breastmilk can promote gut bacterial colonization which enhances their low levels of vitamin K.

Insufficient vitamin K in neonates can lead to vitamin K-responsive hemorrhagic disease. To prevent hemorrhage and to raise prothrombin levels, 1 mg of vitamin K is routinely given intramuscularly. An equal oral dose of vitamin K is absorbed in the intestinal tract in amounts sufficient to prevent bleeding (Haroon et al., 1982), plus the infant is spared the pain of an injection and the risk of nerve damage always possible with any intramuscular injection.

Water soluble. Water-soluble vitamins—ascorbic acid, nicotinic acid, riboflavin, B_{12} (thiamine), and B_6 (pyridoxine)—are readily influenced by the maternal diet. If maternal supplements are taken, the vitamin levels in the milk increase and then plateau (Worthington-Roberts & Williams, 1989). While supplementation is beneficial for undernourished women, it is not necessary if the mother is well nourished and eating a diet that contains foods close to their natural state (Nail, Thomas & Eakin, 1980).

Vitamin B_6 is needed for early development of the baby's central nervous system, and its presence in human milk is critical. A mother eating a vegan diet without meat or dairy products may produce milk deficient in B_6. This was demonstrated by a breastfed infant who developed severe hematologic and neurologic problems which resolved rapidly with B_6 supplementation (Higginbottom, Sweetman & Hyhan, 1978). High pharmacologic doses of vitamin B_6 have been reported to suppress prolactin and thus lactation. However, doses low in nutrition have no effect on plasma prolactin or on breast milk volume. Doses as high 4.0 mg of vitamin B_6 taken as part of a vitamin-B complex supplement should be considered safe for both lactating mother and infant (Andon et al., 1985).

MINERALS

Minerals tend to be highest in human milk in the first few days following birth and, excepting magnesium, decrease slightly in a consistent pattern throughout lactation, with little diurnal or within-feed variation. Maternal age, parity, and diet, even when supplemented, have minimal influence on mineral concentrations in milk, probably because of regulation by maternal body storage levels (Butte et al., 1987; Casey, Neville & Hambridge, 1989; Karra et al., 1986; Freely et al., 1983). Although human milk provides sufficient minerals to support adequate growth and normal serum levels in the full-term infant, they are less than the recommendations established by the National Research Council's Food and Nutrition Board.* Recommended daily allowances are influential guidelines that, when wrong, undermine breastfeeding. The problem is that these standards are interpreted by individuals who are not aware of the high bioavailability of breastmilk constituents. Those who have the power to do so have a responsibility to make revising these standards a priority.

Zinc. The most abundant trace mineral in human milk, zinc is actively transported into the mammary gland. Zinc levels rise to a peak on the second day postpartum and then decline for the duration of lactation (Casey, Neville & Hambridge, 1989). Zinc is eight times more abundant in human colostrum than in mature milk. Krebs and Hambridge (1986) suggest that zinc requirements are based on growth velocity; therefore requirements are relatively high in the very young infant and decrease with increasing age of the infant. Zinc is known to dramatically improve acrodermatitis enteropathica, a rare but serious congenital metabolic disorder that manifests itself in part in severe derma-

*Committee on Dietary Allowances in Washington, D.C.

titis (Evans & Johnson, 1980). Infants with this disorder who continue to receive human milk exhibit no symptoms. The high bioavailability of zinc in human milk is brought about by a zinc-binding ligand that facilitates zinc absorption (Sandstrom et al., 1983).

Abnormally low zinc levels in breastmilk are rare but apparently can sometimes occur in mothers of infants with low birth weights. A slowing growth rate and persistent perioral or perianal rash (with or without diarrhea) in infants who are fed solely breastmilk may be due to zinc depletion (Atkinson et al., 1989).

Iron. Although human milk has only a small amount (0.5–1 mg/L) of iron, breastfed babies are rarely iron deficient. They maintain their iron status at the same level as formula-fed infants receiving iron supplements for up to nine months (Duncan et al., 1985; McMillan, Landaw & Oski, 1976; Siimes et al., 1984; Salmenpera et al., 1986). Breastfed infants are sustained by sufficient iron reserves laid down in utero, plus the high lactose and vitamin-C levels in human milk which facilitate absorption. Also, breastfed infants do not risk loss of iron as do infants fed cow's milk; the latter may experience microhemorrhages of the bowel as a result of mucosal damage by non-human milk (Woodruff, Latham & McDavid, 1977).

For the first few months of life, healthy, full-term infants draw on extensive iron reserves generally present at birth. Normally an infant's hemoglobin level is high (16–22 gm/dL) at birth and decreases rapidly as physiologic adjustment is made to extra-uterine life. At four months of age, normal hemoglobin ranges between 10.2 and 15 gm/dL.

The early introduction of solid foods impairs the efficiency of iron absorption from breastmilk. Iron supplementation is not usually needed and may in fact be detrimental to the breastfeeding baby during the first six months after birth. Excess iron tends to saturate lactoferrin and thereby diminish its anti-infective properties (Bullen, Rogers & Leigh, 1972). Iron supplements taken by the mother will not increase iron levels in her milk but they may produce constipation.

Calcium. Like iron, calcium appears only in small quantities in human milk (20–34mg/100mL). Yet babies absorb 67% of the calcium in human milk

TABLE 5–3 MAJOR COMPONENTS OF HUMAN MILK AND THEIR FUNCTIONS

Component	Function
Amylase	Facilitates infant's digestion of polysaccharides
Ascorbic acid	Antioxidant
Epidermal growth factor	Stimulates epithelial proliferation
Lactose	Major carbohydrate; breaks down into galactose and glucose; enhances absorption of calcium, magnesium, and manganese
Lipase	Hydrolizes fat in infant's intestine; bactericidal activity
Minerals	Regulate normal body functions; little influence from maternal diet
Nonprotein nitrogen	Contains free amino acids necessary for growth
Oligosaccharides	Contribute to bifidus activity and prevent adhesion of microbes to tissue walls
Protein Whey	Contains lactalbumin, lactoferrin, lysozyme, albumin, and immunoglobulins
Taurine	Possible function in brain development and maturation
Thyroxine	Regulates basal metabolic rate; protects against congenital hypothyroidism
Triglycerides	Largest sources of calories for infant; broken down into free fatty acids and glycerol by lipase; types of fat dependent upon maternal diet
Water	Constitutes 87.5% of human milk; provides adequate hydration to infant

compared to only 25% of that in cow's milk. Neonatal hypocalcemia and tetany are more commonly seen in the formula-fed infant because cow's milk has a much higher concentration of phosphorus (a calcium:phosphorus ratio of 1.2:1.0 vs. 2:1 in human milk), which leads to decreased absorption and increased excretion of calcium. Calcium and phosphorus supplements are sometimes given to breastfed infants with low birth weights who should be monitored for hypercalcemia (calcium >11 mg/dL) (Steichen, Krug-Wispe & Tsang, 1987).

Other minerals. Copper levels are highest on the first few days postpartum, decrease for about five to six months, and then tend to remain stable. Magnesium, on the other hand, gradually increases after four to six months postpartum or remains constant (Butte et al., 1987). Selenium is usually higher in human milk than in formula (Smith, Picciano & Milner, 1982). Very little is known about the mechanisms or control of the secretion of trace elements into human milk.

RENAL SOLUTE LOAD

Another unique aspect of human milk is its effect on the renal solute load and on the infant's kidney function and general state of hydration. Human milk has significantly lower levels of calcium, phosphorus, sodium, and potassium than bovine milk. Because of this and the low protein content of human milk, the solute load on the immature kidney of the breastfed infant is approximately one-third that of the infant fed bovine milk. Since excess salts require additional water for excretion, greater obligatory water loss occurs when the infant is not fed human milk. Advances in formula composition have reduced the renal solute load of artificial feeds on the infant. But there is always the possibility of error in preparing formulas, e.g., using excessive amounts of powder which results in a high-protein concentration (Miller & Chopra, 1984). Table 5–3 lists the major components and function of human milk.

ANTI-INFECTIVE PROPERTIES

That breastmilk offers the newborn protection against disease has been recognized for hundreds of years; however, only in the past few decades have investigators begun to identify the specific antiinfective components of human milk that make it a peerless substance for feeding the human infant. Breastmilk has been viewed since ancient times as a living tissue and rightly so. This "white blood" contains enzymes, immunoglobulins, and leukocytes in abundance. It is these components, one frequently enhancing the efficacy of another, that account for most of the unique antiinfective properties of human milk. In some cultures, fresh breastmilk is regularly used as eyedrops to treat conjunctivitis; elsewhere it is common practice to apply breastmilk on the skin to heal cracked nipples.

Several studies that measured the protectiveness

of human milk reaffirm its significance in preventing infections (Cunningham, 1979; Frank et al., 1982; Gullick, 1986; Pullan et al., 1980; Rosenberg, 1989; Victora et al., 1987; Watkins, Leeker & Corkhill, 1979; Kovar et al., 1984). Cunningham (1981) estimated in 1981 that if breastfeeding were universal, 5,000 lives would be saved in the United States annually. The evidence is strongest for gastroenteritis and necrotizing enterocolitis but is likewise convincing for respiratory infections. This protective effect is most striking in communities with poor sewage systems, poverty, and malnutrition (Kramer, 1988). According to the World Health Organization (Snyder & Merson, 1982), more than five million children under the age of five years die annually from gastrointestinal-related disease. Many more suffer from gastrointestinal illness.

Wherever infant morbidity and mortality are high, breastfeeding conclusively helps prevent infantile diarrhea and gastrointestinal infections (Almroth & Latham, 1982; Brown et al., 1989; Clavano, 1982; Goldman et al., 1986; Jason, Niebury & Marks, 1984; Grantham-McGregor & Back, 1972; Habicht, DaVanso & Butz, 1988; Koopman et al., 1985; Kovar et al., 1984; Mata, 1979, 1990; Shoub, 1977). Breastfeeding minimizes diarrhea by both providing protective factors and reducing exposure to other foods or water that may contain enteropathogens. In a review of field studies conducted to identify the effect of breastfeeding on childhood diarrhea in Bangladesh, Glass and Stoll (1989) found that during the first six months of life breastfeeding did protect children against diarrhea. Those children partially breastfed had a greater risk of diarrhea than those who were exclusively breastfed. Although the breastmilk's protective effect is most easily demonstrated in areas of poverty and malnutrition, worldwide data consistently indicates protective effects. In China, Chen, Yu, and Li (1988) showed that, compared with breastfed infants, artificially fed infants are more likely to be admitted to the hospital for gastroenteritis and other conditions. In the Cebu region of the Philippines, giving water, teas, and other liquids to breastfed babies doubles or triples the likelihood of diarrhea (Popkin et al., 1990).

Cunningham (1977, 1979) reviewed hospital and clinical records of children hospitalized in Cooperstown, New York, during the mid-1970s. During their first year, breastfed infants had significantly fewer episodes of illness than those not breastfed. The dif-

ferences remained significant when stratified individually for paternal education, maternal age, presence of older siblings, exposure to day-care centers and parental smoking.

Chandra (1979) prospectively studied 30 breastfed and 30 bottle-fed Canadian babies for two years. Infants exclusively breastfed for the first two months had significantly fewer episodes of diarrhea than infants bottle-fed from birth. Khin-Maung U. et al., (1985) compared clinical outcomes in two groups of children under two years of age with acute diarrhea: one group received oral rehydration solution alone, and the other group breastfed in addition to receiving oral rehydration solution. The breastfed children passed 250 ml less of diarrheal stools and recovered from diarrhea more quickly than children who were not breastfed. The breastfed children also required less oral rehydration solution than those who were not breastfed during the early acute phase of diarrhea. Goldman (1989) states, "The epidemiological evidence indicates that human milk continues to confer protection even if the infant is supplemented. Even partial breastfeeding is better than no breastfeeding at all."

RESPIRATORY ILLNESS

Studies of the protective effects of breastfeeding against respiratory tract infections are less well established and are conflicting (Paine & Coble, 1982; Adebonojo, 1972; Cunningham, 1979; Watkins, Leeker & Corkhill, 1979). Several studies support that breastfeeding helps prevent respiratory infections. When Chen, Yu, and Li (1988) looked for an association between type of feeding and the hospitalization of infants in Shanghai, People's Republic of China, they found that artificial feeding was associated with more frequent hospitalizations for respiratory infections during the first 18 months of life. The effect of artificial feeding was independent of demographic characteristics and socio-educational status. In a careful review of Chen's study, Kramer (1988) concluded that the findings "are convincing and add to the accumulating and now overwhelming evidence that breast-feeding protects against infant and early childhood infection, particularly in non-Western, less industrialized countries."

There is mounting evidence that breastmilk protects against respiratory syncytial virus (RSV) infection (Downham et al., 1976; Duffy et al., 1986; Bell et al., 1988; Holberg et al., 1991; Rahman et al., 1987). Duffy et al. (1986) prospectively studied 197 infants to examine the relationship between mode of feeding and risk of rotavirus infection. Infants exclusively breastfed for at least four months had the lowest attack rates (5%) for rotavirus-related gastroenteritis compared to infants fed formula—or a combination of breastfeeding and formula-feeding. Similar protection has been established for *Haemophilus influenzae* bacteremia and meningitis (Cochi et al., 1986). Downham et al. (1976) compared 115 infants under one year of age who were hospitalized with RSV vs. 162 control infants. A positive breastfeeding history was obtained from 7.0% of the hospitalized infants compared with 27.5% of the control infants—a significant difference.

OTITIS MEDIA

Breastfeeding probably protects against ear infections (otitis media). The reasons are not completely clear; however, immunological factors, the feeding position, and lack of irritation from bovine-based formula may explain it. Saarinen et al. (1982) followed healthy term infants through their first three years of life. Up to six months of age, no infant had otitis media during the period of exclusive breastfeeding, whereas 10% of the babies who were given any cow's milk did. These significant differences persisted up to three years of age. Other studies (Cunningham, 1979; Chandra, 1979; Schaefer, 1971) support an inverse relationship between ear infections and breastfeeding.

In contrast to global evidence that breastfeeding helps to protect infants against health problems, Bauchner, Levanthal, and Shapiro (1986) and others (Leventhal et al., 1986; Sauls, 1979) have challenged that breastfeeding protects infants in developed countries. They point to lack of control for potentially confounding factors, such as low birth weight, parental smoking, crowding, sanitation, and other characteristics of socioeconomic status. These articles, which received wide publicity, were vigorously refuted by Cunningham (1988) who claimed that the critics themselves used flawed methods in coming to their conclusions.

Howie et al. (1990) settled this controversy by examining the effect of breastfeeding on childhood illness in Scotland in a study of a sample that met the methodological criteria set by Bauchner, Leventhal,

and Shapiro (1986). Howie concluded that breastfeeding during the first 13 weeks of life confers protection against gastrointestinal illness beyond the period of breastfeeding itself. In a prospective multicenter study on the effect of breast milk in preventing necrotising enterocolitis, Lucas and Cole (1990) found that the disease was 6–10 times more common in exclusively formula-fed babies as compared to exclusively breastmilk fed babies.

THE IMMUNE SYSTEM

The body's immune system is known as the *systemic immune system*. Another immune system, the *secretory immune system,* invokes the external surfaces of the body (such as the breast) and acts locally. Lymphocytes in the secretory immune system are different from other lymphocytes. Sensitized to antigens found in the gastrointestinal or the respiratory tracts, these lymphocytes travel through mucosal lymphoid tissues (e.g., breasts, salivary glands, bronchi, intestines, and genitourinary tract) where they secrete antibodies.

Most antigens to which a mother has been exposed sensitize lymphocytes migrating to the breast. There they secrete immunoglobulins into the milk—hence, the term secretory IgA or sIgA. These components are further described in a later section of this chapter on "immunoglobulins."

Immunity occurs actively and passively. Maternal antibodies passed to the fetus through the placenta before birth, and through breastmilk after birth, are examples of passive immunity. Poliovirus or rubella immunization of women can also confer passive immunity to the breastfed baby. Passive immunological protection is only temporary since the infant's immune system has not itself responded.

Breastfeeding can also confer long-term protection by stimulating an active immune response. Active immunity is a specific immunity whereby the immune system formulates a long-term memory of exposure to a certain antigen. An example of active immunity is the breastfed infant's common immune response to cytomegalovirus in human milk.

Protective factors in human milk discussed in this chapter are grouped under specific headings: cells (macrophages and lymphocytes), antibodies/immunoglobulins, non-antibody factors, and anti-inflammatory components.

CELLS

Human milk contains two main types of white cells: phagocytes and lymphocytes. (See Fig. 5–4.) Although phagocytes (mostly macrophages) are most abundant (90%), the lymphocyte population (10%) provides significant protective effects to the recipient infant. The concentration of these cells and the predominant cell type varies with the duration of lactation. Following birth the number of these cells is higher than at any other time; they decline progressively thereafter.

Phagocytes. Macrophages are the dominant phagocyte in human milk and are a type of leukocyte. Their action is to engulf and absorb pathogens. Macrophages release IgA although they probably do not synthesize it. Macrophages are both polymorphonuclear (PMN) and mononuclear. Because PMN numbers increase dramatically during inflammation of the breast, they may function to protect the mammary tissue *per se,* rather than to impart protection to the newborn (Buescher & Pickering, 1986). Macrophages also produce complement, lactoferrin, and

lysozymes, which are discussed later in this section. Neutrophils are yet another phagocytic leukocyte. Short-lived but effective, they are first to arrive at an inflamed site such as often occurs during mastitis.

Lymphocytes. Lymphocytes are also leukocytes; they include T-cells, B-cells, and assorted T-cell subsets. The several ways lymphocytes recognize and help to destroy antigens are called cell-mediated immunity. Cell-mediated immunity is important in the destruction of viruses because the cells within which they live shield them from the action of antibodies.

T-cells decrease rapidly in the first week after birth and continue to decline steadily. It has been suggested that T-cells are a special and separate immune component since there is a striking lack of correlation between milk and blood T-cell responses in the same person (Ogra & Ogra, 1979). The role of B-cells is not clear. B-cells may be a discarded and nonfunctional subset of lymphocytes or may have functional capabilities similar to T-cells (Slade & Schwartz, 1987).

Davis, Savitz, and Graubard (1988) suggest that

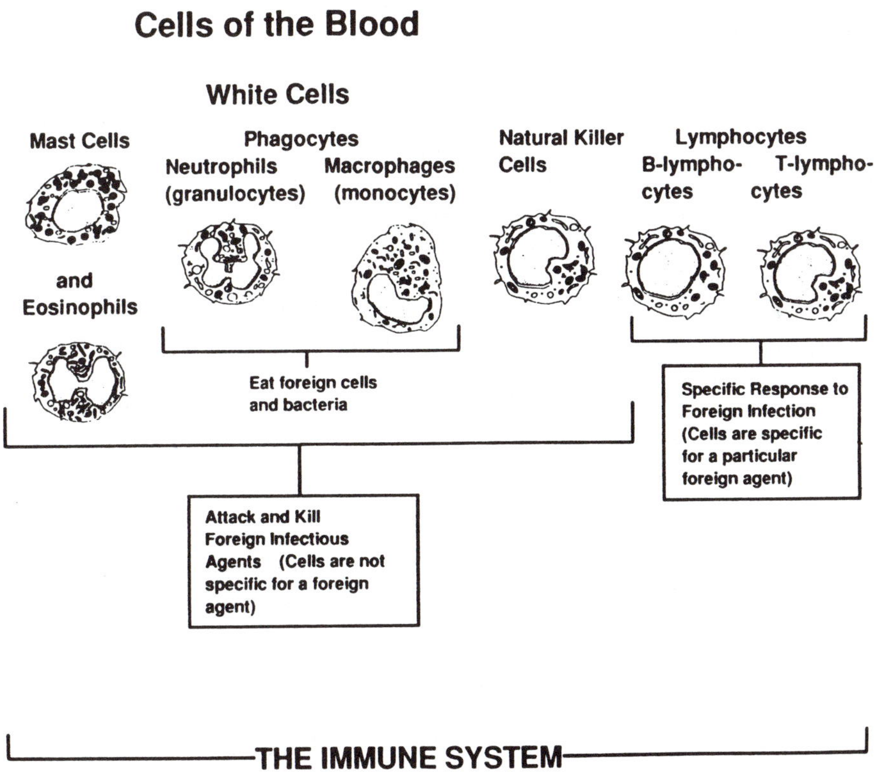

Cells of the Blood

White Cells

FIGURE 5–4 From Fan, H, Conner, R, and Villarreal, L: *The Biology of AIDS,* Boston, 1989, Jones and Bartlett Publishers, Inc., p. 28.

breastfeeding, by increasing resistance to a viral infection during infancy, helps to prevent childhood lymphoma. Certainly their study demonstrates striking protection from this form of childhood cancer in infants breastfed for more than six months. Interaction of the infant's developing immune system with infectious agents could be critical to later immune response to infection or to reactivation of tumors in partial immunodeficiencies.

ANTIBODIES/IMMUNOGLOBULINS

Immunoglobulins are proteins produced by plasma cells in response to an immunogen. Antibodies are immunoglobulins that recognize and act on a particular antigen. There are five types of immunoglobulins: IgG, IgA, IgM, IgE, and IgD. Both IgA and IgE play a critical role in biological specificity of human milk on the recipient infant.

Secretory IgA (sIgA) is the major immunoglobulin in all human secretions. SIgA provides the initial bolus that supplements immunoglobulins transferred earlier across the placenta to the fetus. It is the immunoglobulin most frequently noted in medical literature as having immense immunologic value to the neonate. SIgA, which is both synthesized and stored in the breast, reaches levels up to 5 mg/mL in colostrum; then it decreases to 1 mg/mL in mature milk. As the mother yields more milk, the infant receives more sIgA so that the total dose of sIgA the baby receives throughout lactation is constant or even increases depending on the milk intake.

SIgA synthesis via the secretory immune system described above is an elegant lymphocyte traffic pathway called GALT and BALT (gut-associated or bronchus-associated lymphoid tissue). This pathway leads to the development of lymphoid cells in the mammary gland which produce IgA antibodies after exposure to specific microbial or environmental antigens on the intestinal or respiratory mucosa (Goldman et al., 1983; Okamoto & Ogra, 1989). This transfer of immunologic responsiveness from both BALT and GALT to the mammary glands supports the concept of a common mucosal immune system that is unique (Slade & Schwartz, 1987).

SIgA acts at the intestinal mucosal surface, resisting breakdown by gastrointestinal juices and enzymes; thus it "paints" the intestinal epithelium and blocks adhesion of potential pathogens to mucosal surfaces. Since the infant's own IgA is deficient and

only increases slowly during the first several months after birth, sIgA in human milk provides important passive immunological protection to the digestive tract of newborn infants. SIgA is only minimally absorbed from the intestine: SIgA levels in the feces of breastfed infants are significantly higher than in those of formula-fed infants at the same age (Garza et al., 1987; Jatsyk, Kuvaeva & Gribakin, 1985).

A number of IgA antibodies in human milk which act upon viruses or bacteria that cause respiratory and gastrointestinal tract infections have been reported. These infecting agents include *E. coli, V. cholerae, Clostridium difficile, Salmonella,* rotavirus, poliovirus, *G. lamblia, E. histolytica,* and *Camplylobacter* (Pickering & Kohl, 1986; Ruiz-Palacios et al., 1990). As stated earlier, immunizing breastfeeding women with poliovirus or rubella creates IgA antibodies in milk which specifically target these agents. IgA$_4$ may also play a role in host defense of mucosal surfaces; in some women IgA$_4$ is produced locally in the mammary gland (Keller et al., 1988). In addition to IgA, other Ig classes, including IgD, may be involved in local immunity of the breast. Several investigators (Steel & Leslie, 1985; Bahna, Keller & Heiner, 1982, Litwin, Zehr & Insel, 1990) have demonstrated high levels of locally produced IgD in breast tissues and breastmilk.

As shown in Figure 5–5, clear biological rhythms of protective factors predictably rise and fall as lactation progresses. While the reasons for waxing and waning of various anti-infective components are not always clear, we assume they are adapted to the needs of the infant.

NON-ANTIBODY ANTIBACTERIAL PROTECTION

Non-antibody factors in human milk, an elegant and intricate system, protect the infant against bacterial infection. These factors include lactoferrin, the bifidus factor, lactoperoxidase, oligosaccharides, and complement.

Lactoferrin. Lactoferrin, a potent bacteriostatic iron-binding protein, is abundant in human milk (1–6 mg/mL) but is not present in bovine milk. In the presence of IgA antibody and bicarbonate it readily absorbs enteric iron, thus preventing pathogenic organisms, particularly *E. coli, salmonella,* and *Candida albicans* (Kirkpatrick et al., 1971), from obtaining the iron needed for survival. Because exogenous

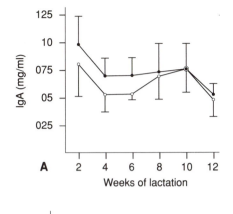

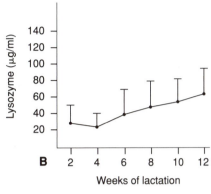

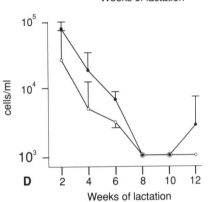

FIGURE 5–5 A longitudinal study of selected resistance factors in human milk of normal American women. **A,** Total (•) and secretory ( ) IgA. **B,** Lysozyme. **C,** Lactoferrin. **D,** Macrophages-neutrophils (•—•) and lymphocytes (—). (Modified from Goldman, AS, et al.: Immunologic factors in human milk during the first year of lactation, *J Pediatr* 100:663, 1982.)

iron may well interfere with the protective effects of lactoferrin, the giving of iron supplements to the healthy breastfed infant must be carefully weighed. Lactoferrin also has been shown to be an essential growth factor for human B- and T-cell lymphocytes (Hashizume, Kuroda & Murakami, 1983).

The bifidus factor.   The intestinal flora of breastfed infants is dominated by gram-positive lactobacilli, especially *Lactobacillus bifidus.* This bifidus factor in human milk, first recognized by Gyorgy (1953), promotes the growth of these beneficial bacteria. Together with the low-protein, phosphate, and buffering capacities of milk, the bifidus factor contributes to the low pH (5–6) of stools. This acid environment discourages replication of enteropathogens such as shigella, salmonella and some *E. coli.*

Lactoperoxidase.   Although levels of the enzyme lactoperoxidase are low, substantial amounts are present in the newborn's saliva. It is thought that IgA in milk enhances the ability of lactoperoxidase to kill *Streptococcus* (Goldman & Goldblum, 1985).

Oligosaccharides.   Oligosaccharides (carbohydrates composed of a few monosaccharides) in human milk help to block antigens from attaching to the epithelium of the gastrointestinal tract. This blocking mechanism prevents the attachment of *Pneumococcus,* which is particularly adhesive (Goldman et al., 1986). The large amount of oligosaccharides in human milk is about 10 times the amount in bovine milk.

Complement.   The complement system is a nonspecific body defense system against inflammation. Although the major component of the *complement* system, C_3, is biologically active in human milk, there is little evidence that it has a significant protective effect (Goldman & Goldblum, 1985).

ANTI-INFLAMMATORY COMPONENTS
Human milk appears to be rich in anti-inflammatory agents and poor in inducers and mediators of inflammation. This is because the major biochemical pathways of inflammatory agents are either absent or poorly represented in breastmilk. Goldman et al.

(1986) have identified anti-inflammatory factors: the protease inhibitors in breastmilk are alpha$_1$-antitrypsin and catalase. The anti-inflammatory effects of these components have not as yet been directly demonstrated in the nursing infant. The specific properties of breastmilk shown to be active against bacteria, viruses and parasites are listed in Tables 5–4, 5–5, and 5–6.

BIOACTIVE COMPONENTS

Hamosh (1985) designates a relatively newly discovered group of substances as "bioactive components." These substances promote growth and development of the newborn by special activities that continue after the infant ingests breastmilk. Most are not available to the infant in commercial infant for-

TABLE 5–4   ANTIBACTERIAL FACTORS FOUND IN HUMAN MILK

Factor	Shown, *in vitro*, to be active against:	Effect of heat
Secretory IgA	*E. coli* (also pili and capsular antigens), *C. tetani, C. diphtheriae, K. pneumoniae, Salmonella* (6 groups), *Shigella* (2 groups), *Streptococcus, S. mutans, S. sanguis, S. mitis, S. salivarius, S. pneumoniae, C. burnetti, H. influenzae* *E. coli* enterotoxin, *V. cholerae* enterotoxin, *C. difficile* toxins, *H. influenzae* capsule	Stable at 56°C for 30 min; some loss (0–30%) at 62.5°C for 30 min; destroyed by boiling
IgM, IgG	*V. cholerae* lipopolysaccharide; *E. coli*	IgM destroyed and IgG decreased by a third at 62.5°C for 30 min
IgD	*E. coli*	
Bifidobacterium bifidum growth z factor	Enterobacteriacea, enteric pathogens	Stable to boiling
Factor binding proteins (zinc, vitamin B$_{12}$, folate)	Dependent *E. coli*	Destroyed by boiling
Complement C1–C9 (mainly C3 and C4)	Effect not known	Destroyed by heating at 56°C for 30 min
Lactoferrin	*E. coli*	Two-thirds destroyed at 62.5°C for 30 min
Lactoperoxidase	*Streptococcus, Pseudomonas, E. coli, S. typhimurium*	Destroyed by boiling
Lysozyme	*E. coli, Salmonella, Micrococcus lysodeikticus*	Some loss (0–23%) at 62.5°C for 30 min; essentially destroyed by boiling for 15 min
Unidentified factors	*S. aureus, C. difficile* toxin B	Stable at autoclaving; stable at 56°C for 30 min
Carbohydrate	*E. coli* enterotoxin	Stable at 85°C for 30 min
Lipid	*S. aureus*	Stable to boiling
Ganglioside (GMI like)	*E. coli* enterotoxin, *V. cholerae* enterotoxin	Stable to boiling
Glycoproteins (receptor-like) + oligosaccharides	*V. cholerae*	Stable to boiling for 15 min
Analogues of epithelial cell receptors (oligosaccharides)	*S. pneumoniae, H. influenzae*	Stable to boiling
Milk cells (macrophages, neutrophils, B and T lymphocytes)	By phagocytosis and killing: *E. coli, S. aureus, S. enteritidis* By sensitized lymphocytes: *E. coli* By phagocytosis: *C. albicans, E. coli* Lymphocyte stimulation: *E. coli* K antigen, tuberculin PPD. Monocyte chemotactic factor production: PPD	Destroyed at 62.5°C for 30 min

From May, JT: Microbial contaminants and antimicrobial properties of human milk, *Microbiol Sci* 5:42–46, 1988.

TABLE 5–5 ANTIVIRAL FACTORS FOUND IN HUMAN MILK

Factor	Shown, *in vitro*, to be Active Against:	Effect of Heat
Secretory IgA	Poliovirus types 1, 2, 3. Coxsackie types A9, B3, B5, echovirus types 6, 9. Semliki Forest virus, Ross River virus, rotavirus, cytomegalovirus, retrovirus type 3, rubella virus, herpes simplex virus, mumps virus, influenza virus, respiratory syncytial virus	Stable at 56°C for 30 min; some loss (0–30%) at 62.5°C for 30 min; destroyed by boiling
IgM, IgG	Rubella virus, cytomegalovirus, respiratory syncytial virus	IgM destroyed and IgG decreased by one-third at 62.5°C for 30 min
Lipid (unsaturated fatty acids and monoglycerides)	Herpes simplex virus, Semliki Forest virus, influenza virus, dengue, Ross River virus, Japanese B encephalitis virus, Sindbis virus, West Nile virus	Stable to boiling for 30 min
Non-immunoglobulin macromolecules	Herpes simplex virus, vesicular stomatitis virus, Coxsackie B4 virus, Semliki Forest virus, retrovirus 3, poliotype 2, cytomegalovirus, respiratory syncytial virus, rotavirus	Most stable at 56°C for 30 min and destroyed by boiling
α_2-macroglobulin (like)	Influenza virus haemagglutinin, parainfluenza virus haemagglutin	Stable to boiling for 15 min
Ribonuclease	Murine leukaemia virus	Stable at 62.5°C for 30 min
Haemagglutinin inhibitors	Influenza and mumps viruses	Destroyed by boiling
Milk cells	Induced interferon: virus or PHA	Destroyed at 62.5°C for 30 min
	Induced lymphokine (LDCF): phytohaemagglutinin (PHA)	
	Induced cytokine: by herpes simplex virus	
	Lymphocyte stimulation: cytomegalovirus, rubella, herpes, measles, mumps, respiratory syncytial viruses	

From May, JT: Microbial contaminants and antimicrobial properties of human milk, *Microbiol Sci* 5:42–46, 1988.

mula. Research on bioactive components is a rapidly growing area of investigation. These bioactive components may play a significant role in child health.

TABLE 5–6 ANTIPARASITE FACTORS FOUND IN HUMAN MILK

Factor	Shown, *in vitro*, to be Active Against:	Effect of Heat
Secretory IgA	*G. lamblia* *E. histolytica* *S. mansoni* *Cryptosporidium*	Stable at 56°C for 30 min, some loss (0–30%) at 62.5°C for 30 min, destroyed by boiling
Lipid (free)	*G. lamblia* *E. histolytica* *T. vaginalis*	Stable to boiling
Unidentified	*T. rhodesiense*	

From May, JT: Microbial contaminants and antimicrobial properties of human milk, *Microbiol Sci* 5:42–46, 1988.

ENZYMES

Mammalian milk contains a large number of enzymes, some of which appear to have a beneficial effect on the development of the newborn. The enzyme content of human milk and bovine milk differ substantially (Hamosh, 1985). For example, lysozyme activity is several thousand times greater in human milk than in bovine milk. The alkaline pH of the stomach of the human infant has a limited effect on the antitrypsin activity of breast milk, thereby protecting children with alpha₁ antitrypsin deficiency against severe liver disease and early death (Udall et al., 1985). Most mammal milks contain many enzymes that appear to be species-specific because of their varying level of activity. A few enzymes discussed below serve a digestive function in the infant or may be important to neonatal development.

Lysozyme. Lysozyme, a major component of human milk whey fraction, has both bacteriocidal and anti-inflammatory action. It acts with peroxide and ascorbate to destroy *E. coli* and some salmonella strains (Pickering & Kohl, 1986).

Lysozyme is much more abundant in human milk (400 ug/mL) than in bovine milk. Instead of slowly declining as lactation progresses, lysozyme activity increases progressively about six months after delivery (Goldman et al., 1982; Prentice et al., 1984b). Why is the lysozme different from other protective factors in this respect? Because many babies begin receiving solid foods at around six months, high levels of lysozyme may be a teleological safeguard against the greater risk from pathogens and diarrheal disease at this time.

Lipase. In order to digest fat, adequate lipase activity and bile salt levels must be present. Pancreatic lipase activity and bile salt concentrations are low in the newborn, especially in the premature. Thus, the newborn depends on two alternate sources of lipase for fat digestion: lingual and gastric lipases. Breastfed infants have an additional substance which digests fats: bile salt-stimulated lipase. This combined activity can effectively complete hydrolysis of ingested fat and compensate for the normal low levels of pancreatic lipase in infants. When human milk is frozen, lipase is not affected; however, heating severely reduces lipase activity (Hamosh, 1986). Several protozoa, *Giardia lamblia*, *Entamoeba histolytica*, and *Trichomonas vaginalis* have been shown *in vitro* to be killed rapidly by exposure to salt-stimulated lipase, which is found only in the milk of humans and mountain gorillas (Blackberg et al., 1980).

Amylase. Amylase is necessary for the digestion of starch. Although amylase is synthesized and stored in the pancreas of the newborn, the infant is around six months old before amylase is released into the duodenum. Human milk contains about 10–60 times as much alpha-amylase as does normal human serum, thus providing an alternate source of this starch-digestive substance. No alpha-amylase is present in bovine, goat, or swine milk, suggesting that this enzyme appeared late in the evolutionary continuum. Hamosh (1985) observed that breastfed infants have fewer problems digesting solid foods than do formula-fed infants, even if these foods are introduced early. Breastfed infants may tolerate the early introduction of solids because of the alpha-amylase provided by breastmilk.

Biotinidase. The enzyme biotinidase regulates the metabolism of biotin. Biotinidase activity in colostrum is about five times higher than in human milk. While the role of biotinidase is not yet known, its high levels in colostrum suggest it might have a special nutritional role in neonates (Oizumi & Hayakawa, 1988).

GROWTH FACTORS

Human milk contains growth-promoting components also known as growth modulators. As with its antiinfective properties, these substances are more pronounced in colostrum than in mature milk. Neither their biologic significance nor their method of action is yet clear. It is not certain, for instance, whether growth factors influence growth and repair of mammary tissue; promote growth and repair cells within the intestines of the neonate; and/or are absorbed from the neonatal gut, enter the circulation of the neonate, and exert an effect upon enteric or target organs (Morriss et al., 1986).

Epidermal growth factor. Epidermal growth factor (EGF), a polypeptide that contains 53 amino acids, is many times more abundant in colostrum and mature milk than it is in serum. There is no diurnal variation nor variation between pre-term and term milk. EGF is also present in other body fluids, including plasma, saliva, and amniotic fluid. It is a major growth-promoting agent in breastmilk (Carpenter, 1980) stimulating growth of mucosal cells and epithelium and thus strengthening the mucosal barrier to antigens. This growth-promotion activity is higher than can be accounted for by insulin and EGF, which suggests there are other growth-promoting factors present (Read et al., 1984; Jansson, Karlson & Westermark, 1985). EGF might also be involved in the development of low-density (LDL) receptors and in cholesterol metabolism. Jensen et al. (1988) speculate that "by extraordinary coincidence, a portion of the lipoprotein LDL receptor on human cells has an amino acid sequence very similar to that of the EGF precursor. These receptors bind and internalize LDL eventually processing the cargo of cholesterol."

Human growth factors I, II, and III. Three polypeptides, called human milk growth factors (HMGF) I, II, and III, have been isolated (Klagsburn, 1978;

Shing & Klagsburn, 1984). HMGF III stimulates DNA synthesis and cellular proliferation, which suggests that it is an epidermal growth factor. Several *in vivo* (Widdowson, Colombo & Artavanis, 1976; Heird, Schward & Hansen, 1984) studies on growth factors in animal milk have shown striking increases in the mass of intestinal mucosa. Morriss et al. (1986) point out that "the presence of growth factors in human milk may influence the growth of target tissues in the suckled infant by provoking an *endogenous hormonal response* that is different from that provoked by ingestion of a proprietary formula." Different growth factors may have overlapping functions, both stimulating cell growth and indirectly affecting the infant's defense mechanism against disease.

HORMONES

Insulin-like growth factor. An insulin-like growth factor (IGF-I) in human milk is thought to have a growth-promoting role. The concentration of this factor in colostrum is about 30 times that in human serum. These high levels (4.1 nmol/L) decrease rapidly (1.3 nmol/L) as colostrum alters to transitional milk (Read et al., 1984) but do not decline further. In fact, Corps et al. (1988) found that the concentration of an insulin-like growth factor in human milk increased (2.5 nmol/L) by the sixth week postpartum.

Thyroxine- and thyrotropin-releasing hormone. Thyroxine is present in human milk in small quantities but is not in commercial formulas. The concentration in colostrum is low, increases by the first week postpartum, and gradually declines thereafter. It has been suggested that thyroxine may stimulate the maturation of the infant's intestine (Morriss, 1985).

Although the thyroxine level is significantly higher in breastfed children than formula-fed children at one and two months of age (Rovet, 1990), reports disagree about whether breastfeeding protects breastfed infants against clinical evidence of congenital hypothyroidism (Bode, Vanjonack & Crawford, 1978; Latarte et al., 1980; Tenore, Parks & Bongiovanni, 1977; Rovet, 1990). Some infants receive sufficient thyroxine in their mother's milk to compensate for hypothyroidism, and thus the symptoms may be masked for several months. Although this does not appear to be true for all infants, the results of thyroid studies after the first week of life

should be interpreted with caution in breastfed infants and should include measurements of both T_4 and thyroid-stimulating hormone (TSH) concentrations.

Cortisol. Cortisol is present in relatively high concentrations in colostrum, declines rapidly by the second day, and remains low thereafter. Two theories have been presented concerning the function of cortisol in the infant. The first is that it controls the transport of fluids and salts in the infant's gastrointestinal tract (Kulski & Hartmann, 1981). The second is that it plays a role in the growth of the infant's pancreas (Morrisset & Jolicoeur, 1980).

Prostaglandins. Prostaglandins, a special group of lipids, are present in most mammal cells and tissues and affect almost every biologic system. Prostaglandins are formed by numerous body tissues and affect many physiologic functions, including local circulation, gastric and mucous secretion, electrolyte balance, zinc absorption, and the release of brush border enzymes. The protective activity of milk lipids is thought to be due to the presence of prostaglandins PGE_2 and PGF_{2a}, which are present both in colostrum and mature milk. Concentrations there are about 100 times greater than their levels in adult plasma (Lucas & Mitchell, 1980). PGE_2 particularly is thought to exert a cytoprotective action (protection against inflammation and necrosis) on the gastric mucosa by promoting the accumulation of phospholipids in the neonatal stomach (Reid, Smith & Friedman, 1980). The full extent of the beneficial effects of prostaglandins in human milk awaits future scientific research.

TAURINE

Taurine, absent in bovine milk, is the second most abundant amino acid in human milk (Raiha, 1985). This unusual amino acid, which may function as a neurotransmitter, plays an important role in early brain maturation (Gaull, 1985). Before 1983, taurine was thought to act only in the conjugation of bile acids. Infants who do not receive taurine in their diet conjugate bile acids with glycine, which less effectively assists absorption of dietary fats. While deleterious effects of low taurine levels are not known in humans, deficiencies have caused retinal problems in cats and monkeys (Jensen et al., 1988). Taurine was added to most commercial formulas when formula-fed infants were found to have plasma taurine levels only half as high as breastfed infants. Concern about lack of taurine in premature infants was especially strong as these infants have smaller bile acid pools and less pancreatic lipase secretion compared with full-term infants (Jarvenpaa et al., 1983; Moore, 1988).

ANTIALLERGENIC PROPERTIES

In 1936 Grulee and Sanford published a classic study which demonstrated for the first time that breastfeeding, compared to feeding with cow's milk, reduced the incidence of eczema seven-fold. There is general agreement that allergies are less common in completely breastfed babies, since foreign food intake is limited to that which is eaten by the mother and secreted into her breastmilk. At the same time this topic is controversial and engenders considerable debate in published literature and in discussions.

The incidence of food-induced allergic disease in children has been estimated to be between 0.3 and 7.5% (Metcalfe, 1984). Heredity is a significant predictor of allergic disease (Savilahti et al., 1987). Sixty percent of all those who will develop atopic eczema do so within the first year of life and 90% do so within the first five years (Hanifin, 1984). Before six to nine months of age, the infant's intestinal mucosa is permeable to proteins; moreover, his own secretory IgA, which will later "paint" the mucosa and bind sensitizing proteins to itself, is not yet functioning effectively.

Bovine milk is probably the most common single allergen. Proteins in bovine milk known to act as allergens include lactoglobulin, casein, bovine serum albumin (BSA), and lactalbumin. Modern processing of formula through heat treatment may have reduced, but certainly not eliminated, the allergic potential of these proteins. The problem is probably increased by the sizable dose of allergens in formula and the large volume of formula ingested. At two to four months of age, for example, a baby consumes his body weight in milk each week. This is the equivalent of nearly seven quarts a day for an adult—truly a macrodose!

Allergy symptoms to cow's milk commonly appear during the first few months of life. Cow's milk most frequently affects the gastrointestinal tract (vomiting, diarrhea, colic, occult bleeding) of allergic infants. It also affects the respiratory tract (runny nose, cough, asthma) and the skin (dermatitis, urticaria). Because the symptoms are varied and nonspecific, the diagnosis is often mistaken or missed (Bahna, 1987).

At birth the IgE system is defective in the potentially allergic infant, and problems arise if this system is activated by allergens. When the introduction of foreign proteins is delayed for four to six months, the baby's own IgA system is permitted to become more fully functional and thus allergic responses may be minimized or entirely avoided. Exclusive consumption of breastmilk facilitates the early maturation of the intestinal barrier; it also provides an exogenous passive barrier to potentially antigenic molecules until the baby's own natural barriers develop. The rationale for delay of solids for the first six months after birth is thus reinforced.

Studies on the effect of breastfeeding on allergic disease are conflicting and some are seriously flawed (Kovar et al., 1984; Kramer, 1988). The majority of studies, however, show that breastmilk has a protective effect against allergies. Kajosaari and Saarinen (1983) followed breastfed Finnish infants of atopic parents for one year. The children who were exclusively breastfed, without supplements or solid foods for six months, had less atopic eczema and food allergy than those who started on solids at three months. Hide and Guyer (1981) conducted a large cohort study of atopic disease in infants and found a small, statistically nonsignificant difference of eczema between breastfed and bottle-fed infants. Jenkins et al. (1984) looked at 46 children with colitis and identified food allergy as a major cause of colitis. In eight children in the study, the onset of colitis occurred soon after starting foods other than breastmilk.

Taylor et al. (1982) reported that increasing duration of breastfeeding (both exclusive and nonexclusive) was associated with decreasing likelihood of eczema at any time during the child's life. Blair (1977) followed children in his London private practice for five years to determine if asthma was affected by infant feeding. More children who had not been breastfed had severe asthma as compared with those who had been breastfed. Twenty years later, the differences were still significant: 64% who had not been breastfed had chronic or recurrent asthma as contrasted with 46% who had been breastfed one week or less and 35% who had been breastfed eight weeks or more. The Italian Collaborative Study (1988) on 303 infants less than one year of age showed that breastfeeding was not more common or of longer duration in controls as compared to cases.

As a result of this conflicting information, not everyone agrees with the recommendation by the American Academy of Allergy and Immunology Committee on Adverse Reaction to Foods that breastfeeding reduces food allergies. After conducting a meta analysis on 22 original research reports on infant feeding and atopic disease, Kramer (1988) decided that errors in research methods preclude definitive conclusions.

Problems in this type of research are manifold: For instance, are those with a family history of atopic eczema more likely to breastfeed because they are aware that it has a protective effect? When the infant is said to breastfeed, does that mean that he receives no other nutriments? A few breastfed infants do develop atopic eczema. Of those who do, according to several well-documented studies, the culprit is often foods ingested by the mother—especially cow's milk (Gerrard et al., 1973; Jakobsson et al., 1985; Chandra et al., 1986). Chandra et al. (1986) completed a prospective study of 109 women with a history of a previous child with atopic disease. By almost completely excluding milk, dairy products, eggs, fish, beef, and peanuts throughout pregnancy and lactation, he documented a significant reduction in the incidence and severity of atopic eczema among breastfed infants of these mothers. Several studies have reported the detection of cow's milk antigen in breast milk (Cavagni et al., 1988; Stuart et al., 1984; Paganelli, Cavagni & Pallone, 1986; Jakobsson et al., 1985; Axelsson et al., 1986). A Danish study (Host, Husby & Osterballe, 1988) showed that early and occasional exposure to cow's milk protein sensitizes neonates so that later even minute amounts of bovine milk protein in human milk may act as booster doses eliciting allergic reactions.

Others disagree that symptoms of allergy in a breastfed infant may be caused by the passage of food antigen into the mother's milk. A Swedish study (Lilja et al., 1989) found no preventive effect on the development of atopic disease in infants up to 18 months of age when their mothers avoided hen's eggs and cow's milk during late pregnancy and the first two months of lactation. Given that immune responses are present in the fetus before the end of the first trimester, and that many other potential allergens were neither assessed nor controlled in this study, such a finding is hardly surprising.

IMPLICATIONS FOR CLINICAL PRACTICE

Human milk is a species-specific fluid with diverse composition which includes non-nutrient substances that protect the infant. While the significance of these non-nutrient components in protecting the infant is well known, their influence on the growth and development of infants is a new field that is just beginning to be explored. The known health benefits and protective effects of breastmilk discussed throughout this text are summarized in Table 5–7.

A thorough understanding of the biologic components of human and bovine milks and of manufactured formulas is essential for a health-care specialist providing lactation assistance. Parents have a right to make an informed decision about how they will feed their infant. When prenatal discussion with the parents and prenatal classes include information about the advantages of immunological protection discussed in this chapter, then the parents can make a truly informed choice.

Very little research has been done on the perception of the mothers themselves about breastmilk. But in a recent qualitative study Bottorff and Morse (1990) revealed that mothers clearly recognize the difference between colostrum and mature breastmilk; however, they rarely use scientific terminology to describe either. Because of the relative thickness of colostrum, some mothers believe it is the "strongest" milk—significant for its "rich" supply of antibodies rather than for its nutritional properties. Breastmilk also frequently was "described by using fat-related terms (e.g., lean, creamy, rich) and evaluated by drawing comparisons to cow's milk and infant formula, as if some similarities should exist between the two."

Given the differences between the growth patterns of breastfed infants and infants fed human-milk substitutes, practitioners need to question using standardized growth charts, which are developed primarily from bottle-fed infants, to evaluate breastfed infants. Otherwise, breastfeeding mothers might be told that their babies are gaining "too slowly" and that their milk production must be insufficient when their babies are obviously healthy in all

TABLE 5–7   PREVENTION OF DISEASE BY HUMAN MILK

Disease	Ameliorating Properties of Human Milk
Sudden infant death	Antiinfectious, antiallergic (Mitchell, 1991)
Gastrointestinal infection	Humoral and cellular antiinfectious factor
Necrotizing enterocolitis	Immunologic factors, macrophages, osmolarity of human milk (Lucas & Cole, 1990)
Neonatal hypocalcemia	Ideal calcium/phosphorus ratio, better calcium resorption
Iron deficiency anemia	Better iron resorption, no blood loss from intestines
Infantile eczema	No species-non-specific proteins
Acrodermatitis enteropathica	More efficient zinc absorption
Vitamin-E deficiency anemia	Sufficient vitamin E in human milk
Chronic constipation	Stools soft
Hypernatremic dehydration	Low mineral and sodium content
Childhood lymphoma	Increases resistance and immunity; strengthens defenses (Davis, Savitz & Graubard, 1988)
Hypertrophic pyloric stenosis	Uncertain; speculate breastfeeding prevents pyloric spasm and edema (Habbick, Khanna & To, 1989)
Liver disease	Protease inhibitors, including antitrypsin, protects children with δ-AT deficiency (Udall et al., 1985)
Otitis media	Antibody protection and/or lack of irritation from cow's milk (Saarinen et al., 1982)
Atopic disease (allergies, asthma)	Inhibits potential antigen molecules from entering neonate by providing passive barrier
Celiac disease	Protects against development of villous atrophy in intestinal mucosa (Auricchio et al., 1983; Logan, 1990)
Crohn's disease	Uncertain (Bergstrand & Hellers, 1983; Koletzko et al., 1989)

From Auricchio, S, et al.: Does breast feeding protect against the development of clinical symptoms of celiac disease in children? *J. Pediatr Gastroenterol Nutr* 2:428–33, 1983; Udall, JN, et al.: Liver disease in antitypsin deficiency, *JAMA* 253:2679–82; Habbick, BF, Khanna, C, and To, T: Infantile hypertropic pyloric stenosis: a study of feeding practices and other possible causes, *CMAJ* 140:401–4, 1989; Davis, MK, Savitz, DA, and Graubard, BI: Infant feeding and childhood cancer, *Lancet* Aug. 13, 1988; Saarinen, UM, et al.: Prolonged breastfeeding as prophylaxis for recurrent otitis media, *Acta Paediatr Scand* 71:567–71, 1982; Kovar, MG, et al.: Review of the epidemiologic evidence for an association between infant feeding and infant health, *Pediatr* 74(suppl.):615–38, 1984; Logan, MF: Coeliac disease, *Lancet* 336:633, 1990; Bergstrand, O, and Hellers, G: Breast-feeding during infancy in patients who develop Chrohn's disease, *Scand J Gastroenterol* 18:903–6, 1983; Lucas, A, and Cole, TJ: Breast milk and neonatal necrotising enterocolitis, *Lancet* 336:1519–23, 1990; Koletzko, S, et al.: Role of infant feeding practices in development of Crohn's disease in childhood, *Br Med J* 298:1617–18, 1989; Mitchell, EA, Scragg, R, Stewart, AW, et al.: Results from the first year of the New Zealand cot death study, *NZ Med J* 104:71–76, 1991.

respects. See Chapter 19 on slow weight gain for a more detailed discussion of this issue.

The high fat (and thus calories) in hindmilk at the end of a feeding implies caution in routinely recommending "switch" nursing (repeated feedings from breast to breast). Although this method is helpful in stimulating milk production, an infant repeatedly switched from breast to breast during feedings must take in up to 140% of the usual amount of milk ingested at any one feeding in order to obtain sufficient calories (Woolridge & Fisher, 1988).

Given the high water content, coupled with the low solute load and mineral content in human milk,

the breastfed infant with free access to this mother's breast needs no additional water even in hot, dry conditions (Almroth, 1978; Brown et al., 1986b). If a breastfeeding infant develops diarrhea, the low mineral level in human milk prevents a rapid osmotic shift of free (extracellular) water; therefore dehydration is less severe and recovery is more rapid than in the artificially fed infant (Khin-Maung-U., 1985).

Hamosh's work (1986) on enzymes supports giving fresh, rather than heat-treated, human milk whenever possible. Due to the action of the bile salt-stimulated lipase, fat in fresh human milk is absorbed to a greater extent than that in pasteurized milk. Mixing mother's milk with formula is perfectly acceptable. It is particularly important for premature infants, who lack digestive enzymes: when fresh human milk is mixed with formula, fat absorption is improved. Ideally, pre-term infants will be receiving high volumes of their own mother's milk or mother's milk enriched with human milk components, both of which sustain excellent growth without the risks of bovine milks.

During the assessment phase of working with a breastfeeding family, the practitioner needs to ask if there is a family history of allergies. If so, encourage the mother to breastfeed for a minimum of nine months and to delay the introduction of solid foods until the baby show signs of readiness. Commercial cow's milk-based formula contains the same allergenic proteins as raw untreated cow's milk. Because of risk of sensitization to these proteins, particularly in babies who have a family history of allergies, even occasional formula supplements can trigger an allergic reaction and should be avoided as long as possible. In addition to preventing allergies, infant malabsorption problems such as celiac disease are lessened when the baby is breastfed and solid foods are delayed (Auricchio et al., 1983; Logan, 1990).

Solid foods are usually started around six months of age as the baby's intestinal enzymes mature and he becomes increasingly capable of digesting complex proteins and starches. When solid foods are introduced into the infant's diet, the mother should introduce only one food at a time at weekly intervals. In this way, the infant can be watched for allergic reactions to individual foods, and those that cause difficulties can be withdrawn from his diet.

In the maternal diet, dairy products particularly are potential allergens to the nursing baby. If the mother notices that a particular food seems to cause an allergic response in her infant, she needs to consider eliminating it from her diet. A case report (Wilson, Self & Hamburger, 1990) describes rectal bleeding in a four-day-old infant who was exclusively breastfed: her mother was drinking four to five glasses of cow's milk per day. While this case is extreme and rare, it demonstrates the potential problems caused when a breastfeeding mother drinks large quantities of cow's milk. Discussion of diet and appropriate substitution should be part of the care provided the mother by the health-care worker offering lactation consultation and support.

SUMMARY

The nutritional components of human milk, combined with its immune and antiallergic properties, make it the ideal foundation for optimal infant health. Allowed to breastfeed at will in response to their own needs, infants generally obtain milk in amounts which satisfy their energy needs and maintain normal patterns of growth. Practical experience has clearly suggested the benefits of breastfeeding. In recent years, scientific data from all parts of the world confirm what the practitioner has long observed.

Commenting on its unique adaptability, Ratner (1981) noted: "Human milk has a remarkable fitness in terms of the demands and needs of the infant. . . . The configuration of elements in the milk are like computer information with a reciprocal fitness between the mother and the infant." Moreover, even in special cases, such as the accelerated energy needs of the premature infant, this adaptability is seen in the greater availability of energy in the pre-term milk. Jensen et al. (1988) poetically describe this reciprocity as "human milk as a carrier of important physiological messages" to the recipient infant.

REFERENCES

Adebonojo, FO: Artificial vs breast-feeding; Relation to infant health in a middle class American community, *Clin Pediatr* 11:25–29, 1972.

Ala-Houhala, M: 25-hydroxyvitamin D levels during breast-feeding with or without maternal or infantile supplementation of vitamin D, *J Pediatr Gastroenterol Nutr* 4:220–26, 1985.

Almroth, SG: Water requirements of breast-fed infants in a hot climate, *Am J Clin Nutr* 31:1154–57, 1978.

Almroth, SG, and Latham, MC: Breast feeding practices in rural Jamaica, *J Trop Pediatr* 28:103–9, 1982.

American Academy of Pediatrics, Committee on Nutrition: Commentary on breastfeeding and infant formulas, including standards for formulas, *Pediatrics,* 57:278–85, 1976.

American Academy of Pediatrics, Committee on Nutrition: Vitamin and mineral supplement needs in normal children in the United States, Pediatrics 66:1015–21, 1980.

Andon, MB, et al.: Nutritionally relevant supplementation of vitamin B_6 in lactating women: Effect on plasma prolactin, *Pediatrics* 76:769–73, 1985.

Arthur, PG, et al.: Measuring short-term rates of milk synthesis in breast-feeding mothers, *Q J Exp Physiol* 74:419–28, 1989.

Arthur, PG, Smith, M, and Hartmann, PE: Milk lactose, citrate, and glucose as markers of lactogenesis in normal and diabetic women, *J Pediatr Gastroenterol Nutr* 9: 488–96, 1989.

Atkinson, SA, et al.: Abnormal zinc content in human milk: Risk for development of nutritional zinc deficiency in infants, *Am J Dis Child* 143:608–11, 1989.

Atkinson, SA, Anderson, G, and Bryan, MH: Human milk: comparison of the nitrogen composition of milk from mothers of premature infants, *Am J Clin Nutr* 33:811–15, 1980.

Auricchio, S, et al.: Does breast feeding protect against the development of clinical symptoms of celiac disease in children? *J Pediatr Gastroenterol Nutr* 2:428–33, 1983.

Axelsson, I, et al.: Bovine β-lactoglobulin in the human milk, *Acta Paediatr Scand* 75:702, 1986.

Bahna, SL: Milk allergy in infancy, *Ann Allergy* 59:131–36, 1987.

Bahna, SL, Keller, MA and Heiner, DC: IgE and IgA in human colostrum and plasma, *Pediatr Res* 16:604, 1982.

Bauchner, J, Levanthal, JM, and Shapiro, ED: Studies of breastfeeding and infection: How good is the evidence? *JAMA* 256:887–92, 1986.

Bell, LM, et al.: Rotavirus serotype-specific neutralizing activity in human milk, *Am J Dis Child* 142:275–78, 1988.

Bergstrand, O, and Hellers, G: Breast-feeding during infancy in patients who develop Crohn's disease, *Scand J Gastroenterol* 18:903–6, 1983.

Blackberg, LD, et al.: The bile salt stimulated lipase in human milk is an evolutionary newcomer derived from a non-milk protein, *FEBS Lett,* 112:51, 1980.

Blair, H: Natural history of childhood asthma: A twenty-year follow-up, *Arch Dis Child* 52:613–19, 1977.

Bode, HH, Vanjonack, WJ, and Crawford, JD: Mitigation of cretinism by breast feeding, *Pediatrics* 62:13, 1978.

Bottorff, JL, and Morse, JM: Mother's perceptions of breast milk, *JOGNN* 19:518–27, 1990.

Brown, KH, et al.: Infant-feeding practices and their relationship with diarrheal and other diseases in Huascar (Lima), Peru, *Pediatrics* 83:31–40, 1989.

Brown, KH, et al.: Lactational capacity of marginally nourished mothers: relationships between maternal nutritional status and quantity and proximate composition of milk, *Pediatrics* 78:909–19, 1986a.

Brown, KH, et al.: Milk consumption and hydration status of exclusively breast-fed infants in a warm climate, *J Pediatr* 108:677–80, 1986b.

Buescher, ES, and Pickering, LK: Polymorphonuclear leukocytes in human colostrum and milk. In Howell, RR, Morriss, FH, and Pickering, LK, eds.: *Human milk in infant nutrition and health.* Springfield, Ill., Charles C Thomas, 1986, pp. 160–73.

Bullen, JJ, Rogers, HJ, and Leigh, L: Iron-binding proteins in milk and resistance to *Escherichia coli* infection in infants, *Br Med J* 1:69–75, 1972.

Butte, NF et al.: Human milk intake and growth in exclusively breast-fed infants, *J Pediatr* 104:187–95, 1984.

Butte, NF, et al.: Macro- and trace-mineral intakes of exclusively breast-fed infants, *Am J Clin Nutr* 45:42–47, 1987.

Butte, NF, Smith, EO, and Garza, C: Energy utilization of breast-fed and formula-fed infants, *Am J Clin Nutr* 51: 350–58, 1990.

Canfield, LM, and Hopkinson, JM: State of the art vitamin K in human milk, *J Pediatr Gastroenterol Nutr* 8:430–41, 1989.

Carpenter, G: Epidermal growth factor is a major growth-promoting agent in human milk, *Science* 210:198–99, 1980.

Casey, CE, and Hambidge, KM: Nutritional aspects of human lactation. In *Lactation: Physiology, Nutrition and Breastfeeding.* New York: Plenum Press, 1983.

Casey, CE, Neville, MC, and Hambidge, KM: Studies in human lactation: secretion of zinc, copper, and manganese in human milk, *Am J Clin Nutr* 49:773–85, 1989.

Cavagni, G, et al.: Passage of food antigens into circulation of breast-fed infants with atopic dermatitis, *Ann Allergy* 61:361–65, 1988.

Chandra, RK: Prospective studies of the effect of breastfeeding on incidence of infection and allergy, *Acta Paediatr Scand* 68:691–94, 1979.

Chandra, RK, et al.: Influence of maternal food antigen avoidance during pregnancy and lactation on incidence of atopic eczema in infants, *Clin Allergy* 16:563–69, 1986.

Chen, Y, Yu, S, and Li, W: Artificial feeding and hospitalization in the first 18 months of life, *Pediatrics* 81:58–62, 1988.

Clavano, NR: Mode of feeding and its effect on infant mortality and morbidity, *J Trop Pediatr* 28:287–93, 1982.

Cochi, SL, et al.: Primary invasive *Haemophilus influenzae* type b disease; a population-based assessment of risk factors, *J Pediatr* 108:887–96, 1986.

Committee on Dietary Allowances: Washington, D.C., 1980, National Academy of Sciences, pp. 46–47.

Corps, et al.: The insulin-like growth factor I content in human milk increases between early and full lactation, *J Clin Endocrinol Metab* 67(1):25–29, 1988.

Cox, S: Why do some babies prefer only one breast at each feed? *Breastfeed Rev* (13):85–86, November, 1988.

Cunningham, A: Congressional hearing on infant feeding practices before the Subcommittee on Domestic Marketing, Consumer Relations, and Nutrition, Washington, D.C., June 22, 1981, U.S. Government Printing Office.

Cunningham, AS: Morbidity in breast-fed and artificially fed infants I, *J Pediatr* 90:726–29, 1977.

Cunningham, AS: Morbidity in breast-fed and artificially fed infants II, *J Pediatr* 95:685–89, 1979.

Cunningham, AS: Studies of breastfeeding and infections. How good is the evidence? A critique of the answer from Yale, *J Hum Lact* 4:54–56, 1988.

Davis, MK, Savitz, DA, and Graubard, BI: Infant feeding and childhood cancer, *Lancet* (2) (8607):265–68, 1988.

Dewey, KG, and Lonnerdal, B.: Milk and nutrient intake of breast-fed infants from 1 to 6 months: Relation to growth and fatness, *J Pediatr Gastroenterol Nutr* 2: 497–506, 1983.

Downham, MA, et al.: Breast-feeding protects against respiratory syncytial virus infection, *Br Med J* 2:274–76, 1976.

Duffy, LC, et al.: The effects of infant feeding on rotavirus-induced gastroenteritis: a prospective study, *Am J Public Health* 76:259–63, 1986.

Duncan, B, et al.: Iron and the exclusively breast-fed infant from birth to six months, *J Pediatr Gastroenterol Nutr* 4:412–25, 1985.

Edidin, DY, et al.: Resurgence of nutritional rickets associated with breast-feeding and special dietary practices, *Pediatrics* 65:232–35, 1980.

Evans, GS, and Johnson, PE: Characterization and quantitation of a zinc-binding ligand and human milk, *Pediatr Res* 14:876–80, 1980.

Fan, H, Conner, R, and Villareal, L: *The Biology of AIDS.* Boston: Jones & Bartlett Publishers, Inc., 1989, p. 28.

Frank, AL, et al.: Breast-feeding and respiratory virus infection, *Pediatrics* 70:239–45, 1982.

Freely, RM, et al.: Calcium, phosphorus, and magnesium contents of human milk during early lactation, *J Pediatr Gastroenterol Nutr* 2:262–67, 1983.

Forman, MR, et al.: Undernutrition among Bedouin Arab infants: the Bedouin Infant Feeding Study, *Am J Clin Nutr* 51:343–39, 1990.

Garza, C, et al.: Changes in the nutrient composition of human milk during gradual weaning, *Am J Clin Nutr* 37:61–65, 1983.

Garza, C., et al.: Special properties of human milk, *Clin Perinatol* 14:11–31, 1987.

Garza, C, Stuff, J, and Butte, N: Growth of the breast-fed infant. In Goldman, AS, Atkinson, SA, and Hanson, LA, eds.: *Human Lactation: The effects of human milk on the recipient infant,* New York, 1986, Plenum Press, pp. 109–21.

Gaull, GE: Significance of growth modulators in human milk, *Pediatr* 75(suppl.):142–45, 1985.

Gebre-Medhin, M, et al.: Breast milk composition in Ethiopian and Swedish mothers: I. Vitamin A and carotine, *Am J Clin Nutr* 29:441–45, 1976.

Gerrard, JW, et al.: Cow's milk allergy: prevalence and manifestations in an unselected series of newborns, *Acta Paediatr Scand* (suppl.)234:1–21, 1973.

Glass, RI, and Stoll, BJ: The protective effect of human milk against diarrhea: A review of studies from Bangladesh, *Acta Paediatr Scand* (suppl.)351:131–36, 1989.

Goldman, S: La Leche League International, Annual Seminar for Physicians. Breastfeeding: a natural world resource, Anaheim, Calif., July, 1989.

Goldman, AS, et al.: Anti-inflammatory properties of human milk, *Acta Paediatr Scand* 75:689–95, 1986.

Goldman, AS, et al.: Immunologic components in human milk during gradual weaning, *Acta Paediatr Scand* 72:133–34, 1983.

Goldman, AS, et al.: Immunologic factors in human milk during the first year of lactation, *J Pediatr* 100:563–67, 1982.

Goldman, AS, and Goldblum, RM: Protective properties of human milk. In Walker, WA, and Watkins, JB, eds., *Nutrition in pediatrics,* Boston, Little, Brown & Co., 1985, pp. 819–28.

Grantham-McGregor, SM, and Back, EH: Breast feeding in Kingston, Jamaica, *Arch Dis Child* 45:404–9, 1972.

Greer, FR, And Marshall, S: Bone mineral content, serum vitamin D metabolite concentrations and ultraviolet B light exposure in infants fed human milk with and without vitamin D_2 supplements, *J Pediatr* 114:204–12, 1989.

Grulee, CG, and Sanford, HN: The influence of breast and artificial feeding on infantile eczema, *J Pediatr* 9:223–25, 1936.

Gulick, EE; The effect of breast-feeding on toddler health, *Pediatr Nurs* 12:51–54, 1986.

Guthrie, HA, Picciano, MF, and Sheehe, D: Fatty acid patterns of human milk, *J Pediatr* 90:39–41, 1977.

Gyorgy, P: A hitherto unrecognized biochemical difference between human milk and cow's milk, *Pediatrics* 11:98–104, 1953.

Habbick, BF, Khanna, C, and To, T: Infantile hypertropic pycoric stenosis: a study of feeding practices & other possible causes. CMAJ 140:401–4, 1989.

Habicht, JP, DaVanso, J, and Butz, WP: Mother's milk and sewage: Their interactive effects on infant mortality, *Pediatrics* 81:456–60, 1988.

Hall, B: Uniformity of human milk, *Am J Clin Nutr* 32:304–12, 1979.

Hamosh, M: Enzymes in human milk. In Howell, RR, Morriss, FH, and Pickering, LK, eds.: *Human milk in infant nutrition and health,* Springfield, Ill., 1986, Charles C Thomas, pp. 67–97.

Hamosh, M: Human milk. In Colon, AR, and Mohsen, Z, eds.: *Pediatric Pathophysiology,* Boston, 1985, Little, Brown & Co., pp. 69–85.

Hanifin, JM: Atopic dermatitis, *J Allergy Clin Immunol* 73:211–22, 1984.

Haroon, Y, et al.: The content of phylloquinone (vitamin K_1) in human milk, cow's milk and infant formula foods determined by high performance liquid chromatography, *J Nutr* 112:1105–17, 1982.

Hartmann, PE: Lactation and reproduction in Western Australian women, *J Reprod Med* 32:543–47, 1987.

Hartmann, PE, and Prosser, CG: Physiological basis of longitudinal changes in human milk yield and composition, *Fed Proc* 43:2448–53, 1984.

Hashizume, S, Kuroda, K, and Murakami, H: Identification of lactoferrin as an essential growth factor for human lymphocytic cell lines in serum-free medium, *Biochem Biophys Acta* 763:377, 1983.

Hayward, I, Stein, MT, and Gibson, MI: Nutritional rickets in San Diego, *Am J Dis Child* 141:1060–62, 1987.

Heird, WC, Schward, SM, and Hansen, IH: Colostrum-induced enteric mucosal growth in beagle puppies, *Pediatr Res* 18:512, 1984.

Hide, DW, and Guyer, BM: Clinical manifestations of allergy related to breast and cows' milk feeding, *Arch Dis Child* 56:172–75, 1981.

Higginbottom, MD, Sweetman, L, and Hyhan, WL: A syndrome of methylmalonic aciduria, homocystinuria, megaloblastic anemia, and neurologic abnormalities in a vitamin B_{12} deficient breast-fed infant of a strict vegetarian, *N Engl J Med* 299:317, 1978.

Holberg, CJ, et al.: Risk factors for respiratory syncytial virus-associated lower respiratory illnesses in the first year of life, *Am J Epidemiol* 133:1135–51, 1991.

Hollis, BW: Individual quantitation of vitamin D_2, vitamin D_3 25-hydroxyvitamin D_2, and 25-hydroxyvitamin D_3 in human milk, *Anal Biochem* 131:211–19, 1983.

Host, A, Husby, S, and Osterballe, O: A prospective study of cow's milk allergy in exclusively breast-fed infants, *Acta Paediatr Scand* 77:663–70, 1988.

Houston, MJ, Howie, PW, and McNeilly, AS: Factors affecting the duration of breast feeding: 1. Measurement of breast milk intake in the first week of life, *Early Hum Dev* 8:49–54, 1983.

Howie, PW, et al.: Protective effect of breast feeding against infection, *Br Med J* 300:11–16, 1990.

Hui, VH: *Human Nutrition Diet Therapy.* Monterey, Calif.: Wadsworth Publishing Co., 1983, p. 351.

Humenick, SS: The clinical significance of breastmilk maturation rates, *Birth* 14(4):174–79, 1987.

Inch, S, and Renfrew, M: Common breastfeeding problems. In Chalmers, I, Enkin, M, and Keirse, MJNC, eds.: *Effective care in pregnancy and childbirth,* Oxford, 1989, Oxford University Press, pp. 1375–89.

Italian Collaborative Study: Cow's milk allergy in the first year of life, *Acta Paediatr Scand,* Suppl. 348, 1988.

Jackson, RL, et al.: Growth of "well-born" American infants fed human and cow's milk, *Pediatr* 33:642, 1964.

Jakobsson, I, et al.: Dietary bovine β-lactoglobulin is transferred to human milk, *Acta Paediatr Scand* 74:342, 1985.

Jansson, L, Akesson, B, and Holmberg, L: Vitamin E and fatty acid composition of human milk, *Am J Clin Nutr* 34:8–13, 1981.

Jansson, L, Karlson, FA, and Westermark, B: Mitogenic activity and epidermal growth factor content in human milk, *Acta Paediatr Scand* 74:250–53, 1985.

Jarvenpaa, A-L, et al.: Feeding the low-birth-weight infant. I. Taurine and cholesterol supplementation of formula does not affect growth and metabolism, *Pediatrics* 71:171–78, 1983.

Jason, JM, Niebury, P, and Marks, JS: Mortality and infectious disease associated with infant-feeding practices in developing countries, *Pediatrics* 74(suppl.):702–27, 1984.

Jatsyk, GV, Kuvaeva, IB, and Gribakin, SG: Immunological protection for the neonatal gastrointestinal tract: the importance of breast feeding, *Acta Paediatr Scand* 74:246–49, 1985.

Jenkins, HR, et al.: Food allergy: the major cause of infantile colitis, *Arch Dis Child* 59:326–29, 1984.

Jensen, RG, et al.: Human milk as a carrier of messages to the nursing infant, *Nutr Today* 23:20–25, 1988.

Juex, G, et al.: Growth pattern of selected urban Chilean infants during exclusive breast feeding, *Am J Clin Nutr* 38:462–68, 1983.

Kajosaari, M, and Saarinen, UM: Prophylaxis of atopic disease by six months' total solid food elimination, *Acta Paediatr Scand* 72:411–14, 1983.

Karra, MV, et al.: Changes in specific nutrients in breast milk during extended lactation, *Am J Clin Nutr* 43:495–503, 1986.

Keller, MA, et al.: IgAG4 in human colostrum and human milk: continued local production or selective transport from serum, *Acta Paediatr Scand* 77:24–29, 1988.

Khin-Maung-U, J, et al.: Effect of clinical outcome of breastfeeding during acute diarrhea, *Br Med J* 290:587–89, 1985.

Kirkpatrick, CH, et al.: Inhibition of growth of *Candida albicans* by iron-unsaturated lactoferrin: relation to host defense mechanisms in chronic mucocutaneous candidiasis, *J Infect Dis* 124:539, 1971.

Klagsburn, M: Human milk stimulates DNA synthesis and cellular proliferation in cultured fibroblasts, *Proc Natl Acad Sci USA* 75:5057–61, 1978.

Koletzko, S, et al.: Role of infant feeding practices in development of Crohn's disease in childhood, *Br Med J* 298:1617–18, 1989.

Koopman, JS, et al.: Infant formulas and gastrointestinal illness, *Am J Public Health* 75:477–80, 1985.

Kovar, MG, et al.: Review of the epidemiologic evidence for an association between infant feeding and infant health, *Pediatrics* 74(suppl.):615–38, 1984.

Kramer, MS: Infant feeding, infection, and public health, *Pediatr* 81:164–66, 1988.

Krebs, NF, and Hambidge, KM: Zinc requirements and zinc intakes of breast-fed infants, *Am J Clin Nutr* 43:288–92, 1986.

Kulski, JK, and Hartmann, PE: Changes in the concentration of cortisol in milk during different stages of human lactation, *Aust J Exp Biol Med Sci* 59:769, 1981.

Kumpulainen, J, et al.: Formula feeding results in lower selenium status than breast-feeding or selenium supplemental formula feeding: a longitudinal study, *Am J Clin Nutr* 45:49–53, 1987.

Lakdawala, DR, and Widdowson, EM: Vitamin D in human milk, *Lancet* 1:167–68, 1977.

Latarte, J, et al.: Lack of protective effect of breast-feeding in congenital hypothyroidism: Report of 12 cases, *Pediatr* 65:703–5, 1980.

Lemons, JA, et al.: Differences in the composition of preterm and term human milk during early lactation, *Pediatr Res* 16:113–17, 1982.

Lepage, G, et al.: The composition of preterm milk in relation to the degree of prematurity, *Am J Clin Nutr* 40:1042–49, 1984.

Leventhal, JM, et al.: Does breastfeeding protect against infection in infants less than 3 months of age? *Pediatr* 78:896–903, 1986.

Lilja, G, et al.: Effects of maternal diet during late pregnancy and lactation on the development of atopic diseases in infants up to 18 months of age—*in-vivo* results, *Clin and Exp Allergy* 19:473–79, 1989.

Litwin, SD, Zehr, BD, and Insel, RA: Selective concentration of IgD class-specific antibodies in human milk, *Clin Exp Immunol* 80:263–67, 1990.

Logan, RF: Coeliac disease, letter, *Lancet* 336:633, 1990.

Lucas, A, and Cole, TJ: Breast milk and neonatal necrotizing enterocolitis, *Lancet* 336:1519–23, 1990.

Lucas, A, and Mitchell, MD: Prostaglandins in human milk, *Arch Dis Child* 55:950, 1980.

McMillan, JA, Landaw, SA, and Oski, FA: Iron sufficiency in breast-fed infants and the availability of iron from human milk, *Pediat* 58:686–91, 1976.

Markestad, T: Plasma concentrations of vitamin D metabolites in unsupplemented breast-fed infant, *Eur J Pediatr* 141:77, 1983.

Mata, L: Breast-feeding, infections and infant outcomes: an international perspective. In Atkinson, SA, Hanson, LA, and Chandra, RK: *Breastfeeding, nutrition, infection and infant growth in developed and emerging countries,* St. John's, Newfoundland, Canada, 1990, ARTS Biomedical Publisher.

Mata, L: The malnutrition-infection complex and its environment factors, *Proc Nutr Soc* 38:29–40, 1979.

May, JT: Microbial contaminants and antimicrobial properties of human milk, *Microbiol Sci* 5:42–46, 1988.

Metcalfe, DD: Food hypersensitivity, *J Allergy Clin Immunol* 73:749–62, 1984.

Miller, SA, and Chopra, JG: Problems with human milk and infant formulas, *Pediatrics* 74 (suppl.):639–47, 1984.

Mitchell, EA, Scragg, R, Stewart, AW, et al: Results from the first year of the New Zealand cot death study, *NZ Med J* 10:71–76, 1991.

Moore, MM: Taurine supplementation; Theoretical and practical considerations, *Pediatr Nurs* 14:489–91, 1988.

Morriss, FH: Method for investigating the presence and physiologic role of growth factors in milk. In Jensen, RG, and Neville, MC: *Human lactation: milk components and methodologies,* New York, 1985, Plenum Press, pp. 193–200.

Morriss, FH, et al.: Relationship of human milk pH during course of lactation to concentrations of citrate and fatty acids, *Pediatrics* 78:458–64, 1986.

Morrisset, J, and Jolicoeur, L: Effect of hydrocortisone on pancreatic growth in rats, *Am J Physiol* 239:295, 1980.

Nail, PA, Thomas, MR, and Eakin, R: The effect of thiamin and riboflavin supplementation on the level of those vitamins in human breast milk and urine, *Am J Clin Nutr* 33:198–204, 1980.

Neville, MC, et al.: Studies in human lactation; milk volumes in lactating women during the onset of lactation and full lactation, *Am J Clin Nutr* 48:1375–86, 1988.

Neville, MC, and Oliva-Rasbach, J: Is maternal milk production limiting for infant growth during the first year of life in breast-fed infants? In Goldman, AS, Atkinson, SA, and Hanson, LA, eds.: *Human lactation 3: The effects of human milk on the recipient infant,* New York, 1987, Plenum Press, pp. 123–33.

Ogra, SS, and Ogra, PL: Components of immunologic reactivity in human colostrum and milk. In Ogra, PL, and Dayton, D, eds.: *Immunology of breast milk,* New York, 1979, Raven Press.

Oizumi, J, and Hayakawa, K: Biotinidase in human breast milk, *Am J Clin Nutr* 48:295–97, 1988.

Okamoto, Y, and Ogra, P: Antiviral factors in human milk: Implications in respiratory snycytial virus infection, *Acta Paediatr Scand* (suppl.)351:137–43, 1989.

Osborn, FR: Relationship of hypotension and infant feeding to the aetiology of coronary disease, *Colleques Int Cont Natl Res CS* 169:93, 1968.

Ostrea, EM, et al.: Influence of breast-feeding on the restoration of the low serum concentration of vitamin E and beta-carotene in the newborn infant, *Am J Obstet Gynecol* 154:1014–17, 1986.

Paganelli, R, Cavagni, G, and Pallone, F: The role of antigenic absorption and circulating immune complexes in food allergy, *Ann Allergy* 57:330–36, 1986.

Paine, F, and Coble, RJ: Breast-feeding and infant health in a rural U.S. community, *Am J Dis Child* 136:36–38, 1982.

Pickering, LK, and Kohl, S: Human milk humoral immunity and infant defense mechanisms. In Howell, RR, Morriss, FH, and Pickering, LK, eds.: *Human milk in infant nutrition and health,* Springfield, Ill., 1986, Charles C Thomas, pp. 123–40.

Popkin, BM, et al.: Breast-feeding and diarrheal morbidity, *Pediatr* 86:874–82, 1990.

Prentice, AM: Variations in maternal dietary intake, birthweight and breastmilk output in the Gambia. In Aebi, H, and Whitehad, R: *Maternal nutrition during pregnancy and lactation,* Hans Huber Publisher, Bern, 1980, pp. 167–83.

Prentice, AM, et al.: Breast-milk antimicrobial factors of rural Gambian mothers, *Acta Paediatr Scand* 73:796–812, 1984a.

Prentice, AM, et al.: The effect of water abstention on milk synthesis in lactating women, *Clin Sci* 66:291–98, 1984b.

Prosser, CG, Saint, L, and Hartmann, PE: Mammary gland function during gradual weaning and early gestation in women, *Aust J Exp Biol Med Sci* 62:215–28, 1984.

Pullan, CR, et al.: Breast-feeding and respiratory syncytial virus infection, *Br Med J* 281(6247):1034–36, 1980.

Rahman, MM, et al.: Local production of rotavirus specific IgA in breast tissue and transfer to neonates, *Arch Dis Child* 62:401–5, 1987.

Raiha, NCR: Nutritional proteins in milk and the protein requirement of normal infants, *Pediatrics* 75(suppl.): 136–41, 1985.

Ratner, H: La Leche League International, Ninth Annual Seminar on Breastfeeding for Physicians, Chicago, July 1981.

Read, L, et al.: Changes in the growth-promoting activity of human milk during lactation, *Pediatr Res* 18:133–38, 1984.

Reeve, LE, Chesney, RW, and De Luca, HF: Vitamin D of human milk: Identification of biologically active forms, *Am J Clin Nutr* 36:122–26, 1982.

Reid, B, Smith, H, and Friedman, Z: Prostaglandins in human milk, *Pediatrics* 66:870–72, 1980.

Roberts, CC, et al.: Adequate bone mineralization in breast-fed infants, *J Pediatr* 99:192–96, 1981.

Rosenberg, M: Breast-feeding and infant mortality in Norway 1860–1930, *J Biosoc Sci* 21:335–48, 1989.

Rovet, JF: Does breast-feeding protect the hypothyroid infant whose condition is diagnosed by newborn screening? *Am J Dis Child* 144:319–23, 1990.

Ruiz-Palacios, GM, et al.: Protection of breast-fed infants against *Campylobacter* diarrhea by antibodies in human milk, *J Pediatr* 116:707–13, 1990.

Saarinen, JM, et al.: Prolonged breast feeding as prophylaxis for recurrent otitis media, *Acta Paediatr Scand* 71:567–71, 1982.

Salmenpera, L, et al.: Folate nutrition is optimal in exclusively breast-fed infants but inadequate in some of their mothers and in formula-fed infants, *J Pediatr Gastroenterol Nutr* 5:283–89, 1986.

Sandstrom, BA, et al.: Zinc absorption from human milk, cow's milk, and infant formulas, *Am J Dis Child* 137: 726–29, 1983.

Sanjurjo, P, et al.: Plasma fatty acid composition during the first week of life following feeding with human milk or formula, *Acta Paediatr Scand* 77:202–6, 1988.

Sauls, JS: Potential effect of demographic and other variables in studies comparing morbidity of breast-fed infants, *Pediatrics* 64:523–27, 1979.

Savilahti, E, et al.: Prolonged exclusive breast feeding and heredity as determinants in infantile atopy, *Arch Dis Child* 62:269–73, 1987.

Schaefer, O: Otitis media and bottle-feeding: An epidemiological study of infant feeding habits and incidence of recurrent and chronic middle ear diseases in Canadian Eskimos, *Can J Public Health* 62:478–89, 1971.

Serdula, MK, Seward, J, and Marks, JS: Seasonal differences in breast-feeding in rural Egypt, *Am J Clin Nutr* 44:405–9, 1986.

Shing, YW, and Klagsburn, M: Human and bovine milk contain different sets of growth factors, *Endocrinology* 115: 273, 1984.

Shoub, BD: A microbiological investigation of acute summer gastroenteritis in Black South African infants, *J Hygiene* 78:377–80, 1977.

Siimes, MA, et al.: Exclusive breast-feeding for nine months: risk of iron deficiency, *J Pediatr* 104:196–99, 1984.

Slade, HB, and Schwartz, SA: Mucosal immunity: The immunology of breast milk, *J Allergy Clin Immunol* 80: 348–58, 1987.

Smith, AM, Picciano, MF, and Milner, JA: Selenium intakes and status of human milk and formula fed infants, *Am J Clin Nutri* 35:521, 1982.

Snyder, JD, and Merson, MH: The magnitude of the global problem of acute diarrhoeal disease; a review of active surveillance data, *Bull WHO* 60:605–13, 1982.

Specker, BL, et al.: Sunshine exposure and serum 25-hydroxyvitamin D concentrations in exclusively breast-fed infant, *J Pediatr* 107:372–76, 1985.

Steel, MG, and Leslie, GA: Immunoglobulin D in rat serum, saliva and milk, *Immunology* 55:571–77, 1985.

Steichen, JJ, Krug-Wispe, SK, and Tsang, RC: Breastfeeding the low birth weight preterm infant. In Lawrence, R: Breastfeeding, *Clin Perinatol* 14:131–71, 1987.

Stuart, CA, et al.: Passage of cow's milk protein into breast milk, *Clin Allergy* 14:533–35, 1984.

Stuff, JE, and Nichols, GL: Nutrient intake and growth performance of older infants fed human milk, *J Pediatr* 115:959–68, 1989.

Taylor, B, et al.: Breast-feeding, bronchitis and admissions for lower-respiratory illness and gastroenteritis during the first five years, *Lancet* 1:1227–29, 1982.

Tenore, A, Parks, JS, and Bongiovanni, AM: Relationship of breast feeding to congenital hypothyroidism. In Chiumello, G, and Laron, Z, eds.: *Recent progress in pe-diatric endocrinology,* London, 1977, Academy Practice, pp. 213–21.

Udall, JN, et al.: Development of the gastrointestinal mucosal barrier. II. The effects of natural versus artificial feeding on intestinal permeability to macromolecules, *Pediatr Res* 19:245–49, 1981.

Udall, JN, et al.: Liver disease in α_1-antitrypsin deficiency, *JAMA* 253:2679–82, 1985.

van der Westhuyzen, J, Chetty, M, and Atkinson, PM: Fatty acid composition of human milk from South African black mother consuming a traditional maize diet, *Eur J Clin Nutr* 42:213–20, 1988.

van Steenbergen, WM, et al.: Energy supplementation in the last trimester of pregnancy in East Java, Indonesia: effect on breast-milk output, *Am J Clin Nutr* 50:274–79, 1989.

Victora, CG, et al.: Evidence for protection by breastfeeding against infant deaths from infectious diseases in Brazil, *Lancet* 2(8554):319–21, 1987.

Wagner, V, and Stockhausen, JG: The effect of feeding human milk and adapted milk formulae on serum lipid and lipoprotein levels in young infants, *Eur J Pediatr* 147:292–95, 1988.

Watkins, CJ, Leeker, SR, and Corkhill, RT: The relationship between breast and bottle feeding and respiratory illness in the first year of life, *J Epidemiol Comm Health* 33:180–82, 1979.

West, KP, et al.: Breast-feeding, weaning patterns, and the risk of xerophthalmia in Southern Malawi, *Am J Clin Nutr* 44:690–97, 1986.

Whitehead, RG, et al.: Factors influencing lactation performance in rural Gambian mothers, *Lancet* 2:178–81, 1978.

Whitehead, RG, and Paul, AA: Infant growth and human milk requirement, a fresh approach, *Lancet* 2:161–63, 1981.

Widdowson, EM, Colombo, VE, and Artavanis, CA: Changes in the organs of pigs in response to feeding for the first 24 hours after birth, II. The digestive tract, *Biol Neonate* 28:272, 1976.

Wilson, JV, Self, TW, and Hamburger, R: Severe cow's milk induced colitis in an exclusively breast-fed neonate, *Clin Pediatr* 29:77–80, 1990.

Wood, CS, et al.: Exclusively breast-fed infants: growth and caloric intake, *Pediatr Nurs* 14(2):117–24, 1988.

Woodruff, CW, Latham, E, and McDavid, S: Iron nutrition in the breast-fed infant, *J Pediatr* 90:36–38, 1977.

Woolridge, MW, and Fisher, C: Colic, "overfeeding," and symptoms of lactose malabsorption in the breast-fed baby: A possible artifact of feed management? *Lancet,* August 13, 1988, pp. 382–84.

World Health Organization and Agricultural Organization of the U.S. (WHO/FAO): *Report of a Joint FAO/WHO ad hoc expert committee,* Rome, 1980 National Academy of Science on Dietary Allowances.

Worthington-Roberts, BS, and Williams, SR: *Nutrition in pregnancy and lactation,* St. Louis, 1989, Times Mirror/The C.V. Mosby Co., pp. 244–322.

6

Drugs and Breastfeeding

JAN RIORDAN

The current rise in the popularity of breastfeeding parallels the rise in the use of drugs, both therapeutic and illegal; therefore health professionals often are asked by lactating mothers about the safety of taking a certain medication. There are three "knowns" about drugs and human milk: first, most drugs pass into breastmilk; second, almost all medication appears in only small amounts in human milk, usually less than one percent of the maternal dosage; and third, very few drugs are contraindicated for breastfeeding women.

The methods used to measure chemicals in breastmilk have changed remarkably in the past two decades. Gas-liquid chromatography, atomic absorption spectrophotometry, and radioimmunoassay have vastly improved our ability to measure drugs in milk; thus, even microscopic amounts can be detected.

As a result, more is known about the effect of maternal drugs on the breastfeeding baby than ever before. At the same time, our improved ability to measure drugs in human milk far exceeds our ability to make clinical judgments about their presence (Roberts, 1984). This easy detection of drugs in human milk, even in minute amounts, is a double-edged sword. On the positive side, it facilitates close monitoring of drug levels in the mother and the infant. Even microscopic amounts of a drug in milk may be clinically significant in the case of a premature infant who is ill, or in the instance of a mother who must take a medication for a long time or in combination with other medications.

On the negative side, the tendency is to recommend that a mother not breastfeed when she must use a medication known to pass into milk. There are

other problems. Many research reports on lactation and drugs are single-case reports which lack the validity of reports based on the experiences of many women. Milk sampling is often not done when the drug is at a steady-state plasma concentration. The daily variability of milk fat is not considered, nor are infant plasma drug concentrations measured (Giacoia & Catz, 1988). A drug can be relegated to the contraindicated list for years based on a single, often faulty, case report (Lederman, 1989).

Despite the availability of information about medication during lactation, too few physicians know much about the effect on the nursling of drugs in breastmilk. They are unduly influenced by the well-known teratogenic effects of drugs taken during pregnancy. This awareness makes them fear the potential of similar toxic effects of drugs in breastmilk. However, the analogy is unwarranted. Whereas the placenta permits drugs to cross over to the fetus, the breast serves as a nearly impermeable barrier. At the same time, too many physicians are concerned about legal repercussions when they order medication for a nursing woman. Because the health of the vulnerable infant is so important, the value of breastfeeding so poorly appreciated, and the climate (in the United States) so litigious, the tendency is to err on the side of caution (Riordan, 1987). The net result is that it is easier and less threatening to recommend weaning than it is to look into the matter and be reassured that medication poses no danger to the baby (Tyree, 1992). The victim of such caution is the breastfeeding woman who, lacking time, energy, and wherewithal to sift through the research literature, succumbs to her physician's advice and weans her infant.

Roberts (1984) warns that a physician should advise weaning only when scientific documentation indicates that a drug will be harmful to the infant:

> It is no longer acceptable for the physician to intervene arbitrarily with the mother's wish to breastfeed her infant merely because maternal drug therapy is clearly indicated. Nor does it seem reasonable to discontinue breast-feeding solely because the drug in question has been implicated in one or two case reports of toxic side-effects in primary recipients.

PASSAGE OF MATERNAL DRUGS INTO BREASTFEEDING INFANTS

Several authors (Wilson, 1981; Atkinson & Begg, 1990) have developed equation models which permit prediction of the concentration of a drug in breast milk; however, the concentration in breastmilk may be, in and of itself, of limited clinical use because so many other maternal and infant factors are involved. For example, a drug present in breastmilk may be destroyed in the infant's gastrointestinal (GI) tract before it is absorbed. Because the drug levels in the nursing baby are usually not measured, we have little information about the actual dose that the infant receives from the milk.

DRUG FACTORS

The amount of drug transported into breastmilk partially depends upon the drug's characteristics. These characteristics include the drug's molecular weight, the degree to which the drug is bound to plasma and milk proteins, its solubility in lipids and in water, the proportion of the drug that is ionized (carries a positive or negative charge) vs. non–ionized, its pH factor, its half-life, and its milk/plasma ratio. Following are simplified, general guidelines for drug factors:

1. *The lower the drug's molecular weight, the more easily it passes through to milk and vice versa.* Drugs with a high (over 200) molecular weight (heparin, insulin, warfarin) are restricted from passing into human milk. Because

of their high molecular weight, they are also not absorbed in the gastrointestinal tract.

2. *The more a drug binds to plasma proteins (is protein-bound) the less likely it freely diffuses through the alveolar membranes into milk.* Conversely, if a drug binds readily to milk proteins in the mother's milk, the drug tends to accumulate in the milk.

3. *The more lipid-soluble a medication or substance, the greater the quantity transferred and the greater the speed of transfer into milk.* Medications with a low-lipid solubility diffuse slowly into milk. Lipid-soluble drugs more readily cross cell membranes by dissolving in the lipid layer, whereas water-soluble drugs must cross cell membranes through pores or openings.

4. *The greater the proportion of a drug in a non-ionized form, the more readily it diffuses across the lipid cellular membrane and into milk.* When a non-ionized molecule enters the milk compartment, it is quickly ionized and back-diffusion is prevented; it becomes "trapped" in this form and accumulates in the milk. This accumulation is reflected in a high M/P ratio.

5. *Drugs that are weak bases (more alkaline) tend to concentrate more in breastmilk. Conversely, drugs that are weak acids do not readily transfer* (Feldman & Pickering, 1986). This is because acids tend to attract bases. Because human milk is usually more acid (7.0–7.4) than plasma (7.4), drugs that are weak bases (lincomycin, erythromycin, antihistamines, alkaloids, and isoniazid) would theoretically be more likely to cross the membranes from plasma into milk than drugs that are weak acids (barbiturates, sulfonamides, penicillins, and diuretics).

6. *The longer the half-life of the drug, the greater the risk of accumulation in the mother and in the infant.* The rate of removal of a drug from the body is known as clearance. *Half-life* ($t_{\frac{1}{2}}$) is another term frequently used to estimate how fast a drug leaves the body. Half-life is the time necessary for the drug serum concentration to decrease by one-half. Half-life is determined by the drug's rates of absorption, metabolism, and excretion from the body. Half-life varies considerably from one drug to another. For instance, penicillin has a serum half-life of less than one hour, whereas that of digitoxin is about one week. A drug with a short half-life is taken more frequently than one with a long half-life. When a

drug is given at a fixed dose, about four or five half-lives are required to achieve *steady–state* serum concentration in which plasma drug levels remain fairly steady.

7. *The higher the milk/plasma ratio, the more the drug is found in milk.* The M/P ratio refers to the concentration of the protein-free fractions in milk and in plasma. For example, the M/P ratio of a particular sulfonamide is 0.08. This means that the level of the medication in the milk is 8% the level of the medication in the plasma. An M/P ratio of 4.0 means that the level of the medication in milk is four times higher than the level in plasma. A medication with an M/P ratio of 1.0 has the same concentration in milk that it does in plasma (Lipkin, 1989). M/P ratios are only estimations but special concern should be given to drugs which have an M/P greater than one (Wilson, 1981).

MATERNAL FACTORS

The amount of medication the mother takes, how often she takes it, and the route of administration affect the magnitude and duration of drug passage into breastmilk. As expected, the higher the dosage, the more the drug transfers into the milk. If the medication is taken right after breastfeeding, the drug has the maximum time to clear the maternal blood. Drugs taken 30 to 60 minutes before a feeding are likely to be at maximum serum levels when the infant feeds. On the other hand, when feedings are frequent (up to 16 times per day in some cultures), timing the dose would make little difference.

The level of a drug in the breastmilk and how soon it appears also depends on where the drug enters the mother's system. Whereas the infant's exposure to the substance is always through the gastrointestinal tract, the drug can enter the mother through one of several routes: orally, intravenously, intramuscularly, topically, or through inhalation. Oral medications have a slower drug action and take longer to reach breastmilk. The intravenous route, which bypasses gastrointestinal barriers to absorption, allows a drug to enter the milk quickly and at higher levels than if the drug were given orally. The intramuscular route also allows quick transfer of drugs because muscles have an abundant blood supply. Generally, topical medications (e.g., skin creams) reach breastmilk more slowly and in lesser amounts than medications administered in other ways.

The mother's and the infant's genetic make-up and health play a role in their response to certain drugs. For instance, some breastfed infants are sensitive to certain drugs, such as caffeine from coffee drunk by the mother, while others feel no effect from it (Yurchak & Jusko, 1976). Finally, if the mother's kidneys or liver function are impaired, normal metabolic pathways which excrete the drug are less effective, and there is greater and/or prolonged transfer of the drug to breastmilk.

INFANT FACTORS

The age and maturity of the breastfeeding infant are important when the health professional weighs the risks and benefits of maternal ingestion of a drug. Because the infant is a dynamic, changing organism, what adversely affects him at one point may not be an issue a week or a month later. Premature infants have immature renal and hepatic systems and are at risk for developing high plasma drug concentrations. The premature infant's liver may be overwhelmed by breakdown products from hemoglobin or from medications administered directly to the infant. As his renal and liver systems develop, the same infant may then be able to handle medication that previously might have triggered harmful consequences. The full-term newborn's developing enzyme systems, the lipid-brain barrier, and renal function are not yet fully developed. Thus, during the first week or so of life for the healthy neonate, and much later for the premature infant, detoxification of chemicals in the milk by either acetylation or oxidation is hampered. A healthy, three-month-old baby whose liver and renal systems have matured is much better equipped to metabolize a drug and has far fewer problems. Moreover, babies tolerate maternal drugs more easily as they get older because they are larger, therefore, the drug is distributed over a larger volume. For example, a male baby in the 50th percentile almost doubles his weight by three months.

The frequency of feedings and volume of breastmilk the infant takes must be considered. The child who is feeding only once or twice a day and taking other nourishment consumes considerably less drug than does a baby who breastfeeds 10 times a day and receives no other form of nourishment. Calculations of infant dose are often made assuming exclusive breastfeeding. Such calculations are helpful because they give the maximum drug transfer. At the same time, they exaggerate the hazard in the case of an infant who takes other nutriments. Also, the presence of a substance in milk does not necessarily mean that it is absorbed in the infant's gastrointestinal tract. Some drugs such as gentamicin, kanamycin, tetracycline, and insulin are absorbed very poorly in the GI tract of infants—and of adults as well.

BREAST AND MILK FACTORS

Most breastmilk is manufactured during feedings; the breast "stores" only a minimal quantity of milk. Therefore, the timing of a drug dose relative to breastfeeding influences how much of the drug will appear in breastmilk. If the infant feeds when the mother's drug serum levels are at a peak (highest) level, the amount of the drug that transfers into her milk (while it is being manufactured) is also higher than if her drug serum levels are at a trough (lowest) level. This is true, in part, because changes in mammary blood flow alter the amount of drug transported to the breast. The blood flow in the breast increases many times over when the breast begins to lactate; high mammary blood flow at the time the drug peaks—or any other time—delivers an even greater quantity of drug to milk (Wilson, 1981; Vorherr, 1978).

Breastmilk composition also affects the ability of the drug to cross the plasma into milk. Colostrum is high in protein and low in lactose, the reverse of mature milk. As milk composition changes, especially its fluctuations in fat content, drug-transport mechanisms also change. In addition, mammary blood pH, permeability of cellular and extracellular membranes within the secretory unit, cellular transport mechanisms in the alveoli, drug metabolism by breast tissue, and a drug's characteristics (such as pH and protein-binding ability) affect the passage of drugs into human milk.

ROUTES OF TRANSPORT

Nature provides a series of barriers that help prevent drugs from getting into human milk. A drug in a mother's bloodstream first passes out of the blood capillary lumen into the mammary interstitium—the connective tissue space surrounding the secretory lobules. In order to pass into the alveolar lumen, it must first penetrate the membranes of the myoepithelial cells and walls of the secretory cells lining the alveolus. It does this either by diffusion through the lipid portion of the membranes or through protein channels in the membranes. There are two main types of diffusion:

passive (movement from higher concentration to lower concentration) and active (movement from lower concentration to higher concentration). Passive diffusion is the more common mechanism. In an alternative route, a drug molecule may travel from the interstitium to the alveolar lumen via small intercellular clefts, bypassing the secretory and myoepithelial cells. Table 6–1 lists the approximate percent of maternal drugs that pass into milk.

TABLE 6–1 PERCENT OF MATERNAL DRUG APPEARING IN BREASTMILK

Drug	Percent (approx.)	Half-life (hr)
Aspirin	0.5	
Cefazolin	0.075	
Cephalexin	0.08	9
Chloramphenical	1.3	4
Chlorpromazine	0.07	12
Digoxin	0.07–0.14	
Diphenylhydantoin	1.4	24
Ethanol	0.25–1.0	2.9
Imipramine	0.1	18
^{131}I	0.1	
Isoniazid	0.75	5.9
Kanamycin	0.05	
Lincomycin	0.025	
Lithium	0.12	22
Methotrexate	0.01	7.2
Nalidixic Acid	0.05	2
Penicillin	0.03	
Phenobarbital	1.5	99
Prednisolone	0.12	8.2
Prednisone	0.04	1.8
Propranolol	0.03	
Rifampin	0.05	3.5
Salicylate	0.18–0.36	
Streptomycin	0.5	
Sulfapyridine	0.12	
Tetracycline	0.03	6–11
Theophylline	4	4.0
Thiouracil	5.0	

Modified from Vorherr, H: Human lactation and breastfeeding. In Larson, BL, ed.: *Lactation: A comprehensive treatise*, vol. 4, New York, 1978, Academic Press. Inc., pp. 181–279; Berlin, CM: The excretion of drugs and chemicals in human milk. In Yaffe, SJ: *Pediatric pharmacology*, New York, 1980, Grune & Stratton, Inc., pp. 137–47; Rivera–Calimlim, L: The significance of drugs in breast milk. In Lawrence, R., ed.: Breastfeeding, *Clin Perinat* 14(1):51–70, 1987.

DRUGS THAT AFFECT MILK VOLUME

A number of drugs inhibit or enhance milk secretion. This effect is achieved by stimulating or suppressing prolactin or by steroid-like activity (Dickey & Stone, 1975). (See Table 6–2.)

Some medications used in the treatment of psychiatric disorders cause an increase in breastmilk production (galactorrhea) by interfering with dopamine release. Since dopamine inhibits prolactin, a decrease in dopamine stimulates lactation. Drugs that interfere with dopamine release include reserpines (Serpasil), rauwolfia derivatives (Raudixin), and phenothiazines (Thorazine, Stelazine, Mellaril).

Metoclopramide (Reglan) is commonly used to treat gastroesophageal reflux and other gastric problems in infants and post-operative nausea. It is routinely ordered for preventing nausea following a cesarean birth. It also is a galactogogue that increases breastmilk volume by stimulating prolactin secretion (Ehrenkranz & Ackerman, 1986; Guzman et al., 1979; Kauppila et al., 1983). Metoclopramide appears to be clinically effective for women who are having problems maintaining an adequate milk supply, and no adverse effects have been reported in infants whose mothers are taking this medication (Sousa, 1975; Gupta & Gupta, 1985; Kauppila et al., 1983; Tanis, A.: Personal communication, 1990). Daily oral doses of 30–45 mg are divided in three doses per day. The average interval between the first dose of metoclopramide and improvement in lactation is about three days (Rimar, 1986). As of now there are no published reports of adverse reactions in nursing mothers.

Ergot alkaloids, such as bromocriptine, inhibit prolactin secretion. Until recently, bromocriptine (Parlodel) was extensively used to suppress lactation postpartum. However, following reports of serious adverse effects (Canterbury et al., 1987; FDA, 1982; Watson et al., 1989) its use is declining. The trend

TABLE 6–2   DRUGS THAT AFFECT MILK VOLUME

Inhibits Milk Production		Enhances Milk Production	
Generic Name	**Trade Name**	**Generic Name**	**Trade Name**
levodopa	Dopar, Larodopa	rauwolfia	Roudisin, Rauval
phenelzine	Nardil	reserpine	Serpasil
tranylcypromine	Parnate	chlorpromazine	Thorazine
ergocryptine	Ergocryptine	perphenazine	Trilafon, Triavil
barbiturates	(numerous)	prochlorperazine	Compazine
apomorphine	Apomorphine	promazine	Sparine
antihistamines	(numerous)	thioridazine	Mellaril
pyridoxine	Vitamin B_6	trifluoperazine	Stelazine
prostaglandin E_2	——	chlorprothixene	Taractan
estrogens	(numerous)	haloperidol	Haldol
androgens	(numerous)	metoclopramide	Reglan
bromocriptine	Parlodel	thiothixene	Navane
alcohol (excessive)	——	amitriptyline	Elavil
		imipramine	Tofranil
		methyldopa	Aldomet
		thyroid releasing hormone (TRH)	Thyroid releasing hormone (TRH)
		insulin	insulin
		oxytocin (nasally)	Syntocinon
		sulpiride	

Taken from: Aono, T, et al.: Effect of sulpiride on poor puerperal lactation, *Am J Obstet Gynecol* 143:927, 1982; Dickey, RP, and Stone, SC: Drugs that affect the breast and lactation, *Clin Obstet Gynecol* 18(2):95–111, 1975; Peterson, RG, and Bowes, WA: Drugs, toxins and environmental agents in breast milk. In Neville, MC, and Neifert, M: *Physiology, nutrition and breast-feeding*, New York, 1983, Plenum Press, pp. 367–403.

for treating postpartum engorgement in mothers who do not intend to breastfeed is once again "old-fashioned" methods: ice, breast binders, analgesics, and sympathy. Other ergot derivatives, ergonovine maleate (Ergotrate) and methylergonovine maleate (Methergen), may be given once or twice to control postpartum bleeding and do not significantly affect milk yields (Bowes, 1980; Jolivet et al., 1978).

Combined (estrogen and progestogen) oral contraceptives may inhibit milk production if estrogen dosage is high (Miller & Hughes, 1970; Koetsawang, Bhiraleus & Chiemprajert, 1972). There is also some evidence that oral contraceptives can slightly lower protein, fat, and minerals in breastmilk (Kader et al., 1969).

GENERAL INFORMATION

The following brief discussion of the safety of drugs for breastfeeding mothers and infants is organized by pharmaceutical classifications. This information is derived from drug reviews cited at the end of the chapter on page 150.

ANALGESICS, NSAID'S AND NARCOTICS
Mild analgesics (acetaminophen, ibuprofen, mefenamic acid, and propoxyphene) are safe during lactation and are preferred to aspirin. While aspirin is still the antiarthritic drug of choice for the breastfeeding mother, her infant should be monitored for increased prothrombin time and signs of bleeding. Ibuprofen (Motrin) is commonly used for menstrual cramps and does not cross into breastmilk in significant quantities. Acetaminophen (Tylenol) is the drug of choice for reducing fever in children. It enters the maternal milk rapidly but the amount of medication the infant takes in is only 0.52% of the lowest recommended infant single dose. A single case of infant rash, apparently from maternal use of acetaminophen, has been reported (Notarianni, Oldham & Bennett, 1987).

Little is known about the effect of intrapartal epidural narcotics on subsequent breastfeeding. Anecdotal reports (LLLI, 1990) that infants of mothers who have had these drugs take longer to latch on to the breast need to be evaluated. If the mother needs narcotic analgesia postpartum, short use does not adversely affect the infant. When narcotics are used repeatedly, the infant should be monitored for drowsiness, poor breastfeeding, and weight loss. Narcotics frequently used postpartum are oxycodone and aspirin (Percodan), propoxyphene (Darvon), codeine, and meperidine (Demerol).

ANTICOAGULANTS
Previously, all anticoagulants were contraindicated for nursing mothers. Newer research indicates that some anticoagulants are not a problem. Warfarin (Coumadin) is present in breastmilk but only in very small amounts. The prothrombin time is usually normal in infants whose mothers are taking warfarin and dicumarol. Heparin does not appear in breastmilk. To be on the safe side, monitoring the infant's prothrombin time is recommended. The baby is given vitamin K (Mephyton) if needed. Phenindione (Hedulin, Dindevan) is contraindicated when the mother is breastfeeding because it has been reported to cause bleeding in breastfed infants.

ANTICONVULSANTS
Common medications used to treat seizure disorders are phenytoin (Dilantin), carbamazepine (Tegretol, Primidone, Mysoline) and phenobarbital. Carbamazepine transfers into milk in high levels but no adverse effects on breastfeeding infants have been reported. Phenobarbital and phenytoin (Dilantin) transfer into milk in insignificant amounts and are generally considered safe for the breastfeeding mother to use. If the mother takes high doses of phenobarbital, however, her baby may become drowsy. Short-acting phenobarbiturates (secobarbital, pentobarbital) are preferred to long-acting ones, because they appear in lower concentration in milk.

ANTIHISTAMINES
Antihistamines specifically compete with histamine, a naturally occurring amine that causes allergy symptoms. The secondary action is an anti-cholingeric or atropine-like action that results in inhibition of secretions, blurred vision, fast heart rate, urinary retention, and constipation. Practicing clinicians consistently report that mothers taking antihistamines often have a marked decrease in milk production shortly after taking the medication, often an over-the-counter

(OTC) cold preparation. Frequently used antihistamines include diphenhydramine (Benadryl), brompheniramine (Dimetane), methdilazine (Tacaryl), and tripelennamine (Pyribenzamine).

ANTIMICROBIALS

Most antibiotics are relatively safe for the breastfeeding mother. A general rule of thumb is that if an antibiotic can be given directly to an infant, it can also be taken by the nursing mother. With the exception of cephalexin (Keflex), cephalothin (Keflin), oxacillin (Prostaphlin), and nystatin (Mycostatin), antibiotics transfer into milk. Because any oral antibiotic changes the gastrointestinal flora and mucosa, the infant's stools may loosen and change in color. Since antibiotics predispose the mother and the infant to candidiasis, monitoring for this problem is advised.

The breastfeeding baby may develop sensitization to the antibiotics the mother is taking. A strong family history of drug sensitization should be taken into account when deciding whether a mother should take antibiotics and related drugs (Roberts, 1984). Allergies may be a problem. We saw a case in which the mother, who was highly allergic to penicillin, developed a rash and hives on her breasts from nursing her baby who was on ampicillin. The mother resolved her allergic response by giving her baby the ampicillin immediately after nursing instead of before the feeding. Chloramphenicol has relatively high concentration in milk. Most physicians avoid using tetracycline because it can discolor teeth during the formative years. The infant receives such a minute amount through breastmilk, however, that the possibility of this happening is remote.

Quinolones are synthetics that differ chemically from other antibiotics. Ciprofloxacin (Cipro), a new drug, is reportedly effective in treating a wide variety of infections. At therapeutic doses in children, arthropathies have been associated with quinolones; since quinolones can be excreted into human milk and attain concentrations comparable to or exceeding those of maternal serum, Stoukides (1991) recommends that these drugs be avoided in the breastfeeding period.

Metronidazole (Flagyl) should be given in a single 2-gm dose and breastfeeding should be interrupted for 12 hours following the dose. Such a plan interrupts breastfeeding for only 12 hours rather than a week (Erickson, Oppenheim & Smith, 1981). Sulfa drugs should not be taken by the mother during the first month of the infant's life because of the risk of neonatal jaundice. Sulfa drugs may be used after the first month of life; short-acting sulfonamides are preferred to long-acting ones.

ANTIFUNGALS

Nystatin (Mycostatin), miconazole (Monistat), and clotrimazole (Lotrimin, Mycelex) are antifungals used in the treatment of superficial infections. They are used topically and orally for treating fungal infections of the breastfeeding woman and her infant. Nystatin is the main therapeutic agent to control infections caused by *Candida albicans,* including thrush and diaper rash in infants. It is poorly absorbed in the gastrointentional tract, skin, or mucous membranes, and is used for a local effect. It can be given directly to the infant. Miconazole is a relatively new synthetic antifungal agent. About 50% of

TABLE 6-3   ANTIFUNGALS USED IN TREATING SUPERFICIAL INFECTIONS

Drug Name	Preparations	Usual Dosage
clotrimazole (Lotrimin, Myclex)	Creams, solutions, vaginal cream	Skin cream: apply 2 times/day Vaginal cream: 100 mg 4 times/day for 7 days or (if not pregnant) 200 mg 4 times/day for 3 days
miconazole (Monistat)	Creams, lotions, vaginal cream, and vaginal suppositories	Skin cream or lotion: apply 3–4 times/day Vaginal cream or suppository: 100 mg/day for 7 days
nystatin (Mycostatin, Nilstat)	Oral Use: suspensions or tablets Topical Use: powders, solutions, creams, ointment, and vaginal suppositories	Adults: 1,5000,000U to 2,400,000U/day divided in 3–4 doses Infants: 400,000U/day to 800,000U/day divided in 3–4 doses Use for 48 hours after symptoms disappear

miconazole is absorbed from the gastrointestinal tract and is widely distributed into body tissues and fluids. Clotrimazole has been used safely for more than a decade to treat vaginal yeast infection or candidiasis and is highly effective with minimum risk. Only small amounts of clotrimazole are absorbed systemically. Recently the FDA approved clotrimazole as an over-the-counter (OTC) drug.

BRONCHODILATORS

Ephedrine, epinephrine and cromolyn (Intal) are destroyed in the infant's gastrointestinal tract. Although relatively safe for breastfeeding infants, theophylline tends to accumulate in infants, who should be monitored for irritability and insomnia. Nursing women who take theophylline should avoid eating chocolate, another source of theophylline. Use of an inhaler minimizes the amount of theophylline passed into breastmilk.

CARDIOVASCULAR DRUGS

Digoxin is considered safe during lactation if maternal serum levels are carefully monitored. Many mothers who have toxemia and hypertension in pregnancy wish to breastfeed. Beta-blockers, atenolol, nadolol, and propranolol are relatively safe for these mothers to use while breastfeeding unless the infant has impaired renal or liver function. Methyldopa increases milk volume but no adverse effects have been reported.

DIURETICS

Furosemide (Lasix) is not excreted in breastmilk. Thiazide diuretics (Hydrodiuril Esidrix, Oretic) are relatively safe but can potentially cause dehydration in the infant and reduce maternal milk production. The infant should be weighed regularly and the number of wet diapers noted.

LAXATIVES

Laxatives are given routinely postpartum. Bulk-forming laxatives such as metamucil are considered a "natural" laxative; they are preferable to irritant cathartics (Peri-Colace, Ducolax) which stimulate intestinal peristalsis and inhibit the reabsorption of water in the large intestine. While there may be some concern about the possibility of dehydration,

Peri-Colace and Ducolax are frequently taken by breastfeeding mothers, apparently without ill effects. Mothers should be taught that use of a stimulant cathartic for more than one week may cause the large intestine to lose its tone.

NEUROPSYCHOTROPICS

Medications given for mental disorders are usually given over a long period of time; therefore they have a greater potential for accumulating than other medications. At the same time, drug levels are easily monitored by measuring serum drug levels (peak and trough) in both the mother and the infant. Tricyclic antidepressants such as desipramine are often used to treat postpartum depression. Negligible amounts pass into breastmilk.

Lithium is listed as "contraindicated" on the most recently published Drug List from the American Academy of Pediatrics Committee on Drugs (AAP, 1989). (See the special appendix on p. 153 at the end of this chapter.) However, since publication its author (Roberts, 1990) now contends that breastfeeding mothers should be able to take lithium with careful monitoring. In discussing lithium and breastfeeding, Schou (1990) agrees that "accumulating evidence points strongly to the beneficial effects of breastfeeding for both child and mother, mentally and physically, and it is an open question whether the gain outweighs the losses when breastfeeding is avoided. Supported by husband and physician, the mother must make her own choice."

Diazepam (Valium), a tranquillizer, is a commonly prescribed psychotherapeutic agent. High doses have been associated with infant lethargy, drowsiness, and jaundice. Ayd (1973) warned that competition for glucuronic acid by diazepam may result in hyperbilirubinemia in breastfed infants of Valium-treated mothers.

As discussed earlier, some psychotherapeutic medications increase the mother's milk supply. A mother should be forewarned that she may have more milk as a result of taking such a medication.

ORAL CONTRACEPTIVES

Combined (estrogen and progestin) oral contraceptives, especially those with more than 50 µg estrogen significantly decrease milk output and are contraindicated during lactation (Peralta et al., 1983;

Croxato et al., 1983). Progestin-only oral contraceptives have no effect on breastmilk and are not contraindicated during lactation, particularly if they are started when lactation is well established and the lowest effective dose is used. The amount of steroids absorbed by the breastfeeding infant of a mother using oral contraceptives is small and appears to have no long-term effects on children (Nilsson et al., 1986).

HERBS

Herbs, especially herbal teas, are currently very popular. Herbs have been used since antiquity for a variety of purposes, especially for medicinal purposes and the restoration of health.

Fleiss (1988) estimates that more than 30 herbs are considered to be powerful galactagogues. Perhaps the most widely known is foenugreek, the principal ingredient in the legendary "Lydia Pinkham's Vegetable Compound." Ixbut, an herb from Guatemala, is used to help women increase their breastmilk. Cascara and senna are two herbal remedies not recommended for the breastfeeding woman because they can cause the baby to have diarrhea. Sage acts like estrogen; therefore, it can reduce milk production. In South India, jasmine flowers suppress lactation when fashioned into a bra-like "wreath" over engorged breasts (Shrivastav et al., 1988). Similarly, in Australia, raw cabbage leaves placed on the breasts are routine treatment for engorgement (Scott, personal communication, 1988).

Since herbs are drugs, albeit in a natural rather than purified form, breastfed infants can have a reaction if the mother is ingesting herbs just as they might from any drug. In a Canadian report (Koren et al., 1990), a mother had taken ginseng in high doses during her pregnancy and while breastfeeding. Her full-term baby boy was noted to have thick black pubic hair, hair over his forehead and swollen red nipples. Although this case cannot establish ginseng as the cause of neonatal hirsutism, the reversal of hair growth after the mother discontinued taking ginseng suggested a cause-and-effect relationship.

CLINICAL IMPLICATIONS

Pharmaceuticals commonly taken by childbearing women include antibiotics, antidepressants, thyroid preparations, oral contraceptives, and over-the-

---

BREASTFEEDING MOTHERS NEEDING MEDICATIONS: QUESTIONS TO ASK

1. **What did your physician tell you when he ordered this medication for you?**
   Identify the medical reason for taking the medication and the doctor's opinion about whether the mother should continue breastfeeding. Phrased this way, the question captures how the mother reacted and her feelings about what she has been told.
2. **What is the drug's name, what is the prescribed dosage and scheduled time the drug is supposed to be taken?**
   This should yield basic information for evaluating the drug's action, excretion rate, and possible effect on infant and/or the mother's milk supply.
3. **How old is your baby and how often are you breastfeeding?**
   The infant's maturity makes a difference in its ability to metabolize drugs—the older the baby, the better. It may be possible to schedule taking the drug at certain times during the day that avoid peak plasma and milk drug levels—minimizing the amount of drug the baby receives through the milk. Usually, the best time to take the medication is right after feeding.
4. **Do you know how to hand express or use a breast pump?**
   If the mother must interrupt breastfeeding, this gives her options. Sometimes feedings need to be interrupted for only a few hours, or for a day or two so that hand expression avoids the expense and bother of renting or purchasing a pump. Reassure her that her milk production will continue if she expresses her milk regularly.

counter (OTC) medications for colds and minor respiratory problems. When a mother calls and asks whether she can continue to breastfeed while she takes a certain drug, the lactation consultant (LC) faces the dilemma (as well as the legal implications) of being asked a "medical" question.

While the final decision must be made by the woman and her physician, the LC can be an invaluable source of information and provide up-to-date information about studies done on the safety of a particular drug when breastfeeding. Many available drug lists provide the needed information. The most current recommendations regarding drugs and breastmilk from the Committee on Drugs of the American Academy of Pediatrics are presented at the end of this chapter (see p. 153) along with a partial list of articles on drugs and breastfeeding (see p. 150).

When using literature provided by drug manufacturers such as the information sheets in the medication packet, keep in mind the following caveat: pharmaceutical houses protect themselves legally by taking the "guilty unless proven innocent" approach. Unless there is documentation proving otherwise, many medications are "not recommended for breastfeeding." General pharmacology textbooks take a similar conservative stance, warning readers that nursing mothers should not take *any* medications.

The first task is to find a discussion of the drug in question in current drug literature. To simplify the search, first identify the *generic* name of the drug. The generic name is the drug's chemical or official name as opposed to its *trade* or *brand* name. For example, ampicillin is the generic name of an antibiotic. Ampicillin is manufactured by several pharmaceutical companies, and sold under a trade name such as Amoxil, Omnipen, or Amcill. Trade names are capitalized; generic names are in lower case. Most drug lists use the generic name followed by its popular trade names. Generic names of drugs are given with their common trade names on pp. 159–160 in the AAP Committee on Drugs appendix at the end of this chapter.

Non-prescription, over-the-counter (OTC) drug sales rise each year. They are frequently combination drugs. Popular OTC drugs include analgesics (ibuprofen, acetaminophen, and aspirin); antihistamines (diphenhydramine and chlopheniramine) for colds and sinus conditions; bronchodilators (ephedrine); antacids; and cathartics. Generally OTC drugs are compatible with lactation; however, many antihistamine preparations dramatically decrease the milk supply, particularly in the very early breastfeeding period or when the baby is nursing infrequently (three times a day or less). The clinical care plan described in Table 6–4 opposite describes a typical situation.

The many OTC cold preparations which have long-acting or sustained action are advertised to "last" 12 hours. Fillers are added to the drug to produce a timed release so that the mother cannot excrete it all within a 12-hour period. Such drugs will be long acting for the infant as well; these preparations increase the potential for accumulation in both the mother and the infant.

Scheduling the best time of day for a mother to take medication minimizes the amount of drug the infant receives. If a mother is taking penicillin with a known half-life of one hour, the infant theoretically receives the least amount of penicillin through her milk if she nurses her baby *just before* taking the medication, when serum levels are likely to be at their lowest. Whenever the mother takes a medication over a long period of time, the timing of the medication in relation to feeding her baby is less important because the concentration of the drug in her serum remains relatively stable.

At least one drug appears to make breastmilk taste bitter. In one case (Smolek-Houghton, 1984), after a nursing mother took an OTC antihistamine, her toddler refused to breastfeed, spitting out her milk. The mother stopped taking the drug and the toddler promptly resumed nursing again.

Health professionals have a formidable responsibility when it comes to making decisions about drugs and breastfeeding. On the one hand, physicians are anxious (and rightly so) about their legal risk if something adverse happens. On the other hand, if the doctor recommends weaning, the result can be disastrous. Abrupt weaning can be so traumatic that many women painfully recall the experience in vivid detail decades later—sometimes with hostility toward the physician if they realize that weaning was not necessary. The infant who is weaned even temporarily is at greater risk of infection and may develop allergies or other severe health problems. The following example illustrates, in the extreme, what may happen when breastfeeding is interrupted because of maternal medication.

Diagnosed as having a urinary tract infection and started on a sulfonamide medication, a breastfeed-

TABLE 6–4 CLINICAL CARE PLAN

A 30-year-old mother is feeding her four week-old-old male infant exclusively with breastmilk. After taking Coricidin (sustained action) and Drixoral for a severe head cold, her milk suddenly "dries up."

Assessment	Interventions	Rationale
Sudden decrease in milk supply following ingestion of Coricidin and Drixoral (OTC drugs) for head cold	Determine drug components of Coricidin and Drixoral to identify chemical agent possibly causing problem	Certain medications inhibit lactation
	Advise to discontinue OTC medications since both contain antihistamines and sympathomimetics	Antihistamines dry all body secretions including breastmilk; sympathomimetics may interfere with prolactin release
	Encourage rest, fluids, and foods high in vitamin C for duration of head cold	Enhances body's ability to "fight" cold; liquifies secretions
	Encourage to breastfeed more often—at least 6–8 times/day	Builds milk supply and helps maintain nutritional and hydration needs
	If necessary, supplement infant with extra stored mother's milk or formula until milk supply returns to normal	Infants require frequent and adequate nutriments for growth
Mother unsure and confused; she wonders if she has lost her milk "forever"	Reassure mother that following excretion of the medications from her system, her milk supply will return to normal in a day or two	There is little risk of nipple confusion developing at 4 weeks Half-life of Coricidin is 12 hours; therefore the drug should clear in about 2 days

ing mother was told to discontinue breastfeeding for the duration of the therapy (ten days). Already discouraged because she had needed to pump her breasts earlier when her infant was jaundiced, the mother felt overwhelmed and decided to give up breastfeeding. Later the physician's office called to say that her urine culture was negative, but that she should continue the drug as a precautionary measure. Shortly after discontinuing breastfeeding, her infant developed vomiting, diarrhea, and later ec-

---

GENERAL GUIDELINES FOR BREASTFEEDING AND MEDICATION USE

- Use a medication only if it is absolutely necessary. Consider alternative non-drug therapies.
- Delay starting the medication (if there is a choice) until the infant is more mature and better able to detoxify and metabolize drugs that might be transported through the milk.
- Take the lowest dose possible for the shortest time possible.
- Choose a drug that transfers the least amount into breastmilk, using its reported milk/plasma ration as a guide. Avoid drugs with an M/P greater than or equal to 1.
- Avoid a drug with a long half-life, if possible.

- Avoid sustained release preparations.
- Schedule taking the medication so that the lowest amount gets into the milk—usually immediately after a feeding or before the infant has a long sleep period.
- Observe for any untoward reaction, such a fussiness, rash, colic, or change in feeding or sleeping habits. If any of these occur, the physician should be notified and given information about all of the drugs used by the mother.
- Teach expression or provide a breast pump and instructions for its use if the mother must take a contraindicated drug for a short time.

zema. The parents and physician desperately switched from one formula to another to find one the infant could tolerate. The infant developed periods of apnea and was placed on a home apnea monitor between hospitalizations. Ultimately, more complications developed, and an ileostomy was performed. Desperate, the mother began relactating while she collected fresh breastmilk donated by other women; eventually she was able to sustain the infant on her milk. This child is now reasonably healthy, but still cannot tolerate cow's milk and is allergic to many other foods (Riordan & Riordan, 1984).

Finally, the LC may find herself in a "tug-of-war" between the mother and the physician about the safety of taking a medication. I found myself in this situation when a breastfeeding mother called me for help. She was ordered by her psychiatrist to take an antidepressant and to wean her baby immediately. Several drug lists showed the drug in question to be considered safe for breastfeeding. I relayed this information to the family. The psychiatrist held firm. Following several heated discussions between the mother and her psychiatrist, the mother relented and weaned.

While there are no easy answers which resolve this kind of problem, the story points out that the LC, acting as a client advocate and using reliable information, can only advise or recommend but can't force a decision.

MATERNAL ADDICTION

According to a 1985 survey by the National Institute on Drug Abuse, about 70 million Americans have used an illegal substance such as cocaine, marijuana, or heroin on at least one occasion (National Institute on Drug Abuse, 1986). Persons with the highest rate of use are those between 18 and 25 years old. Thirty percent of women between 18 and 34 years of age reported using an illicit drug in the past year (Johnson, 1987). Most breastfeeding women do not use illegal drugs but some do. While there are a multitude of illegal drugs, this discussion is limited to those most commonly used.

Marijuana is so widely used today that it is probably the most commonly used illegal drug among breastfeeding women. In a 1985 survey (Johnson, 1987) 21% of women 18 to 25 years old reported use within the past month. Braude et al. (1987) estimate

that 5–15% of pregnant women use or have used marijuana. Marijuana purportedly impairs DNA and RNA formation in laboratory animals (Nahas & Panon, 1976) but there have been no reports of infant health problems solely from maternal use of marijuana during lactation or pregnancy. There have, however, been anecdotal reports of marijuana-induced drowsiness in breastfeeding infants. Tetrahydrocannabinol, the active ingredient in marijuana, is readily absorbed from the gastrointestinal tract and metabolized by the baby (Perez & Wall, 1982). Sidestream from marijuana cigarettes inhaled by the infant increases his exposure to the drug.

Thus the dilemma arises: should a woman be advised not to breastfeed it she refuses to give up her recreational use of marijuana? Obviously, smoking marijuana is not wise; the optimal situation is for the mother to be free of all drugs while breastfeeding. However, because there is little evidence that marijuana causes serious harm, it is probably better for the occasional marijuana user to continue to breastfeed rather than wean her baby. On the other hand, no infant should *ever* have to inhale passive smoke from marijuana or any cigarette, cigar, or pipe.

Cocaine use in the United States has dramatically increased in the past several years. More recently, a cheaper and even more popular form of cocaine known as "crack" has emerged. Cocaine harms the fetus and the nursing infant. Because it is highly lipid-soluble and readily crosses biologic membranes, its use by a breastfeeding mother can have serious effects.

Chasnoff, Lewis, and Squires (1987) reported a case in which a mother who was a cocaine user brought her two-week-old infant girl to a hospital emergency room. The baby was extremely irritable, and was frequently startled by minimal stimulation. She also exhibited dilated pupils, vomiting, and tachycardia, all symptoms of cocaine intoxication. Intravenous fluids were started and breastfeeding was discontinued. Milk samples were negative for cocaine and its metabolites by 36 hours after the mother's last cocaine use. The infant's urine was negative by 60 hours after the last breastfeeding. The baby fully recovered and was discharged home with the parent under court supervision. Another infant reportedly developed apnea and seizures from direct ingestion of cocaine which her mother had used as a topical anesthetic for sore nipples (Chaney,

Fronke & Wadlington, 1988). These reports are the basis for legal action of child abuse against breastfeeding women who use cocaine.

The recommendation is clear: cocaine should *never* be used when breastfeeding. Those who do not only risk the health of their child, but also legal action against them which may result in the removal of the child from their custody.

SUBSTANCE ABUSE

AMPHETAMINES

Amphetamines readily transfer into breastmilk; levels are three times higher than those in the mother's plasma. Despite these high levels, a case report (Steiner et al., 1984) of a mother taking high doses of amphetamines recounts that a nursing infant had no adverse effects and developed normally. A large study of more than 100 breastfeeding women taking amphetamines failed to detect any adverse changes in the behavior of their infants (Ayd, 1973).

ALCOHOL

Alcohol affects the central nervous system of both the breastfeeding mother and infant. When taken in sufficient quantity it can potentially inhibit milk ejection. The effects of alcohol on the breastfeeding baby appear to be directly related to the quantity that the mother ingests. When the lactating woman drinks lightly, the amount of alcohol the baby receives is commonly thought not to be harmful but may have a mildly sedative effect. While "social" drinking is usually not considered a problem for breastfeeding women, a troubling study by Little et al. (1989) showed that the motor development of breastfed infants may be slower when the mother drinks alcohol. This decline in motor skills was related to how much the mother drank even after more than 100 variables were controlled, including smoking and general drug use. Mental development was not affected.

Binkiewicz, Robinson, and Senior (1978) reported a case of a mother who chronically drank large amounts of alcohol while breastfeeding her four-month-old baby. The alcohol content in her breastmilk was 100 mg/dL. The child appeared to have pseudo-Cushing's Syndrome; he was obese and had a moon-shaped facial appearance. After the mother stopped drinking, these characteristics disappeared.

ENVIRONMENTAL CONTAMINANTS

The great concern—perhaps the tragedy of our age—is the ever increasing contamination of our planet. A global problem shared by all countries, industrial pollution of air and water respects no boundaries. The threat that a mother's milk may no longer be safe causes justifiable public alarm and outcry.

Understandably, our information about toxic substances in breastmilk is derived from animal studies or case reports rather than from controlled human studies. While human milk appears to be a useful medium for monitoring organochlorine pesticides (Niessen et al., 1984; Stacey, Perriman & Whitney, 1985), there is little evidence that contaminants in human milk cause harm to the nursling. While numerous toxins can enter breastmilk, the major contaminants are pesticides (DDT, DDE, chlordane, heptachlor), other organohalogen compounds (PCBs, PBBs, dioxin, benzofurans, benzene hexachloride), and radioactivity. Polybrominated biphenyls (PBBs) are chemical compounds similar to polychlorinated biphenyls (PCBs) and dichloro diphenyl trichlorethane (DDT).

Laug, Kunze, and Prickett (1951) published a report on DDT levels in human milk which exceeded that permitted by WHO and the U.S. Code of Federal Regulations. The widespread use of DDT was halted in 1972 when its FDA registration was withdrawn. The first widespread alarm over breastmilk contamination occurred in 1973, when Michigan farm animals were contaminated with polybrominated biphenyl compounds (PBBs) that were accidentally mixed with their feed. Breastfeeding mothers living on the contaminated Michigan farms were advised to wean their infants. Later, Rogan (1983) found no difference in the levels of PCBs in the milk of women exposed to PCBs and those not exposed to a given spill.

Dioxin is another name for a series of chemicals called polychlorinated dibenzodioxins or PCDDs. Women exposed to these herbicides have high levels of the toxin during their first lactation but lower levels with subsequent lactation. Overweight women have somewhat lower PCDD levels while underweight women have slightly higher levels (Ahlborg, Waern & Hakanssan, 1987). Mothers eating food contaminated with mercury have not been associated with toxicity in their breastfeeding infants, even though the infants had high serum levels of mercury (Amin-Zaki et al., 1974).

The effect of nuclear pollution on breastmilk has been studied following the massive release of radioactivity at the Chernobyl nuclear power plant. Following the 1986 explosion at Chernobyl, radioactive fallout occurred throughout many areas of western Europe. Radioactive levels in cow's milk and in leafy vegetables were sufficiently high that these foods were banned for consumption by pregnant women and children. DeLallo and colleagues (1987) measured the ^{131}I concentrations in human milk from women in two hospitals in Rome and from a milk bank in Rome for the first seven months after the explosion. Gori et al. (1988) examined samples of human placenta and human milk in Italy for one year after the accident to determine radioactive levels. Placental levels climbed rapidly. Although levels in human milk increased, the increase was much lower from the start, and it continued at a substantially slower rate. Radioactivity in human milk was about one-third the level found in placentas.

Shortly after the DeLallo report, Lindemann and Christensen (1987) reported their findings from Norway, Sweden, and Austria. In Sweden, identical amounts of ^{137}I were found in both cow's milk and human milk. In Austria, the amount in human milk

was only one-tenth that found in cow's milk. In Norway, the total amount of radioactive cesium in cow's milk never exceeded 60 Bq/L. The accepted upper limit of radioactive cesium in milk and/or babyfood is 370 Bq/kg. Radioactive cesium has a biologic half-life of 70 to 110 days. Since the amount in human milk was negligible, these investigators also concluded that "there was never any danger for the breast-fed infants.... If a similar accident should occur, the infants may safely be nursed but the mothers should take care and be advised when using local vegetables, meat, fish, and milk products" (Lindemann & Christensen, 1987). All of these reports document that radioactive levels rose much higher in cow's milk than in human milk, probably because of the bovine diet of plant foods. These authors concluded that the concentrations in human milk were low enough that they did not present a threat to the nursing infant.

A massive release of radioactivity occurred in the United States during the mid-1940s. A nuclear weapons plant in Hanford, Washington, poured so much radioactive iodine into the air that children living nearby were exposed to massive and cumulative doses (Church, 1990). Presumably, infants in the area were being breastfed. No known studies were done on the milk of mothers in the area nor on the breastfed children who are now adults; consequently, long-term outcomes related to breastfeeding are unknown.

CLINICAL IMPLICATIONS

Generally, if the mother has been detoxified and is narcotic free, she should be encouraged to breastfeed. A woman on an average methadone maintenance dose will theoretically excrete only about 57 μg/day in her first five weeks, which is considered a trace amount not harmful to her infant (Ostrea, Chavez & Stryker, 1978; Beeley, 1986; White & White, 1984) and may minimize withdrawal symptoms to the infant.

According to one study (Ostrea, Chavez & Stryker, 1978), when these mothers were under care and supervision, their children's mental and psychomotor development was within normal limits up to two years of age. Although the drug-dependent mother needs more support and guidance, fears of the addicted mother's unstable lifestyle, potential for child abuse, and/or neglect have been overrated. Others disagree about this mother's ability to function and provide adequate care for her infant. Kantor (1978) considers the addicted mother a poor risk for parenting even though she is receiving help. In the United States, it is becoming more common for grandmothers and others to take over parental care when addicted women voluntarily relinquish their children.

The desire to mother and to breastfeed can be a powerful motivator to stay off drugs—at least for a while. It is not at all uncommon for a drug user to give up her drug habit during pregnancy and lactation—the experience of childbearing is a "high" in itself. For some, this is their one opportunity to "be normal" even if temporarily, and give something of themselves. Williams (1990) interviewed women who had been addicted to heroin for more than 15 years. Children were central to the lives of these women. Several described how they had stopped drug use when they they were pregnant but then resumed their habits after their children were born.

While environmental pollution is worsening, there are few reports of either short- or long-term adverse effects on infants from pollutants in mother's milk. In discussing environmental pollutants and breastfeeding with medical researchers, Rogan (1990) projected that even under the worst conditions a breastfed child would lose only two days of life from exposure to such pollutants in human milk if he lived a normal life span. If the baby is weaned to formula or cow's milk, these foods also carry the risk of toxicity from lead or other contaminants. Eventually, the child eats the same foods as the rest of the family and is equally exposed to any contaminants in them. The risk of pollution exists for everyone, not just breastfeeding babies.

While most lactating women are at minimal risk for contamination of their milk, there are exceptions depending on where one lives and works. The risk is greater in an agricultural area where chemicals are sprayed, particularly by aerial spraying; or in an industrial area where chemicals are used; or near contaminated water (such as the Great Lakes). There are ways for women to minimize pollutant contamination (Bartmess, 1988; Stacey, Perriman & Whitney, 1985; Drijver et al., 1988). Lactating women should take care to:

- avoid fresh-water fish from waters known to be contaminated

- wash and peel nonorganic vegetables and fruits thoroughly before eating
- eat low-fat foods and cut fat from meats
- avoid using pesticides in the home or on the lawn
- avoid a "crash" diet, thereby preventing the sudden release of toxins from body fat into breastmilk
- avoid contact with wood preservatives containg pentachlorophenol
- avoid fatty meat and fatty fish in the diet to minimize the amount of animal fat
- avoid buildings or homes treated for termites with dieldrin.

Even using lanolin as a nipple ointment is suspect. Pesticide residues in lanolin have been found in Australia and the United States (Copeland, Raebel & Wagner, 1989). A mother who is concerned about environmental contamination can contact the local Department of Health and the Environmental Protection Agency, Human Effects Monitoring Branch in the Office of Pesticide Programs for information about a milk analysis (Lauwers & Woessner, 1990). While analysis of the level of contaminants in breastmilk may be helpful, the results are of limited value unless the clinical history (including exposure events and chronic illness) justifies them. Another problem is unreliability of onetime results. A Norwegian study (Bakken & Seip, 1976) showed a dramatic variance of insecticide levels in the same mother's milk at different times. While breastfeeding is still considered "safe," active efforts to diminish contaminants in our environment, and subsequently in human milk, must continue.

SUMMARY

The issue which pervades this chapter is the widespread use of drugs. More drugs are used in the management of human illness and for recreational purposes than ever before. There is a dangerous tendency to believe that drugs are the answer to any problem. Perhaps this is a notion left over from times when infectious diseases were the major health problem—even though infectious diseases are reduced primarily through public health measures such as improved sanitation. We forget that many illnesses are self-limiting, causing only minor discomforts that subside with or without drugs. For example, a tense new mother taught to use progressive relaxation techniques or meditation avoids exposing her infant to a chemical tranquilizer. In some cases, maternal drug treatment can be delayed until after the infant has weaned on his own. In essence, the question should not be, "Can this medicated mother be allowed to breastfeed?" but rather "Does this mother really need to be medicated?"

The question of drugs and breastfeeding also depends on belief systems. If the involved health professionals believe that breastfeeding is important, they will make every effort to find a safe way for a mother to continue breastfeeding. If they do not value it, they probably will not make the effort and recommend that the mother wean. The same is true for breastfeeding during recreational drug use: there are those who believe that the lactating woman must make a clear choice between taking drugs or breastfeeding her baby; others prefer to weigh the risks and benefits of each individual situation.

More and more foreign substances in milk will continue to be found as analytic tools are improved. The problem now lies with evaluating this information and translating it into practical and safe action, while respecting the wishes (and rights) of women who bear children and desire to breastfeed. We need better surveillance systems that will alert us to potential problems before the child is exposed to drug or environmental toxins. Health-care providers can help reduce these risks by staying current with new research findings and by teaching parents methods for avoiding unnecessary exposure.

REVIEWS OF DRUGS IN HUMAN MILK

Briggs, GG, et al.: *Drugs in pregnancy and lactation,* Baltimore, 1983, The Williams & Wilkins Co.

Kirksey, A, and Groziak, SM: Maternal drug use: evaluation of risks to breast-fed infants, *Wld Rev Nutr Diet* 43:60–79, 1984.

Lauwers, J, and Woessner, C: *Chemical agents and breast milk,* Garden City Park, New York, 1990, Avery Publishing Group, Inc.

Lawrence, R: *Breastfeeding: A guide for the medical profession,* 3rd ed., St. Louis, 1989, The C.V. Mosby Co., pp. 518–95.

O'Brien, TE: Excretion of drugs in human milk, *Am J Hosp Pharm* 31:844–54, 1974.

Riordan, J: Drugs in breastmilk. In Pagliaro, LA, and Pagliaro, AM, eds.: *Problems in pediatric drug therapy,*

Hamilton, Ill., 1987, Drug Intelligence Publ., pp. 194–258.

Roberts, R: *Drug Therapy in infants,* Philadelphia, 1984, W.B. Saunders Co., pp. 346–83.

White, GJ, and White, MK: Breastfeeding and drugs in human milk, *Vet Hum Toxicol* 26 (suppl.):1–26, 1984.

Wicklund, S: Special report: Drugs for two in lactation, *AJN* 82:68–70, 1982.

Wilson, J: *Drugs in breast milk,* Balgowlah, South Australia, 1981, ADIS Press.

REFERENCES

Ahlborg, GG, Waern, F, and Hakansson, H: Interactive effects of PCDDs and PCDFs occurring in human mother's milk, *Chemosphere* 16: 1701–6, 1987.

American Academy of Pediatrics, Committee on Drugs: The transfer of drugs and other chemicals into human milk, *Pediatrics* 84:924–36, 1989.

Amin-Zaki, L, et al.: Studies of infants postnatally exposed to methylmercury, *J Pediatr* 85:81–84, 1974.

Aono, T, et al.: Effect of sulpiride on poor puerperal lactation, *Am J Obstet Gynecol* 143:927–32, 1982.

Atkinson, JC, and Begg, EJ: Prediction of drug distribution into human milk from physicochemical characteristics, *Clin Pharmacokinet* 18:151–67, 1990.

Ayd, FJ: Excretion of psychotropic drugs in human breast milk, *Int Drug Ther Newslett* 8:33–35, 1973.

Bakken, AR, and Seip, M: Insecticides in human breast milk, *Acta Paediatr Scand* 65:535–39, 1976.

Bartmess, JE: The risk of polychlorinated dibenzodioxins in human milk, *J Hum Lact* 4:105–7, 1988.

Beeley, L: Drugs and breastfeeding, *Clin Obstet Gynecol* 13:24–51, 1986.

Berlin, CM: The excretion of drugs and chemicals in human milk. In Yaffe, SJ: *Pediatric pharmacology,* Philadelphia, 1983, Grune & Stratton, Inc., pp. 137–47.

Binkiewicz, A, Robinson, MJ, and Senior, B: Pseudo-Cushing syndrome caused by alcohol in breast milk, *J Pediatr* 93:965–67, 1978.

Bowes, WA: The effect of medications on the lactating mother and her infant, *Clin Obstet Gynecol* 23:1073–79, 1980.

Braude, MC, et al.: Perinatal effects of drugs of abuse, *Fed Proc* 46:2446–53, 1987.

Canterbury, RJ, et al.: Postpartum psychosis induced by Bromocriptine, *South Med J* 80:1463–64, 1987.

Chaney, NE, Franke, J, and Wadlington, WB: Cocaine convulsions in a breast-feeding baby, *J Pediatr* 112:134–35, 1988.

Chasnoff, IJ, Lewis, DE, and Squires, L: Cocaine intoxication in a breast-fed infant, *Pediatrics* 80:836–38, 1987.

Church, GJ: There was death in the milk, *Time,* p. 28, July 23, 1990.

Copeland, C, Raebel, MA, and Wagner, SL: Pesticide residue in lanolin (letter), *JAMA* 261:242, 1989.

Croxato, HB, et al.: Fertility regulation in nursing women: IV. Long-term influence of a low-dose combined oral contraceptive initiated at day 30 postpartum upon lactation and infant growth, *Contraception* 27:27–37, 1983.

DeLallo, E, et al.: Radioactivity in breast milk in central Italy in the aftermath of Chernobyl (letter), *Acta Paediatr Scand* 76:530–31, 1987.

Dickey, RP, and Stone, SC: Drugs that affect the breast and lactation, *Clin Obstet Gynecol* 18:95–111, 1975.

Drijver M, et al.: Determinants of polychlorinated biphenyls (PCBs) in human milk, *Acta Paediatr Scand* 77:30–36, 1988.

Ehrenkranz, TA, and Ackerman, BA: Metoclopramide effect on faltering milk production by mothers of premature infants, *Pediatrics* 78:614–20, 1986.

Erickson, SH, Oppenheim, GL, and Smith, GH: Metronidazole in breast milk, *Obstet Gynecol* 57:48–50, 1981.

Feldman, S, and Pickering, LK: Pharmacokinetics of drugs in human milk. In Howell, RR, Morriss, FH, and Pickering, LK: *Human milk in infant nutrition and health*, Springfield, Ill., 1986, Charles C Thomas, Publisher, pp. 256–78.

Fleiss, P: Herbal remedies for the breastfeeding mother, *Mothering*, Summer, 1988, pp. 68–70.

Giacoia, GP, and Catz, CS: Drug therapy in the lactating mother, *Postgrad Med* 83:211–18, 1988.

Gori, G, et al.: Radioactivity in breast milk and placentas during the year after Chernobyl, *Am J Obstet Gynecol* 159:1232–34, 1988.

Gupta, AP, and Gupta, PK: Metoclopramide as a lactogogue, *Clin Pediatr* 24:269–72, 1985.

Guzman, V, et al.: Improvement of defective lactation by using oral metoclopramide, *Acta Obstet Gynec Scand* 58:53–55, 1979.

Johnson, EM: Substance abuse and women's health, *Public Health Rep* (suppl.)101:42–48, 1987.

Jolivet, A, et al.: Effect of ergot alkaloid derivatives on milk secretion in the immediate postpartum period, *J Gynecol Obstet Biol Reprod* (Paris) 1:129–34, 1978.

Kader, A, et al.: Biochemical and experimental studies on lactation, III. Clinical changes induced in human milk by gestagens, *Am J Obstet Gynecol* 105:978–85, 1969.

Kantor, GK: Addicted mother, addicted baby: a challenge to health care providers, *MCN* 3:281–84, 1978.

Kauppila, A, et al.: A dose response relation between improved lactation and metoclopramide, *Lancet* 1(8231):1175–77, 1983.

Koetsawang, S, Bhiraleus, P, and Chiemprajert, T: Effects of oral contraceptives on lactation, *Fertil Steril* 23:24–28, 1972.

Koren, G, et al.: Maternal ginseng use associated with neonatal androgenization (letter), *JAMA* 264:1866, 1990.

La Leche League International, Discussion Session with Speakers, International Annual Physicians Seminar, Boston, 1990.

Laug, EP, Kunze, FMN, and Prickett, CS: Occurrence of DDT in human fat and milk, *Arch Ind Hyg* 3:245–46, 1951.

Lauwers, J, and Woessner, C: *Chemical agents and breast milk*, Garden City Park, New York, 1990, Avery Publishing Group, Inc., pp. 3–6.

Lederman, SA: Breast milk contaminants: Maternal medications, *Clin Nutr* 8(3):131–38, 1989.

Lindemann, R, and Christensen, GC: Radioactivity in breastmilk after the Chernobyl accident (letter), *Acta Paediatr Scand* 76:981–82, 1987.

Lipkin, GB: Drug therapy in maternal care. In Spencer, RT, et al.: *Clinical pharmacology and nursing management*, 3rd ed. Philadelphia, 1989, J.B. Lippincott Co., pp. 1132–70.

Little, RE, et al.: Maternal alcohol use during breast-feeding and infant mental and motor development at one year, *N Engl J Med* 321:425–30, 1989.

Miller, GH, and Hughes, LR: Lactation and genital involution effects of a new low-dose oral contraceptive on breastfeeding mothers and their infants, *Obstet Gynecol* 35:44–50, 1970.

Nahas, G, and Panon, W, eds.: *Marihuana: chemistry, biochemistry, and cellular effect*, New York, 1976, Springer-Verlag, New York, Inc.

Nation, RL, and Hotham, N: Drugs and breast-feeding, *Med J Aust* 146:308–13, 1987.

National Institute on Drug Abuse: *Drug abuse statistics 1985 population estimates*, Washington D.C., 1986, Alcohol, Drug Abuse, and Mental Health, United States Public Health Service.

Niessen, KH, et al.: Chlorinated hydrocarbons in adipose tissue of infants and toddlers: inventory and studies on their association with intake of mothers' milk, *Eur J Pediatr* 142:238–43, 1984.

Nilsson, S, et al.: Long-term follow-up of children breastfed by mothers using oral contraceptives, *Contraception* 34:443–57, 1986.

Notarianni, LJ, Oldham, HG, and Bennett, PN: Passage of paracetamol into breast milk and its subsequent metabolism by the neonate, *Br J Clin Pharmacol* 24:63–67, 1987.

Ostrea, EM, Chavez, DJ, and Stryker, JC: *The care of the drug dependent woman and her infant*, Lansing, Mich., 1978, Michigan Department of Public Health.

Peralta, O, et al.: Fertility regulation in nursing women: V: Long-term influence of a low-dose combined oral contraceptive initiated at day 90 postpartum upon lactation and infant growth, *Contraception* 27:27–37, 1983.

Perez, RM, and Wall, ME: Presence of Δ^9 tetrahydrocannabinol in human milk, *N Engl J Med* 307:819–20, 1982.

Peterson, RG, and Bowes, WA: Drugs, toxins and environmental agents in breast milk. In Neville, MC, and Neifert, M: *Lactation: Physiology, nutrition and breast-feeding*, New York, 1983, Plenum Press, pp. 367–403.

Postpartum hypertension, seizures, strokes reported with bromocriptine, *FDA Bull* 14(1):3, 1982.

Rimar, JM: Metoclopramide for enhancing lactation, *MCN* 11:93, 1986.

Riordan, J: Drugs in breastmilk. In Pagliaro, LA, and Pagliaro, AM, eds.: *Problems in pediatric drug therapy*, Hamilton, Ill., 1987, Drug Intelligence Publ., pp. 194–258.

Riordan, J, and Riordan, M: Drugs in breastmilk: Is the risk exaggerated? *AJN* 84:328–32, 1984.

Rivera-Calimlim, L: The significance of drugs in breast

milk. In Lawrence, R, ed.: Breastfeeding, *Clin Perinatol* 14:51–70, 1987.

Roberts, RJ: *Drug therapy in infants*, Philadelphia, 1984, W.B.Saunders Co., pp. 346–83.

Roberts, RJ: Drugs and breastfeeding: an overview, A presentation made to La Leche League International, Seminar for Physicians, Boston, July 12–13, 1990.

Rogan, RJ: Chromatographic evidence of polychlorinated biphenyl exposure from a spill, *JAMA* 249:1057–58, 1983.

Rogan, W: *Should the presence of carcinogens in breastmilk discourage breastfeeding?* International Society for Research on Human Milk and Lactation, 1990, Ambulatory Pediatric Association Annual Meeting, Anaheim, Calif., 1990.

Schou, M: Lithium treatment during pregnancy, delivery, and lactation: an update, *J Clin Psychiatry* 51(10):410–13, 1990.

Shrivastav, P, et al.: Suppression of puerperal lactation using jasmine flowers, *Aust NZ Obstet Gynaecol* 28:68–71, 1988.

Smolek-Houghton, M: My milk connoisseur, *La Leche League News* 26(3):50,1984.

Sousa, PLR: Metoclopramide and breast-feeding, *Br Med J* 1:512, 1975.

Stacey, Cl, Perriman, WS, and Whitney, S: Organochlorine pesticide residue levels in human milk, Western Australia, 1979–1980, *Arch Environ Health* 40(2):102–8, 1985.

Steiner, E, et al.: L Amphetamine secretion in breast milk, *Eur J Clin Pharmacol* 27:123–24, 1984.

Stoukides, CA: Quinolone antibiotics and breastfeeding, *J Hum Lact* 7:143–44, 1991.

Tyree, DJ: Perinatal medications and breastfeeding, *J Hum Lact* 8:87–90, 1992.

Vorherr, H: Human lactation and breastfeeding. In Larson, BL, ed: *Lactation: A comprehensive treatise*, vol. 4, New York, 1978, Academic Press Inc., pp. 181–279.

Watson, DL, et al.: Bromocriptine Mesylate for lactation suppression: A risk for postpartum hypertension? *Obstet Gynecol* 74:573–76, 1989.

White, GJ, and White, MK: Breastfeeding and drugs in human milk, *Vet Human Toxicology* 26 (suppl.):1–26, 1984.

Williams, AB: Reproductive concerns of women at risk for HIV infection, *J Nurs Midwif* 35:292–98, 1990.

Wilson, J: *Drugs in breast milk*, Balgowlah, South Australia, 1981, ADIS Press.

Yurchak, AM, and Jusko, WJ: Theophylline secretion into breast milk, *Pediatrics* 57:518–20, 1976.

ADDITIONAL REFERENCES

Berlin, CM: Drugs and chemicals: exposure of the nursing mother, *Clin Pharm* 36:1089–97, 1989.

Lederman, SA: Breast milk contaminants: Substance abuse, infection, and the environment, *Clin Nutr* 8(3):120–30, 1989.

Palma, PA, and Adcock, EW: Human milk and breast-feeding, *Am Fam Phys* 24:173–81, 1981.

Rogan, WJ, Bagniewska, A and Damstra, R: Pollutants in breast milk, *N Engl J Med*, June 26, vol 302:1450–53, 1980.

AMERICAN ACADEMY OF PEDIATRICS

Committee on Drugs

Transfer of Drugs and Other Chemicals Into Human Milk

Since the first publication of this statement,[1] much new information has been published concerning the transfer of drugs and chemicals into human milk. This information, in addition to other research published before 1983, makes a revision of the previous statement necessary. In this revision, lists of the pharmacologic or chemical agents transferred into human milk and their possible effects on the infant or on lactation, if known, are provided (Tables 1 to 7). The fact that a pharmacologic or chemical agent does not appear in the Tables is not meant to imply that it is not transferred into human milk or that it does not have an effect on the infant but indicates that there are no reports in the literature. These tables should assist the physician in counseling a nursing mother regarding breast-feeding when the mother has a condition for which a drug is medically indicated.

The following questions should be considered when prescribing drug therapy to lactating women. (1) Is the drug therapy really necessary? Consultation between the pediatrician and the mother's physician can be most useful. (2) Use the safest drug; for example, acetaminophen rather than aspirin for oral analgesia. (3) If there is a possibility that a drug may present a risk to the infant (eg, phenytoin, phenobarbital), consideration should be given to measurement of blood concentrations in the nursing infant. (4) Drug exposure to the nursing infant may be minimized by having the mother take the medication just after completing a breast-feeding and/or just before the infant has his or her lengthy sleep periods.

Data have been obtained from a search of the medical literature. Because methodologies used to quantitate drugs in milk continue to improve, this current information will require continuous updating. Brand names are listed in Table 8 in accordance with the current *AMA Drug Evaluation,* the *USAN* and *USP Dictionary of Drug Names.* The reference list is not inclusive of all articles published.

Physicians who encounter adverse effects in infants fed drug-contaminated human milk are urged to document these effects in a communication to the AAP Committee on Drugs and the US Food and Drug Administration. Such communication should include: the generic and brand name of the drug, the maternal dose and mode of administration, the concentration of the drug in milk and maternal and infant blood in relation to time of ingestion, the age of the infant, and the method used for laboratory identification. Such reports may significantly increase the pediatric community's fund of knowledge regarding drug transfer into human milk and the potential or actual risk to the infant.

ACKNOWLEDGMENT

We thank Linda Harnden for her work in reference identification, document retrieval, and manuscript preparation.

Drugs cited in Tables 1 to 7 are listed in alphabetical order by generic name.

Reprint requests to Publications Department, American Academy of Pediatrics, 141 Northwest Point Blvd, PO Box 927, Elk Grove Village, IL 60009–0927.
PEDIATRICS (ISSN 0031 4005). Copyright © 1989 by the American Academy of Pediatrics. **RE9160**

TABLE 1.   Drugs That Are Contraindicated During Breast-Feeding

Drug	Reported Sign or Symptom in Infant or Effect on Lactation	Reference No.
Bromocriptine	Suppresses lactation	2
Cocaine	Cocaine intoxication	3
Cyclophosphamide	Possible immune suppression; unknown effect on growth or association with carcinogenesis; neutropenia	4, 5
Cyclosporine	Possible immune suppression; unknown effect on growth or association with carcinogenesis	6
Doxorubicin*	Possible immune suppression; unknown effect on growth or association with carcinogenesis	7
Ergotamine	Vomiting, diarrhea, convulsions (doses used in migraine medications)	8
Lithium	1/3 to 1/2 therapeutic blood concentration in infants	9–11
Methotrexate	Possible immune suppression; unknown effect on growth or association with carcinogenesis; neutropenia	12
Phencyclidine (PCP)	Potent hallucinogen	13
Phenindione	Anticoagulant; increased prothrombin and partial thromboplastin time in 1 infant (not used in USA)	14

* Drug is concentrated in human milk.

TABLE 2.   Drugs of Abuse That Are Contraindicated During Breast-Feeding*

Drug	Effect	Reference No.
Amphetamine	Irritability, poor sleep pattern	15
Cocaine	Cocaine intoxication	3
Heroin		16
Marijuana	Only one report in literature; no effect mentioned	17
Nicotine (smoking)	Shock, vomiting, diarrhea, rapid heart rate, restlessness; decreased milk production	18–20
Phencyclidine	Potent hallucinogen	13

* The Committee on Drugs believes strongly that nursing mothers should not ingest any of these compounds. Not only are they hazardous to the nursing infant but they are detrimental to the physical and emotional health of the mother.
† Drug is concentrated in human milk.

TABLE 3.   Radiopharmaceuticals That Require Temporary Cessation of Breast-Feeding*

Drug	Recommended Alteration in Breast-Feeding Pattern	Reference No.
Gallium-67 (^{67}Ga)	Radioactivity in milk present for 2 wk	21
Indium-111 (^{111}In)	Small amount present at 20 h	22
Iodine-125 (^{125}I)	Risk of thyroid cancer; radioactivity in milk present for 12 d	23
Iodine-131 (^{131}I)	Radioactivity in milk present 2–14 d depending on study	24–27
Radioactive sodium	Radioactivity in milk present 96 h	28
Technetium-99m (^{99m}Tc), ^{99m}Tc macroaggregates, ^{99m}TcO$_4$	Radioactivity in milk present 15 h to 3 d	29–34

* Consult nuclear medicine physician before performing diagnostic study so that a radionuclide with the shortest excretion time in breast milk can be used. Before study, the mother should pump her breast and store enough milk in freezer for feeding the infant; after study, the mother should pump her breast to maintain milk production but discard all milk pumped for the required time that radioactivity is present in milk.

TABLE 4.   Drugs Whose Effect on Nursing Infants Is Unknown but May Be of Concern

Drug	Effect	Reference No.
Psychotropic drugs	Special concern when given to nursing mothers for long periods of time	35
Antianxiety		
Diazepam	None	36, 37
Lorazepam	None	38
Prazepam*	None	39
Quazepam	None	40
Antidepressant		
Amitriptyline	None	41, 42
Amoxapine	None	43
Desipramine	None	44, 45
Dothiepin	None	46
Doxepin	None	47
Imipramine	None	44
Trazodone	None	48
Antipsychotic		
Chlorpromazine	Galactorrhea in adult; drowsiness and lethargy in infant	49, 50
Chlorprothixene	None	51
Haloperidol	None	52, 53
Mesoridazine	None	54
Chloramphenicol	Possible idiosyncratic bone marrow suppression	55, 56
Metoclopramide*K	None described; potent central nervous system drug	57, 58
Metronidazole	In vitro mutagen; may discontinue breast-feeding 12–24 h to allow excretion of dose when single-dose therapy given to mother	59, 60
Tinidazole	See Metronidazole	61

* Drug is concentrated in human milk.

TABLE 5.   Drugs That Have Caused Significant Effects on Some Nursing Infants and Should Be Given to Nursing Mothers With Caution*

Drug	Effect	Reference No.
Aspirin (salicylates)	Metabolic acidosis (dose related); may affect platelet function; rash	62–64
Clemastine	Drowsiness, irritability, refusal to feed, high-pitched cry, neck stiffness (1 case)	65
Phenobarbital	Sedation; infantile spasms after weaning from milk containing phenobarbital, methemoglobinemia (1 case)	66–70
Primidone	Sedation, feeding problems	66, 67
Salicylazosulfapyridine (sulfasalazine)	Bloody diarrhea in 1 infant	71

* Measure blood concentration in the infant when possible.

TABLE 6.   Maternal Medication Usually Compatible With Breast-Feeding*

Drug	Reported Sign or Symptom in Infant or Effect on Lactation	Reference No.
Anesthetics, Sedatives		
Alcohol	Drowsiness, diaphoresis, deep sleep, weakness, decrease in linear growth, abnormal weight gain; maternal ingestion of 1 g/kg daily decreases milk ejection reflex	18, 72–74
Barbiturate	See Table 5	
Bromide	Rash, weakness, absence of cry with maternal intake of 5.4 g/d	75
Chloral hydrate	Sleepiness	76
Chloroform	None	77
Halothane	None	78
Lidocaine	None	79
Magnesium sulfate	None	80
Methyprylon	Drowsiness	81
Secobarbital	None	82
Thiopental	None	83
Anticoagulants		
Bishydroxycoumarin	None	84
Warfarin	None	85
Antiepileptics		
Carbamazepine	None	86, 87
Ethosuximide	None; drug appears in infant serum	86, 88
Phenobarbital	See Table 5	66–70, 86
Phenytoin	Methemoglobinemia (1 case)	68, 86, 89
Primidone	See Table 5	66, 67, 86
Thiopental	None	69, 83
Valproic acid	None	86, 90, 91
Antihistamines, decongestants, and bronchodilators		
Dexbrompheniramine maleate with *d*-isoephedrine	Crying, poor sleep patterns, irritability	92
Dyphylline†	None	93
Iodides	May affect thyroid activity; see Miscellaneous, iodine	94
Pseudoephedrine†	None	95
Terbutaline	None	96
Theophylline	Irritability	97, 98
Triprolidine	None	95

TABLE 6.—Continued

Drug	Reported Sign or Symptom in Infant or Effect on Lactation	Reference No.
Antihypertensive and cardio-vascular drugs		
Acebutolol	None	99
Atenolol	None	100
Captopril	None	101
Digoxin	None	102, 103
Diltiazem	None	104
Disopyramide	None	105, 106
Hydralazine	None	107
Labetalol	None	108
Lidocaine	None	79
Methyldopa	None	109
Metoprolol†	None	100
Mexiletine	None	110
Minoxidil	None	111
Nadolol†	None	112
Oxprenolol	None	113, 114
Procainamide	None	115
Propranolol	None	116–118
Quinidine	None	119
Timolol	None	114
Verapamil	None	120
Antiinfective drugs (all anti-biotics transfer into breast milk in limited amounts)		121
Acyclovir†	None	122
Amoxicillin	None	123
Aztreonam	None	124
Cefadroxil	None	123
Cefazolin	None	125
Cefotaxime	None	126
Cefoxitin	None	126
Ceftazidine	None	127
Ceftriaxone	None	128
Chloroquine	None	129–131
Clindamycin	None	132
Cycloserine	None	133
Dapsone	None; sulfonamide detected in infant's urine	131, 134
Erythromycin†	None	121
Ethambutol	None	133
Hydroxychloroquine†	None	135, 136
Isoniazid	None. acetyl metabolite also secreted; ? hepatoxicity	133, 137
Kanamycin	None	133
Moxalactam	None	138
Nalidixic acid	Hemolysis in infant with glucose--6-phosphate deficiency (G-6-PD)	139
Nitrofurantoin	Hemolysis in infant with G-6-PD	140
Pyrimethamine	None	131, 141
Quinine	None	142
Rifampin	None	133
Salicylazosulfapyridine (sulfasalazine)	See Table 5	71, 143, 144
Streptomycin	None	133
Sulbactam	None	145
Sulfapyridine	Caution in infant with jaundice or G-6-PD, and in ill, stressed, or premature infant. Appears in infant's urine.	143, 144

TABLE 6.—Continued

Drug	Reported Sign or Symptom in Infant or Effect on Lactation	Reference No.
Sulfisoxazole	Caution in infant with jaundice or G-6-PD, and in ill, stressed, or premature infant. Appears in infant's urine	146
Tetracycline	None; negligible absorption by infant	147, 148
Ticarcillin	None	149
Trimethoprim/sulfamethoxazole	None	150, 151
Antithyroid drugs		
Carbimazole	Goiter	152
Methimazole (active metabolite of carbimazole)	None	153
Propylthiouracil	None	154
Thiouracil	None mentioned; drug not used in USA	155
Cathartics		156, 157
Cascara	None	157
Danthron	Increased bowel activity	158
Senna	None	159
Diagnostic agents		
Iodine	Goiter; see Miscellaneous, iodine	94
Iopanoic acid	None	160
Metrizamide	None	161
Diuretic agents		
Bendroflumethiazide	Suppresses lactation	162
Chlorothiazide, hydrochlorothiazide	None	163, 164
Chlorthalidone	Excreted slowly	165
Spironolactone	None	166
Hormones		
^{3}H-norethynodrel	None	167
19-norsteroids	None	168
Clogestone	None	169
Contraceptive pill with estrogen/progesterone	Rare breast enlargement; decrease in milk production and protein content (not confirmed in several studies)	170–177
Estradiol	Withdrawal, vaginal bleeding	178
Medroxyprogesterone	None	169
Prednisolone	None	179
Prednisone	None	180
Progesterone	None	181
Muscle relaxants		
Baclofen	None	182
Methocarbamol	None	183
Narcotics, nonnarcotic analgesics, anti-inflammatory agents		
Acetaminophen	None	184–186
Butorphanol	None	187
Codeine	None	186, 188
Dipyrone	None	189
Flufenamic acid	None	190
Gold salts	None	191–194
Hydroxychloroquine	None	135, 136
Ibuprofen	None	195, 196
Indomethacin	Seizure (1 case)	197, 198
Mefenamic acid	None	199
Methadone	None if mother receiving ≤20 mg/24 h	200, 201

TABLE 6.—Continued

Drug	Reported Sign or Symptom in Infant or Effect on Lactation	Reference No.
Morphine	None	142
Nefopam	None	202
Phenylbutazone	None	203
Piroxicam	None	204
Prednisolone, prednisone	None	179, 180
Propoxyphene	None	205
Salicylates	See Table 5	62–64
Suprofen	None	206
Tolmetin	None	207
Stimulants		
Caffeine	Irritability, poor sleep pattern, excreted slowly; no effect with usual amount of caffeine beverages	98, 208–212
Vitamins		
B_1 (thiamin)	None	213
B_6 (pyridoxine)	None	214–216
B_{12}	None	217
D	None; follow infant's serum calcium if mother receives pharmacologic doses	218–220
Folic acid	None	221
K_1	None	222, 223
Riboflavin	None	213
Miscellaneous		
Acetazolamide	None	224
Atropine, scopolamine	None	188
Cimetidine†	None	226
Cisapride	None	225
Cisplatin	Not found in milk	7
Domperidone	None	227
Iodine (povidone-iodine/ vaginal douche)	Elevated iodine levels in breast milk, odor of iodine on infant's skin	94
Metoclopramide	See Table 4	57, 58
Noscapine	None	228
Pyridostigmine	None	229
Tolbutamide	? Jaundice	230

* Drugs listed have been reported in the literature as having the effects listed or no effect. The word "none" means that no observable change was seen in the nursing infant while the mother was ingesting the compound. It is emphasized that most of the literature citations concern single case reports or small series of infants.
† Drug is concentrated in human milk.

TABLE 7. Food and Environmental Agents and Their Effect on Breast-Feeding

Agent	Reported Sign or Symptom in Infant or Effect on Lactation	Reference No.
Aflatoxin	None	231
Aspartame	Caution if mother or infant has phenylketonuria	232
Bromide (photographic laboratory)	Potential absorption and bromide transfer into milk; see Table 6, Anesthetics, sedatives	233
Cadmium	None reported	234
Chlordane	None reported	235
Chocolate (theobromine)	Irritability or increased bowel activity if excess amounts (16 oz/d) consumed by mother	98, 236
DDT, benzenehexachlorides, dieldrin, aldrin, hepatachlorepoxide	None	237, 243
Fava beans	Hemolysis in patient with glucose-6-phosphate deficiency (G-6-PD)	244

TABLE 7.—Continued

Agent	Reported Sign or Symptom in Infant or Effect on Lactation	Reference No.
Fluorides	None	245, 246
Hexachlorobenzene	Skin rash, diarrhea, vomiting, dark urine, neurotoxicity, death	247, 248
Hexachlorophene	None; possible contamination of milk from nipple washing	249
Lead	Possible neurotoxicity	250, 251
Methyl mercury, mercury	May affect neurodevelopment	252–254
Monosodium glutamate (MSG)	None	255
Polychlorinated biphenyls and polybrominated biphenyls	Lack of endurance, hypotonia, sullen expressionless facies	256–260
Tetrachlorethylene-cleaning fluid (perchloroethylene)	Obstructive jaundice, dark urine	261
Vegetarian diet	Signs of B_{12} deficiency	262

TABLE 8. Trade Names of Generic Drugs*

Generic	Trade	Generic	Trade
acebutolol	Sectral	danthron	Dorbane, Modane
acetaminophen	Tylenol, Tylenol Extra Strength, Tempra, Phenaphen	dapsone desipramine dexbrompheniramine	Norpramin, Pertofrane Drixoral, Disophrol,
acetazolamide	Diamox	maleate with	Chronotab
amitriptyline	Elavil, Endep	d-isoephedrine	
amoxapine	Asendin	diazepam	Valium
amoxicillin	Amoxyl	dicumarol	
amphetamine (dexamphetamin)	Dexedrine	digoxin diltiazem	Lanoxin, SK-Digoxin Cardizem
aspartame	Nutrasweet	dipyrone	Novaldin
atenolol	Tenormin	disopyramide	Norpace
aztreonam	Azactam	domperidone	
baclofen	Lioresal	dothiepin	Prothiaden
bendroflumethiazide	Naturetin	doxepin	Adapin, Sinequan
bromocriptine	Parlodel	doxorubicin	Adriamycin
butorphanol	Stadol	dyphylline	Dilor
captopril	Capoten	ergotamine tartrate with caffeine	Cafergot
carbamazepine	Tegretol		
carbimazole	Neo-mercazole	estradiol	Estrace
cefadroxil	Duricef	ethambutol	Myambutol
cefazolin	Ancef, Kefzol	ethosuximide	Zarontin
cefotaxime	Claforan	flufenamic acid	Arlef
ceftazidime	Fortaz	gold sodium thiomalate	Myochrysine
ceftriaxone	Rocephin	haloperidol	Haldol
chloramphenicol	Chloromycetin	hydralazine	Apresoline
chloroquine	Aralen	hydrochlorothiazide	Hydrodiuril
chlorothiazide	Diuril, Chlotride	hydroxychloroquine	Plaquenil
chlorpromazine	Thorazine	ibuprofen	Motrin
chlorprothixene	Taractan	imipramine	Tofranil, SK-Pramine, Imavate
chlorthalidone	Hygroton, Combipres		
cimetidine	Tagamet	indomethacin	Indocin
cisapride	Benzamide	iopanoic acid	Telepaque
cisplatin	Platinol	isoniazid	INH
clemastine	Tavegil, Tavist	kanamycin	Kantrex
clindamycin	Cleocin	labetalol	Normodyne, Trandate
cyclophosphamide	Cytoxan	lidocaine	Xylocaine
cycloserine	Seromycin	lorazepam	Ativan

TABLE 8.—Continued

Generic	Trade	Generic	Trade
medroxyprogesterone	Provera	propoxyphene	Darvon, SK65, Dolene
mefenamic acid	Ponstel	propranolol	Inderal
mesoridazine	Lidanar	propylthiouracil	Propacil
methadone	Westadone	pseudoephedrine	Actifed
methimazole	Tapazole	pyrimethamine	Daraprim
methocarbamol	Robaxin	pyridostigmine	Mestinon
methotrexate (amethopterin)	Folex	quazepam	Dormalin
		quinine	Quine
methyprylon	Noludar	rifampin	Rifamycin, Rifadin, Rimactane
metoclopramide	Reglan		
metoprolol	Lopressor	salicylazosulfapyridine	Azulfidine
metrizamide	Amipaque	secobarbital	Seconal, Seco-8
metronidazole	Flagyl	senna	Senokot
mexiletine	Mexitil	spironolactone	Aldactone
minoxidil	Loniten	sulbactam	Unasyn
monosodium glutamate	MSG, Accent, Adolph's Meat Tenderizer	sulfisoxazole	Gantrisin
		suprofen	Suprol
moxalactam	Moxam	terbutaline	Bricanyl, Brethine
nadolol	Corgard	tetracycline	Achromycin, SK-Tetracycline
nalidixic acid	NegGram		
nefopam	Acupan	theophylline	Theo-Dur, Elixophyllin, Slo-Phyllin, Bronkodyl
nitrofurantoin	Furadantin, Nitrofor, Macrodantin		
		thiopental	Pentothal
³H-norethynodrel	Envoid	thiouracil	Thiouracil
noscapine	Tusscapine	ticarcillin	Timentin
oxprenolol		timolol	Blocadren, Timoptic
phenindione	Hedulin, Eridione	tolbutamide	Orinase, SK-Tolbutamide
phenylbutazone	Azolid, Butazolidin		
phenytoin	Dilantin	tolmetin	Tolectin
piroxicam	Feldene	trazodone	Desyrel
prazepam	Centrax	trimethoprim with sulfamethoxazole	Bactrim, Septra, Septra DS
prednisolone	Delta-Cortef, Sterane		
prednisone	Deltasone, Meticorten, SK-Prednisone	triprolidine	Actifed
		valproic acid	Depakene
primidone	Mysoline	verapamil	Calan
procainamide	Pronestyl	warfarin	Coumadin, Panwarfin

* For convenience, one or more examples of the trade name are given.

REFERENCES

1. American Academy of Pediatrics, Committee on Drugs. The transfer of drugs and other chemicals into human breast milk. *Pediatrics.* 1983;72:375–383
2. Kulski JK, Hartmann PE, Martin JD, et al. Effects of bromocriptine mesylate on the composition of the mammary secretion in non-breast-feeding women. *Obstet Gynecol.* 1978;52:38–42
3. Chasnoff IJ, Lewis DE, Squires L. Cocaine intoxication in a breast-fed infant. *Pediatrics.* 1987;80:836–838
4. Wiernik PH, Duncan JH. Cyclophosphamide in human milk. *Lancet.* 1971;1:912
5. Amato D, Niblett JS. Neutropenia from cyclophosphamide in breast milk. *Med J Aust.* 1977;1:383–384
6. Flechner SM, Katz AR, Rogers AJ, et al. The presence of cyclosporine in body tissue and fluids during pregnancy. *Am J Kidney Dis.* 1985;5:60–63
7. Egan PC, Costanza ME, Dodion P, et al. Doxorubicin and cisplatin excretion into human milk. *Cancer Treat Rep.* 1985;69:1387–1389
8. Fomina PI. Untersuchungen uber den Ubergang des aktiven agens des Mutterkorns in die milch stillender Mutter. *Arch Gynecol.* 1934;157:275
9. Schou M, Amdisen A. Lithium and pregnancy, III: lithium ingestion by children breast-fed by women on lithium treatment. *Br Med J.* 1973;2:138
10. Tunnessen WW Jr, Hertz C. Toxic effects of lithium in newborn infants: a commentary. *J Pediatr.* 1972;81:804–807
11. Sykes PA, Quarrie J, Alexander FW. Lithium carbonate and breast-feeding. *Br Med J.* 1976;2:1299
12. Johns DG, Rutherford LD, Leighton PC, et al. Secretion of methotrexate into human milk. *Am J Obstet Gynecol.* 1972;112:978–980
13. Kaufman KR, Petrucha RA, Pitts FN Jr, et al. PCP in amniotic fluid and breast milk: case report. *J Clin Psychiatry.* 1983;44:269–270
14. Eckstein HB, Jack B. Breast-feeding and anticoagulant therapy. *Lancet.* 1970;1:672–673
15. Steiner E, Villen T, Hallberg M, et al. Amphetamine secretion in breast milk. *Eur J Clin Pharmacol.* 1984;27:123–124
16. Cobrinik RW, Hood RT Jr, Chusid E. The effect of maternal narcotic addiction on the newborn infant: review of literature and report of 22 cases. *Pediatrics.* 1959;24:288–304
17. Perez-Reyes M, Wall ME. Presence of tetrahydrocanna-

binol in human milk. *N Engl J Med.* 1982;307:819–820

18. Bisdom W. Alcohol and nicotine poisonings in nurslings. *JAMA.* 1937;109:178

19. Ferguson BB, Wilson DJ, Schaffner W. Determination of nicotine concentrations in human milk. *Am J Dis Child.* 1976;130:837–839

20. Luck W, Nau H. Nicotine and cotinine concentrations in the milk of smoking mothers: influence of cigarette consumption and diurnal variation. *Eur J Pediatr.* 1987;146:21–26

21. Tobin RE, Schneider PB. Uptake of ^{67}Ga in the lactating breast and its persistence in milk: case report. *J Nucl Med.* 1976;17:1055–1056

22. Butt D, Szaz KF. Indium-111 radioactivity in breast milk. *Br J Radiol.* 1986;59:80

23. Palmer KE. Excretion of ^{125}I in breast milk following administration of labelled fibrinogen. *Br J Radiol.* 1979;52:672–673

24. Honour AJ, Myant NB, Rowlands EN. Secretion of radio-iodine in digestive juices and milk in man. *Clin Sci.* 1952;11:447

25. Karjalainen P, Penttila IM, Pystynen P. The amount and form of radioactivity in human milk after lung scanning, renography and placental localization by ^{131}I labelled tracers. *Acta Obstet Gynecol Scand.* 1971;50:357–361

26. Bland EP, Crawford JS, Docker MF, et al. Radioactive iodine uptake by thyroid of breast-fed infants after maternal blood-volume measurements. *Lancet.* 1969;2:1039–1041

27. Nurnberger CE, Lipscomb A. Transmission of radioiodine (I^{131}) to infants through human maternal milk. *JAMA.* 1952;150:1398

28. Pommerenke WT, Hahn PF. Secretion of radioactive sodium in human milk. *Proc Soc Exp Biol Med.* 1943;52:223

29. O'Connell MEA, Sutton H. Excretion of radioactivity in breast milk following ^{99}T$_c$m-Sn polyphosphate. *Br J Radiol.* 1976;49:377–379

30. Berke RA, Hoops EC, Kereiakes JC, et al. Radiation dose to breast-feeding child. *J Nucl Med.* 1973;14:51–52

31. Vagenakis AG, Abreau CM, Braverman LE. Duration of radioactivity in the milk of a nursing mother following 99^{m}Tc administration. *J Nucl Med.* 1971;12:188

32. Wyburn JR. Human breast milk excretion of radionuclides following administration of radiopharmaceuticals. *J Nucl Med.* 1973;14:115–117

33. Pittard WB III, Merkatz R, Fletcher BD. Radioactive excretion in human milk following administration of technetium Tc 99m macroaggregated albumin. *Pediatrics.* 1982;70:231–234

34. Maisels MJ, Gilcher RO. Excretion of technetium in human milk. *Pediatrics.* 1983;71:841–842

35. American Academy of Pediatrics, Committee on Drugs. Psychotropic drugs in pregnancy and lactation. *Pediatrics.* 1982;69:241–244

36. Patrick MJ, Tilstone WJH, Reavey P. Diazepam and breast-feeding. *Lancet.* 1972;1:542–543

37. Cole AP, Hailey DM. Diazepam and active metabolite in breast milk and their transfer to the neonate. *Arch Dis Child.* 1975;50:741–742

38. Summerfield RJ, Nielson MS. Excretion of lorazepam into breast milk. *Br J Anaesth.* 1985;57:1042–1043

39. Brodie RR, Chasseaud LF, Taylor T. Concentrations of N-descyclopropylmethylprazepam in whole-blood, plasma, and milk after administration of prazepam to humans. *Biopharm Drug Dispos.* 1981;2:59–68

40. Hilbert JM, Gural RP, Symchowicz S, et al. Excretion of guazepam into human breast milk. *J Clin Pharmacol.* 1984;24:457–462

41. Bader TF, Newman K. Amitriptyline in human breast milk and the nursing infant's serum. *Am J Psychiatry.* 1980;137:855–856

42. Erickson SH, Smith GH, Heidrich T. Tricyclics and breast feeding. *Am J Psychiatry.* 1979;136:1483–1484

43. Gelenberg AJ. Single case study: amoxapine, a new anti-depressant appears in human milk. *J Nerv Ment Dis.* 1979;167:635–636

44. Sovner R, Orsulak PJ. Excretion of imipramine and desipramine in human breast milk. *Am J Psychiatry.* 1979;136:451–452

45. Stancer HC, Reed KL. Desipramine and 2-hydroxydesepramine in human breast milk and the nursery infant's serum. *Am J Psychiatry.* 1986;143:1597–1600

46. Rees JA, Glass RC, Sporne GA. Serum and breast milk concentrations of dothiepin. *Practitioner.* 1976;217:686

47. Kemp J, Ilett KF, Booth J, et al. Excretion of doxepin and N-desmethyldoxepin in human milk. *Br J Clin Pharmacol.* 1985;20:497–499

48. Verbeeck RK, Ross SG, McKenna EA. Excretion of trazodone in breast milk. *Br J Clin Pharmacol.* 1986;22:367–370

49. Polishuk WZ, Kulcsar SA. Effects of chlorpromazine on pituitary function. *J Clin Endocrinol Metab.* 1956;16:292

50. Wiles DH, Orr MW, Kolakowska T. Chlorpromazine levels in plasma and milk of nursing mothers. *Br J Clin Pharmacol.* 1978;5:272–273

51. Matheson I, Evang A, Fredricson Overo K, et al. Presence of chlorprothidone and its metabolites in breast milk. *Eur J Clin Pharmacol.* 1984;27:611–613

52. Stewart RB, Karas B, Springer PK. Haloperidol excretion in human milk. *Am J Psychiatry.* 1980;137:849–850

53. Whalley LJ, Blain PG, Prime JK. Haloperidol secreted in breast milk. *Br Med J.* 1981;282:1746–1747

54. Ananth J. Side effects in the neonate from psychotropic agents excreted through breast-feeding. *Am J Psychiatry.* 1978;135:801–805

55. Havelka J, Hejzlar M, Popov V. Excretion of chloramphenicol in human milk. *Chemotherapy.* 1968;13:204–211

56. Smadel JE, Woodward TE, Ley HL Jr, et al. Chloramphenicol (Chloromycetin) in the treatment of tsutsugamushi disease (scrub typhus). *J Clin Invest.* 1949;28:1196

57. Gupta AP, Gupta PK. Metaclopramide as a lactogogue. *Clin Pediatr.* 1985;24:269–272

58. Kauppila A, Arvela P, Koivisto M, et al. Metaclopramide and breast-feeding: transfer into milk and the newborn. *Eur J Clin Pharmacol.* 1983;25:819–823

59. Erickson SH, Oppenheim GL, Smith GH. Metronidazole in breast milk. *Obstet Gynecol.* 1981;57:48–50

60. Heisterberg L, Branebjerg PE. Blood and milk concentrations of metronidazole in mothers and infants. *J Perinat Med.* 1983;11:114–120

61. Evaldson GR, Lindgren S, Nord CE, et al. Tinidazole milk excretion and pharmacokinetics in lactating women. *Br J Clin Pharmacol* 1985;19:503–507

62. Clark JH, Wilson WG. A 16-day-old breast-fed infant with metabolic acidosis caused by salicylate. *Clin Pediatr.* 1981;20:53–54

63. Levy G. Salicylate pharmacokinetics in the human neonate. In Morselli PL, ed. *Basic and Therapeutic Aspects of Perinatal Pharmacology.* New York, NY: Raven Press; 1975:319

64. Fakhredding J, Keshavarz E. Salicylate excretion in breast milk. *Int J Pharmaceutics.* 1981;8:285

65. Kok THHG, Taitz LS, Bennett MJ. Drowsiness due to clemastine transmitted in breast milk. *Lancet.* 1982;1:914–915

66. Nau H, Rating D, Hauser I, et al. Placental transfer and pharmacokinetics of primidone and its metabolites phenobarbital, PEMA and hydroxyphenobarbital in neonates and infants of epileptic mothers. *Eur J Clin Pharmacol.* 1980;18:31–42

67. Kuhnz W, Koch S, Helge H, et al. Primidone and pheno-

barbital during lactation period in epileptic women: total and free drug serum levels in the nursed infants and their effects on neonatal behavior. *Dev Pharmacol Ther.* 1988;11:147–154

68. Finch E, Lorber J. Methaemoglobinaemia in the newborn: probably due to phenytoin excreted in human milk. *J Obstet Gynaecol Br Emp.* 1954;61:833

69. Tyson RM, Shrader EA, Perlman HH. Drugs transmitted through breast milk, II: barbiturates. *J Pediatr.* 1938;13:86–90

70. Knott C, Reynolds F, Clayden G. Infantile spasms on weaning from breast milk containing anticonvulsants. *Lancet.* 1987;2:272–273

71. Branski D, Kerem E, Gross-Kieselstein E, et al. Bloody diarrhea—a possible complication of sulfasalazine transferred through human breast milk. *J Pediatr Gastroenterol Nutr.* 1986;5:316–317

72. Binkiewicz A, Robinson MJ, Senior B. Pseudo-cushing syndrome caused by alcohol in breast milk. *J Pediatr.* 1978;93:965–967

73. Cobo E. Effect of different dose of ethanol on the milk-ejecting reflex in lactating women. *Am J Obstet Gynecol.* 1973;115:817–821

74. Kesaniemi YA. Ethanol and acetaldehyde in the milk and peripheral blood of lactating women after ethanol administration. *J Obstet Gynaecol Br Comm.* 1974;81:84–86

75. Tyson RM, Shrader EA, Perlman HH. Drugs transmitted through breast milk, III: bromides. *J Pediatr.* 1938;13:91–93

76. Lacey JH. Dichloralphenazone and breast milk. *Br Med J.* 1971;4:684

77. Reed CB. A study of the conditions that require the removal of the child from the breast. *Surg Gynecol Obstet.* 1908;6:514

78. Cote CJ, Kenepp NB, Reed SB, et al. Trace concentrations of halothane in human breast milk. *Br J Anaesth.* 1976;48:541–543

79. Zeisler JA, Gaardner TD, DeMesquita SA. Lidocaine excretion in breast milk. *Drug Intell Clin Pharm.* 1986;20:691–693

80. Cruikshank DP, Varner MW, Pitkin RM. Breast milk magnesium and calcium concentrations following magnesium sulfate treatment. *Am J Obstet Gynecol.* 1982;143:685–688

81. Shore MF. Drugs can be dangerous during pregnancy and lactations. *Can Pharmaceut J.* 1970;103:358

82. Horning MG, Stillwell WG, Nowlin J, et al. Identification and quantification of drugs and drug metabolites in human breast milk using GC-MS-COM methods. *Mod Probl Paediatr.* 1975;15:73

83. Andersen LW, Qvist T, Hertz J, et al. Concentrations of thiopentone in mature breast milk and colostrum following an induction dose. *Acta Anaesthesiol Scand.* 1987;31:30–32

84. Brambel CE, Hunter RE. Effect of dicumarol on the nursing infant. *Am J Obstet Gynecol.* 1950;59:1153

85. Orme ML'E, Lewis PJ, deSwiet M, et al. May mothers given warfarin breast-feed their infant? *Br Med J.* 1977;1:1564–1565

86. Nau H, Kuhnz W, Egger JH, et al. Anticonvulsants during pregnancy and lactation. *Clin Pharmacokinet.* 1982;7:508–543

87. Pynnonen S, Kanto J, Sillanpaa M, et al. Carbamazepine: placental transport, tissue concentrations in foetus and newborn and level in milk. *Acta Pharmacol Toxicol.* 1977;41 244–253

88. Koup JR, Rose JQ, Cohen ME. Ethosuximide pharmacokinetics in a pregnant patient and her newborn. *Epilepsia.* 1978;19:535–539

89. Mirkin B. Diphenylhydantoin: placental transport, fetal localization, neonatal metabolism, and possible teratogenic effects. *J Pediatr.* 1971;78:329–337

90. Alexander FW. Sodium valproate and pregnancy. *Arch Dis Child.* 1979;54:240

91. Von Onruh GE, Froescher W, Hoffmann F, et al. Valproic acid in breast milk: how much is really there? *Ther Drug Monit.* 1984;6:272–276

92. Mortimer EA Jr. Drug toxicity from breast milk? *Pediatrics.* 1977;60:780–781

93. Jorboe CH, Cook LN, Malesic I, et al. Dyphylline elimination kinetics in lactating women: blood to milk transfer. *J Clin Pharmacol.* 1981;21:405–410

94. Postellon DC, Aronow R. Iodine in mother's milk. *JAMA* 1982;247:463

95. Findlay JWA, Butz RF, Sailstad JM, et al. Pseudoephedrine and triprolidine in plasma and breast milk of nursing mothers. *Br J Clin Pharmacol.* 1984;18:901–906

96. Lindberg C, Boreus LO, DeChateau P, et al. Transfer of terbutaline into breast milk. *Eur J Respir Dis.* 1984;65:87–91

97. Yurchak AM, Jusko WJ. Theophylline secretion into breast milk. *Pediatrics.* 1976;57:518–520

98. Berlin CM Jr. Excretion of the methylxanthines in human milk. *Semin Perinatol.* 1981;5:389–394

99. Boutroy MJ, Bianchetti G, Dubruc C, et al. To nurse when receiving acebutolol: is it dangerous for the neonate? *Eur J Clin Pharmacol.* 1986;30:737–739

100. Liedholm H, Melander A, Bitzen P-O, et al. Accumulation of atenolol & metoprolol in human breast milk. *Eur J Clin Pharmacol.* 1981;20:229–231

101. Devlin RG, Fleiss PM. Captopril in human blood and breast milk. *J Clin Pharmacol.* 1981;21:110–113

102. Loughnan PM. Digoxin excretion in human breast milk. *J Pediatr.* 1978;92:1019–1020

103. Levy M, Granit L, Laufer N. Excretion of drugs in human milk. *N Engl J Med.* 1977;297:789

104. Okada M, Inoue H, Nakamura Y, et al. Excretion of diltiazem in human milk. *N Engl J Med.* 1985;312:992–993

105. MacKintosh D, Buchanan N. Excretion of disopyramide in human breast milk. *Br J Clin Pharmacol.* 1985;19:856–857

106. Hoppu K, Neuvonen PJ, Korte T. Disopyramide and breast feeding. *Br J Clin Pharmacol.* 1986;21:553

107. Liedholm H, Wahlin-Boll E, Hanson A, et al. Transplacental passage and breast milk concentrations of hydralazine. *Eur J Clin Pharmacol.* 1982;21:417–419

108. Lunell HO, Kulas J, Rane A. Transfer of labetalol into amniotic fluid and breast milk in lactating women. *Eur J Clin Pharmacol.* 1985;28:597–599

109. White WB, Andreoli JW, Cohn RD. Alpha-methyldopa disposition in mothers with hypertension and in their breast-fed infants. *Clin Pharmacol Ther.* 1985;37:387–390

110. Lownes HE, Ives TJ. Mexiletine use in pregnancy and lactation. *Am J Obstet Gynecol.* 1987;157:446–447

111. Valdivieso A, Valdes G, Spiro TE, et al. Minoxidil in breast milk. *Ann Intern Med.* 1985;102:135

112. Devlin RG, Duchin KL, Fleiss PM. Nadolol in human serum and breast milk. *Br J Clin Pharmacol.* 1981;12:393–396

113. Sioufi A, Hillion D, Lumbroso P, et al. Oxprenolol placental transfer plasma concentrations in newborns and passage into breast milk. *Br J Clin Pharmacol.* 1984;18:453–456

114. Fidler J, Smlth V, DeSwiet M. Excretion of oxprenolol and timolol in breast milk. *Br J Obstet Gynaecol.* 1983;90:961–965

115. Pittard WB III, Glazier H. Procainamide excretion in human milk. *J Pediatr.* 1983;102:631–633

116. Levitan AA, Manion JC. Propranolol therapy during pregnancy and lactation. *Am J Cardiol.* 1973;32:247

117. Karlberg B, Lundberg D, Aberg H. Excretion of propranolol in human breast milk. *Acta Pharmacol Toxicol.* 1974;34:222–224

118. Bauer JH, Pape B, Zajicek J, et al. Propranolol in human plasma and breast milk. *Am J Cardiol.* 1979;43:860–862

119. Hill LM, Milkasian GD Jr. The use of quinidine sulfate throughout pregnancy. *Obstet Gynecol.* 1979;54:366–368

120. Anderson P, Bondesson U, Mattiasson I, et al. Verapamil and norverapamil in plasma and breast milk during breast feeding. *Eur J Clin Pharmacol.* 1987;31:625–627

121. Matsuda S. Transfer of antibiotics into maternal milk. *Biol Res Pregnancy Perinatol.* 1984;5:57–60

122. Lau RJ, Emery MG, Galinsky RE. Unexpected accumulation of acyclovir in breast milk with estimation of infant exposure. *Obstet Gynecol.* 1987;69:468–471

123. Kafetzis DA, Siafas CA, Georgakopoulos PA, et al. Passage of cephalosporins and amoxocillin into the breast milk. *Acta Paediatr Scand.* 1981;70:285–288

124. Fleiss PM, Richwald GA, Gordon J, et al. Aztreonam in human serum and breast milk. *Br J Clin Pharmacol.* 1985;19:509–511

125. Yoshioka H, Cao K, Takimoto M, et al. Transfer of cefazolin into human milk. *J Pediatr.* 1979;94:151–152

126. Dresse A, Lambotte R, Dubois M, et al. Transmammary passage of cefoxitin: additional results. *J Clin Pharmacol.* 1983;23:438–440

127. Blanco JD, Jorgensen JH, Castaneda YS, et al. Ceftazidine levels in human breast milk. *Antimicrob Agents Chemother.* 1983;23:479–480

128. Kafetzis DA, Brater DC, Fanourgakis JE, et al. Ceftriaxone distribution between maternal blood and fetal blood and tissues at parturition and between blood and milk postpartum. *Amtimicrob Agents Chemother.* 1983;23:870–873

129. Soares R, Paulini E, Pereira JP. Da concentracao e eliminacao da cloroquina atraves da circulacao placentaria e do leite materno, de pacientes sob regime do sal cloroquinado. *Rev Bras Malariol Doencas Trop.* 1957;9:19–27

130. Ogunbona FA, Onyeji CO, Bolaji OO, et al. Excretion of chloroquine and desethylchloroquine in human milk. *Br J Clin Pharmacol.* 1987;23:473–476

131. Edstein MD, Veenendal JR, Newman K, et al. Excretion of chloroquine, dapsone and pyrimethamine in human milk. *Br J Clin Pharmacol.* 1986;22:733–735

132. Smith JA, Morgan JR, Rachlis AR, et al. Clindamycin in human breast milk. *Can Med Assoc J.* 1975;112:806

133. Snyder DR Jr, Powell KE. Should women taking antituberculosis drugs breast-feed? *Arch Intern Med.* 1984;144:589–590

134. Dreisbach JA. Sulphone levels in breast milk of mothers on sulphone therapy. *Lepr Rev.* 1952;23:101–106

135. Ostensen M, Brown ND, Chiang PK, et al. Hydroxychoroquine in human breast milk. *Eur J Clin Pharmacol.* 1985;28:357

136. Nation RL, Hackett LP, Dusci LJ, et al. Excretion of hydroxychloroquine in human milk. *Br J Clin Pharmacol.* 1984;17:368–369

137. Berlin CM Jr, Lee C. Isoniazid and acetylisoniazid disposition in human milk, saliva and plasma. *Fed Proc.* 1979;38:426

138. Miller RD, Keegan KA, Thrupp LD, et al. Human breast milk concentration of moxalactam. *Am J Obstet Gynecol.* 1984;148:348–349

139. Belton EM, Jones RV. Haemolytic anaemia due to nalidixic acid. *Lancet.* 1965;2:691

140. Varsano I, Fischl J, Sochet SB, et al. The excretion of orally ingested nitrofurantoin in human milk. *J Pediatr.* 1973;82:886–887

141. Clyde DF, Shute GT, Press J. Transfer of pyrimethamine in human milk. *J Trop Med Hyg.* 1956;59:277

142. Terwilliger WG, Hatcher RA. The elimination of morphine and quinine in human milk. *Surg Gynecol Obstet.* 1934;58:823

143. Jarnerot G, Into-Malmberg MB. Sulphasalazine treatment during breast feeding. *Scand J Gastroenterol.* 1979;14:869–871

144. Berlin CM Jr, Yaffe SJ. Disposition of salicylazosufapyridine (Axulfidine) and metabolites in human breast milk. *Dev Pharmacol Ther.* 1980;1:31–39

145. Foulds G, Miller RD, Knirsch AK, et al. Sulbactam kinetics and excretion into breast milk in postpartum women. *Clin Pharmacol Ther.* 1985;38:692–696

146. Kauffman RE, O'Brien C, Gilford P. Sulfisoxazole secretion into human milk. *J Pediatr.* 1980;97:839–841

147. Tetracycline in breast milk. *Br Med J.* 1969;4:791

148. Posner AC, Prigot A, Konicoff NG. Further observations on the use of tetracycline hydrochloride in prophylaxis and treatment of obstetric infections. In Welch H, Martilbanez F, eds. *Antibiotics Annual: 1954–1955.* New York, NY: Medical Encyclopedia Inc; 1955:594

149. Von Kobyletzki D, Dalhoff A, Lindemeyer H, et al. Ticarcillin serum and tissue concentrations in gynecology and obstetrics. *Infection.* 1983;11:144–149

150. Arnauld R. Etude du passage de la trimethoprime dans le lait maternel. *Ouest Med.* 1972;25:959

151. Miller RD, Salter AJ. The passage of trimethoprim/sulphamethoxazole into breast milk and its significance. Proceedings of the 8th International Congress of Chemotherapy, Daikos GK, ed. Athens, Greece: Hellenic Society for Chemotherapy. 1974;1:687–691

152. Cooper DS. Antithyroid drugs: to breast-feed or not to breast-feed. *Am J Obstet Gynecol.* 1987;157:234–235

153. Cooper DS, Bode HH, Nath B, et al. Methimazole pharmacology in man: studies using or newly developed radioimmunoassay for methimazole. *J Clin Endocrinol Metab.* 1984;58:473–479

154. Kampmann JP, Johansen K, Hansen JM, et al. Propylthiouracil in human milk: revision of dogma. *Lancet.* 1980;1:736–737

155. Kay GA, Jandorf BJ. Thiouracil: its absorption, distribution, and excretion. *J Clin Invest.* 1944;23:613–627

156. Lewis JH, Weingold AB. The use of gastrointestinal drugs during pregnancy and lactation. *Am J Gastroenterol.* 1985;80:912–923

157. Tyson RM, Shrader EA, Perlman HH. Drugs transmitted through breast milk, I: laxatives. *J Pediatr.* 1937;11:824–832

158. Greenhalf JO, Leonard HSD. Laxatives in the treatment of constipation in pregnant and breast-feeding mothers. *Practitioner.* 1973;210:259–263

159. Werthmann MW, Krees SV. Quantitative excretion of Senokot in human breast milk. *Med Ann DC.* 1973;42:4–5

160. Holmdahl KH. Cholecystography during lactation. *Acta Radiol.* 1955;45:305

161. Ilett KF, Hackett LP, Paterson JW. Excretion of metrizamide in milk. *Br J Radiol.* 1981;54:537–538

162. Healy M. Suppressing lactation with oral diurtics. *Lancet.* 1961;1:1353

163. Werthmann MW Jr, Krees SV. Excretion of chlorothiazide in human breast milk. *J Pediatr.* 1972;81:781–783

164. Miller EM, Cohn RD, Burghart PH. Hydrochlorothiazide disposition in a mother and her breast-fed infant. *J Pediatr.* 1982;101:789–791

165. Mulley BA, Parr GD, Pau WK, et al. Placental transfer of chlorthalidone and its elimination in maternal milk. *Eur J Clin Pharmacol.* 1978;13:129–131

166. Phelps DL, Karim A. Spironolactone: relationship between concentrations of dethioacetylated metabolite in human serum and milk. *J Pharm Sci.* 1977;66:1203

167. Laumas KR, Malkani PK, Bhatnagar S, et al. Radioactivity in the breast milk of lactating women after oral administration of ^{3}H-norethynodrel. *Am J Obstet Gynecol.* 1967;98:411–413

168. Pincus G, Bialy G, Layne DS, et al. Radioactivity in the

milk of subjects receiving radioactive 19-norsteroids. *Nature.* 1966;212:924–925

169. Zacharias S, Aguilera E, Assenzo JR, et al. Effects of hormonal and nonhormonal contraceptives on lactation and incidence of pregnancy. *Contraception.* 1986;33:203–213

170. Nilsson S, Mellbin T, Hofvander Y, et al. Long-term followup of children breast-fed by mothers using oral contraceptives. *Contraception.* 1986;34:443–457

171. Nilsson S, Nygren KG. Transfer of contraceptive steroids to human milk. *Res Reprod.* 1979;11:1–2

172. American Academy of Pediatrics, Committee on Drugs. Breast-feeding and contraception. *Pediatrics.* 1981;68:138–140

173. Barsivala VM, Virkar KD. The effect of oral contraceptives on concentration of various components of human milk. *Contraception.* 1973;7:307

174. Borglin NE, Sandholm LE. Effect of oral contraceptives on lactation. *Fertil Steril.* 1971;22:39–41

175. Curtis EM. Oral contraceptive feminization of a normal male infant: report of a case. *Obstet Gynecol.* 1964;23:295

176. Kora SJ. Effect of oral contraceptives on lactation. *Fertil Steril.* 1969;20:419–423

177. Toaff R, Ashkenazi H, Schwartz A, et al. Effects of oestrogen and progestagen on the composition of human milk. *J Reprod Fertil.* 1969;19:475–482

178. Nilsson S, Nygren KG, Johansson EDB. Transfer of estradiol to human milk. *Am J Obstet Gynecol.* 1978;132:653–657

179. McKenzie SA, Selley JA, Agnew JE. Secretion of prednisolone into breast milk. *Arch Dis Child.* 1975;50:894–896

180. Katz FH, Duncan BR. Entry of prednisone into human milk. *N Engl J Med.* 1975;293:1154

181. Diaz S, Jackanicz TM, Herreros C, et al. Fertility regulation in nursing women, VIII: progesterone plasma levels and contraceptive efficacy of a progesterone-releasing vaginal ring. *Contraception.* 1985;32:603–622

182. Eriksson G, Swahn CG. Concentrations of baclofen in serum and breast milk from a lactating woman. *Scand J Clin Lab Invest.* 1981;41:185–187

183. Campbell AD, Coles FK, Eubank LLK, et al. Distribution and metabolism of methocarbamol. *J Pharmacol Exp Ther.* 1961;131:18

184. Berlin CM Jr, Yaffe SJ, Ragni M. Disposition of acetaminophen in milk, saliva, and plasma of lactating women. *Pediatr Pharmacol.* 1980;1:135–141

185. Bitzen PO, Gustafsson B, Jostell KG, et al. Excretion of paracetamol in human breast milk. *Eur J Clin Pharmacol.* 1981;20:123–125

186. Findlay JWA, DeAngelis RL, Kearney MF, et al. Analgesic drugs in breast milk and plasma. *Clin Pharmacol Ther.* 1981;29:625–633

187. Pittman KA, Smyth RD, Losada M, et al. Human perinatal distribution of butorphanol. *Am J Obstet Gynecol.* 1980;138:797–800

188. Sapeika N. The excretion of drugs in human milk—a review. *J Obstet Gynaecol Br Commw.* 1947;54:426

189. Zylber-Katz E, Linder N, Granit L, et al. Excretion of dipyrone metabolites in human breast milk. *Eur J Clin Pharmacol.* 1986;30:359–361

190. Buchanan RA, Eaton CJ, Koeff St, et al. The breast milk excretion of flufenamic acid. *Curr Ther Res.* 1969;11:533–538

191. Bell RAF, Dale IM. Gold secretion in maternal milk. *Arthritis Rheum.* 1976;19:1374

192. Blau SP. Metabolism of gold during lactation. *Arthritis Rheum.* 1973;16:777–778

193. Gottlieb NL. Suggested errata. *Arthritis Rheum.* 1974;17:1057

194. Ostensen M, Skavdal K, Myklebust G, et al. Excretion of gold into human breast milk. *Eur J Clin Pharmacol.* 1986;31:251–252

195. Townsend RJ, Benedetti T, Erickson SH, et al. A study to evaluate the passage of ibuprofen into breast milk. *Drug Intell Clin Pharm.* 1982;16:482

196. Townsend RJ, Benedetti TJ, Erickson SH, et al. Excretion of ibuprofen into breast milk. *Am J Obstet Gynecol.* 1984;149:184–186

197. Eeg-Olofsson O, Malmros I, Elwin CE, et al. Convulsions in a breast-fed infant after maternal indomethacin. *Lancet.* 1978;2:215

198. Fairhead FW. Convulsions in a breast-fed infant after maternal indomethacin. *Lancet.* 1978;2:576

199. Buchanan RA, Eaton CJ, Koeff ST, et al. The breast milk excretion of mefenamic acid. *Curr Ther Res.* 1968;10:592–597

200. Blinick G, Inturrisi CE, Jerez E, et al. Methadone assays in pregnant women and pregnancy. *Am J Obstet Gynecol.* 1975; 121:617–621

201. Blinick G, Wallach RC, Jerez E, et al. Drug addiction in pregnancy and the neonate. *Am J Obstet Gynecol.* 1976;125:135–142

202. Liu DTY, Savage JM, Donnell D. Nefopam excretion in human milk. *Br J Clin Pharmacol.* 1987;23:99–101

203. Leuxner E, Pulver R. Verabreichung von irgapyrin bei Schwangeren und Wochnerinnen. *MMW.* 1956;98:84

204. Ostensen M. Piroxicam in human breast milk. *Eur J Clin Pharmacol.* 1953;25:829–830

205. Kunka RL, Venkataramanan R, Stern RM, et al. Excretion of propoxyphene and norpropoxyphene in breast milk. *Clin Pharmacol Ther.* 1984;35:675–680

206. Chaikin P, Chasin M, Kennedy B, et al. Suprofen concentrations in human breast milk. *J Clin Pharmacol.* 1983;23:385–390

207. Sagraves R, Waller ES, Goehrs HR. Tolmetin in breast milk. *Drug Intell Clin Pharm.* 1985;19:55–56

208. Tyrala EE, Dodson WE. Caffeine secretion into breast milk. *Arch Dis Child.* 1979;54:787–800

209. Hildebrandt R, Gundert-Remy V. Lack of pharmacological active saliva levels of caffeine in breast-fed infants. *Pediatr Pharmacol.* 1983;3:237–244

210. Berlin CM Jr, Denson HM, Daniel CH, et al. Disposition of dietary caffeine in milk, saliva, and plasma of lactating women. *Pediatrics.* 1984;73:59–63

211. Ryu JE. Caffeine in human milk and in serum of breast-fed infants. *Dev Pharmacol Ther.* 1985;8:329–337

212. Ryu JE. Effect of maternal caffeine consumption on heart rate and sleep time of breast-fed infants. *Dev Pharmacol Ther.* 1985;8:355–363

213. Nail PA, Thomas MR, Eakin R. The effect of thiamin and riboflavin supplementation on the level of those vitamins in human breast milk and urine. *Am J Clin Nutr.* 1980;33:198–204

214. Roepke JLB, Kirksey A. Vitamin B_6 nutrature during pregnancy and lactation, I: vitamin B_6 intake, levels of the vitamin in biological fluids, and condition of the infant at birth. *Am J Clin Nutr.* 1979;32:2249–2256

215. Greentree LB. Dangers of vitamin B_6 in nursing mothers. *N Engl J Med.* 1979;300:141–142

216. West KD, Kirksey A. Influence of vitamin B_6 intake on the content of the vitamin in human milk. *Am J Clin Nutr.* 1976;29:961–969

217. Samson RR, McClelland DBL. Vitamin B_{12} in human colostrum and milk: quantitation of the vitamin and its binder and the uptake of bound vitamin B_{12} by intestinal bacteria. *Acta Paediatr Scand.* 1980;69:93–99

218. Cancela L, LeBoulch N, Miravet L. Relationship between the vitamin D content of maternal milk and the vitamin D status of nursing women and breast-fed infants. *J Endocrinol.* 1986;110:43–50

219. Rothberg AD, Pettifor JM, Cohen DF, et al. Maternal-infant vitamin D relationships during breast-feeding. *J Pediatr.* 1982;101:500–503

220. Greer FR, Hollis BW, Napoli JL. High concentrations of vitamin D_2 in human milk associated with pharmacologic doses of vitamin D_2. *J Pediatr.* 1984;105:61–64

221. Retief EF, Heyns ADuP, Oosthuizen M, et al. Aspects of folate metabolism in lactating women studied after ingestion of ^{14}C-methylfolate. *Am J Med Sci.* 1979; 277:281–288

222. Dyggve HV, Dam H, Sondergaard E. Influence on the prothrombin time of breast-fed newborn babies of one single dose of vitamin K_1, or synkavit given to the mother within 2 hours after birth. *Acta Obstet Gynecol Scand.* 1956;35:440

223. Kries RV, Shearer M, McCarthy PT, et al. Vitamin K_1 content of maternal milk: influence of the stage of lactation, lipid composition, and vitamin K_1 supplements given to the mother. *Pediatr Res.* 1987;22:513–517

224. Soderman P, Hartvig P, Fagerlund C. Acetazolamide excretion into human breast milk. *Br J Clin Pharmacol.* 1984;17:599–600

225. Hofmeyr GJ, Sonnendecker EWW. Secretion of the gastrokinetic agent cisapride in human milk. *Eur J Clin Pharmacol.* 1986;30:735–736

226. Somogyi A, Gugler R. Cimetidine excretion into breast milk. *Br J Clin Pharmacol.* 1979;7:627–629

227. Hofmeyr GJ, van Iddekinge B. Dompridone and lactation. *Lancet.* 1983;1:647

228. Olsson B, Bolme P, Dahlstrom B, et al. Excretion of noscapine in human breast milk. *Eur J Clin Pharmacol.* 1986;30:213–215

229. Hardell L-I, Lindstrom B, Lonnerholm G, et al. Pyridostigmine in human breast milk. *Br J Clin Pharmacol.* 1982;14:565–567

230. Moiel RH, Ryan JR. Tolbutamide (orinase) in human breast milk. *Clin Pediatr.* 1967;6:480

231. Wild CP, Poinneau FA, Montesano R, et al. Aflatoxin detected in human breast milk by immunoassay. *Int J Cancer.* 1987;40:328–333

232. Stegink LD, Filer LJ Jr, Baker BL. Plasma, erythrocyte and human milk levels of free amino acids in lactating women administered aspartame or lactose. *J Nutr.* 1979;109:2173–2181

233. Mangurten HH, Kaye CI. Neonatal bromism secondary to maternal exposure to a photographic laboratory. *J Pediatr.* 1982;100:596–598

234. Radisch B, Luck W, Nau H. Cadium concentrations in milk and blood of smoking mothers. *Toxicol Lett.* 1987;36:147–152

235. Miyazaki T, Akiyama K, Kaneko, et al. Chlordane residues in human milk. *Bull Environ Contam Toxicol.* 1980;25:518–523

236. Resman BH, Blumenthal HP, Jusko WJ. Breast milk distribution of theobromine from chocolate. *J Pediatr.* 1977;91:477–480

237. Wolff MS. Occupationally derived chemicals in breast milk. *Am J Ind Med.* 1983;4:259–281

238. Egan H, Goulding R, Roburn J, et al. Organo-chlorine pesticide residues in human fat and human milk. *Br Med J.* 1965;2:66

239. Quinby GE, Armstrong JF, Durham WF. DDT in human milk. *Nature.* 1965;237:726

240. Bakken AF, Seip M. Insecticides in human breast milk. *Acta Paediatr Scand.* 1976;65:535–539

241. Adamovic VM, Sokic B, Smiljanski MJ. Some observations concerning the ratio of the intake of organochlorine insecticides through food and amounts excreted in the milk of breast-feeding mothers. *Bull Environ Contam Toxicol.* 1978;20:280–285

242. Savage EP, Keefe TJ, Tessari JD, et al. National study of chlorinated hydrocarbon insecticide residues in human milk, USA, I: geographic distribution of dieldrin, heptachlor, heptachlor epoxide, chlordane, oxychlordane, and mirex. *Am J Epidemiol.* 1981;113:413–422

243. Wilson DJ, Locker DJ, Ritzen CA, et al. DDT concentrations in human milk. *Am J Dis Child.* 1973;125:814–817

244. Emanuel B, Schoenfeld A. Favism in a nursing infant. *J Pediatr.* 1961;58:263–266

245. Simpson WJ, Tuba J. An investigation of fluoride concentration in the milk of nursing mothers. *J Oral Med.* 1968;23:104–106

246. Esala S, Vuori E, Helle A. Effect of maternal fluorine intake on breast milk fluorine content. *Br J Nutr.* 1982;48:201–204

247. Dreyfus-See G. Le passage dans le lait des aliments ou medicaments absorbes par de nourrices. *Rev Med Interne.* 1934;51:198–200

248. Ando M, Hirano S, Itoh Y. Transfer of hexachlorobenzene from mother to newborn baby through placenta and milk. *Arch Toxicol.* 1985;56:195–200

249. West RW, Wilson DJ, Schaffner W. Hexachlorophene concentrations in human milk. *Bull Environ Contam Toxicol.* 1975;13:167–169

250. Rabinowitz M, Leviton A, Needleman H. Lead in milk and infant blood: a dose-response model. *Arch Environ Health.* 1985;40:283–286

251. Sternowsky JH, Wessolowski R. Lead and cadmium in breast milk: higher levels in urban vs rural mothers during the first 3 months of lactation. *Arch Toxicol.* 1985;57:41–45

252. Koos BJ, Longo LD. Mercury toxicity in the pregnant woman, fetus, and newborn infant: a review. *Am J Obstet Gynecol.* 1976;126:390–409

253. Amin-Zaki L, Elhassani S, Majeed MA, et al. Studies of infants postnatally exposed to methylmercury. *J Pediatr.* 1974;85:81–84

254. Pitkin RM, Bahns JA, Filer LA Jr, et al. Mercury in human maternal and cord blood, placenta, and milk. *Proc Soc Exp Biol Med.* 1976;151:565–567

255. Stegink LD, Filer LJ Jr, Baker GL. Monosodium glutamate: effect on plasma and breast milk amino acid levels in lactating women. *Proc Soc Exp Biol Med.* 1972;140:836–841

256. Miller RW. Pollutants in breast milk: PCBs and cola-colored babies. *J Pediatr.* 1977;90:510–511. Editorial

257. Rogan WJ, Bagniewska A, Damstra T. Pollutants in breast milk. *N Engl J Med.* 1980;302;1450–1453

258. Wickizer TM, Brilliant LB, Copeland P, et al. Polychlorinated biphenyl contamination of nursing mothers in Michigan. *Am J Public Health.* 1981;71:132–137

259. Brilliant LB, Van Amburg G, Isbister J, et al. Breast milk monitoring to measure Michigan's contamination with polybrominated biphenyls. *Lancet.* 1978;2:643–646

260. Wickizer TM, Brilliant LB. Testing for polychlorinated biphenyls in human milk. *Pediatrics.* 1981;68:411–415

261. Bagnell PC, Ellenberger HA. Obstructive jaundice due to a chlorinated hydrocarbon in breast milk. *Can Med Assoc J.* 1977;117:1047–1048

262. Higginbottom MC, Sweetman L, Nyhan WL. A syndrome of methylmalonic aciduria, homocystinuria, megaloblastic anemia and neurologic abnormalities in a vitamin B_{12} deficient breast-fed infant of a strict vegetarian. *N Engl J Med.* 1978;299:317–323

7

Viruses in Human Milk

There is considerable evidence that the antibodies, interferon, and white blood cells in human milk play a vital role in protecting the suckling young from infections due to viruses (Pass, 1986). At the same time, a variety of animal and human viruses can be transmitted through mothers' milk. Since breastmilk is a highly cellular fluid and viruses are intracellular (that is, they live within the cell) the passage of viruses through milk is possible. For example, transmission of cytomegalovirus (CMV) through breastmilk is common. This transmission provides a natural vaccine that confers active immunity which protects the infant against infection. New evidence shows that breastfeeding also enhances the infant's immune response to vaccination with *Haemophilus influenza* type-b vaccine and with Bacille Calmette-Guérin (BCG) vaccine (Pabst & Spady, 1989, 1990).

HUMAN IMMUNODEFICIENCY VIRUS

Human Immunodeficiency Virus (HIV) and Acquired Immune Deficiency Syndrome (AIDS) are the most serious threat to worldwide public health since the polio epidemics earlier in this century. The African continent accounts for more than one-half of an estimated worldwide total of eight million virus carriers. The number of AIDS cases in the developed world began to explode sometime in the late 1970s, particularly in the U.S. male homosexual population. Formerly considered a "gay" or drug abuser's disease in the developed world, AIDS is also becoming a woman's disease as the number of HIV-infected women grows each year. Approximately 75% of women diagnosed as HIV-positive are in their childbearing years (CDC, 1989). About one-

JAN RIORDAN

half of women with AIDS have used drugs parenterally. One-fourth are sexual partners of men who have used drugs illegally (CDC, 1990). This last group is the fastest growing. Contaminated blood transfusions account for several thousand cases of AIDS; of those infected directly by transfusion, about one-third are women (CDC, 1989). Many children are also infected. As of July 1, 1990, 2,380 cases of pediatric AIDS were reported in the United States; most of these children were transplacentally infected by their mothers (Davis, 1990a).

As a result, health professionals working with childbearing women can expect to see infected women clients in increasing numbers (Fekety, 1989). While there are more uninfected than infected babies of HIV-positive mothers, the urgency for lactation consultants to have up-to-date and accurate information about HIV is clear.

Whether the HIV-positive mother should breastfeed is controversial and the subject of heated debate. Internationally, public policy makers differ in their recommendations about HIV infection and breastfeeding. WHO/UNICEF has made the recommendations outlined on p. 168.

At the time of this writing, it is standard medical practice to advise HIV-positive women living in developed countries (with a safe water supply and sanitation system) not to breastfeed. The Centers for Disease Control (CDC, 1985) has advised that no HIV-infected woman should breastfeed—in order to avoid postnatal transmission to a child who may not have been infected in utero. Recommendations from

167

WHO 1987 RECOMMENDATIONS

1. Breastfeeding should continue to be promoted, supported and protected in both developing and developed countries. The overall immunological, nutritional, psychosocial and child-spacing benefits of breastfeeding to infants and their mothers continue to be important factors in determining the overall health of mother and child.

2. If, for whatever reason, the biological mother cannot breastfeed or her milk is not available, and the use of pooled human milk is considered, the report of isolation of HIV in breastmilk should be taken into account. Pasteurization at 56°C for 30 minutes is reported to inactivate the virus. Further research on the effectiveness of different methods of pasteurization, however, is needed. As an additional precaution, the possibility of screening donors (in accordance with WHO criteria on HIV screening) should be considered, especially in areas where the prevalence of HIV infection is known to be high. Similarly, if for whatever reason, the biological mother cannot breastfeed, or her milk is not available, and where wet-nursing is the next obvious choice, care may need to be taken in selecting the wet nurse, bearing in mind her possible HIV infection status and that of the infant who is to be fed.

From World Health Organization, *Wkly Epidem Rec*, no. 33, Aug. 14, 1987; reprinted by permission.

---

the United Kingdom are similar to those of the CDC. The American Academy of Pediatrics Task Force on Pediatric AIDS (AAP, 1988) recommends that "in the United States and other countries where safe nutrition other than breast-feeding is available, HIV-infected mothers should be advised against breastfeeding their infants to avoid that possible route of HIV infection."

The CDC recommendations have been criticized on several grounds. All of the published accounts of HIV transmission by breastfeeding are anecdotal reports by physicians or parents. None are controlled

studies that are conclusive (Baumslag, 1987, 1988; Jelliffe & Jelliffe, 1988). Furthermore, if an HIV-infected infant is not breastfed, he is deprived of vitally needed maternal antibodies in his mother's milk, a natural form of immunization. Without the passive protection conferred by breastmilk, the high-risk infant is denied immunologic protection by human milk to ward off opportunistic infection (Minchin, 1987). The CDC's worldwide influence is likely to result in fewer mothers in developing countries choosing to breastfeed and, subsequently, the unnecessary deaths of thousands of infants. Options that make sense in one situation may be fatal in another situation where dangerous water supplies, poor sanitation, and poverty prevail (Armstrong, 1988; Smith, 1988).

Kennedy et al. (1990) propose a mathematical model for estimating infant mortality in developing countries both in the presence and absence of breastfeeding. They estimate that deaths due to HIV infection through breastfeeding could be between 1,000 and 19,000. By contrast, deaths due to diseases of infancy caused by not breastfeeding would range from 10,000 to 75,000 in a year's time. Another decision-analysis model demonstrated that in communities where the HIV prevalence rate among mothers reaches 40%, breastfeeding should still be recommended in the absence of HIV screening, unless HIV transmission via breastmilk surpasses 30% (Heymann, 1990).

The first case implicating breastmilk transmission of AIDS was reported by Ziegler, Cooper, and Johnson in 1985. An infant with eczema tested positive for HIV antibodies months after having been breastfed for six weeks. The mother had received a postpartum transfusion from a donor who subsequently developed AIDS. It was assumed that the mother seroconverted (serum changed from HIV-negative to HIV-positive) after she received the blood, although an infection before birth could not be excluded since she had not been tested earlier. Entry of the virus through the infant's eczematous lesions was also not excluded as a possible route of transmission. It is not clear whether the infant was exclusively breastfed. Soon after the publication of this report, the CDC published its recommendations based on this case and the finding of free HIV virus in specimens of cell-free breastmilk from three HIV-positive women (Thiry et al., 1985). Their recommendation was made even though the presence of HIV within cells is considered necessary before the virus can be transmitted (Levy, 1988). Later, in 1988, HIV in human milk was detected by electron microscope (Goudsmit et al., 1988), which supported the notion that breastmilk could carry the virus.

Thus far several published cases (LePage et al., 1987; Colebunders et al., 1988; Weinbreck et al., 1988; Ziegler, Cooper & Johnson, 1985; Ziegler et al., 1988) implicate human milk in transmitting HIV. In the majority of these reported cases, the mothers received a contaminated blood transfusion after delivery and presumably became infected at that time. It was assumed that they infected their infants through their breastmilk. None of the milk of any of these mothers was tested for HIV. In one case (Ziegler et al., 1988), both the mother and her breastfed infant had a seroconverting illness at 11 months postpartum, having shared intravenous needles two months earlier. In another case, in Kinshasa, Zaire, the child was found to be HIV-1 seropositive at 11 months of age after being breastfed by his infected aunt when his own mother died (Colebunders et al., 1988).

TRANSMISSION

There are no data available on the incidence of HIV transmission by breastfeeding, but the relative risk of breastfeeding compared with intrauterine transmission is considered to be low. Prospective studies comparing the transmission rates between breastfed and bottle-fed infants conclude that there does not appear to be a high risk associated with HIV transmission via breastmilk (Mok et al., 1987; Senturia et al., 1987; Stanback et al., 1988; Belec et al., 1990). Oxtoby (1988) showed that in a study of 11 U.S. infants of HIV-positive mothers breastfeeding their babies for up to seven months, only five of the infants became infected. This is similar to the rate of infection for babies who were formula-fed.

This pattern is worldwide. The infants of HIV-infected mothers in several European countries were followed for over a year in a European Collaborative Study (1988). Of 271 children, 24% became infected. The researchers found no evidence that either method of delivery or breastfeeding influenced transmission rates. In another study, Tozzi, Pezzotti, and Greco (1990) collected data from the Italian National Registry of AIDS to determine the interplay of breastfeeding on the incubation time of AIDS in vertically infected children. The median incubation time for developing AIDS for bottle-fed children was 9.7 months, while for breastfed children it was 19.0 months.

Belec et al. (1990) point out that the blood transfusion cases may have led to overestimation of the risk of transmission through milk because these mothers breastfed during the seroconversion stage, when they were highly infectious.

There are other transmission possibilities not yet explored in the literature. For example, blood from cracked nipples or from rupture of capillaries in the breast may possibly transmit HIV to the breastfeeding infant. The risk of transmitting HIV through breastmilk remains theoretical at this point; perhaps similar to the risk of transmission through saliva. HIV has been found in saliva; yet families of HIV-positive people are not advised to forgo kissing, even though there are other ways of showing affection.

Transmission is referred to as being either *vertical* (from the infected mother to the fetus or newborn) or *horizontal* (person to person via exchange of body fluids). An infected mother has about a 30% chance of vertically passing the virus to her baby either transplacentally or during delivery (Davis, 1990a, 1990b). In most cases, transmission appears to occur close to or at delivery (Ehrnst et al., 1991). No cases of transfusion-acquired AIDS have been reported in children transfused since the initiation of mandatory donor screening for HIV antibody in the spring of 1985. AIDS can be transmitted by transfusion of blood when the donor is in the early stages of HIV infection, and is seronegative, but this is rare (Rogers, 1987). Women with newly acquired infections or with advanced HIV disease may be more likely to have transmitted the infection to their babies *in utero* and prior to breastfeeding (Davis, 1990a).

TESTING

Human immunodeficiency viruses are one of the envelope viruses known as retroviruses. Standard tests for HIV (enzyme immunoassay and the Western blot test) do not detect the virus but rather the presence of antibodies to HIV. Unfortunately *all* babies born to infected mothers have high HIV antibody levels; therefore testing would be expected to result in a positive outcome in both infected and uninfected infants. Occasionally a child with a positive viral culture will test negative for antibodies. Polymerase chain reaction (PCR) is a new test to detect HIV. PCR technology allows scientists to produce large quantities of genetic material (DNA) from minute amounts (PCR, 1988) and may avoid some of the problems that have plagued the old testing methods.

COURSE OF DISEASE

Children born to HIV-positive mothers who do not become infected and remain clinically well gradually lose their antibodies and seroconvert back to HIV-negative before 15 to 18 months (AAP, 1988; Holman, 1989). Most other maternal antibodies in the infant are undetectable by six months; it is not clear why HIV antibodies persist. Most infants who become permanently infected with HIV appear normal at birth but develop symptoms within four to six months of life as they lose the passive protection of maternal antibodies (Falloon et al., 1989). These children often fail to thrive and have hepatomegaly, splenomegaly and lymphadenopathy, chronic diarrhea, and recurrent bacterial infections. Developmental disabilities and neurologic dysfunction are common. Since babies lack a developed immune system, the progression of infection and disease may be more rapid than in the adult.

An infected mother goes through several stages typical of adult HIV infection (Cohn, 1989). The seronegative stage begins with HIV infection and usually lasts from 6–12 weeks, although it may last up to 14 months. No detectable levels of anti-HIV antibody are present at first; therefore an infected mother may not develop detectable antibody levels for six months or more after exposure. Next, seroconversion occurs with symptoms, including fever, malaise, and lymphadenopathy. At this point the mother will test positive in a standard blood test for HIV. After seroconversion, the infected individual can feel and look perfectly well for prolonged periods, from several months to seven years. During the later stages of the disease, HIV symptoms of persistent lymphadenopathy gradually advance to later symptoms of oral candidiasis, weight loss, thrombocytopenia, *Pneumocystitis carinii* pneumonia, and ultimately death.

CLINICAL IMPLICATIONS

A vast amount of AIDS research is being conducted, especially in the United States, where millions of dollars have been allocated to researchers. Some of the investigations are promising. Several studies (Begin,

1989; Isaacs & Thormar, 1990; McDougal, 1991) suggest that human milk lipids inactivate enveloped viruses and that certain fatty acids found in human milk are efficient antiviral agents. In testing antiviral activity of human milk, Isaacs and Thormar (1990) showed that all enveloped viruses exposed to antiviral milk lipids or milk stomach contents were inactivated, including HSV-1, CMV, and HIV-1. New drugs, namely zidovudine (Retrovir, AZT) help delay or prevent the development of clinical AIDS in HIV-positive mothers and children.

A risk-factor assessment of mothers through personal interviews helps identify high-risk mothers, yet this screening is not always successful. Mothers later identified as HIV-positive are not always picked up through a voluntary screening program (Sperling et al., 1989). All women who are seropositive for HIV are advised to defer pregnancy as it is suspected that pregnancy accelerates HIV disease (Gloeb, O'Sullivan & Efantis, 1988; Fekety, 1989; Cohn, 1989). Pregnant women who are HIV-positive will most likely begin pregnancy as asymptomatic carriers and develop additional symptoms as the pregnancy progresses. While the usual recommendation for women who are seropositive is to defer pregnancy, Fekety (1989) reports three realities in practice: "Clients who have tested positive prior to the pregnancy fail to effectively contracept; clients whose sero status is unknown until early pregnancy testing is performed do not elect, for a host of reasons, to terminate the pregnancy; or prenatal testing may be delayed to a point in gestation where termination, even if desired, is not possible."

While transmission of AIDS through breastmilk is a rare event and the current data are conflicting, it appears possible that such transmission may occur—especially with highly infectious mothers. Most health professionals strongly advise mothers at risk for AIDS not to breastfeed.

The primary concern of women at risk for AIDS is not about breastfeeding but about infecting their unborn children. Most of the at-risk women interviewed by Williams (1990) were sure they would transmit AIDS to their unborn children, rejecting current professional information that less than 20–40% of infants born to HIV-infected women will become infected. They greatly fear the results of antibody testing. One woman in the study was so afraid of being told her test results that she continued her pregnancy without that information.

HIV-infected women come from all walks of life; some are not drug abusers or prostitutes and are victims themselves. Whatever the direct cause of their illnesses, their lives are shattered by finding out they are HIV-positive, which may be disclosed when their babies are born or when their spouses become ill or die. Often they feel dirty, useless, unwanted, and unlovable (Wofsy, 1987). While they desperately need help from family, friends, and other support groups, they are isolated because HIV is a "secret" disease. They suffer profound grief over the loss of their health, their sexuality, their chance to have more children and their ability to safely breastfeed. Counseling and the development of a support group are essential to the care of at-risk mothers. When offering counseling, it is essential to recognize that children are central to many of these women's lives and they are reluctant to forgo childbearing. At the same time concern for their children is a powerful motivator for dramatically changing behavior (Williams, 1990).

Practitioners who work with human milk and/or with breastfeeding women are rightly concerned about their own protection. In 1987, the CDC published a document that recommended precautions to be used when handling blood and body fluid for all patients regardless of their status of infection. These universal precautions apply to blood and other body fluids that contain visible blood—for example, semen and vaginal secretions. Universal precautions *do not apply* to human breast milk unless it contains visible blood (MMWR, 1988). Occupational exposure to human breastmilk has not been implicated in the transmission of HIV. Only when personnel are frequently exposed to breastmilk—for instance while working in human milk banks—should health-care workers regularly wear gloves.

Gloves are not needed when touching the breasts, e.g., in breast assessment. Nor are they usually necessary for handling breastmilk. However, if the health-care worker is in daily contact with human milk, she may choose to wear gloves (CDC, 1987). Gloves are routinely worn during delivery and for newborn care until the infant has been washed and dried, as well as for a suckling assessment. Vigorous handwashing—both before and after any physical contact with a client or with any body fluid—is standard practice for infection control and should be done consistently to prevent transmission of *any* infection in the mother, the child, and the health-care worker. As discussed in Chapter 22, pasteurization is now advised for all pooled breast milk and should eliminate any risk of transmission of HIV, making HIV-antibody screening of donors unnecessary (Eglin and Wilkinson, 1987).

HERPES SIMPLEX

Herpes simplex (HSV), caused by *herpes virus hominus,* is a common viral infection in humans. HSV is most serious during pregnancy and in the neonate. It is one of a group of infections known as TORCH (**T**oxoplasmosis, **R**ubella, **C**ytomegalovirus, **H**erpes) for which cord blood is routinely screened. Herpetic lesions can erupt anywhere on the body, including the breast or the genital area, usually as a result of direct contact. The infection may be either primary or recurrent. Diagnosis is made either by culture of the lesion or by drawing serum antibody titers.

The painful mucocutaneous blisterlike vesicles of herpes can appear from a few hours to up to 20 days after exposure. After the lesions heal, the virus enters a dormant phase and resides in the nerve ganglia in the affected area. Usually the primary infection is the most severe and appears to be triggered by stress or a rundown physical state. Neonatal HSV infection is usually acquired when the newborn passes through an infected genital tract; congenital infection is responsible for the most serious illness in neonates (Oxtoby, 1988). A cesarean section is routinely done when any active herpes lesions are present at the time of delivery. The seriousness of HSV infection appears to be age-related. Neonates may become seriously ill; beyond the first few weeks of the neonate's life, however, there are few adverse consequences. Despite the high prevalence of genital herpes in the general population, the incidence of neonatal herpes is low, about 1 in 10,000 births.

It is doubtful that neonatal herpes is transmitted through human milk. Transmission during breastfeeding, if it occurs, is most likely from direct contact with the herpes vesicle on the breast (Quinn & Lofberg, 1978; Pass, 1989; Oxtoby, 1988; Sealander & Kerr, 1989; Sullivan-Bolyai et al., 1983).

Sealander and Kerr (1989) report a case of a nursing toddler transmitting herpes simplex virus to the mother through breastfeeding. In this case, the child's oral lesions (on the inner aspect of the lower lip) caused painful blisters on the mother's nipples. Culture of the child's oral lesions and the mother's nipple lesions were positive for HSV. Following one week's cessation of breastfeeding, during which she was given oral acylclovir—200 mg five times a day for five days—the mother resumed breastfeeding. The authors recommended that whenever a young child develops oral HSV lesions, the mother should be asked if she is breastfeeding in order that the risk of contracting herpes simplex from her child can be explained, and appropriate intervention offered.

Sullivan-Bolyai and colleagues (1983) reported a case of a mother with a maternal breast lesion identified as herpes simplex Type I. Although her infant experienced an uneventful nursery course and was discharged from the hospital at two days of age, the mother reported developing a "skin sore" on the areola of her left breast during her postpartum stay. On the fourth day of life, the baby appeared to have pustules in the corner of his mouth and on his chin. On days six and seven, herpes simplex virus was isolated from the mouth of the infant; on day seven, the virus also was isolated from the mother's breast lesions. The infant died at 11 days of age. This case points out the need to avoid direct infant contact with a herpes simplex virus lesion. While the mother's milk may be free of the virus, the lesion itself is not.

Although HSV can occasionally be cultured from breastmilk, this appears to be rare (Oxtoby, 1988). HSV has not been isolated in any of the CMV studies which used culture techniques appropriate for HSV (Pass, 1986b); no role in transmitting infection in the absence of a local HSV lesion has been demonstrated. Breast lesions are seldom the first clinical evidence of herpes in the family (Sullivan-Bolyai et al., 1983). The primary herpetic lesion can be manifested in other family members who then pass it on: the father who transmits it while making love to the mother or a sibling who kisses a baby brother or sister. Therefore, transmission can be from mother-to-infant or from infant-to-mother; or some other family member can infect the infant who then passes the virus onto his mother during feedings.

Providing there are no breast lesions, the newborn of a mother with HSV, if he is healthy, may breastfeed and be with the mother in her room; however, scrupulous hand washing, gowning, and covering of any lesions must be practiced to prevent possible cross-contamination. The mother does not need to wear rubber gloves while breastfeeding.

Treatment is usually directed toward symptomatic relief and prevention of a secondary infection since there is no known cure for herpes (see Table 7–1). Two antiviral drugs are specifically indicated for herpes simplex infections: acyclovir (Zovirax) and vidarabine. Acyclovir can be given orally (Sealander & Kerr, 1989), applied topically, or given intravenously (usually in treating neonatal HSV). Vidarabine is given by intravenous infusion as an alternative to acyclovir treatment (Spencer et al., 1989). Cleansing with povidone-iodine (Betadine) solution is thought to help prevent a secondary infection and applying Burow's solution (aluminum acetate) may relieve some of the discomfort. Vitamin C or lysine and lysine supplements are frequently suggested to prevent recurrence; however, their effectiveness is unknown (Olds, London & Ladewig, 1988).

CHICKENPOX (HERPES ZOSTER)

Since chickenpox (varicella-herpes zoster), an acute communicable disease, can occur during the reproductive years, a women may develop this infection while she is breastfeeding. If the mother has had chickenpox, breastfeeding should continue since the antibodies in her milk confer passive immunity to her baby against chickenpox. This passive immunization may even prevent the breastfed baby from having symptoms of chickenpox (Berman, 1982). If this baby does develop chickenpox, the course of his disease is usually mild. The incubation period is from 11 to 21 days but may be as long as 25 days. Lesions begin on the neck or trunk and spread to the face, scalp, mucous membranes, and extremities. Lesions first appear as small, flat, red blotches that progress to raised vesicles which form crusts over a period of from two to four days. If the mother has never had chicken pox, she will have no antibodies in her breastmilk to help protect the baby against chickenpox. A mother who develops chicken pox several days before she delivers her baby presents a special, complex medical case that can be potentially life-threatening.

Two cases of varicella-herpes zoster are described by Frederick, White, and Braddock (1986). In the first case, a 33-year-old mother developed classic herpetiform lesions on her left back and side. The breast was not involved. Expressed milk obtained within 24 hours of the appearance of the lesions re-

TABLE 7–1   CLINICAL CARE PLAN FOR BREASTFEEDING MOTHER WITH HERPES SIMPLEX INFECTION

Problem	Intervention	Rationale
Seropositive for HSV	Encourage continued breastfeeding unless breast lesions are present	Infant receives protective antibodies
Herpes No breast lesion	Wash hands thoroughly with soap before breastfeeding	Helps prevent spreading infection
	Caution against touching baby or breast after touching lesion from any site	Shedding occurs
	Avoid tub bath with infant; use universal precautions (hospital staff)	Shedding occurs
Breast lesion present	Discourage breastfeeding from affected breast; use breast pump to maintain comfort and milk supply; sterilize pump part coming in contact with breast after each use	To prevent infant's direct contact with lesion
Pain	Tylenol	Analgesia
	Burrow's solution topically	Soothing effect
	Imagery	Distraction by focusing
Feelings of shame	Reassure that HSV occurs frequently	Mothers tend to blame themselves
Secondary infection	Cleanse lesion with Betadine	Antibacterial
Recurrence	Take Vitamin C	Possibly prevents recurrence
	Anti-viral medication as prescribed	

vealed no varicella-herpes zoster virus. Breastfeeding continued from both breasts, with slight position changes to avoid direct infant contact with the lesions. The infant remained healthy throughout the course of the mother's illness.

The second case involved a 21-year-old mother who developed chickenpox at 40 weeks' gestation after contracting the illness from her older child. No prior history of chickenpox was noted and she developed severe pulmonary problems due to varicella pneumonia. Following an emergency cesarean section, her healthy infant was treated prophylactically with zoster immune globulin and parenteral acyclovir. The mother was isolated; her infant was not put to breast because of her extensive cutaneous lesions and the danger of neonatal varicella infection from contact with the mother. During the mother's isolation, the baby remained healthy. Milk production was established and sustained through breast pumping for three weeks until the mother chose not to continue pumping. Milk samples obtained during her three-week hospitalization revealed no evidence of the virus. Frederick, White, and Braddock (1986) concluded that milk from a mother with varicella-herpes zoster virus is safe and may continue to be provided during the course of the illness.

CYTOMEGALOVIRUS

Cytomegalovirus (CMV), another herpes virus, is probably the most prevalent infection in the TORCH group. Almost one-half of all adults have antibodies for CMV, evidence of an infection at some point in their lives. The incidence of CMV antibody in young children is highest in developing countries and in countries where communal child care and breastfeeding are common (Yow et al., 1987). The virus can be found in the breast, genital tract, urine, and pharynx and is transmitted by any close contact. As with other herpes viruses, it remains in host cells indefinitely. CMV can be transmitted through human milk; in fact, breastfeeding has proven to be an important means of conveying passive immunity to CMV. The incidence of infection, approximately 20%, has epidemiological importance (Dworsky et al., 1983). Breastfed children thus immunized to CMV by breastfeeding are protected later in life from symptomatic infection and from primary infection during pregnancy, which can cause intrauterine tissue damage (Pass, 1986b).

In a prospective study, Dworsky et al. (1983) studied CMV in 58 postpartum mother-baby pairs. Consumption of infected breast milk led to infection in the majority of the infants. All infected infants chronically shed cytomegalovirus; however, no infant had any sequelae. There is no evidence of disease in full-term infants who develop CMV infection from breastfeeding. Premature infants, particularly if they are seronegative, are at risk for serious illness if they acquire CMV; therefore, premature infants should receive banked human milk from seronegative donors only.

RUBELLA

Because rubella in the first trimester of pregnancy causes serious birth defects, the uninformed person might be unduly concerned that rubella in human milk likewise is deleterious. Although the rubella virus can be passed through maternal milk lymphocytes to the infant, there is no evidence that the baby who acquires rubella in this manner becomes ill (Losonsky et al., 1982). Like CMV, transmission of maternal antibodies against rubella is beneficial to the infant by serving as a natural vaccine.

If the mother is immunized postpartum, the breastfeeding infant will develop antibodies to rubella but will not show symptoms of the disease. Buimovici-Klein and colleagues (1977) describe a case where the mother developed a rash, glandular swelling and fever 12 days after postpartum vaccination. The infant had no clear antibody response; however, one year later when the child was immunized, his antibody response suggested that he had sometime earlier acquired the virus. In another case (Klein, Byrne & Cooper, 1980) a breastfeeding mother developed a rubella-like rash eight days after a normal delivery. Eighteen days before the onset of the rash, she had been in close contact with a person with a clinically diagnosed case of rubella. The newborn girl was followed for signs of rubella. The mother stopped breastfeeding for the first two days of her rash, but resumed without incident on the third day. Her daughter remained clinically well, without sign of infection for the next six weeks.

HEPATITIS B

Hepatitis B virus (HBV) causes a systemic illness that involves the liver, with symptoms ranging from none to mild flu-like symptoms to a fulminating illness.

HBV is usually transmitted by contact with infected blood, body secretions, or through transfusion of contaminated blood. Contamination of the mucous membranes during birth or sexual intercourse is another method of transmission. Although less than 10% of all infants born to HBV-positive mothers are infected transplacentally, an infant exposed to hepatitis in the birth canal has a high probability of acquiring the infection. Medical and birthing centers routinely screen for HBV from umbilical cord blood. Indicators of HBV are the presence of HBeAg in the blood, serologic testing for antibody to the surface antigen (HBsAg), and the newly developed hepatitis B virus-DNA probe (HBV-DNA).

Infants born to an HBV-positive mother, already exposed to maternal blood, amniotic fluid, and vaginal secretions during delivery, may breastfeed. The neonate should receive Hepatitis B Immune Globulin (HBIG) within 12 hours after birth followed by a series of injections of HBV vaccine: the first during the first week, the second at one month, and the third at six months (Larson, 1987; Olds, London & Ladewig, 1989). All infants should have pediatric follow-up, including repeated screening for HBsAg to rule out chronic carriers.

Several investigators have examined the risk to the breastfeeding infant if the mother is infected. Lee, Ip, and Wong (1978) found that following immunization of 447 infants born to mothers who were positive for the Hepatitis B antigen, infection was somewhat higher in the infants born vaginally compared with those delivered by cesarean section (24.9% vs. 10%). At birth, none of the newborns delivered by cesarean, compared with 13 of the 67 infants born vaginally, were positive for HBV-DNA. The investigators concluded that the risk of infection to the infants was lessened if cesarean section was performed. Follow-up with administration of passive antibodies from HBIG vaccine further reduces the risk of the high-risk infants.

Tseng, Lam, and Tam (1988) report that there is no evidence that breastfeeding will increase the risk of HBV infection in infants, regardless of whether they have been immunized. There were no differences in the rate of development of antigenemia or immunity against hepatitis B between the breastfed and bottle-fed babies during the first year of life, and almost all infants were HBsAb-positive at one year of age regardless of how they were fed. They concluded that there was "no valid contraindication for breastfeeding in infants born to HBsAg-positive mothers," especially if the infants were immunized soon after birth. Beasley et al. (1975) concur, concluding that "breast-feeding is not an important means of transmission from mother to child," and that cord-blood positive infants were probably infected *in utero* and thus are not susceptible to post-delivery infection.

DeMartino et al. (1987) followed 47 breastfed and 112 formula-fed infants born to mothers who were positive for HBsAg. No difference was observed between the groups regarding the percentage of infants who seroconverted. Seven months after birth, the formula-fed infants did develop transient but significantly higher anti-HBs antibody levels compared with the breastfeeding infants. The authors speculate about the suppressive factors in human milk and orally induced tolerance (55% of the milk samples were found to have detectable HBsAg) that may contribute to this suppression.

Breastfeeding does not increase the rate of infection among infants. Moreover, in areas of high prevalence of hepatitis B and environmental exposure, lack of breastfeeding places the infant at greater risk of contracting the disease. Krugman's review (1985) of viral hepatitis concludes that passive immunization of HBIG is an appropriate approach to take when caring for infants and children who are at risk for contracting the infection. He notes that there is little risk of hepatitis to the infant from breastmilk and that breastfeeding should not be discouraged.

IMPLICATIONS FOR CLINICAL PRACTICE

A viral infection in the mother rarely, if ever, indicates the need to terminate breastfeeding (see Table 7–2). From a practical standpoint, the infant has already been exposed to the virus, usually transplacentally and during the birth process. The only antibody protection that is available to the infant is from his mother's milk as a result of her infection. If the mother is well enough to care for her baby and the infant does not require special care, mother and baby should stay in the same hospital room. Concern of health-care providers should be directed, not at mothers known to have an infection, but at those with an unidentified infection.

For the breastfeeding mother with a viral disease, isolation precautions should be taken by the mother while in the hospital. If the infant's mother is positive for Hepatitis B or other viruses, scrupulous hand washing and gowning are routinely practiced to prevent possible cross-contamination. While antiseptic soaps for handwashing kill organisms more effectively, no data show that infection rates are any different when plain vs. antiseptic soap is used. The mother does not need to wear rubber gloves while breastfeeding. The most effective ways to prevent the spread of infections among neonates, parents, and staff is to maintain body substance precautions and to teach others to do so as well (Larson, 1987).

A new mother is already under stress. The news that she has a viral infection, which may or may not

TABLE 7–2 VIRUSES IN MILK

Virus	Transmission through Milk	Associated Disease	Breastfeeding
Cytomegalovirus	Proven	None	Permitted Protective effect
Herpes Simplex	Probably not	Disseminated herpes possible in neonate	Permitted if no breast lesions
Rubella	Proven	None	Encouraged Protective effect
Hepatitis B Virus	Unknown	Unknown	Permitted if infant and mother have HBIG and HbsAg
HIV	Possibly	AIDS	Not in developed countries
Chickenpox	Probably not	None apparent	Permitted

From Pass, RF: Viral Contamination of Milk. In Goldman, AS, Atkinson, SA, and Hanson, A, eds., *Human Lactation 3: The Effects of Milk on Recipient Infant,* New York, 1986b, Plenum Press, pp. 279–87.

be considered a sexually transmitted disease, may bring pain, anger, and guilt. These feelings can be compounded by a fear that she should not breast-feed her baby. Encouraging the mother to express her fears, answering her questions, and then supporting her desires is a vital contribution to her care and well-being.

SUMMARY

Toward the end of pregnancy, the fetus receives passive immunity from the mother; the baby, therefore, is born with his mother's immunities. Breastfed infants acquire additional antibodies to influenza, mumps, and chickenpox, as well as other viruses—either through the mother's clinical exposure or through immunization. This passive immunity lasts from three to six months and protects the infant from childhood diseases. Concern about the risk of viral transmission through breastmilk appears limited to HIV. Thus, for all other viral infections, breastfeeding should continue except in the case of a mother who has a herpes simplex lesion on her breasts.

The possibility of HIV transmission by human milk has had a negative effect on breastfeeding that is yet unmeasured. In developing countries where artificial feeding is often lethal, this effect is a major concern. Kennedy et al. (1990) offer a modification to the CDC recommendations on HIV and breastfeeding. This modification would change the recommendations so that "breastfeeding is discouraged in a seropositive mother who is in an advanced stage of the disease or in the rare case of a woman who has had a known, recent, seropositive transfusion. If breastfeeding were discouraged only in such specific cases, the life-giving benefits of breastfeeding, especially in developing countries, could be maintained."

Unfortunately, the specter of HIV transmission through human milk has had a devastating effect on human milk banking in many parts of the world, because of the fear of transmitting HIV and other viruses and because of the extra trouble and cost of pasteurization. From a teleological standpoint, it is difficult to accept the spectre of a fatal infection conferred by breastmilk—the fluid of life and growth—particularly in the face of questionable evidence that it may occur.

REFERENCES

American Academy of Pediatrics Task Force on Pediatric AIDS: Perinatal human immunodeficiency virus infection, *Pediatrics* 82:941–44, 1988.

Armstrong, H: AIDS and human milk: How worried should we be? *J Hum Lact* 4:57, 1988.

Baumslag, N: AIDS and breastfeeding: Panic or logic? (editorial), *Breastfeeding Abstr,* 4:7, 1988.

Baumslag, N: Breast-feeding and HIV infection, *Lancet* 2(8555):401, 1987.

Beasley, RP, et al.: Evidence against breast-feeding as a mechanism for vertical transmission of hepatitis B, *Lancet* 2:740, 1975.

Begin, M: Possible role of polyunsaturated fatty acids in the pathogenesis of AIDS, *Arch AIDS Res* 4:93–104, 1989.

Belec, L, et al.: Antibodies to human immunodeficiency virus in the breast milk of healthy, seropositive women, *Pediatrics* 85:1022–26, 1990.

Berman, A: Varicella and breastfeeding (letter), *J Fam Pract* 15:617, 620, 1982.

Buimovici-Klein, E, et al.: Isolation of rubella virus in milk after postpartum immunization, *J Pediatr* 6:939–41, 1977.

Centers for Disease Control: *HIV/AIDS Surveillance Report,* AIDS program, Atlanta, May 12, 1989.

Centers for Disease Control: *HIV/AIDS Surveillance Report,* AIDS program, Atlanta, April, 1990.

Centers for Disease Control: Recommendations for assisting in the prevention of perinatal transmission of human T-lymphatic virus type III lymphadenopathy-associated virus and acquired immunodeficiency virus, *MMWR* 34:7211–32, 1985.

Centers for Disease Control: Recommendations for prevention of HIV transmission in health care settings, *MMWR* 36 (suppl. no. 25), 1987.

Centers for Disease Control: Update: Universal precautions for prevention of transmission of human immune deficiency virus, Hepatitis B virus, and other bloodborne pathogens in health-care settings, *MMWR* 37:378-87, 1988.

Cohn, JA: Virology, immunology, and natural history of HIV infection, *J Nurs Midwif* 34:242–52, 1989.

Colebunders, R, et al.: Breastfeeding and transmission of HIV, *Lancet* 2:(8626/8627):1487, 1988.

Davis, MK: Clinical recommendations concerning viral transmission in human milk—cause for concern or unjustified panic? La Leche League International, Annual Physicians Seminar, Boston, 1990a.

Davis, MK: The role of human milk in human immunodeficiency virus infection. In Atkinson, SA, Hanson, LA, and Chandra, RK, eds.: *Breastfeeding, nutrition, infection and infant growth in developed and emerging countries,* St. John's, Newfoundland, Canada, 1990b, ARTS Biomedical Publisher, pp. 151–60.

de Martino, MM, et al.: Different degree of antibody response to Hepatitis B Virus Vaccine in breast- and formula-fed infants born to HBsAg-positive mothers, *J Pediatr Gastroenterol Nutr* 6:208–11, 1987.

Dworsky, MY, et al.: Cytomegalovirus infection of breast milk and transmission in infancy, *Pediatrics* 72:295–99, 1983.

Eglin, RP, Wilkinson, AR: HIV infection and pasteurization of breast milk, *Lancet* 1(8541):1093, 1987.

Ehrnst, A, et al.: HIV in pregnant women and their offspring: evidence for late transmission, *Lancet* 338:203–7, 1991.

European Collaborative Study: Mother-to-mother transmission of HIV infection, *Lancet* 2(8619):1039–42, 1988.

Falloon, J, et al.: Human immunodeficiency virus infection in children, *J Pediatr* 114:1–30, 1989.

Fekety, SE: Managing the HIV-positive patient and her newborn in a CNM service, *J Nurs Midwif* 34:253–58, 1989.

Frederick, IB, White, RJ, and Braddock, SW: Excretion of varicella-herpes zoster virus in breast milk, *Am J Obstet Gynecol* 154:1116–17, 1986.

Gloeb, DJ, O'Sullivan, MJ, and Efantis, J: Human immunodeficiency virus in women. 1: The effects of human immunodeficiency virus on pregnancy, *Am J Obstet Gynecol* 159:756–61, 1988.

Goudsmit, J, et al.: *Virological and electron microscopic evidence for postnatal HIV transmission via breast milk.* Presented at Fourth International Conference on AIDS, Stockholm, June 12–16, 1988, Abstract 5099.

Heymann, SJ: Modeling the impact of breast-feeding by HIV-infected women on child survival, *Am J Public Health* 80:1305–9, 1990.

Holman, S: Epidemiology and transmission of HIV infection in women, *J Nurs-Midwif* 34:233–41, 1989.

Isaacs, CE, and Thormar, H: Human milk lipids inactivate enveloped viruses. In Atkinson, SA, Hanson, LA, and Chandra, RK, eds.: *Breastfeeding, nutrition, infection and infant growth in developed and emerging countries,* St. John's, Newfoundland, Canada, 1990, ARTS Biomedical Publisher, Canada, pp. 161–74.

Jelliffe, DB, and Jelliffe, EF: HIV and breastmilk: Nonproven alarmism, *J Trop Pediatr* 34:142, 1988.

Kennedy, KI, et al.: Do the benefits of breastfeeding outweigh the risk of postnatal transmission of HIV via breastmilk? *Trop Doc* 20:25–29, 1990.

Klein, EB, Byrne, T, and Cooper, LZ: Neonatal rubella in a breast-fed infant after postpartum maternal infection, *J Pediatr* 97:774–75, 1980.

Krugman, S: Viral hepatitis: 1985 update, *Pediatr Rev* 7(1):3–10, 1985.

Larson, E: Trends in neonatal infections, *JOGNN* 16:404–9, 1987.

Lee, AK, Ip, HM, and Wong, VC: Mechanisms of maternal-fetal transmission of hepatitis B virus, *J Infec Dis* 138:668–71, 1978.

LePage, P, et al.: Postnatal transmission of HIV from mother to child, *Lancet* 2(8555):400, 1987.

Levy, JA: The transmission of AIDS: the case of the infected cell, *JAMA* 259:3037–38, 1988.

Losonsky, GA, et al.: Effect of immunization against rubella on lactation products. I. Development and characterization of specific immunologic reactivity in breast milk, *J Infec Dis* 145:661–66, 1982.

McDougal, JS: Pasteurization of human breast milk and its effect on HIV infectivity, The Human Milk Banking Association of North America, *Newsletter No. 7,* Winter, 1991.

Minchin, M: *AIDS and infant feeding: what are the choices?* Melbourne, Australia, 1987, The Bean Machine.

Mok, JQ, et al.: Infants born to mothers seropositive for HIV: preliminary findings from a multicenter European study, *Lancet* 1:1164–68, 1987.

Olds, S, London, ML, and Ladewig, PA: *Maternal-newborn nursing,* 3rd ed., Menlo Park, Calif., 1988, Addison-Wesley Publishing Co. pp. 237–38.

Oxtoby, MJ: Human immunodeficiency virus and other viruses in human milk: placing the issues in broader perspective, *Pediatr Infec Dis* 7:825–35, 1988.

Pabst, HF, et al.: Effect of breast-feeding on immune response to BCG vaccine, *Lancet* 1:295–97, 1989.

Pabst, HF, and Spady, DW: Effect of breast-feeding on antibody response to conjugate vaccine, *Lancet* 1(336):269–70, 1990.

Pass, RF: Transmission of viruses through human milk. In Howell, RR, Morriss, FG, and Pickering, LK, eds.: *Human milk in infant nutrition and health,* Springfield, Ill., 1986a, Charles C Thomas, Publisher, pp. 205–23.

Pass, RF: Viral Contamination of Milk. In Goldman, AS, Atkinson, SA, and Hanson A, eds.: *Human Lactation 3: The Effects of Milk on Recipient Infant,* New York, 1986b, Plenum Press, pp. 279–87.

Pass, RF: *Viruses in human milk,* La Leche League International, 17th Annual Seminar for Physicians, Anaheim, Calif., July 11, 1989.

PCR: A new test for HIV: Clinical News, *AJN* 88:1172, 1988.

Quinn, PT, and Lofberg, JV: Maternal herpetic breast infection: another hazard of neonatal herpes simplex, *Med J Aust* 2:411–12, 1978.

Rogers, MF: *Transmission of human immunodeficiency virus infection in the United States,* Report of the Surgeon General's Workshop on Children with HIV infection and their families, USDHHS Publ. No. HRS-D-MC 87–1, 1987, pp. 17–18.

Sealander, JY, and Kerr, CP: Herpes simplex of the nipple: Infant-to-mother transmission, *Am Fam Phys* 39:111–13, 1989.

Senturia, UD, et al.: Breast-feeding and HIV infection, *Lancet* 2:400–401, 1987.

Smith, EJ: AIDS and Breast Milk, *JOGNN* 17:160, 1988.

Spencer, RT, et al.: *Clinical pharmacology and nursing management* (3rd ed.), Philadelphia, 1989, J.B. Lippincott Co., pp. 252–55.

Sperling, RS, et al.: Umbilical cord blood serosurvey for human immunodeficiency virus in parturient women in a voluntary hospital in New York City, *Obstet Gynecol* 69:285–8, 1989.

Stanback, M, et al.: *Breastfeeding and HIV transmission in Haitian children,* presented at Fourth International Conference on AIDS, Stockholm, June 12–16, 1988, Abstract 5101.

Sullivan-Bolyai, JS, et al.: Disseminated neonatal herpes simplex virus type 1 from a maternal breast lesion, *Pediatrics* 71:455–57, 1983.

Thiry, L, et al.: Isolation of AIDS virus from cell-free breast milk of three healthy virus carriers, *Lancet* 2(8583):981, 1985.

Tozzi, AE, Pezzotti, P, and Greco, D: Does breast-feeding

delay progression to AIDS in HIV-infected children? (letter to the editor), *AIDS* 4:1493–94, 1990.

Tseng, RYM, Lam, CWK, and Tam, J: Breastfeeding babies of HBsAg-positive mothers, *Lancet* 2(8618):1032, 1988.

Weinbreck, P, et al.: Postnatal transmission of HIV infection, *Lancet* 1(8583):482, 1988.

WHO/UNICEF: *Breastfeeding in the 1990's: Review and implications for a global strategy,* Technical meeting, Geneva, June 25–28, 1990.

Williams, AB: Reproductive concerns of women at risk for HIV infection, *J Nurs Midwif* 35:292–98, 1990.

Wofsy, CB: *Intravenous drug abuse and women's medical issues,* Report of the Surgeon General's Workshop on Children with HIV infection and their Families, USDHHS Publ. No. HRS-D-MC 87–1, 1987, pp. 32–33.

Yow, MD, et al.: Acquisition of cytomegalovirus infection from birth to 10 years; a longitudinal serologic study, *J Pediatr* 110:37–42, 1987.

Ziegler, JB, et al.: *Breastfeeding and transmission of HIV from mother to infant.* In IV International Conference on AIDS, Stockholm, 1988 Swedish Ministry of Health and Social Affairs, Abstract 5100, book 1.

Ziegler, JB, Cooper, DA, and Johnson, RO: Postnatal transmission of AIDS-associated retrovirus from mother to child, *Lancet* 1:896–97, 1985.

ADDITIONAL READINGS

Seltzer, V: Breast-feeding and the potential for human immunodeficiency virus transmission, *Obstet Gynecol* 75:713–15, 1990.

World Health Organization: Breast-feeding/breastmilk and human immunodeficiency virus (HIV), *Wkly Epidem Rec* 62:245–46, 1987.

SECTION

THREE

Prenatal and Perinatal Periods

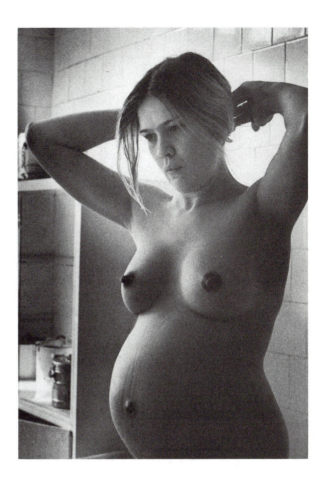

Most infants are born at or near term and are healthy. Some babies are not. Although they represent a small percentage of the total, babies born preterm represent special challenges for their mothers and the care-givers assisting them. Too often, breastfeeding succumbs to the technologically based decisions designed to help the baby survive in the short term—but which do not also consider his needs or those of his mother in the long term. Jaundice is an outcome of early extrauterine life. How it is managed can influence the breastfeeding course, often negatively and unnecessarily. Some babies grow poorly when breastfed. Is this a problem deriving from the mother, the baby, or both? And how can it be resolved without compromising the breastfeeding relationship? Finally, although not premature, some breastfeeding babies become ill. How does this affect breastfeeding? These questions and others are answered in these chapters by highlighting the needs of the breastfeeding baby and how they can be met—even in situations that do not at first appear to be conducive to continued breastfeeding.

8

Breastfeeding Education

Debi Leslie Bocar and Linda Shrago

Education is the cornerstone supporting the entire framework of lactation and breastfeeding. This chapter provides the health-care provider with tools to fashion meaningful educational experiences for breastfeeding families and colleagues. Two types of programs are addressed: those aimed at assisting families in having a positive breastfeeding experience, and those designed to increase the knowledge base of the health-care providers so that they can effectively assist with breastfeeding. Because education permeates all activities in the field of breastfeeding, isolating the educational component is an enormous challenge. This chapter addresses a broad range of educational issues—from theory to practical application. An overview of research related to breastfeeding education is provided, along with strategies for teaching adult learners.

In traditional societies, an inexperienced mother turns to her mother, aunts, or grandmothers for emotional support during childbearing and breastfeeding. Breastfeeding "education" involves a lifelong immersion in a culture in which seeing a baby at breast is a normal, welcomed sight. Even though formal breastfeeding and parental education is common in many parts of the world, it is still only a replacement for a time-honored family function.

The dramatic decrease in breastfeeding in industrialized societies during the first half of the twentieth century reduced the number of mothers who could share their breastfeeding experiences. Over time, expectant mothers were less likely to see an infant breastfeed or to know someone who could provide practical assistance. Geographic mobility further isolated young families from traditional support networks. Into the vacuum came alternative support systems for the few women who chose to breastfeed.

Self-help groups such as La Leche League International, Nursing Mothers Association of Australia, and childbirth education groups began to organize. They flourished worldwide, providing accurate information, practical assistance and emotional support for breastfeeding families using a mother-to-mother approach.

As breastfeeding initiation rates rose, health-care systems began to offer formal breastfeeding assistance. Hospitals, clinics, health maintenance organizations, and medical practice groups increasingly offer classes of all types to parents, siblings, and grandparents. While the primary purpose of these programs is educational, they are also effective public relations techniques for attracting families to those institutions. In an era in which health-care agencies are increasingly competitive, patient/client education can be an effective marketing strategy.

Recent shifts in the U.S. health-care industry directly affect breastfeeding education. Third party reimbursement rewards birth settings where patients are discharged quickly; yet when families leave the hospital or birthing center within hours or days after birth, teaching opportunities are abbreviated.

LEARNING PRINCIPLES

Learning is most effective when individuals are ready to learn—that is, when they feel a need to know something (Redman, 1988). "Teachable moments" refer to those periods when learners perceive the need for information and skills. Motivation is further enhanced when the material to be learned is organized in a manner that makes it meaningful to the learner. Activities which are novel and interesting to learners are equated with a continued motivation to learn. Active, rather than passive, participation is associated with more meaningful and permanent learning (Darkenwald & Merriam, 1982). Bloom (1956) reported that learning is often divided into three domains: (1) cognitive skills (gathering information, linking concepts, problem solving); (2) psychomotor skills (listening to instructions, observing skills, repetitive practice, mastery of skill performance); and (3) affective learning (modifying attitudes, values, and preferences). Breastfeeding education involves each of these domains.

Learning methods should also be considered when planning teaching strategies (Dunn, 1979). Some participants learn primarily through auditory perceptions; they listen intently and remember what they hear. Others learn best visually and retain information about what they see. These learners benefit from visual aids and printed materials. A third mode of learning is kinesthetic or psychomotor learning. Kinesthetic learners benefit from touching and handling equipment. Most learners use all three modalities with one or two modes being their preferred

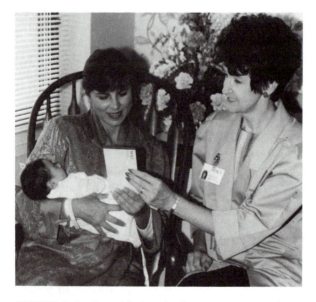

FIGURE 8–1 Pamphlets and other written materials reinforce one-to-one teaching. (Courtesy Shira L. Bocar.)

style. Therefore, when teaching about breast pumps, learning is strengthened by discussion coupled with showing slides which demonstrate how pumps work, plus having the learners manipulate the pumps themselves.

Since success is predictably more motivating than failure, dividing tasks and information into easily mastered segments keeps the adult motivated to continue the program. Learners respond to specific descriptions of their positive performance. Praise enhances feelings of self-confidence and conveys respect for the learner.

ADULT EDUCATION

Adult learners differ widely from children in their learning styles. Unlike children, who are required to attend school, adults are self-directed when they choose to attend educational activities (Knowles, 1980). Adults perceive time as one of their most valued and scarce assets, and they are not willing to spend it in meaningless activity (Dolphin & Holtzclaw, 1983). Education programs must, therefore, demonstrate a clear applicability to the adult's "real life." For example, a discussion of the anatomy of the breast and the physiology of breastfeeding is more meaningful when related directly to practical skills, such as latch-on techniques and how often to feed the baby.

Adult learners have a variety of experiential backgrounds and motivations for participating in educational programs than do children. They appreciate and expect to be accorded respect as unique individuals. Assisting adults in identifying their own personal learning goals and providing feedback about their progress towards achieving these goals enhances self-directed learning.

There are several factors that enhance a positive learning climate for adult learners. Lighting, temperature, seating, the availability of writing surfaces furnished with paper and pencils, and the ability to view learning materials comfortably have a tremendous impact on learning (Darkenwald & Merriam, 1982). Adults appreciate physical comfort and knowing where drinks, food, and restroom facilities are located.

Adult education programs tend to be a social as well as a learning activity, since they afford opportunities to become acquainted with other adults. It is a good idea to structure break periods with refreshments to encourage socializing. Adults enjoy sharing informal learning activities with others, and successful programs encourage adults to have fun as they learn. Adults also expect teachers to value student opinions about the usefulness of learning activities. By requesting informal verbal feedback or formal written evaluations from students, instructors elicit important data to modify and improve the program.

TEACHING STRATEGIES

Good teaching involves organizing learning experiences that keep the participant's interest and use the facilitator's time efficiently. The lecture format yields an efficient use of the instructor's time; however, it requires that participants remain passive, and it is associated with decreased retention. An effective strategy is to *vary the teaching format.* Team presentations, small group discussions, demonstrations, role-playing, question-and-answer sessions with teacher-led or student-led questioning, observations and comments by participants, group projects, and individualized instruction modules are effective ways to break the monotony of lecture presentations.

Each teaching session should include an *introduction, learning experience, and conclusion/summary.* A fundamental axiom is to "explain what you're going to teach, teach, and then describe what you have taught." When using the lecture format remember to:

- use a conversational tone (avoid reading notes word for word)
- vary speech (infection, speed, and tone)
- wear bright, interesting clothing
- move around while lecturing and use gestures for emphasis
- use visual aids liberally (slides, charts, models, portions of videotapes/films)
- use humor
- demonstrate psychomotor tasks (appropriate for groups of less than 25)
- encourage the audience to participate with questions and comments
- schedule breaks every 50 minutes for maximum retention.

Charts, slides, line drawings, and role-playing are useful in dividing a psychomotor skill, such as positioning and latch-on, into understandable steps. Follow this with a video or film presentation of the skill. The facilitator must always preview audio-visual materials and be knowledgeable about equipment operation so that each learner's time is used efficiently. The three boxed checklists on the following pages offer suggestions regarding audio-visual presentations, a comparison of audio-visual formats, and development of slide presentations.

Learners retain information and psychomotor skills more effectively if they incorporate the information they have received and practice their new skills (Kozier & Erb, 1987). Return demonstrations in which learners

---

TIPS FOR A SUCCESSFUL AUDIO-VISUAL PRESENTATION

- Arrange for all necessary equipment (projectors, screens, video equipment, tape recorder, pointer, light stick, podium light, chart stands) well in advance of the presentation.
- Identify light switches and sound control panels; make certain that a responsible person is available to operate them.
- Set up and test all equipment. Have a back-up plan for all equipment. Always have spare projector bulbs.
- Adjust the volume of the public announce-

ment system so that persons in the back of the room can hear easily.
- Tape extension cords and cables to the floor to reduce the likelihood of an accident.
- Adjust the location of the slide projector so that images fill the entire screen and can be seen clearly by all participants.
- Adjust the position of the television monitor(s) so that videos can be seen by all participants.

Box continues

- Adjust the lighting in the room so that there is no glare on the screen.
- Adjust the lighting in the room to enhance the visual presentation and still allow for taking notes.
- Arrange equipment so that it does not block the view of the screen(s).
- When showing part of a video or film, preset the tape or film to the place where it is to begin.
- Meet with the equipment operator and review the audio-visual component of the presentation; explain what the operator will need to do during the presentation (e.g., change slide trays, press "play" on the video player).
- Make certain that the equipment operator is knowledgeable about general procedures and can solve common problems (e.g., adjust the focus, sound volume, release a jammed slide).
- Avoid using super-capability (140-slot) slide trays; they often jam when slides are warped or slightly frayed.
- Always screen visuals before the presentation (unmarked slides are especially prone to being placed backwards and/or upside down).
- Avoid facing the audio-visuals when speaking or standing between them and the audience. Audio-visuals which are presented effectively greatly enhance teaching. Learners are frustrated when audio-visuals are poorly presented or the instructor talks about a wonderful audio-visual that is not available. Adequate planning and preparation are the best insurance for an effective presentation.

AUDIO-VISUAL FORMATS

Slides:
- can be "worth a thousand words"
- are easily stored and transported
- are flexible; there is infinite variety in how they can be sequenced
- are relatively inexpensive
- can be operated by remote control, which enhances presentation

Transparencies:
- are easy to make and the least expensive of all the media options
- are easily damaged
- are difficult to combine with slide presentations
- may require a second person at the projector
- are limited to charts and words (photographs do not reproduce well)
- appear to be less professional than other formats

Videotape:
- is excellent for demonstrating live-action psychomotor skills (e.g., positioning mother and baby for breastfeeding)
- is easily transported and stored
- is excellent for home use and for reinforcing information
- may be expensive; equipment rental or purchase is expensive
- must be sophisticated; lesser quality video productions are rarely appreciated

16mm Film:
- has been replaced largely with video formats
- is expensive
- requires a projector which is more complicated to operate than a video machine

Slide-Tape/Sound-Filmstrip:
- has been replaced largely with video formats
- can be adapted (the slide portion) for class presentations

DEVELOPING A SLIDE PRESENTATION

Seek assistance from a professional audio-visual consultant during the early stages of presentation planning.

- Identify key concepts to be emphasized.
- Keep the content simple; one idea/per slide.
- Make sure that all lettering is large enough to be read in the back of the room.
- Insist that all lettering, artwork, and photography be of professional quality.
- Use simple graphs and drawings; avoid complicated, detailed artwork that is more suitable for print publications.

- Use multiple colors to maintain interest.
- Choose photographs that are sharp, clear, visually appealing, uncluttered, and convey a single key point.
- Limit each slide to one step of a complex task.
- Include photographs that are several feet away from the subject, within a few feet of the subject, and very close to the subject.
- Select only those photographs that illustrate the presentation; avoid using unnecessary slides.
- Remember that well-selected photographs help viewers to see how information can be used in their lives.

---

repeat the teacher's demonstration provide opportunities for reinforcing correct execution. This increases learner confidence. Clarifying suggested actions facilitates correct performance of a skill.

Evaluation of the learning experience should be a joint effort by both learner and instructor. Attainment of goals and enjoyment of the learning process are important criteria for evaluating success. Adults want recognition for their efforts and appreciate awards of completion (e.g., certificates, ceremonies, public listings). Suggestions for creating a positive climate for adult learners are summarized in the boxed list below.

CREATING A POSITIVE CLIMATE FOR ADULT LEARNERS

- Greet each person warmly; demonstrate genuine concern for each one as a unique individual.
- Use first names of participants (if appropriate).
- Assist participants in identifying their own learning needs.
- Recognize and value participants' rich experiential backgrounds.
- Arrange an attractive learning "package"; emphasize the usefulness and practical application of instructional topics.
- Provide a structural overview so that participants will know where they are in a program.
- Organize activities in increments to increase the likelihood of success.
- Give explicit instructions so that participants clearly understand what they are being asked to do.

- Provide specific, immediate feedback following each activity.
- Respect participants who do not perceive a topic as meaningful.
- Respect participants' rights not to take part in all educational activities.
- Recognize the importance of body language and nonverbal communication.
- Provide tangible rewards/recognition (e.g., certificates of completion).
- Recognize the social/recreational aspect of adult learning by providing refreshments and a relaxed atmosphere during breaks.
- Assist participants in focusing on their own activities, resourcefulness, and increased self-sufficiency.

PARENT EDUCATION

Facilitating the learning experience for parents requires an understanding of the tasks of adulthood (Darkenwald & Merriam, 1982). Families seeking breastfeeding assistance are couples involved in a major life change: the acquisition of the parental role. There are four stages of transition into parenthood: anticipatory, formal, informal, and personal (Bocar & Moore, 1987). During the *anticipatory stage,* before the birth of the infant, expectant parents benefit from realistic information about infant care. It is important for parents to understand that, in the first weeks after the baby is born, they will experience loss of sleep, fatigue, and episodes of crying (by baby, mom, and possibly dad). In this phase, parents should be encouraged to:

- form realistic expectations of infant care
- identify responsibilities they can relinquish in order to devote time and energy to infant care
- learn practical aspects of infant care (including psychomotor experiences with dolls, or infants if possible)
- begin to identify philosophical approaches to child care (such as how they will respond to a crying infant)
- learn about typical emotional responses to new parenthood so that their experiences can be placed in perspective
- review previous personal success experiences to support self-confidence
- socialize with other new families to increase opportunities for incidental learning and for developing a support network.

The *formal stage* begins with the birth of the infant. Parents are often surprised at their intense feelings about the responsibilities of parenthood. While forming attachment bonds with their infant, they are simultaneously achieving parental roles. Attachment is enhanced if parents have rooming-in privileges which enable them to get acquainted with their baby (Anderson, 1989). Health-care providers can also use the infant's given name frequently to personalize the infant.

Parental care-taking behavior is often characterized by rigidity as parents seek to perform psychomotor tasks "the one best way." They are often overwhelmed if given too many equally attractive alternatives in child care. They may become noticeably frustrated if they receive conflicting information during this phase of role acquisition. New parents often feel awkward and inadequate because they lack experience and confidence in care-taking skills. They often equate their performance of infant care with their ability to parent effectively. During this stage, new parents are extremely vulnerable to implied judgment of their care-taking abilities. They are quite sensitive to nonverbal communication regarding their performance. Health-care providers and experienced parents are particularly powerful role models as the self-image of the new parents emerges. The most persistent feelings during such role transition are those of inadequacy and lack of self-confidence (Crummette, 1975).

New parents benefit from simple, concrete instructions divided into easily mastered segments. Specific, positive feedback about their performance, coupled with an expression of confidence by someone whose opinion is important to them, can greatly enhance their self-confidence. During this time of emotional transition new parents tend to be fatigued, and feelings of being overwhelmed are common. New parents need frequent assistance in placing their experiences in perspective.

The *informal stage* begins when parents begin to feel that they have mastered child-care tasks. Coopersmith (1967) notes that self-confidence increases as a person accrues successful experiences. Several weeks or months are required by most parents to amass adequate successful experiences so that they can proceed to the informal stage of role acquisition. Health-care providers are in a unique position to enhance parental self-confidence by providing enthusiastic praise of performance and reviewing positive experiences. The relatively restrictive behavior of the formal stage is replaced by a willingness to consider options. Behavior becomes more spontaneous and there is less fear of imperfection. A reassuring environment which supports experimentation and provides stimulation through a variety of role models enables parents to progress to the final stage of parental role acquisition.

During the *personal stage* behaviors are further modified so that a parental role style evolves which is consistent with the parents' personalities. Relinquishing the fantasy of being the "perfect parent" frees parents to develop a unique set of behaviors with which they are comfortable. Support groups and classes provide ideal social settings in which parents can share their personal child-care techniques and approaches with other parents, thus integrating their new parental role into their personalities.

BREASTFEEDING EDUCATION FOR PARENTS

Because breastfeeding is considered instinctive by many mothers and health-care providers, the need for knowledge about the process often remains unrecognized. Yet, as mothers encounter difficulties and abandon breastfeeding for readily available alternatives, the need for knowledge and expert assistance becomes more obvious.

It is not enough to promote breastfeeding. Health-care providers should assist mothers to have positive breastfeeding experiences by increasing their knowledge of the practical aspects of the management of breastfeeding. Because there is a large volume of information needed by mothers who have had little or no experience with breastfeeding, it is appropriate to present content in small segments over time.

Breastfeeding education programs usually have three purposes:

- to influence or to support prenatal decision-making regarding infant feeding choice
- to provide practical information on management of lactation at the onset of the breastfeeding experience
- to provide on-going support after the initiation of breastfeeding.

THE INFANT FEEDING DECISION

Pregnancy is an appropriate time to support a mother's decision to breastfeed, to add to the information she already has about breastfeeding, and to encourage undecided expectant mothers to consider breastfeeding. Because of the influence of the mother's partner and other family members, breastfeeding education programs should speak to these support persons by encouraging their attendance at classes and group meetings and providing educational materials specifically directed to them.

Breastfeeding education programs provided early in pregnancy need to describe the benefits of breastfeeding to mothers as well as to infants

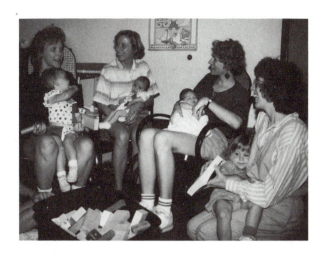

FIGURE 8–2   La Leche League meeting: adult learning in action. (Courtesy Debi Leslie Bocar.)

(Switzky, Vietz & Switzky, 1979; Newton & Newton, 1950, 1967). An awareness of the values in a particular culture is essential. For instance, the primary reason given by women for selecting breastfeeding in certain cultures is its contraceptive effect (Kocturk, 1988). In other cultures, breastfeeding is selected primarily for the protective health benefits it affords the infant (Kocturk, 1988).

Breastfeeding programs designed to influence the decision to breastfeed must address maternal concerns—including those related to convenience, modesty, participation of the father in infant care, as well as incorporation of breastfeeding into the mother's lifestyle, her return to employment, plus any previous negative experiences with breastfeeding by the mother or her peers, *and* contraceptive considerations (Grassley & Davis, 1978; Jones, 1987; Young & Kaufman, 1988).

In summary, educational programs instigated early-on in pregnancy need to provide adequate information so that expectant parents can make an informed choice regarding infant feeding. In addition, these programs should address specific maternal concerns, include support persons, and identify additional resources for information.

PRACTICAL INFORMATION FOR EARLY BREASTFEEDING

Toward the end of pregnancy, breastfeeding education appropriately focuses on the basics of breastfeeding initiation and management during the early days and weeks following the baby's birth. The site where mothers receive prenatal care is optimal for access to expectant mothers and their support persons. Classes can be offered at times convenient to these families. Pamphlets and videos can be utilized by patients while they are waiting for appointments. Health-care providers can also assess and add to the patients' knowledge during the appointment. Free-standing classes can be provided by institutions and health-care professionals in the community—hospitals, clinics, libraries, childbirth education programs, breastfeeding support groups, and lactation consultants.

The content of breastfeeding classes offered during pregnancy should include information necessary to initiate breastfeeding—e.g., timing of the first breastfeeding, positioning and assisting the infant to latch-on to the breast, prevention of nipple trauma, management of engorgement, assessment of the adequacy of milk intake, and establishing, maintaining, and increasing milk supply. See the boxed outlined below for suggested topics to cover in prenatal classes on breastfeeding. A variety of techniques can be used, including formal or informal classes, videos, and printed materials. Educational programs, however well developed, augment rather than replace the responsibility of the health-care professional for *individualized* assessment and one-on-one teaching specific to each breastfeeding family.

It is important *not* to assume that supplying information about breastfeeding management is sufficient to assure breastfeeding success. Mothers still need expert assistance during the hours and days

---

RECOMMENDED TOPICS FOR PRENATAL BREASTFEEDING CLASSES

Early Pregnancy Class

Making the feeding choice
  Importance of the decision
  Reasons mothers choose to breastfeed
    Health benefits (mother and baby)
    Closeness with baby
    Convenience
    Cost savings
  Reasons mothers choose to bottle-feed
    Return to work
    Father's involvement in feeding
    Modesty
Discuss feeding choice with baby's father, read materials, ask questions, learn about resources for assistance
Getting ready for breastfeeding
  Identify myths and discuss factual information
  Assess nipple protractility; treat flat/inverted nipples
  Avoid placing drying agents, including soap, on nipples
  Select bras/clothing
  Assist with mental preparation (reading, dialogue with partner, family members, physician, employer, care-giver)

Later Pregnancy Class

  Getting started with breastfeeding

Breastfeed soon after birth
Breastfeed every 2–3 hours
Discuss the risks of artificial feeding (occasional and exclusive)
Avoid overuse of pacifier/swaddling
Point out that keeping baby with its mother is helpful in learning to respond to baby's early cues
Assess baby's readiness to feed (rooting and mouth opening reflexes, eye contact, hand-to-mouth motions)
Provide alerting and consoling techniques
Positioning and latch-on
Prevention of nipple trauma; treatment of sore nipples
Prevention of engorgement; treatment of engorgement
Milk ejection reflex: how it works, when it works
Milk supply
  Importance of colostrum
  Principle of milk production in response to milk removal
  Relation between fullness and milk supply: when fullness is less obvious, the milk supply is not diminished
The feasibility of combining maternal employment with breastfeeding

RECOMMENDED TOPICS FOR CLASS ON BREASTFEEDING THE FIRST WEEK OF LIFE

Physiologic frequency of breastfeeding
  In response to infant's early hunger cues
  At intervals not greater than 3 hours (daytime)
  Minimum of 8 feedings/24 hours
  Avoid prolonging feeding intervals with pacifiers, complements or supplements.
  Alerting or rousing baby

Latch-on
  Positioning mother and infant
  Adequate mouth opening (avoiding inappropriate latch-on)
  Assess areolar grasp
Assessing milk intake
  Sustained suckling and swallowing
  Infant satiety cues
  Minimum of 8 feedings/24 hours
  ≥3 bowel movements/24 hours (after 5 days of life)
  ≥ 6 urinations/24 hours

Milk supply
  Adequate milk supply continues after obvious fullness subsides
  Milk supply is:
  –increased by greater frequency and duration of breastfeeding (if infant swallowing occurs)
  –enhanced by maternal rest/relaxation
  –hindered by giving complements or delaying feeding by using pacifiers

Nipple care
  Correct any trauma at latch-on
  Switch to alternate breast during feeding when swallowing ceases
  Air-dry nipples
  Avoid creams, soap, other drying agents

Breast fullness and engorgement
  Avoid long intervals (> 3 hours) between daytime feedings
  Soften areola, if necessary, to avoid traumatic latch-on
  Apply cool compresses to reduce edema

Milk ejection reflex
  Not all women perceive sensations in the first two weeks
  Evidenced by infant's sustained suckling and swallowing

Special circumstances
  Cesarean birth
  Physiologic jaundice

Returning home
  Realistic expectations in the first month (sleepy baby, abundant milk supply)
  Avoid overstimulating infant and increasing parental fatigue
  Simplify household responsibilities; accept help from family and friends
  Sibling adjustment

Maternal nutrition
  Weight loss should be gradual and steady; will occur more rapidly if the mother is breastfeeding frequently
  Nutritional requirements; fluid requirements; food myths
  Medications, caffeine, alcohol, drugs of abuse, smoking

Enjoying baby
  Basic needs include food, warmth, safety, human contact, stimulation
  Fear of spoiling vs. meeting infant's needs

When to seek assistance
  Severe nipple soreness after 7 days
  Inadequate bowel or urine output, continuous breastfeeding without infant satiety
  Mother is concerned that breastfeeding is not going well
  Identification of resources
    Someone who has had a positive breastfeeding experience
    Hotline or warmline telephone counseling
    Mother-to-mother support group
    Lactation consultant or other knowledgeable health-care worker

immediately following birth to acquire experiential skills. Dr. Audrey Naylor, Director of Wellstart in San Diego, California, says, "Successful breastfeeding requires more than words of encouragement. It requires a continuum of skilled services designed to enhance the synchronous breastfeeding duet learned by the mother-infant couple" (Riordan, 1983).

While mothers can have a very positive breastfeeding experience within the birth setting with the assistance of knowledgeable and enthusiastic health-care providers, breastfeeding duration is strongly influenced by situations that the mother encounters after she returns home.

Anticipatory guidance can be provided in the hospital or birth setting through education programs. Given the mother's limited stamina and inability to retain large quantities of new information, care should be taken not to overwhelm families with the sheer volume of material. Prioritize the content of classes in the birth setting—from most important to least important. For example, information that relates to continuing breastfeeding and insuring infant well-being is "most important," while information that pertains to returning to employment and weaning can be covered at a later time.

When special circumstances such as prematurity, multiple births, congenital anomalies, or infant neurologic impairment affect the initiation of breastfeeding, the learning needs of the parents are complicated by the emotional ramifications of the experience. Families with special needs benefit from individualized teaching and assistance, as well as educational materials and on-going group support specific to their needs.

CONTINUING SUPPORT
FOR BREASTFEEDING FAMILIES

The sharp decline in breastfeeding in the early weeks postpartum (Bloom et al., 1982; Yeung et al., 1981) demonstrates the need mothers have for assistance and follow-up. A systematic program to assure contact with the new breastfeeding mother can be a powerful influence on breastfeeding duration. Where feasible, telephone contact is ideal. Home visits or early return visits to a clinic are also helpful. Each mother should be able to identify at least one resource for information, support, and assistance. The breastfeeding mother needs information about:

- assessing and managing her milk supply
- preventing and healing sore nipples
- correcting the source of nipple trauma
- managing engorgement
- consoling the infant
- determining proper maternal nutrition
- incorporating the infant and breastfeeding into the family lifestyle
- managing plugged ducts and/or mastitis if they occur
- breastfeeding through maternal or infant illness
- continuing breastfeeding after returning to work
- expressing and storing breastmilk
- noting normal infant developmental milestones (such as teething) and assessing their effect on breastfeeding
- weaning techniques and weanling foods.

In addition to information and assistance with solving breastfeeding challenges, mothers need support and encouragement to continue breastfeeding. Family, peers, and community resources should be her primary sources of support. However, health-care professionals have a role to play in assessing and augmenting or creating support systems.

Fathers are often the most influential support persons in the early breastfeeding period (Beske & Garvis, 1982; Auerbach, 1984). Fathers benefit from suggestions of specific ways by which they can support their partners. They can help the mother achieve a comfortable breastfeeding position; provide nutritional support and household assistance; burp and console the infant; monitor the mother's fatigue level; limit visitors; and show delight in the decision to breastfeed.

As breastfeeding continues, the baby is a powerful source of positive feedback for the mother (Beske & Garvis, 1982). The baby who thrives on mother's milk, and who is healthy and contented, is obvious validation of the unique nourishment the mother provides.

However, even the evidence of a healthy infant and the encouragement of health-care providers may be insufficient to overcome lack of support among peers and the community. In industrialized cultures in particular, where artificial feeding has been the cultural norm for some time, breastfeeding support may be inversely related to the age of the infant. Assisting mothers to become a part of formal or informal support systems, or even creating an on-going support system, is an appropriate focus for the health-care professional who wishes to encourage continued breastfeeding. Ideally, mothers are able to iden-

---

RECOMMENDED TOPICS FOR AN ON-GOING BREASTFEEDING SUPPORT CLASS

- Milk supply concerns
  Assessing adequacy of infant's intake; appetite spurts; increasing milk supply
- Infant weight gain: expected gain and normal variations
- Father's special contributions
  Support for mother; relationship with baby
- Nighttime needs of infants and parents
  Realistic expectations; minimizing sleep disruption
- Parenting
  Comforting babies; infant developmental milestones; mother-baby separation; sibling adjustment; role of grandparents and other relatives
- Sexuality
  Fatigue; spontaneity; sexual and nutritional functions; milk leaking; episiotomy and/or cesarean incision healing; vaginal lubrication; lactational amenorrhea and contraception
- Maternal nutrition
- Obstructed ducts and mastitis
  Prevention; signs, symptoms, and treatment
- Thrush
- Employed breastfeeding mothers
  Feasibility of combining breastfeeding and employment; feeding options; negotiating with employer; dealing with co-workers; child care; managing time; expressing and storing breastmilk; methods of giving breastmilk to infant; maintaining and increasing milk supply
- Starting weaning foods
  American Academy of Pediatrics recommendations
- Weaning
  When and how; extended breastfeeding
- Keeping breastfeeding in perspective

---

tify at least one mother they know who enjoyed breastfeeding and can give them practical assistance.

EFFECTIVENESS OF BREASTFEEDING EDUCATION

Breastfeeding education programs are prominent strategies to promote breastfeeding initiation and duration. However, education programs cannot be considered a panacea. Research shows that some education programs have little or no influence on initiation and duration of breastfeeding.

The money available for education programs is often limited, as is staff availability and access to patients. Therefore, it is appropriate to scrutinize the effectiveness of breastfeeding education programs in order to utilize limited resources productively.

Breastfeeding initiation. Some studies indicate that professionals have little influence on the feeding decisions made by expectant mothers (Aberman & Kirchhoff, 1985; Auerbach, 1984; Baranowski et al., 1983; Beske & Garvis, 1982; Bryant, 1982; Gulick, 1982; Lawrence, 1984; Sullivan & Jones, 1986). More influential are the baby's father, peers, and the maternal grandmother (Aberman & Kirchhoff, 1985;

Baranowski et al., 1983; Beske & Garvis, 1982; Bryant, 1982; Sullivan & Jones, 1986).

The influence of health-care professionals may be minimized by the timing of their contact with expectant parents, which usually occurs only during pregnancy. How the mother will feed her baby is a decision that often is made prior to conception (Birenbaum, Fuchs & Reichman, 1989; Ekwo & Olson, 1983; Kaplowitz & Olson, 1983) or very early in pregnancy (Beske & Garvis, 1982). Therefore, educational efforts may need to target future parents prior to conception, through elementary and secondary school systems, the mass media, churches, community organizations, and other influential institutions.

A striking finding of one study was that information from books and pamphlets provided the greatest influence on feeding choice (Beske & Garvis, 1982). The implications of this are particularly important when one considers the inaccuracies in printed materials and the fact that many are designed to promote breastmilk substitutes.

The reported minimal influence of health-care providers on breastfeeding decisions also may reflect the fact that in many cases infant feeding is not discussed with patients. Health-care providers may be reluctant to encourage breastfeeding for fear of contributing to feelings of guilt a mother may experience if she chooses not to breastfeed. However, such concerns do not negate the responsibility to provide families with accurate and complete information so they can make an informed choice. Ethical questions arise when information is withheld from clients. In addition, mothers who choose not to breastfeed do not necessarily experience guilt about their choice, as documented by Brown et al. (1960).

Health-care professionals have a responsibility to provide accurate information and to *actively* encourage the decision to breastfeed, just as they encourage other health-optimizing choices—such as early prenatal care, appropriate nutrition, use of car restraint systems, immunizations, and avoidance of smoking, alcohol, and drugs of abuse. A *neutral* attitude toward feeding choice is inappropriate, as it implies an equivalence of breastmilk and its substitutes. It also communicates to mothers that their efforts to breastfeed are unimportant.

In a study described by Collins et al. (1984), participants in a WIC program were no more likely to select breastfeeding than those not enrolled in the program. WIC participants were more likely to describe formula as "just as good" as breastmilk. Conversely, Young and Kaufman (1988) reported an increase in breastfeeding initiation among a low-income group of expectant mothers who attended prenatal education classes. Education programs have been shown to be effective in increasing parental knowledge, but not necessarily in influencing attitudes about breastfeeding (Kaplowitz & Olson, 1983; Kistin et al., 1990).

Breastfeeding duration. Various studies support the effectiveness of breastfeeding education, expert assistance in the birth setting, and/or postpartum support in increasing breastfeeding duration

(Wiles, 1984; Hall, 1978; Whitley, 1978; Ladas, 1972; Cohen, 1980; Young & Kaufman, 1988; Palti et al., 1988). However, other studies demonstrate their lack of effectiveness (Hewat & Ellis, 1986). In a study reported by Wiles (1984), primiparous women who received prenatal breastfeeding education reported a significantly higher frequency of success in breastfeeding at one month postpartum than did primiparous women who did not receive prenatal education. Auerbach (1985) found that breastfeeding duration was increased when WIC staff were educated in breastfeeding management and when a lactation consultant saw mothers at least once. Telephone or home follow-up visits also have been reported to increase breastfeeding duration (Houston & Howie, 1981).

Hewat and Ellis (1986) suggest that mothers benefit from realistic guidance about breastfeeding, and not just information that stresses its positive aspects. They identify variables which influence the initiation and maintenance of breastfeeding. These include the mother's priorities related to beliefs, values, and goals; the congruence of her expectations to actual experiences; her physical recovery; her interpretation of infant behavior; the type of support she receives; and infant characteristics such as feeding frequency, temperament, and physical attributes.

Various programs have been designed to promote the decision to breastfeed and to influence its duration. Components and the effectiveness of these programs are summarized in Table 8–1.

Education programs may play an important role in influencing breastfeeding experiences, but they are only one part of a larger milieu. More research is needed to identify which characteristics of an education program are most effective. These may vary in different cultures and among individuals. The following five-point checklist summarizes principles that may be applicable in a variety of settings.

FIVE PRINCIPLES OF BREASTFEEDING EDUCATION PROGRAMS

1. Content and timing of teaching coincides with parents' readiness to learn (prior to conception, during pregnancy, immediately postbirth, later postpartum).
2. Information is prioritized and presented in easily understood and easily mastered segments.
3. Anticipatory guidance is practical and realistic.
4. Printed material and other media reinforce and augment rather than replace individualized assessment and teaching.
5. Breastfeeding support resources are identified.

TABLE 8-1   EFFECTIVENESS OF BREASTFEEDING EDUCATION PROGRAMS

Author/Year	Interventions	Effectiveness
Breastfeeding Initiation		
Birenbaum, Fuchs & Reichman, 1989	Prenatal breastfeeding class	Not increased
Brimblecome & Cullen, 1977	Education of midwives and health visitors	Increased
Collins et al., 1984	Enrollment in WIC program	Not increased
Young & Kaufman, 1988	Prenatal breastfeeding class	Increased
Palti et al., 1988	Prenatal breastfeeding information, nipple assessment and treatment of retracted nipples, postpartum follow-up	Increased
Sloper et al., 1975	Education of maternity nursing staff, discontinuation of routine complementary feeds	Increased
Breastfeeding Duration		
Auerbach, 1985	Prenatal contact with lactation consultant	Increased
Cohen, 1980	Postpartum teaching	Increased
De Chateau et al., 1977	Education of fathers	Increased
Ellis & Hewat, 1984	In-hospital breastfeeding class, in-hospital support from an expert clinician	Not increased
Hall, 1978	Slide-tape presentation, pamphlet	Not increased
Hall, 1978	Slide-tape presentation, pamphlet, nursing staff support, telephone follow-up	Increased
Houston & Howie, 1981	Telephone follow-up, home visits	Increased
Palti et al., 1988	Prenatal breastfeeding information, nipple assessment and treatment of retracted nipples, postpartum follow-up	Increased
Whitley, 1978	Prenatal breastfeeding class	Increased
Wiles, 1984	Prenatal breastfeeding class	Increased
Young & Kaufman, 1988	Prenatal breastfeeding class	Increased

METHODS AND TECHNIQUES

THERAPEUTIC COMMUNICATION

Communication is a process whereby we transmit information, thoughts, ideas, and feelings. It is often categorized into two types: verbal (spoken or written) and nonverbal. Although both types of communication may occur concurrently, experts estimate that between 65% (Haber & Hoskins, 1987) and 90% (Kozier & Erb, 1987) of messages received are nonverbal.

Nonverbal communications not only portray a persons's feelings, they indicate how people are *coping* with their feelings (Bolton, 1979). Many psychologists believe that "how" words are spoken—i.e., the rate of speech, tone of voice, pitch, inflection, volume, rhythm, pauses and silence—conveys more reliable information than actual words. Nonlanguage vocalizations such as sighing, gasping, sobbing, moaning, grunting, and laughing also communicate significant messages.

Body motion and posture along with facial expressions are important sources of nonverbal messages (Haber & Hoskins, 1987) and communicate self-image, mood, and state of health. The face not only discloses specific emotions, its intensity can telegraph the importance of a topic. Eye contact can communicate the amount of trust and acceptance between people and the level of interest and involvement. In Western societies, direct eye contact usually communicates a high level of interest and implies positive regard for another person. Mutual eye contact conveys a willingness to maintain communication. Eye contact is often averted or avoided when a person feels weak, defenseless, or embarrassed (Kozier & Erb, 1987). Hand movement and gestures convey messages such as anxiety, impatience, avoidance, indifference, relaxation, and confidence (Scheflen & Scheflen, 1972).

Phases of interaction are punctuated with body movements. Initially, participants in a class may keep some physical distance. As the working phase begins, they move more loosely and even lean toward each other. Empathy and understanding are conveyed by mirroring another person's posture and/or body position. Desire to terminate an interaction is indicated by stretching, averting eye contact, straightening papers, closing a briefcase, or standing in preparation for leaving (Bolton, 1979).

Touch is another powerful way we communicate. A hand placed on the shoulder conveys compassion and support. In Western cultures, touch validates the spoken message. As with all nonverbal communication, it must be used with sensitivity, always considering how it can affect individuals, always using it within a cultural context. Appearance, including physical characteristics and manner of dress, acts as a nonverbal message which confirms or contradicts verbal messages. Choice of clothing, adornments, and grooming practices are highly personal and convey social and financial status, religion, and group association.

Core dimensions of facilitative communication include empathy, unconditional acceptance, respect, genuineness, concreteness, and immediacy (Haber & Hoskins, 1987). *Empathy* indicates interest and a sense of caring when the care-giver attempts to understand the other person's feelings and perceptions of reality. *Unconditional acceptance* is demonstrated when the person is regarded as a unique and valued individual. *Respect* conveys a belief in the person's ability to solve problems and to assume responsibility. *Genuineness* is the ability to be honest and authentic with another person. *Concreteness* is being specific, succinct, and clear when communicating. *Immediacy* is focusing in the present and relating both the past and the future to current concerns.

There are two types of therapeutic communication skills: attending skills and responding skills. *Attending skills* include active listening which uses all of the senses. Therapeutic listening is an active process that requires energy and concentration. Egan (1982) has outlined five ways to convey physical attending skills:

- face the other person squarely
- maintain comfortable eye contact
- lean toward the other person to convey interest and involvement
- maintain an open posture in which neither arms nor legs are crossed
- remain relatively relaxed.

Sitting with a family, rather than standing above one or more of its members, decreases feelings of condescension. People often perceive that more time is spent with them when the health-care provider sits rather than stands. Focusing complete attention on the speaker and identifying themes and patterns in the family's message provides the basis for responding effectively.

Responding skills include:

- reflecting, restating, and paraphrasing
- clarifying and validating
- asking open–ended questions
- focusing
- stating observations and sharing interpretations
- identifying strengths and building hope
- summarizing

Reflecting, restating, and paraphrasing help the listener to convey understanding of the initial message. Reflecting the feelings implied in a message helps families identify underlying themes in the primary message. Clarifying identifies areas of confusion and enables the listener to request more information. Validating confirms that the restated message is what the person meant to communicate.

Questions or statements that are *open-ended* often yield significant information by encouraging parents to express themselves fully. Open-ended questions typically start with "how" or "tell me about." For example, if a mother is asked *where* she is having breast tenderness, the answer will probably relate only to the site. But if she is asked to tell you *about* the tenderness, you may be given information about its location, intensity, and duration. As more specific information is needed, questions begin with "who," "what," "when," "where," "how much" and "how often." *Close-ended* questions usually start with "are," "is," "do," and "does." Such questions can also be answered with a "yes" or "no" and yield the least amount of information. For example, "Is your breast tender?" (Lauwers & Woessner, 1989).

Asking too many questions in sequence or in an interrogating manner (such as "why" questions) is threatening. Balancing questioning with other therapeutic skills promotes the family's problem-solving abilities by involving the family in clarifying the problem, generating resolution strategies, and evaluating the outcome. Focusing keeps the communication goal-directed, specific, and concrete. Focusing on central issues and returning to the main topic keeps the interaction purposeful rather than rambling.

Stating observations and sharing interpretations provides constructive feedback to families about how their messages are perceived. Identifying strengths helps families focus on their positive qualities. Indicating that a family's specific concerns are common experiences helps place the concern in perspective and builds hope that there is a solution. It is extremely important not to discount or trivialize a family's concerns in an attempt to decrease their anxiety. Personal concerns are valid and must be treated with respect. The intent is to offer empathy, genuine concern, and assistance in problem solving.

Summarizing unifies pieces of information into themes of content and feeling. By highlighting the most significant information they have shared, families are more easily able to participate in the problem-solving process.

Barriers to effective communication include changing topics abruptly; moralizing or being judgmental; criticizing; quickly giving rigid directions or orders (rather than developing a plan with suggestions and recommendations); questioning excessively; offering trite expressions and meaningless cliches; and giving glib or unwarranted reassurance.

SMALL GROUP DYNAMICS

Formal classes and various educational media have the potential for providing information to large numbers of people. However, there are valuable benefits to participation in small groups, whether for education, support, or a combination of the two.

Tubbs (1984) defines a group as two or more people who interact and influence each other, accomplish common goals, and derive satisfaction from maintaining membership in the group. The ideal group size ranges from 2–15 people, with the best outcome resulting in groups with 8–12 members. After a review of the literature, Tubbs (1984) concluded that subgroups with 7–10 group members are optimal; more than 10 people in a subgroup decreases productivity.

Small groups have the advantage of many opportunities for interaction among group members. This allows a free flow of information and encouragement among participants' as different questions are asked and new topics are raised. Such groups may meet the individual's need for companionship, knowledge, and identity. Discussion in a small group is more likely to meet participants' needs since they usually feel more comfortable asking questions and changing the topic than when they are in a large group. The group setting can be a powerful agent for behavior change. Additionally, group discussions enhance peer support, decision-making, and decrease dependence on health-care professionals (Ross, 1982).

An informal, relaxed setting encourages participation. The group leader is responsible for ensuring that needed content is presented within an accepting, flexible framework. She needs to be expert in the subject content area and skilled in group dynamics. Familiarity with the different roles played by group members (initiator, elaborator, evaluator, coordinator, encourager, harmonizer, compromiser, aggressor, recognition-seeker, confessor, dominator) enhances the group leader's effectiveness in moving the group in a fruitful direction (Sampson & Marthas, 1981).

While the group may have to actively guide the discussion initially, the goal is to act as a resource for information, encouraging participants to develop their own creative and problem-solving abilities (Nichols & Edwards, 1988). When participants share their personal experiences, it enhances learning and increases self-worth as individuals' efforts are reinforced and supported by the group.

A variety of techniques can be used by a group leader/facilitator to enhance the group process. These include the following: support, confrontation, advice and suggestions, summarizing, clarifying, probing and questioning, repeating, paraphrasing, highlighting, reflecting, interpretation and analysis, and listening (Sampson & Marthas, 1981). Concrete examples of communication techniques, which were recorded at a La Leche League meeting, are listed in Table 8–2.

TABLE 8–2 COMMUNICATION TECHNIQUES

Positive communication	Example
1. Accepting	"I can understand the way you feel . . ."
2. Giving recognition	"You really tried, didn't you?"
3. Offering self	Introductions by each woman and telling about personal experience.
4. Giving broad openings	"Is there something we haven't mentioned that you'd like to discuss?"
5. Making observations	"She sure seems to be healthy despite her problems . . ."
6. Encouraging descriptions and perceptions	"Didn't you have some of the same experiences she had?"
7. Encouraging comparison	"Was this something like . . ."
8. Reflecting feelings	"It bothers you then, to nurse when your relatives are around?"
9. Focusing and relating	"You seem to be tuned in to this already . . ."
10. Giving information	Numerous nutritional tips and information given.
11. Seeking clarification	"Do you mean you like using the blender better than the grinder?"
12. Summarizing and encouraging evaluation	"When I feed my family better, they don't seem to have as many colds . . . Does anyone else feel this way?"

From Riordan, J: *A Practical Guide to Breastfeeding,* St. Louis, 1983, The C.V. Mosby Co., p. 106.

EDUCATIONAL MATERIALS

Written materials and audio-visual materials can be invaluable aids in reinforcing teaching content. One study indicates that adult learners retain only about 30% of the information they hear. A multimodal approach (seeing and hearing) increases retention to 50% (Becton & Dickenson, 1981). However, learning retention is always shorter under stress. After the physical and emotional stress of childbirth, families benefit from educational materials that reinforce verbal teaching. Written educational materials should only be used to *reinforce* teaching and cannot effectively *replace* individualized teaching.

Materials must be scrutinized closely for their accuracy to determine that no outdated information is included. Information must be consistent. New parents are frustrated by conflicting recommendations. Since nonverbal messages have a more profound impact on behavior than verbal instructions (Pease, 1984), materials must be carefully evaluated for correctness of maternal-infant positioning and latch-on (Shrago & Bocar, 1990). Discrete breastfeeding should be modeled in cultures where public exposure of the breasts is discouraged or considered taboo.

Educational materials aimed at promoting breastfeeding should include practical tips for successful breastfeeding as well as resources for additional information. It is a disservice to enthusiastically expound the benefits of breastfeeding without providing practical assistance to help families meet their breastfeeding goals.

Materials should be attractively packaged. Families from a variety of socioeconomic backgrounds have access to sophisticated printed materials and commercial television programs; they expect similar quality in materials about breastfeeding. Pamphlets must be inviting, easy to read, and organized for scanning (with bold headings and generous amounts of white space). Too many words on a page can overwhelm a reader. Pictorial learning is superior to verbal learning for recognition and recall (Redman, 1988). Pictures and drawings make materials more interesting. Riordan (1985) identifies readability, relevancy, and reliability as important components when evaluating breastfeeding literature.

More materials are not always better. If families are bombarded with thick stacks of pamphlets and materials, the likelihood of their use is decreased. A few carefully selected pamphlets can convey the idea that breastfeeding is uncomplicated and enjoyable.

Pamphlets and short audio-visual programs are preferable to lengthy materials that attempt to cover the gamut of breastfeeding experiences. Brief, focused materials should address the issues the family perceives as meaningful and which they are motivated to learn. This concept applies especially to families in special circumstances (such as prematurity, birth anomalies, and relactation). Books that are divided into small segments and have detailed indexes help families locate needed information.

The source of materials must be considered in evaluating educational materials. Organizations whose purpose is to promote human milk substitutes cannot be expected to genuinely promote breastfeeding. Underlying messages may communicate that bottle-feeding is the cultural norm and that breastfeeding is difficult, complicated, uncomfortable, immodest, and inconvenient. There is often an explicit message that *when* families begin using formula, the product of that company is optimal. Auerbach identifies techniques sometimes used in written materials which may leave a negative impression about breastfeeding (Auerbach, 1988).

In 1981, the World Health Organization adopted the International Code of Marketing of Breast Milk Substitutes (WHO 34.22, 1981), often referred to as the WHO Code. The Code was designed to apply to all countries and restricts advertising and promotion of products through health-care facilities. No words or pictures idealizing artificial feeding should be included in materials given to childbearing families. Most health-care facilities in the United States do not comply with the WHO Code. Individual health-care providers can make a personal commitment to abide by the Code provisions by not providing materials produced by infant formula companies. The WHO Code provisions are given in Chapter 1.

Giving families material that contains incorrect and/or misleading information, conflicting messages, and subtle themes that undermine breastfeeding may be more detrimental than giving them no such written material. Riordan notes in her review of breastfeeding pamphlets that the price of some "free" pamphlets is one's credibility (Riordan, 1985).

The target audience should be considered when evaluating educational materials. Materials must be written at a reading level the reader can understand— all too often, they are written at too high a level. The FOG index is a useful tool in assessing reading levels (Gunning, 1968). There are also computer software programs that determine reading levels.* Visual materials are more effective if they depict families with ethnic, socioeconomic, and/or cultural backgrounds

that are similar to the target audience. For example, teen-age mothers respond most favorably to visuals of adolescent mothers.

Lactation consultants review current educational materials relating to breastfeeding in each issue of the *Journal of Human Lactation,* the official journal of the International Lactation Consultant Association. The reviews provide valuable information for screening materials for their appropriateness in specific settings. Supplements to the *Journal of Human Lactation* have compiled reviews of breastfeeding books and films (Flashner, 1988, 1989).

Excellent breastfeeding education materials are available from a variety of companies. A list of resources for ordering materials about breastfeeding is provided in Appendix 8–1 at the end of this chapter. The following outline summarizes criteria for evaluating educational materials.

ADAPTING EDUCATION MATERIALS FOR SPECIAL GROUPS

In the United States, women who have low incomes, who are poorly educated, or who are members of particular ethnic groups initiate and sustain breastfeeding at rates less than one-half of those prevailing nationally (Hendershot, 1980, 1984; Leeper, Milo & Collins, 1983; Rassin et al., 1984; Biegelson, Cowell & Goldberg, 1986; Forman et al., 1985; Hirschman & Butler, 1981; Martinez & Dodd, 1983; Smith et al., 1982). Although poverty and ethnic values play a role in breastfeeding, research indicates that *maternal educational level* is the most consistent predictor of both incidence and duration of breastfeeding. Through its predictive power, education is a potentially potent force influencing breastfeeding initiation, duration, the quality of the experience, and the infant's health (Hanson & Bergstrom, 1990).

In the United States, poorly educated mothers are likely to be economically disadvantaged; yet they have breastfeeding concerns similar to those of more affluent mothers: modesty, partner participation, lifestyle changes, contraception, and fear of difficulty or pain. In addition, they are influenced by the relative absence of peer models and social support. Women with minimal education may lack self-confidence, control over their lives, and assertiveness skills that are likely to enhance their success at breastfeeding.

If the teacher or leader of a breastfeeding class is

Readability Estimation (BertaMax Software Co.; Cost: $50)

CRITERIA FOR EVALUATING EDUCATIONAL MATERIALS

Content

- Accurate, reliable information based on valid research reports?
- Accepted principles of anatomy and physiology?
- Up-to-date recommendations?
- Consistency between narrative and visuals?
- Simple, uncomplicated approach?
- Relevant to a family's learning needs?

Presentation

- Attractive, inviting?
- Appropriate reading level?
- Organized for easy scanning—bold headings, short paragraphs, ample amounts of white space?
- Generous use of appropriate pictures, drawings, and graphs that are consistent with the narrative?
- Visuals depict families from similar backgrounds of audience?
  - Peer age
  - Socioeconomic status
  - Cultural and ethnic representation
- Appropriate length?
  - Short video segments, pamphlets address specific concerns

  - More complete resource with distinct subtopics, indexed for easy use

Promotional Materials

- Enthusiastically discusses benefits of breastfeeding?
- Includes risks of bottle-feeding?
- Culturally appropriate breastfeeding is modelled?
- Includes practical tips for successful breastfeeding?
- Provides information for additional resources?

Source of Materials

- Carefully scrutinized for underlying messages?
- Is breastfeeding presented as complicated, uncomfortable, immodest, inconvenient?
- Have materials from companies that produce human milk substitutes been assessed carefully for their hidden messages?
- Breastfeeding is not subtly undermined?
- Formula products are not promoted?
- Meets with compliance of WHO Code, which precludes health-care providers from distributing materials provided by formula companies?

from a different socioeconomic and/or ethnic group than the mothers she is teaching, she may have a difficult time being accepted as a peer in whom the mothers can confide and trust. An example is a white, highly educated, articulate, and well-dressed woman leading an inner-city group of black or Hispanic mothers in a WIC program. A group leader or class instructor should be cognizant of dress and vocabulary differences to prevent these issues from becoming barriers to acceptance. Trained peer counselors, such as those associated with La Leche League International, or graduates of the Cook County, Illinois, Hospital Peer Counseling Program, are one solution to this potential problem.

It is imperative that the educator understand cultural variations (Taylor, 1985), which can include elaborate food proscriptions, sexual restrictions,

and acceptable intervals for breastfeeding. Consulting the literature, keen observation of nonverbal communication, questioning knowledgeable people within the culture or subculture, and an open, accepting attitude can help the nurse or LC to work effectively within various cultural contexts. Printed materials and audio-visual resources need to portray members of the population served, address concerns unique to that group, and be written at an appropriate literacy level (Doak, Doak & Root, 1985).

Adolescents' concerns regarding breastfeeding are influenced by their developmental stage (Yoos, 1985). The primary focus of the young adolescent is the self. Self-consciousness and modesty may be so pronounced that the young mother may be reluctant to consider breastfeeding. Typical concerns of North

American adolescent mothers include issues of modesty, sexuality, mobility, lifestyle, peer approval, the wish to return to school, and the attitude of the baby's father. In some cases, peer role models exert a strong influence in favor of breastfeeding (Radius & Joffe, 1988). Adolescents are typically interested in having new experiences; some teen-age mothers show interest in breastfeeding because they do not want to miss the "novel" experience of breastfeeding.

Parents who have delayed childbearing, whether by choice or as a result of infertility, have unique concerns. Incorporating an infant and breastfeeding into their established lifestyles is not easy, and they may require frequent reassurance. On the positive side, older parents have the advantages of varied life experiences, and perhaps wisdom and patience which enhance parenting skills. They may need assistance to locate peers with whom they can relate. The older mother may need reassurance that the ability to breastfeed does not decrease with increasing maternal age.

THE TEAM APPROACH

A team approach to breastfeeding education enhances the learning experiences of childbearing families. Health-care providers cannot simply promote breastfeeding; they must provide specific information to enhance breastfeeding success. It is crucial that each team member presents consistent information. Acquisition of the parental role is enhanced when new parents are given specific, concrete recommendations (Bocar & Moore, 1987). Conflicting information frustrates the patient and erodes new parents' trust in the health-care system.

The health-care team is responsible for a comprehensive approach. The fragmented care that often typifies women's health care today is not conducive to effective breastfeeding education. Families need a thorough understanding of the dynamics of breastfeeding. Consistent information shared by a variety of providers on multiple occasions strengthens the impact of each breastfeeding education encounter. Each family has varying breastfeeding goals. Health-care providers can assist families to meet *their* goals based on informed decisions.

Each member of the team must be aware of the content discussed by other members to avoid unintentional contradiction. Documenting what has been discussed with teaching checklists and care plans allows the educator to build on that foundation and to reinforce key points. Networking among local and regional colleagues provides many opportunities to improve educational programs and to avoid the omission of key topics. Each health-care provider develops a unique relationship with a breastfeeding family and can make unique contributions to the family's education.

Perinatal nurses. Perinatal nurses possess minimum competencies related to breastfeeding education and provide breastfeeding education along with many other types of health education. Perinatal nurses usually provide assistance with early breastfeeding. Nurses may be certified as breastfeeding educators, lactation educators, lactation counselors, or possess other titles that indicate their completion of a study of breastfeeding basics.\

Dieticians. Dieticians' responsibilities include nutritional counseling for childbearing families. They can describe the influence of breastfeeding on maternal and infant nutrition needs. Many dieticians working with breastfeeding families are employed by WIC programs and other community health settings.

Childbirth educators. Childbirth educators develop rapport with breastfeeding families during their multi-session childbirth classes. They provide invaluable anticipatory guidance by including

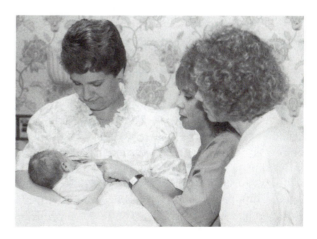

FIGURE 8–3 Perinatal nurse learning new skills from lactation consultant. (Courtesy Debi Leslie Bocar.)

breastfeeding information in general childbirth education programs. Following childbirth, families frequently seek breastfeeding assistance from the childbirth instructors with whom they already have rapport.

Lactation consultants. Lactation consultants are health-care providers whose primary focus is providing breastfeeding assistance. Lactation consultants provide a variety of specialized services—including individual consultations for unusual breastfeeding situations; care plans developed in collaboration with other health-care providers; breastfeeding class sessions; and instruction in the use of specific breastfeeding products. They also serve as a resource for information and data, develop special programs or projects related to breastfeeding, and conduct research. (See Chapter 20 on work strategies.)

LLLI leaders and support groups. Mother-to-mother support groups create an invaluable social support network for breastfeeding families. Practical tips and much incidental learning about parenting are derived from these important support groups. The largest and most effective self-care group for breastfeeding support is La Leche League International (LLLI). Founded in 1956, LLLI's core service is mother-to-mother support and information provided through small neighborhood-based groups. Topics of monthly group meetings include: (1) the advantages of breastfeeding to mother and baby; (2) the arrival of the baby; (3) the art of breastfeeding and overcoming difficulties; and (4) nutrition and weaning.

Leaders are available between meetings for individual assistance and problem solving. The relaxed, friendly interchange between women with common interests in breastfeeding, childbearing, and childrearing is a basic strength of this highly successful organization. The organization is effective in meeting the educational and support needs of middle-class women in 46 countries. More than 9,000 volunteer leaders are estimated to serve over 100,000 families in the United States each year.

LLLI's Peer Counseling Program was developed in 1986 to meet the needs of socioeconomically disadvantaged families in the United States. The program educates mothers from low-income areas and provides accurate information and assistance to their peers. Some childbirth education groups in the United States have developed additional mother-to-mother breastfeeding support groups. There are also peer support groups in many other countries. See Appendix G at the end of the book for a listing of these organizations.

Physicians. Physicians can serve as powerful breastfeeding promoters. Their support of breastfeeding can be a potent force in a family's decision to begin and continue breastfeeding (Graffy, 1992). Physicians often refer families to lactation consultants for time-intensive treatment of breastfeeding difficulties or follow-up.

HEALTH-CARE PROVIDER EDUCATION

Most educational programs in medicine, nursing, and nutrition prepare students to be generalists (Crowder, 1981; Hayes, 1981). Additional study and clinical experience are necessary to develop expertise in the specific field of lactation. Recognition of the need for additional education is demonstrated by the emergence of programs that prepare practitioners to assist breastfeeding families.

It is necessary to distinguish between programs that prepare participants to be peer counselors, breastfeeding educators, and lactation consultants. In all categories, there is a wide range of knowledge and expertise. In general, peer counselors and breastfeeding educators are prepared to provide education and assistance relating to the management of normal lactation. They are also prepared to identify and refer more complicated breastfeeding situations. Lactation consultants have more extensive education in lactation and are prepared to assist breastfeeding families in complex situations. Various programs are available to prepare practitioners in the area of lactation management. Table 8–3 summarizes lactation education programs in the United States.* Addresses of these programs can be found in Appendix 8–1 at the end of this chapter.

*Curriculum outlines for basic educational programs for breastfeeding educators and lactation consultants are available from La Leche League International, Illinois; Lactation Consultant Services, Oklahoma; The Lactation Institute, California; Breastfeeding Support Consultants, Pennsylvania; and UCLA Extension, Department of Health Sciences, California. (See Appendix 8–1 for addresses.)

TABLE 8–3 LACTATION EDUCATION PROGRAMS IN THE UNITED STATES

Program	Target students	Prerequisites	Practice goal	Approximate cost and length of program
La Leche League Leader; LLLI	Breastfeeding mothers	Breastfed at least one infant; natural weaning; supports LLLI philosophy	Mother-to-mother support; provision of current information	One year; $60 + texts
Peer Counselor; LLLI	Breastfeeding mothers	Breastfed at least one infant	Breastfeeding assistance and support to minority, low-income or other communities with low incidence of breastfeeding	One year; $170–$450
Certified Breastfeeding Educator; Lactation Consultant Services	Nurses, nutritionists, childbirth educators	None	Assist breastfeeding mothers in normal situations	12 hours of lectures; role-play; discussion; written exam; $200–$250
Lactation Educator Training Program; UCLA Extension, Dept. of Health Science Division of Nursing	Practicing, certified professionals in MCH field	License to practice	Assist breastfeeding families in private practice or institutional clinical setting	10 weeks of lectures or 5-day intensive program; clinical and written components, $725
Lactation Consultant Program; UCLA Extension Dept. of Health Science Division of Nursing	Nurses and nutritionists	Must be licensed health-care worker	Assist families in normal and complex breastfeeding situations	10-week lecture program plus 9 months of supervised clinical work; $1,600
Certified Lactation Specialist; The Lactation Institute and Pacific Oaks College	Professional and non-professional practioners in lactation	For B.A.: 60 units lower division college course work; for M.A.: bachelor's degree	Assist mothers with complicated breastfeeding problems; teach professionals	B.A. or M.A. degree: 38–40 units + 900 clinical hours + research; $12,000
Certified Lactation Educator; The Lactation Institute and Pacific Oaks College	Professional and non-professional practitioners in lactation	None	Teach breastfeeding education classes to parents; assist breastfeeding mothers with basic breastfeeding management	30 hours of lectures; 15 hours of clinical work; $600
Wellstart; Lactation Management Education Program	Pediatricians, obstetricians, perinatal nurses	None	Trains mostly non-U.S. health-care professionals; modify hospital practices; solve local infant nutrition problems; develop promotional campaigns	Domestic Course Work: 14 days, International Course Work: 1 month
Lactation Program Women's and Children's Services, Presbyterian/St. Luke's Medical Center Denver, Colorado 80218	Health-care professionals	License to practice	Clinical management of common and complex breastfeeding education	1–3 weeks; $1,000/week
Lactation Specialist Programs; Evergreen Hospital Medical Center, Kirkland, Washington	Nurses, physicians, others assisting breastfeeding families	None	Parent education; clinical assistance in unusual situations	$325
National Capital Lactation Center	Health care professionals and others interested in breastfeeding assistance	None	Assisting breastfeeding families in normal and complicated breastfeeding circumstances	$350; 5 days

BREASTFEEDING CLASS TEACHING TIPS

Tip A

Divide women and men into separate groups. Ask them to write down their concerns about childbirth and breastfeeding, or ask them to list the advantages and disadvantages of breastfeeding. Then have them assemble together and ask their partners to discuss the similarities and differences of their perceptions.

Tip B

In prenatal classes, use dolls and pillows to allow mothers to practice positioning infants at the breast. Pretend to cue the infant by eliciting a mouth opening reflex and assist each mother in lifting her breast to center her nipple over her baby's tongue as she pulls her baby close for latch–on.

Although a mother needs to quickly pull her infant close to her breast to avoid incremental latch–on, emphasize the gentle nature of breastfeeding. Prenatally, the goal is to increase the mother's confidence in this new psychomotor activity through actual practice. How the skill is described also influences her perception of breastfeeding.

ALWAYS provide specific, positive feedback regarding each mother's practice. Gentle suggestions can be made after focusing on what she is performing correctly. When making suggestions, it is important to describe what she is doing correctly; add "AND you might try." Avoid using "but" after a positive remark. "But" tends to negate the previous phrase.

Tip C

Emphasize specific activities that fathers, grandmothers, and siblings can do to assist mothers to breastfeed. For example, discuss alerting and consoling techniques for bringing an infant to an appropriate state for breastfeeding. Have participants brainstorm to develop a list of ways that family members can participate in care-taking activities (bathing, diapering, playing) not related to feeding.

Tip D

When discussing different breast pumps, have models available for mothers to operate. Inflated balloons are helpful for inserting in the pump flange so that mothers can see how suction is exerted on the breast. Always remind mothers that the balloons are much more elastic than breast tissue.

Tip E

When discussing nipple–areolar distortion with pathologic engorgement, use a partially inflated balloon with tip simulating a well everted nipple. Compress the back of the balloon with one hand to demonstrate swelling in the nipple–areolar junction during pathologic engorgement. Then use the other hand to demonstrate an areolar softening technique while simultaneously releasing the compression at the back of the balloon. As the nipple becomes more everted, participants can see how latch–on is facilitated with a softened areolar–nipple area.

STAFF EDUCATION

When developing and presenting staff educational programs, the core components of the teaching process should focus on five steps:

1. Assess the learning needs of the participants.

2. Assess participants' motivation and readiness to learn.

3. Plan and develop learning objectives, curriculum content, and teaching methods.

4. Implement teaching strategies and assist participants in focusing attention on learning tasks.

LEARNING NEEDS SURVEY FOR HEALTH-CARE PROVIDERS

A breastfeeding education program is being planned for the staff. Please complete this questionnaire to identify what topics are important to you in your clinical practice. Please use this key to indicate the importance of each topic.

1—Very Important, discuss thoroughly
2—Somewhat Important, discuss moderately
3—Not Very Important, discuss minimally

_____ Informed Decision Regarding Infant Feeding
_____ Breastfeeding Basics (Overview of How Breastfeeding Works)
_____ Prenatal Breast Assessment
_____ Techniques to Assist with Positioning and Latch–on
_____ Management of Difficult Latch–on
_____ Nipple Trauma and Engorgement (Prevention and Management)
_____ Special Maternal Situations Including Cesarean Births
_____ Premature/Critically Ill Infants
_____ Psychosocial Concerns of New Parents
_____ Jaundice Related to Breastfeeding
_____ Nutrition for Lactating Mothers
_____ Medications, Smoking, Substance Abuse Related to Lactation
_____ Sexuality, Contraception and Breastfeeding
_____ AIDS and Breastfeeding
_____ Discharge Planning/Anticipatory Guidance, Family Concerns
_____ Assessing Breastfeeding Adequacy
_____ Employed Mothers, Expression and Storage of Breastmilk
_____ Supplementation (Including Nipple Confusion and Finger-Feeding)
_____ Weaning
_____ Applying Knowledge in Clinical Practice (Effecting Change)

Please list additional topics of interest.

5. Evaluate the outcome of teaching activities.

Staff managers are often aware of learning deficits in the clinical staff through feedback from families and other health-care providers. In addition to administrative input regarding learning needs, potential participants of the educational program should be involved in assessing their own learning needs. Their involvement in the planning stage will enhance their belief that the program will benefit them in their clinical practice. The sample questionnaire above is an example of an assessment tool for gauging learning needs which can be distributed to staff and managers to obtain input for planning programs.

CONTINUING EDUCATION

Professional staff may attend educational programs either because their employer requires attendance or because they need to attend a certain number of continuing education offerings to maintain their professional registration and/or certification (extrinsic motivation). But if participants are there because they want to be (intrinsic motivation), they are self-directed learners who have identified their learning goals, and are enthusiastic about learning. Relating the curriculum content directly to a clinician's practice is a key strategy for arousing and maintaining interest in the program.

Providing continuing education credit for programs developed for health-care providers offers an additional incentive to participate; it also provides recognition for their educational efforts. Each professional organization has specific criteria for obtaining continuing education credit for such activities. Appendix 8–1 includes the names and addresses of professional organizations that confer continuing education credit. The composition of the target audience will determine the organizations with which continuing education credit applications are completed.

Four obstacles to adult learning and how they are related to learning activities with health-care providers must be considered when developing such an educational program: (1) lack of confidence; (2) sensitivity to failure; (3) poor self-image and (4) resistance to change (Staropoli & Waltz, 1978). Providing a structured overview of the program, clearly identifying what is expected of the participants, and reassuring the learners that they will be able to perform assigned activities help alleviate these common obstacles.

Teaching strategies are similar to those used with breastfeeding families. Health-care providers are generally action oriented; they do not enjoy being passive participants. They also appreciate frequent breaks since they are rarely sedentary in their employment settings.

Evaluating professional educational programs should include the health-care providers' own assessment of the usefulness of the program to their clinical practices. This information is invaluable in modifying future programs; it also helps convey the goal of clinical applicability and communicates respect for participants as valuable individuals.

CURRICULUM DEVELOPMENT

Assessing learning needs is mandatory when working with adult learners. There must be a "match" between what the learner needs to know and what the teacher presents. If the teacher erroneously assumes that learners already possess a high level of knowledge, learners can be frustrated because the information is too complex. Conversely, learners may be offended if the instructor assumes they have minimal knowledge. Accurate assessment is essential in providing relevant information.

To assess levels of knowledge when working with small groups, the facilitator can ask non-threatening

questions—such as, "What are some of the myths about breastfeeding you have heard?" In larger class settings, the content cannot be customized to each participant. Asking participants at the beginning of class what specific topics they would like to discuss helps assess their learning needs and involves them in establishing the curriculum. If the topics are written on the blackboard as they are suggested, and each topic is crossed off as it is addressed, the participants are more likely to feel that their learning needs are respected.

In addition to the participants' perceived learning needs, critical breastfeeding knowledge and skills must be identified and included in the curriculum. Posner and Rudnitsky (1982) describe five organizational models that aid in ordering curriculum content:

1. The *chronological* model presents information in the order of its usual occurrence. Thus, prenatal nipple assessment precedes a discussion of the importance of early breastfeeding opportunities, which in turn precedes an explanation of positioning and latch-on techniques.

2. The *utilization* model presents information when participants are likely to need it. Therefore information on breastmilk expression techniques precedes discussion of the storage of breastmilk.

3. Organizing content from *simple to complex* is also a helpful strategy. A lecture on simple infant cuing and latch-on techniques precedes one on difficult latch-on management. Preventive strategies for avoiding problems are covered before moving on to the management of existing problems. Thus, a discussion on preventing nipple trauma precedes one on the treatment of sore nipples.

4. *Moving from the general to the specific* places information in perspective. Discussing the concept of nutritional supplementation precedes an explanation of specific techniques for supplementation.

5. *Proceeding from the known to the unknown* is helpful when relating new tasks to those already known, making the new task seem less difficult. For example, when teaching an alternative breastfeeding position, explain that cuing and latch-on are completed in the same manner as with a previous position.

EXAMPLES OF BEHAVIORAL OBJECTIVES

Wrong

The participant will understand the relationship between breastfeeding and jaundice.

(Note: the student's "understanding" is not observable.)

Right

The learner will list three types of neonatal jaundice and will describe the relationship of each type to breastfeeding.

Not Observable

Understand, know, appreciate learn, perceive, recognize, be aware of, comprehend, grasp the significance of, gain a working knowledge of

Observable

State, list, define, identify, describe, compare, critique, rate, demonstrate, plan, design, choose, discuss, match, relate, categorize, distinguish between, select, locate, define

---

DESCRIPTION OF A SAMPLE CONTINUING EDUCATION PROGRAM

Program title: Optimal timing of the first breastfeeding

Description: The optimal timing of the first breastfeeding experience will be considered, examining the significance of infant behavioral cues, potential risks of test feeds, and properties of colostrum.

Objectives:

1. Describe feeding readiness cues in the neonate during the first hours after birth.
2. Describe the risk/benefit ratio of test feeds for normal, term infants who are breastfed.
3. List three advantages of colostrum for an infant's initial feeding.

(Three objectives can usually be adequately covered in one hour.)

Teaching Methodology: Lecture, slides

Instructor: Jane Doe, IBCLC

Bibliography:
Brazelton, TB: *Infants and Mothers: Differences in Development,* New York, 1986, Dell Publishing Co., Inc.
Brazelton, TB: *A neonatal behavioral assessment scale,* Philadelphia, 1973, J.B. Lippincott Co.
Emde, R, et al.: Human wakefulness and biological rhythms after birth, *Arch Gen Psychiatry* 32:780–83, 1975.
Lawrence, RA: *Breastfeeding: A Guide for the Medical Profession,* 3rd ed., St. Louis, 1989, The C.V. Mosby Co.
Oren, J, et al.: Effects of the components of breast milk on mucosal enzyme activity of the newborn small intestine, *Pediatr Res* 21:126–30, 1987.
Richard, L, Alade, MO: Effect of delivery room routines on success of first breast-feed. *LANCET* 336(8723): 1105–7, 1990.
Weaver, LT, et al.: Milk feeding and changes in intestinal permeability and morphology in the newborn, *J Pediatr Gastroenterol Nutr* 6:351–58, 1987.
Widstrom, AM, et al. Gastric suction in healthy newborn infants: Effects on circulation and developing feeding behavior, *Acta Paediatr Scand* 76:566–72, 1987.
Yagi, H, et al.: Epidermal growth factor in cow's milk and milk formulas, *Acta Paediatr Scand* 75:233–35, 1986.

The importance of a topic should be reflected in the time given to it, taking into consideration how frequently the information will be used. For example, positioning and latch-on are fundamental to breastfeeding success and so deserve a more thorough discussion than adoptive nursing, which is relevant to a much smaller group of learners.

As we discussed earlier, too much information at one time is overwhelming and prioritizing teaching is critical. Basic physiologic requirements (e.g., adequacy of the infant's nutrient intake) help guide prioritization. Health-care providers also must be aware of additional family resources and defer some teaching for later health visits. Thus, when a family is in the birth setting, the health-care provider may remind the mother that breastfeeding can continue when she is employed outside the home. However, specific techniques for doing so will be taught *after* breastfeeding is established.

DEVELOPING LEARNER OBJECTIVES

When developing education programs for health-care professionals, it is useful to clearly identify what the learner is expected to master. Writing behavioral objectives is one concrete way of identifying learning goals. A behavioral objective states what the student will be able to *do* at the end of the session (American Nurses' Association, 1984).

THE CHANGE PROCESS

Educating expectant families and breastfeeding mothers is a good beginning point for breastfeeding support. However, in order for mothers to have positive breastfeeding experiences, it is also necessary that practices in the birth setting assist, rather than hinder, early breastfeeding. Specific hospital practices have been identified which are detrimental to the establishment of lactation. These include mother-infant separation, delay in initial breastfeeding, prelacteal feeds, complementary or supplementary bottle-feeding, prolonged intervals between feedings, and failure to give individual breastfeeding assistance. Changing such practices is essential to achieving goals of increasing breastfeeding success.

An understanding of the change process can help accomplish a complex change, which though desirable, may nevertheless be resisted. According to Nyberg (1980), "planned change is a conscious, deliberate attempt to apply new knowledge in order to modify behavior or practices." The change agent must not only identify the desired outcome but must also consider "how" to make the change.

Change is inevitable. Planned, rather than haphazard, change is characteristic of a professional approach. Planned change is characterized by a well defined, valued goal and a systematic problem-solving approach. The change process has been conceptualized by various authors and is summarized in Table 8–4.

Assessing and planning for change are the most critical and the most time-consuming components of the change process. However, implementation is often the most challenging aspect because of the human tendency to resist change. Resistance to change is not inherently bad. It enables individuals and society to avoid destabilization and inefficiency which could result from trivial or nonbeneficial change. Resistance also stimulates the change agent to convincingly support and modify, if necessary, recommended innovation.

Lewin concluded that when any proposed change is introduced, there will be driving forces which favor the change and resisting forces which oppose it (Lewin, 1951). Resistance to change can stem from threatened self-interest, inaccurate perceptions of the intended change, objective disagreement with the change, psychological reaction, or low tolerance for change (New & Couillard, 1981).

Numerous techniques are available for dealing with resistance to change. These include participation, coercion, manipulation, education, use of an external agent, incentives, supportive behavior, and gradual introduction (New & Couillard, 1981). Strategies, either singly or in combination, need to be individualized to each situation. Common mistakes in attempting to implement change include ambiguous objectives, poorly defined strategies, and the use of a limited number of change techniques.

An important strategy for change is to recruit the support of powerful people within the organization. The change agent should not "own the project." Rather, the change agent should involve a variety of participants in the change process—from initial assessment through planning, implementation, and evaluation. People are more likely to support, rather than sabotage, a project which they helped create.

The change process can be broken down into specific steps. The identification of these steps can help accomplish desired change. The following list identifies the steps in the change process.

TABLE 8–4   THE PROCESS OF CHANGE: A COMPARISON OF FOUR THEORIES

CONCEPTUALIZATION OF THE CHANGE PROCESS

Lewin	Rogers	Havelock	Lippitt
Change has three basic stages: 1. Motivation to create change occurs. 2. New responses are developed based on collected information. 3. New ideas are integrated and stabilized into the value system.	Change has antecedents that include the background of the individuals involved as well as the environment.	Emphasis is on the planning stages, which takes the greatest time but where significant changes occur.	Emphasizes problem-solving and interpersonal aspects; multitheoretical approach including motivation, behavior systems, development and learning theories.

STEPS IN THE CHANGE PROCESS

Lewin	Rogers	Havelock	Lippitt
1. Unfreezing (Disequilibrium)	1. Awareness 2. Interest	1. Building a relationship 2. Diagnosing the problem 3. Acquiring the relevant resources	1. Diagnosis of the problem 2. Assessment of the motivation and capacity for change 3. Assessment of the change agent's motivation and resources
2. Moving	3. Interest 4. Evaluation 5. Trial adoption	4. Choosing the solution 5. Gaining acceptance	4. Selecting progressive change objectives 5. Choosing the appropriate role of the change agent
3. Refreezing (Equilibrium)	6. Adoption accepted or rejected	6. Stabilization and self-renewal	6. Maintenance of the change 7. Termination of a helping relationship

Adapted from Welch (1979).

THE CHANGE PROCESS

1. Assess the current situation/program/practice.
2. Identify the problem.
3. Recruit interdisciplinary support from task force.
4. Select target objective(s).
5. Select criteria to measure outcome(s).
6. Assess the likelihood that the system and personnel will change.
7. Select the course of action from among available options.
8. Develop a flow chart with a sequence of actions and target the time frame necessary to move the system from the present state to the desired state.
9. Assign specific individuals to carry out each action.
10. Create peer support group.
11. Provide support, coordination, and supervision to ensure performance of assignments.
12. Evaluate the process and outcome(s).
13. Revise the plan.
14. Accept the change.
15. Evaluate the effects of the change.

An example of the change process drawn from a clinical setting involves a large suburban hospital in the United States, in which an extensive computer system was introduced. Some nurses resisted the system because their typing skills were limited. Others resisted using the system for patient care plans because they perceived that it impaired their freedom to individualize care. Strategies used to deal with resistance included coercion (previous charting options were removed); participation (nurses collaborated on developing standard care plans); education (classes were provided that taught staff members how to use the new system); gradual introduction (only one program at a time was begun); and supportive behavior (staff members taught each other).

How professionals approach colleagues with proposed changes can affect how new ideas are received. A nonthreatening approach is to focus on improving patient care. It is helpful to point out the vulnerability of new parents. They become frustrated when encountering inconsistent recommendations from health-care providers whom they regard as knowledgeable authorities. That frustration negatively influences parents' perceptions of the institution.

In order to facilitate change when presenting new ideas, credibility is important. This requires preparation involving thorough review and sharing of relevant literature, references, articles, and texts. It is best to identify specific recommendations rather than to present vague goals. Role-playing with a supportive person can help identify possible responses and barriers which the change agent may encounter and offers an opportunity for brainstorming and experimentation in a nonthreatening setting.

"Constructive confrontation" of colleagues is an approach in which one shares information and seeks input from another person in a way that respects that person's expertise. It helps to create a conducive time and place for discussion; it is essential to be thoroughly prepared. Body language should reflect confidence rather than defensiveness or belligerence. The presenter should describe the problem situation with a patient-centered focus and avoid casting blame. The person or group addressed by the change agent should be asked to consider reference materials as they apply to the identified problem. A time is then set to meet again for further discussion. With the patient's optimal care as a shared goal, there need be no winner or loser among professional colleagues. Sharing, discussing, and asking for feedback demonstrate a belief in the abilities of one's colleagues and help elicit mutual respect.

A SAMPLE SUPPORT PROGRAM

Many organizations and institutions in the United States have developed exemplary programs for breastfeeding education. Some of the programs focus on client education, others on professional education. Some have a two-pronged focus.

The Breastfeeding Resource Center at Mercy Health Center in Oklahoma City, Oklahoma, provides comprehensive breastfeeding education for families and health-care providers. Approximately 150 infants are born at the center each month. The majority of the population is comprised of well-educated, two-parent families.

Prenatally, families may attend six hours of structured classes that provide a broad base of information about breastfeeding. A lactation consultant presents material using a variety of teaching strategies—including slides, video tapes, demonstrations with a doll and breast model, and group discussion. Mothers practice positioning techniques with dolls to increase their psychomotor confidence and retention of critical information. Fathers and support persons are encouraged to attend the prenatal classes. Books and videos on a variety of breastfeeding topics are available for loan or purchase from the health center.

Perinatal staff nurses who have completed a breastfeeding educator certification program respond to questions and provide breastfeeding assistance. Additionally, families may attend a 45-minute class taught by a lactation consultant in which individual concerns can be addressed and validated. These sessions are lively; a mother is often eager to ask questions and clarify points now that she is breastfeeding her baby. If the mother cannot attend the class, she may view a video of the class and then ask questions. If a mother has a special breastfeeding situation, a lactation consultant is available for individual consultations.

After leaving the birth setting, families can use the telephone "warmline" staffed by lactation consultants. Any family in the community may make an appointment for an out-patient consultation. The lactation consultant collaborates with the family's physician in developing the care plan and follow-up. Telephone follow-up and return consultation visits, if indicated, are continued until the problem is resolved and a written summary of the consultation and follow-up care is sent to the physician.

Breastfeeding products (breast shells, supplemental nutrition systems, breastpump purchase or rental) are available through the Breastfeeding Resource Center. Personalized instruction and written information are provided with all rented or purchased products. All education materials are evaluated for use in the breastfeeding program. If no appropriate materials are identified, or if information unique to the health center is needed, materials are developed.

Perinatal staff development is another facet of the breastfeeding education program. Nurses have attended a minimum of 12 hours of breastfeeding education programs, taken part in a role-playing demonstration of positioning and difficult latch-on management, and passed a 50-item multiple-choice exam on breastfeeding assistance. Participants who successfully complete the minimal competencies are designated as certified breastfeeding educators. They are prepared to assist with common breastfeeding circumstances as they provide comprehensive perinatal care. An orientation system for new employees includes breastfeeding assistance as a mandatory competency.

Semiannual inservice programs and research updates keep the staff alerted to recent advances in breastfeeding. Staff input is requested for help in selecting discussion topics. The results of quality assurance audits and feedback from patient follow-up care are also shared with nursing staff. Lactation consultants are available as a staff resource; for example, they might conduct a literature search on a specific topic. Staff are invited to attend informal journal club programs to discuss the clinical applicability of current literature. Periodic programs for medical personnel increase the consistency and comprehensiveness of curriculum content.

Lactation consultants develop and revise standards of care and nursing care plans related to breastfeeding using nursing and medical staff input. A triage tool for assistance and a list of referral criteria are available for staff, as well as a breastfeeding resource book which contains pertinent journal articles and summaries of management strategies. Bulletin postings display recent articles and protocols.

Lactation consultants participate in quality assurance projects with periodic chart audits and problem-oriented audits. Quality assurance projects, patient satisfaction surveys, and direct oral and written feedback from breastfeeding families provide data for evaluating the breastfeeding education programs. Research in clinical management of breastfeeding is conducted within the program. Site visits and program or project consultations are available for institutions and organizations seeking to develop a comprehensive breastfeeding education program.

Help with breastfeeding extends to the health center's employees as well. Prenatal breastfeeding classes and one-on-one consultations are free. A breastfeeding support room is available to employees 24 hours a day. It includes an electric breast pump, rocking chair, foot rest, sink and restroom facilities, refrigerator, telephone, audio tape player, and picture frames for mothers' photographs of their infants.

SUMMARY

Breastfeeding families need to be empowered for self-sufficiency. Empowerment can result when health-care providers furnish information in an accurate, well-organized manner so that families can recognize the importance of the information on their lives. Thus, breastfeeding families are empowered by knowledge; they assist health-care providers in identifying the family's goals and in problem solving in order to increase parental self-confidence and self-reliance. These activities are most effective in conjunction with health-care practices that promote breastfeeding success.

While providing information to families and assisting with problem solving are components of empowerment, removing specific barriers to breastfeeding also is essential. Strategies that promote breastfeeding success include: facilitating early, frequent breastfeeding; encouraging rooming-in; providing early assistance and follow-up; avoiding routine formula supplementation; teaching families the signs of adequate nutritional intake by the infant; and instructing families about the relationship between milk removal from the breast and continued milk production. Applying principles of the change process can assist health-care providers in promoting practices that improve breastfeeding success.

Underestimating a family's desire to breastfeed may be an unrecognized barrier to success. This is particularly true with such groups as adolescent mothers, single mothers, mothers from ethnic minority populations, or mothers who are employed outside the home. Health-care providers tend to underestimate a family's interest in such information. One study (Waitzkin, 1985) found that physicians spent little time informing their patients and that they underestimated the patient's desire for information.

Developing and presenting educational programs for health-care providers who assist breastfeeding families requires significant time and energy. One needs to remember the ripple effect from staff education; enormous numbers of breastfeeding families benefit from the enhanced knowledge of health-care providers.

A successful education program—regardless of its subject matter—entails positive experiences for both the learner and teacher. Identifying the components of effective breastfeeding programs can assist health-care providers who are involved in planning, implementing, and evaluating breastfeeding education.

REFERENCES

Aberman, S, and Kirchoff, KT: Infant-feeding practices: Mothers' decision-making, *JOGN Nurs* 14:394–98, 1985.

American Nurses' Association: *Standards for Continuing Education in Nursing,* Kansas City, Mo., 1984, The Association.

Anderson, GC: Risk in mother–infant separation postbirth, *Image* 21:196–99, 1989.

Auerbach, KG: Beyond the issue of accuracy: evaluating patient education materials for breastfeeding mothers, *J Hum Lact* 4:108–10, 1988.

Auerbach, KG: The effect of lactation consultant contact on breastfeeding duration in a low-income population, *Neb Med J* 70:341–46, 1985.

Auerbach, KG: Employed breastfeeding mothers: Problems they encounter, *Birth* 11:17–20, 1984.

Baranowski, T, et al.: Social support, social influence, ethnicity and the breastfeeding decision, *Soc Sci Med* 17:1599–1611, 1983.

Becton, LG, and Dickenson, CC: Patient comprehension profiles: Recent findings and strategies, *Pat Couns Health Educ* 2:101–6, 1981.

Beske, EJ, and Garvis, MS: Important factors in breast-feeding success, *MCN* 7:174–79, 1982.

Biegelson, D, Cowell, C, and Goldberg, D: Breast-feeding practices in a low-income population in New York City: A study of selected health department child health stations, *J Am Diet Assoc* 86:90–91, 1986.

Birenbaum, E, Fuchs, C, and Reichman, B: Demographic factors influencing the initiation of breast-feeding in an Israeli urban population, *Pediatrics,* 83:519–23, 1989.

Bloom, BS: *Taxonomy of educational objectives,* New York, 1956, David McKay Co., Inc., pp. 7–8.

Bloom, K, et al.: Factors affecting the continuance of breastfeeding, *Acta Paediatr Scand* (Suppl.) 300:9–14, 1982.

Bocar, DL, and Moore, K: *Acquiring the parental role: a theoretical perspective*/(Unit 16), Lactation Consultant Series, Garden City Park, N.Y., 1987, Avery Publishing Group, Inc., pp. 2–11.

Bolton, R: *People skills: How to assert yourself, listen to others, and resolve conflicts,* New York, 1979, Simon & Schuster, Inc., pp. 79–83.

Brimblecombe, FSW, and Cullen, D: Influences on a mother's choice of method of infant feeding, *Public Health, London* 91:117–26, 1977.

Brown, F, et al.: Studies in choice of infant feeding by primiparas: I. Attitudinal factors and extraneous influences, *Psychosom Med* 22:421–29, 1960.

Bryant, CA: The impact of kin, friend, and neighbor networks on infant feeding practices, *Soc Sci Med* 16:1757–65, 1982.

Cohen, SA: Postpartum teaching and the subsequent use of milk supplements, *Birth Fam J* 7:163–67, 1980.

Collins, TR, et al.: Perceptions and knowledge of breast-feeding among WIC and non-WIC pregnant women in Alabama, *Ala J Med Sci* 21:145–48, 1984.

Coopersmith, S: *The antecedents of self–esteem,* San Francisco, 1967, W.H. Freeman, pp. 37–38.

Crowder, DS: Maternity nurses' knowledge of factors promoting successful breastfeeding: A survey of two hospitals, *JOGN Nurs* 10:28–30, 1981.

Crummette, BD: Transitions in motherhood, *MCN* 4:65–74, 1975.

Darkenwald, GG, and Merriam, SB: *Adult education: foundations of practice,* New York, 1982, Harper & Row, Publishers, Inc.

Doak, CC, Doak, LG, and Root, JH: *Teaching Patients With Low Literacy Skills,* Philadelphia, 1985, J.B. Lippincott Co., pp. 35–41.

Dolphin, P, and Holtzclaw, BJ: *Continuing education in nursing: strategies for lifelong learning,* Reston, Va., 1983, Reston Publishing.

Dunn, R: Learning—A matter of style, *Educ Lead* 36:430–32, 1979.

Egan, G: *The skilled helper: model, skills and method of effective helping,* 2nd ed., Monterey, Calif., 1982, Brooks/Cole Publishing Co., pp. 60–61.

Ekwo, EE, Dusdieker, LB, and Booth, BM: Factors influencing initiation of breast-feeding, *Am J Dis Child* 137:375–77, 1983.

Ellis, DJ, and Hewat, RJ: Factors related to breastfeeding duration, *Can Fam Phys* 30:1479–84, 1984.

Flashner, C, ed.: Breastfeeding books for new mothers: a reader's guide, *J Hum Lact* (suppl. 2) 4:2–19, 1988.

Flashner, C, ed.: Breastfeeding films for new mothers: a viewer's guide, *J Hum Lact* (suppl. 3) 5:1–27, 1989.

Forman, MR, et al.: Exclusive breast-feeding of newborns among married women in the United States: The National Natality Surveys of 1969 and 1989, *Am J Clin Nutr* 42:864–69, 1985.

Graffy, J: Breastfeeding: The GD's role. *Practitioner* 236:322–24, 1992.

Grassley, J, and Davis, K: Common concerns of mothers who breast-feed, *MCN* 6:347–51, 1978.

Gulick, E: Informational correlates of successful breastfeeding, *MCN* 7:370–75, 1982.

Gunning, R: *The technique of clear writing* (Rev ed.), New York, 1968, McGraw-Hill Book Co., pp. 38–40.

Haber, J, and Hoskins, PP: *Comprehensive psychiatric nursing,* 3rd ed., New York, 1987, McGraw-Hill Book Co.

Hall, ET: *The hidden dimension,* Garden City, N.Y., 1969, Doubleday & Co. Inc., p. 45.

Hall, JM: Influencing breastfeeding success, *JOGN Nurs* 7:28–32, 1978.

Hanson, LA, and Bergstrom, S: The link between infant mortality and birth rates—the importance of breastfeeding as a common factor, *Acta Paediatr Scand* 79:481–89, 1990.

Havelock, R: *The Change Agent's Guide to Innovation in Education.* New Jersey: Educational Technology Publications, 1973.

Hayes, B: Inconsistencies among nurses in breastfeeding knowledge and counselling, *JOGN Nurs* 10:430–33, 1981.

Hendershot, G: Trends in breastfeeding, *Advance Data* 59:1–5, 1980.

Hendershot, GE: Trends in breast-feeding, *Pediatrics* 74 (Suppl.): 591–602, 1984.

Hewat, RJ, and Ellis, DJ: Similarities and differences between women who breastfeed for short and long duration, *Midwifery* 2:37–43, 1986.

Hirschman, C, and Butler, M: Trends and differentials in breast feeding: an update, *Demography* 18:39–54, 1981.

Houston, MJ, and Howie, PW: Home support for the breast feeding mother, *Midwife, Health Visitor Comm Nurse* 17:378–80, 1981.

Joffe, A, and Radius, SM: Breast versus bottle; Correlates of adolescent mothers' infant feeding practices, *Pediatrics* 79:689–95, 1987.

Jones, DA: The choice to breast feed or bottle feed and influences upon that choice: A survey of 1525 mothers, *Child Care Health Dev* 13:75–85, 1987.

Kaplowitz, DD, and Olson, CM: The effect of an education program on the decision to breastfeed, *J Nutr Educ* 15:61–65, 1983.

Kistin, N, et al.: Breast-feeding rates among black urban low-income women: effect of prenatal education, *Pediatrics* 86:741–46, 1990.

Knowles, M: *The Modern Practice of Adult Education,* New York, 1980, Cambridge Univ. Pr.

Kocturk, T: Advantages of breastfeeding according to Turkish mothers living in Istanbul and Stockholm, *Soc Sci Med* 27:405–10, 1988.

Kozier, B, and Erb, G: *Fundamentals of nursing: concepts and procedures,* 3rd ed., Menlo Park, Calif., 1987, Addison-Wesley Publishing Co., Inc.

Ladas, AK: Information and social support as factors in the outcome of breastfeeding. *J Appl Behav Sci* 8:110–14, 1972.

Lauwers, J, and Woessner, C: *Counseling the nursing mother,* 2nd ed., Garden City Park, N.Y., 1989, Avery Publishing Group, Inc., p. 13.

Lawrence, RA: Practices and attitudes toward breastfeeding among medical professionals, *Pediatrics* 70:912–20, 1984.

Leeper, J, Milo, T, and Collins, T: Infant-feeding and maternal attitudes among mothers of low-income, *Psychol Rep* 53:259–65, 1983.

Lewin, K: *Field Theory in Social Science,* New York, 1951, Harper & Row, Publishers, Inc.

Lippitt, R: *Dynamics of Planned Change,* New York, 1969, Crowell Publishing Co.

Martinez, GA, and Dodd, DA: 1981 milk feeding patterns in the United States during the first 12 months of life, *Pediatrics* 71:166–70, 1983.

New, JR, and Couillard, NA: Guidelines for introducing change, *J Nurs Admin* 11:17–21, 1981.

Newton, N, and Newton, M: Psychological aspects of lactation, *N Engl J Med* 277:1179–88, 1967.

Newton, N, and Newton, M: Relationship of ability to breastfeed and maternal attitudes toward breastfeeding, *Pediatrics* 5:869–75, 1950.

Nichols, FH, and Edwards, MR: Are your group process skills up to par? *Nurs Health Care* 9:205–8, 1988.

Nyberg, J: Probing the change process, *Superv Nurs* 11:31–33, 1980.

Palti, H, et al.: Evaluation of the effectiveness of a structured breast-feeding promotion program integrated into a maternal and child health service in Jerusalem, *Is J Med Sci* 24:342–48, 1988.

Pease, A: *Signals,* New York, 1984, Bantam Bks., Inc., pp. 6–7.

Posner, GJ, and Rudnitsky, AN: *Course design: a guide to curriculum development for teachers,* 2nd ed., New York, 1982, Longman Publishing Group, pp. 108–17.

Radius, SM, and Joffe, A: Understanding adolescent mothers' feelings about breastfeeding: A study of perceived benefits and barriers, *J Adoles Health Care* 9:156–60, 1988.

Rassin, DK, et al.: Incidence of breast-feeding in a low socioeconomic group of mothers in the United States: Ethnic patterns, *Pediatrics* 73:1321–37, 1984.

Redman, BK: *The process of patient education,* 6th ed., St. Louis, 1988, The C.V. Mosby Co.

Riordan, J: *A Practical Guide to Breastfeeding,* St. Louis, 1983, The C.V. Mosby Co.

Riordan, J: Readable, relevant, reliable: the three "R's" of breastfeeding pamphlets, *Breastfeeding Abstr* 5:5–6, 1985.

Rogers, C: The necessary and sufficient conditions of personality change, *J Consult Psychol* 22:95–110, 1957.

Ross, HS: Group discussion methods, *Pat Educ News,* February, 1982.

Sampson, EE, and Marthas, M: *Group Process for the Health Professions,* New York, 1981, John Wiley & Sons, Inc.

Scheflen, AE, and Scheflen, A: *Body language and social order,* Englewood Cliffs, N.J., 1972, Prentice Hall, pp. 40–41.

Shrago, LC, and Bocar, DL: The infant's contribution to breastfeeding, *JOGNN* 19:209–15, 1990.

Sloper, K, McKean, L, and Baum, JD: Factors in influencing breast-feeding, *Arch Dis Child* 50:165–70, 1975.

Smith, JC, et al.: Trends in the incidence of breastfeeding for Hispanics of Mexican origin and Anglos on the US-Mexico border, *Am J Public Health* 72:59–61, 1982.

Starapoli, CJ, and Waltz, C: *Developing and evaluating educational programs for health care providers,* Philadelphia, 1978, F.A. Davis Co., p. 11.

Sullivan, J, and Jones, LC: Breastfeeding adoption by low-income black women, *Health Care Wom Int* 7:295–309, 1986.

Switzky, LT, Vietz, P, and Switzky, NN: Attitudinal and demographic predictors of breastfeeding and bottlefeeding behavior by mothers of 6 week old infants, *Psychol Rep* 45:3–14, 1979.

Taylor, MM: *Transcultural aspects of breastfeeding*-USA (Unit 2), Lactation Consultant Series, Garden City Park, N.Y., 1985, Avery Publishing Group, Inc.

Tubbs, SL: *A Systems Approach to Small Group Interaction,* Reading, Mass., 1984, Addison-Wesley Publishing Co., Inc.

Waitzkin, H: Information giving in medical care, *J Health Soc Behav* 26:81–101, 1985.

Welch, LB: Planned Change in nursing: the theory, *Nurs Clin North Am* 14:307–21, 1979.

Whitley, N: Preparation for breastfeeding: A one year follow-up of 34 nursing mothers, *JOGN Nurs* 7:44–48, 1978.

Wiles, LS: The effect of prenatal breastfeeding education on breastfeeding success and maternal perception of the infant, *JOGN Nurs* 13:253–57, 1984.

Yeung, DL, et al.: Breastfeeding: Prevalence and influencing factors, *Can J Public Health* 72:323–30, 1981.

Yoos, L: Developmental issues and the choice of feeding method of adolescent mothers, *JOGN Nurs* 14:68–72, 1985.

Young, SA, and Kaufman, M: Promoting breastfeeding at a migrant health center, *Am J Public Health* 78:523–25, 1988.

Appendix 8–1   Providers of Lactation Education in the United States

Provider	Program
The Breastfeeding Connection 618 N. Wheaton Ave. Wheaton, IL 60187 708–665–6848 or 708–420–2172	Breastfeeding conferences
Breastfeeding Consultants, Inc. 219 Dickinson Ave. Swarthmore, PA 19081 215–543–5990 or 215–543–5995	Workshops for lactation consultants
Breastfeeding Support Consultants (BSC) 1009 Schoolhouse Road Pottstown, PA 19464 215–326–6551	Correspondence course; workshops for lactation consultants; texts and pamphlets
Health Education Associates (HEA) 8 Jan Sebastian Way (Unit 13) Sandwich, MA 02563 508–888–8044	Breastfeeding workshops; book; pamphlets; visual aids
International Lactation Consultant Association (ILCA) 201 Brown Ave. Evanston, IL 60202–3601 708–260–8874	Annual international conference for lactation consultants; publishes *Journal of Human Lactation*
La Leche League International (LLLI) 9616 Minneapolis Ave. Franklin Park, IL 60131 312–455–7730	Yearly Physicians' Seminar; lactation consultant workshops; international conference; books; pamphlets; reference library; breastfeeding aids; publishes lactation consultant series and *Breastfeeding Abstracts*
Lactation Associates 254 Conant Road Weston, MA 02193 617–893–3553	Breastfeeding workshops; educational materials; reference books
Lactation Consultant Services 11320 Shady Glen Road Oklahoma City, OK 73162 405–722–2163	Workshops for breastfeeding educators; conferences
Lactation Institute 16161 Ventura Blvd., Suite 223 Encino, CA 91436 818–995–1913	Lactation specialist training; teaching tools; pamphlets; lactation consultant charting forms, teaching doll; reference books
Lactation Program Women's and Children's Services Presbyterian-St. Luke's Medical Center 1719 E. 19th St. Denver, CO 80218 303–869–1888	Clinical preceptorships; conferences; milk bank; newsletter
Lactation Seminars 11170 Delta Circle Boca Raton, FL 33428 407–482–2670	Workshops and conferences
Lactation Specialist Programs Evergreen Hospital Medical Center 12040 NE 126th St. Kirkland, WA 98034 206–899–2680	Clinical preceptorships; workshops; conferences

(continued)

Appendix 8–1   Providers of Lactation Education in the United States (*cont*.)

Provider	Program
Lectures Unlimited 2240 Willow Road Homewood, IL 60430 708–206–1880	Workshops and conferences
National Capital Lactation Center 3800 Reservoir Road NW Washington, DC 20207 202–784–6455	
UCLA Extension Department of Health Sciences Division of Nursing 10995 Le Conte Ave., Room 614 Los Angeles, CA 90024 310–825–9187	Lactation educator training; lactation consultant training
Wellstart Lactation Management Education Program 4062 First Ave. San Diego, CA 92103 619–295–5192	On-site clinical training for physicians and nurses; mostly international participants

9

The Breastfeeding Process

KATHLEEN G. AUERBACH
JAN RIORDAN
BETTY ANN COUNTRYMAN

Helping new mothers during the lactation process is a rewarding and important experience for the nurse or lactation consultant (LC). With a basic understanding of the anatomy and physiology of the breast and of the nutritional and immunologic properties of breastmilk, the health-care worker can contribute greatly to a mother's breastfeeding experience. However, the care provider also must be prepared to offer practical assistance supported by relevant research findings and to meet the urgent needs of mothers with little or no breastfeeding experience—as well as the needs of mothers, who despite previous breastfeeding experience, are still anxious about doing it. Emphasis on confident self-care is a major goal.

What the mother learns about breastfeeding and caring for herself and her baby in the medical office or the hospital or clinic will affect her breastfeeding relationship for a long time, and may influence how she feeds not one but all of her children. Recognizing that many women who initiate breastfeeding wean after two months or even sooner, we realize the necessity for self-care skills. Self-care, the guiding framework for this book, can be defined as "the practice of activities that individuals personally initiate and perform on their own behalf in maintaining life, health, and well-being" (Orem, 1980). In the self-care approach to breastfeeding, the nurse or other care provider educates, assists, encourages, and nurtures the mother and her family toward effective use of their own resources for achieving an optimal breastfeeding experience. As Rubin so clearly demonstrated, the maternal role, far from being intuitive, is learned (Rubin, 1961, 1967a, 1967b).

The self-care orientation is congruent with the current recognition of consumer participation and partnership in health care. Self-care education is based on the parent's perceived needs, not needs identified by the health-care provider. It is especially appropriate for maternal-infant care nursing—a field in which, unlike in other areas of nursing, clients are usually healthy. In no other area of health care is the consumer's involvement in her own care more rewarding to assist and to observe.

PREPARATION FOR BREASTFEEDING

Preparation for breastfeeding is often given a great deal of importance in discussions which address the mass market. The best preparation for any mother is to learn as much about breastfeeding as possible before she embarks on her own personal lactation adventure. Gaining this knowledge can be accomplished in any number of ways. She may choose to take a prenatal breastfeeding class. The best classes are usually offered by independent lactation consultants or by community-based breastfeeding support groups such as La Leche League International or the Nursing Mothers Association groups. Additionally, both LLLI and NMA groups offer ongoing support and are not dependent on a single institution. Thus, they are less likely to include questionable recommendations that stem from the practices or routines of a particular hospital or clinic.

Some physicians in pediatrics or family practice also offer breastfeeding classes in their offices. These classes usually are part of doctors' regular services, which cover the prenatal through the immediate postbirth period. Breastfeeding classes are also offered by hospitals as a way of encouraging parents to use their facility. In still other cases, breastfeeding is the topic for one or two sessions of a multiweek childbirth preparation or parenting class.

In addition to a class, mothers can prepare by reading books about breastfeeding. The trick to learning about breastfeeding through reading is in the proper choice of the reading material. Information by reputable authors is best; the recommendations of knowledgeable reviewers may be quite valuable. While many brochures and book-length materials are available, not all are accurate or up-to-date. Reading material prepared by propriety formula companies or companies that make infant feeding equipment, for example, often leave the impression that breastfeeding is difficult and requires the use of supplemental infant formula. Such material may also imply that weaning from the breast will occur early.

Another way to prepare for breastfeeding is for a prospective mother to chat with one or more women who have breastfeeding experience. If they also share the same career or live in the same neighborhood, they may become a mutual resource for finding a pediatrician, or a reputable babysitting service, as well as comparing breastfeeding experiences. The experienced breastfeeding mother who acts as a mentor to the less experienced woman can teach her the usual how-to-do-it information. She also can respond to the new mother's concerns and feelings and advise her on aspects of breastfeeding that are more difficult to address in written form or in a less personal setting.

BREAST AND NIPPLE PREPARATION

While learning about breastfeeding from books is important, physical preparation is another matter. For example, prenatal preparation of nipple tissue, a frequent recommendation, is based upon a faulty assumption: that the nipple and breast tissue *require* treatment when preparing for breastfeeding. On the contrary, the mother who makes no such efforts will be just as ready to breastfeed as the mother who spends time and effort attempting to condition her breasts (Whitley, 1974; Brown & Hurlock, 1975).

Some mothers are told to attempt to express colostrum, to roll their nipples and/or to condition the nipple through the use of friction. There is no need to express colostrum prior to the birth of the baby. The mother with a history of pre-term labor should *avoid* stimulating her breasts through expression or nipple rolling. The latter technique in particular may stimulate labor contractions (Elliot & Flaherty, 1984; Capeless & Mann, 1984; Oki et al., 1987). Colostrum is produced throughout the pregnancy and need not be expressed to determine its presence. In some mothers, colostrum spontaneously leaks during sexual intercourse and late in pregnancy when nipples rub against clothing. Nipple rolling, too, is unnecessary to prepare the breasts for breastfeeding, although women learn how quickly the nipples respond to stimulation when they do so. During pregnancy, the breasts begin making milk and the nipples become more elastic, which may explain why women characterize their nipples as "flat" or "inverted" at the beginning, but not at the end, of pregnancy.

If the nipple remains flat or retracted, nipple rolling may stimulate a greater degree of eversion than might otherwise be observed; however, the negative pressure exerted by the baby in the act of suckling will have the same effect. How the nipple looks when the baby is not suckling bears little resemblance to its appearance in the baby's mouth, nor is it necessary for the nipple to be everted when not in the baby's mouth. Hoffmann's exercises for nipple inversion and/or flatness have no noticeable impact on the appearance of the nipple (Hoffmann, 1953). For women who have never handled their breasts except in a sexual context, occasional nipple rolling, Hoffman's exercises, and other manipulations may help them to view their breasts in a more matter-of-fact manner. For that reason, such preparation may be helpful. One study (Gulick, 1982) found that women who practiced nipple care during pregnancy had better overall success with breastfeeding than women who did not handle their breasts. The reason may be that they were more committed to breastfeeding than those who made no effort to prepare, coupled with a psychological comfort level that developed during pregnancy.

It is a fallacy to assume that nipple tissue, with stimulation—or use by the baby—will become "toughened" (Auerbach, 1990). Such a term implies a reduction in sensitivity; but the nipple must be sensitive to the baby's stimulation if it is to send the correct messages to the brain which trigger milk production and milk ejection.

Two studies suggest that prenatal preparation of the breasts may be helpful in preventing nipple soreness and engorgement. Atkinson (1979) compared 22 primigravidas who used nipple rolling and friction on one breast, while the other breast served as the control. The amount of pain experienced during breastfeeding in the treated (experimental) nipple was significantly less compared with that in the control nipple. Nine years later, Storr (1988) used a similar design to study 25 women who used nipple rolling, friction, and breast massage on one breast, while the other served as the control. While nipple tenderness and breast engorgement were decreased in the prepared, massaged breast, Storr discussed possible bias influencing the findings of her study. Every subject said she believed that prenatal nipple conditioning would decrease her nipple tenderness. Furthermore, all the mothers were fully aware which breast was conditioned and massaged and which one was not.

Rubbing with a towel—in fact, any source of friction—serves only to remove the oils that keep the nipple tissue supple. Washing with soap also tends to dry the skin and increase tenderness. Thus, if the nipples appear functional and are not inverted, the best preparation is to do as little as possible. Involving the breasts and nipples in lovemaking—except when the mother has a history of pre-term labor (Salmon et al., 1986)—washing without soap, and providing occasional brief exposure to sun and air are sufficient to prepare the nipples for breastfeeding (Riordan, 1980a).

The most important organ in breastfeeding is the mother's brain. When it receives signals from the nipple and breast, milk production and ejection will occur. Mothering is more learned than instinctive (Rubin, 1967a, 1967b), and a mother's best "teacher" is her own baby. When reaffirmed as a person and supported in her early efforts to breastfeed, a mother will have most of what she needs to assume her new role and relish the unique joys it will provide her.

THE BIRTH PLAN AND FEEDING PLAN

The prospective mother in the United States must purchase her health care; it is her right to get what she pays for. Frequently, expectant parents identify issues of importance to them, develop a birth plan, and use this plan to discuss with their midwife or physician their goals for the birth of their baby.

Using the same principles, parents may devise a feeding plan. Breastfeeding is the means by which the infant receives optimal nutrition. The infant's right to this milk must be preserved and protected, even if the baby is not immediately able to receive this milk. The family's wishes as they relate to breastfeeding need to be understood by health-care workers at the outset, particularly when the mother is apt to give birth in a setting away from her own home. The feeding plan on p. 218 addresses issues to be included in an infant feeding plan in a hospital setting.

In some institutions, specific elements in the feeding plan may be more difficult to implement than in other settings. For example, where glucose and artificial formula feedings are considered routine and where parental consent is not usually obtained prior to their use, provisions that restrict feeding to the breast alone will require that hospital care-givers furnish a kind of care they may be unaccustomed to giving. It is the responsibility of the parents to speak for the infant who is unable to voice his preference.

EARLY FEEDINGS

Following birth, continuing assessment of the mother's physical condition and psychosocial status is essential. The optimal time for initiating breastfeeding depends on these factors, as well as on the mother's informed choice, and will not, of course, be the same for all individuals. If the birth process has been relatively uncomplicated, the mother should be encouraged to breastfeed immediately after birth and regularly thereafter.

There are several reasons why early and frequent breastfeeding promotes an optimal level of functioning for both the infant and the mother:

1. Suckling stimulates uterine contractions, aids in the expulsion of the placenta, and helps control excessive maternal blood loss.

FEEDING PLAN

- The mother's chart will indicate that she plans to breastfeed her baby.
- The baby's chart will be similarly marked to indicate that the baby is to be breastfed.
- The mother indicates the degree to which she expects to receive assistance with breastfeedings during her stay in the hospital and from whom she expects to receive such assistance. If her doctor employs an LC, that individual needs to have hospital privileges in order to see the physician's patients while they are in the hospital. It is appropriate to ask if the physician's LC can see patients in the hospital.
- The mother indicates whether she is willing to allow the baby to be fed by someone other than herself at any time during the hospital stay and whether she will provide her own milk for someone else to feed. She also specifies how her milk is to be given and under what conditions this may occur.
- The mother indicates what fluids other than human milk she will allow her baby to receive during the hospital stay, how such fluids are to be given, and under what conditions this may occur.
- If a family history of allergies has been identified (in a sibling of the new baby, his mother, his father, or other relative), that fact should be noted on the mother's chart and on the baby's chart; recommendations relating to the risks of using fluids other than human milk should be noted accordingly.
- The mother indicates whether she expects the baby to be housed exclusively with her in her room and under what conditions, if any, the baby may be housed elsewhere.
- The mother indicates the frequency with which she expects to breastfeed her baby and under what circumstances, if any, she will not breastfeed the baby.
- The mother indicates whether she will provide her own milk to her baby in the event the baby is unable to suckle directly, and whether she will arrange to provide fresh unrefrigerated, fresh refrigerated, fresh frozen, or deep-frozen human milk in containers acceptable to the hospital where her newborn is cared for.

Each of the above points should be in writing, thereby providing a record of parental expectations about optimal care. A written feeding plan protects the parents, the out-patient care-givers, and all hospital staff members who work with the family by providing a clear understanding of the preference and expectations of the parents with regard to the care and feeding of their child. It also serves to generate discussions between the care-givers and the parents about how their baby will be fed, as well as the advantages and disadvantages of each chosen element in the plan.

---

2. The infant's suckling reflex is most intense during the first 20–30 minutes after birth. Delaying gratification of this reflex can make it more difficult for the baby to learn to suckle later on (Eppink, 1969; Anderson et al., 1982).

3. The infant promptly begins to receive the immunologic advantages of colostrum.

4. The infant's digestive peristalsis is stimulated, thereby promoting elimination of the by-products of hemoglobin breakdown. Jaundice is more likely to occur when feeding and peristalsis are delayed.

5. Breast engorgement is minimized or prevented by the early and frequent removal of milk from the ducts and sinuses of the breast (Newton, 1961).

6. Lactation is accelerated, plus early and frequent intake of breastmilk lessens infant weight loss after birth.

7. Attachment and bonding are enhanced at a time when both the mother and the infant are in a heightened state of readiness.

If there are no intervening complications, the first breastfeeding should take place right after the infant's birth. After the airway has been cleared, the infant can be placed in the mother's arms to breastfeed. Several studies have demonstrated that mother-infant body contact is as effective as supplemental heat in maintaining the healthy newborn's temperature (Hill & Shronk, 1979; Britton, 1980). The placenta is normally expelled soon after birth, often before the infant is put to breast for the first time; but if a delay occurs, breastfeeding may hasten detachment and expulsion.

With the mother propped on her side and a pillow at her back for support, the baby may suckle in the delivery room. If the mother delivers in a birthing suite, so much the better. The ambience and homey comforts of the setting encourage early breastfeeding. When the father is present, he can share the enjoyment of these first moments together and help position the mother and infant in a comfortable chair or in the birthing bed.

Newborns often suckle minimally at this time; frequently they only lick or nuzzle the nipple. Given ample opportunity, however, they will attempt to move up the mother's trunk and suckle strongly and at length (Widstrom et al., 1987). Regardless of the baby's initial suckling behavior, this interaction is advantageous because it stimulates uterine contractions, promotes colonization of harmless bacteria on the nipple, and possibly helps to protect the infant from pathogenic bacteria (Klaus & Kennell, 1982)—a very pleasant method of infection control. Explaining to the mother that her baby will take hold of the breast later and that "nuzzling" is normal behavior will help her to see this activity as a positive response rather than as disinterest or "rejection" of the breast.

Sometimes the first breastfeeding takes place after the mother and her newborn are transferred from the delivery area to their room. Wherever it may be, if the mother is awake and oriented, it is best that she put her baby to breast as soon as possible. The optimal time for this first feeding is within two hours after birth, since during this period the baby is usually in an alert state and later falls asleep. (See Table 9–1.)

Women breastfeed for a longer duration if feedings are initiated early (Salariya, Easton & Cater, 1978; Ekwo, Dusdieker & Booth, 1983; Goodine & Fried, 1984; Quandt, 1985; Woolridge, Greasley & Silpisornkosol, 1985; Winikoff et al., 1986; Anlar, Anlar & Tonyali, 1988). The first several feedings have an imprinting effect. A positive, satisfying experience gets breastfeeding off to the right start, and

TABLE 9–1 FIRST-DAY SLEEP PATTERNS OF NEONATES BORN IN HOSPITAL

Infant State	Time Period
Alert and eager	Birth–2 hours
Light and deep sleep	2–20+ hours
Increasing wakefulness*	20–24 hours

*Often includes a cluster of 5–10 feeding episodes over 2–3 hours followed by a 4–5 hour deep sleep.

parents often recall this experience in great detail many years later. A care-giver's unhurried nurturing approach helps to establish rapport with the mother. It is important to explain to the first-time mother that breastfeeding is not as automatic for her as the suckling and rooting reflexes are for her baby. Yet the experience is new to the baby, too, and the first few times at breast offer opportunities for each to learn from the other. Early breastfeedings may be optimized in the following ways:

1. *Arrange for privacy.* Concentrating on learning a new skill is easier when it is not attempted in public. Shut the door of the mother's room or pull the curtains around her bed if she wishes. Suggest that she cleanse her *hands* with soap and rinse them.

2. Work with the mother to *find the most comfortable position* and make sure there are several pillows available. Women who have had a cesarean birth often find it more comfortable to breastfeed while sitting in a comfortable chair with low arms. Almost always, the *least* comfortable position is leaning back in the bed, as if in a lounge chair. At the first feeding, arrange pillows on her lap, behind her back, and under her arm and shoulder on the side on which the baby is to nurse. If the mother is in bed, raise the back of the bed to high Fowler's position with plenty of pillows for additional support. The experienced breastfeeder, or the mother who must remain flat because epidural or other anesthesia has been administered during labor or birth, may lie on her side with pillows at her back and between her knees.

3. *Work with the mother at her eye level.* If she is in a chair, kneel down; if she is in bed, pull up a chair; or, if the bed is electronically operated,

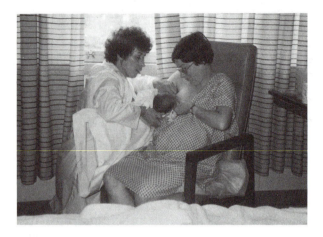

FIGURE 9–1   Lactation consultant assisting mother at eye-level during first breastfeeding.

raise the bed to bring her to your eye level. When an individual is engaging in *any* kind of new activity, anyone standing higher than the learner provokes anxiety in the learner.

4. Help to *position the baby's head so that it is snuggled securely in the mother's arms and rotated toward her.* This permits the mother to easily maintain eye contact with her baby. By cradling the infant's upper thigh or the buttock of his lower leg with her arm, the mother can change the baby's position with ease.

5. *Ask the mother to support her breast with her hand,* keeping her thumb well above the areola and the rest of her fingers below and under the breast. This is sometimes called the "C-hold." In this position, the mother is able to lift the breast and to guide her nipple in any direction as she assists the baby in taking more of the areola in his mouth. By lifting her breast slightly, she can easily maintain the infant's airway. (See Fig. 9–2.)

6. Help the mother position her baby so that his nose is at the level of the mother's nipple. Ask the mother to brush her nipple lightly against the baby's lower lip. *When the infant opens his mouth wide (rooting reflex) in response to this stimuli, signal the mother to bring it to her breast in one quick movement of her hand or forearm, slipping the nipple in towards the upper part of his wide open mouth.* Bringing the baby to the breast at the exact moment that his mouth is at its widest gape is desirable because it maximizes the amount of breast tissue he grasps. The baby's lower lip should be flanged outward and his nose resting against the surface of the breast so that he can easily breathe. (See Fig. 9–3.)

7. Explain that for these early feedings, *her infant should be offered both breasts at each feeding to stimulate the need-supply response.* In some cases, the neonate will suckle only one breast well before falling asleep. As long as each breast is offered frequently (at least every two hours), single-breast feeds of whatever duration the baby wishes are an appropriate option until the baby shows a desire for both breasts (Woolridge, Ingram & Baum, 1990). Suggest that the

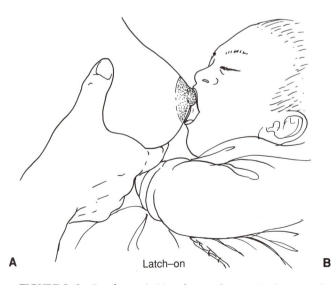

A   Latch–on

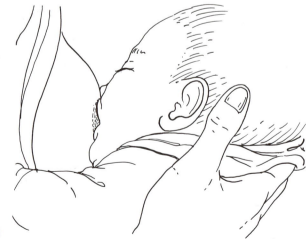

B

FIGURE 9–2   Latch-on. **A,** Mouth gaped open. **B,** Grasping breast.

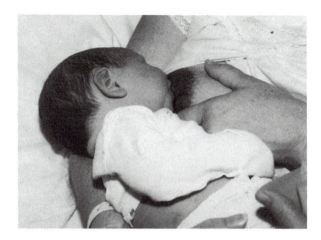

FIGURE 9–3   The "C" hold.

mother feed until she becomes relaxed to the point of sleepiness—a delightful side effect of oxytocin secretion (Mulford, 1990)—or until she notes cues from the infant suggesting satiety (suckling activity ceases or he falls asleep). The length of the feedings is up to her; she need not watch a clock.

8. If the mother elects to end a feeding before her baby has slipped off the breast or pushed the nipple out of his mouth, *teach her how to break the infant's suction on the breast* by placing her finger in the corner of his mouth between his gums.

Occasionally an otherwise healthy newborn will not latch on to his mother's breast nor suckle even after several attempts. Most nurses and lactation consultants have witnessed the frustrating situation in which a distraught mother repeatedly tries to breastfeed her neonate for the first time. The baby's lack of interest may be due to labor-related or postbirth narcotics, to the infant's neurological immaturity, or to inappropriate timing by those who attempt to promote suckling before the baby is rousable and shows active interest.

Although the epidural has been called the "cadillac of obstetrical anesthesia" and allows the mother to be awake during a cesarean birth, Standley, Klein, and Soule (1974) showed that infants of mothers receiving epidurals (lidocaine, tetracaine, mepivicaine, and bupivicaine) were more irritable and less mature in motor activity than controls. Unfortunately, in this study, no distinction was made among the drugs used. Rosenblatt et al. (1981) found dose-related reduced motor organization, poor self-quieting skills, and a decrease in visual skills and alertness among infants whose mothers receive epidural bupivicaine. The lack of careful studies identifying the short- and long-term effects, if any, of maternal medications on suckling behavior in the neonate is one of many areas of lactation and breastfeeding in need of further research.

Most maternal and infant problems will solve themselves with time: meanwhile, the infant should not go without nourishment or fluids for a long period. We recommend the following guidelines for intervention when the infant does not latch-on to the breast soon after birth.

INTERVENTION GUIDELINES WHEN NEONATE DOES NOT LATCH-ON TO THE BREAST FOLLOWING BIRTH

If the infant has not latched-on to the breast by 12 hours following birth (or after two to three feeding attempts), the following interventions are appropriate:

• Continue to put the infant at the breast at least eight times/day.
• Ask the mother to pump her breast in order to stimulate her milk supply after each feeding attempt.
• Give the infant pumped breastmilk using a regular syringe, peridontal syringe, or other feeding-tube device—or by finger feeding. (See "Instructions for Finger-Feeding a Neonate," which follow.)
• Alternate syringe feedings with putting the infant on the breast while continuing feedings using a #5 French gavage tube attached to the syringe or a feeding-tube device, if necessary.
• Continue to alternate syringe feedings with regular breastfeedings for 48 hours.
• Supplements should be human milk or formula, not glucose or sterile water.

INSTRUCTIONS FOR FINGER-FEEDING A NEONATE*

- Make sure that your hands are clean and your nails are short before you begin finger-feeding. In some institutions, wearing a rubber glove or finger cott is required when the baby is finger-fed by someone other than the mother or father. Babies do not always respond well to the feel or taste of rubber in their mouths. If the baby refuses to suck when finger-feeding is attempted, and the person finger-feeding is wearing a glove or a finger cott, assume that the baby is rejecting the glove or cott, not the attempt at finger-feeding.

- Place the baby in the football or cradle position, or prop him high in your lap. This may require the use of a pillow in your lap while your legs are elevated on a footstool in order to keep the baby comfortably in place. If you are using a dropper or syringe, both hands will be needed.

- When using a dropper, avoid squeezing the milk into the baby's mouth. This can cause gagging, aspiration, and other problems, particularly if the baby is not ready to suck when the milk is squeezed into his mouth. A more appropriate approach is to drip a drop or two into the baby's mouth so that the taste of the milk results in the baby starting to suck.

- When using a feeding tube device that can be worn around the neck, the tube can be held or taped to the finger. If tape is used, it should be placed back far enough on the finger and tube so that the tape is not drawn into the baby's mouth. Fluid can loosen the tape.

- When using a feeding tube device, a medium tube is appropriate in most cases involving a normal full-term neonate. However, small or large tubing may be necessary, depending on the baby's sucking response and his overall condition. In cases in which the baby's suck is very poor, and the goal is to present as much milk with as little effort by the baby as possible, both tubes of the same size (e.g., the smallest tubing), can be used at the same time.

- Select a finger that is about the same size as the breadth of the mother's nipple.

- Slide the finger in so that the pad side touches the baby's hard palate and nail bed rests on his tongue. Your finger should be in the baby's mouth past the alveolar ridge (gum line), but not so deep in his mouth that you trigger the gag reflex. In most instances, the baby will begin suckling as soon as he feels the finger pad on the hard palate.

- If the baby is suckling appropriately, the person who is finger-feeding the baby will feel a pulling sensation along the nail bed with each exertion of negative pressure (suckle), as if the nail is being pulled deeper into the baby's mouth, and feel a reduction of such pressure when the baby swallows. The suck-swallow pattern will be rhythmic.

- Record the amount of human milk (or formula) that the baby takes with each finger-feeding. Neonates should be offered 1–2 ounces with each such feeding. Many times, the baby will take some but not all of this amount. By offering a bit more than you expect the baby will take, you prevent him from sucking air through the tube after he has drained all of the milk from the container.

- Record the baby's response to finger-feeding, including his willingness to do so, his suck pattern, the duration of rhythmic suckling, the presence (if any) of nonrhythmic suckling, and any difficulties the baby exhibited.

- After showing the mother how to finger-feed, help her to learn how to do so, particularly if you anticipate that the baby may need more finger-feedings, or they are likely to occur when you are not available to assist.

*Derived from Walker, M: *Breastfeeding Premature Babies* (Unit 14), Lactation Consultant Series, Garden City Park, N.Y., 1991, Avery Publishing Group, Inc., p. 23.

HYPOGLYCEMIA

Hypoglycemia, a deficiency of blood glucose, is partially a matter of definition. Whether a baby is considered to have low blood sugar depends on the laboratory values the physician uses as a criterion for hypoglycemia. Before deciding what is abnormal, it must first be established what is normal. On the basis of research findings from a large sample of well, term infants, Heck and Erenberg (1987) recommend that hypoglycemia in full-term infants be defined as serum glucose concentration of less than 30 mg/dL in the first day of life or less than 40 mg/dL in the second day of life. According to another study (Sexson, 1984), if the higher level of 40 mg/dL is used, 20.6% of well, term infants would be considered hypoglycemic and unnecessarily receive glucose water.

Hypoglycemia is most often a concern for the infant of a mother with diabetes, a postmature neonate, or a small-for-gestational-age infant. The infant of a diabetic mother is most apt to experience hypoglycemia shortly after birth because the newborn continues to produce high levels of insulin, which deplete the blood glucose, within hours after birth. The degree of infant hypoglycemia usually is in proportion to the success achieved in controlling the mother's blood sugar during pregnancy. Symptomatic neonates are given 10% to 15% glucose intravenously immediately after birth until the baby stabilizes.

Postmature infants also need early frequent breastfeedings to normalize their glucose levels. Lethargy and poor feeding in these babies may contribute to increased hypoglycemia; thus, any interest shown in feeding should be followed by immediate, unrestricted access to the breast as often as the baby wishes. Most postmature neonates, after a first breastfeed, show increased interest in subsequent breastfeeding, thus reducing the risk of continued hypoglycemia.

The newborn who is small for its gestational age is also at risk for hypoglycemia. Prompt first breastfeeding followed by very frequent nursing thereafter is usually sufficient to bring the baby's blood glucose level to normal. In some cases poor feeding may require a supplement, but this practice need not continue once the baby is nursing well.

Whenever glucose feeds are offered to the neonate, whether as a routine or in an attempt to resolve a problem such as hypoglycemia, the health-care worker needs to be mindful of the negative effects such feedings have on infant interest in breastfeeding and effective suckling at the breast. Unless nonhuman milk is used, any fluid (such as sterile water or glucose) that is substituted for breastfeedings will result in a lower calorie feed and subsequent greater early weight loss than is likely to occur from colostrum-to-mature milk feedings (Glover & Sandilands, 1990). Such a reduction in caloric intake must be considered a risk to avoid if possible. If deemed essential, limit such feedings to as few as possible.

Problems which are most likely to be of concern in the early days of breastfeeding relate to method of birth, breast engorgement, sore nipples, and other perceived problems that usually disappear quickly. This next section focuses on breastfeeding events during the early postpartum period. In a summary of research on breastfeeding problems during the first week postpartum, Kearney, Cronenwett, and Barrett (1990) found that mothers voiced concerns about the following issues: sore nipples, insufficient or inadequate milk supply, infant sleepiness, infant fussiness, maternal fatigue, and too-frequent feeding. (See also Humenick and Van Steenkiste, 1983; Chapman et al., 1985; Mogan, 1986; and Graef et al., 1988.) In all cases, we note fallacies in assuming that all such concerns will be experienced by all women and discuss how each might be prevented or resolved if they do occur.

CESAREAN BIRTHS

Cesarean birth has been implicated in reducing the likelihood of breastfeeding in the United States, although similar findings have not been found in other countries (Padawer et al., 1988; Victora et al., 1990). Such a finding may be related to various factors. For example, an unexpected and unplanned cesarean delivery is usually a major disappointment for the mother. In addition, recovery from major surgery takes more time, is more painful, and represents additional risks compared to an uneventful vaginal birth. A woman may interpret such a birth as a reflection on her adequacy as a woman. To the degree that she feels violated, the shock of the cesarean birth may also reflect on her self-esteem. Some Asian women consider a cesarean birth to be a form of mutilation (Taylor, 1985).

Often the mother who has an unplanned cesarean

birth may be more anxious about herself as a woman and more fearful that she will fail at breastfeeding because she perceives that she failed with birthing (Pietz, 1989). "From the waist up, I felt like a success; from the waist down, a failure!" In these few words one mother summed up the feelings of guilt, frustration, and loss of self-esteem that a cesarean mother may experience. The sensitive care-giver can assist the mother to see that breastfeeding is not another proving ground, but rather an affirmation of her femininity, a experience that she need not forgo because she had an operative delivery.

The type of labor and birth medication influences how soon mother and baby begin breastfeeding. The attachment process is often delayed for mothers who have delivered by cesarean because they need extra time to recover before they can move into mothering and breastfeeding. Crawley, Hedahl, and Pegg (1983), as well as Lie and Juul (1988) found that mothers who had epidural rather than general anesthesia for surgery not only held and breastfed their babies sooner, but nursed longer than women who had general anesthesia. This finding held with elective vs. emergency cesarean.

Early lactation failure occurs more frequently following cesarean birth. Ellis and Hewat (1984) indicate that inconsistent hospital assistance, plus lack of a support system (Grossman et al., 1990) after the cesarean, may play a role in such untimely weaning. The mother's commitment to breastfeeding plays a substantial role despite unexpected birth outcomes. A greater commitment to breastfeeding, regardless of the manner of birth, results in longer duration of breastfeeding (Janke, 1988). When mothers give birth to premature infants, and the birth is by cesarean section, they are significantly *more* likely to provide milk for the pre-term baby than are women who have given birth vaginally. Difficulties appear to strengthen a committed mother's resolve to breastfeed. More recently, Kearney, Cronenwett, and Reinhardt (1990) report the impact of cesarean delivery on the time of first breastfeeding. Mothers giving birth by cesarean had a later first breastfeeding, and expressed less satisfaction with the birth experience, than did those who delivered vaginally. The delayed first breastfeeding, however, did not affect breastfeeding duration.

In working with a mother who has had a cesarean birth, the nurse or the lactation consultant needs to assess the mother's degree of physical comfort and awareness. If she is not fully conscious, she is not ready to put her baby to breast. If the mother is alert and able to hold her baby, however, she can begin breastfeeding.

The mother should be asked how she wants to hold her infant. Some mothers, particularly those still receiving intravenous pain medication or those who have had a narcotic epidural, are quite comfortable holding their babies in the cradle position. Others are hesitant to hold the baby at all until they have been reassured that they can do so without touching or placing any pressure near their abdominal incision. (See Fig. 9–4.) Suggest that if the mother holds her baby in a football (clutch) position she will avoid the sensitive incision area. (See Fig. 9–11.)

The baby born by cesarean birth may be lethargic, particularly if the birth followed a long period of exposure to analgesia or anesthesia in labor. If so, explain to the mother that a delay in feeding will not deter breastfeeding; rather, her milk supply will be established slightly later than it would following a vaginal birth (Moon & Humenick, 1989). If, as a result of early bottle-feedings, the mother is concerned about infant nipple confusion, reassure her that some babies are affected by this to a greater degree than others, but that it can be overcome. Observation of the baby at the breast will enable the lactation consultant or nurse to evaluate the extent to which the baby has been affected by bottle-feedings and to offer appropriate help to restore suckling at breast during subsequent feedings.

As the mother progresses through her postpartum course, breastfeeding will sometimes be satisfying; at other times not. When she is very tired, for example, she may be easily frustrated if the baby does not readily take the breast or suckle enthusiastically. At other feedings, the new mother will be gratified to find that she and her baby need little or no assistance—proof that each is learning to work with the other. The mother may need an occasional reminder that both she and her baby are learning a new skill; she should expect that some feedings will go better than others. The goal is not to have a perfect breastfeeding each time, but rather many opportunities for each to learn about—and from—the other. This uneven pattern from one feeding to another characterizes early feeding behavior following both vaginal and cesarean births.

Epidural morphine and other narcotics given following cesarean birth relieve pain so effectively that

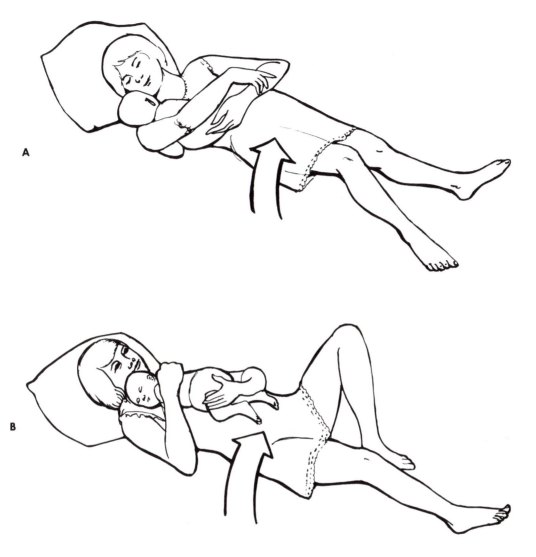

FIGURE 9–4   **A** and **B**, Transferring infant to other breast following a cesarean birth. (Concept from K. Frantz and B. A. Kalmen.)

many women are up and about within hours of delivery (Rimar, 1986). A longer postpartum hospital stay following a cesarean birth enables a woman to benefit from direct assistance for a somewhat longer period. The effect of epidural narcotics—such as fentanyl given before birth—on the neonate's suckling is not known.

Another unknown is the effect of antihistamines, which are used to relieve generalized itching, a common reaction in a mother who has had epidural morphine following a cesarean birth or a birth in which she has sustained a severe tear. Trimeprazine tartrate (Temaril) is a phenothiazine. Since phenothi-

azines usually increase milk supply, theoretically, this class of medications should not affect breastfeeding. Furthermore, they are not considered harmful to the infant. Benadryl (diphenhydramine) is also used; sometimes it is mixed with Narcan or Nubaine to counteract pruritis in the mother. Diphenhydramine (see Chapter 6) appears to decrease the milk supply; therefore, its use should be avoided and an alternate drug should be selected instead.

As the pain of her incision decreases, the mother can be instructed and assisted in the use of positions other than the football hold. By the second or third day postpartum, side-lying is generally comfortable,

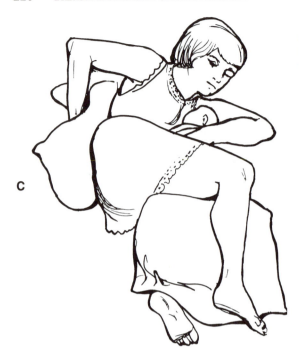

FIGURE 9–4   **C,** Transferring infant to other breast following a cesarean birth.

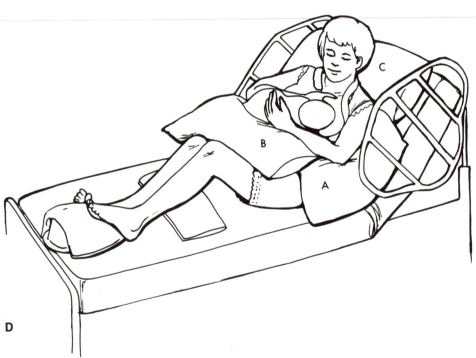

FIGURE 9–4   **D,** Comfortable position for breastfeeding especially for women who have delivered by cesarean section. (Concept from K. Frantz and B. A. Kalmen.)

especially if the mother is adequately supported with pillows at her back and beneath her abdomen. Encouraging the mother to decide when she would like to nurse the baby in the cradle position will help her to see herself as being in charge of at least *this* aspect of her own progress. Just as with a vaginal birth, frequent feedings stimulate milk production after a cesarean. This should be emphasized to the mother as a means of helping her to feel that she shares yet another similarity with women whose births were what she expected but did not experience.

BREAST FULLNESS VS. ENGORGEMENT

Maternal engorgement is a major issue in most discussions of early breastfeeding. Such preoccupation stems from many factors, not the least of which is the assumption that the condition is normal; that is, that it occurs in all breastfeeding women. Most published materials continue to present the condition as a norm or an *indication* of early lactation. This assumption is, in part, incorrect. While the gradual build-up of fluid in the breasts following parturition is a welcome sign of breast milk, breast engorgement and breast fullness are two different matters. The nearly universal experience of transient breast fullness does not prevent the infant from feeding; however, clinical engorgement usually precludes breastfeeding. The distinction between breast fullness and breast engorgement may be seen in Newton and Newton's (1948) operational definitions of these two conditions, from which many later discussions derive. However, often such discussions do not note that the Newtons' definitions provide a four-step progression, beginning with mild fullness, which, if mishandled, can result in severe breast engorgement. (See Table 9–2.)

As noted in Table 9–2, with breast fullness, the mother's breast tissue remains compressible, thus enabling the infant to suckle comfortably and efficiently, without risk of trauma to the breast or nipple tissue. Breast fullness rarely lasts more than 24 hours, during which time breastfeeding can continue without discomfort. The mother with breast fullness should be encouraged to view this state as a transitory indication of an increase in milk production which will begin to regulate to meet the baby's needs as the infant suckles. She should be encouraged to offer the breast frequently to reduce the likelihood that breast fullness will become breast engorgement.

TABLE 9–2 DIFFERENCES BETWEEN BREAST FULLNESS AND BREAST ENGORGEMENT

Systemic Characteristics	Breast Fullness	Breast Engorgement*
Onset of symptoms	2–4 days	2–10 days
Site	Bilateral	Bilateral
Swelling	Generalized	Generalized
Heat	Occasional	Generalized
Pain	None–rare	Generalized
Palpation of breast	Soft	Hard
Breast tenderness	None	Generalized
Body temperature	<38°C	>38.4°C
Maternal symptoms	Feels well	Breast tightness, discomfort

*Derived in part from Lawrence, RA: *Breastfeeding: A guide for the medical profession*, St. Louis, 1989, The C.V. Mosby Co., p. 209.

Breast engorgement, by contrast, is often the consequence of mismanagement of the normal state of transient breast fullness caused by the delay and/or restriction in duration and frequency of breastfeeding. Such delay or restriction allows milk stasis to occur. The infant then finds it difficult or impossible to grasp the severely engorged breast. When the baby is unable to suckle, the mother's discomfort mounts, and her breast and nipple tissue may be so significantly stretched that even leaking cannot occur. Under such conditions, further trauma to the tissue is apt to occur when a vigorous baby attempts unsuccessfully to grasp and draw the nipple and areola into his mouth. Numbness and tingling of the mother's hand and arm may occur with severe engorgement because of pressure on brachial plexus nerves in the axilla (Simkin, 1988).

A fever of unknown origin in a mother during the first week postpartum is another sign of breast engorgement. If she is breastfeeding, how often and how long her infant is suckling should be assessed. If the baby feeds less often than eight times in 24 hours and for less than an *average* of 15 minutes per feeding, it is not enough. If the mother is unable to increase the number of feedings, she may obtain relief with the judicious use of hand expression or an electric breast pump set on intermittent *minimum* pressure. Under no circumstances should a mother whose breasts are engorged be allowed to use an electric breast pump that does not provide *intermittent* minimum pressure. Pumping should also be limited to a maximum duration of 10 minutes to avoid traumatizing the distended breast tissues.

If the woman is not breastfeeding and her breasts are engorged, she needs instruction in gentle breast massage and the use of warm showers followed by cool compresses to reduce her discomfort while her body is ceasing to produce milk. Washcloths or small towels, wrung out in water and folded, serve as inexpensive, moist compresses and are less time consuming than showers. Immersing her breasts in a basin of tepid water also may work well if the mother takes care to avoid a backache. Wearing a tight-fitting breast binder is unnecessary and should be avoided in the interests of reducing the risks of iatrogenically induced mastitis.

The United States Food and Drug Administration (FDA press release, September, 1989) recommends against the use of bromocriptine and related dopamine receptor antagonists when the need for medication is minimal. Less than 10% of women have been found to need drug therapy to control symptoms of breast engorgement when they do not breastfeed. The serious side effects of bromocriptine—including stroke (Watson, et al., 1989), myocardial infarction (Ruch & Duhring, 1989), puerperal seizures (Rothman, Runch & Dreyer, 1990), and postpartum psychosis (Canterbury et al., 1987)—support its avoidance. In addition, women who have received lactation suppressants often report significant rebound engorgement after withdrawal of the medication. Usually rebound engorgement occurs after the mother has left the hospital, so the likelihood that she will be seen by a knowledgeable health-care worker is reduced.

A nipple shield is sometimes offered in a well-meaning attempt to reduce engorgement. However, a nipple shield neither reduces engorgement nor enables the neonate to suckle effectively. While pressure from the rubber teat of the shield against the roof of the baby's mouth activates the suck response, the severely engorged breast will not be milked since the negative pressure created by the baby's suckling serves only to compress the rubber nipple shield. In addition, using a nipple shield that has inner bumps, or striations of rubber on the flange surrounding the nipple to "stimulate" the breast, only causes additional trauma to already tender, bruised tissue.

Moon and Humenick (1989) identified several factors that increase the risk of breast engorgement. They found that supplementing the breastfeeding infant with other feeds contributes to breast engorgement, while allowing breastfeedings to last as long as the mother and baby wish decreases breast engorgement. There is wide variation in the length of a feeding. Between the fifth and seventh day postpartum, a baby may spend from 7 to 30 minutes at the breast. The mean is about 17 minutes (Howie, Houston & Cook, 1981). Breast changes are also related to the timing of the first feed; mothers feeding soon after birth are more likely to have full breasts sooner than mothers whose first feeding is delayed. Mothers have fewer breast changes following a cesarean birth than a vaginal birth because of the usual pattern of delayed breastfeeding among women who have experienced a cesarean birth. (See Table 9–3.) Moreover, primiparous women are more likely to have early breast engorgement and to breastfeed for a shorter duration than multiparous women. This probably reflects greater sensitivity in primiparous

TABLE 9–3   KEY FACTORS RELATED TO BREAST ENGORGEMENT

	Vaginal Birth	Cesarean Birth	Primiparous Mother	Multiparous Mother
Number of hours before first feeding	–.26^*	–.52**	–.44**	–.07
Number of times to breast in 48 hours	.12	.36*	.49**	–.07
Cumulative duration of feedings in 48 hours	–.51**	–.78	–.66**	–.64**

^ = correlation
* = p<.05>.10
** = p<.05

Derived from Moon, JL, and Humenick, SS: Breast engorgement: contributing variables and variables amenable to nursing intervention, *JOGNN* 18:309–15, 1989.

Dear Nurse:

IF I AM A HEALTHY, FULL TERM BABY,

1. Please don't give me any water bottles, formula, or pacifiers.
2. I eat "on demand" or q 2–3 hr., whichever comes first, a.m. & p.m.
3. I may be allowed to sleep one 4–5 hr. period at night—if I have already had 8 feedings that day.
4. My mom allows "bunching" (i.e., frequent feedings) whenever I want it.
5. My mom feeds me from both breasts at each feeding for as long as I want. (Mom won't get sore as long as my grasp of her nipple is correct.)
6. My mom wants to feed me 8–12 times in 24 hrs.
7. THANK YOU FOR HELPING ME GET OFF TO A GOOD START!

_____Mother's signature
Reprint with Permission & Credit
Lactation Consultants of Cincinnati

Jo Williams   Susan Mueller
(513) 251–3176   (513) 542–2576
© 1988

From Williams, J, and Mueller, S: A message to the nurse from the baby, *J Hum Lact* 5:19, 1989. Reprinted with permission.

women to breast changes, even minor ones. The notice shown above can be posted on the baby's crib in the hospital as a reminder not to feed supplements to the infant.

SORE NIPPLES

Transient nipple soreness appears to be normal for the breastfeeding mother in the early postpartum period. It occurs in a majority of breastfeeding mothers in the first week postpartum, peaks between the third and the sixth day, and then recedes (Chapman et al., 1985; deCarvalho, Robertson & Klaus, 1984; Gosha & Tichy, 1988; Gunther, 1945; Hewat & Ellis, 1987; Riordan, 1985; Ziemer et al., 1990).

If nipple soreness increases or lasts beyond the first week, a number of factors may be responsible.

Pain is a warning that something is wrong; since breastfeeding is a two-person activity, it is imperative to consider both partners when assessing possible causes of protracted nipple pain and trauma. (See the list highlighted below.)

Recent research findings indicate what is known at this time. For example, deCarvalho and colleagues (1984) found that early breastfeeding discomfort was related neither to the frequency nor to the duration of feedings. In their sample of mothers, nipple pain peaked at three days postpartum and declined rapidly thereafter. Hewat and Ellis (1987) also found that feeding frequency was unrelated to nipple pain and trauma. They confirmed that skin color, hair color, or prenatal nipple preparation did not make a difference in preventing tenderness. Furthermore, the application of human milk or colostrum rather than a commercial lanolin preparation made no difference in the pain levels reported. Ziemer et al. (1990) discovered that 96% of the women in their study reported nipple pain and that skin color is not associated with nipple pain.

Infant suckling patterns can contribute to nipple tenderness in the mother, particularly if the baby's first suckling has been conditioned by a rubber teat from bottle-feeding or a pacifier (Newman, 1990; Riordan, 1980b). Another factor that has recently been "rediscovered" is the effect of a frenulum attached too near the tip of the tongue as a cause of nipple or areolar abrasions (Berg, 1990; Marmet, Shell & Marmet, 1990; Notestine, 1990; Wilton, 1990). Careful evaluation of the infant at the breast, therefore, will include asking the mother how the breast feels when the baby is suckling as well as an examination of the frenulum. The following assessments also should be made:

1. *What do the baby's cheeks look like?* The baby's cheeks should round outward if he is suckling effectively. When the cheeks are drawn inward, causing "dimpling," it is an indication that the baby may be tongue sucking rather than stimulating the maternal milk-ejection response. Thus, the baby is not receiving milk.
2. *Where is the baby's tongue?* Pull the corner of the baby's mouth slightly away from the breast while the baby is suckling. The tongue should be visible under the areolar tissue and nipple, and forward over the baby's gumline. If the tongue is not visible, it may be curled back-

---

SOME CAUSES OF SORE NIPPLES

Maternal issues

Unrelieved negative pressure

Secondary or pathologic breast engorgement

Flat or retracted nipples

Breaking suction improperly

Sensitivity to nipple creams, lotions or oils

Delayed healing of cracks or abrasions from use of creams, soaps, ointments, or oils

Improper or excessive use of breast pumps

Using nipple shields

Prolonged exposure to wet nursing pads or to moisture build-up in poorly vented milk cups (breast shells)

Thrush (Johnstone & Marcinak, 1990)

Lack of nipple exposure to light and air

Infant issues

Improper infant positioning at breast

Disorganized or dysfunctional infant suckling

Thrush (Johnstone & Marcinak, 1990)

Derived from Walker, M, and Driscol, JW: Sore nipples: the new mother's nemesis, *MCN* 14:260–65, 1989.

---

wards. If the tongue does not extend over the gumline and the mother complains of pain when the baby is nursing, check for a short frenulum or one whose attachment prevents the tongue from extending forward sufficiently to allow effective suckling.

3. *What do you hear when the baby is suckling?* Listen to the baby. A baby who is breastfeeding effectively will make a swallowing sound that is sometimes very quiet, but which will occur after one to three sucks. Additionally, no "slurping" sounds should be heard; this is usually an indication that the baby is sucking his own tongue or is not creating a complete seal around the areola.

4. *How tight is the baby's seal on the breast?* Check the suction of the baby on the breast. If a good seal is formed, the mother may need to insert her finger into the side of the baby's mouth to effect removal without causing pain. If the baby easily falls from the breast when he appears to be suckling actively, the seal is inadequate.

The baby is only one member of the breastfeeding partnership. The mother's breasts need to be inspected too. Simply noting the position of bruises on the breast may indicate the cause of the problem. For example, if too much of the top of the areola, and too little of the bottom, is drawn into the baby's mouth, stretching and cracking of nipple tissue on the underside of the breast is likely. If the mother complains about nipple tenderness, ask her to visualize a clock face superimposed on her breast and indicate where there is a bruise or a crack. If the baby suckles too low on the breast or too close to the tip of the nipple, trauma is most likely to occur between 10 to 12 o'clock and 4 to 6 o'clock positions on the right breast; on the left breast, the areas of maximum tenderness will occur between 12 to 2 o'clock and 6 to 8 o'clock positions. Simply bringing the baby closer to the mother's body so that the tip of his nose brushes the mother's breast tissue is usually all that is needed to enable the tender areas to heal. (See Fig. 9–5.)

In cases where both a crack and a bruise are evident, bathing the crack with fresh expressed milk will aid healing and prevent bacterial infection. Usually, the crack will close and scab over prior to the disappearance of the bruise.

Unfortunately, hospital personnel often advise limiting the duration of feedings to prevent or treat sore nipples. Hospital staff rarely see the mother after discharge and, with today's brief hospital stays, they may continue to hold the erroneous belief that restriction of time at the breast is a good preventive measure. In reality, putting a time limit on the length of each feeding has several negative effects. First, it

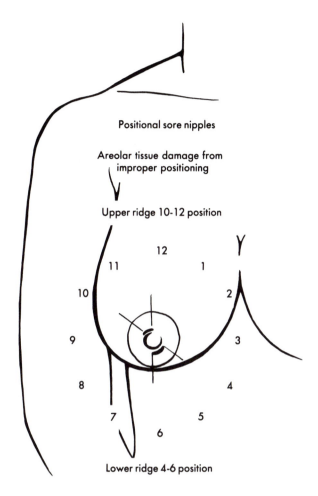

Positional sore nipples

Areolar tissue damage from improper positioning

Upper ridge 10-12 position

Lower ridge 4-6 position

FIGURE 9–5   Imagine the face of a clock superimposed on right breast. Soreness usually develops in the crescent around the perimeter of the nipple at 10 to 12 o'clock position and below the perimeter of the nipple at 4 to 6 o'clock position. With the left breast, maximal potential for soreness is, similarly, at 12 to 2 o'clock and 6 to 8 o'clock positions.

simply delays nipple soreness (Whitley, 1974). Second, short feedings prevent the baby from receiving the creamy hind milk. Finally, if the feed is very short, it may end before the milk ejection occurs; that is particularly true in the early feedings after birth when the let-down reflex may take several minutes to begin.

Nipple ointments are commonly used for sore nipples. There is little evidence that ointments or creams have a salutary effect either on nipple healing or on soreness, although they are still widely recommended and sold (especially lanolin-based oint-

ments). Newton (1952) investigated the effect of hydrous lanolin and vitamin A&D preparation and reported no significant reduction of nipple soreness when compared to the use of plain water. Brown and Hurlock (1975) evaluated Massé cream using three groups of women: those who prepared their breasts prenatally using nipple rolling, those who expressed colostrum, and those who applied Massé cream. No significant differences among the three treatment groups were found. Riordan (1985) compared postpartum mothers who used lanolin cream, tea bags and no treatment; she demonstrated that these treatments neither prevented nor reduced nipple soreness.

Some nipple treatments are, in fact, potentially harmful. Some institutions have discontinued using lanolin for breastfeeding mothers since pesticides have been found in Australian and U.S. samples (Rosanove, 1987; Copeland, Raebel & Wagner, 1989). Other investigators consider the levels of pesticides in the lots tested to be low and not hazardous (Morse, 1989). Marx et al. (1985) found increased serum concentrations of vitamin E in breastfeeding babies after six days of ingesting milk from their mothers who were applying vitamin E to their nipples.

The mini-guide on pp. 232–233 describes many of the commonly used agents for nipple soreness. In considering each item's use, the care provider needs to keep in mind that two people are exposed to the product in question whenever it is used on the mother's nipples. What may be appropriate use for the mother may expose the infant to unnecessary risk. If the product must be removed completely from the nipple to avoid infant exposure, the care provider needs to consider if such action is self-defeating for the mother and/or if some other element might be more appropriate.

Nicholson (1986) investigated three separate treatments for cracked nipples: expressing milk and not breastfeeding while the cracked nipple was healing; using a nipple shield during breastfeeding; and continuing breastfeeding while receiving assistance designed to improve the baby's position on the breast. She found no significant differences in outcome. Gosha and Tichy (1988) provided new mothers with a breast shell designed with multiple air holes and found that postpartum nipple pain was unaffected by its use.

Some practitioners (Pevarski, 1991) claim that

Commonly Used Agents for Sore Nipples

Name	A&D Ointment (Schering Corp., Galloping Hill Rd., Kenilworth, NJ 07033; 201–558–4000; 1–800–526–4099)
Description	Ointment in a tube
Ingredients	Anhydrous lanolin, petrolatum, fragrance, mineral oil, fish liver oil, and cholecalciferol
Comments	For *external use* only. In case of ingestion, contact a poison control center. There are no vitamins in this ointment.

Name	Bag Balm (Dairy Association, Inc., Lyndonville, VT 05851; 802–626–3610)
Description	Stiff yellow ointment
Ingredients	Petrolatum, lanolin, 8-hydroxyquinoline sulfate, sanitas, and water
Comments	A fungistat and bacteriocide for farm use. *Not for internal use* since 1969 because it causes cancer in laboratory animals.

Name	Eucerin Cream (Beiersdorf, PO Box 5529, Norwalk, CT 06856; 203–853–8008)
Description	Cream in a jar
Ingredients	Petrolatum, mineral oil, mineral wax, wool wax alcohol, methylchloroiso-thisazo-linone-methylisothiazolinone
Comments	For *external use* only.

Name	Mammol Ointment (Abbott Laboratories, Pharmaceutical Products Division, North Chicago, IL 60064; 708–937–7069)
Description	Ointment
Ingredients	Bismuth subnitrate, caster oil, anhydrous lanolin, ceresin wax
Comments	Advertised as a dressing for nipples of nursing mothers. However, instructions advise washing and drying nipples before and after use. **Warning**: Subnitrate may be reduced by bacteria in the bowel of infants to yield nitrate, which causes methemoglobinemia after absorption.

Name	Massé Cream (Ortho Pharmaceutical Corp., Raritan, NJ 08869; 201–524–0400)
Description	Cream in a tube
Ingredients	Glyceryl stearate, glycerin, cetyl alcohol, peanut oil, sorbitan stearate, stearic acid, polysorbate 60, sodium benzoate, propylparaben, methylparaben, potassium hydroxide
Comments	Advertised for pre- and postnatal nipple care. However, instructions advise cleansing the breasts before and after each nursing with a clean cloth and water. Contraindicated in mastitis and breast abscess. While most of the ingredients are innocuous, the glycerin is rapidly metabolized and can cause hyperglycemia. The cetyl alcohol is a laxative, and aspiration of peanut oil can cause severe and fatal bronchitis in small children.

Name	Moist towelettes, generic (while not "an agent for nipple soreness," some hospital staffs ask mothers to wipe their nipples with these.)
Description	Premoistened towelettes
Ingredients	Benzalkonium chloride 1:750, alcohol 20%
Comments	A germicide and sanitizer for surface cleaning. Toxic to laboratory animals. For preoperative disinfection of unbroken skin. Rinse thoroughly after use. For *external use* only.

Box continues

Name	Rotersept (Fair Laboratories, Ltd., United Kingdom)
Description	Antiseptic spray
Ingredients	Chlorhexidine gluconate, propellant gas, alcohol, acetone
Comments	Persistent antimicrobial effect against gram-negative and gram-positive bacteria. **Warning**: Avoid contact with eyes, ears, and mucous membranes. Effect of acetone is similar to anesthetic effect of ethyl alcohol. For *external use* only.
Name	USP Lanolin (Merck "Lanum") (Merck, Sharp, and Dohme, Division of Merck and Co., Inc., West Point, PA 19486; 215–661–5000)
Description	Tube or cream
Ingredients	Hydrous lanolin
Comments	Highly allergenic wool derivative. Analysis of a range of lanolin creams revealed all contained organophosporous pesticide residue including diazinon.
Name	USP Modified Lanolin ("Lansinoh") (Lansinoh Laboratories, Oak Ridge, TN 37830; 1–800–292–4794)
Description	Jar (1.5 ounce)
Ingredients	100% anhydrous, modified lanolin
Comments	Hypoallergenic. Estimated to contain under 1.5 ppm of combined impurities. No caution required for use on open wounds or where ingestion may occur.
Name	Vitamin E (generic)
Description	Vitamin capsules, oil, gelatin, or cream
Ingredients	Vitamin E in suspension; capsules = 400 IU each
Comments	U.S. recommended daily allowance for Vitamin E in infants is 5 IU/day. Effect of increased serum concentrations of Vitamin E is unknown.

References providing information on one or more of the above products:
Derived from *Drug Evaluations*, 6th ed., Chicago, 1986, American Medical Association Department of Drugs, Division of Drugs and Technology, in cooperation with the American Society for Clinical Pharmacology and Therapeutics; Gosselin, RE, Smith, RP, and Hodge, HC: *Clinical Toxicology of Commercial Products*, 5th ed., Baltimore, 1984, The Williams & Wilkins Co.; *Handbook of Nonprescription Drugs*, 7th ed. Washington, D.C., 1982, American Pharmaceutical Association; Marx, CM, et al.: Vitamin E concentrations in serum of newborn infants after topical use of vitamin E by nursing mothers, *Am J Obstet Gynecol* 152:668–70, 1985: Monheit, BM, and Luke, BG: Pesticides in breastmilk—a public health perspective, *Common Health Stud* 14:269–73, 1990; Morse, J: The hazards of lanolin, *Am J Mat-Child Nurs* 14:204, 1989; *Physician's Desk Reference for Non-Prescription Drugs*, 11th ed., Oradell, N.J., 1990, Medical Economics Co., Inc.; Po, ALW: *Non-prescription Drugs*, London, 1982, Blackwell Scientific Publications; Rosanove, R: Dangers of the application of lanolin (letter), *Med J Aust* 146:232, 1987; Spannraft, E: A hidden source of Vitamin E, *Am J Mat-Child Nurs* 14:204, 1989; *Springhouse Drug Reference*, Springhouse, Pa., 1988, Springhouse Publishing Co.

placing tea bags on sore and cracked nipples promotes healing and relieves pain (Jennie Pevarski, Roanoke, Virginia; personal communication, 1991). Tea, which contains tannic acid (an astringent), is a traditional home remedy for many skin problems. Astringents act by precipitating proteins at the surface of the cell and reducing the permeability of the membrane without killing the cell. Secretions are inhibited and the local inflammatory response is reduced. However, Riordan (1985) found no difference in the effect of tea bags and lanolin when they were compared.

The value of these studies may be limited since few took into account other contributing variables, such as the positioning of mother and infant for breastfeeding, cleansing the breast prior to feeding, and restricting the duration of suckling. In two cases, duration of breastfeeding was found *not* to increase the likelihood of nipple pain. These and other negative findings point the way toward eliminating routines that do not stand up to the scrutiny of careful investigation. See the clinical care plan for sore nipples in Table 9–4.

It is clear that we still know too little about the causes of nipple pain and trauma. For example, clinicians have long observed that the position of the infant at breast improves maternal comfort and infant suckling; yet there are still no studies that substantiate the role of positioning.

TABLE 9–4 CLINICAL CARE PLAN FOR SORE NIPPLES NURSING DIAGNOSIS: COMFORT, ALTERATION IN

Assessment	Interventions	Rationale
Nipples slightly red and chapped in light-skinned mother; appear shiny in very dark-skinned mother.	Reassure mother that discomfort is temporary and condition will improve.	Breast is sensitive at start of breastfeeding. Many mothers have some early nipple sensitivity.
Mother complains of soreness at latch-on or at start of pumping. Soreness subsides when milk-ejection reflex occurs.	Discontinue if soap or antiseptic is being used to clean breasts. Air-dry the nipples by leaving bra flaps down.	Maintains natural skin oils. Furnishes sufficient air to dry nipples.
Wincing as infant grasps breasts (or draws nipple into mouth).	"Fan" blow-dryer set on "warm air" over nipple right after feeding. Sit in sun or under 60-watt bulb, briefly exposing nipples. Use all-cotton bra. Remove any plastic liners. Massage breast to milk-ejection reflex to stimulate flow.	Softens nipple/breast before latch-on.
	Place crushed ice in plastic bag (covered by washcloth) to nipples.	Cold relieves discomfort.
Nipple sticks to bra or breast pad.	Moisten bra or breast pads before removing. Change pads more frequently.	Avoids removing keratin layer of skin.
Mother using breast cream.	Discontinue using cream and note any change.	
Crescent-shaped abrasions above and/or below the nipple. Nipple tip is blanched after suckling episode Discomfort and pain throughout feeding	Review position, making sure infant's mouth is open wide before latching-on and baby is held high on mother's chest wall with entire body facing mother. Reposition as necessary	Infant is gumming and pinching nipple and/or sliding up and down because of poor positioning.
Baby's tongue is retracted behind lower gum.	Draw infant in sufficiently so that breast is positioned deep in the baby's mouth.	Tongue retraction prevents normal perfusion to nipple.
	Bring tongue forward. Pull baby's lower lip out if it is drawn inward while feeding. Show mother alternative nursing positions.	Pressure on other areas of nipple allows healing of abraded areas.
Bright pinkish-red extending beyond nipple/areola. Mother complains of pain that extends throughout feeding.	Apply anti-fungal medication to nipples. Treat infant for thrush. Treat family for candidiasis.	Prompt treatment alleviates problem. Candidiasis spreads with warm, moist contact among family members.

LEAKING

Leaking is most likely to occur in the first month of breastfeeding, when infant needs and maternal responses are not yet well attuned to one another and when daily variability of feeding frequency and duration is greatest. A variety of stimuli may cause the mother's breasts to leak milk. The sound of her own or another's baby stirring or crying is a common stimulus. The scent of her baby's clothes, thinking about her baby, the sound of a breast pump (if she has been using one regularly), listening to music she has heard while breastfeeding, or seeing or using the chair she has used while breastfeeding often stimulate milk let-down or leaking.

Leaking varies greatly among mothers with respect to stimuli, amount of leaked milk, and the length of time the leaking continues. While most women will experience some leaking in the early weeks of breastfeeding, the amount of milk that drips is usually small and declines over time. Other mothers report leaking for a considerably longer period and/or leaking milk in quantities sufficient to soak a cloth diaper. Mothers need instruction in ways to reduce spontaneous milk release. Gentle pressure for a few seconds on a leaking breast is usually sufficient to cue it to retain milk until an "official" feeding. When modesty is not an issue, pressure can be applied with fingers or the palm of the hand. In a public setting, pressing the upper arm or elbow against the breast while touching one's earlobe or earring will usually be interpreted by others as an attempt to scratch one's ear or adjust an earring. When the mother feels her milk letting down, crossing both arms over her chest and pressing gently for 5–10 seconds usually stops the leaking. Only another breastfeeding mother is likely to recognize the maneuver as a means of halting inadvertent leaking. Leaking milk in the early postpartum period may serve as a "safety valve," since many women who have recurrent mastitis often report never having spontaneously dripped or leaked milk.

INSUFFICIENT MILK SUPPLY

Insufficient milk supply seems to be a major concern of many new mothers during the first few weeks postpartum; it is the reason given by many, especially in the United States, for early weaning and for supplementation. Although many women *fear* that they will not be able to produce enough milk to feed their babies (Tully & Dewey, 1985), the notion that many women have an insufficient milk supply is unsubstantiated. Some argue that mammalian survival has depended on sufficient milk production to enable the young of the species to survive. If milk insufficiency occurred frequently, the survival of the species would be in jeopardy. A recent study found that in 51 mother-infant pairs in Sweden, 55% of the mothers experienced "transient lactation crises, emanating mostly from a perception of breast milk insufficiency" (Hillervik-Lindquist, Hofvander & Sjölin, 1991). However, there was no difference in the milk intake during the crisis period compared to one week later. Although the babies of the mothers in the crisis group had lower weight at 2,3,4, and 9 months than the control group, neither group was below the NCHS (National Center for Health Statistics) mean for expected growth at those time periods. The authors concluded that insufficiency of breast milk may be a perceived problem, but that it is not reflected in actual reduction of milk production or in subsequent poor infant growth (Hillervik-Lindquist, Hofvander & Sjölin, 1991). Newman (1986) is one who suggests that milk insufficiency is mostly a nonproblem, generated in part by societal ignorance of normal breastfeeding and in part by iatrogenic elements that make breastfeeding difficult. His point is buttressed by the knowledge that the problem of insufficient milk is culturally bound. For example, it is milk *oversupply*, not undersupply, that is a major problem for breastfeeding women in Australia and New Zealand.

Before insufficient milk supply can be assumed to exist, a wide variety of factors which the mother may perceive as evidence of insufficient milk need to be ruled out. For example, if the mother does not know that breastfed infants need to feed frequently, she may conclude that her baby's need to do so indicates that she has insufficient milk. The reality is that the baby is not being offered the breast frequently enough. Milk production is a reflection of breast stimulation, as seen in the high levels of milk yield by women with twins and triplets (Saint, Maggiore & Hartmann, 1986; Hartmann, 1987).

In addition, infants typically have a sleep-wake cycle that includes a tendency for wakefulness in the late afternoon and evening (Emde, Gaensbauer & Harmon, 1976). This wakeful, sometimes fussy period at the end of the day may be particularly trying for the inexperienced mother who is unsure of her ability to breastfeed and unaware that wakefulness and frequent feeding at these times are entirely normal and do not reflect poor mothering skills (Riordan, 1990).

According to Walker (1989), the mother may complain of any one or more of the following:

The Baby
- is restless or irritable during or between feedings
- acts "hungry all the time," sucks his fists or blanket, moves his head rapidly from side to side at the breast
- comes off the nipple frequently
- cries or is fussy constantly, is difficult to console, is fussy right after a feeding
- has feedings that are excessively long
- takes formula from a bottle right after a feeding

- falls asleep at breast
- nurses less than 15 to 20 minutes on either or both breasts, leading the mother to believe she does not have enough milk.

The Mother

- does not feel the milk-ejection reflex as she thinks she should
- reports that her breasts feel soft before each feeding, not just afterwards
- cannot express much milk (or less than at previous times)
- has been told that frequent feedings indicate a decreased milk supply
- was told not to put baby to breast because of cracked nipples
- reports that her breasts did not enlarge or become tender during pregnancy; that she did not become engorged; or that she is concerned about previous breast surgery.

Others have noted that breastfeeding failure can occur after a mother has had significant stress (Ruvalcaba, 1987), as following the 1985 Mexican earthquake, after breast biopsy (Day, 1986), and when the mother is a smoker (Matheson, 1989; Woodward & Hand, 1988). These reports emphasize the need to rule out as many factors as possible which might have a direct or indirect influence on milk production before assuming that primary breast insufficiency exists.

A very few women may have a true low milk supply from congenital insufficient glandular tissue. In one of the first published discussions of the syndrome, Neifert, Seacat, and Jobe (1985) describe three cases. All of the women in the study had marked differences in breast size and/or shape. The authors infer that a lack of glandular tissue, a rare occurrence, explained the mothers' inability to produce sufficient quantities of milk in the face of a vigorously suckling infant and frequent feedings. If such a rare phenomenon is encountered, there is no need to discontinue breastfeeding. Rather, the mother can use a tube-feeding device to deliver additional nutrition to the infant while he is at the breast. In a later study, Neifert and colleagues (1990) found that women with an insufficient milk supply were more likely to report minimal breast enlargement during pregnancy and when their milk came in, compared with women who had adequate milk. Among the sample of women in this study, however, about 7%

had previous breast surgery, a much higher proportion than is normally found in breastfeeding populations.

The number of women with primary breast insufficiency is unknown. While it appears to exist in a few women, there is danger of this diagnosis as an explanation for conditions that render breastfeeding difficult or encourage women to distrust that their bodies can nourish their infants. Rather, effort should be made to identify and correct all other possible causes.

Further complicating the picture is the possibility that the mother's milk supply may decline as a secondary response to dysfunctional or ineffective suckling by the infant (Shrago & Bocar, 1990). Desmarais and Browne (1990) offer a detailed discussion of the ways in which the clinician can separate the responsibility of the baby from that of the mother, so as to improve to optimal level the milk production potential of the mother while preserving the nutritional integrity of the growing infant. They, like Hill and Humenick, also note the many ways in which factors unrelated to the mother's glandular tissue or the baby's ability to suckle can interfere with the way mother and baby interact. Hill and Humenick (1989) have proposed a conceptual model describing insufficient milk supply as well as some potential antecedents and indicators. (See Fig. 9–6.)

Metoclopramide (Reglan) given orally for several days is an option for treating a low milk supply. Clinicians have found metoclopramide to be very helpful for mothers of premature babies in rapidly building a good milk supply (and the mother's confidence). To date, no adverse effects have been observed in short-term use of the drug; however, long-term use may be associated with maternal depression.

BREAST MASSAGE

Massage has been used extensively and effectively during the childbearing period. It relieves the discomforts of labor and is often used for infant stimulation. Massage of the lactating breasts is common in many parts of the world and is often used to relieve engorged breasts. A lesser-known but time-honored practice which spans several cultures is breast massage to stimulate milk production and drainage.

A special technique, Alternate Breast Massage, wherein the mother alternately massages each

POTENTIAL
DETERMINANTS

INDICATORS

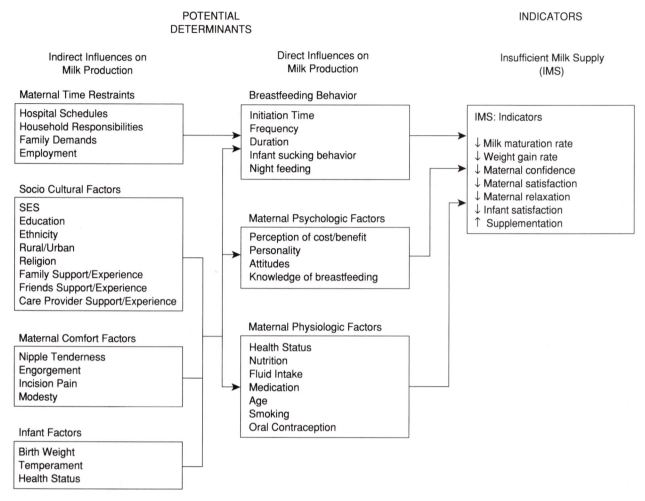

FIGURE 9–6   Insufficient milk supply: potential determinants and indicators. (From Hill, PD, and Humenick, SS: Insufficient milk supply, *Image* 21:145–48, 1989.)

breast, was developed by Iffrig (1968) and later tested by Bowles, Stutte, and Hensley (1988). The mother massages the base of her breast when she observes the infant begin rapid, shallow suckling movements. She then alternates massage with the infant's suckling. Infants of mothers using such breast massage have been reported to gain more weight than other infants whose mothers did not practice this technique (Bowles, Stutte & Hensley, 1988).

In Japan, one popular breast massage technique is the Oketani method, named after the nurse-midwife who developed it. This massage involves an elaborate sequence in which the entire breast is raised from the chest wall, pulled, and twisted. Then, each breast is milked for one minute and the technique is repeated for 15 minutes on each breast. Many Japanese, including physicians, are convinced that it effectively increases the milk supply and relieves plugged ducts (Riordan, 1990). Cantlie, a Canadian physician, uses breast massage to strip the milk ducts of mothers with mastitis, thereby promoting healing (Cantlie, 1988).

Massaging the mother's back to relieve discomfort from engorgement or to relax her if she has difficulty letting down her milk is an acupressure technique La Leche leaders have recommended for years. The mother sits in a chair and someone standing behind her uses the knuckles of a fist to briskly rub from the base of the mother's neck to the bottom of her shoulder blades on both sides of her spine.

TOO MUCH MILK

In the United States, little attention has been paid to those women who make more milk than their babies need. Women who breastfeed their infants at will, without concern for frequency and duration of feedings, have noted that milk production may exceed the baby's need (Rattigan, Ghisalberti & Hartmann, 1981). Feeding technique may account for oversupply. In some cases, switching the baby from the first breast before he has shown that he wishes to go to the next breast has been offered as an explanation for overfeeding (Woolridge & Fisher, 1988). The subsequent colicky behavior in the baby has often been characterized as "overactive let-down reflex" (Andrusiak & Larose-Kuzenko, 1987).

A more recent examination (Woolridge, Ingram & Baum, 1990) of the nutrient intake comparing feedings using one breast instead of two found that babies receive slightly less milk when breastfed from only one breast per feeding, but that total fat intake obtained was slightly higher with single breastfeedings. The authors urged that mothers allow their babies to set the breastfeeding pattern, which will vary throughout the course of the breastfeeding. Based on a description of "overactive let-down reflex" by Andrusiak and Larose-Kuzenko (1987), the clinician should be aware that this "embarrassment of riches" can cause the baby to wean early. Choking and having to struggle with a fast, abundant flow of milk at each feeding is simply too difficult for some babies to handle.

Women with overabundant milk supplies often have a moment of intense pain as the milk-ejection reflex occurs. One of the authors of this chapter has found that the following step-by-step approach is effective in reducing the mother's milk supply sufficiently to make her more comfortable and to enable the baby to suckle more comfortably:

1. Encourage the mother to offer only one breast at each feeding; if the second breast becomes uncomfortably full, express just enough milk to reduce ductal pressure. (Vigorous pumping should be avoided.) Remind the mother that her baby is not in danger of weight loss. Often these infants are well above average weight levels at the time the mother seeks help.
2. Position the baby so that he is straddling the mother's leg, directly facing the breast, with his head slightly above the mother's nipple. Ask the mother to lean back slightly, as if in a lounge chair, and support the baby at the breast. The mother may wish to slip a towel under the breast to catch any dripping or leaking milk. Because the mother is leaning back, excess milk is more likely to drip out of the baby's mouth rather than make him choke. Some women find that lying on their side to nurse is also helpful, using a diaper or towel to catch the excess.
3. If the baby stops nursing and wants to return to the breast in less than one hour, use the same breast that was used at the previous feeding.
4. Ask the mother to take a deep breath and count to 10; then breathe deeply and make a conscious effort to relax during the first milk-ejection reflex. In many cases, the first ejection consists exclusively of forceful sprays; thereafter, sprays appear to be less forceful. Some mothers have found that the initial sprays of milk are so overwhelming that they should be allowed to escape into a towel. The baby is then put to breast after the first spray has subsided to drips.
5. Advise the mother to burp the baby frequently, particularly if she hears continuing loud gulping throughout the feeding. However, in the upright position, the baby is less prone to struggle in order to stay ahead of the milk flow.
6. Encourage the mother to avoid expressing milk unless absolutely necessary for comfort.

Within a week, the mother's milk supply will generally diminish sufficiently so that the baby can breastfeed comfortably with a minimum of burping, little or no choking, and a resumption of comfort suckling. In some cases, babies of mothers with too much milk are never able to engage in comfort suckling until the milk supply has been reduced. Such babies may be offered the comfort of a pacifier. Once the milk supply has been reduced, the baby may again suckle at both breasts, without subsequent difficulties. As always, be mindful of the importance of following the baby's lead.

CLOTHING

Clothing needs in the puerperium are simple. Mothers need to be concerned with ease of laundering as well as comfort and convenience for breastfeeding. A dress that closes in the back has no place in the breastfeeding mother's wardrobe—unless she can guarantee that she will not need to feed the baby or experience any leaking while she is wearing it!

Increasingly, clothing stores carry garments specifically designed for the breastfeeding mother. Designs today include hidden zippers, snaps, velcro closures, and buttons which cleverly hide openings that are incorporated into darts, seams, pockets, or other fashion details.

Cotton tends to be cooler in warm months and warmer in cool months; in addition, it allows greater flow of air to the skin. Wrinkles are less likely with some of the cotton-synthetic blends. Two-piece outfits that enable the blouse to be pulled up from the waist offer breastfeeding mothers easy access to the breasts while also allowing them to maintain modesty. Many experienced mothers are well aware that breastfeeding "from the waist up" rather than "from the neck down" enables them to nurse their babies in virtually any setting. Light-colored, patterned clothes (rather than dark solid colors) camouflage telltale leaking (Phillips, 1989).

Cotton bras—100% cotton, if possible—tend to be more comfortable than those made of synthetic materials. Bras with plastic liners or so-called "moisture barriers" should be avoided; they keep the skin damp and contribute to tenderness. Pads worn in a bra will absorb leaking milk, but pads with plastic backing or a "moisture barrier" should not be used because they hold moisture and create an ideal environment for candidiasis. Cup closures should be easy to manage with one hand. In most stores, the pregnant mother can not only obtain a personalized fitting but can test whether the openings are easy to manage prior to purchasing a bra. Some bras have front openings that enable the mother to remove the bra from both breasts if she prefers the greater freedom this affords. Small-breasted women unused to wearing a bra often find that the lightweight bras made of multi-stretch material provide adequate support. Lactating women should always be cautioned against wearing underwire bras during the course of breastfeeding. Underwires tend to constrict and compress the milk ducts and predispose breastfeeding mothers to recurrent plugged ducts or mastitis.

INFANT CARE

CRYING AND COLIC

An infant cries to signal a need. That need may be for suckling, comfort, a diaper change, or a change of position. Most parents go to their infants when they hear the baby cry and make every possible effort to comfort the child. The baby whose cries are responded to quickly soon learns to trust his parents (or care-givers). The baby who is responded to quickly generally stops crying sooner than the infant who is allowed to cry for some time (Barr & Elias, 1988). Prompt response reduces the baby's stress level and enhances the parents' enjoyment of the baby and their new role as parents. The hospital-based care-giver who assists new parents has a unique opportunity to help them interpret their baby's crying and learn the importance of meeting the baby's needs promptly (Riordan, 1980b). In time, as the baby learns to distinguish between stress factors and the parents learn to interpret the baby's signals, the specific cause of the baby's distress will be more easily recognized and dealt with.

Unlike other cries, colic is usually characterized by a high-pitched wail or scream, a sign that the baby is in pain. Colic is the result of sudden spasmodic abdominal cramping. Often the baby draws up his knees and, in some cases, his abdomen will be distended. Some infants experience colic only once or twice a day—at about the same time each day. With others, the colic occurs after nearly every feeding and gradually disappears in three to four months.

Reasons for colic abound. Explanations, many of which relate to feeding, include the following:

- allergies to cow's milk-based formula (Lothe, Lindberg & Jakobsson, 1982; Lifschitz et al., 1988; Bishop, Hill & Hosking, 1990) or to some element in the lactating mother's diet
- overfeeding, especially if bottle-feeding, although breastfeeding infants are also susceptible (Woolridge & Fisher, 1988)
- Underfeeding, especially if the baby is not offered feeds frequently and is allowed to cry until it is "time" to feed
- "too rich" or "too weak" milk
- too much fat, sugar, or protein (especially if the baby receives artificial milk)
- too large or too small holes in the bottle teat
- excessive swallowing of air, especially if the baby is bottle-fed or poorly positioned at the breast
- temperament of the baby (Barr, et al., 1989)
- smoking on the part of the mother (Said, Patois & Lellouch, 1984; Woodward & Hand, 1988; Matheson, 1989)
- anxious mother who interprets all crying as a sign of hunger (Taubman, 1988)—which often

leads her to stop breastfeeding in the mistaken belief that her emotional state has somehow affected her milk and her baby's ability to digest it.

Bottle-feedings of artificial bovine- or vegetable-based baby milk may at times be responsible for colic (Jenkins et al., 1984; Chandra, Puri & Hamed, 1989; Working Group on Cow's Milk Protein Allergy, 1988; Høst, Husby & Osterballe, 1988). Sometimes, breastfeeding techniques may be the culprit. For example, correcting poor positioning will reduce the likelihood of the baby's swallowing air while suckling if this is the problem. If the colicky baby is fully breastfed, the mother's diet should be reviewed. If she drinks large quantities of cow's milk, a diet which eliminates all dairy products for at least one week is indicated (Jakobsson & Lindberg, 1978, 1983; Jakobsson et al., 1985). The mother begins by eliminating all dairy products and foods containing dairy products from her diet. If this is the cause of the baby's distress following feedings, she will note a marked change in the baby's behavior within three to four days. Without the offending bovine-milk proteins in the mother's milk, the baby remains comfortable after each breastfeeding. At the end of the first week of the elimination of dairy food, if the mother confirms that the baby is better, she can begin to reintroduce dairy products slowly into her diet. She might be encouraged to try the following approach:

- *First week:* eliminate all dairy products. Calcium is available in foods other than those in the dairy group. (If the mother is concerned about her calcium intake, she may use calcium tablets.)
- *Second week:* reintroduce only hard cheeses—such as cheddar and Swiss—or yogurt in small quantities.
- *Third week:* reintroduce soft cheeses—such as gouda, brie, and American, as well as cottage cheese and cream cheese—in small quantities.
- *Fourth week:* reintroduce butter, ice cream, and milk in cooked form.
- *Fifth week:* reintroduce cow's milk in small quantities.

Usually, while reintroducing dairy products into her diet, the mother will discover how much, and in what form, the baby can tolerate her intake of these foods. She should be encouraged to ingest only those dairy products to which the baby does not react. It is essential to wait several weeks or months—depending on the baby's reaction—before challenging the baby with an increase of dairy products in the mother's diet.

Occasionally, a week of elimination may not be sufficient to detect and remove the offending proteins. Clyne and Kulcyzcki (1991) note that bovine IgG levels were markedly higher in the milk of mothers of colicky babies than in the milk of mothers whose babies were not colicky. They noted that bovine IgG has a prolonged half-life, and that its presence in high levels may require a longer period of elimination than is usually suggested for short dietary trials. If a mother is herself sensitive to cow's milk, the lactation consultant may ask her to extend her elimination of dairy products somewhat longer to determine whether the baby's colic is caused by her dietary intake.

While cow's milk appears to be the single most frequent offender in a mother's diet, other foods have also been implicated (Cant, Marsden & Kilshaw, 1985; Chandra et al., 1986; Cavagni et al., 1988). They include beef, eggs, wheat (and related glutens like nuts), as well as high-acid fruits and vegetables (Chandra et al., 1986). Often, babies who develop colic in response to foods in the breastfeeding mother's diet exhibit allergic symptoms when exposed to the same foods later in life (Kajosaari & Saarinen, 1983; Pittschieler, 1990).

While restrictive diets often help to reduce colic in the infant, medications such as atropine and phenobarbital are generally ineffective; in some cases they have been found to be harmful (O'Donovan & Bradstock, 1979).

FREQUENT FEEDINGS

Breastfeeding babies need frequent feedings. This is often cause for alarm in uninformed mothers, particularly those who have bottle-fed a previous infant. The breastfed infant feeds more frequently and in patterns that differ from those of the artificially fed infant, who is regulated more by external factors, including both the clock and the relatively less digestible curds of artificial baby milk.

When access to the mother is not restricted after birth, the breastfeeding neonate exhibits a pattern similar to that illustrated in Table 9–1. The initial alertness and eagerness of the baby to suckle (Anderson et al., 1982) is followed by progressively deeper sleep, and then increased wakefulness and interest in nursing. During this period of increased wakefulness, the baby may want to feed frequently, alternating between relatively short periods of light sleep and quiet wakefulness (Williams & Mueller, 1989). Mothers may interpret these "cluster feedings" as indicators that the baby is not getting any milk or an insufficient amount. However, they actually constitute a series of mini-feedings, snacks, or courses in a larger banquet that is part of a single breastfeeding episode. A cluster of mini-feeds is usually followed by a period of deep sleep on the part of the infant, during which time the mother should be encouraged to catch up on her own sleep.

This period of deep sleep following cluster feedings is particularly important to the infant. Babies whose mothers have received medication in labor may engage in their first cluster of mini-feedings 20 to 24 hours after birth. The time lag may reflect the effect of the mother's medication on the neonate. Often this phenomenon occurs late at night, or in the very early morning hours when the mother may be urged to sleep or to let others take care of the baby. If a baby is born at home or in an institutional setting where he is not removed from the mother's room, cluster feedings usually occur much earlier, often within one or two hours after birth, thereby "cementing" suckling behavior sooner. These feedings are followed by a period of deep sleep, after which the infant breastfeeds frequently, but with more regular spacing between suckling episodes.

If the baby is denied access to the mother when the cluster feedings are most likely to occur, this behavior may not occur until *after* the mother is home. If she is not told to expect it, she may be concerned that her milk production is not meeting the baby's needs and think that she should supplement. In truth, what both mother and baby need is time to get to know one another and to practice their new skills.

SUCKLING PATTERN

The pattern of normal infant suckling has been discussed earlier in this book. Neonates housed with their mothers immediately after birth quickly learn to suckle and show increasing facility with each subsequent feeding. In general, term infants demonstrate a well-organized sequence of suckling behaviors, including bringing the hand to the mouth, rooting and suckling within the first hour after birth (Widstrom et al., 1987). Delays in getting the baby to breast (Taylor, Maloni & Brown, 1986), including those caused by routine suctioning of gastric fluids, can disrupt this pattern of behavior. Another potential disruption is suctioning the infant's nares with a DeLee mucus trap after birth. The suction tends to cause the infant to have nasal edema and "stuffiness." Because the baby's airway is somewhat obstructed, the baby does not feed well (breast or bottle) until the swelling subsides.

Matthews' (1988) Infant Breastfeeding Assessment Tool (see Chapter 21) can be used to evaluate infant suckling over several feedings and is a useful instrument to show mothers that their babies are learning with each feeding and are becoming more efficient at obtaining milk. This tool focuses on the baby's readiness to feed (arousability), rooting pattern, fixing or latching-on behavior, and actual suck pattern. It reminds the mother that what her baby does is both complex and predictable and that he needs lots of opportunities to practice, just as she needs many opportunities to learn how to hold and position the baby for optimal breastfeeding. The ease of using this tool means that the mother can evaluate for herself what occurs at each feeding. The nurse caring for the mother may also find the tool useful, for it breaks down the infant's suckling behavior into four discreet though related elements; each is easily identifiable and requires no intervention to evaluate. In addition, since the baby's suckling must be done at the mother's breast, the lactation consultant or nurse must observe the feeding, thereby providing an opportunity to offer the mother praise and encouragement about how well the nursing couple is doing. Positive feedback is essential in preparing the mother to continue breastfeeding after she is discharged home to an environment where breastfeeding may or may not be positively reinforced.

STOOLING PATTERNS

As discussed earlier, the stools of the breastfed newborn go through several changes and can be used as an indicator of milk intake. These changes are easily observed and occur at predictable intervals. (See Table 9–5.) Black tarry stools (meconium) are passed in the first several days. With each succeeding

TABLE 9–5 CHARACTERISTIC STOOL CHANGES OVER TIME

Time Period	Type of Stool	Number Per Day	Amount
0–6 days	Meconium, transitional, milk stool	2+	Scant to copious
7–28 days	Milk stool	5–10+	Scant
29+ days	Milk stool	1 every 4–12 days*	Copious

*Occasionally infants may go as long as 3–4 weeks between copious stools.

milk feeding, the stool gradually lightens in color and becomes less sticky and more liquid. Thus the transitional stools appear. The totally breastmilk stool is yellow and generally very soft or liquid. At times, it may contain small curds, while at other times, it has a mushy consistency and is greenish-yellow to mustard-yellow. As the color changes, an odor develops that is sweeter and not as strong as that of the artificially fed infant. It has been likened to a "yeasty" odor rather than the predominantly bile odor of the formula-fed infant.

In addition to changes in stool color, the frequency of the stool also changes. Stooling usually begins shortly after birth and continues two more times daily during the first week of life. Often these relatively infrequent, mostly meconium stools are copious and explosive. As their frequency increases, the amount of stool passed each time declines. After the first week, when the infant passes some stool during or immediately after nearly every breastfeeding, the amount of liquid yellow stool may be no more than a stain on the diaper rather than a gush that leaks out. The liquid nature of the totally breastfed infant's stool—as well as its greater frequency—are neither a cause for concern nor an indication of diarrhea. Grandmothers, and other helpers whose experience has been with artificially fed infants, need to be reassured that these are normal stool patterns for the breastfed infant.

Throughout the first month, most infants stool very frequently (Weaver, Ewing & Taylor, 1988). The new mother may find that she needs to change her baby's diaper at every feeding or at least every other feeding.

After the first month to six weeks of life, however, the totally breastfed baby's stool pattern changes again. The frequency of stooling gradually declines and the volume of stool passed increases each time. The color of the stool remains the characteristic mus-

tard-yellow color, and the odor remains the same as well. Many infants stool only once every 4 to 12 days on average (Weaver, Ewing & Taylor, 1988). With a baby who is obviously thriving, the long period between stools in the second and later months after birth is not a cause for concern, provided that the infant's abdomen remains soft and he seems content and alert (Riordan, 1990).

Whenever artificial formula is offered, the stools change. The stool becomes darker in color, more formed, and has more odor. Curds are usually larger than in the stool of the totally breastfed baby, and the frequency of the stool varies. While the totally breastfed infant passes very frequent, scanty stools during the first month of life, the bottle-fed infant tends to pass larger, more copious and odorous, but less frequent stools. While the totally breastfed infant passes copious stools very infrequently after the fourth week of life, the bottle-fed infant tends to pass larger and more odorous stools more frequently. As the volume of artificial formula increases in the diet of the breastfeeding baby, the stools reflect this intake.

The same is true when solid foods are added. Generally, the odor of the breastfed baby's stool becomes more noticeable as solid food is added to the baby's diet. Early occasional meals of solid foods which represent only a small proportion of the infant's total daily intake will not cause a marked change in the stool pattern. As the proportion of solid foods increases, however, the stooling occurs two or three times per day, and the odor, color and consistency reflect what the baby has ingested. In some cases, portions of undigested food may be visible in the stool. An example is peas, the casing of which may appear virtually unchanged in the stool. If the infant is growing well, the appearance of such food particles in the stool is not a cause for concern.

STOOLING AS AN INDICATION OF A PROBLEM

The newborn who does not stool may have an organic problem that needs to be ruled out. Hirschsprung's Disease and cystic fibrosis are two such examples. The newborn who does not stool frequently in the first month of life, but who is growing well in all parameters (head circumference, height, and weight), may be one of those relatively rare individuals who adopts an infrequent stool pattern earlier than usual. Occasionally, some element in the mother's diet may contribute to an unexpected stool pattern. The authors are aware of one infant whose stools were hard and occurred only every five to six days—until his mother stopped taking prenatal multivitamins with extra iron.

Generally, an infant who is stooling fewer than four times a day *and* who is not gaining weight appropriately needs to be evaluated; infrequent stooling in such cases may be an early sign of inadequate milk intake (Auerbach & Eggert, 1987) or inadequate intake of the hindmilk which tends to stimulate stooling. (See also Chapter 19 on slow weight gain.)

MULTIPLE INFANTS

Breastfeeding more than one infant at a time is entirely possible. Mothering and nursing multiples, however, requires greater organization by the mother than caring for a single baby or two babies of different ages (Sollid et al., 1989). Driscoll and Walker (1985) suggest that the mother of twins may wish to keep a chart of daily activities, especially those related to the babies' feeding. The chart might record which breast each baby used at the latest feeding, in order to remind the mother to switch the babies so that each uses both breasts at subsequent feedings. This will avoid stimulating only one breast by the more vigorous twin. The mother may also wish to record nursing positions from time to time so that she does not have to rely on her memory. Wet diapers, stools, and other pertinent information may be logged. Finally, if vitamin or mineral supplements are being given, she may wish to record the amount and to note what has been administered to each twin.

Term or near-term twins have needs that are the same as full-term singletons; the mother's needs, however, are likely to be greater. In hospital and during the early weeks at home, the mother of multi-

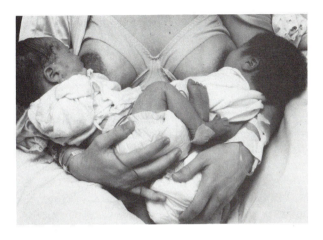

FIGURE 9–7 Breastfeeding term twins.

ples needs the assistance of at least one other pair of hands. She also needs more pillows! Fortunately, nature has taken care to ensure that two babies can suckle—even simultaneously—if they wish. (See Figs. 9–7 and 9–8.)

When twins, triplets or quadruplets are born prematurely, the infants' needs relating to their prematurity take precedence over the mother's desire to breastfeed, but she can begin to provide breast milk for her babies with the assistance of hand expression or a breast pump. Needs, problems and solutions vary with each situation. One lactation consultant recently assisted two mothers who had quadruplets and pumped for many weeks before all the babies were on the breast. Mother A gave birth to her quads

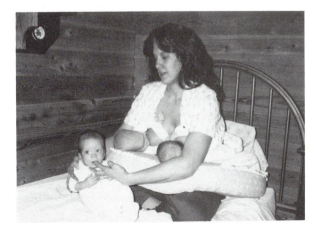

FIGURE 9–8 Breastfeeding triplets. (Courtesy Jane Bradshaw.)

at 34 weeks. She took the first baby home one week after birth, feeding from a bottle; direct nursing did not occur until almost five weeks later. The second and third babies went home at five weeks postpartum; one was a good nurser from the start, the other a very poor nurser. The fourth baby went home after eight weeks of hospitalization for respiratory distress; however, within one week he was breastfeeding. This mother nursed, as well as pumped and fed, one or more babies with a bottle for at least eight weeks. Her youngest quad never breastfed well; he required breastfeedings and bottle-feedings for most of the breastfeeding course. The mother weaned all four babies at around seven months of age.

Mother B gave birth to quadruplets near term; three of her babies went home together around one week of age. All three were nursing and receiving some supplementary bottles when they went home. The fourth baby was nearly one month old when he went home. He was nursing poorly at the time. The first three babies weaned themselves about the time of their first birthday, while the remaining quad weaned at 14–15 months. This mother pumped milk, in addition to nursing, until her babies were almost 10 months old. She returned to work for 10-hour shifts on the weekends when her babies were five months old; she chose to continue pumping in order to provide human milk for the babies when she was at work and to maintain her supply when she was home. (Personal communication, Virginia H. Brackett; Evanston, Illinois.)

With multiples one baby is usually ready to go to the breast before the other(s). This gives the mother an opportunity to learn to nurse one baby before she needs to handle two—or more! When breastfeeding is begun, following days or weeks of pumping, the mother may need to be reminded that it will take time before she is able to fully breastfeed. Storr (1989) describes the approach of one mother of triplets who used interim bottle-feedings with each baby while she gradually increased her milk supply. Milk production *will* increase to meet the needs of multiple infants (Saint, Maggiore & Hartmann, 1986). While some mothers of twins begin by nursing both babies simultaneously, they may not continue this approach, preferring instead to devote their attention to one baby at a time—at least during feedings!

Dietary needs of the mother of multiple infants are greater than for the mother of a single breastfeeding infant. Certainly, the mother of multiples needs additional on-going assistance with household chores as she spends more time and energy meeting the needs of her babies.

An important consideration for the care-giver is to remain sensitive to the need of the mother to attach or bond to each baby individually. The attachment process is more likely to be disrupted when more than one infant is born, particularly if the twin or triplet birth was a surprise or not discovered until very shortly before birth. Assisting the mother to see and relate to each baby as a separate individual, rather than as part of a multiple unit, is important. It can begin when the care-giver points out unique qualities in each baby as she helps the mother to get to know her offspring.

REFUSING THE BREAST

Although it may occur throughout the breastfeeding course, seven to nine months of age is a time at which some infants suddenly refuse to breastfeed. While the mother may think the infant has weaned himself, this is not necessarily the case. The abruptness of the infant's refusal to breastfeed is usually the mother's best clue to what is known as a "breastfeeding strike." Normal weaning seldom occurs so rapidly.

Most mothers who have experienced such refusal believe the strike is a signal of the baby's distress, dissatisfaction, or confusion associated with feedings—and an attempt by the baby to exert some control. Situations in which the older breastfeeding infant suddenly refuses to nurse occur when the mother:

- attempts to get the baby on a new feeding schedule
- leaves the infant with a bottle (even breastmilk) when he is unaccustomed to it
- rebukes the baby (understandably) for biting her breast, usually early in the teething period
- leaves the baby for several days.

When the baby refuses the breast, efforts to encourage resumption of breastfeeding may take several days. During this time, the mother needs to spend more time with the baby, carrying him more and offering a great deal of skin-to-skin contact. It is

Lactation History and Risk Assessment

G ____   P ____   EDC _____   Age _____

FEEDING CHOICE:
Breast ____
Breast/Formula ____
Undecided ____

PHYSICAL EXAM:
NIPPLES: Flat ____
              Inverted ____
              Other ____
              WNL ____
BREASTS   Size increase during pregnancy?
              Yes ____   No ____
              Other _____

HISTORY:
Previous breastfeeding experience?   Yes ____   No ____
How long _____
Did you want to breastfeed but were unable to for some reason?
Yes ____   No ____
Why? _____

Did you have any of the following (check all that apply):
____ Sore nipples
____ Cracked and/or bleeding nipples
____ Not enough milk
____ Breast infection
____ Baby did not gain weight well

Did you stop nursing before you really wanted to?
Yes ____   No ____
Why? _____

RISK FACTORS (check all that apply):
____ Multiple gestation
____ Diabetes
____ History of pre-term infant
____ Breast surgery

Medications (prescription and nonprescription) taken:
_____
_____
Medical condition: _____
_____

Derived from Dodgson, J: Early identification of potential breastfeeding problems; originally published in *J Hum Lact* 5:80–81, 1989.

generally useless to attempt to put the baby to breast while he is awake; mothers are often more successful offering the breast to the baby while he is dropping off to sleep or just waking. The health-care provider or family member may support the mother by helping her to sort out the circumstances surrounding the baby's refusal, by encouraging her to maintain her milk supply, and by assuring her that the problem does not lie with her.

CLINICAL IMPLICATIONS

Assessment is a critical first step in working with a client. Lactation consultants often find that identifying problems a client had with a previous infant may often be helpful. For instance, if the mother has sore nipples with an earlier baby, the care-giver may need to reassure the concerned or anxious mother that a similar condition need not recur. Dodgson (1989) urges that risk assessment be used to identify women for whom the anticipated course of lactation may hold special worries. (See boxed material on p. 245.)

DISCHARGE PLANNING

Early discharge from the hospital, a fact of life today for new mothers and their neonates, has had a major impact on postpartum care. Mothers and infants often return home in the first 24–48 hours after a vaginal birth and four days or sooner after a cesarean birth. There are distinct advantages to early discharge. It promotes parent-infant attachment, lessens exposure to nosocomial infections, reduces the length of time when hospital routines can interfere with early breastfeeding, and saves health-care costs. Studies of early discharge outcomes indicate no increase in maternal or infant morbidity (Norr & Nacion, 1987; Harrison, 1990).

Yet drawbacks to early discharge do exist—it may negatively influence the mother's feeling of competence in her mothering (Waldenstrom, Sundelin & Lindmark, 1987). Simultaneously, it markedly reduces time to teach beginning breastfeeding skills and the opportunity to assess how well the mother has learned certain aspects of her new role, plus how well the baby is breastfeeding. Driscoll (1989/90) states that babies are being discharged after having been breastfed only a few times or having minimally passed meconium; likewise, mothers are being discharged with limited referrals to community re-

sources and with no help at home. Such abandonment contributes to later difficulties if the mother does not know to whom to turn for assistance. Often the result is early, unnecessary weaning and a feeling that she has failed herself and her baby.

Hospital maternity services and other health-care providers are now beginning to do something about this problem with follow-up telephone calls and home visits (Brucker & MacMullen, 1985; see also Jansson, 1985).

The goal of discharge planning is twofold: to *prevent common problems* and *to provide emotional support* (Page-Goertz, 1989). With such a brief time in the hospital, the mother needs a care-giver who imparts as much basic information as possible without overwhelming her. She also needs reinforcement of her self-confidence in her role as a new mother. These two goals are mutually reinforcing and, as the care-giver instructs the mother in the prevention of problems, she is in a position to simultaneously enhance the new mother's self-esteem and self-confidence.

In endeavoring to prevent the most common problems that may arise, three priorities need to be addressed: positioning the baby at the breast, understanding basic feeding techniques, and recognizing signs of the need for intervention. These subjects are discussed in turn below.

POSITIONS

Prior to hospital discharge, the new mother needs to know ways to position her neonate. The three most frequently taught techniques are the Madonna (cradle or cross-chest), the football (or clutch), and the side-lying positions. Before discharge, the mother should have more than one opportunity to practice each position with assistance and to demonstrate that she can place her baby in each position without assistance.

Each position has its positive and negative elements. The mother who is informed about each position and has practiced each prior to discharge will be more likely to select the position that works best for her at different times. (See Table 9–6.)

BASIC FEEDING TECHNIQUES

In teaching basic feeding techniques, priority needs to be given to the following points:

- *Feed the baby frequently (8 or more feedings in a 24-hour period).* Using a visual aid to demon-

TABLE 9–6   POSITIVE AND NEGATIVE ELEMENTS OF INFANT FEEDING POSITIONS

Infant Positioning Options	Positive Elements	Negative Elements
Madonna [cross-chest or cradle] position	Most frequently pictured. Most often used by experienced mothers.	Often most difficult to master. Baby's head tends to wobble around on the mother's arm. Mother may feel she has minimal control over baby's head. Sometimes difficult to keep baby's head close to the breast and/or appropriately high on mother's chest wall.
Football [clutch] position	Provides most complete control of the baby's head. An excellent option following cesarean birth or tubal ligation. Easily accomplished with a small baby [SGA or pre-term].	Least frequently pictured in books. Least familiar to care-givers. Some mothers are not comfortable holding their babies in this manner.
Side-lying position	Often expected to be used before breastfeeding in a chair. Enables the mother to rest more completely than is possible if she is sitting up.	Not always taught in hospital. Mothers often fear smothering baby in this position. Rarely practiced as often as the Madonna position.

strate the size of the newborn's stomach is an excellent way to illustrate why the neonate needs frequent feedings—his stomach is simply too small to hold large quantities at a time! Additionally, the small curd formed by human milk is more easily digested than the large curd formed by artificial baby milks. The breastfeeding infant, therefore, is less likely to experience a sense of fullness for an extended period.

- *Offer both breasts at each feeding without time restriction,* allowing the baby to finish the first breast before moving on to the second breast. After breastfeeding becomes established, it may not be necessary to use both breasts at each feeding.
- *Avoid the use of artificial teats, pacifiers (dummies), supplemental infant formula, water or glucose feeds for the first two to four weeks.* Telling the mother *why* these practices can interfere with early, effective breastfeeding will give her the ammunition she may need to fend off well-meaning, but uninformed, attempts to "assist" her with these unnecessary feedings.
- *Identify various ways in which the mother can recognize that her infant is getting sufficient milk:* These include listening for and identifying

the infant's swallows (Lau & Henning, 1989). Another way, particularly in the first month, is noting the number of stools (several after the first week) and the frequency of voiding (at least six to eight cloth diaper changes and at least four paper diaper changes) in a 24-hour period. When paper diapers are used, one technique many mothers have found helpful is to place a piece of white tissue in the bottom of the paper diaper. The tissue wrinkles when it becomes wet, serving as a cue to the mother that, even though the paper diaper feels dry, it needs to be changed.

SIGNS THAT INTERVENTION IS NEEDED

Seven signs that indicate a need for health-care intervention include the following:

1. The infant is putting out scant or no urine.
2. The infant has infrequent stools (fewer than four per day by the end of the first week of life).
3. The baby is lethargic (difficult or impossible to waken for feedings).
4. The baby is extremely fretful (never contented after any feedings).
5. No swallowing is felt or heard during feedings.

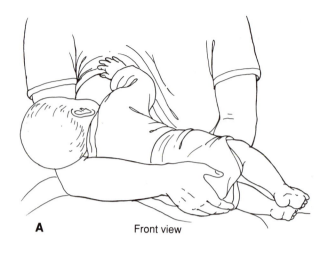

A Front view

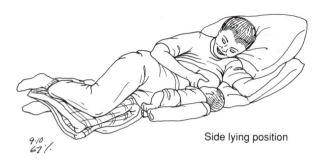

Side lying position

FIGURE 9–10   Side-lying position.

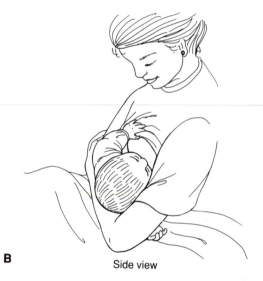

B Side view

FIGURE 9–9   Madona cradle position. **A,** Front view. **B,** Side view.

6. Nipple soreness has become more intense even though it existed earlier; or it suddenly develops when it was previously absent.
7. The mother's breasts are clinically engorged and very painful, making it difficult or impossible for the baby to breastfeed.

At discharge, the parents may be given clear, simply written materials that provide step-by-step information and are individualized as much as possible. Walker (1989) suggests that Polaroid photographs of positioning and other techniques may be helpful, depending on the situation. The hospital care-giver should establish a definite plan for follow-up: make a

phone call to the mother at a specific time post discharge or provide her with the phone numbers of the hospital "warm milk" line and of lactation consultants or La Leche League leaders in the area. Public health, home health or nurse case-manager follow-

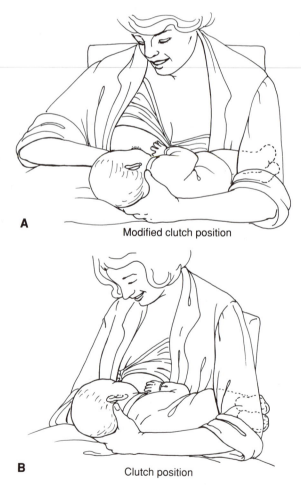

A Modified clutch position

B Clutch position

FIGURE 9–11   **A,** Football or clutch position. **B,** Side or modified clutch hold.

ups are other options in some communities. In many countries other than the United States, new mothers are routinely visited by midwives and home health visitors. The optimal time for a follow-up visit or call is about five to seven days after birth. This is an especially crucial period because enough time has passed to make an accurate evaluation of the mother's milk supply and the infant's intake. By this time, too, the mother has probably passed the peak of transient sore nipples and, if things are progressing normally, is beginning to feel comfortable with breastfeeding. Five to seven days is also about the midpoint between discharge and the baby's first scheduled visit to the physician. This is a critical period that remains unaddressed by the U.S. health-care system.

SUMMARY

Consumer advocacy, the expectations of parents, childbirth education, early hospital discharge, frequent cesarean births, and new technologies are all forces that affect birthing and early breastfeeding. In recent years, the emphasis has changed from a management approach to support and education of childbearing families for their own self-care. No longer do we view the mother and her infant as separate entities; rather we care for them as a natural single unit. Many hospitals now boast a family-centered birthing unit (a.k.a. family birthplace, single-room maternity care, new-life center) where the mother and infant are cared for together in one room. Birthing rooms today look much like a bedroom, with a comfortable recliner chair for the mother's support person; hook-ups for medical equipment are concealed behind wall prints and other decorations. A prime benefit of this kind of mother-baby care is that families receive more comprehensive, coordinated care which facilitates breastfeeding.

Unfortunately, institutional concern for the family with a newborn usually stops at discharge. The transition process after discharge is a neglected element in the prospective payment system. Who is to look after these families during this vulnerable period in their lives? Follow-up care in the home is a basic necessity that requires political action by professionals and families. It should not be looked upon as a luxury.

Breastfeeding is sometimes perceived as a complicated skill instead of a natural function. New mothers need to be reassured that they can enjoy an uncomplicated breastfeeding experience and that common concerns can be easily managed without complicated technologies or frequent visits to the doctor's office (Arthur, Hartmann & Smith, 1987). Guidance given by the knowledgeable health provider not only assures the infant of a healthy start in life, but also provides valuable lifelong health education for the family. The effort expended may be great, but the rewards are myriad.

REFERENCES

Anderson, GC, et al.: Development of sucking in term infants from birth to four hours postbirth, *Res Nurs Health* 5:21–27, 1982.

Andrusiak, F, and Larose-Kuzenko, M: *The effects of an overactive let-down reflex* (Unit 13), Lactation Consultant Series, Garden City Park, N.Y., 1987, Avery Publishing Group, Inc.

Anlar, Y, Anlar, B, and Tonyali, A: Some factors influencing the time of lactation, *J Trop Pediatr* 34:198, 1988.

Arthur, PG, Hartmann, PE, and Smith, M: Measurement of the milk intake of breast-fed infants, *J Pediatr Gastroenterol Nutr* 6:758–63, 1987.

Atkinson, L: Prenatal nipple conditioning for breastfeeding, *Nurs Res* 28:448–51, 1979.

Auerbach, KG: Breastfeeding fallacies: their relationship to understanding lactation, *Birth* 17:44–49, 1990.

Auerbach, KG, and Eggert, LD: The importance of infant suckling patterns when a breast-fed baby fails to thrive (letter), *J Trop Pediatr* 33:156–57, 1987.

Barr, RG, and Elias, MF: Nursing interval and maternal responsivity: effect on early infant crying, *Pediatrics* 81:529–36, 1988.

Barr, RG, et al.: Feeding and temperament as determinants of early infant crying/fussing behavior, *Pediatrics* 84:514–21, 1989.

Berg, KL: Two cases of tongue-tie and breastfeeding, *J Hum Lact* 6:124–26, 1990.

Bishop, JM, Hill, DJ, and Hosking, CS: Natural history of cow milk allergy: clinical outcome, *J Pediatr* 116:862–67, 1990.

Bowles, BC, Stutte, PC, and Hensley, J: Alternate massage in breastfeeding, *Genesis* 9:5–9, 1988.

Britton, G: Early mother-infant contact and infant temperature stabilization, *JOGN Nurs* 9:84–86, 1980.

Brown, MS, and Hurlock, JT: Preparation of the breast for breastfeeding, *Nurs Res* 24:448–51, 1975.

Brucker, MC, and MacMullen, NJ: Bridging the gap between hospital and home, *Child Today* 14:19–22, 1985.

Cant, A, Marsden, RA, and Kilshaw, PJ: Egg and cow's milk hypersensitivity in exclusively breast fed infants with eczema, *Br Med J* 291:932–35, 1985.

Canterbury, RJ, et al.: Postpartum psychosis induced by bromocriptine, *South Med J* 80:1463–64, 1987.

Cantlie, HB: Treatment of acute puerperal mastitis and breast abscess, *Can Fam Phys* 34:2221–25, 1988.

Capeless, EL, and Mann, LI: Use of breast stimulation for antepartum stress testing, *Obstet Gynecol* 64:641–45, 1984.

Cavagni, G, et al.: Passage of food antigens into circulation of breast-fed infants with atopic dermatitis, *Ann Allergy* 61:361–65, 1988.

Chandra, RK, Puri, S, and Hamed, A: Influence of maternal diet during lactation and use of formula feeds on development of atopic eczema in high risk infants, *Br Med J* 299:228–30, 1989.

Chandra, RK, et al.: Influence of maternal food antigen avoidance during pregnancy and lactation on incidence of atopic eczema in infants, *Clin Allergy* 16:563–69, 1986.

Chapman, J, et al.: Concerns of breast-feeding mothers from birth to 4 months, *Nurs Res* 34:374–77, 1985.

Clyne, PS, and Kulcyzcki, A: Human breast milk contains bovine IgG. Relationship to infant colic? *Pediatrics* 87:439–44, 1991.

Crawley, MS, Hedahl, KJ, and Pegg, S: Women's perceptions of vaginal and cesarean deliveries, *Nurs Res* 32:10–15, 1983.

Copeland, CA, Raebel, MA, and Wagner, SL: Pesticide residue in lanolin (letter), *JAMA* 261:242, 1989.

Day, TW: Unilateral failure of lactation after breast biopsy, *J Fam Pract* 23:161–62, 1986.

de Carvalho, M, Robertson, S, and Klaus, MH: Does the duration and frequency of early breastfeeding affect nipple pain? *Birth* 11:81–84, 1984.

Desmarais, L, and Browne, S: *Inadequate weight gain in breastfeeding infants: assessments and resolutions* (Unit 8), Lactation Consultant Series, Garden City Park, N.Y., 1990, Avery Publishing Group, Inc.

Dodgson, J: Early identification of potential breastfeeding problems, *J Hum Lact* 5:80–81, 1989.

Driscoll, JW: Early discharge, *Childbirth Educ* (Winter), 1989/90; pp. 37–47.

Driscoll, JW, and Walker, M: *Breastfeeding your twins,* Weston, Mass., 1985: Lactation Associates.

Ekwo, EE, Dusdieker, LB, and Booth, BM: Factors influence initiation of breastfeeding, *Am J Dis Child* 137:375–77, 1983.

Elliott, JP, and Flaherty, JF: The use of breast stimulation to prevent postdate pregnancy, *Am J Obstet Gynecol* 149:628–32, 1984.

Ellis, DJ, and Hewat, RJ: Factors related to breastfeeding duration, *Can Fam Phys* 30:1479–85, 1984.

Emde, RN, Gaensbauer, TJ, and Harmon, RJ: *Emotional expression in infancy, Psychological Issues,* Monograph 37, New York, 1976, International Universities Press, Inc.

Eppink, H: Experiment to determine a basis for nursing decisions in regard to initiation of breastfeeding, *Nurs Res* 18:292, 1969.

Frantz, KB, and Kalmen, BA: Breastfeeding works for cesareans, too, *RN* 42:39, 1979.

Glover, J, and Sandilands, M: Supplementation of breast-feeding infants and weight loss in hospital, *J Hum Lact* 6:163–66, 1990.

Goodine, LA and Fried, PA: Infant feeding practices: pre- and postnatal factors affecting choice of method and the duration of breastfeeding, *Am J Public Health* 75:439–44, 1984.

Gosha, JL, and Tichy, AM: Effect of a breast shell on postpartum nipple pain: an exploratory study, *J Nurs-Midwif* 33:74–77, 1988.

Graef, P, et al.: Postpartum concerns of breast-feeding mothers, *J Nurs-Midwif* 33:62–66, 1988.

Grossman, LK, et al.: The infant feeding decision in low and upper income women, *Clin Pediatr* 29:30–37, 1990.

Gulick, E: Informational correlates of successful breast-feeding, *MCN* 7:370–75, 1982.

Gunther, M: Sore nipples: causes and prevention, *Lancet* 2:347–51, 1945.

Harrison, LL: Patient education in early postpartum discharge programs, *MCN* 15:39, 1990.

Hartmann, PE: Lactation and reproduction in Western Australian women, *J Reprod Med* 32:543–47, 1987.

Heck, LJ, and Erenberg, A: Serum glucose levels in term neonates during the first 48 hours of life, *J Pediatr* 110:119–22, 1987.

Hewat, RJ, and Ellis, DJ: Comparison of the effectiveness of two methods of nipple care, *Birth* 14:41–45, 1987.

Hill, PD, and Humenick, SS: Insufficient milk supply, *Image* 21:145–48, 1989.

Hill, ST, and Shronk, LK: The effect of early patient-infant contact on newborn body temperature, *JOGN Nurs* 8:287–90, 1979.

Hillervik-Lindquist, C, Hofvander, Y, and Sjölin, S: Studies on perceived milk insufficiency III. Consequences for breast milk consumption and growth, *Acta Paediatr Scand* 80:297–303, 1991.

Hoffmann, JB: A suggested treatment for inverted nipples, *Am J Obstet Gynecol* 66:346, 1953.

Høst, A, Husby, S, and Osterballe, O: A prospective study of cow's milk allergy in exclusively breast-fed infants, *Acta Paediatr Scand* 77:663–70, 1988.

Howie, PW, Houston, MJ, and Cook, A: How long should a breast feed last? *Early Hum Dev* 5:71–77, 1981.

Humenick, S, and Van Steenkiste, S: Early indicators of breast-feeding progress, *Iss Compr Pediatr Nurs* 6:205–15, 1983.

Iffrig, MC: Nursing care and success in breastfeeding, *Nurs Clin North Am* 3:347–49, 1968.

Jakobsson, I, and Lindberg, T: Cow's milk as a cause of infantile colic in breastfed infants, *Lancet* 2:437–39, 1978.

Jakobsson, I, and Lindberg, T: Cow's milk proteins cause infantile colic in breast-fed infants: a double-blind crossover study, *Pediatrics* 71:268–71, 1983.

Jakobsson, I, et al.: Dietary bovine B-lactoglobulin is transferred to human milk, *Acta Paediatr Scand* 74:342–45, 1985.

Janke, JR: Breastfeeding duration following cesarean and vaginal births, *J Nurs-Midwif* 33:159–64, 1988.

Jansson, P: Early postpartum discharge, *AJN* 85:547–50, 1985.

Jenkins, HR, et al.: Food allergy: the major cause of infantile colitis, *Arch Dis Child* 59:326–29, 1984.

Johnstone, HA, and Marcinak, JF: Candidiasis in the

breastfeeding mother and infant, *JOGNN* 19:171–73, 1990.

Kajosaari, M, and Saarinen, UM: Prophylaxis of atopic disease by six months' total solid food elimination, *Acta Paediatr Scand* 72:411–14, 1983.

Kearney, MH, Cronenwett, LR, and Barrett, JA: Breast-feeding problems in the first week postpartum, *Nurs Res* 39:90–95, 1990.

Kearney, MH, Cronenwett, LR, and Reinhardt, R: Cesarean delivery and breastfeeding outcomes, *Birth* 17:97–103, 1990.

Klaus, KH, and Kennell, JH: *Parent-infant bonding,* 2nd ed., St. Louis, 1982, The C.V. Mosby Co., pp. 78–79.

Lau, C, and Henning, SJ: Noninvasive method for determining patterns of milk intake in the breast-fed infant, *J Pediatr Gastroenterol Nutr* 9:481–87, 1989.

Lawrence, RA: *Breastfeeding: A guide for the medical profession,* St. Louis, 1989, The C.V. Mosby Co.

Lie, B, and Juul, J: Effect of epidural vs. general anesthesia on breastfeeding, *Acta Obstet Gynecol Scand* 67:207–9, 1988.

Lifschitz, CH, et al.: Anaphylactic shock due to cow's milk protein hypersensitivity in a breast-fed infant, *J Pediatr Gastroenterol Nutr* 7:141–44, 1988.

Lothe, L, Lindberg, T, and Jakobsson, I: Cow's milk formula as a cause of infantile colic: a double-blind study, *Pediatrics* 70:7–10, 1982.

Marmet, C, Shell, E, and Marmet, R: Neonatal frenotomy may be necessary to correct breastfeeding problems, *J Hum Lact* 6:117–21, 1990.

Marx, CM, et al.: Vitamin E concentrations in serum of newborn infants after topical use of vitamin E in nursing mothers, *Am J Obstet Gynecol* 152:668–70, 1985.

Matheson, I: The effect of smoking on lactation and infantile colic, *JAMA* 261:42–43, 1989.

Matthews, MK: Developing an instrument to assess infant breastfeeding behaviour in the early neonatal period, *Midwifery* 4:154–65, 1988.

Mogan, J: A study of mothers' breastfeeding concerns, *Birth* 13:104–8, 1986.

Moon, JL, and Humenick, SS: Breast engorgement: contributing variables and variables amenable to nursing intervention, *JOGNN* 18:309–15, 1989.

Morse, J: Letter to the editor, *MCN* 14:204, 1989.

Mulford, C: Subtle signs and symptoms of the milk ejection reflex, *J Hum Lact* 6:177–78, 1990.

Neifert, MR, Seacat, JM, and Jobe, WE: Lactation failure due to insufficient grandular development of the breast, *Pediatrics* 76:823–28, 1985.

Neifert, M, et al.: The influence of breast surgery, breast appearance and pregnancy-induced changes on lactation sufficiency as measured by weight gain, *Birth* 17:31–38, 1990.

Newman, J: Breast-feeding: the problem of "not enough milk," *Can Fam Phys* 32:571–74, 1986.

Newman, J: Breastfeeding problems associated with the early introduction of bottles and pacifiers, *J Hum Lact* 6:59–63, 1990.

Newton, M: Human lactation. In Kon, SK, and Cowie, AT, eds.: *Milk The Mammary Gland and its Secretion,* Vol. 1, New York, 1961, Academic Press, Inc.

Newton, M: Nipple pain and nipple damage: problems in management of breast feeding, *J Pediatr* 41:411–23, 1952.

Newton, M, and Newton, N: The let-down reflex in human lactation, *J Pediatr* 33:698–704, 1948.

Nicholson, WL: Cracked nipples in breastfeeding mothers: a randomised trial of three methods of management, *Breastfeed Rev* 9:25–27, 1986.

Norr, KF, and Nacion, K: Outcomes of postpartum early discharge, 1960–1986: a comparative review, *Birth* 14:135–41, 1987.

Notestine, GE: The importance of the identification of ankyloglossia (short lingual frenulum) as a cause of breastfeeding problems, *J Hum Lact* 6:113–15, 1990.

O'Donovan, JC, and Bradstock, AS: Failure of conventional drug therapy in management of infantile colic, *Am J Dis Child* 133:999, 1979.

Oki, EY, et al.: The breast-stimulated contraction stress test, *J Reprod Med* 32:919–23, 1987.

Orem, DE: *Nursing: concepts of practice,* 2 ed., New York, 1980, McGraw-Hill Book Co.

Padawer, JA, et al.: Women's psychological adjustment following emergency Cesarean versus vaginal delivery, *Psychol Women Q* 12:25–34, 1988.

Page-Goertz, S: Discharge planning for the breastfeeding dyad, *Pediatr Nurs* 15:543–44, 1989.

Phillips, V: *Successful Breastfeeding,* 6th Ed., Numawading, Victoria, Australia, 1991, Nursing Mothers' Association of Australia.

Pietz, CL: The emotional impact of breastfeeding after a cesarean, *Int J Child Educ* 4:20–21, 1989.

Pittschieler, K: Cow's milk protein-induced colitis in the breast-fed infant, *J Pediatr Gastroenterol Nutr* 10:548–49, 1990.

Quandt, SA: Biological and behavioral predictors of exclusive breastfeeding duration, *Med Anthrop* 8:139–51, 1985.

Rattigan, S, Ghisalberti, AV, and Hartmann, PE: Breast milk production in Australian women, *Br J Nutr* 45:243–49, 1981.

Rimar, JM: Epidural morphine for analgesia following a cesarean, *MCN* 11:345, 1986.

Riordan, J: *A Practical Guide to Breastfeeding,* Boston, 1990, Jones and Bartlett Publishers, Inc.

Riordan, J: The effectiveness of topical agents in reducing nipple soreness of breastfeeding mothers, *J Hum Lact* 1:36–41, 1984.

Riordan, J, and Countryman, BA: Basics of breastfeeding, Part IV: Preparation of breastfeeding and early optimal functioning, *JOGN Nurs* 9:273–83, 1980a.

Riordan, J, and Countryman, BA: Basics of breastfeeding, Part V: Self-care for continued breastfeeding, *JOGN Nurs* 9:357–66, 1980b.

Rosanove, R: Dangers of the application of lanolin (letter), *Med J Aust* 146:232 (Feb. 16), 1987.

Rosenblatt, DB, et al.: The influence of maternal analgesia on neonatal behavior. II: Epidural bupivacaine, *Br J Obstet Gynaecol* 88:407–13, 1981.

Rothman, KJ, Runch, DP, and Dreyer, NA: Bromocriptine and puerperal seizures, *Epidemiology* 1:232–38, 1990.

Rubin, R: Attainment of the maternal role. I. Processes, *Nurs Res* 16:237–41, 1967a.

Rubin, R: Attainment of the maternal role. II. Models and referrants, *Nurs Res* 16:342–46, 1967b.

Rubin, R: Basic maternal behavior, *Nurs Outlook* 9:683–86, 1961.

Ruch, A, and Duhring, JL: Postpartum myocardial infarction in a patient receiving bromocriptine, *Obstet Gynecol* 74:448–51, 1989.

Ruvalcaba, RHA: Stress-induced cessation of lactation, *West J Med* 146:228–30, 1987.

Said, G, Patois E, and Lellouch, J: Infantile colic and parental smoking, *Br Med J* 289:660, 1984.

Saint, L, Maggiore, P, and Hartmann, PE: Yield and nutrient content of milk in eight women breast-feeding twins and one woman breast-feeding triplets, *Br J Nutr* 56:49–58, 1986.

Salariya, EM, Easton, PM, and Cater, JI: Duration of breast-feeding after early initiation and frequent feeding, *Lancet* 2:1141–43, 1978.

Salmon, YM, et al.: Cervical ripening by breast stimulation, *Obstet Gynecol* 67:21–24, 1986.

Sexson, WR: Incidence of neonatal hypoglycemia: A matter of definition, *J Pediatr* 105:149–50, 1984.

Shrago, L, and Bocar, D: The infant's contribution to breastfeeding, *JOGNN* 19:209–15, 1990.

Simkin, P: Intermittent brachial plexus neuropathy secondary to breast engorgement, *Birth* 15:102–4, 1988.

Sollid, DT, et al.: Breastfeeding multiples, *J Perinat Neonat Nurs* 3:46–65, 1989.

Standley, K, Klein, RP, and Soule, AB: Local-regional anesthesia during childbirth and newborn behavior, *Science* 180:634–35, 1974.

Storr, GB: Breastfeeding premature triplets: one woman's experience, *J Hum Lact* 5:74–77, 1989.

Storr, GB: Prevention of nipple tenderness and breast engorgement in the postpartal period, *JOGNN* 17:203–8, 1988.

Taubman, B: Parental counseling compared with elimination of cow's milk or soy milk protein for the treatment of infant colic syndrome: a randomized trial, *Pediatrics* 81:756–61, 1988.

Taylor, MM: *Transcultural aspects of breastfeeding—USA* (Unit 2), Lactation Consultant Series, Garden City Park, N.Y., 1985, Avery Publishing Group, Inc., pp. 18–19.

Taylor, PM, Maloni, JA, and Brown, DR: Early suckling and prolonged breast-feeding, *Am J Dis Child* 140:151–54, 1986.

Tully, J, and Dewey, KG: Private fears, global loss: a cross-cultural study of the insufficient milk syndrome, *Med Anthrop* 8:225–43, 1985.

Victora, CG, et al.: Caesarean section and duration of breast feeding among Brazilians, *Arch Dis Child* 65:632–34, 1990.

Waldenstrom, U, Sundelin, C, and Lindmark, G: Early and late discharge after hospital birth: breastfeeding, *Acta Paediatr Scand* 76:727–32, 1987.

Walker, M: *Breastfeeding Premature Babies* (Unit 14), Lactation Consultant Series, Garden City Park, N.Y., 1991, Avery Publishing Group, Inc.

Walker, M: Management of selected early breastfeeding problems seen in clinical practice, *Birth* 16:148–58, 1989.

Walker, M, and Discoll, JW: Sore nipples: the new mother's nemesis, *MCN* 14:260–65, 1989.

Watson, DL, et al.: Bromocriptine mesylate for lactation suppression: a risk for postpartum hypertension? *Obstet Gynecol* 74:573–76, 1989.

Weaver, LT, Ewing, G, and Taylor, LC: The bowel habit of milk-fed infants, *J Pediatr Gastroenterol Nutr* 7:568–71, 1988.

Whitley, N: Preparation for breastfeeding: a one-year follow-up of 34 nursing mothers, *JOGN Nurs* 7:44–48, 1974.

Widstrom, A-M, et al.: Gastric suction in healthy newborn infants, *Acta Paediatr Scand* 76:566–72, 1987.

Williams, J, and Mueller, S: A message to the nurse from the baby, *J Hum Lact* 5:19, 1989.

Wilton, JM: Sore nipples and slow weight gain related to a short frenulum, *J Hum Lact* 6:122–23, 1990.

Winikoff, B, et al.: Dynamics of infant feeding: mothers, professionals, and the institutional context in a large urban hospital, *Pediatrics* 77:357–65, 1986.

Woodward, A, and Hand, K: Smoking and reduced duration of breast-feeding, *Med J Aust* 148:477–78, 1988.

Woolridge, MW, and Fisher, C: Colic, "overfeeding," and symptoms of lactose malabsorption in the breast-fed baby: a possible artifact of feed management? *Lancet* 2:382–84, 1988.

Woolridge, MW, Greasley, V, and Silpisornkosol, S: The initiation of lactation: the effect of early versus delayed contact for suckling on milk intake in the first week postpartum. A study in Chiang Mai, Northern Thailand, *Early Hum Dev* 12:269–78, 1985.

Woolridge, MW, Ingram, JC, and Baum, JD: Do changes in pattern of breast usage alter the baby's nutrient intake? *Lancet* 336(8712):395–97, 1990.

Working Group on Cow's Milk Protein in Allergy: Cow's milk allergy in the first year of life, *Acta Paediatr Scand* (Suppl.) 348:2–14, 1988.

Ziemer, MM, et al.: Methods to prevent and manage nipple pain in breastfeeding women, *West J Nurs Res* 12:732–44, 1990.

10

Breastfeeding the Pre-Term Infant

Paula P. Meier
Henry H. Mangurten

In the United States, more than one-half of mothers who want to breastfeed their pre-term infants will have abandoned lactation efforts prior to their infant's discharge from the high-risk nursery (Ehrenkranz et al., 1985; Pereira et al., 1984; Richards et al., 1986). Although mothers of pre-term infants have stated repeatedly that breastfeeding is the one thing they can do for their pre-term infants when other care-taking activities have been assumed by professionals, they cite numerous in-hospital obstacles to successful breastfeeding. Among these are inconsistencies in information and support provided by hospital staff, availability of equipment for milk expression, and absence of a private place to express milk and breastfeed their infants (Ehrenkranz & Ackerman, 1986; Ehrenkranz et al., 1985; McCoy et al., 1988; Richards et al., 1986). Additionally, mothers report that they receive inadequate and conflicting information about methods for feeding the pre-term infant at breast during the in-hospital and postdischarge periods.

Historically, breastfeeding and the artificial feeding of mothers' milk (e.g., gavage and medicine dropper) were standard practices in the premature infant stations of the United States during the 1920s and 1930s (Lundeen, 1939, 1954, 1959). Breastfeeding for pre-term infants was supported both for the recognized health benefits, and because safe alternatives to breastfeeding were unavailable postdischarge. Mothers of pre-term infants were supervised in this technique by the nursery nurses. Pre-term infants began feeding at the mother's breast when they weighed approximately four pounds. Commonly, a healthy, full-term infant was positioned at one breast and allowed to suckle, electing the milk-ejection reflex. Once the mother's milk began to flow freely, the nurse positioned the pre-term infant at the other breast. The rationale for this practice was that the pre-term infant could exert minimal energy by suckling postejection milk.

Although little research-based data are available to explain the decline in breastfeeding for pre-term infants over subsequent decades, it is reasonable that the causes parallel those cited for term infants. This period in the history of the United States coincides with "Scientific Motherhood," which was characterized by a decline in breastfeeding and increasing involvement of the physician in the management of infant feeding (Apple, 1987). It is likely that an entire generation of neonatal nurses was unexposed to the art and science of supporting breastfeeding for pre-term infants.

The current low incidence of breastfeeding success among mothers of pre-term infants in the United States reflects the paucity of research-based interventions to facilitate breastfeeding for this population. Although the incidence of breastfeeding success for pre-term infants is reportedly higher in Scandinavian countries, even researchers there report an inverse relationship between gestational age and duration of breastfeeding (Haggkvist, 1990; Meberg, Willgraff & Sande, 1982; Verronen, 1985). Many physicians and nurses still feel that breastfeeding is "too stressful" for pre-term infants and are not comfortable with the "inexactness" of feeding volumes and schedules. Additionally, family members, consumer groups, and some health professionals make recommendations about breastfeeding pre-term infants based on standards for full-term, healthy babies. Both approaches demonstrate that, until recently, little research was available to guide breastfeeding decisions for pre-term infants. The management of breastfeeding for pre-term infants should be guided by a health practitioner who has expertise in both lactation and the clinical care of high-risk infants. Such a practitioner is able to individualize interventions based on research findings in order to meet the needs of breastfeeding mothers and their pre-term infants.

In this chapter research-based interventions for management of breastfeeding for pre-term infants are reviewed within a four-phase temporal model. The four phases of this model include: (1) expression and collection of mothers' milk; (2) gavage feeding of expressed mothers' milk (EMM); (3) in-hospital breastfeeding sessions; and (4) postdischarge consultation. This model was developed through ongoing content analysis of breastfeeding records maintained for 132 mothers of pre-term/high risk infants for a 12-month period from 1989 to 1990. Of the 132 mothers who received these breastfeeding interventions in a Level III neonatal intensive care unit (NICU), 72% were still breastfeeding at the time of the infant's discharge from the hospital. Thus, the model can be considered effective in preventing breastfeeding failure during the in-hospital period for mothers of pre-term infants. Central to this model is a health-care provider, preferably an experienced NICU nurse, who coordinates a breastfeeding plan with each mother and involves other care providers as appropriate. For purposes of this chapter, this role will be referred to as the NICU breastfeeding specialist.

PHASE ONE: EXPRESSION AND COLLECTION OF MOTHERS' MILK

THE DECISION TO BREASTFEED

Every mother who has an infant admitted to the NICU should be considered a breastfeeding "candidate" until she has indicated otherwise. This approach will assure that each mother receives an initial consultation from the NICU breastfeeding specialist, who can answer the mother's questions about the benefits and mechanics of breastfeeding as they relate to her infant's special condition.

Although most mothers will have decided whether to breastfeed or bottle-feed during pregnancy, some mothers who give birth to very premature infants may not have made a final feeding decision at the time of the infant's NICU admission. When an infant is born prematurely or with other clinical problems, a mother who had intended to bottle-feed may elect to breastfeed—at least for a short time, so that the infant receives the unique immunological and nutritional benefits of mothers' milk. In a recent study, in-depth interviews were conducted with 20 mothers of pre-term infants at one month following infant discharge from the NICU in order to describe the maternal experience of breastfeeding a pre-term infant in the postdischarge period (Kavanaugh, personal communication, 1992). Although the focus of this study did not include eliciting information about the decision to breastfeed, many mothers shared their feelings about this decision. At least one-half of them reported that their decision to breastfeed was motivated not by the desire to breastfeed, per se, but rather by the fact that they felt the associated health benefits were important to their pre-term infants.

This finding has important implications for NICU personnel. Mothers who are indecisive about breastfeeding should be encouraged to initiate milk expression for two reasons. First, it is physiologically easier to stimulate lactation in the early postpartum period than it is several days later (Lawrence, 1989; Neifert & Seacat, 1988). Second, the milk produced in early lactation, especially colostrum, contains antiinfective properties that are most beneficial to the infant (Atkinson & Kaufman, 1986; Neifert & Seacat, 1988; AAP, 1980a, 1980b). Mindful of these two principles, mothers who are indecisive should be encouraged to begin milk expression, knowing that they can discontinue efforts later if they wish. Meanwhile, pre-term infants can receive EMM for the length of time which their mothers elect to breastfeed. Although many of these mothers will continue to feed infants directly at the breast, some will not. Mothers in the latter group should be commended and assured that infants received unique health benefits from the early mothers' milk.

INITIAL BREASTFEEDING CONSULTATION

During the initial consultation with the mother of a pre-term infant, the NICU breastfeeding specialist should recommend a schedule for milk expression, arrange to have a breast pump made available for post-discharge use, and explain the NICU policies with respect to bacteriologic surveillance of EMM. This conversation should be held in a private place, such as the mother's postpartum room or the parent room in the NICU. If convenient, the NICU breastfeeding specialist can also assess the mother's breasts and her use of in-hospital breast pump equipment.

DEVELOPING A MILK EXPRESSION SCHEDULE

The milk expression schedule should reflect an understanding of the mother's physical condition as well as the presence of supports and barriers to milk expression in the mother's environment. Ideally, the milk expression schedule for a mother of a pre-term infant should parallel the frequency with which a term, healthy infant breastfeeds—e.g., 8 to 12 times daily. Early, frequent feeding for term infants has been demonstrated to result in greater maternal milk supply, greater infant weight gain, and earlier maturation of mothers' milk (De Carvalho et al., 1983; Drewett & Woolridge, 1979; Howie et al., 1981; Humenick, 1987). In the absence of data which specifically address the ideal frequency of milk expression for the mother of a pre-term infant, these guidelines are appropriate. Once the mother has established a milk supply, the frequency of milk expression may be decreased on an individual basis.

Numerous maternal and environmental considerations may preclude such a frequent milk expression schedule for some mothers of pre-term infants. The mother may have had complications of pregnancy which necessitate longer periods of rest than are compatible with this schedule. Second, if mothers spend lengthy time travelling to and from the NICU after they have been discharged, this plan must be modified, because they may not have access to breast pump equipment every two to three hours. Finally, the presence of small children or other household demands must be considered. It is important that the NICU breastfeeding specialist and the mother develop a workable plan that incorporates the physiologic principles of early and frequent milk expression in the postpartum period.

SECURING A SUITABLE BREAST PUMP

The initial consultation with the mother needs to include making plans for obtaining a suitable breast pump for in-home use. The commercial products that are available for rental and purchase are reviewed in Chapter 11. Without exception, mothers of pre-term infants should be encouraged to rent an electric breast pump for use in the home. Many mothers should purchase a double-pump collecting kit in order to optimize prolactin levels and decrease pumping times (Neifert & Seacat, 1985). Although most mothers of NICU infants could benefit from the double-pump collecting kit, it should be the standard of care for the following mothers: (1) those with infants weighing less than 1500 grams; (2) those whose infants will be unable to feed directly at the breast for at least two weeks; and (3) those with multiple births. Mothers should be informed that, with few exceptions, pumping will continue for at least two weeks after the infant has been discharged from the NICU.

Under optimal conditions, the NICU breastfeeding specialist will have worked with the hospital to contract for breast pump rentals and purchases. The underlying principle is that the NICU refers breastfeeding mothers to an agency or rental depot in exchange for services which benefit those mothers. For example, the contracting agency which receives NICU referrals might then be expected to provide the following services: (1) delivery of the pump to the NICU at no additional charge to the parent; (2) direct billing of third parties for reimbursement of pump expenses, including providing documentation from the neonatologist that the infant's condition necessitates mothers' milk; (3) securing pumps from other agencies or the manufacturers within 24 hours, in the event that all pumps in the referral agency have been rented; and (4) complimentary pickup of the pump from the mother's home when she no longer needs it. Agencies that typically provide such services might include an affiliated home health agency, a local pharmacy, a hospital gift shop, or rental depot.

Unless a parent requests otherwise, the NICU breastfeeding specialist should assume responsibility for contacting the referral agency. This relieves the mother or extended family of the burden of an additional phone call at a stressful time and allows the NICU breastfeeding specialist to consolidate all

NICU referrals into one or two phone calls daily. The mother should be told that information about third-party reimbursements will be provided to the referral agency, unless the mother prefers that this information not be shared. Such an agreement has obvious benefits for both the mother and the referral agency. The mother has an appropriate pump and collecting equipment delivered to the NICU without numerous phone calls and insurance inquiries, and the referral agency enjoys the volume of business provided by an NICU, making additional services and competitive rates possible.

EXPLAINING NICU POLICIES ABOUT
BACTERIOLOGIC SURVEILLANCE
OF MOTHERS' MILK

Depending upon the specific NICU, policies may have been established for bacteriologic surveillance of EMM. Although the data are not conclusive with respect to a culturing protocol for pre-term infants, certain principles are universal. First, it is well known that term infants ingest a variety of bacteria during breastfeeding and that no adverse consequences have been reported for this population (Eidelman & Szilagyi, 1979). However, these data cannot be generalized for small, pre-term infants who have compromised immunologic systems and who do not receive milk directly from the breast. Case studies of pre-term infants who have developed adverse consequences

from ingestion of contaminated EMM have been reported in the literature (Botsford et al., 1986; Donowitz et al., 1981; O'Donovan & O'Brien, 1985; Ryder et al., 1977). Thus, it is appropriate for an NICU to have developed protocols for maternal breast care and for bacteriologic surveillance of EMM.

The amount of bacteria in EMM that can be ingested by the pre-term infant is unknown, so standards for acceptable milk vary in the literature (AAP, 1980b; Meier & Wilks, 1987). Two fairly universal criteria are that the EMM should have an absence of all bacteria other than normal skin flora, and that skin flora should be present in minimal concentrations, usually 10^2 to 10^4 colony-forming units per milliliter (Meier & Wilks, 1987). Achievement of these standards requires that mothers incorporate bacteria-reducing techniques during milk expression. These techniques are summarized in Fig. 10–1.

For infants who are particularly susceptible to infection from *staphylococcal epidermidis*, mothers may be asked to clean the nipple and areola with mild soap prior to each expression of milk (Meier & Wilks, 1987; Wilks & Meier, 1988). While this intervention seldom renders milk sterile, it does significantly reduce the colony counts of microorganisms (Costa, 1989). There are no research-based data to demonstrate that use of soap for nipple cleansing is associated with nipple pain or dryness. Additionally, use of soap for nipple cleansing is usually a short-term intervention for these mothers. The alternative

---

☐ Wash your hands thoroughly with soap and water. Take care to clean under and around the fingernails.

☐ Assemble sterile milk collection equipment beside the pump. Take care not to touch the inside of the collecting bottle, flange, or the bottom of the lid. Also take care not to cough or sneeze near equipment.

☐ Hand express and discard the first 10 cc (about two teaspoons) of milk from each breast.
Cleanse the nipples and areolae as follows:

• Wet 4 sterile gauze wipes with sterile water*
Apply a few drops of pHisoDerm soap to two of the wipes. Use these to clean the nipples and areolae. (Begin with the nipple itself, then work outward in a circular fashion until the areola is cleansed)

*The materials are provided by the hospital.

• Use the other two moistened wipes to rinse off the soap.
(Again, rinse the nipple first and then work outward.)

• Dry the nipples and then the areolae with dry sterile gauze.

☐ Place the collecting device over one breast, and begin to use the pump. In doing so, take care not to touch the inside of the flange or your nipple area.

☐ When the breast is emptied, pour your milk from the collecting device to the sterile container for milk storage. Do not touch the inside of the storage container or the inside of its lid. Place the collecting device over the other breast and repeat as instructed above.

☐ Label the storage container with your baby's name, the date, and time; immediately freeze or refrigerate the container, depending on the plan you discussed with the nurse.

FIGURE 10–1 Mothers' instruction for milk expression.

to reducing the concentration of *staphylococcal epidermidis* in EMM usually involves feeding sterile formula to these small, susceptible infants.

The NICU breastfeeding specialist should explain the milk expression technique, and the reasons for the special precautions, so that it is understood by the mother. The mother should be assured that her basic hygiene is not being questioned; rather, she is being asked to reduce the bacteria normally present on her nipple and areola to a level that is "abnormally" low. This approach will facilitate the mother's compliance, and will reduce the likelihood that she feels her personal hygiene is being scrutinized.

The NICU breastfeeding specialist, in consultation with the neonatologist, should develop an individualized plan for bacteriologic surveillance of each mother's EMM; this should be communicated to the mother as early as possible during the infant's hospitalization. For infants at minimal risk of infection, the plan may be to obtain EMM cultures until a result has been returned which reflects that the mother is exercising appropriate expression technique—and then to discontinue routine cultures. For infants at greater risk of infection, initial EMM cultures should be obtained. In addition there should be a plan for continued surveillance, e.g., once weekly for a certain period of time.

In the absence of conclusive studies that support a particular option for a particular infant, each NICU should establish protocols that reflect the following research-based principles:

- Expressed mothers' milk is almost never sterile and contains *staphylococcal epidermidis*, which may be pathogenic for small pre-term infants (Meier & Wilks, 1987; Wilks & Meier, 1988).
- The smaller, sicker pre-term infant has a compromised immune system and may be more susceptible to bacteria in EMM.
- Continuous infusion of EMM permits bacterial growth in already colonized milk.
- EMM which has not been frozen contains optimal antiinfective properties that would have been destroyed or reduced by freezing; therefore if fresh EMM is administered, the infant may be able to tolerate slightly greater concentrations of skin flora.

Thus, infants at greatest risk would be those very small, clinically unstable pre-term infants who receive frozen EMM by continuous gavage infusion. For these infants, bacteriologic cultures should be performed at least weekly. Larger, clinically stable pre-term infants who receive bolus gavage feedings accompanied by breastfeedings constitute minimal risk. In most instances, bacteriologic cultures are unnecessary for this group of infants. Finally, cultures should always be obtained as a component of a sepsis evaluation in an infant who has received EMM by gavage feedings. If sepsis is suspected or must be eliminated as a diagnosis for an infant, EMM cultures should be as routine as those for blood, urine, or cerebral spinal fluid.

STORAGE OF EXPRESSED MOTHERS' MILK

Expressed mothers' milk should be placed in sterile, airtight containers which are easily handled by the nurses who will prepare the milk for gavage or bottle feedings. Standard, over-the-counter "nurser" bags are unsuitable for milk storage in the NICU, because the EMM is difficult to defrost and handle without contaminating the contents. Graduated plastic feeders with twist-on, airtight caps are ideal for EMM storage. No definitive guidelines are available for the length of time EMM can remain refrigerated until it is fed to the infant. However, a conservative policy based on available literature (AAP, 1980b) is that fresh or previously frozen EMM should be fed to pre-term infants within 24 hours of refrigeration. Ideally, if a mother is available to express milk just prior to each feeding, freezing and/or refrigeration of EMM can be avoided entirely. This approach is optimal in minimizing bacterial growth and maximizing antiinfective properties of milk received by the infant.

PHASE TWO: GAVAGE FEEDING OF EXPRESSED MOTHERS' MILK

Most small pre-term infants receive mothers' milk by gavage infusion until they have demonstrated the ability to feed orally. Infants who receive EMM by gavage infusion are generally smaller and less stable clinically than other pre-term infants. Issues to be addressed for these small infants who receive gavage feedings of EMM include: optimal method for administration of EMM; the adequacy of EMM for pre-term infant growth; the use of human milk fortifiers;

and principles concerning "contaminants" in EMM fed to small pre-term infants.

METHODS OF GAVAGE ADMINISTRATION OF EMM

Depending upon the NICU, infants will receive continuous or intermittent gavage infusions of milk. In previously published research, intermittent bolus gavage feedings have been associated with adverse short-term physiologic and biochemical responses, e.g., apnea, bradycardia, and hypoxemia (Churella, Bachhuber & MacLean, 1985; Eckburg et al., 1987; Herrell, Martin & Fanaroff, 1980; Krauss et al., 1978; Lefrak-Okikawa, 1988; Mukhtar & Strothers, 1982). Thus, policies in many NICUs stipulate that small pre-term infants, who tend to be most prone to these responses, be fed by continuous nasogastric (CNG) infusion, which theoretically is not accompanied by such responses. However, a series of studies have documented nutrient loss and bacterial growth in EMM administered by the CNG route (Botsford et al., 1986; Brooke & Barley, 1978; Greer, McCormick & Loker, 1984; Lemons et al., 1983; Stocks et al., 1985).

Nurses have noted anecdotally that the lipid fraction of EMM adheres to the infusion syringe and tubing during CNG feedings. The phenomenon of lipid loss during slow-infusion gavage feedings has been confirmed by numerous published studies (Brooke & Barley, 1978; Greer, McCormick & Loker, 1984; Lemons et al., 1983; Stocks et al., 1985). This finding is extremely significant for clinical management of small pre-term infants, because the lipid component of EMM represents its greatest caloric source. If lipids adhere to the infusion syringe and tubing, infants may receive a more dilute, low-calorie milk and subsequently demonstrate suboptimal growth. In general, there is an inverse relationship between infusion rate and lipid loss during gavage feedings, with little or no lipid loss occurring during intermittent bolus feedings (Greer, McCormick & Loker, 1984). Placement of the infusion syringe in a semi-upright position results in delivery of EMM with minimal lipid losses (Narayan, Singh & Harvey, 1984); however, lipids can potentially adhere to the infusion tubing once EMM has left the syringe. Minimizing the size of the infusion tubing lumen may reduce lipid loss during CNG feedings (Brennan-Behm, personal communication, 1992). In a recent unpublished study, less lipid loss was demonstrated during simulated CNG feedings of EMM using small lumen

(0.6 mL) rather than standard lumen (5.00 mL) tubing. Although the differences in lipid loss were significantly different for the two types of tubing, marked lipid loss occurred for both types of infusion tubing. The results of this study suggest that EMM should not be administered by slow infusion methods if the lipid complement is to be preserved.

Another disadvantage of administering EMM by CNG infusion is that the bacteria in EMM multiply rapidly in the infusion syringe and tubing when EMM remains at room or incubator temperature for prolonged periods of time (Botsford et al., 1986; Lemons et al., 1983). Thus, frequent changes of syringe and tubing are essential in preventing significant bacterial growth in EMM. If EMM is administered by CNG infusion, the literature would suggest that syringe and tubing be changed completely at least every four hours, and more frequently for infants who might be particularly susceptible to infection (Botsford et al., 1986; Lemons et al., 1983).

Such frequent changes of infusion apparatus make volumetric infusion systems with lengthy infusion tubing undesirable for CNG feedings. Such systems require 20 to 30 mL of EMM to prime the tubing; changing the tubing every four hours would result in a tremendous wastage of EMM, as well as the sizeable expense of replacing volumetric sets. Nurses report anecdotally that routine changing of volumetric tubing is frequently circumvented in the clinical setting by changing the tubings every 24 hours, while flushing them with sterile water every four to eight hours between changes. Although this approach may reduce the expense of volumetric tubing, it is inadequate from the perspective of controlling bacteriologic growth in EMM. Flushing the infusion tubing with sterile water may cleanse the tubing, but does not sterilize already contaminated tubing. Thus, bacteria remain in the tubing and continue to grow from one flushing to the next. In an unpublished study, bacterial growth in EMM administered by volumetric infusion was measured in a clinical setting in which tubing was changed every 24 hours and flushed every four hours (Loebel & Gennardo, personal communication, 1989). This study was discontinued because results demonstrated that the bacterial growth in EMM under these conditions was so great that continuing the study was considered unethical. In fact, for the majority of infants, the bacterial growth reached a level that was "too high to quantify" after four to eight hours of infusion.

Thus, two major clinical implications concerning method of gavage infusion of EMM can be delineated. First, whenever possible, infants should be fed EMM by intermittent bolus infusion. The rate of administration should be sufficiently slow to minimize or prevent adverse consequences of rapid gastric filling. Second, for those infants who must receive CNG infusion of EMM, selected safeguards are required. These include:

- routine bacteriologic surveillance of EMM, so that EMM contains only skin flora in concentrations not exceeding 10^3 cfu/mL
- infusing the EMM at the highest possible rate deemed safe for the infant, in order to minimize bacterial growth and nutrient loss
- use of a syringe pump placed at a 45° angle and small lumen infusion tubing to minimize nutrient loss
- daily measurement of the lipid content of EMM by creamatocrit (Lucas et al., 1978; Lemons, Schreiner & Gresham, 1980) at the distal end of the infusion system, in order to estimate the caloric value of EMM that is actually received by the infant
- changing syringe and tubing every four hours to minimize bacterial growth.

ADEQUACY OF EXPRESSED MOTHERS' MILK AND THE USE OF HUMAN MILK FORTIFIERS

In the early 1970s, results of studies conducted with animals suggested that the feeding of mothers' milk to pre-term infants may prevent the development of necrotizing enterocolitis (Pitt, 1979). A recent study supports this protective effect (Lucas & Cole, 1990). As a consequence, many neonatal units established donor milk banks so that pre-term infants could be fed mothers' milk. The early reports from these practices suggested that pre-term infants did not gain weight as rapidly on donor human milk as they did when they were fed formula, which raised the issue as to what constituted "optimal" extrauterine weight gain (Davies, 1977; Davies & Evans, 1978; Fomon, Ziegler & Vazquez, 1977; Gaull, Raiha & Rassin, 1979; Heird, 1977). A major issue in the research literature at the time was whether donor milk contained adequate amounts of protein to support optimal brain growth in pre-term infants.

Although the question of whether pre-term milk differed in composition was first raised in 1969 (Stevens, 1969), this problem received extensive investigation during the late 1970s. Studies suggested that milk produced by mothers who delivered pre-term infants differed in composition from milk produced by mothers who delivered at term. Specifically, pre-term milk was found to have higher concentrations of protein, sodium, calcium, lipids, and selected anti-infective properties. This difference in composition was consistent with the unique nutritional needs of pre-term infants. Generally, these differences disappear over the first month of lactation, at which time pre-term milk resembles term milk in composition. These compositional differences have been summarized in a review by Atkinson and Kaufman (1986).

The significance of differences in pre-term milk has been the subject of considerable debate. It has been proposed that the consistency in composition of pre-term milk and the pre-term infant's growth needs represent yet another "species-specific" advantage of breastfeeding. Another plausible theory is that compositional differences in pre-term milk are due to greater permeability of the immature mammary gland (Atkinson & Kaufman, 1986).

Although the research literature supports the existence of compositional differences between pre-term and term milk, the clinician must remember that considerable variability exists in samples of mothers' milk; these differences are present between and within individual mothers. Additionally, the available research does not differentiate between "compositional" inadequacies of milk and the loss of nutrients in the milk through gavage feeding. Thus, it is important that each mother's milk be evaluated with respect to her own infant's nutritional needs. It is a widely accepted view that mother's milk alone may not be adequate for optimal nutrition in very low-birth-weight infants.

Human milk has been recommended with increasing frequency for pre-term and low-birth-weight infants; however, recent clinical and research experience have suggested certain inadequacies in mothers' milk for some infants. A number of problems have been identified which warrant the use of human milk fortifiers. These include nutritional inadequacy characterized by slower growth rate (Gross et al., 1980); hypoproteinemia (Ronnholm, Sipila & Siimes, 1982) and hyponatremia (Al-Dahhan et al., 1984); and osteopenia of prematurity with diminished bone mineralization (Sagy et al., 1980).

The typical profile of an infant who may require such fortification is the extremely pre-term (i.e., less than 25 to 26 weeks of gestation) and/or very low-birth-weight (i.e., less than 900 to 1000 grams) infant who initially requires aggressive ventilation and other treatment for hyaline membrane disease, patent ductus arteriosus, or pulmonary edema, followed by the development of bronchopulmonary dysplasia. This infant often also experiences enteric feeding intolerance, fluid intolerance, and electrolyte depletion secondary to chronic use of diuretics.

As a result of extensive studies of growth, biochemical status, and mineral metabolism of such infants, a number of human milk fortifiers have been developed. Enfamil Human Milk Fortifier is a powder available in 0.95-gram packets. This fortifier is appealing because it provides supplemental nutrients without displacing milk volume, thus allowing for greater intake of human milk itself. However, the theoretical hazard exists of delivering excessive amounts of protein and minerals to the infant, depending on the nutrient content of the milk itself.

Similac Natural Care liquid human milk fortifier is available in four-ounce bottles. In contrast to the powdered form, this fortifier may dilute the higher level of nutrients present in the expressed milk of some mothers because it is mixed in a ratio with the amount of human milk to be given to the baby. In addition, the liquid fortifier contributes to the infant's total volume of intake, thus diminishing the actual amount of human milk ingested.

Both commercially available fortifiers contain cow milk's protein with a whey-to-casein ratio of 60:40. The Enfamil fortifier contains very little fat. Similac Natural Care contains a mixture of medium-chain and long-chain triglycerides. If human milk and Similac Natural Care are mixed, the lipase in the milk may enhance hydrolysis of fats in the fortifier in vivo. The net effect would be improved fat absorption in the pre-term patient.

The composition of Enfamil fortifier and Similac Natural Care are listed in the Table 10–1. Also listed are final compositions of pre-term milk reconstituted with each of the fortifiers.

The importance of human milk fortifier in the nutrition of low-birth-weight and pre-term infants cannot be overemphasized. However, it should be stressed that this should not be used routinely in all babies (Gross, 1987). In particular, larger, more stable, healthier pre-term infants who are started on en-teric feedings early and who are easily weaned from intravenous nutrition may not be candidates for human milk fortifiers. The use of fortifiers may be particularly helpful in improving calcium and phosphorous intake, which may be inadequate during the feeding of human milk alone (Rowe et al., 1979). The addition of either fortifier should provide enough calcium and phosphorous to approach the recommended requirements. It should also be noted that neither fortifier provides significant quantities of iron (Thompson & McClead, 1987). Therefore, additional supplemental iron should be presented on an as-needed basis. Both fortifiers also contain vitamins. It is important to take this into account when prescribing fortifiers in order to avoid excessive vitamin intake.

GUIDELINES FOR ADMINISTRATION
Enfamil Human Milk Fortifier:

- Add 4 packets of fortifier to each 100 mL of human milk (or 1 packet to each 25 mL of human milk).
- Add fortifier immediately before feeding, followed by thorough mixing. Any mixture of fortifier and milk left over after the feeding should be discarded.
- Iron supplementation at 2–3 mg/kg/day should be started between two weeks and 12 months of age.
- Fat-soluble vitamin intake should be calculated for any infant over 2 kilos who is still receiving fortified milk in order to avoid chronic high vitamin ingestion.
- Serum electrolytes and urea nitrogen should be monitored twice per week until stable, followed by weekly monitoring thereafter.

Fortifier should be discontinued prior to discharge from the nursery.

Similac Natural Care Human Milk Fortifier:

- Shake the bottle of fortifier thoroughly to resuspend the minerals.
- Alternate feedings of human milk and fortifier, or mix human milk and fortifier in a 50:50 ratio immediately before feeding (a 25:75 ratio of human milk to fortifier may be advisable for infants with osteopenia of prematurity).

TABLE 10-1   COMPOSITION OF PRE-TERM (PT) MILK, FORTIFIERS, AND FORTIFIERS ADDED TO MILK

Nutrients	PT Milk (at 14 days) 100 mL	Enfamil Fortifier 4 pkts	PT Milk + Enfamil Fortifier[1] 100 mL	Similac Natural Care 100 mL	PT Milk + Similac Natural Care[2] 100 mL
Calories	67	14	81	81	75
Carbohydrate, gm	6.4	2.7	9.1	8.6	7.5
Protein, gm	1.9	0.7	2.6	2.2	2.1
Fat, gm	3.8	0.05	3.8	4.4	4.1
Ca, mg	28	60	88	170	99
P, mg	15	33	48	85	50
Mg, mg	3	4	7	10	7
Na, mg	32	7	39	38	35
K, mg	69	15.6	85	112	91
Cl, mg	54	17.7	72	71	63
Fe, mg	0.1	–	0.1	0.3	0.2
Zn, mcg	375	310	685	1200	788
Cu, mcg	52	80	132	200	126
Vit A, IU	44	780	824	550	297
Vit E, IU	0.6	3.4	4.0	3	1.8
Vit C, mg	4.2	24	28.2	30	17.1
Vit D, IU	2.2	260	262.2	120	61.1
Vit K, mcg	1.5	9.1	10.6	10	5.8
Vit B_1, mg	0.016	0.187	0.203	0.2	0.11
Vit B_2, mg	0.036	0.25	0.286	0.5	0.27
Niacin, mg	0.147	3.1	3.247	4.0	2.07
Vit B_6, mg	0.01	0.193	0.203	0.2	0.11
Vit B_{12}, mcg	0.03	0.21	0.24	0.45	0.24
Folic Acid, mcg	5.2	23	28.2	30	17.6
Pantothenic Acid, mg	0.184	0.79	0.974	1.5	0.84

[1]PT Milk + Enfamil Fortifier = 100 mL pre-term milk mixed with 4 packets Enfamil fortifier.
[2]PT Milk + Similac Natural Care = 50 mL pre-term milk mixed with 50 mL Similac Natural Care.
Modified from Thompson, M, and McClead, RE: Human milk fortifiers, *J Pediatr Perinat Nutr* 1:65–74, 1987.

- Any mixture of fortifier and milk left over after the feeding should be discarded.
- Supplemental vitamin D should be administered as needed, depending on the infant's volume of intake and bone mineralization. (Infants weighing 1–2 kilos who are taking 120–140 kcal/kg/feeding should be given 200 international units of supplemental vitamin D per day to achieve recommended requirements.)
- Iron supplementation at 2–3 mg/kg/day should be started between two weeks and two months of age.

- Serum electrolytes should be monitored biweekly until stable, followed by weekly monitoring thereafter.
- Fortifier should be discontinued before discharge from the nursery.

CONTAMINANTS IN EXPRESSED MOTHERS' MILK TO BE FED TO PRE-TERM INFANTS

Although the presence of contaminants in mothers' milk was discussed in Chapter 6, certain principles must be considered prior to gavage administration of EMM containing contaminants to pre-term infants. Recommendations issued by the Committee on Drugs of the American Academy of Pediatrics concerning the transfer of drugs and other chemicals into human milk (AAP, 1989) are included on pp. 153–165 of this book. This document is a valuable reference, and should be used to guide decision-making regarding feeding of EMM to pre-term infants. However, the breastfeeding specialist and neonatologist will need to adapt the principles and drug lists to the individual mother-infant situation.

For example, a drug that is considered "safe" if present in EMM for full-term, healthy infants may not be equally "safe" for a 750-gram, 26-week-old infant, depending upon the maternal dosage and clinical condition of the infant. Thus, the breastfeeding specialist, in consultation with the neonatologist, should approach on an individual basis each situation in which a mother is receiving a medication or has other environmental contaminants in her milk. Of particular concern is whether the pre-term infant can tolerate the concentration of drug that is likely to be ingested in EMM and whether he can metabolize it effectively. In selected instances, obtaining infant serum levels of the drug may be indicated in managing the infant feeding.

Other lactation support personnel should refrain from advising a mother who is expressing milk for her pre-term infant about the appropriateness of ingesting a specific medication, without first consulting with the NICU breastfeeding specialist and neonatologist. The mother can be told that a particular medication is considered safe during breastfeeding for term infants, but certain precautions may be necessary for the milk to be fed to a pre-term infant. In all such instances, the mother should be encouraged to discuss her concerns about any medications, smoking, or alcohol ingestion with the NICU breastfeeding specialist or the neonatologist.

A pre-term infant may receive EMM by gavage infusion for several weeks before oral feedings are initiated. Providing appropriate interventions within this phase is essential in sustaining mothers through the difficult period of pumping milk for their infants. Mothers report that seeing their infants grow and recover from illnesses while receiving EMM by gavage is an extremely important phase of breastfeeding for them (Kavanaugh, personal communication, 1992). Thus, it is important that the NICU follow established, research-based policies for feeding of EMM by gavage in order to insure adequate infant growth and protection from infection, as well as maternal perseverance with milk expression.

PHASE THREE: IN-HOSPITAL BREASTFEEDING MANAGEMENT

In the past, breastfeeding practices for pre-term infants have been guided by tradition and untested assumptions rather than by research (McCoy et al., 1988; Meier, 1988; Meier & Anderson, 1987; Meier & Pugh, 1985; Walker, 1990). In most NICUs, breastfeeding for pre-term infants was delayed until a critical weight had been achieved and infants demonstrated the ability to consume entire bottle-feedings without distress. Unfortunately, this timing usually coincided with infant discharge from the NICU, so that mothers had little opportunity to practice breastfeeding in the NICU environment. Additionally, by this time many infants had developed latching-on and sucking mechanisms conducive to feeding from a bottle rather than breastfeeding. Thus, the withholding of breastfeedings until infant discharge was imminent has been identified as a major barrier to in-hospital breastfeeding success (Gotsch, 1990; McCoy et al., 1988).

Another barrier to in-hospital breastfeeding success is not providing mothers with an adequate environment to feed their pre-term infants. Many NICUs do not have a private room where mothers can breastfeed; if such a room exists, a nurse may not be available to remain with the mother during the feeding. Results from a recent study of 20 mothers of pre-term infants which was conducted in the home one month postdischarge emphasized the importance of having a private place to breastfeed in the hospital (Kavanaugh, personal communication, 1992). When asked what was different about breastfeeding in the NICU and at home, mothers emphasized that they wanted a private, quiet place to breastfeed while infants were hospitalized. However, they qualified this response by reporting that they did not want to be left alone in a "parent" room or a "breastfeeding" room. They wanted to be able to take their infant away from the NICU environment, while a knowledgeable nurse assisted them with lactation and assured them that they were doing the "right things" and that their infants were "okay."

Although participants received in-hospital breast-feeding support in an NICU with parent rooms for breastfeeding, not all mothers had access to them at all times. Occasionally, these rooms were occupied with several breastfeeding mothers, which forced some mothers to feed elsewhere. On other occasions, when the breastfeeding specialist was not available to assist mothers, they were asked to breastfeed in the NICU with a screen for privacy. In such instances, some mothers commented that it was "more comfortable" to feed by bottle.

Phase III of this model includes research-based interventions for management of in-hospital breast-feeding sessions and is divided into two sections: early and late breastfeeding sessions. The goals of early breastfeeding sessions are positioning the infant correctly at breast and physiologic stability during feeding, whereas the goal of later breastfeeding sessions is the infant's consuming adequate volumes of milk in order to prepare for discharge.

SCIENTIFIC BASIS FOR EARLY BREASTFEEDING SESSIONS

Clinicians frequently offer three reasons for delaying breastfeeding for pre-term infants: (1) the infant is too small; (2) the infant doesn't bottle-feed well enough to breastfeed; and (3) accurate measurement of intake is impossible during breastfeeding. Results from a series of published and more recent ongoing studies suggest that these criteria for delaying initial breastfeeding experiences are not research based (McCoy et al., 1988; Meier, 1988; Meier & Anderson, 1987; Meier et al., 1990) and should not be used in NICU protocols that delineate breastfeeding readiness.

The infant is too small. No published research has been located in which infant weight has been related to readiness or ability to breastfeed. In contrast, in many countries outside the United States, early breastfeeding for very small pre-term infants is the standard of care (Anderson, Marks & Wahlberg, 1986; Meberg, Willgraff & Sande, 1982; Pearce & Buchanan, 1979; Singh, 1979). For the most part, reports reflect observation of practices, rather than controlled studies that focused on measurable infant outcomes. However, these reports add credibility to available data that pre-term infants are capable of breastfeeding at lower weights than is currently practiced in the United States.

At Helsingborg Hospital in Sweden, Persson (1990) has conceptualized and implemented early breastfeeding for pre-term infants in the form of a program that begins with skin-to-skin contact for very small infants and terminates with the pre-term infants' consuming all feedings at breast. The phases of this process are depicted in Fig. 10–2. This gradual introduction to breastfeeding differs considerably from models of care in the United States because of differences in health-care policies for the two countries. For example, in Sweden, parents receive 18 months of paid parental leave following the birth of an infant; this leave can be used by one parent, or can be divided between the two parents. This policy makes it possible for mothers to spend 8 to 10 hours daily in the hospital with their pre-term infants, while fathers care for other children and see to household duties. Persson has modified the nursery environment at Helsingborg Hospital in numerous ways to accommodate parents who want to come and spend long periods of time with their pre-term infants (Persson; personal communication, 1991). The model of care is characterized by parents providing care to the infant (e.g., administration of gavage feedings while the infants suckle at breast) and nurses providing care and support to parents. Additionally, pre-term infants are reportedly discharged at larger weights than is typical in the United States, and discharge is contingent upon infants' consuming all daily feedings by breast. Successful breastfeeding during this time is measured by the infants' demonstrating an acceptable daily weight gain.

In the United States and Canada, most NICUs still include a minimum infant weight as a criterion for initiating breastfeeding. This minimum weight criterion varies among clinical units, but is usually within the range of 1600 to 1800 grams. Mean weight for pre-term infants to begin breastfeeding in a series of research studies by Meier and colleagues (McCoy et al., 1988; Meier, 1988; Meier & Anderson, 1987; Meier & Pugh, 1985) was 1350 grams, with infants as small as 1100 grams doing so. In a separate, ongoing study, the relationship between infant weight and gestational age to volume of intake during breast-feeding was correlated. Results indicated that infant weight and gestational age were not related to volume of intake: several pre-term infants consumed greater volumes of milk at breast during feedings when they were smaller and less mature than during later feedings. Thus, neither the literature nor research

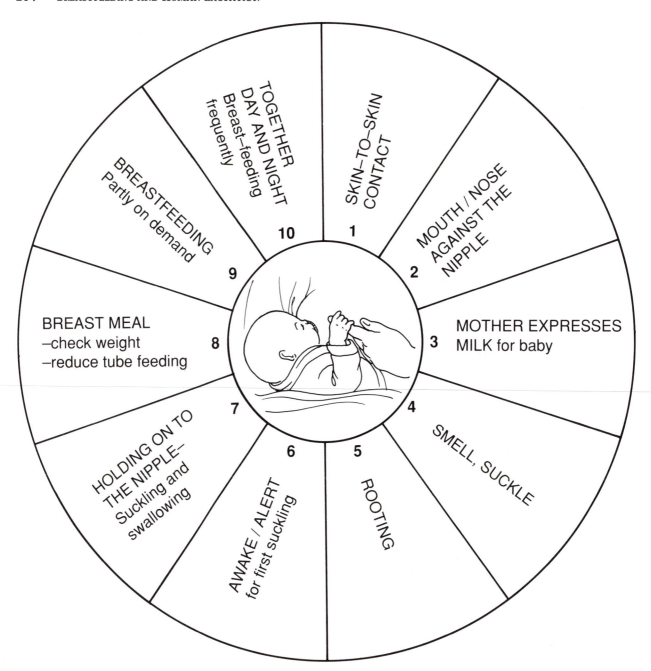

FIGURE 10–2 The starting process for breastfeeding of premature infants. (Courtesy of Berlith Persson, Helsingborg Hospital, Sweden.)

currently being conducted support the use of infant weight as a criterion for initiation of breastfeeding.

The infant doesn't bottle-feed well enough to breastfeed. It is widely assumed that breastfeeding is more stressful or requires more energy than does bottle-feeding. However, no published research has been located which supports this assumption. Several studies for term and pre-term infants have demonstrated that oral feeding with a bottle results in physiologic and biochemical changes—including hypoxemia, hypercarbia, reduced minute volume, apnea, bradycardia, and cyanosis (Bodefeld et al., 1979; Daniels et al., 1990; Garg et al., 1988; Guille-minault & Coons, 1984; Jain et al., 1987; Mathew & Bhatia, 1989; Mathew, 1988; Mathew, Clark & Pron-ske, 1985; Mathew et al., 1985; Mathew, 1991; Meier, 1988; Meier & Anderson, 1987; Rosen, Glaze & Frost, 1984; Wilson et al., 1981; Shivpuri et al., 1983). These adverse consequences are so universal that clinicians have come to consider them as a "nor-mal" response to bottle-feeding.

On the contrary, research conducted with pre-term infants who served as their own controls for bottle-feeding and breastfeeding sessions suggests that these same consequences do not occur during breastfeeding. In two separate studies, pre-term infants weighing less than 1500 grams at the time of first oral feedings served as their own controls for se-quential bottle-feedings and breastfeedings from the time of the first feeding until discharge from the NICU (Meier, 1988; Meier & Anderson, 1987; Meier et al., 1991). In the first study (Meier, 1988; Meier & Anderson, 1987), infants demonstrated a more stable pattern of transcutaneous oxygen pressure during breastfeeding than bottle-feeding. (See Fig. 10–3.) In the second study (Meier et al., 1991), mean values of oxygen saturation were higher for breastfeeding than bottle-feeding—both during and following the feeding sessions. When these find-ings are interpreted in perspective with previously published studies of bottle-feeding, the probable conclusion is that breastfeeding is less physiologi-cally stressful than bottle-feeding for pre-term in-fants.

An explanation for the differences in physiologic and biochemical responses for the two feeding methods is that infants coordinate the mechanisms

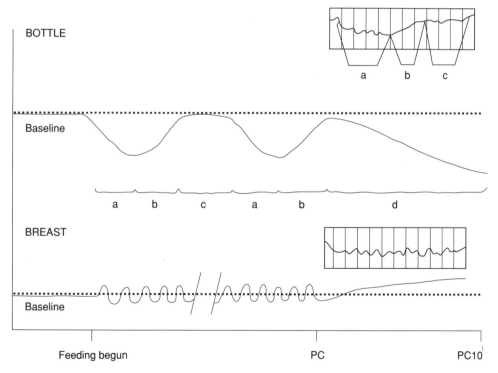

FIGURE 10–3   Schematic of typical tcPO$_2$ patterns during bottle and breastfeeding. Note in bottle feeding (BoF) (a) decline, (b) recovery, (c) plateau, (d) decline between end of feed-ing (PC) and 10 minutes postfeeding (PC10). Both schematics have been magnified some-what for clarity. Also note interruption in the breastfeeding (BrF) line to show that BrFs were generally longer than BoFs. Insets are from actual tcPO$_2$ recordings.

of sucking, swallowing, and breathing differently for breastfeeding and bottle-feeding. Apparently, breast-feeding interrupts breathing less than bottle-feeding, as exemplified by the relatively stable patterns of ox-ygenation during breastfeeding. This hypothesis is currently being studied by Meier and associates for pre-term infants who serve as their own research controls for the two feeding methods. The study of suckling during breastfeeding has been made possi-ble by recent research that has validated a new, non-invasive instrument for this purpose (de Monterice, personal communication, 1992).

Accurate measurement of intake is impossible during breastfeeding. The most commonly used estimate of intake during breastfeeding in the clini-cal setting is the test-weighing technique. Test-weighing involves weighing the infant pre- and postfeed under identical conditions; estimated vol-ume of intake (in mL) is calculated by subtracting the prefeed from the postfeed weight (in grams), where 1 gram = 1 mL of intake (Woolridge et al., 1985). Prior to the use of electronic scales for test-weighing, the procedure was known to be inaccurate, with ex-amples in the research literature in which estimates of intake were as great as 100% different from actual volume of intake (Coward, 1984; Culley et al., 1979; Whitfield, Kay & Stevens, 1981). However, several research reports have documented the accuracy of the test-weighing technique for term infants when electronic scales are used (Coward, 1984; Neville et al., 1988; Woolridge et al., 1985).

A single study has established test-weighing as an accurate estimate of intake for small pre-term infants who consume considerably smaller volumes of milk than term infants (Meier et al., 1990), making accu-rate estimation of intake more difficult. In this study, 50 clinically stable pre-term infants who weighed be-tween 1088 grams and 2440 grams were studied during bottle-feeding. Each infant was test-weighed on a mechanical scale and an electronic scale pre- and postfeed by one research assistant. Each infant was bottle-fed a prescribed volume of intake by a dif-ferent research assistant. Each research assistant was blind to the other's measurement. Results demon-strated the accuracy of test-weighing measurements for the electronic, but not for the mechanical scale. Mean absolute differences between actual and esti-mated volumes of intake were 1.97 and 9.00 mL for the electronic and mechanical scales, respectively. These data support the use of test-weighing with an electronic scale for both clinical and research pur-poses in pre-term infants.

Although the accuracy of the test-weighing tech-nique has been demonstrated for pre-term infants, nurses and physicians in many NICUs still have not incorporated this measurement into standard breastfeeding management for pre-term infants. There continues to be the widespread assumption that test-weighing will make the mother nervous or anxious, or in some way interfere with the breast-feeding relationship. There are no research-based data to support this assumption. On the contrary, newer, ongoing research findings suggest that moth-ers want to know how much milk their infants have consumed at breast (Kavanaugh, personal com-munication, 1992). Mothers report that not knowing their infants have consumed at least the volume of milk prescribed for that feeding is stressful for them. They express concerns about infant satiety and growth rates; they do not want these responses compromised by in-hospital breastfeeding experi-ences. With test-weighing, mothers can be assured that breastfeedings will be complemented as neces-sary.

Opposition to test-weighing for pre-term infants includes some clinicians' statements that test-weigh-ing is not necessary to estimate volume of intake. In-stead, these clinicians propose that volume of intake can be estimated accurately by observing the feeding session for maternal milk ejection, sucking and swal-lowing by the infant, and indications of infant sati-ety. The accuracy of clinical indicators in estimating volume of intake for pre-term infants has been ad-dressed in one study (Fleming, personal communi-cation, 1992.) In this study, 10 pre-term infants were observed during two breastfeeding sessions, spaced one week apart, by a certified lactation consultant (CLC). The CLC estimated volume of intake con-sumed using clinical indicators. These estimates of intake were compared with test-weights, completed by a graduate nursing student, who had not ob-served the feeding sessions. The clinical estimates and the test-weights were compared for all the feed-ing sessions. Subsequent statistical analysis demon-strated unacceptably large differences between these two measures, with greater differences occur-ring for higher intake. Thus, the use of clinical indi-cators cannot be assumed to provide an accurate estimate of intake during breastfeeding for pre-term infants.

Small pre-term infants frequently demonstrate sucking and swallowing in the presence of maternal milk ejection without measurable intake. This may be due to the pre-term's relatively weak suction pressures, which fail to sustain milk flow. Thus, audible swallowing may result from occasional drops of milk or mere buccal secretions. Similarly, often recommended clinical indicators of satiety, e.g., appearing sleepy or rejecting subsequent attempts at placement at breast, occur routinely in pre-term infants in the absence of measurable intake.

While routine test-weighing is not recommended for healthy, term infants, it should be the standard of care for smaller pre-term infants. It is extremely important to know the volume of milk that pre-term infants consume during breastfeeding so that other fluids, e.g., supplemental gavage feedings or parenteral fluids, can be adjusted accordingly. Additionally, test-weighing need not be a stressful procedure for mothers if the rationale for it is presented appropriately. The mother needs to understand that the reason for test-weighing during early breastfeeding sessions is to allow the clinician to alter other sources of fluids precisely. Test-weighing should not be presented as a determinant of whether or not a breastfeeding session is "successful." On the contrary, mothers should understand before the feeding that small pre-term infants often do not consume measurable volumes of milk initially—and that adequate intake is not the goal of early feedings. Additionally, mothers should be told that the volume of intake during early breastfeeding sessions does not predict the volume of intake that an infant will consume later, or at the time of discharge from the NICU.

MANAGING EARLY BREASTFEEDING SESSIONS
As previously mentioned, the goals of early breastfeeding sessions are for the infant to achieve proper positioning at breast and to remain stable physiologically. Interventions within this phase of breastfeeding support include: determining readiness to breastfeed; positioning the infant at breast; and monitoring and documenting responses to breastfeeding.

Determining readiness to breastfeed. No universally accepted criteria or tools are available for determining readiness of a pre-term infant to feed orally, either by bottle or breast. However, many NICUs still use criteria for determining readiness to breastfeed that are inconsistent with current research findings. For example, a minimum infant weight and the ability to consume oral feedings by bottle are inappropriate criteria and should not be used to determine the readiness to breastfeed. Additionally, initiating breastfeeding at the time an infant is moved from an incubator to an open bassinet is not a research-based criterion. Previous studies have demonstrated that pre-term infants maintain their body temperatures, or become warmer, during breastfeeding, provided that they are clothed and swaddled (Meier, 1988; Meier & Anderson, 1987). Thus, criteria which should not be used in protocols to define the readiness to breastfeed are infant weight, ability to bottle-feed, or type of thermal support that an infant requires.

Many NICUs incorporate a "maturity" criterion for determining readiness to feed orally by breast or bottle, based upon a critical period for the coordination of sucking and swallowing. Although it is widely assumed that coordination of the suck-swallow reflexes occurs at 34 to 35 weeks of gestation, no research studies could be located to document this assumption. The most closely related and commonly cited study used to document this assumption was conducted by Gryboski (1969), in which sucking and swallowing were studied during bottle-feeding for larger (1700 grams to 2500 grams) pre-term infants. In this study, Gryboski differentiated between "immature" and "mature" sucking bursts. For "immature" sucking bursts, swallowing preceded or followed relatively short sucking bursts, whereas for "mature" sucking bursts, multiple swallows occurred within longer sucking bursts. In all instances, swallowing inhibited respiration. However, the coordination of sucking and swallowing at 34 to 35 weeks of gestation was not addressed in this study.

Results from previous studies conducted by Meier and associates (Meier, 1988; Meier & Anderson, 1987; Meier & Pugh, 1985), in which pre-term infants served as their own controls for breastfeedings and bottle-feedings, suggest that the ability to coordinate sucking, swallowing, and breathing may occur earlier for breastfeeding than for bottle-feeding. Many clinically stable infants demonstrate the ability to latch onto the breast and organize sucking into short bursts (two to five sucks) and pauses at 32 weeks of gestation, even though these infants may have been much smaller and sicker at birth. However, on only isolated occasions has the organization of sucking into short bursts during breastfeeding been observed in infants of less than 32 weeks of gestation. Gestational age, in isolation, is a poor predictor of readiness to breastfeed, because considerable variability exists among infants—e.g., some infants can feed at 32 weeks, whereas others are not ready until 36 weeks (McCoy et al., 1988; Meier & Anderson, 1987).

Other criteria to determine breastfeeding readiness are more anecdotal rather than research based. Although an infant should be stable clinically, the interpretation of this criterion must be individualized to the infant. For example, a 1350-gram infant who tolerates bolus gavage feedings, but who experiences occasional apnea and bradycardia during sleep, is "clinically stable" for purposes of breastfeeding. However, if the same infant demonstrated protracted bradycardia in response to gavage feedings, breastfeedings should be delayed.

Additionally, the infant should demonstrate the ability to coordinate sucking and swallowing of secretions during nonnutritive sucking with minimal changes in the cardiorespiratory response. It is widely recognized that swallowing interrupts breathing during oral feeding (Ardran, Kemp & Lind, 1958a, 1958b; Weber, Woolridge & Baum, 1986; Wilson et al., 1981; Woolridge, 1986); therefore one of the most important assessments to make prior to introducing breastfeeding or bottle-feeding is whether the infant can coordinate the swallow-breathe mechanism.

Clinically, a crude assessment of this coordination can be done just prior to an infant's receiving a bolus gavage feeding. A pacifier can be inserted into the infant's mouth to stimulate nonnutritive sucking, and a bedside cardiorespiratory monitor can be used to evaluate this response. Typically, as the infant begins to suck on the pacifier, the baseline heart rate will increase slightly, and respirations will become irregular. As the infant continues to suck, the nurse should note the number of sucks per burst, as well as whether the sucks are rhythmic in nature. As the infant swallows secretions, which can be assessed visually or by cervical auscultation of swallowing (Vice et al., 1990), the heart rate may decrease slightly and a few seconds of apnea may follow. An immature infant will demonstrate wide variability in cardiorespi-

ratory patterns, ranging from tachycardia (greater than 20 beats per minute above baseline) with sucking, to clinically detectable apnea and bradycardia during swallowing of secretions. Oral feeding of any type should be delayed for an infant who responds in this manner.

Obviously, a research-based clinical tool is needed to enable the nurse and physician to make decisions about readiness to feed; development of such a tool is a research priority. Until the time that such a tool is available, many NICUs can alter policies in a very simplistic manner so as to greatly enhance breastfeeding success and minimize resistance from those who are skeptical about early breastfeeding. This approach includes initiating breastfeeding according to the criteria currently being used for initiating bottle-feeding, and delaying bottle-feedings for at least one week while the infant learns to breastfeed. For example, if an NICU policy specifies that bottle-feedings are introduced at 34 weeks of gestation when an infant weighs a minimum of 1500 grams, these criteria can be used for determining readiness to breastfeed. The goal of this intervention is to introduce the pre-term infant to breastfeeding before bottle-feeding, according to whatever criteria are currently used for bottle-feeding. As breastfeeding advocates within the staff become successful with this approach, they will gain support from colleagues about initiating breastfeeding at lower infant weights and earlier gestational ages.

Positioning the infant at breast. A primary goal of early breastfeedings is correct positioning of the pre-term infant in order to enable effective sucking. The mother should be seated comfortably in a chair or sofa so that her feet touch the ground. At least two pillows will be necessary: one for her lap to support the infant and one under the arm to help support the breast at which the infant is feeding. The mother should be asked if she has a particular preference for which breast she would like to begin with; most mothers have a preference, either because "they get more milk" from one breast, or because one feels more natural to them.

The mother can prepare the breast by cleansing it with sterile water and a gauze pad, while the nurse holds the infant. Then, the mother can support the breast by encircling the outer aspect with her "same side" hand (right hand to right breast, left hand to left breast) and exerting a very mild backward, downward pressure on the upper aspect of the breast just behind the areola. Then the nurse can position the pre-term infant on the mother's lap, chest-to-chest. The mother's free arm can be brought around the back of the infant, with the hand encircling the infant's head. (See Fig. 10–4.) Then, the infant's head can be moved toward the breast with the mother brushing the nipple over the infant's lips.

The infant may spontaneously open his mouth and latch onto the breast. This is most likely to happen if the infant has not become accustomed to the artificial nipple and if the mother's nipples elongate to facilitate the infant's latching-on. If the infant does not latch onto the breast spontaneously, the breastfeeding specialist can assist the infant after several tries by placing an index finger on the mandible and gently pressing it downward to generate maximum jaw excursion. Mothers should be dis-

couraged from trying to manipulate, elongate, or compress the nipple into the infant's mouth. This technique is seldom successful and does not allow the infant to learn proper latching-on behavior. Once the infant is placed at breast, his cheeks, jaw, tongue, and other oral structures should not be manipulated or stimulated. The only exception might be the mother's gently stroking the infant's cheek or mandible if she desires.

For mothers with large breasts and areolae, a variant on this technique is recommended. These mothers can support the breast in two hands, with thumbs on the upper aspect of the breast and the remaining fingers on the lower aspect of the breast. The breastfeeding specialist can support and direct the infant's head toward the breast, and facilitate infant latching-on. (See Fig. 10–5.) For some mothers, this position is the only one that facilitates latch-on for the first several breastfeeding sessions. It requires that a second person be available to assist the mother at all times.

Once an infant has demonstrated the ability to latch-on effectively using the position described above, the football hold may be introduced. This position, like the cross-chest position, allows the mother to control extraneous movements of the infant's head. For most mothers, it also permits better visibility of the infant, making it the preferred position for many mothers. However, most pre-term infants latch-on and continue sucking more effectively in the cross-chest position and consume more milk from one breast than the other throughout hospitalization.

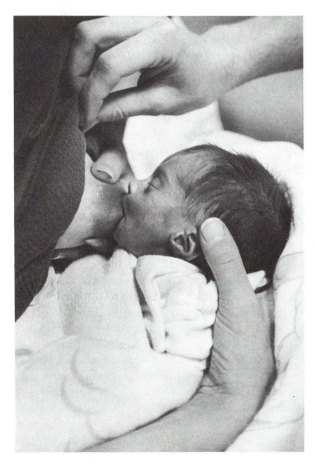

FIGURE 10–4   Head support and latching-on for a small, pre-term infant.

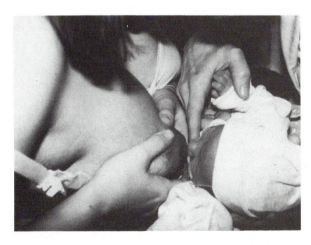

FIGURE 10–5   Use of both hands to support the large breast with flattened nipples for breastfeeding a pre-term infant.

Monitoring infant responses to breastfeeding. Frequently nurses comment that physicians or other colleagues are not supportive of early breastfeeding sessions for pre-term infants. However, this resistance may be tempered if nurses approach early breastfeedings as scientifically as they do other aspects of pre-term infant care. Thus, selected infant responses should be monitored noninvasively and documented during early breastfeeding sessions. Specifically, the following responses should be monitored: heart rate, respiratory rate, oxygen saturation or transcutaneous oxygen pressure, and body temperature. Additional factors to be evaluated include sucking pattern, volume of intake, and duration of the feeding session. If the cardiorespiratory or oxygen saturation monitor has a trend recorder, the breastfeeding specialist should make hard-copy trend recordings to share with primary nurses and neonatologists. These measures will document physiologic stability and will assist in the identification of "fatigue-related" responses should they occur.

It is essential to recognize individual infant differences with respect to readiness and ability to breastfeed. Research-based data support the principle that pre-term infants are able to coordinate sucking, swallowing, and breathing functions earlier for breastfeedings than for bottle-feedings. However, the data also demonstrate that mean volume of intake during these early breastfeedings is minimal, but that the range for volume of intake is quite high. Therefore, test-weights should be performed to determine volume of intake during early breastfeedings. Some type of crude assessment of coordination of swallowing and breathing should be performed prior to initiating breastfeeding for pre-term infants. This is especially important for infants whose mothers have demonstrated a milk-ejection reflex which produces very high rates of milk flow.

Although no universally accepted tool is available for determining readiness to breastfeed, each NICU should establish (or eliminate) criteria based on the principles outlined in this section. Correct positioning of the pre-term infant for breastfeeding is essential for both optimal breastfeeding behaviors and for physiologic stability. In any event, routine noninvasive monitoring of physiologic stability should be incorporated into the standards of practice for management of early breastfeedings.

Later breastfeedings. The transition from early to later breastfeedings is gradual rather than dichotomous, and depends more upon infant responses to the feeding situation than to characteristics such as weight and maturity. The goal of later breastfeeding sessions is to develop interventions that allow the infant to consume adequate volumes of milk from the breast in anticipation of discharge. This goal replaces the goal of physiologic stability once the infant has demonstrated the ability to consume measurable volumes of milk while maintaining stable physiologic indices.

Interventions within this phase of breastfeeding support include routine performance and evaluation of test-weights; transition to cue-based feeding schedules; and selected techniques for intake-related problems. Ideally, these interventions will help prepare the mother and infant for breastfeeding success in the postdischarge period.

Performing and evaluating test-weights. Although the importance of test-weighing was discussed previously with respect to early breastfeeding, it has an equally important function in the management of later breastfeeding sessions. Under optimal conditions nutritive intake will have occurred within one week of beginning early breastfeeding sessions, as measured by test-weighing. Measurable nutritive intake in excess of five ml suggests that the mother has experienced milk ejection in response to infant sucking at the breast. Provided that the infant consumed the milk without physiologic compromise, interventions from this point on will focus on optimizing intake over the remainder of the hospitalization.

In an ongoing study of 35 pre-term infants in whom serial test-weights were measured three times weekly from initial feeding to discharge, results demonstrated that mean volume of intake increased progressively from earlier feedings to later ones. However, in this study volume of intake was extremely variable, both within and between infants, and was not related to infant weight, maturity, duration of the feeding session, or volume of comparable gavage or bottle-feedings. These data support the use of routine test-weighing to determine volume of intake and demonstrate that pre-term infants, like term infants, do not consume a "set" volume of milk at each breastfeeding session (Bowen-Jones, Thompson & Drewett, 1982; Drewett & Woolridge, 1979; Howie et al., 1981; Lucas, Lucas & Baum, 1981).

Thus, test-weights should be evaluated on an individual basis for each infant. Ideally, volume of intake during breastfeeding should approximate that consumed by the infant during gavage or bottle-feeding and should demonstrate a trend of increasing volume over time. If an infant consumes an inadequate volume of milk at each breastfeeding over several days, the breastfeeding specialist should determine the cause for the inadequate intake. First, the volume of milk consumed during breastfeeding by the infant should be compared to the volume of milk that the mother expresses with the breast pump. This assessment will assist in identifying a low maternal milk supply, for which specific interventions can be initiated. Commonly, the mother will have expressed more milk with a breast pump than the infant will have consumed at the breast.

The consumption of less milk by the infant during breastfeeding than the mother expresses with a breast pump indicates that milk transfer to the infant is compromised. This can be due to problems with maternal milk ejection or to the infant's sucking pattern. Most of the time, the breastfeeding specialist can observe a feeding and make this distinction, which is important in planning the appropriate intervention. Asking a mother whether she feels the milk ejecting during breastfeeding may not be a reliable method of diagnosing milk ejection. Many mothers of pre-term infants deny sensing milk ejection during breast pumping and breastfeeding, even when rapid milk flow from the opposite breast is visible to an observer.

To consume an adequate volume of milk, the pre-term infant must sustain a sucking pattern that permits milk transfer once milk ejection has occurred. This requires that the sucking burst has matured to include several sucks, and that the duration of pauses between bursts has diminished. This sucking pattern coincides with maturation of the infant and is highly variable. Some infants demonstrate such a pattern by 33 weeks of gestation, whereas others still have not done so by 38 weeks of gestation. Frequently, the pre-term infant will suckle for several minutes before milk ejection occurs and then fall asleep shortly after a bout of nutritive sucks. This type of sucking pattern does not allow the infant to consume large volumes of milk, but appears to be a normal maturational phase that precedes the ability to consume larger volumes.

Thus, serial test-weights are essential in allowing the breastfeeding specialist to evaluate the progress of later breastfeeding sessions. Many mothers become concerned when their 1500-gram infants do not consume volumes comparable to those that they receive by gavage or bottle; they want to know what will happen if this is still the trend at discharge. These mothers should be reassured that small volumes of intake are normal, especially until milk ejection and mature infant sucking patterns are synchronized. The breastfeeding specialist and other support personnel can emphasize that this pattern of intake seldom persists at the time of infant discharge, but in the event it should, appropriate postdischarge interventions will be prescribed.

Transition to cue-based feeding schedules. Little is known about the appropriateness of cue-based vs. scheduled feedings for pre-term infants, especially for infants who are breastfed. Results from two published studies suggest that pre-term infants may benefit from cue-based rather than scheduled bottle-feedings (Collinge et al., 1982; Horton, Lubchenco & Gordion, 1952); however, both studies were conducted with relatively small sample sizes and deserve a larger clinical trial. Data from research with term infants suggest that infants consume more milk and grow at faster rates when fed frequently and on cue (De Carvalho et al., 1983). Thus, when both sets of studies are considered, it seems probable that pre-term infants can breastfeed on cue as they approach term, at least on a modified basis. In most NICUs pre-term infants are fed every three hours until they reach a critical weight, at which time feedings are instituted every four hours. In some instances, pre-term infants are maintained on feedings every three hours until discharge. Based on the research with term infants during breastfeeding, and pre-term infants during bottle-feeding, it seems reasonable that pre-term infants can be placed on a modified "cue-based" schedule for breastfeeding at approximately 35 to 36 weeks of gestation. The modified NICU policy might include minimum and maximum intervals that should elapse between feedings, e.g., two to five hours, with no fewer than six feedings daily. This will permit the infant longer intervals between feedings to consolidate sleep and shorter intervals between feedings as hunger cues are demonstrated.

It is often assumed that the pre-term infant can self-regulate sleep and feeding behaviors in the same manner as does a term infant, but these assumptions have not been tested. On the contrary, in numerous clinical examples the pre-term infant's need for sleep overrides the ability to feed, with resultant poor weight gain or dehydration. Thus, the transition of a pre-term infant from a three-hour to a cue-based feeding schedule must be individualized and monitored carefully until the clinician is comfortable that the infant will consume an adequate volume of milk. For this reason, the ideal time to effect such a transition is while the infant is in the hospital rather than at the time of discharge.

NICU policies that support a cue-based schedule in the hospital are also more conducive to mothers' needs. Clinically, mothers have expressed confusion over what appear to be conflicting messages. They report that their infants are fed large volumes of milk by bottle every four hours in the hospital, but at the time of discharge they are told by the neonatologist or nurse to feed their infants on demand. The mothers have had no experience with "demand" feedings and are frequently not sure what "demand" means with respect to their infants. However, if this plan is instituted during the last week or two of an infant's hospitalization, mothers would have the opportunity to observe their infants awaken in response to hunger, and perhaps to sleep for extended periods of time. Mothers could put this behavior within the perspective of "normal" for their individual infants. This approach will alert the clinician to potential intake-related problems prior to discharge, and will make the transition from hospital to home an easier one for breastfeeding mothers.

Selected techniques for intake-related problems. Most intake-related problems for pre-term infants who breastfeed fall into two categories: improper positioning on the breast and suboptimal milk transfer from mother to infant. Although these problems will present during the in-hospital period, they may not resolve until the infant has been discharged.

Improper latching-on to the breast can often be prevented if breastfeeding is introduced earlier than, or at the same time as, bottle-feedings for pre-term infants. Breastfeeding necessitates that the infant open his mouth wider than for bottle-feedings, and that he exercise greater excursion of the mandible with each suck. Thus, for small infants with small mouths latching onto the breast can be problematic. The infants who experience the greatest difficulty with correct latching-on are those whose mothers

have large areola and flat nipples. The infant's attempts to latch-on to such breasts result in the nipple slipping out of the mouth with the first suck. Both mother and infant become frustrated with repeated attempts at latching-on.

The NICU breastfeeding specialist should explain the problem honestly and thoroughly to the mother. She should be told that the relatively flat nipple may make initial breastfeeding efforts frustrating, but that as the strength of the infant's suck increases he will be able to "draw" the nipple into the mouth and retain it in position during nutritive sucking. Unfortunately, for many pre-term infants this degree of suction usually coincides with reaching 38 to 40 weeks of gestation, at which time most infants will have been discharged. Thus, the mother should be prepared for the experiences ahead, but should be reassured that most infants gradually adapt to feeding at breasts with flat nipples.

Techniques to elongate the nipple for the infant represent an initial intervention. These include wearing breast shells, manual elongation, and use of the electric pump. The infant may require assistance at lowering the mandible during latch-on. A soft, pliable breast shield has been used effectively for these mothers, especially when the pre-term infant has repeatedly demonstrated a suck too weak to retain the nipple in his mouth during feeding. Many pre-term infants consume adequate volumes of milk from the breast with a breast shield, and gradually make the transition to the breast postdischarge (Kavanaugh, personal communication, 1992).

Problems with milk transfer have been described previously, but selected interventions may assist the pre-term infant who consumes measurable, but inadequate volumes of milk. First, an immature pattern of sucking, in which the infant sucks in short bursts and long pauses, will correct itself as the infant matures and as the maternal milk ejection becomes synchronized with initial sucks at the breast. Mothers should be reassured that this is a normal process. Clinical experience suggests that most infants with an immature pattern of sucking consume adequate volumes of milk from the breast at between two weeks and one month postdischarge (Kavanaugh, personal communication, 1992). Complemental feedings can be provided in the interim.

Less frequently, an infant will demonstrate a mature sucking pattern characterized by longer bursts and shorter pauses, but will suck for only a few minutes at a session. Because the sucking pattern is mature, an intervention that has worked successfully with these infants is to apply the breast pump to one breast while the infant feeds at the other. The stimulation of the breast pump will maintain the milk flow, encouraging the infant to continue feeding. A supplemental nurser will also work effectively for this type of infant.

A frequently asked question is whether bottle-feeding should be avoided entirely for pre-term infants who are breastfeeding, especially those who have selected problems with intake. Alternative methods of feeding—with a cup, syringe and tubing—or finger-feeding have been recommended (Walker, 1990) and used in selected instances. However, no published research demonstrating the safety of these devices could be located. Of particular concern is whether the infant experiences greater physiologic compromise from these devices than from a feeding with a bottle. This type of study needs to be completed before wide-scale implementation of alternative feeding devices occurs.

A related approach is to withhold bottles and maintain the breastfed pre-term infant on gavage feedings when the mother is not available to breastfeed. Although this may be advisable during the first week that breastfeedings are being introduced, it should not be done routinely as infants grow and mature. Gavage feedings—and the insertion and retention of gavage feeding tubes—are not without risk to the infant and should not be done as standard practice (Greenspan et al., 1990; Heldt, 1988; Stocks, 1980; Van Someren et al., 1984). Occasionally a mother may request that her infant receive gavage feedings when she is not present to breastfeed. This request can be honored provided that the mother is committed to breastfeeding for at least three-fourths of daily feedings and that she understands the risks of gavage feedings.

Finally, it is important to note that most mothers of pre-term infants do not object to alternating bottle-feedings and breastfeedings while their infants are hospitalized. The mothers report that transition of the infant from gavage to all oral feedings (bottle or breast) is a step toward discharge and represents a major milestone in their infant's progress (Kavanaugh, personal communication, 1992). By this stage of a pre-term infant's hospitalization, many mothers will already have decided that "once they are home" they will manage breastfeeding in their own way. Usually this means that they perceive they will have sufficient control over feeding decisions, plus access to the infant in order to "make it work." However, even predischarge many mothers of pre-term infants often plan to have the father or another family member administer expressed milk by bottle at least once or twice daily. Reasons for this vary from ensuring adequate intake to wanting the infant to be able to feed by both methods. Thus, the significance of bottle-feeding seems to be perceived somewhat differently for mothers of pre-term infants than is suggested in the consumer support literature for term infants. This difference must be considered when the NICU staff or other breastfeeding support personnel counsel the mother about withholding bottle-feedings to facilitate breastfeedings.

Interventions for later breastfeeding sessions are focused on preparing the mother and pre-term infant so that the infant consumes an adequate volume of milk during breastfeeding postdischarge. An essential intervention within this phase is the performance and evaluation of serial test-weights to determine the individual infant's pattern of intake in-hospital. Second, the available data support the institution of a modified cue-based breastfeeding schedule for pre-term infants. Such a schedule is consistent with maternal needs and provides practitioners with information about an individual infant's integration of sleep and feeding patterns.

PHASE FOUR: POSTDISCHARGE CONSULTATION

The final phase of the four-phase model for supporting breastfeeding is postdischarge consultation. No previously published research could be located addressing postdischarge management of breastfeeding for pre-term infants. In the past, few mothers in this country were successful at continuing breastfeeding throughout the in-hospital period, so only small numbers of these mothers breastfed postdischarge.

SCIENTIFIC BASIS FOR POSTDISCHARGE BREASTFEEDING MANAGEMENT

As a part of an ongoing four-phase model for breastfeeding support a plan to ensure that infants would consume an adequate volume of milk postdischarge was instituted. Along with individualized instructions about intake, a telephone consultation schedule was established. The research team telephoned the mother approximately 48 hours postdischarge, and 48 hours after that. Mothers were asked to telephone a member of the research team after the first pediatric visit, which was within one week postdischarge. Additionally, mothers were encouraged to contact a member of the research team for any reason at any time after discharge.

A supplementation/complementation plan that had been individualized for each mother and infant was reviewed in the days preceding discharge. In general, the plan included three general categories: those infants who did not require supplementation; those infants who might require supplementation; and those who required supplementation. The first group of infants, on the basis of demonstrated patterns of intake in-hospital, did not require routine supplementation. To fall within this category, an infant should have consumed a minimum of 40 to 45 ml of mothers' milk at breast fairly consistently during the week preceding discharge. The second group included those infants who, if they were to feed 10 to 12 times daily, would not require supplementation. However, if they fed only six, seven, or eight times daily, they would not receive enough milk. Infants in this category consumed from 20 to 35 mL of mothers' milk at breast fairly consistently during the week preceding discharge. Additionally, for this group the reason for the limited intake should be related to milk transfer, rather than to a primary problem with maternal milk supply. The third group of infants required supplementation, at least on a temporary basis. These infants consumed less than 20 ml of mothers' milk at breastfeeding sessions during the week preceding discharge. Different options for providing supplements and complements were discussed with each mother, and a plan was agreed upon prior to infant discharge. Mothers were reminded to use the electric breast pump after breastfeedings to ensure that the breasts were stimulated adequately and that the milk supply would be maintained.

While in-hospital, each of these mothers had received several hours of individualized, research-based breastfeeding intervention. Thus, the research team predicted that most mothers would not experience major breastfeeding problems postdischarge.

However, this was not the case. When mothers were telephoned according to the above schedule, most reported at least one major breastfeeding problem, which they did not feel was sufficiently significant to "bother" the research team. Instead, they had either asked a friend or family member for advice or had decided upon a way to manage the problem themselves, e.g., administering supplemental bottles. In all cases, the mothers were anxious to talk and ask questions when contacted by a member of the research team. Thus, the average time of these postdischarge telephone conversations was 45 minutes; maximum times reached one hour and 15 minutes.

In this study mothers reported that their major concern related to whether their infants were consuming enough milk at breast. This concern was not limited to mothers whose infants had consumed minimal or borderline volumes of milk during the in-hospital period, but included mothers whose infants had routinely consumed 60 to 80 ml in the NICU. When mothers sought advice from traditional consumer groups or from pediatricians, it usually fell within one of two categories: advice that was appropriate for term infants, and advice based on the assumption that adequate intake during breastfeeding was not possible for pre-term infants. Individuals and groups which supported breastfeeding tended to make recommendations for feeding based on principles of ensuring adequate intake for term infants. Mothers were encouraged to breastfeed on demand, to wake infants frequently for feeding, and to keep them awake long enough to feed from both breasts. One mother was told by a consumer support organization to awaken her pre-term infant each hour to breastfeed, since he consumed such small volumes of milk. These recommendations do not reflect knowledge of the pre-term infant's ability to feed or the need for sleep; they could seriously compromise infant growth and/or hydration. Pediatricians and family members who were generally less knowledgeable about breastfeeding reflected the opinion that all pre-term infants needed routine supplementation of breastfeedings. Thus, mothers were encouraged to supplement or complement breastfeedings on a routine basis "just to be sure" the infant consumed enough milk.

The preliminary information acquired from this study indicated that the postdischarge period was extremely stressful for mothers who were breastfeeding pre-term infants. A second study was conducted to learn more about the experiences of mothers who breastfeed a pre-term infant in the postdischarge period (Kavanaugh, personal communication, 1992). Major findings from this study include an understanding of maternal concerns about breastfeeding a pre-term infant, as well as the type of advice and support received from family, friends, and professionals.

Based on the results from this study, concern about adequacy of infant intake during breastfeeding was nearly universal. It might be suggested that this is a concern of ALL breastfeeding mothers, whether or not infants were born pre-term. However, the data from this study highlight the unique vulnerability of mothers who are responsible for the continued growth of infants who have been small and sick—and who were weighed every day while they were hospitalized. One mother reported that "weight was the basis for everything," including decisions about nutrition, transfer within the nursery, transition to a bassinet, and discharge. She emphasized that "weight" was no less of a concern for her postdischarge.

Mothers reported a number of approaches for managing the anxiety associated with not knowing how much milk infants had consumed during breastfeeding. The most commonly used approach was administering supplemental bottles of expressed milk. Many mothers sought out advice from friends and professionals who would support this decision. When asked how they determined that their infants were not consuming an adequate volume of milk during breastfeeding, the mothers' responses were extremely diverse. Most striking was the contrast in how mothers perceived infant sleep patterns. One mother decided her infant needed additional milk because he awoke every two hours to breastfeed, whereas another mother made the same decision because her infant "slept too much," i.e., for four-hour stretches. Repeatedly, mothers wanted some objective way of knowing how much an infant had consumed during breastfeeding. They frequently said how reassuring it was to bottle-feed, because they could see how much milk their infants had consumed.

The second finding involved maternal perception of support for breastfeeding. Analyses of the data revealed that this support fell within two categories: technical and mechanical assistance with breastfeeding, and general encouragement and reassurance.

Mothers consistently reported that breastfeeding assistance was provided by a member of the research team and gave examples of interventions that were provided by the team, e.g., positioning, use of a nipple shield, and answers to questions postdischarge. The other category of "general" support was provided by in-hospital nurses, neonatologists, social workers, friends, family members, and pediatricians. Mothers described this support as "encouraging me to stick with it," "telling me what a good thing I'm doing for my baby," and "reassuring me that everything will be fine." When additional questions were asked about the latter category of support, mothers could think of no specific assistance or advice that these people had provided. However, the fact that these people were supportive of the mothers' efforts was extremely important in their decision to continue breastfeeding.

RESEARCH-BASED PROTOCOLS FOR THE POSTDISCHARGE PERIOD

Although more research is needed to facilitate breastfeeding in the postdischarge period, the results of these studies can guide some aspects of pre- and postdischarge breastfeeding support. First, an individualized plan for breastfeeding management should be developed during the week preceding discharge of the infant from the NICU. This plan should be developed by the NICU breastfeeding specialist and the mother and should be reviewed by the neonatologist. The plan should reflect patterns of intake at breast during the in-hospital period using criteria outlined in this section. An overall principle should be that it is more important for a pre-term infant to be adequately hydrated and grow appropriately than it is to nourish the infant entirely by breastfeedings. Thus, the plan should allow for liberal complementation/supplementation.

Second, the mother should be "given permission" to supplement and/or complement breastfeedings as she perceives necessary. She can be told that there is no reason, based on in-hospital assessments, that her infant requires additional milk: however, experience suggests that many mothers feel the need to administer extra milk. Such permission is essential if the mother is to feel comfortable in contacting the breastfeeding specialist postdischarge. Results from the previously mentioned studies suggest that mothers are reluctant to seek assistance from the breastfeeding specialist if they have deviated significantly from the established plan.

Third, frequent telephone consultation and occasional home visits are essential in the first week postdischarge. This follow-up could be provided by a number of professionals, but should reflect an understanding both of the discharge plan and the unique needs of pre-term infants. Maternal counseling should not be based on principles appropriate for term infants. Not only will this be unsuccessful at alleviating maternal anxiety, but it may compromise infant growth.

Less is known about the fourth phase of breastfeeding support for pre-term infants than the other phases—primarily because so few mothers have continued to breastfeed their pre-term infants. The available data suggest that this period is one of extreme vulnerability for mothers and that most of the advice that they receive is inappropriate for breastfeeding pre-term infants. Although a few specific clinical recommendations were made, this aspect of care requires additional research focused on determining which interventions in the postdischarge period are effective in preventing breastfeeding failure.

SUMMARY

In this chapter a four-phase temporal model for supporting breastfeeding for mothers of pre-term infants is described. Central to this model is the designation of an NICU breastfeeding specialist who has expertise in lactation processes and in the clinical care of pre-term infants. The primary responsibility of this specialist is to develop an individualized breastfeeding plan which incorporates appropriate research findings. Other personnel, including neonatologists, pediatricians, NICU nurses, and lactation consultants should participate in providing care within this model according to individual expertise. Although considerably more research is needed within each of the phases of the model, research-based recommendations for clinical protocols are provided.

REFERENCES

Al-Dahhan, J, et al.: Sodium homeostasis in term and pre-term neonates. III Effect of salt supplementation, *Arch Dis Child* 59:945–50, 1984.

American Academy of Pediatrics: Encouraging breast feeding, *Pediatrics,* 65:657–58, 1980a.

American Academy of Pediatrics: Human milk banking, *Pediatrics* 65:854–57, 1980b.

American Academy of Pediatrics Committee on Drugs: Transfer of drugs and other chemicals into human milk, *Pediatrics* 84:924–36, 1989.

Anderson, GC, Marks, EA, and Wahlberg, V: Kangaroo care for premature infants, *AJN* 86:807–9, 1986.

Apple, RD: *Mothers and medicine: A social history of infant feeding 1890–1950,* Madison, Wis., 1987, University of Wisconsin Press.

Ardran, GM, Kemp, FH, and Lind, J: A cineradiographic study of bottle feeding, *Br J Radiology* 31:11–22, 1958a.

Ardran, GM, Kemp, FH, and Lind, J: A cineradiographic study of breast feeding, *Br J Radiology* 31:156–62, 1958b.

Atkinson, SA, and Kaufman, KJ: Lactational performance and milk composition in relation to duration of pregnancy and lactation. In Hamosh, M, and Goldman, AS, eds.: *Human Lactation 2: Maternal and Environmental Factors,* New York, 1986, Plenum Press, pp. 103–19.

Bodefeld, E, et al.: Continuous tcPO$_2$ monitoring in healthy and sick newborn infants during and after feeding. In Huch, A, Huch, R, and Lucey, JF, eds.: *Continuous transcutaneous blood gas monitoring,* New York, 1979, Alan R. Liss, Inc.

Botsford, KB, et al.: Gram-negative bacilli in human milk feedings: Quantitation and clinical consequences for premature infants, *J Pediatr* 109:707–10, 1986.

Bowen-Jones, A, Thompson, C, and Drewett, RF: Milk flow and sucking rates during breast feeding, *Dev Med Child Neurol* 24:626–33, 1982.

Brooke, OG, and Barley, J: Loss of energy during continuous infusions of breast milk, *Arch Dis Child* 53:344–45, 1978.

Churella, HR, Bachhuber, WL, and MacLean, WC: Survey: Methods of feeding low-birth weight infants, *Pediatrics* 76:243–49, 1985.

Collinge, JM, et al.: Demand vs. scheduled feedings for premature infants, *JOGN Nurs* 11:362–67, 1982.

Costa, KM: A comparison of colony counts of breast milk using two methods of breast cleansings, *JOGNN* 18:231–36, 1989.

Coward, WA: Measuring milk intake in breastfed babies, *J Pediatr Gastroenterol Nutr* 3:275–79, 1984.

Culley, P, et al.: Are breastfed babies still getting a raw deal in hospital? *Br Med J* 2:891–93, 1979.

Daniels, H, et al.: Infant feeding & cardiorespiratory maturation, *Neuropediatrics* 21:9–10, 1990.

Davies, DP: Adequacy of expressed breast milk for early growth of preterm infants, *Arch Dis Child* 52:96–301, 1977.

Davies, DP, and Evans, TJ: Nutrition and early growth of preterm infants, *Early Hum Dev* 2:383–92, 1978.

De Carvalho, M, et al.: Effect of frequent breastfeeding on early milk production and infant weight gain, *Pediatrics* 72:307–11, 1983.

Donowitz, LG, et al.: Contaminated breast milk: A source

of Klebsiella bacteremia in a newborn intensive care unit, *Rev Infec Dis* 3:716–20, 1981.

Drewett, RF, and Woolridge, M: Sucking patterns of human babies on the breast, *Early Hum Dev* 3:315–20, 1979.

Eckburg, JJ, et al.: Effects of formula temperature on post-prandial thermogenesis and body temperature of premature infants, *J Pediatr* 111:588–92, 1987.

Ehrenkranz, RA, et al.: Breast feeding and premature infant: Incidence and success (abstracted), *Pediatr Res* 19:99A (Abstract 530), 1985.

Ehrenkranz, RA, and Ackerman, BA: Metoclopramide effect on faltering milk production by mothers of premature infants, *Pediatrics*, 78:614–20, 1986.

Eidelman, AI, and Szilagyi, G: Patterns of bacterial colonization of human milk, *Obstet Gynecol* 53:550–52, 1979.

Fomon, SJ, Ziegler, EE, and Vazquez, H: Human milk and the small premature infant, *Am J Dis Child* 131:463–67, 1977.

Garg, M, et al.: Clinically unsuspected hypoxia during sleep and feeding in infants with bronchopulmonary dyplasia, *Pediatrics* 81:635–42, 1988.

Gaull, E, Raiha, N, and Rassin, D: Nutrition and the early growth of preterm infants, *Early Hum Dev* 3:373–78, 1979.

Gotsch, G: *Breastfeeding your premature baby,* Franklin Park, Ill., 1990, La Leche League International.

Greenspan, JS, et al.: Neonatal gastric intubation: Differential respiratory effects between nasogastric and orogastric tubes, *Pediatr Pulm* 8:254–58, 1990.

Greer, FR, McCormick, A, and Loker, J: Changes in fat concentration of human milk during delivery by intermittent bolus and continuous mechanical pump infusion, *J Pediatr* 105:745–49, 1984.

Gross, SJ, et al.: Bone mineralization in preterm infants fed human milk with and without mineral supplementation, *J of Pediatr* 111:450–58, 1987.

Gross, SJ, et al.: Nutritional composition of milk produced by mothers delivering preterm, *J Pediatr* 96:641–44, 1980.

Gryboski, JD: Suck and swallow in the premature infant, *Pediatrics* 43:96–102, 1969.

Guilleminault, C, and Coons, S: Apnea and bradycardia during feeding in infants weighing > 2000 grams, *J Pediatr* 104:932–35, 1984.

Haggkvist, AP: *What factors influence the breast feeding prevalence of mothers to premature babies?* Proceedings of the Child International Conference of Maternity Nurse Researchers, Gateborg, Sweden, June, 1990.

Heird, WC: Feeding the premature infant: Human milk or an artificial formula? *Am J Dis Child* 131:468–69, 1977.

Heldt, G: The effect of gavage feeding on the mechanics of the lung, chest wall, and diaphragm of preterm infants, *Pediatr Res* 24:55–58, 1988.

Herrell, N, Martin, RJ, and Fanaroff, A: Arterial oxygen tension during nasogastric feeding in the preterm infant, *J Pediatr* 96:914–16, 1980.

Horton, FH, Lubchenco, LO, and Gordion, HH: Self-regulation feeding in a premature nursery, *Yale J Biol Med* 24:263–72, 1952.

Howie, PW, et al.: How long should a breast feed last? *Early Hum Dev* 5:71–77, 1981.

Humenick, SS: The clinical significance of breastmilk maturation rates, *Birth*, 14:174–79, 1987.

Jain, L, et al.: Energetics and mechanics of nutritive sucking in the preterm and term neonate, *J Pediatr* 111:894–98, 1987.

Krauss, AN, et al.: Pulmonary function following feeding in low-birth-weight infants, *Am J Dis Child* 132:139–42, 1978.

Lawrence, RA: *Breastfeeding: A guide for the medical profession,* 3rd ed., St. Louis, 1989, The C.V. Mosby Co.

Lefrak-Okikawa, L: Nutritional management of the very low birth weight infant, *J Perinat Neonat Nurs* 2:66–77, 1988.

Lemons, JA, Schreiner, RI, and Gresham, EL: Simple method for determining the caloric and fat content of human milk, *Pediatrics*, 66:626–28, 1980.

Lemons, PM, et al.: Bacterial growth in human milk during continuous feeding, *Am J Perinat* 1:76–80, 1983.

Lucas, A, and Cole, TJ: Breast milk and neonatal necrotising enterocolitis, *Lancet* 336:1519–23, 1990.

Lucas, A, Lucas, PJ, and Baum, JD: Differences in the pattern of milk intake between breast and bottle fed infants, *Early Hum Dev* 5:195–99, 1981.

Lucas, A, et al.: Creamatocrit: Simple clinical technique for estimating fat concentration and energy value of human milk, *Br Med J* 1:1018–20, 1978.

Lundeen, EC: Feeding the premature baby, *AJN* 39:3–11, 1939.

Lundeen, EC: Newer trends in the care of premature infants, *Nurs Wrld* 133:1959.

Lundeen, EC: Prematures present special problems: Basic factors in nursing care, *Mod Hosp* April: 60–65, 1954.

Mathew, OP: Breathing patterns of preterm infants during bottle feeding: role of milk flow, *J Pediatr* 119:960–65, 1991.

Mathew, OP: Nipple units for newborn infants: A functional comparison, *Pediatrics* 81:688–91, 1988.

Mathew, OP, and Bhatia, J: Sucking and breathing patterns during breast- and bottle-feeding in term neonates, *Am J Dis Child* 143:588–92, 1989.

Mathew, OP, Clark, ML, and Pronske, MH: Apnea, bradycardia, and cyanosis during oral feeding in term neonates, *J Pediatr* 106:857, 1985.

Mathew, OP, et al.: Breathing pattern and ventilation during oral feeding in term newborn infants, *J Pediatr* 106:810–13, 1985.

McCoy, R, et al.: Nursing management of breast feeding for preterm infants, *J Perinat Neonat Nurs* 2:42–55, 1988.

Meberg, A, Willgraff, S, and Sande, HA: High potential for breast feeding among mothers giving birth to pre-term infants, *Acta Paediatr Scand* 71:661–62, 1982.

Meier, PP: Bottle and breast feeding: Effects on transcutaneous oxygen pressure and temperature in preterm infants, *Nurs Res* 37:36–41, 1988.

Meier, PP, and Anderson, GC: Responses of preterm infants to bottle and breast feeding, *MCN* 12:420–23, 1987.

Meier, PP, and Pugh, EJ: Breast feeding behavior of small preterm infants, *MCN* 10:396–401, 1985.

Meier, PP, and Wilks, SO: The bacteria in expressed mothers milk, *MCN* 12:420–23, 1987.

Meier, PP, et al.: Bottle and breastfeeding: Physiologic effects on preterm infants (abstract), *Neon Netw* 10:78, 1991.

Meier, PP, et al.: The accuracy of test-weighing for preterm infants, *J Pediatr Gastroenterol Nutr* 10:62–65, 1990.

Mukhtar, AI, and Strothers, JK: Cardiovascular effects of nasogastric tube feeding in the healthy preterm infant, *Early Hum Dev*, 6:25–30, 1982.

Narayan, I, Singh, B, and Harvey, D: Fat loss during feeding of human milk, *Arch Dis Child* 59:475–77, 1984.

Neifert, MA, and Seacat, J: *Milk yield and prolactin rise with simultaneous breast pump:* Abstract from the Ambulatory Pediatric Association Annual Meeting, Washington, D.C., May 7–10, 1985.

Neifert, MA, and Seacat, J: Practical aspects of breastfeeding the premature infant, *Perinatol-Neonatol* 12:24–30, 1988.

Neville, MC, et al.: Studies in human lactation: Milk volumes in lactating women during the onset of lactation and full lactation, *Am J Clin Nutr* 48:1375–86, 1988.

O'Donovan, P, and O'Brien, N: Group B Beta haemolytic disease in preterm twins associated with the ingestion of infected breast milk: A case report, *Irish J Med Sci* 154:158–59, 1985.

Pearce, JL, and Buchanan, LF: Breast milk and breastfeeding in very low birthweight infants, *Arch Dis Child* 54:897–99, 1979.

Pereira, GR, et al.: Breastfeeding in neonatal intensive care: Beneficial effects of maternal counseling, *Perinatol-Neonatol* 8:35–42, 1984.

Persson, B: *Kangaroo method: The key to alternative premature care,* Proceedings of the Third International Conference of Maternity Nurse Researchers, Goteborg, Sweden, 1990, Nordic School of Public Health, p. 51.

Pitt, J: Breast milk and the high risk baby: Potential benefits and hazards, *Hosp Pract* 14:81–86, 1979.

Richards, MT, et al.: Breastfeeding the VLBW infant: Successful outcome and maternal expectations, *Pediatr Res* 20:388A (Abstract No. 1385), 1986.

Ronnholm, KA, Sipila, I, and Siimes, MA: Human milk protein supplementation for the prevention of hyponatremia without metabolic imbalance in breast milk-fed, very low-birth-weight infants, *J Pediatr* 101:243–47, 1982.

Rosen, CL, Glaze, DG, and Frost, JD: Hypoxemia associated with feeding in the preterm infant and full-term neonate, *Am J Dis Child* 138:623–27, 1984.

Rowe, JC, et al.: Nutritional hypophosphatemic rickets in a premature infant fed breastmilk, *N Engl J Med* 300:293–96, 1979.

Ryder, RW, et al.: Human milk contaminated with Salmonella Kottbus, *JAMA* 238:1533–34, 1977.

Sagy, M, et al.: Phosphate-depletion syndrome in a premature infant fed human milk, *J Pediatr* 96:683–85, 1980.

Shivpuri, CR, et al.: Decreased ventilation in preterm infants during oral feeding, *J Pediatr* 103:285–89, 1983.

Singh, M: Early discharge of low-birthweight babies, *Trop Geog Med* 31:565–69, 1979.

Stevens, LH: The first kilogram: The protein content of breast milk of mothers of babies of low birth weight, *Med J Aust* 2:555–57, 1969.

Stocks, J: Effect of nasogastric tubes on nasal resistance during infancy, *Arch Dis Child* 55:17–21, 1980.

Stocks, RJ, et al.: Loss of breast milk nutrients during tube feeding, *Arch Dis Child* 60:164–66, 1985.

Thompson, M, and McClead, RE: Human milk fortifiers, *J Pediatr Perin Nutr* 1:65–74, 1987.

Van Someren, V, et al.: An investigation into the benefits of resiting nasoenteric feeding tubes, *Pediatrics* 74:379–83, 1984.

Verronen, P: Breastfeeding of low birth weight infants, *Acta Paediatr* Scand 74:495–99, 1985.

Vice, FL, et al.: Cervical auscultation of suckle feeding in newborn infants, *Dev Med Child Neurol* 32:760–68, 1990.

Walker, M: *Breastfeeding premature babies.* In Auerbach, KG, ed.: Lactation Consultant Series (Unit 14), Garden City Park, N.Y., 1990, Avery Publishing Group, Inc., pp. 1–38.

Weber, F, Woolridge, MW, and Baum, JD: An ultrasonographic study of the organization of sucking and swallowing by newborn infants, *Dev Med Child Neurol* 28:19–24, 1986.

Whitfield, MF, Kay, R, and Stevens, S: Validity of routine clinical test-weighing as a measure of intake in breastfed infants, *Arch Dis Child* 56:919–20, 1981.

Wilks, SO, and Meier, PP: Helping mothers express milk suitable for preterm and high-risk infant feeding, *MCN* 13:121–23, 1988.

Wilson, SL, et al.: Coordination of breathing and swallowing in human infants, *J Appl Physiol* 50:851–58, 1981.

Woolridge, MW: The "anatomy" of infant sucking, *Midwifery* 2:164–71, 1986.

Woolridge, MW, et al.: Methods for the measurement of milk volume intake of the breast-fed infant. In Jensen, RG, and Neville, MC, eds.: *Human Lactation: Milk components and methodologies,* New York, 1985, Plenum Press, pp. 5–20.

11

Breast Pumps
and Other Technologies

Marsha Walker

Kathleen G. Auerbach

Special devices have been used for hundreds of years to help breastfeeding mothers overcome various problems. Examples of someone—or something—other than a baby removing milk from the breasts are cited in medical literature as early as the mid-1500s (Fildes, 1986). Before breast pumps or other instruments were used to withdraw milk from the breasts, children, young puppies, or birth attendants were enlisted to do the job. By the 1500s the medical literature included discussions of "sucking glasses." These devices allowed women to remove milk themselves and were recommended for relieving engorgement or expressing milk when the nipples were damaged or when mastitis was present. Sucking glasses were also thought to help evert flat and inverted nipples. For the most part, vacuum was generated by mouth, and the devices were made of glass. (See Fig. 11–1.) Women could use a glass, glass vial, or glass bottle heated with very hot water and applied to the breast in order to draw out milk. French breast pumps in the 1700s resembled pipes but were made of different materials.

As technology advanced, so did breast pump ma-

terials and design. Combinations of materials such as brass, wood, glass, and rubber were used to make pumps like the syringe pump (Fig. 11–2), the long-handled lever pump (Fig. 11–3) and the glass and rubber "bicycle horn" pump, all circa 1830. The reasons why women chose to express milk also changed. Today women pump their breasts for short periods of time to solve acute problems and for extended periods in order to continue to provide human milk for their babies while they are employed or following a pre-term birth.

CONCERNS OF MOTHERS

Most mothers want a pump that works efficiently and comfortably at a reasonable cost. (See boxed copy.) The amount of milk pumped and the time it takes to pump are the two issues most frequently mentioned by mothers when they are choosing or using a breast pump.

Pump satisfaction, however, is highly individual. In an informal survey of more than 200 mothers, a pump was rated highly if it: (1) worked quickly—less than 20 minutes total; (2) obtained two or more ounces of milk from each breast; and (3) did not cause pain. The mothers in the survey suggested pumping techniques to speed the process and to increase the volume of milk per pumping session. Many mothers expressed the most milk before or after the first morning feeding when the breasts

---

CONCERNS OF MOTHERS

Mothers want pumps to be:
- Efficient
- Comfortable
- Accessible
- Affordable
- Easy to clean
- Easy to use

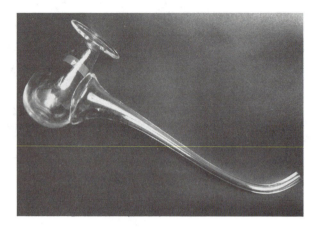

FIGURE 11–1   An American sucking glass circa 1870.

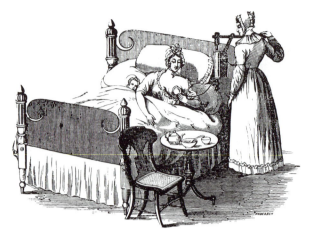

FIGURE 11–3   Expressing breastmilk with a long handled lever pump, c. 1830.

were reported to be most full (and intramammary pressure was the highest); later volumes steadily decreased throughout the day. Many mothers mentioned that if they were not relaxed, or if they were uncomfortable or felt rushed, their output dropped by one-third to one-half the usual amount.

DRAWING THE BREASTS.

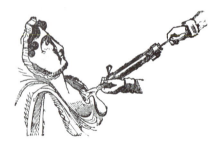

Where the breast is hard, swollen and painful, from inflammation, or the nipple sore from excoriation, the application of this instrument is attended with more ease to the patient than any other means, and she may without difficulty use it herself, by which she can regulate its action agreeably to her own sensations. The flat surface of the glass should be smeared with oil before it is put on, and the bulb preserved in a dependant position to receive the fluid. During the operation the small aperture in the brass socket must be closely covered with the finger, which being removed, admits air into the glass and causes it to be detached from the breast whenever it may be desired.

FIGURE 11–2   Expressing the breasts with a syringe pump, c. 1830.

The majority of mothers used one or more techniques to increase pumping efficiency. The two most frequently mentioned techniques were eliciting the milk-ejection reflex *before* starting to pump and massaging the breast *while* pumping. Both techniques increased pumping speed and milk output. Some mothers were able to double the amount pumped by using both of these techniques at each pumping session.

STIMULATING THE MILK-EJECTION REFLEX

There is a vast amount of research and literature in the dairy industry supporting the importance of eliciting the milk-ejection reflex before starting to pump. Premilking stimulation of the udder increases serum oxytocin levels (Merrill et al., 1987) and results in shorter "machine on" time and a higher average rate of milk flow (Sagi, Gorewit & Zinn, 1980; Dodd & Griffin, 1977; Goodman & Grosvenor, 1983; Gorewit et al., 1983). In the second edition of *Dairy Science,* Petersen (1950) cites a number of factors which contribute to poor milking: undue excitement at milking time; improper stimulation for the letdown of milk; too long an interval between stimulation of let-down and the beginning of milking; too slow milking; and incomplete withdrawal of milk. Petersen makes five observations regarding proper milking techniques which parallel many of the recommendations professionals make, as well as many of the pumping techniques mothers have discovered on their own. Women are not the same as cows, but it should be understood that animal models of lactation often provide a frame of reference from which similarities can be drawn and applied. Petersen recommended:

1. Avoid undue excitement at milking time—"for the best response the cow must be relaxed and enjoy being milked." Many women in the survey mentioned using specific relaxation techniques and visual imagery before and during pumping. Feher et al. (1989) report using a guided relaxation audio tape to increase milk output during breast pumping among mothers of pre-term infants. Newton and Newton (1948) describe the adverse effect of a painful or distracting stimulus during nursing on the milk-ejection reflex.

2. Elicit the milk-ejection reflex first, one to two minutes before pumping begins; massaging with a hot, wet cloth before milking is the most effective stimulus for let-down. Mothers in the survey reported using hot compresses, showers and breast massage before pumping to obtain the best results. Some reported that they were most successful if they pumped one side while the baby nursed on the other breast (as with pumping in dairy cattle when all teats are milked simultaneously), or if the baby elicited the milk-ejection reflex first and they then pumped, or if they hand expressed first and then used the pump.

3. Massage each quarter of the udder during mechanical milking. Massaging during pumping was mentioned by the mothers in the survey as markedly increasing milk yield. There is evidence that breast massage may increase fat content and milk yield when a baby is at breast. Bowles, Stutte, and Hensley (1987/1988) and Stutte, Bowles, and Morman (1988) found that infants gained greater amounts of weight—and mothers experienced little nipple pain or painful engorgement—when the breasts were massaged by quadrant in an alternating pattern with the baby's suckling bursts.

4. When hand milking, avoid point compression and digging in with the finger tips, which is likely to cause injury. The Marmet method of hand expression (Marmet & Shell, 1979) cautions against this technique when a mother is hand expressing her milk.

5. Remove the milking machine as soon as the milk stops flowing. Stopping the pump when the milk stops flowing reduces injury to the tissue. Many mothers noted that when the milk flow slowed this was the signal to switch to the other breast. Some mothers mentioned that pain was the cue for this switch, indicating a change in the pressure gradient. Auerbach (1990b) found that protracted pumping times did not significantly increase milk yield beyond a certain point: "The participants in this study who pumped (sequentially or simultaneously) longer than 16 minutes averaged total milk volumes of 55cc or less."

The dairy literature includes many recommendations which are applicable to human breast pumping. Even the modern electric breast pumps designed for mothers have similarities to the agricultural milking units. The Whittlestone pump has incorporated the design of the double chambered teat cups. The suction and rest phases of a milking unit are either 60/40 or 70/30 (percentage of suction to percentage of rest per cycle). There are usually 60 cycles generated per minute (a calf generates about 120 cycles), and negative pressure is around 375mm Hg (similar to the pressure seen in many breast pumps, including hand pumps).

Breast pumps must also be easy to clean, afford-

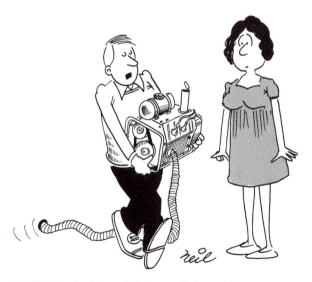

FIGURE 11–4 "They didn't actually have a breast pump. . . ." (Courtesy of Neil Matteson.) © 1984, Marion Books, Wooend, Victoria, Australia.

able, and accessible. When recommending a pump, the care-giver should give a specific name and several places where to find it. Hospital or medical supply houses may have pumps originally designed as chest aspirators which are not as suitable for milk expression as those specifically designed for that purpose. Many mothers in the survey complained of the extra expense incurred if their pump broke (common with the battery pumps) and required replacement. Of 97 battery pumps used in the survey, 24 broke or stopped generating suction and had to be replaced (a 25% breakage rate). The life of a battery-operated pump is considered to be about 16 weeks (4 months) by some companies, which is a much shorter period than many employed mothers require. Batteries are a major expense for mothers who pump regularly; many purchase an A/C adapter to economize. The cost of the accessory kit and daily rental charges for an electric pump can be expensive, even with a long-term rental contract. Some insurance carriers and health maintenance organizations cover the cost of pump rentals only while a baby is hospitalized. The parents must then assume the expense after discharge.

Several mothers in the survey purchased a hand pump solely on the basis of cost. Some were dissatisfied and purchased a second, more expensive pump that worked better. Pump prices vary considerably depending upon the type of store or organization which sell them. Some breastfeeding programs provide breast pumps at cost to their clients. Many hospitals give breastfeeding mothers a high quality hand pump upon discharge rather than formula packs. The boxed list on p. 283 summarizes recommendations for mothers using a breast pump.

HORMONAL CONSIDERATIONS

When milk expression using a pump is necessary, the device used must be efficient enough to activate prolactin and oxytocin release and to efficiently remove milk from the breasts.

PROLACTIN

A steady rise in prolactin during pregnancy prepares the breasts for lactation (Neville, 1983). Prolactin levels will only remain high after the first weeks postpartum if the baby is put to breast, or in the absence

of breast stimulation by an infant, if a pump is used to mechanically maintain prolactin cycling (Noel, Suh & Franzt, 1974; Weichert, 1980; Howie et al., 1980; de Sanctis et al., 1981; Whitworth et al., 1984). Basal prolactin levels and the magnitude of the sucking-induced rise in prolactin normally decrease over time as lactation extends beyond three to four months (Whitworth, 1988). This occurs regardless of the frequency of feeding (Battin et al., 1985; Johnston & Amico, 1986) and regardless of whether breast pump stimulation has replaced the sucking infant (Leake et al., 1983).

According to Whitworth (1988), "Postpartum, the response threshold [of prolactin] is maintained by frequent suckling, which both releases prolactin and ensures that prolactin-release mechanisms remain responsive to future suckling stimuli." Early and frequent breast stimulation causes the mother's serum prolactin levels to rise, which in turn increases milk production. Because of this physiologic sequence, three suggestions should be kept in mind by the clinician if the mother is using a pump during the immediate postpartum period:

1. In the absence of a baby at breast (because of prematurity, maternal or infant illness, early separation), the breasts need to be stimulated eight or more times every 24 hours. A common mistake is to pump only once or twice during the day and never at night, when prolactin levels are at their peak. A faltering milk supply in the following weeks may be attributed to the lack of sufficient prolactin receptors and infrequent breast stimulation while lactation is being established.

2. Prevent painful overdistention of the breasts (secondary engorgement). As alveolar pressure rises, lactation suppression begins. Painful engorgement lasting longer than 48 hours can potentially decrease the milk supply. Therefore, if a baby cannot keep up with a suddenly increased milk supply, the mother should manually express her milk or pump her breasts. When milk production begins in the absence of a baby, pumping frequency may need to be temporarily increased to prevent involution of the alveoli caused by the back-up pressure of milk and the build up of suppressor peptides which down regulate milk volume (Akre, 1989).

3. Assuming that early breastfeeding has a critical

General Pumping Recommendations

1. Read the instructions on the use and cleaning of a pump before expressing milk with any product.
2. Hands should be washed before each pumping session.
3. Frequency: For occasional pumping, pump during, after or between feedings, whichever gives the best results. Most mothers tend to express more milk in the morning. For working mothers, pumping should occur on a regular basis for the number of nursings that are missed. For premature or ill babies who are not at breast, the number of pumpings should total eight or more in 24 hours. Initiation of pumping should be delayed no longer than six hours following birth unless medically indicated. This assures appropriate development and sensitivity of prolactin receptors. More frequent pumping will avoid the build-up of excessive backpressure of milk during engorgement.
4. Duration: With single-sided pumping, optimal duration is 10 to 15 minutes with an electric pump and 10 to 20 minutes with a manual pump. If double pumping with an electric or two battery-operated pumps, 7 to 15 minutes is optimal. Encourage mothers to tailor these times to their own situation.
5. Technique:
   –Elicit the milk-ejection reflex before using any pump.
   –Use only as much suction as is needed to maintain milk flow.
   –Massage the breast in quadrants during pumping to increase intramammary pressure.
   –Allow enough time for pumping to avoid anxiety.
   –Use inserts or different flanges if needed to obtain the best fit between pump and breast.
   –Avoid long periods of uninterrupted vacuum.
   –Stop pumping when the milk flow is minimal or has ceased.

Recommendations for Specific Types of Pumps

1. Avoid pumps that use rubber bulbs to generate vacuum.
2. Cylinder pumps:
   –When "O" rings are used, they must be in place for proper suction.
   –Gaskets must be removed *after each use* for cleaning to avoid harboring bacteria in the pump.
   –The gasket on the inner cylinder may be rolled back and forth to restore it to its original shape.
   –The pump stroke may need to be shortened as the outer cylinder fills with milk.
   –The user may need to empty the outer cylinder once or twice during pumping.
   –Hand position should be palm up with the elbow held close to the body.
3. Battery-operated pumps:
   –Use alkaline batteries.
   –Replace batteries when cycles per minute decrease.
   –Interrupt vacuum frequently to avoid nipple pain and damage.
   –Use an A/C adapter when possible, especially if the pump generates fewer than six cycles per minute.
   –Consider renting an electric pump for pumping that will continue for longer than one or two months.
   –Use two pumps simultaneously if pumping time is limited or to increase the quantity of milk obtained.
   –Choose a pump in which the vacuum can be regulated.
   –Massage the breast by quadrants during pumping.
4. Semiautomatic pumps:
   –Vacuum may be easier to control if the mother does not lift her finger completely off the hole but rolls it back and forth rhythmically so that the vacuum is efficient but not painful.
5. Automatic electric pumps:
   –Use the lowest pressure setting that is efficient.
   –Use a double setup (simultaneous pumping) when time is limited in order to increase a milk supply, as well as for prematurity, maternal or infant illness, or other special situations.

period during which frequent nipple stimulation and milk removal are necessary for a plentiful milk supply in later weeks, the clinician should offer management guidelines with this in mind, especially if mother and baby are separated. Always keep in mind Whitworth's (1988) reminder: "Postpartum, the response threshold [of prolactin] is maintained by frequent suckling, which both releases prolactin and ensures that prolactin-release mechanisms remain responsive to future suckling stimuli."

OXYTOCIN

Oxytocin is the hormone responsible for the milk-ejection reflex. By acting on the myoepithelial processes, oxytocin causes shortening of the ducts without constricting them, thus increasing the milk pressure. Cobo et al. (1967) measured milk ejection by recording intraductal mammary pressure using a catheter placed in a mammary duct. Values were measured at 0.19 plus or minus 0.04 in^2/min and from 0 to 25 mm Hg on recording paper. Ductal contractions last about a minute and occur at about 4 to 10 contractions every 10 minutes. Caldeyro-Barcia (1969) reported that intramammary pressure rose 10mm Hg after five days postpartum with oxytocin release. Drewett, Bowen-Jones, and Dogterom (1982) and McNutley et al. (1983) have shown by minute-to-minute blood sampling that oxytocin occurs in impulses at about one-minute intervals. Thus oxytocin release is pulsatile and variable with intermittent bursts. These pressure changes cease when suckling stimulation ends. Oxytocin also responds in the same way to prenursing stimuli and mechanical nipple stimulation by a breast pump. The milk-ejection reflex, initiated by oxytocin release, serves to increase the intraductal mammary pressure and maintain it at sufficient levels to overcome the resistance of the breast to the outflow of milk.

PUMPS

MECHANICAL MILK REMOVAL

A pump does not pump, suck, or pull milk out of the breast. It works by reducing resistance to milk outflow from the alveoli, allowing the internal pressure of the breast to push out the milk. The milk-ejection reflex produces an initial rise in the intramammary

pressure; because of the pulsatile nature of oxytocin release and its short half-life, periodic rises in ductal pressure maintain the pressure gradient over a period of time.

The classic work on breast pumps was done by Einar Egnell (1956) in 1956; it was based on research in dairy cattle and Egnell's own experiments with a pump which created periodic and limited phases of negative pressure. Egnell assumed that the milk-secreting alveoli of the breast and the cow udder were similar, even though the two organs are anatomically different and do not drain in the same way. He described how the quantity of milk secreted is regulated by the counterpressure it exerts. This counterpressure rises as milk fills the available space; secretion ceases when the pressure reaches 28mm Hg. Egnell's pump created a maximum negative pressure of 200mm Hg below atmospheric pressure (760mm Hg). He based this setting on previous research done with an Abt pump (on human mothers), which produced 30 periods of negative pressure per minute and was reported to rupture the nipple skin in every third breast. Egnell placed his settings well below this level to avoid damaging the human nipple. He calculated the difference between the pressure-filled alveoli and his pump's negative pressure as 760+28−560=228mm Hg. He maintained that it was the pressure within the breast that activated milk outflow.

Egnell's original pump operated in four phases per cycle (a cycle lasts from one initiation of suction to the next initiation of suction): (1) period of increasing suction which is relatively short; (2) decreasing period of suction; (3) resting phase; and (4) slight amount of positive pressure when the decreased suction phase is finished. Egnell contended that mechanical pumping was safer than manual expression because he feared that the "high" positive pressure generated by "squeezing" the breast could damage the alveoli and ducts. He also speculated that manual expression would leave too much milk in the breast, a common concern in the dairy industry. However, in countries where manual expression is the only method used to obtain mothers' milk when the baby is unavailable, increased breast damage has not been reported.

EVOLUTION OF PUMPS

Although the design of breast pumps continues to evolve and there are dozens of new products, many pump manufacturers still use Egnell's pressure settings as a guide. However, many hand-operated pumps are capable of generating more suction than his calculations. As breastfeeding rates increased and reasons for pumping changed, mothers and professionals demanded products that were safe, efficient, and effective in maintaining a good milk supply. The breast pump market has exploded in recent years, particularly in the United States; there are now "bicycle horn" type pumps and chest aspirators as well as a bewildering array of other devices from which to choose.

Pumps can be classified in different ways. In this chapter, three broad classifications are discussed: hand pumps which generate suction manually; battery-operated pumps with small motors which generate suction from power supplied by batteries; and electric pumps in which suction is created by various types of electric motors. Other miscellaneous pumps are also described. (See Table 11–1.) (See also the Appendix at the end of this chapter.)

HAND PUMPS

REVIEW OF RESEARCH

Hand pumps are popular, relatively inexpensive, and readily available. Much information on the efficiency of hand pumps is anecdotal; some pumps work quite well, while others suffer from poor suction, cylinders which pull apart during pumping, and user fatigue from the repeated motions necessary to work the pumps. A few studies have examined the efficiency of hand pumps, as well as their ability to influence prolactin levels, the volume of milk, and its fat and energy content. These studies are difficult to compare because study design and methodology vary widely. The results may depend on single or random milk samples, as well as measurement of milk components obtained at different postpartum times.

Green et al. (1982) evaluated four methods of milk expression, measuring the milk volume obtained as well as fat content with the Evenflo (bulb), Egnell electric pump, Loyd-B hand pump, and manual expression. Six mothers with exclusively breastfed, full-term infants, who were two weeks of age at the time of the study, provided milk samples obtained after 10 minutes of pumping. The percentage of fat content was similar for the four methods,

but the Egnell pump obtained the largest volume of milk. Between the two hand pumps evaluated, the Loyd-B obtained the most milk.

Johnson (1983) evaluated eight pumps in eight categories (pressure; pressure control; nipple cup, size and shape; volume; ease of handling; ease of cleaning; visual feedback; and cost) and observed their use by more than 1,000 mothers. The Egnell electric, Kaneson, and Loyd-B pumps scored the highest in overall user satisfaction. The Gomco (continuous vacuum electric), Davol and Binter (glass bicycle horn) pumps scored lowest, while the Evenflo (bulb) and Ora'lac (mouth suction) pumps were frequently ineffective. The Kaneson and Loyd-B were the highest ranking hand pumps, but no description is given of pumping techniques, days postpartum when pumping occurred, volume of milk pumped, or how long the mothers pumped.

Wennergren, Wiqvist, and Wennergren (1985) studied two manual pumps, the Medela and the Arta Plast (a European cylinder pump similar to the Kaneson). This two-part study asked 13 primiparae and 13 multiparae to evaluate the two pumps during their hospital stay following childbirth. The preferred pump was then used by 30 mothers for a one-month period at home. The Medela manual pump was rated higher by primiparae during their hospital stay and was used for the second part of the study. It was highly rated for relief of engorgement, hypergalactia, and for occasional pumping. Nine out of 12 mothers were highly satisfied when the pump was used for increasing a low milk supply. The authors concluded that a manual pump can be used to provide efficient milk stimulation. The study is limited in that only two pumps were evaluated during the early period of milk production and only one pump was used for the bulk of the study period.

Boutte et al. (1985) compared the Egnell electric pump and the Medela manual pump in nine full-term mothers for one month postpartum. Twenty-four hour pooled milk samples were evaluated for volume, fat, and energy content. The volume of milk collected by the two pumps was similar, but the energy content of milk obtained by the Egnell electric pump was greater than with the Medela manual pump. Because similar volumes of milk with significantly different energy concentrations were found, the authors suggest that collection method is an important consideration when energy content or other nutrient levels are of interest.

TABLE 11–1 TYPES AND BRANDS OF PUMPS

Hand Operated	Battery Operated	Small Semiautomatic Electric	Large Semiautomatic Electric	Large Automatic Electric	Miscellaneous
Rubber bulb Barum Davol Evenflo Goodyear	Evenflo Gentle Expressions (*Grabam-Field, Inc.,* formerly *Health Team*) Lact-B (*Ameda/Egnell*) Mag Mag (*Omron Marshall Products, Inc.*) Medela	Gerber Kadan (*D.A. Kadan, Inc.*) Mada (Mada Medical Products, Inc.) Nurture III (*Bailey Medical Engineering*) Schuco-Vac	Gomco Schuco-Vac White River	Ameda/Egnell Lactina (Medela, Inc.) Medela The Rose (*Grabam-Field, Inc.*) White River Whittlestone (Trigon Industries, Ltd.)	Juice Jar Ora'lac Venturi (water powered)
Unavailable or cannot locate: **Rubber bulb** Au Natural (*Luminscope Co.*) Le Pump (*Labron Scientific Corp.*) New Mothers Way (*JAC Instrument Co.*) **Squeeze handle** Avent (*Cannon Babysafe, Ltd.*) Mother's Touch (*Amede/Egnell*) Loyd-B (*Lopuco Ltd.*)	**Cannot locate:** Natural Choice (Crystal Medical Products)	Cannot locate: Axicare Mary Jane			

Cylinder

Ameda/Egnell

Evenflo

Happy Family
*(International Design/
Manufacturing, Inc.)*

Infa *(Sassy, Inc.* formerly
Monterey Labs)

Kaneson

Medela Manualectric

Precious Care
(Gerber Products Co.)

Ross Deluxe
*(private label for Happy
Family Ross Laboratories)*

Sears

White River

287

Grams (1988) reports comments from 268 women on 12 pumps (Medela Manualectric, Kaneson, Loyd-B, Faultless, and Evenflo bulb hand pumps; Medela, Egnell and White River large electric pumps, plus the Gerber small electric model; Gentle Expressions, Mag Mag, and Egnell Lact-B battery-operated pumps). Top rated were the Medela Manualectric, Kaneson, and Loyd-B hand pumps, and the Medela and Egnell electric models. The other pumps got mixed reviews. However, all the mothers did not use all 12 pumps and then compare their effectiveness; thus these grouped data are of limited value.

Zinaman et al. (1992) studied differences in the volume of milk obtained and prolactin stimulation by various types of breast pumps, as well as by the mother's own baby, in 23 women who were 28 to 42 days postpartum. Their results showed that the double setup (in which both breasts are pumped simultaneously) electric pumps did better in stimulating prolactin levels than battery or manual pumps, or hand expression, when only one breast was stimulated at a time. The White River electric pump was reported to stimulate the highest prolactin levels, cycling at 40 times per minute. Milk volumes were highest with the White River electric pump. Lowest milk volume was with hand expression and the Gentle Expressions battery pump, which produced 6 to 10 cycles per minute. When mothers rated their satisfaction with the pumps, the White River electric rated as one of the more uncomfortable to use. It is important to note that comparison of double pumping to a single baby or sequential pumping of one breast at a time may account for the results of this study. Another test of pump desirability would be to control for breast stimulation by using mothers of twins when comparing double pumping—or use other double pump setups or two pumps simultaneously.

The various types of hand pumps rely on differing mechanisms to generate suction.

Rubber bulb.   Barum, Davol, Evenflo, and Goodyear models are still available or occasionally seen in use. Au Natural, Le Pump, New Mothers Way, and Nurture pumps could not be found on the market and their manufacturers could not be located. Squeezing and releasing a rubber bulb generates a vacuum in these pumps. In most "bicycle horn" pumps, the rubber bulb is attached directly to the collection container. Some manufacturers have separated the bulb from the collection container by modifying the angle at which it is attached to the pump or by adding a length of tubing. These modifications are thought to reduce the high potential for bacterial contamination of the bulb caused by the easy backflow of milk. Backflow risk is reduced when the bulb is separated from the collection container. Vacuum control on these pumps is extremely difficult, thus increasing the likelihood of nipple pain and damage. Even with the use of a blood pressure-type bulb, vacuum control is left to chance. The "bicycle horn" pumps are inexpensive, but collect only about one-half ounce of milk at a time and must be emptied frequently. The other pumps collect milk in a bottle. Mothers often complain of nipple pain during pumping and low milk yields, especially if they have used these pumps for more than a few weeks.

Squeeze-handle pumps.   Avent, Mother's Touch (one-hand Ameda/Egnell), and Loyd-B pumps are all available.

Squeezing and releasing a handle creates suction in these pumps. The Loyd-B pump has a small trigger for vacuum release. The milk is collected in a glass baby food jar or in a standard baby bottle. Two sizes of stoppers accommodate the opening of the collection container used. The earlier version of the Loyd-B used a glass shield; two sizes of plastic shields are now available. A small length of tubing connects the pump handle with the collection container. The Mother's Touch (one hand) and Avent models have pump handles which attach directly to the bottles. The Loyd-B has been used for almost 20 years by mothers who have sometimes found it awkward to operate, although it is efficient in milk extraction and effective in maintaining the milk supply over time. Some mothers remark that larger hands are required or that their hand tires over time. The Avent pump is a new entry in the U.S. market. Few mothers have reported using it. The Mother's Touch (one-hand Ameda/Egnell) pump is also new to the market. These pumps are easily cleaned but their operation may present difficulties for women with hand or arm problems, such as Carpal Tunnel Syndrome. The hand and wrist can tire easily with repeated use.

Cylinder pumps.   Ameda/Egnell, Evenflo, Happy Family (also privately labeled as the Ross Deluxe by

Ross Labs), Infa, Kaneson, Medela Manualectric, Precious Care, Sears, and White River pumps are all available on the market. Chico, Craftco, Crystal, Mary Jane, and Nuk models could not be located on the market, nor could their manufacturers or distributors be found.

All of these pumps, except the Medela and Evenflo, consist of two cylinders. The outer cylinder generates vacuum as it is pulled away from the body. The inner cylinder with the flange is placed against the breast; a gasket at the other end helps form a seal with the edge of the outer cylinder. Gaskets may need to be replaced occasionally if they dry out, shrink, or lose their ability to form a seal. Gaskets can harbor bacteria and must be removed during cleaning, contrary to some user instructions. When placing the gasket back on the cylinder, roll it back and forth over the cylinder to help restore the shape. Some pumps come with extra gaskets. Small plastic or silicone inserts can be placed in the inner opening to custom fit the pump to the breast. Silicone liners are available for some pumps; these are designed to collapse against the breast during the suction phase in order to to provide external positive pressure. These pumps are lightweight, not too expensive, and easily cleaned.

The Medela Manualectric pump is the only hand-operated pump that has adjustable vacuum settings and automatically interrupts suction at about 220mm Hg, when the outer cylinder reaches the end of the outward stroke. The Medela Manualectric and the Evenflo Natural Mother both use a bottle to collect milk. Some pumps also provide an extra cylinder for milk storage or have an angled rather than a straight flange. Some mothers report that the angled flange does not work as well as the straight pumps. As the outer cylinder fills with milk, the gasket is repeatedly dunked in the milk. Mothers who express more than three ounces of milk at a time may have to empty these pumps more than once in a single pumping episode. The instructions for the Ameda/Egnell pump caution mothers to shorten the outward stroke as the outer cylinder fills in order to avoid immersing the gasket repeatedly. Efficiency of use varies from brand to brand. The Medela Manualectric and the Ameda/Egnell can also be adapted for use on the larger electric pumps. Table 11–2 summarizes information on the currently available manually operated pumps.

BATTERY-OPERATED PUMPS

Ameda/Egnell Lact-B, Evenflo, Gentle Expressions, Mag Mag, Mag Mag Advanced, and Medela pumps are currently available. The Natural Choice model by Crystal could not be found, nor could its manufacturer or distributor be located.

These pumps use a small motor with two AA 1.5-volt batteries to generate suction. The Evenflo pump uses two size "C" batteries. The Gentle Expressions pump has a dial to raise or lower the vacuum level. It also has a small cup that can be placed in the collection container that is attached to the motor unit. Called a "trainer cup," it reduces the amount of air in the system, thereby increasing the vacuum. The Ameda/Egnell model has a lever with higher and lower settings for vacuum adjustment, but its motor can block the view of the collection bottle. The Mag Mag pump has no vacuum adjustment dial. The Mag Mag Advanced pump has a vacuum-control dial and a removable inner collecting bottle for milk storage. Vacuum can take 30 seconds to reach its maximum level and is regulated by how frequently the vacuum is interrupted. Most of these pumps have a button or bar to press in order to release the vacuum periodically and simulate the rhythm of a nursing baby. All take varying periods of time for the recovery of suction following each release. This limits the number of suction/release cycles per minute to as few as six and may require relatively long periods of vacuum application to the nipple. To compensate for this, some mothers leave the suction on for much longer than the pump instructions recommend. Times of 30 to 60 seconds were mentioned by several mothers in one survey. Four women never interrupted the suction during the entire pumping session because they could not get the milk flow restarted following vacuum interruption.

Several pumps have A/C adapters to decrease battery use. A major complaint about these pumps is their short battery life. This affects pumping efficiency because fewer cycles are generated as the batteries wear down. Batteries may need to be replaced as frequently as every second or third use. Rechargeable batteries are an option but they usually require charging each night and may not produce as many cycles per minute as alkaline batteries. A/C adapters usually allow the maximum number of cycles per minute that the motor can produce. Maximum suction after each vacuum release will often continue

TABLE 11–2 MANUALLY OPERATED PUMPS

Type	Brand	Vacuum Source	Flange	Contamination	Risks of Use/Comments
Bicycle horn	Barum Davol Goodyear Evenflo	Squeezing and releasing a rubber bulb makes vacuum control very difficult.	One size. No adapters. Barum is made of glass.	Easy backflow of milk into rubber bulb. Bulb is difficult to clean or sterilize and can harbor bacteria. Potential for contamination is high.	No instructions. Less than $\frac{1}{2}$-oz reservoir. Must be emptied frequently. Potential for tissue and vascular damage is very high. Poor efficiency is reported from users.
Other rubber bulbs	**Not Available:** Au Natural Le Pump New Mothers Way Nurture	Squeezing and releasing a rubber bulb. Bulb is separated from collection container by a tube or angled flange. Vacuum control is very difficult.	Nurture has a silicone flange. One size, no adapters.	Rubber bulb still harbors bacteria even after boiling. Lower potential for backflow of milk and subsequent contamination.	Milk is collected in a bottle. Users report slow, inefficient milk removal. Tissue damage potential is high.
Squeeze handle	Avent Ameda/Egnell Loyd-B	Squeezing and releasing a handle generates suction. Loyd-B has a trigger for vacuum release. A short length of tubing connects handle to collection container (baby food jar or bottle). Others have handles that attach directly to standard bottle. Vacuum control moderate to somewhat difficult.	Loyd-B has two sizes, glass, and plastic. Avent has a thin membrane that fits over the flange.	Contamination risk lower than with rubber bulb pumps. Pumps are easy to clean. Reduced potential for backflow of milk.	Avent new to the United States with few reports on use. Loyd-B can be awkward and tire the hands. Its trigger can be hard to reach but is reported to be effective. Ameda/Egnell is new to market. Tissue damage potential is lower than for rubber-bulb pumps.
Cylinder (piston)	Ameda/Egnell Evenflo Happy Family Infa Kaneson Medela Gerber/Precious Care Ross Deluxe Sears White River **Not available:** Chico Craftco Crystal Mary Jane Nuk	Movement of outer cylinder away from the body. Vacuum is easier to control but can become excessive if not properly instructed. Medela automatically releases suction at end of outward stroke (220mm Hg) and has three vacuum settings. Its collection container is a bottle separated from the handle unit. Evenflo has a swivel handle separated from the collection bottle. May need to roll gasket back and forth several times when reattaching it to inner cylinder following cleaning to restore its original shape and efficiency. This will improve suction. Evenflo has a suction valve to increase vacuum.	Hard plastic with two silicone or two plastic adapters and two sizes of flanges. Gerber/Precious Care has soft plastic flange. Happy Family has two angled flanges. Sears angled soft flange can be rolled back to adjust for different size breasts. White River has silicone flange.	Contamination potential is lower; however, gasket must be removed during cleaning to prevent bacteria from collecting under it.	Potential for tissue damage is moderate, as high levels of vacuum can be generated unless mothers are properly instructed. The outer cylinder can come off during the outward stroke on some pumps. Some types of gaskets can lose their seal from repeated boiling or cleaning. Some come with extra gaskets, all of which must be oriented properly for optimum suction. "O" rings must be in place on the pumps that use them for a tight seal. Efficiency varies among these as they are not all the same.

decreasing in amount throughout the pumping session. In contrast, the Medela battery pump automatically produces 32 cycles per minute with alkaline batteries, 30 cycles per minute with rechargeable batteries and 42 cycles per minute with the A/C adapter.

Battery pumps require only one hand to operate, are lightweight, and popular with mothers employed outside the home. Some mothers use two battery-operated pumps simultaneously to decrease pumping time when they are on a tight schedule. Mothers who plan on several months of pumping while at work may consider a long-term rental contract for an electric pump, since battery replacement can be very expensive—as can artificial formula if it must be used to substitute for breast milk. See Table 11–3 for a summary of information on battery-operated breast pumps.

ELECTRIC PUMPS

Small semiautomatic pumps—Gerber, Kadan, Mada, Nurture III, and Schuco-Vac—are available. Axicare and Mary Jane brands could not be found on the market nor could their distributors be located. Large semiautomatic pumps, including Gomco, Schuco-Vac, and White River are available. Of the large automatic pumps, Egnell Lact-E, Lactina (Medela), Medela, and White River models are available. The Rose and Whittlestone models are not available in the United States.

Various types of electric motors are used in this group of pumps to generate suction. Semiautomatic pumps require the mother to cycle suction by using her finger to cover and uncover a hole in the flange base. By alternately covering and uncovering the hole with her finger, she creates a pumping rhythm designed to simulate the pattern of a suckling baby. These pumps maintain a constant negative pressure. Some lack a dial or mechanism to adjust the amount of suction. The actual amount of vacuum delivered to the nipple is determined by the degree of closure of the hole in the flange base. Many mothers learn to roll their finger three-quarters of the way off the hole rather than to lift the finger completely, in order to allow the pump to generate vacuum faster for the subsequent cycle by preventing complete interruption of vacuum. However, too much negative pressure, or negative pressure applied for too long a period, increases the risk of damage to the nipple and underlying vascular structures. The initiation of suction places the greatest pressure on the nipple; thus it is most desirable that a pump generate suction quickly.

Automatic electric pumps are designed to cycle pressure rather than to maintain it. Because Egnell observed nipple damage when cycles were two seconds long (30 per minute), manufacturers have increased the number of cycles so that they more closely simulate that of a nursing baby. Pressure setting parameters on these large pumps also mimic that of an infant. Mean sucking pressures of most full-term infants range from –50 to –155 with a maximum of –220mm Hg (Caldeyro-Barcia, 1969). In pumps that have a preset pulsed suction (automatic pumps), there is a 60/40 ratio. Negative pressure is applied for 60% of the cycle. Forty percent of the cycle is the resting phase. For example, the U.S. model of the Medela electric pump is set so that each cycle lasts 1.15 seconds (suction + rest); 52 cycles are generated per minute. In Europe, with the same pump, 48 cycles occur each minute because of the difference in the frequency of the electric voltage. The Egnell automatic pump generates 50 cycles per minute in the United States at 60 Hz and 42 cycles per minute in Europe at 50 Hz. The maximum pressure that these pumps will generate at their normal (high) setting is 220mm Hg. By comparison, the Nurture III semiautomatic pump produces 220 mm Hg after about 2.5 seconds using a single collecting kit (approximately 24 cycles per minute). With the double collecting kit, this same pump takes about 3.25 seconds to achieve this level, generating about 18 cycles per minute.

Negative pressure is a function of the volume of air in the accessory kit. Negative pressure increases as the bottle fills with milk. The pressure generated varies with different size bottles (collecting containers) and from one manufacturer to another. When double pump setups are used (two collecting containers simultaneously), the potential for very low negative pressure exists if the containers are empty; negative pressure increases as the bottles fill. Some accessory kits attempt to compensate for this in order to keep the pressure levels constant (*Rental Roundup*, 1986b). For example, the Medela Manualectric accessory kit has a valve head and membrane that separate the collection containers from the power source, thereby creating a closed system. Thus, the

TABLE 11-3 BATTERY-OPERATED PUMPS

Brand	Vacuum	Flange/Adapter	Contamination/ Cleaning	Risks of Use	Comments
Evenflo	2 C-size batteries; suction level selector; swivel handle.	Silicone flange with two silicone adapters.	Must avoid tilting the unit to prevent backflow into motor.	Nipple pain or damage can occur with all battery-operated pumps unless instructions are given which stress the importance of frequent interruption of vacuum, massaging while pumping, and eliciting the milk-ejection reflex before applying suction. Batteries must be fresh to generate near the maximum number of cycles per minute. A/C adapter will allow maximum number of cycles per minute.	All of these pumps suffer from a short battery life and work best with alkaline batteries. Most also have A/C adapter capabilities. These may be a good choice for mothers with an abundant milk supply and a quick milk-ejection reflex. These are usually not a good choice for mothers with slow or erratic milk ejection, sore nipples, or low milk supply.
Gentle Expressions	2 AA-size, 1.5-volt batteries; dial to adjust vacuum; small cup inserted into bottle to increase suction.	Hard plastic flange; two silicone inserts; "Lactostim" silicone liner.	Easily cleaned; fluid can be drawn into motor which eliminates vacuum.		
Lact-B Ameda/Egnell	2 AA-size batteries; vacuum control lever with bar or press to interrupt vacuum.	Hard plastic flange; "Flexi-flange" silicone liner.	Foam filter can be washed if milk is pulled into suction unit.		
Mag Mag	2 AA-size batteries; no vacuum adjustment; takes 30 seconds to reach maximum vacuum.	Hard plastic flange with 2 inserts.			
Mag Mag Advanced	Vacuum adjustment.	Insert with ridges.			
Medela	Automatically interrupts vacuum.	Hard plastic flange.		Nipple damage potential is low because pump generates 32 cycles per minute.	New to the market. May be a better choice for mothers who pump on a regular basis. May stimulate and maintain a milk supply better because of the higher number of cycles per minute.
Could not be located: Natural Choice (Crystal Medical)					

292

amount of air in the system remains constant regardless of the amount of fluid in the collection container. If a mother is using an accessory kit or pump without a similar feature, she can compensate by using a smaller collection bottle (Vol-u-feeders fit on some pumps), turning down the vacuum as the bottle fills, emptying the bottle more frequently, or cycling the suction more frequently on the hand, battery-operated, or semiautomatic pumps.

Several of the electric pumps have been adapted to allow pumping both breasts at the same time. Neifert and Seacat (1985) reported the experiences of 10 mothers who were two to seven months postpartum. The women alternated between sequentially pumping each breast for 20 minutes and then pumping both breasts simultaneously for 10 minutes. Milk yield was about the same with both techniques but was obtained in one-half the time with lower pump suction (320mm Hg vs. 260mm Hg) when pumping was simultaneous. They also found a significantly higher prolactin rise with double pumping. This is similar to Tyson's (1977) report of a doubling in prolactin rise when two infants were put to breast simultaneously and the findings of Saint, Maggiore, and Hartmann (1986), who reported larger milk volumes in mothers of twins (up to double that of singleton mothers). Auerbach (1990b) made a study of 25 mothers with babies between 5 and 35 weeks of age. She investigated the amount of milk obtained with single and double pumping, whether it takes longer to pump with a single setup compared to a double setup, and whether the milk fat varies between the two methods of pumping. Results showed that highest milk yields occurred with single pumping over 10 to 15 minutes. With double pumping, maximum milk volumes were seen in 7 to 12 minutes. The maximum yield overall occurred with double pumping. Milkfat concentrations were only slightly higher for double pumping sessions with no time limits. However, the mothers preferred double pumping three to one. Mothers' preferences regarding pumping regimens usually predicted how they obtained the highest yields.

Most electric pumps have hard plastic shields or flanges, except for the White River and Whittlestone brands. The White River electric pump (and all other White River products) uses a flexible silicone flange to achieve a degree of positive pressure and massage over a larger area of the areola and breast. Hughes et al. (1989) made a study comparing three pumps,

manual expression, and infant sucking. They showed that the White River double setup pump generated a 117% rise over baseline prolactin levels compared to a singleton baby at breast and other pumps used sequentially on one breast at a time. When prolactin was measured in mL/serum/hour, this pump yielded 2107mL/serum/hour, which is statistically similar to levels stimulated by a nursing baby. This pump is capable of generating very high vacuum levels, but the flange is designed to help distribute pressure over a wider area of the breast, thus avoiding nipple damage which might otherwise occur. Mothers have reported that the flange will occasionally pinch the nipple as it collapses.

The Whittlestone Breastmilker is a New Zealand pump with a double-pumping flange design based on milking techniques used by the dairy industry. The early mechanical milking devices used on domestic animals consisted of a single-chambered teat cup attached to a vacuum source which withdrew milk by simple suction (Woolford & Phillips, 1978). This design was inefficient, and the cows objected to the discomfort. A teat cup is now used which consists of a metal case lined with soft rubber. The milking apparatus produces a regular collapsing of the rubber liner against the teat to cause stimulation. The Whittlestone breast cups consist of a solid casing attached to a pulsating vacuum source. A foam pad in the cup case is held in place by a liner. When negative pressure occurs in the cup case, the liner moves against the pad, and the nipple and areola are drawn down into the conical portion of the liner (Whittlestone, 1978). Mothers report that this pump is comfortable and efficient.

Johnson (1983) measured several aspects of flanges, including the diameters of the outer opening (flare), inner opening, depth of flare, and length of shank. She measured negative pressure at the inner opening of the flange and reported that the smaller the nipple cup the greater the pressure exerted on the tip of the nipple. The larger and deeper flanges may provide greater stimulation of the areolar region of the breast. Zinaman (1988) repeated the same measurements on 11 manual pumps, four battery pumps, and seven electric pumps. When comparing these measurements among pumps highly rated in the other studies, diameter of the flange ranged from 60 to 69mm, depth ranged from 25 to 30mm, and the inner opening was between 21 and 26mm for the manual pumps. The Schuco-Vac pump has the smallest inner opening—6mm (1/4″)—and generates relatively high vacuum levels; it was also reported to cause noticeable discomfort in many women. A woman with a large or wide nipple may have difficulty with a flange that has a small opening or a narrow slope.

Because one size of flange does not fit all breasts, many manufacturers either provide two sizes of flanges, soft plastic or silicone flexible flanges, or small inserts that are placed at the level of the inner opening to narrow the diameter. The Ameda/Egnell pump has a silicone "Flexiflange" that lines the entire flange, as does the Gentle Expressions pump which features the "Lact-Stim." Inserts and silicone liners placed in the flanges are designed to provide a better fit between pump and breast. In general, the pump is more likely to be effective when it fits the anatomic configuration of the breast. To help with this fitting process, many health professionals who have access to autoclaving or similar sterilizing facilities offer mothers the opportunity to try several different brands of breast pumps in order to ascertain optimal fit before they purchase or rent a pump. Table 11–4 summarizes some features of electric breast pumps. See also Tables 11–5 and 11–6 for technical information.

MISCELLANEOUS PUMPS

JUICE JAR BREAST PUMP

This concept is reminiscent of the bottles mentioned in the beginning of this chapter. A 1-1/2-quart jar is filled with hot water and then emptied. The nipple/areola are inserted into the jar's opening, and a cool wash cloth is rubbed around the outside of the jar. As the hot air in the jar cools, it creates a gentle suction. Leaning over the jar may be uncomfortable for some women and the water must be reheated for each breast. It is an inexpensive method of obtaining milk and may be helpful for women with sore nipples. However, it is time consuming (Rees, 1977).

ORA'LAC

This pump generates suction by the mother sucking on a plastic, tube-like straw. It is the modern plastic version of the early sucking glasses. A second tube is attached to the flange and a saliva trap prevents sa-

liva from entering the bottle. It takes only one hand to operate and can be used even when the mother is lying down. The amount of suction varies and may not be efficient enough for regular pumping. It takes practice to use and may work better for women who have a large milk supply and an easily elicited milk-ejection reflex.

VENTURI BREAST PUMP

The Venturi pump (Fig. 11–5) generates a vacuum as a stream of running water passes through the faucet attachment. The faster and harder the water flows, the more suction is generated. A hole in the flange base is covered and uncovered to generate and release the vacuum. Unless the water is saved and re-used, this method of pumping wastes a lot of water. The mother must have access to a sink with running water in order to use the pump. The parts are inexpensive (Sponsel, 1983).

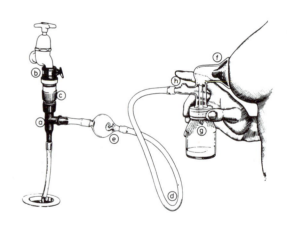

FIGURE 11–5 Venturi water-powered breast pump (*a*) connected to water tap via universal screw on adaptor (*b*), which may be left in place, and click on connector (*c*) (Hozelock UK, Ltd.), which allows easy removal of pump between feeds. Tubing (*d*) transmits suction to milking apparatus, and safety trap (*e*) prevents backflow of water vapour. Breast cup (*f*) is applied to areolar skin, and evacuation of milk bottle and breast cup achieved when valve (*h*) is occluded by mother's finger. Expressed milk enters bottle via internal channel (*g*). Pulsatile sucking action is created by repeated light touch and release of finger valve. From Sponsel, W: Simple and effective breast pump for nursing mothers, *Br Med J* 286:1680, 1983.

TABLE 11–4 ELECTRICALLY OPERATED PUMPS

Type	Brand	Vacuum	Flanges	Contamination/Cleaning	Risks/Comments
Small semiautomatic	Gerber	Continuous vacuum, cycled by covering and uncovering hole in collection funnel; vacuum not adjustable.	Hard and soft flanges; small, angled flange can be uncomfortable.	Vacuum release hole positioned in funnel permitting milk to flow over mother's finger. Increases risk of bacteria entering milk.	Moderate potential for nipple pain. Strength of suction in these pumps is regulated by the degree of closure of the mother's finger over the hole in the flange base.
	Kadan (D.A. Kadan)	Continuous vacuum; vacuum not adjustable.	Hard flange.	Has overflow bottle.	Very high suction; very noisy.
	Mada	Continuous vacuum; vacuum not adjustable.	Hard flange.	Has overflow bottle.	
	Nurture III	Adjustable vacuum; continuous suction.	Hard plastic; no adapters.	Backflow guard in imported French accessory kit.	Capable of simultaneous pumping.
	Schuco-Vac	Continuous vacuum; vacuum not adjustable.	Hard plastic flange; inner opening not entirely circular.		Very short electric cord.
Could not be located for evaluation:	Axicare Mary Jane				
Large semiautomatic	Gomco	High continuous vacuum.	Small inner opening of flange.		Poor markings on vacuum control knob; glass flange and collection container.
	Schuco-Vac	High continuous vacuum; vacuum adjustable.	Narrow opening of glass flange.		Capable of simultaneous pumping; high pressures best controlled by interrupting vacuum every 1–2 seconds. Occasional mother reports pinching of nipple.
	White River	Continuous vacuum; vacuum adjustable.	Flexible silicone flange distributes vacuum over larger area of breast.		All have potential for nipple damage if vacuum is not cycled quickly. Vacuum increases as collection containers fill.

295

TABLE 11–4 ELECTRICALLY OPERATED PUMPS (*continued*)

Type	Brand	Vacuum	Flanges	Contamination/Cleaning	Risks/Comments
Large automatic	Ameda/Egnell	Preset pulsed suction; adjustable vacuum.	Flexi-shield silicone liner can take up room in hard plastic flange.	Overflow safety basket located in accessory kit contains a seal and ball that blocks backflow of milk. No longer uses overflow bottle.	Capable of simultaneous pumping.
	Lactina (Medela)	Has rechargeable battery option; preset suction; adjustable vacuum.	Uses same accessory kit as other Medela electric pump.		Capable of simultaneous pumping.
	Medela	Preset pulsed suction; adjustable vacuum.	Hard flanges with inserts.	Accessory kit has hydrophobic filter that inhibits overflow. No longer uses overflow bottle.	Capable of simultaneous pumping.
	White River	Preset pulsed suction; adjustable vacuum	Flexible flange.		Capable of simultaneous pumping.
Not available in the United States					
	The Rose (Graham-Field)	Preset pulsed suction; adjustable vacuum.	Uses Gentle Expressions bottle as the accessory kit.		Generates about 16 cycles per minute.
	Whittlestone	Preset pulsed suction.	Cup cases with foam pads.		Capable of simultaneous pumping.

TABLE 11-5 SELECTED TECHNICAL DATA ON PUMPS*

Type/Brand	Range of Maximum Pressure Empty (mm Hg)	Pressure With 1 Ounce (mm Hg)	Pressure With 2 Ounces (mm Hg)	Cycles Per Minute	Double Setup Empty (mm Hg)	Double Setup 1 Ounce (mm Hg)	Double Setup 2 Ounces (mm Hg)
Manual							
Rubber bulb							
Barum	120			Erratic			
Davol	76–229			Erratic			
Evenflo	81–127			Erratic			
Cycles per minute depend on number and speed of squeezes on rubber bulb.							
Squeeze handle							
Avent	200–260	200–260	200–260	Variable			
Ameda/Egnell (one hand)	340	300–340	300–340	Variable			
Loyd-B	380–650	620	620	Variable			
Cycles per minute depend on number and duration of squeezes.							
Cylinder							
Ameda/Egnell	380–420 430 with Flexi-Shield	460–500	Spillage with 2 oz during testing	Variable			
Evenflo	60–120	40–100	80–140	Erratic (because of differing number of pulls to reach maximum pressure)			
Happy Family (also private label Ross Labs)	320	250	340	Variable			
Infa	400	380–500	Spillage with 2 oz during testing	Variable			
Kaneson	420–440	480–500	460–480 (spillage)	Variable			
Medela	L 120–140	140–480	160–180	Variable			
Manualectric	M 140–180	180–220	200–220				
	H 235–250	240–270	260–280				
Sears	360	380	440	Variable			
White River	240–320	180–260	200–260	Variable			

Cycles per minute will vary depending on number and duration of outward strokes.

TABLE 11-5 SELECTED TECHNICAL DATA ON PUMPS (*continued*)

Type/Brand	Range of Maximum Pressure Empty (mm Hg)	Pressure With 1 Ounce (mm Hg)	Pressure With 2 Ounces (mm Hg)	Cycles Per Minute	Double Setup Empty (mm Hg)	Double Setup 1 Ounce (mm Hg)	Double Setup 2 Ounces (mm Hg)
Battery							
Evenflo	L 40–94	70–90	60–95	10–28			
	M 90–140	120–140	95–140				
	H 160–180	160–200	160–220				
Gentle Expression	L 20	40	20	9–13			
	M 140	180	140				
	H 180	180	180				
Gentle Expression with small insert cup	L 20						
	M 220						
	H 280						
Lact-B	L 40–100	40–100	40–100	5–15			
Ameda/Egnell	M 140–170	140–180	160–185				
	H 140–180	140–180	160–185				
Mag Mag	110	110	120	15			
Mag Mag Advanced	L 60	60	60	13 (with A/C adapter)			
	M 120	120	140				
	H 260	260	260				
Medela	L 60	60	60	42 (with A/C adapter)			
	M 140	160	160				
	H 200	200	200				

Cycles per minute depend on how frequently and how long the vacuum is interrupted and how fast the vacuum can regenerate following interruption. Cycles are also influenced by the type of battery, whether the batteries are partially worn down, and whether or not an A/C adapter is used.

Electric

Small semiautomatic

Type/Brand	Range of Maximum Pressure Empty (mm Hg)	Pressure With 1 Ounce (mm Hg)	Pressure With 2 Ounces (mm Hg)	Cycles Per Minute	Double Setup Empty (mm Hg)	Double Setup 1 Ounce (mm Hg)	Double Setup 2 Ounces (mm Hg)
Gerber	20	20	40	18			
Kadan	580	580	580	11			
Nurture III	L 120–180	140–180	140–190	9–20	L 160–220	160–220	180–220
	M 160–200	160–200	180–220		H 200–250	195–250	200–260
	H 180–220	200–220	200–240				
Schuco-Vac	120	200	180	52			

Cycles per minute depend on how frequently and how long the vacuum is interrupted and how fast the vacuum can regenerate following interruption.

Large semiautomatic

Schuco-Vac	L 260	360	280	10–12	L 300–320	320	300–320
	M 360	350	360		M 380	360–390	340–360
	H 360	360	360		H 400–440	440–460	380–460
White River	L 370–400	300–400	390–420	12–42			
	M 440–460	460–470	460–480				
	H 320–540	540–560	540–560				

Large automatic

Ameda/Egnell	L 140–180	160–190	170–200	42–52	L 100–120	100–130	100–140
	M 200–250	200–240	220–270		M 120–150	140–160	140–170
	H 320–340	340–360	360–400		H 180–200	200–220	220–240
Medela	L 140	160	160–210	46	L 210–220	220–260	220–260
	M 160	160–170	160–210		M 220–270	240–270	240–270
	H 160	160–180	160–210		H 240–280	240–270	240–280
The Rose	L 40–120	80–120	80–130	16			
	M 160–220	180–240	180–240				
	H 300–320	300–340	300–340				

*All results are approximate. Hand-held vacuum gauge made by MacDaniel Controls, Inc.

TABLE 11–6 SELECTED SPECIFICATIONS OF PUMPS[1,2,3]

Type/Brands	Flange Outer Opening (Inches)	Flange Inner Opening (Inches)	Flange Depth of Flare (Inches)	Capacity of Collection Container (Ounces)	Variable Vacuum Control
Manual					
Rubber bulb					
Barum	2½	7/8	5/8	1	No
Davol	2½	2⅜	7/8	2½	No
Evenflo	2 9/16	1⅛	1	5	No
Squeeze handle					
Avent	2 15/16	1	1	9	No
Ameda/Egnell (one hand)	2⅗	3/4	1⅛	4¾	No
Loyd-B	2¼	7/8	1/8	3–4	No
Cylinder					
Ameda/Egnell	3⅛	7/8	7/8	3	No
Evenflo	3⅝	1	1¼	4	No
Happy Family (also Ross Labs)	2¾	1	3/8	3	No
Infa	2⅜	1	1/2	4	No
Kaneson	2¼	1	3/4	3	No
Medela Manualectric	2¾	7/8	1	5	Yes
Sears	3½	1	1¼–2⅛ (angled)	3.5	No
White River	3	3/4	1	4.5	No
Battery					
Evenflo	3⅝	1	1¾	4	Yes
Gentle Expressions	2½	1	1/2	4	Yes
Lact-B	2¾	1	3/4	7	Yes
Mag Mag	2½	1⅛	1/2	7	No
Mag Mag Advanced	2⅘	1	9/10	4	Yes
Medela	3⅛	1	1⅜	5	Yes

Electric					
Small semiautomatic					
Gerber	2¼	1	3/4	4	No
Kadan	2⅝	7/8	1⅜	5	No
Nurture III	2⅜	1	3/4	4	Yes
Schuco-Vac	3	1	1¼	4.5	No
Large semiautomatic					
Schuco-Vac	2½	1/4	1¾	4–8	Yes
White River	3	3/4	1	8	Yes
Large automatic					
Ameda/Egnell	2¼	3/4	7/8	8	Yes
Medela	2¾	7/8	1	7	Yes
The Rose	2½	1	1/2	4	Yes
White River	3	3/4	7/8	4–8	Yes

1. All measurements are approximate.
2. Johnson, C: An evaluation of breast pumps currently available on the American market, *Clin Pediatr* 22:40–45, 1983.
3. Zinaman, M: Breast pumps: ensuring mothers' success, *Contemp Obstet Gynecol* 32:55–62, 1988.

CLINICAL IMPLICATIONS REGARDING BREAST PUMPS

Concerns of health professionals vary considerably from those of mothers. (See boxed list below.)

Clinical concerns regarding breast pumps typically center around safe collection techniques and the maintenance of low bacteria counts in the expressed milk. Of equal importance are choosing the right pump for each individual situation, providing appropriate pumping instructions, and tempering all this with a consideration of the emotional toll that pumping can sometimes exact.

The professional literature is replete with reports of bacterial contamination of breastmilk and breast pumps. Factors related to nipple cleansing, hand washing, collection technique, type of pump, feeding method of pre-term infants, pump cleaning routines, and gestational age of the baby have all been identified as contributing to concern over high bacteria counts in expressed milk. Expressed breast milk is not sterile; there is considerable disagreement over what constitutes an acceptable bacteria count, especially if the recipient of the milk is a pre-term infant. Caution must be exercised in reviewing the literature on contaminated human milk because certain institutional practices may actually increase the likelihood of problems with expressed milk.

With the increased use of both hand and electric pumps in the 1970s, many reports described contaminated milk as one source of bacteremia, but the reports lacked conclusive epidemiology. Hand expression of breastmilk showed lower bacteria counts than breastmilk obtained by manual or electric pumps when pumps first began to be commonly used. Donowitz et al. (1981) reported an outbreak of Klebsiella-caused bacteremia in a neonatal intensive care unit. The electric breast pump was grossly contaminated and lacked proper bacterial surveillance. Once gas sterilization of pump parts was required between each mother's use of the equipment, the problem disappeared. However, all five affected babies in the report were fed milk by the nasoduodenal route, which delivers the milk directly to the small bowel, thus bypassing the protective action of gastric acid in the stomach. Four of the five infants had received broad spectrum antibiotic therapy prior to the contaminated feedings, and therefore received contaminated milk in a bowel with altered protective gastrointestinal flora. Such a practice predisposes an infant to infection given even small challenges of bacteria.

Gransden et al. (1986) reported an outbreak of *Serratia marcescens* in a NICU via inadequately disinfected breast pumps (Kaneson manual and Egnell electric models). Kaneson pump parts (after being washed) were soaked in a solution of hypochlorite. Egnell pump parts were washed with the metal parts soaked in a solution of 0.5% chlorhexidine in 70% ethyl alcohol. The pumps were soaked for 1.5 hours in a 1% hypochlorite solution, and the solution was changed every 24 hours. Bacteria were isolated from the soaked pump parts as well as from the hypochlorite solution itself. When the Egnell pump parts were autoclaved and the Kaneson pumps were washed at 80° C, the problem was resolved. Often, the available chlorine in these chemical solutions is readily inactivated by small amounts of organic matter. The original disinfection technique in this study had several faults, including failure to dismantle the hand pump completely, failure to remove the rubber gasket, and failure to totally immerse the pump components.

Moloney et al. (1987) reported isolation of *Serratia marcescens, Staphylococcus aureus* and *Streptococcus faecalis* from hand and electric breast pumps. The pumps were disinfected in a hypochlorite solution as in the previous study. That there are infection risks from electrically operated breast pumps is well known. With proper surveillance and sterilizing by autoclaving, gas (ethyline oxide), or high temperature washing—rather than chemical sterilization—the risk of overgrowth and transmis-

---

CONCERNS OF PROFESSIONALS

Professionals should always be aware of:

- the appropriate pump for each situation
- pumps that allow the safe collection of milk
- techniques for expressing milk with low bacteria counts
- appropriate pumping instructions
- the emotional toll of expressing milk (especially on a long-term basis).

sion of pathogenic bacteria can be substantially reduced. If pumps or pump parts are heat sensitive, consideration should be given to using pumps that do not depend on chemical sterilization.

Asquith, Sharp, and Stevenson (1985) compared Medela hand and electric pumps to manual expression in order to measure the amount of bacterial contamination. They found that boiling the personal use kits for 10 minutes worked well. The disposable kits were washed in hot soapy water and used for only one day. In some hospitals a fresh sterile kit is used for each pumping session.

Other approaches to reducing the bacterial count in expressed breastmilk have included expressing techniques and various breast/nipple cleansing routines. Asquith et al. (1984) noted that the bacterial content of milk is high when expression is first begun regardless of collection technique. Asquith and Harod's earlier work (1979) recommended that stripping and discarding the first 10mL of expressed milk would decrease total bacteria counts. The 1984 work observed that bacterial contamination was high within the first 24 hours after birth or after initiation of pumping, whether or not the first 10ml were discarded. Asquith and colleagues (1984) suggest that delayed expression of breastmilk is associated with high bacterial counts of nonnursing mothers of NICU infants: "Milk stasis and breast engorgement may provide an opportunity for bacteria, including 'normal flora' or pathogenic species, to incubate in the breast." Their recommendations for mothers of hospitalized newborns include initiation of expression as soon as possible on a frequent and regular basis, thereby avoiding excessive engorgement, and the discarding of the first 10mL of milk with each pumping. Some mothers may only get 10 mL of colostrum or milk at first, so care should be taken to determine the necessity of discarding this early milk.

Pittard et al. (1991) found no difference in the number of heavily contaminated ($> 10,000$ colony-forming units/mL) milk cultures when a clean vs. a sterile collection container was used, or when manual vs. mechanical collection techniques were employed. They did not observe increased levels of bacteria in the initial milk removed from the breast.

According to Meier and Wilks (1987), acceptable bacteria levels in expressed breastmilk are difficult to define and vary between healthy full-term infants and pre-term, high-risk babies. Healthy term infants can tolerate some pathogens and relatively high levels of nonpathogenic bacteria ($> 10^4$ colony-forming units/mL of milk). Pre-term or high-risk infants with immature immune systems who are not nursing directly from the breast may be at greater risk from the same level of bacterial growth. The investigators' criteria for acceptable bacteria levels for pre-term infants is the absence of any pathogens and a maximum concentration of 10^4 colony-forming units/mL. Mothers in their study were instructed in hand washing, especially under and around the fingernails. The nipples and areolae were cleaned with pHisoDerm soap before each pumping session. Increased nipple soreness was not noticed in this study but the number of weeks of pumping was not specified. Using these guidelines, 74 out of 84 expressed milk specimens had concentrations of $<10^4$ cfu/mL. It is not known whether this type of cleansing increases the risk for problems—other than topical soreness, such as dry areolar skin which is susceptible to breakdown and infection, or a change in the pH of the skin which affects the secretions of the glands of Montgomery.

Costa (1989) showed significantly lower bacterial counts when pre-term mothers washed their nipples and areolae with pHisoDerm soap prior to each pumping session. Although she noticed no skin breakdown with this routine, it is unknown what adverse affects would be encountered from using this soap six to eight times a day over an extended period of time.

Wilks and Meier (1988) describe guidelines for care of hospital breast pump equipment that include scrubbing collection kits and tubing with instrument cleaning solution after each use as well as autoclaving each item. The exterior of the pump should be cleaned with antiseptic solution each day and the pump cultured monthly. They also describe other factors which may influence the amount of nonpathogens that a pre-term baby can tolerate. These include the baby's clinical condition; the use of bolus feedings every two hours rather than continuous feedings; the use of refrigerated rather than frozen milk to retain active antiinfective properties; and feeding the baby directly from the breast as much as possible in order to receive unaltered antiinfective properties, thereby further decreasing the risk of infection.

Nwankwo et al. (1988) showed that colostrum inhibited bacterial growth more than mature milk—term colostrum even more so than pre-term colostrum. At room temperature (27–32° C/74–96°F) mature milk from term mothers could be stored without significant increase in bacterial counts for six hours. Pre-term milk could be stored for four hours at room temperature before bacterial counts exceeded 10^4 cfu/mL, or became significantly higher than initial counts at the time of expression. Colostrum was obtained within six days of delivery and mature milk at six weeks or more postpartum. The authors suggest caution in the storage of pre-term milk. This should also be kept in mind for situations of continuous vs. bolus tube feedings.

Each year many pumps change or add features (especially the electric ones) that reduce the chance of milk backflow and contamination. Some models now have filters in the pump: some use overflow bottles and others have filters and/or protection against overflow in the accessory kit. When choosing a pump for milk collection for pre-term babies, the professional should know if the pump or accessory kit guard against contamination. For example, the Medela pump has a valve with a silicone membrane in the accessory kit which prevents milk from backing up into the system. Milk is diverted into the cap, which has holes that force the milk to visibly leak out of the bottle. If milk bypassed this mechanism (for example, if the collection container tipped over) milk would contact the overflow filter. The pump would continue to run but no suction would be delivered to the breast. This filter has a weave to one micron, functioning as a bacterial filter. Should a mother inadvertently rent or use a contaminated pump, this filter would prevent blow back of bacteria during the positive pressure phase. The accessory kit of the Egnell electric pump has a seal and basket device that sits in the collection container to prevent milk from backflowing into the tubing. The large Schuco-Vac model has no device in the accessory kit to prevent backflow but has a bacterial filter just outside the air intake port on the pump. If a pump depends on an overflow bottle, it is mandatory that the bottle be used at each pumping session and that it be properly cleaned after each use.

Concern over bacterially safe breastmilk is only one aspect of managing milk expression to be considered when mothers and infants are separated. Forte, Mayberry, and Ferketich (1987) collected data from 51 mothers of hospitalized neonates, noting that more than 50% of the sample identified the need for additional information about breastfeeding upon hospital discharge. Some mothers received no written guidelines before or after discharge and lacked information on pumping frequency, how to increase milk production, and pumping and storage techniques. Women in this sample used hand expression (12%), a manual pump (17%), an electric pump (55%), and an electric pump in combination with other methods (16%). Of these mothers, 35% pumped only two to four times in 24 hours, 41% expressed five to six times, and 24% pumped seven to eight times in 24 hours. The number one reason for discontinuing breastmilk collection was obtaining insufficient milk—followed by the complaint that pumping was too time consuming. Over one-half of the women delayed expression until 2 to 5 days postpartum. Only 33% of the mothers identified hygienic practices to be important in the collection of breastmilk. These findings from four different hospitals show the prevalance of practices which are unlikely to promote an optimal supply of bacterially safe breastmilk. According to Forte, Mayberry, and Ferketich (1987), "A lack of perceived support may reduce the number of mothers who are attempting to maintain lactation."

Morse and Bottorff (1988) observed 61 nursing mothers and their emotional experiences related to expressing milk. Many were surprised that the ability to express their milk was not automatic. They often found verbal and written instructions unclear and confusing; many learned by trial and error. Mothers in this study stressed that "instructions for one mother did not necessarily work for all." Some were embarrassed and others were frustrated when they obtained only small amounts of milk. While success with expression increased a mother's self-confidence, women who perceived expression to be an important aspect of breastfeeding, but who were unable to express milk, displayed heightened feelings of inadequacy. The authors suggest modifying how expression is taught to include not only explicit how-to's but also the encouragement of private exploratory practice and the use of humor by the instructor (when appropriate) to reduce embarrassment.

Many mothers have only the instructions which come with the pump to use as a guide in learning milk expression and handling. These instructions vary widely in their recommendations on pumping techniques and even on the cleaning of the pump. Further confusion is possible if a mother uses more than one type of pump, especially if she fails to read all of the instructions carefully.

It is interesting to note that the concerns of mothers were rarely addressed in the professional literature on breast pumps and milk expression. Clinicians must remember that the best pump will do little for a mother whose emotional needs are not met and who lacks the guidelines necessary to use the equipment properly for optimal results. See Table 11–7 for a selected comparison of pump instructions. These are taken directly from the literature provided with the pumps and can vary considerably.

SAMPLE GUIDELINES FOR PUMP RECOMMENDATIONS AND PUMPING TECHNIQUES

The health-care professional needs to base pumping recommendations on many factors and take into account each mother's situation. For example: the mother whose premature infant is under 30 weeks of gestation and is not taking oral feedings needs very different instructions than a mother who is pumping during her hours of employment, or a woman who is only occasionally expressing milk. This mother of the premature infant needs a pump which:

- promotes physiologic prolactin cycling
- obtains milk with a high energy content
- has an easily controlled vacuum
- permits the vacuum to be applied for short periods of time to avoid tissue damage
- produces high milk yields
- is easy to use
- is heat resistant for high-temperature sterilization
- works fairly quickly
- is durable (will not stop working or break easily)
- is economical
- will be accessible.

A reasonable option for long-term pumping is an electric pump with a double collecting kit leased on a long-term basis. The mother should begin pumping as soon after the birth as possible and do so at least eight times in 24 hours.

The mother of a healthy two-to-three-month-old infant who is returning to full-time employment outside the home may have different needs. While battery pumps are popular, using an A/C adapter will help increase efficiency and decrease the cost of replacement batteries. This mother might also consider a long-term lease on an electric pump. If this mother chooses to use a manually operated cylinder pump, instructions should include proper hand positioning in order to avoid developing lateral epicondylitis, a.k.a. tennis elbow (Williams, Auerbach & Jacobi, 1989). These instructions emphasize shoulder adduction, with the elbow lying against the body, the forearm in supination (turned up), and the wrist slightly flexed. A mother with carpal tunnel syndrome—or other hand, wrist, arm or shoulder problems—may need to use an electric pump rather than a manual or battery-operated pump to avoid exacerbation of her symptoms.

A mother who expresses only small amounts of milk or who has a low milk supply should be advised to elicit the milk-ejection reflex—by allowing baby suckling, looking at a picture of her baby, listening to guided relaxation tapes, or slow chest breathing before applying the pump—and to massage the breast by quadrants throughout the pumping session. She may need to sit in a quiet area that permits relaxation with a minimum of interruptions. Pumping the first thing in the morning or on the opposite breast while the baby is nursing may also prove helpful. In the absence of an abundant milk supply and reliable milk-ejection reflex the use of a battery-operated pump may not prove to be the best choice.

COMMON PUMPING PROBLEMS

The most common pumping problems seen by clinicians are sore nipples, small amounts of milk obtained per pumping session, and erratic or delayed milk-ejection reflex associated with long-term pumping (Walker, 1987). *Sore nipples* caused by breast pumps are commonly seen in clinical practice. Sore nipples can be minimized by using the lowest amount of vacuum that works to obtain milk; applying vacuum only after the breast has begun to release its milk; interrupting the vacuum frequently to avoid or decrease pain while still maintaining milk flow; switching from side to side frequently as the milk flow slows (when using single-sided pumping); ensuring proper flange fit with an inner opening that is not too small for the nipple entering it or too large to be ineffective; and pumping for shorter periods of time.

TABLE 11–7 SELECTED USER INSTRUCTIONS

Hand Pumps

Cylinder	Elicit Milk Ejection Before Pumping	Massage Breast	Sterilizing	Technique	Cleaning	Sanitizing	Miscellaneous
Evenflo Natural Mother	Yes	Yes	3–5 minutes in boiling water.	Nipple in exact center; move handle in and out in a steady rhythmic motion. Can increase suction by inserting suction valve. Interrupt suction at end of outward stroke.	Warm soapy water, rinse well. Dishwasher safe in top rack. Leave seal on during cleaning.		Hand position pronated in picture.
Ross Deluxe (Happy Family)	Yes	Yes—before pumping.	No	Slowly push and pull cylinder back and forth; when flow decreases massage and repeat.	Remove gasket during cleaning; use hot soapy water; rinse well. Safe in upper rack of dishwasher, except for gasket and sealing disk.		Hand position supine; flared end of basket must point up.
Sears Naturally Soft	Yes	Yes—before pumping to decrease pumping time.	No	Move outer cylinder to and from breast; as outer cylinder fills shorten pump stroke.	Clean with warm water and mild detergent.	Sanitize in boiling water for ten seconds after cleaning. Before first use boil for ten seconds.	Rinse nipples with plain water; flared end of gasket faces breast; hand supine.
Medela	No	No	Prior to first use and before first use in the morning. Disassemble and boil for 20 minutes.	Slow rhythmic intervals; pull piston full length of cylinder with every stroke.	After each use wash in lukewarm soapy water and rinse well.		Breast cleaned with damp cloth prior to pumping; hand supine with elbow close to body.
Ameda/ Egnell	No	No	Can be boiled briefly prior to first use. Sterilize in upper rack of dishwasher.	Pull pump cylinder slowly down.	No—gasket can be left on during cleaning.	No	

Kaneson	Yes—to decrease pumping time.	Yes—for two minutes to promote let down.	Sterilize in boiling water for 5 minutes before first use. Rubber gasket may remain on.	Nipple in center of adapter, outer cylinder moved away from body. As milk fills outer cylinder shorten length of stroke to avoid gasket coming in contact with milk.	After each use rinse with warm water and clean with mild detergent.	Hand supine.
Infa	Yes	Yes—for a minute or two to stimulate milk flow.	Pre-sterilize all parts in boiling water 3–4 minutes.	Slowly pull the outer cylinder creating suction with a gentle pumping action.	Wash in warm soapy water after each use; dishwasher safe.	Assembly instructions do not include how to attach gasket.
White River Squeeze-handle manual						
Loyd-B	No	No	With shield in stopper, boil for 15 minutes.	Center nipple in shield; pump to comfort level; leave under vacuum 30–45 seconds then release. Hold and release in this cycle for 3 minutes each side twice.	No	
Avent	Yes—by hand expressing.	No	Sterilize by boiling.	Pump gently, occasionally holding handle down for 2-3 seconds to maintain vacuum.	Wash in warm soapy water.	Clean the breast.
Ameda Egnell (one hand)	Yes—warm wet compresses.	Yes—light circular massage.	Sterilize before use by boiling for 20 minutes.	Adjust speed and intensity of hand movements to control vacuum.	After use large parts can go in dishwasher; small parts hand washed.	Attachment for electric pump not packed in all kits.

TABLE 11-7 SELECTED USER INSTRUCTIONS (*continued*)

	Elicit Milk Ejection Before Pumping	Massage Breast	Sterilizing	Technique	Cleaning	Sanitizing	Miscellaneous
Battery Operated							
Evenflo Sof-Touch Ultra	Yes—to promote easier milk flow and prevent soreness.	Yes—for 1–2 minutes	Before first use sterilize in boiling water for 3–5 minutes.	Nipple in exact center; allow suction to increase to a comfortable level. Depress and release button to comfort.	Wash in warm soapy water and mild detergent; rinse well.		Has A/C adapter.
Ameda/Egnell Lact-B	No	No	Sterilize in boiling water for 20 minutes before first and after each use; or place in upper rack of dishwasher.	4–6 seconds of suction followed by 1–2 second interruption to elicit let down and for entire pumping session.	Wash in soapy water after each use.		Cautions that continuous suction may hurt the breast.
Mag Mag	No	Massage during pumping for better suction.	Sterilize in top rack of dishwasher or boil for 3–5 minutes.	Allow suction to build for as long as 30 seconds. Release button for 1–2 seconds.			
Mag Mag Advanced	Yes	Yes—for more fluent suction.	Stir boil for 3–5 minutes.	Determine comfortable suction; release button pushed for 2–3 seconds.	Hand wash all parts; or place in top rack of dishwasher.		Four raised areas in hard nipple adapter claimed to stimulate milk glands. Caution about tilting pump because of danger of milk flowing down into motor. Can flush motor with backed-up milk.
Gentle Expressions	Yes—or can nurse baby on one side while pumping the other.	Yes—to encourage let down.	Before first use; hot soapy water; rinse; boil 5–15 minutes to sterilize; dishwasher safe.	Center the nipple; use the suction-release button frequently after adjusting the suction regulator for comfort.	Wash and sanitize after each use.		

Medela (Mini electric)	No	No	No instructions.	Relax and alternate between breasts.	Disassemble and clean all parts separately.		Clean breast with damp cloth prior to pumping. As batteries wear down, vacuum held longer causing possible discomfort. Reduce vacuum level and replace batteries.
Small semiautomatic electric							
Precious Care	Yes—to decrease pumping time.	Yes—to push milk down into ducts.		Center the nipple; cover vacuum-release hole and release the vacuum to suit your comfort. Some mothers leave the vacuum steady while others create a pulsing or sucking action by covering and uncovering the hole.	After use clean with mild detergent and sanitize for 10 seconds in boiling water.	Before first use wash in hot water and mild detergent; then sanitize in boiling water for 10 seconds.	Rinse nipples with clear water. Allow unit to run for 45 seconds before using.
Nurture III	No—towel soaked in warm water and applied to breasts helps with let down.	No	Begin pumping with low setting; tap hole to make and break suction; vary time interval during which finger covers hole. To further control suction, roll finger back and forth over tap hole rather than lifting it off completely.		Wash before use.		Can also pump both sides simultaneously.
Schuco Model #400	No	No	Disinfect once a day in boiling water for 2–3 minutes.	Center the nipple; regulate pressure by partially or fully covering the vent hole of the suction bell with finger; cover and open vent hole for natural suction.	Clean with water and rinse before each use. Clean after each use, add a few drops of soap to water for cleaning.		Drink fluids as much as possible to stimulate production of milk. Use only a 4-oz collection container and empty at 3½ oz.

TABLE 11–7 SELECTED USER INSTRUCTIONS (*continued*)

	Elicit Milk Ejection Before Pumping	Massage Breast	Sterilizing	Technique	Cleaning	Sanitizing	Miscellaneous
Large Semiautomatic Electric							
Mada #174	No	No	Before first use boil for 20 minutes.	Close and open aperture for repeated suction and relaxation by lifting finger or partially closing and opening hole.	After each use; warm soapy water, rinse in lukewarm water.		If mother does not get milk after several minutes of initial pumping, stop and try again in 20 minutes.
Schuco-Vac Easy Flow Expressor	No	No	No	Center breast shield; press index finger on control to seal. Hold finger over fingertip control for 10–20 seconds and release for 2–5 seconds.	No	No	Should soreness or irritation occur, discontinue use and consult a physician.
Large automatic electric							
White River	Yes—to encourage milk to move down to milk sinuses.	Yes—before and when pumping begins.	To sterilize boil for 20 minutes.	Moisten flexible flange with water; center nipple in flange; cover and release the valve 7 times per 5 seconds.			
Medela	No	No	Prior to first use and before first use in the morning; boil for 20 minutes.	Adjust vacuum to personal comfort.	After each use wash in lukewarm soapy water.		Breast and surrounding area should be cleaned with damp cloth.
Ameda/Egnell	No	No	Can disinfect by boiling for at least 20 minutes.	Adjust pressure to personal comfort.	After use wash in warm soapy water.		
The Rose				Place on low suction to begin and increase to comfortable level.			

Data in this chart have been derived directly from instructional inserts provided with the pumps by the manufacturers.

Obtaining only *small amounts of milk per pumping session* occurs most often when the milk-ejection reflex has not been elicited. Mothers complain that the milk drips but does not spray out and that it takes more than 45 minutes to accumulate one-half to one ounce. As a result of this frustration, pump vacuum levels are often increased and left on for long, uninterrupted periods of time. This contributes more to sore nipples than to increased milk yields. To elicit the milk-ejection reflex, some mothers have reported using a hot shower or hot compresses, having their partner massage their breasts, or establishing a pumping routine (activities performed prior to each pumping session that elicit milk flow). Increasing fluid intake does not usually increase milk yield. Some mothers pump whenever they experience a spontaneous milk ejection. Timing pumping sessions may also help, particularly if some women find it difficult to obtain much milk immediately after the baby has fed. Pumping midway between feedings may help this situation. Morning pumping sessions also tend to yield more milk. Mothers who are employed full-time report that pumping sessions early in the week also tend to yield more milk than pumping sessions later in the week (Auerbach & Guss, 1984).

It is easy to blame the pump, but other factors also affect milk flow. Morse and Bottorff (1988) state, "Understanding the complex feelings towards expressing and the experimental nature of learning to express has important implications for the way that expression is taught." *An erratic or delayed milk-ejection reflex* is common when a mother must respond to a mechanical device rather than her baby, particularly when she is first learning to use a pump. If the milk-ejection reflex is not triggered quickly, the nipples and breast tissue are exposed to high levels of vacuum over an inefficient pressure gradient. This can result in low milk yields, sore nipples, and frustration with the pumping process. While pumps are capable of eliciting milk ejection and their instructions often advise applying the pump for this purpose, some women will have difficulty releasing their milk. This may be caused by inhibitory messages received by the hypothalamus. Embarrassment, tension, fear of failure, pain, fatigue, and anxiety may block the neurochemical pathways required for milk ejection. If these factors appear to interfere with milk ejection, ask the mother how she feels about pumping. A negative attitude does little to

contribute to milk flow. One mother, when offered the option of double pumping, said it made her feel like a cow. Single-sided pumping was more appealing to her. Once the clinician knows the mother's feelings and attitudes about pumping, guidelines can be individually created for each situation.

Some guidelines are necessary for expression techniques as well. Breast massage and hand expressing may be the best method for some mothers but not others. Some mothers use Syntocinon (synthetic oxytocin) for short-term assistance. One mother who found Syntocinon helpful for a couple of days kept the empty bottle in her medicine cabinet. Reaching for the bottle, or just thinking of the bottle on the shelf, resulted in milk ejection for weeks after its use had been discontinued.

It is not unusual for the milk-ejection reflex to take longer to trigger as the lactation course increases. This is common both with a baby at breast and with long-term pumping. What works early in lactation may change over time. Some mothers report improved results later in lactation, after they change to a different pump or use a different flange which may fit the breast better.

Expressing milk has different meanings for each mother. Some see it as a way to continue providing breastmilk in their absence, especially in families with a history of allergies. Other mothers view pumping as part of a grief-like reaction which is reinforced every two to three hours when they must use a pump in the absence of a baby at breast. Sound pump recommendations, pumping instructions based on a clear understanding of the anatomy and physiology of the breast, and knowledge of the lactation process will enable many women to give their infant the best possible nutritional and emotional start.

NIPPLE SHIELDS

Nipple shields appear in the medical literature as early as the mid-1600s. Scultetus describes shields made of silver and used so that "... nurses may suckle the infants without trouble which, when children were breast-fed until long after their front teeth were cut, must have been very necessary" (Bennion, 1979). Shields were first used to evert flat nipples and protect nipples from the cold and rubbing against clothing between feedings. Shields were made of lead (which caused brain damage in babies), wax, wood, gum elastic, pewter, tin, horn, bone, ivory, silver, and glass. The gum elastic shield in Fig. 11–6 was used for babies to nurse on. Maygrier (1833) states that, "This mode is difficult and generally the child is unwilling."

The design of nipple shields has changed little since the 1500s. By the 1800s rubber shields began appearing. The Maw's shield (Fig. 11–7) was constructed with a rubber lining, a glass shank, and a rubber teat. In the 1980s this design was still used with a glass or plastic shank and a rubber teat (Davol). Rubber versions of the silver and wood shields also began appearing. The early shields were composed of thick rubber with a firm nipple cone (The Mexican Hat, Macarthy's Surgical, Ltd.). One U.S. version, the Breast-Eze, was a modified rubber

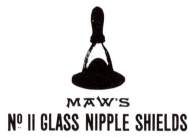

MAW'S
No II GLASS NIPPLE SHIELDS
FITTED WITH
Teat and India-Rubber Lining, 1 - each.

FIGURE 11–7 Nipple shield and breast glass, circa 1864.

nipple on a rubber base with thick rubber ribs lining the inside to help "stimulate" the breast. This design was reported to be very painful to use. The rubber shields gradually became thinner (Evenflo) and were replaced with thin latex (Lewin Woolf, Griptight, Ltd.) and silicone (Cannon Babysafe) seen today. (See Fig. 11–8.)

Shields are currently used during feedings to assist baby and/or mother to:

- latch onto flat nipples
- latch onto nipples which are everted but which the baby does not actively draw into his mouth
- latch-on when he has experienced difficulty from the previous use of artificial nipples
- latch onto an engorged breast in which the nipple is surrounded by noncompressible areolar tissue
- ease feeding when a weak, disorganized, or dysfunctional suck is present (in the case of special babies with neurological problems, following pre-term birth, or Down syndrome)
- protect sore or damaged (cracked) nipples during a breastfeeding
- prevent sore nipples (claimed by manufacturers but not proven).

While the idea of protecting the nipple may be made in good faith, the ramifications of nipple shield use can be both destructive to the course of lactation and risky to the health of the baby (Desmarais & Browne, 1990).

REVIEW OF LITERATURE

Woolridge, Baum, and Drewett (1980) studied the effect of the all rubber shield (Macarthy-Mexican

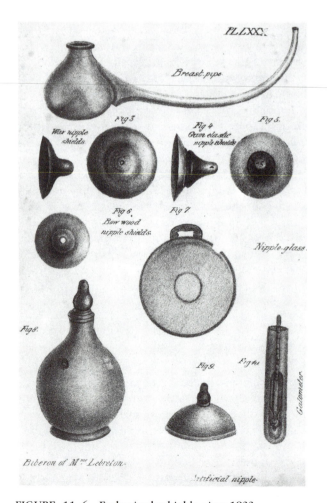

FIGURE 11–6 Early nipple shields, circa 1833.

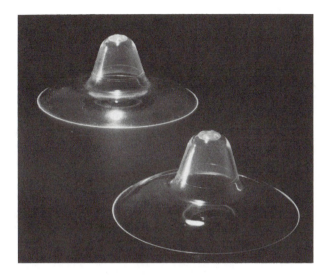

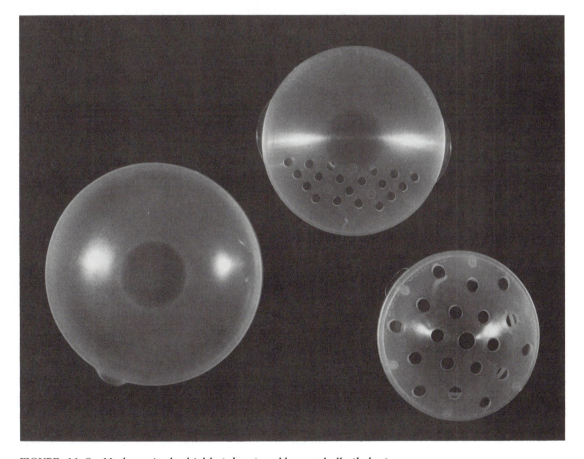

FIGURE 11–8 Modern nipple shields (*above*) and breast shells (*below*).

Hat) and a thin latex shield on the sucking patterns and milk intake of five-to-eight-day-old babies of mothers with problem-free lactation experiences. The Macarthy-Mexican Hat reduced milk transfer by 58% and changed infant sucking patterns by increasing the sucking rate and the time spent pausing. This is a pattern typically seen when milk flow decreases. The thin latex shield reduced milk intake by 22% and had no significant effect on sucking patterns. This thin shield was being tested as part of an apparatus in a new system for measuring milk flow and composition during breastfeeding. The babies observed in this study had no difficulty latching onto mothers' nipples, and no nipple soreness was reported by the mothers in the study. Theoretically, if these problems existed, milk transfer and sucking patterns could be further compromised with the use of any shield.

Using the same thin latex shield, Jackson et al. (1987) showed a 29% decrease in milk transfer during their study of nutrient intake in healthy, full-term newborns.

Amatayakul et al. (1987) measured plasma prolactin and cortisol levels in mothers—with and without a thin latex nipple shield in place. They found that prolactin and cortisol levels were unaffected by the shield but that milk transfer was decreased by 42% when the shield was in place during feedings. They postulate that this effect on milk volume is attibutable to an interference with oxytocin release.

Auerbach (1990a) studied changes in milk volume both with and without the use of a thin silicone shield (Cannon Babysafe). Twenty-five mothers used a breast pump (Medela electric model) to provide milk samples, which prevented any change in infant sucking patterns from affecting milk volume amounts. Milk volume was significantly reduced when a shield was in place. Seventy-one percent of the total milk obtained was recorded when no shield was used. Pumping without a shield resulted in mean volumes five to seven times greater than when a shield was in place.

RISKS

Besides reducing milk volume transfer, all shield designs have drawbacks and can cause more serious problems than the original problem which they were meant to alleviate.

All rubber shield. Before recommending the use of all rubber shields, remember that they can:

- interfere with positioning baby properly at breast
- present a firm nipple portion which can be inserted into baby's mouth rather than being drawn in by the infant, thus reducing the likelihood that the baby will learn correct latch-on to the breast
- change the sucking pattern to a nonnutritive mode (typically seen when milk flow decreases at the end of a breastfeeding)
- reduce stimulation of the nipple/areolar complex, potentially interfering with prolactin and oxytocin release
- temporarily or permanently reduce the milk-producing capacity of the breasts, and contribute to slow, low, or no weight gain in the baby— resulting in acute dehydration, failure to thrive, and weaning
- prevent proper extension of the nipple back into the baby's mouth (Minchin, 1985)
- pinch the nipple and areola causing abrasion, pain, skin breakdown, and internal trauma to the breast
- create nipple shield addiction (DeNicola, 1986), after which the baby will not feed at breast without the shield in place
- predispose the nipple to damage when the baby is put to breast without the shield, as he may chew rather than suckle
- relay the message to the mother that she or her baby may not be good enough to feed her baby unless a barrier is placed between the two.

Standard bottle nipples or bottle nipples attached to a glass or plastic base. In addition to the problems listed above, these types of shields place the baby and his mouth one to two inches away from the mother's nipple, significantly altering positioning at breast. This does not permit compression of the milk sinuses or skin-to-skin stimulation of the nipple/areolar complex and may alter prolactin cycling. Milk may pool in the base which holds the artificial nipple and never reach the baby—or simply leak out the sides.

Latex and silicone shields. These are extremely thin, flexible shields shaped like the rubber shields. Only the nipple portion is firm, about two cm long with four holes in the tip. Because the silicone is so thin, more stimulation reaches the areola and milk volume is not as seriously depleted as with the other designs (Auerbach, 1990a).

RESPONSIBILITIES

The health-care professional has the following responsibilities regarding breastfeeding women and nipple shields:

1. Understand the risks of using such a device. Hospital-based providers must be aware of the previously mentioned long-term consequences when shields are given to mothers. Research-based hospital protocols should clearly state the rationale behind avoiding the use of shields.

2. Assess the situation before recommending a shield (Auerbach, 1989). Shields used as a quick fix to assure infant feedings before early discharge act as "band-aid therapy." They cover up the problem without addressing the cause. Identify and take steps to correct the problem rather than issuing a shield as the initial therapy. The following boxed chart summarizes alternatives to shield use.

3. Employ informed consent (Kutner, 1986) if a mother wishes to use a shield and sensitize providers to its risks. A consent form should be signed by the mother, the father (if available), and the provider who is recommending the shield. This will assure that everyone knows the risks of using a shield, as well as how to use it so that its dangers are mini-

---

ALTERNATIVES TO NIPPLE SHIELD USE

Situation	Management
Sore or cracked nipples	Observe and correct maternal and infant positioning. Document a correct nutritive suckling pattern and tongue placement of baby at breast. Assist baby to latch-on with a wide open mouth if necessary, and hand express colostrum or milk to prevent build-up of negative pressure.
Flat or retracted nipples	Roll and shape the nipple prior to feeding. Pump briefly before each feeding to evert nipples. Wear breast shells between feedings
Engorgement	Hand express to increase compressibility of areolar tissue, followed by use of an electric pump if necessary prior to feedings for easier latch-on.
Difficulty or failure of baby to latch onto the breast	In addition to the above, or if the baby requires more assistance, incentives at breast to promote latch-on should be attempted, i.e., feeding tube device, syringe, or dropper to place or dribble fluid into or near the baby's mouth. Finger-feeding can be done by either parent to establish appropriate nutritive suckling patterns.

mized. A consent form used in this manner also serves as a teaching aid to professionals who are unaware of potential long-range problems. A copy should be given to the mother, another copy is retained in the medical record, and a third copy is sent to the pediatrician.

The consent form should specify the reason the shield has been recommended. It should clarify that the shield is for temporary use; warn that continuous use at each feeding can cause a decreased milk supply, low weight gain and acute dehydration; note that the baby's weight needs to be monitored twice a week; and state that the mother may need to pump milk to maintain an adequate supply.

4. Realize that the risks of nipple shield use have legal implications for the hospital and/or professional who recommends them. A malpractice case has already been lodged against a nurse and her employing hospital after a nipple shield was dispensed without warning the parents of the potential consequences of its use (Bornmann, 1986).

5. Provide proper instructions and referrals if a shield is used as an interim recommendation to assist with breastfeeding. **Written** instructions should include how to use a silicone shield with the tip of the shield snipped off. The mother should understand that shield use is temporary and that it should be discontinued as soon as possible. It can be used to assist with latch-on and removed when baby has established rhythmic nutritive suckling. The baby should be put directly to breast as much as possible and may accept the breast better when in a state of light sleep. If a mother is discharged from the hospital using a shield, a community referral must be made to a lactation consultant or the nurse practitioner at the pediatrician's office for daily follow-up. Weight checks may need to be obtained twice a week. The pediatrician should be alerted to the problem which required use of the shield in the first place and should be aware of suggestions for discontinuing its use.

WEANING FROM A SHIELD

Weaning a baby from a shield can be a lengthy process. If a thick rubber shield is being used or a bottle nipple has been placed over the mother's nipple, switch to a thin silicone shield immediately. Cut off the tip of the shield to allow more milk to flow to the baby. Use the shield for a few seconds first, then remove it and allow the baby to feed directly on the mother's breast. This may help draw flat nipples out far enough for the baby to grasp without the shield (Auerbach, 1987). A feeding tube can be secured to the outside or inside of the shield with a supplement running to promote latch-on and deliver expressed breastmilk or formula to a calorie-deprived baby. Sometimes a quick removal of the shield, with the supplement delivered by a tube taped to the areola under the shield, orients the baby to breast quickly.

Ongoing assessment and management to eliminate the original cause for use of the shield should continue. Rarely, a situation may arise in which a shield can temporarily be used to eliminate the need to wean the baby from breast. The author has used a silicone shield with a mother who presented with weeping eczema on the areola of her right breast. The mother had been advised to wean because the orange discharge would "make the baby sick." Instead of weaning, she began pumping that breast, which exacerbated the damage to the areola, and suffered much pain with each pumping session. After referral, we secured a thin silicone shield (Cannon Babysafe) on which the baby nursed at each feeding; pumping the right breast was discontinued. The shield was thoroughly cleaned between uses while cortisone therapy resolved the eczema. The baby went back to the involved nipple/areola with no problems.

Postpartum units which are reluctant to discontinue stocking nipple shields may benefit from a product evaluation form describing the drawbacks of shields, along with copies of documentation from the breastfeeding literature (Shrago, 1988).

The occasional use of thin silicone shields may be appropriate but cannot replace thorough assessment of the presenting problem.

BREAST SHELLS

Breast shells are two-piece plastic devices worn over the nipple and areola to evert flat or retracted nipples. Historically, these shells were called nipple glasses (Item #7, Fig. 11–6) and were used to protect the mother's clothing from leaking milk, or applied if the mother had "too much" milk. Some brands are still marketed as a device for catching leaked milk between feedings. Currently, shells are not recommended for this use, although many mothers find them helpful for collecting drip milk from one breast while nursing or pumping on the opposite side. Some clinicians also recommend their use for engorgement, as their gentle pressure encourages milk to leak. The milk collected between feedings must be discarded because of potential high bacteria counts. If drip milk is collected during a feeding or pumping session, it can be stored as usual.

Inverted nipples are identified when the areola is compressed behind the base of the nipple and the nipple retreats into the surrounding skin. Lawrence (1989) calls this a "tied nipple," which is caused by the presence of the original invagination of the mammary dimple. Prenatally, breast shells are worn for increasingly longer periods throughout the day and removed at night. The constant gentle pressure around the base of the nipple is thought to release the adhesions anchoring the nipple, thus allowing it to protrude when the baby latches onto the breast. Shells can be worn between feedings after the baby is born if nipple flattening or retraction is identified postpartum or if the nipples still need correction.

Several brands of shells are available, all of which have a dome that is placed over a base through which the nipple protrudes when worn under a bra. Depending on the brand, the dome may have one or many ventilation holes. The domes with only one or two holes may not provide adequate air circulation to the nipple and areola. The retained moisture and heat (especially in hot weather) can create a miniature greenhouse effect which promotes soreness and skin breakdown. Extra holes can be drilled in the top of the dome. Some brands have many holes in the dome to help with this problem. The Ameda/Egnell shells have absorbent pads which are placed in the bottom of the shell under the areola to absorb leaked milk and moisture. (See Fig. 11–8.) It is not known whether this padding provides a reservoir for bacterial buildup. They also have a pad which is placed between the shell and skin to decrease skin irritation or discomfort. The Medela shell is well ventilated and somewhat narrower than the Egnell shell. A breast pad may be worn between the shell and bra with the Medela shell as there are vent holes in the bottom of the dome as well.

RECOMMENDATIONS FOR USE

Prenatal use of breast shells is suggested for nipples that appear retracted or severely flattened. When instructing the expectant mother in the prenatal use of breast shells, advise her to:

- wear the shells for one or two hours a day, gradually increasing the time until they are worn all day; remove the shells before going to bed, wash them well, rinse and air dry overnight
- in hot weather, or if moisture build-up occurs, remove the shells for 20 minutes at a time, two or three times a day and dry the shells well
- if the nipple does not fit completely through the hole in the base, use a brand with a larger opening or a less sloping base.

When instructing a mother in their use postpartum, advise her to:

- wear the shells for 30 minutes prior to each feeding or for the entire time between feedings, whichever gives the best results
- use only the drip milk that collects during a feeding or pumping session; discard any milk that is collected between feedings
- wear shells to relieve excess milk build-up in the lactiferous sinuses by inducing slow leaking
- wash the shells in hot, soapy water and rinse well before using them in order to collect drip milk if they have been worn between feedings
- remove the shells at bedtime or for naps so that areas of the breast do not become obstructed
- use shells whose domes are well ventilated
- obtain a snug fitting shell; if painful rings occur on the areola, consider changing to a larger bra or increase the cup size of the bra.

FEEDING TUBE DEVICES

Feeding tube devices, both noncommercial and commercial, are a recent addition to the options for help in special breastfeeding situations. Judicious use of these devices enables many mothers and babies to breastfeed who otherwise would have lost this unique opportunity.

DESCRIPTION

Feeding tube devices consist of some kind of container to hold breastmilk or formula and a length of thin tubing that runs from the container to the mother's nipple. The tube is secured in place by paper tape and as the baby suckles at breast supplement is simultaneously delivered. Providing milk in this manner may be a novel idea to both the mother and her nurse or physician. Careful explanations need to be provided regarding the mechanism of use and the expected outcomes. Reactions to the use of these devices are related to the attitudes people have about infant feeding. Bottle-feeding and breastfeeding are not the same thing, just as formula and breastmilk are quite different. An explanation that the device is generally a temporary aid in establishing the baby at breast while assuring adequate nutrition is usually helpful for all concerned.

There are several commercial devices on the market as well as noncommercial devices that can be constructed from bottles or syringes and tubing.

Lact-Aid (USA). Developed in 1971 for nursing the adopted baby, the Lact-Aid device created a breastfeeding experience for those mothers and babies who previously had no choice in terms of feeding methods. It is a closed system consisting of a pre-sterilized, disposable four-ounce bag to hold milk—with a cap through which a length of fine tubing extends to the nipple. The bag hangs around the mother's neck on a cord. Air is squeezed out of the bag to facilitate milk flow. Powdered or meat-based formulas will not flow readily through the device.

Supply Line (Australia). In Australia, this device uses two 140-mL feeding bottles worn around the neck in a pouch with a double length of tubing. The tubing is threaded through a hole in the bottle lid.

D-I-Y Nursing Supplementer (UK). A regular bottle and nipple are used with a length of tubing inserted through the nipple into the bottle. The mother must hold the bottle and regulate the flow by changing the height of the bottle.

Axi-Care Nursing Supplementer (UK). The Axi-Care device uses a plastic bottle, tubing and a roller clamp (as on an IV setup) to control supplement

flow. Reports indicate that the bottle will sometimes collapse as it is not a completely vented system.

Supplemental Nutrition System (USA) Medela, Inc. The SNS device consists of a six-ounce plastic bottle with a cap through which a length of tubing is secured to each breast. This two-tube unit allows the tubing to be set up on both breasts at the same time and comes with three different sizes of tubing. It is a vented system with a cap which has notches for pinching off both tubes while setting up the unit and securing one tube while the baby is feeding from the other side. Flow rates are influenced by the size of the tubing used (small, medium, large), the height of the bottle, and whether or not the opposite tube is pinched off during the feeding.

SITUATIONS FOR USE

Feeding tube systems can be recommended and used in many situations where other measures have failed or in order to prevent further complications.

Infant sucking problems. Babies with weak, disorganized, or dysfunctional sucking are candidates for feeding tube systems. This includes:

- hyperactive or hypoactive infants
- infants with Down syndrome
- pre-term infants
- infants with cardiac problems
- infants with cleft lip and/or palate
- infants who have experienced perinatal asphyxia
- nipple-confused infants
- neurologically impaired infants
- infants with low, slow, or no weight gain—or weight loss—due to ineffective suckling
- lethargic infants in the hospital who are at risk for decreased stooling, increased bilirubin levels or supplementation with sugar water using an artificial nipple.

Maternal situations. Several groups of mothers can benefit from the use of feeding tube devices, including:

- adoptive nursing (induced lactation) mothers (Auerbach & Avery, 1981; Sutherland & Auerbach, 1985)
- mothers who are relactating (i.e., inducing a

milk supply after a separation or interruption of breastfeeding (Bose et al., 1981; Auerbach & Avery, 1980)

- mothers who have had breast surgery, especially breast reduction mammaplasty that included moving the nipple
- mothers who suffer from primary lactation insufficiency, i.e., not enough functional breast tissue to support a full milk supply (Neifert & Seacat, 1985)
- mothers with severe nipple trauma
- mothers who have recently discontinued short-term medications contraindicated for a nursing infant
- mothers who are suffering from an illness or undergoing surgery or hospitalization
- mothers who have flat or inverted nipples and a baby who cannot latch-on.

METHOD OF USE

Generally, the goals of using a feeding tube device involve maintaining a mother's milk supply, delivering sufficient or extra nutrients to the baby, and creating a behavior modification situation which shapes the baby's suckling pattern to one suitable for obtaining milk from the breast (or prevents the suckling pattern from changing). These devices allow feedings to be done at breast when formerly, in certain situations, bottles with artificial nipples were used. Because these devices are used only in special situations, it is imperative that the professional who recommends their use follow-up closely—daily if necessary—to assure adequate milk intake by the baby, correct use by the mother, and weaning from the device when it is appropriate to do so.

In order for a baby to use a feeding tube at breast, he must be able to latch-on and execute some form of suckling. For babies who are unable at first to do this because of complete nipple confusion, strong extensor positioning, hypotonia, or lethargy, finger-feeding with the device can be used as an interim measure (Bull & Barger, 1987). The mother can place a tube on the pad of her index finger or whichever finger is closest in size to her nipple. She allows the baby to draw the finger into his mouth. Correct suckling will cause the milk to flow and reward the desired behavior. This is a teaching technique that only rewards correct suckling; no milk is removed if the baby bites the finger like an artificial nipple. This also allows the father or other care-giver to feed the baby. Finger-feeding in this manner will prevent improper suckling patterns from being reinforced and move the baby to breast faster than if artificial nipples were used to feed the baby.

CLINICAL IMPLICATIONS REGARDING FEEDING TUBE DEVICES

In-hospital situations—such as the infant's reluctance to latch-on, poor or frustrating feedings, few wet diapers, inefficient feedings at breast with minimal intake, increased bilirubin levels, and inability to establish baby at breast before discharge—may benefit from the assistance of a feeding tube device. Edgehouse and Radzyminski (1990) describe a device made from a 20cc- or 30cc-syringe and 12″ tubing formed from a butterfly needle. The tubing is taped in place on the areola at each feeding and serves as a "coaxer," delivering colostrum, breastmilk, water, or formula to effect latch-on and suckling. If the baby cannot cause fluid to flow at first, the plunger can be depressed slightly as an incentive. A nurse or lactation consultant should remain with the mother at each feeding until efficient suckling and swallowing is documented without the device.

Feeding problems associated with early introduction of artificial nipples, pacifiers, delayed first feedings, limited number and duration of feedings, or separation routines (especially at night) can confuse or delay the proper suckling of the baby at breast. Artificial nipples require a different pattern of sucking. Some babies cannot differentiate between the two different modes of suckling and fail to remove milk from the breast. When given bottles with artificial nipples, the condition worsens. Newman (1990) describes an alternative to supplementing with bottles. He uses a feeding bottle filled with expressed breastmilk or formula and a 36″ length of #5 feeding tube. The bottle is set on a table at the level of the baby's head, and the tubing is taped in place on the breast. He uses this to prevent or treat hypoglycemia and to effect latch-on so that artificial nipples can be avoided during a temporary situation. If the baby refuses the breast, if the infant and mother are separated, or if the mother's nipples are so sore that she cannot put the baby to breast, then the tube is placed on the pad of the index finger for finger-feeding.

Finger-feeding can be used to take the edge off the baby's hunger before putting him to breast. The author's feeding plan to establish these babies at breast involves finger-feeding for a few minutes to establish correct and rhythmic sequencing of a suck-swallow pattern. This is followed by putting the baby to breast and repeating the process for a period of time (determined by the mother and baby) at each feeding, until either the mother or baby become frustrated or the baby latches-on and feeds. These practice sessions at breast may last no longer than 10 minutes before the feeding at breast ends and the feed is completed by fingerfeeding with a tubing device.

When a baby will latch onto the breast but is unable to suckle properly or long enough to maintain good intake and weight gain, a tube feeding device can be used with a written feeding plan provided to the mother. Consistency of use is important in establishing the baby at breast and in reducing the mother's confusion in using the device. (See the case study on p. 321.)

OTHER CONSIDERATIONS

When considering employing feeding tube devices, the clinician should note the following guidelines:

1. They can be used as a temporary assist to establish the baby at breast but are generally not necessary if the baby is gaining weight adequately.
2. In situations of adoptive nursing, breast reduction surgery, primary lactation insufficiency, and certain genetic, anatomic or neurologic problems in an infant, these feeding devices may require long-term use with or without breast pumping.
3. Feeding tubes are not always easy to use, either physically or psychologically, for the mother. Not all women will accept their use or use them as instructed.
4. Close follow-up is mandatory with short- or long-term use.
5. Because the baby controls the flow, he will not aspirate or be overwhelmed by the fluid he receives. When he swallows or releases the vacuum, the milk flows backward and the baby must initiate another suck to start the flow. If he cannot initially do this, the bottle or bag of sup-

plement can be squeezed or the plunger of the syringe can be pushed slightly. The milk will not continuously drip or flow as with a bottle and artificial nipple.
6. Risks of use include "addiction" to the device by the clinician, mother, and/or baby. The mother and baby should be weaned from the device as quickly as is appropriate. Some mothers may have difficulty believing that they can support a milk supply without the device and not trust themselves to provide for the baby. The clinician should avoid routine use of tube feeding devices except where necessary. Some clever babies learn to suck only on the tube, in which case it should be placed so it does not extend beyond the end of the mother's nipple. If the baby has become accustomed to the feel of the tubing, it can be moved to the corner of his mouth and gradually removed. One mother finally taped a one inch length of the tube to her areola and withdrew it after her baby latched-on.
7. The "football-hold" position may be easier to use at first because the mother has greater control of the infant's head.
8. A gavage setup with a #5 feeding tube can also be used as a feeding device.
9. Tubing from a butterfly needle can also be used as it is smaller and softer than gavage tubing.
10. A baby can also be fed by dropper, spoon, cup, or bowl if tubing is not available.
11. If a mother needs a tube feeding device but cannot afford to buy a commercial one, it can be loaned to her and the tubing replaced with each new user.
12. Powdered formulas and special formulas may clog the smaller tubes if the formula is not mixed well.
13. If special formulas are used, larger sizes of tubing may be necessary to prevent clogging.
14. The device should be rinsed in cold water after each use and then filled with warm soapy water which is squeezed through the tubing and rinsed well. Sterilization can be done once a day, usually by placing it in boiling water for 20 minutes. In the hospital some of the devices can be steamed or autoclaved (*Rental Roundup*, 1986a).
15. Feeding in public may be more difficult or obvious. The mother may prefer to use alternatives to tube feeding when she is away from home.

CASE STUDY
FEEDING TUBE DEVICE FOR BABY CARA

Three-week-old baby Cara was referred after failing to regain her birthweight and showing a loss of two ounces at a three-week weight check. She had been readmitted into the hospital after discharge for two days of phototherapy when her bilirubin levels reached 17mg/dL on day four. During her two-day stay, Cara was taken off breastmilk and fed formula every three hours by bottle and artificial nipple. Cara's mother pumped her milk after being told it was contributing to the infant's jaundice. She froze it for use at a later date. Cara's mother described feedings at the breast prior to phototherapy as taking at least one hour, followed by Cara's fussiness when removed from the breast. After discharge, Cara would frequently refuse the breast, and her wet diaper count fell to five in each 24 hours. Fearing that she was not getting enough milk, Cara's mother began giving her one bottle of formula in the early evening, which was quickly increased to two bottles per day. Pediatric advice called for topping off each feeding with a bottle of formula.

This perpetuated a downward cycle of poor feeding at breast and a decreased milk supply. Upon observing a breastfeeding session, it was noted that the baby had a large resolving cephalohematoma from a vacuum extraction delivery. Digital examination of Cara's mouth revealed that she bunched her tongue in the middle, but a rhythmic suck with a cupped tongue was established with gentle massage of the tongue and hard palate. At breast, Cara displayed 8 to 10 nonnutritive sucks before one nutritive suck and swallow. With the milk-ejection reflex, this changed to a 4 to 1 ratio but soon reverted back to 8 to 10 sucks for each swallow. Alternate massage (massage and compression of the breast during the pauses between sucking bursts) improved this ratio somewhat but not enough to significantly increase milk intake. A Supplemental Nutrition System was recommended because of the weight loss of the baby and distress of the mother.

The feeding plan included the following protocols:

- Feed 8 to 10 times each 24 hours.
- Fill the supplementer with three to four ounces of breastmilk or formula.
- Use middle-size tubes with the bottle at a level above the breasts.
- Tape the tubes in place so that they extend to the end of the nipple.
- Use the supplementer at each feeding for three days and obtain a weight check.
- If the weight gain was good and the sucking has improved, run the supplementer to the end of each feeding; obtain another weight check in three days. If the sucking has not improved, the supplementer will continue to be used with each feeding.
- Keep a log and record at each feeding how much supplement was offered and how much the baby took. Note the weekly changes in amounts, record the number of wet diapers and bowel movements each 24 hours, and note when the breasts begin to feel fuller and more supplement is being left in the device. Also record the weight of the baby at each check and note when stool reverts to a predominantly breastmilk consistency and color.
- When the growth rate is appropriate and the supplement has decreased, change to the smallest size tube. Run the supplementer at the end of every other feeding if weight gain continues to be appropriate.
- Pump the breasts if no breast changes have been observed in three days of use at each feeding and if supplement is still being completely drained after one week.
- Finger-feed with the two large tubes if Cara does not feed well at breast, if more feedings are necessary than the mother can initially cope with, or if she will not be available for a feeding.

16. For long-term use with the SNS device, some mothers may want two or three of the plastic bottles with lids so they can be prefilled with breastmilk or formula for the day. If using other devices, a backup set of tubing or bags or bottles should be available.

17. Mothers may appreciate contact with other women who have used such a device for support and understanding of the conflicting feelings they may experience at different times during the use of the device.

SUMMARY

Just as the health-care professional must base recommendations for use of breast pumps on various factors, the same holds true for the temporary use of other breastfeeding technologies. Too often, a breastfeeding mother may see a device advertised as an aid to breastfeeding and assume that she needs to use it. If she then attempts to do so without thoroughly understanding its risks and benefits, actual and presumed, she could unwittingly interfere with the lactation course and/or the baby's ability to breastfeed. This is particularly true if she obtains the device from a person or institution which lacks a specialist in lactation management.

Nipple shields are most apt to be used when they are not necessary—in part because of their wide availability and in part because of their attractiveness in busy hospitals or practices, where health-care workers offer the devices because they appear to "make the baby nurse." As noted in this chapter, however, the design of the nipple shield can, in some cases, cause sore nipples when they did not previously exist. In nearly all cases, some change in the infant's suckling pattern results from the frequent use of a nipple shield. Thus, when a health-care provider considers offering the device to a mother, careful instructions and emphasis on the temporary nature of the use of the device must be offered.

Breast shells are less easily misused because they must be removed in order for the baby to feed. However, collecting milk in the cups without careful attention to the cleanliness of the shell and the time period over which the drip milk was obtained can create other problems—not the least of which is offering the baby contaminated milk.

Feeding tube devices are more complex and therefore potentially more off-putting than either breast shells or nipple shields. Mothers who insist upon using the device because they are convinced that their own milk supplies are inadequate to support appropriate infant growth need careful follow-up. Too often, the mother misinterprets the instructions or reads only enough to know how to put the device together and to clean it. The manner in which the device should be used is rarely completely understood from a single reading of the instructions that accompany the device. Health-care providers or counselors who recommended the inappropriate use of feeding tube devices can potentially interrupt the breastfeeding relationship or cause further problems. In addition, observation and assessment of the mother and infant as they breastfeed both with and without the device is a necessity if the health-care provider is to make appropriate recommendations for an optimal outcome. In most cases, the nature of the problem that requires assistance of a tube feeding device is such that the mother's anxiety level is high and the need to provide additional nutrition for the baby is critical. The lactation consultant, nurse, or other health-care worker can expect that working with such a mother and baby will be time consuming and will require many more hours of follow-up time than is the case for other situations.

In all cases where a breastfeeding device is used, the benefits of the device must be weighed against the risks of interfering in the breastfeeding relationship—just as bottle-feeding represents a risk of varying degrees for different mothers and their babies. Anticipating the emotional response of mothers to devices and discussing them in a straightforward manner will assist the health-care provider in determining whether and when to suggest a particular device, as well as how to help the mother stop using it when it is no longer necessary. As with all other care, the use of a breastfeeding device of any kind must first be found to "do no harm"; thereafter its benefits must outweigh the risks it represents in order for the breastfeeding relationship to truly be supported.

REFERENCES

Akre, J, ed.: Infant feeding:the physiological basis, *Bull WHO* (suppl.) 67: p. 22, 1989.
Amatayakul, K, et al.: Serum prolactin and cortisol levels

after suckling for varying periods of time and the effect of a nipple shield, *Acta Obstet Gynecol Scand* 66:47–51, 1987.

Asquith, M, and Harod, J: Reduction of bacterial contamination in banked human milk, *J Pediatr* 95:993–94, 1979.

Asquith, M, Sharp, R, and Stevenson, D: Decreased bacterial contamination of human milk expressed with an electric breast pump, *J Calif Perin Assoc* 4:45–47, 1985.

Asquith, M, et al.: The bacterial content of breast milk after early initiation of expression using a standard technique, *J Pediatr Gastroenterol Nutr* 3:104–7, 1984.

Auerbach, KG: *Breastfeeding techniques and devices,* Lactation Consultant Series Unit 17, Garden City Park, N.Y., 1987, Avery Publishing Group, Inc.

Auerbach, KG: The effect of nipple shields on maternal milk volume, *JOGNN* 19:419–27, 1990a.

Auerbach, KG: Sequential and simultaneous breast pumping: a comparison, *Int J Nurs Stud* 27:257–65, 1990b.

Auerbach, KG: Using nipple shields appropriately, *Rental Roundup* 6:4–5, 1989.

Auerbach, KG, and Avery, JL: Induced lactation: a study of adoptive nursing by 240 women, *Am J Dis Child* 135:340–43, 1981.

Auerbach, KG, and Avery, JL: Relactation: a study of 366 cases, *Pediatrics* 65:236–42, 1980.

Auerbach, KG, and Guss, E: Maternal employment and breastfeeding: a study of 567 women's experiences, *Am J Dis Child* 138:958–60, 1984.

Battin, D, et al.: Effect of suckling on serum prolactin, luteinizing hormone, follicle-stimulating hormone, and estradiol during prolonged lactation, *Obstet Gynecol* 65:785–88, 1985.

Bennion, E: *Antique medical instruments,* Berkeley, Calif., 1979, University of California Press, p. 271.

Bornmann, P: *Legal considerations and the lactation consultant—USA,* Lactation Consultant Series Unit 3, Garden City Park, N.Y., 1986, Avery Publishing Group, Inc.

Bose, C, et al.: Relactation by mothers of sick and premature infants, *Pediatrics* 67:565–68, 1981.

Boutte, C, et al.: Comparison of hand- and electric-operated breast pumps, *Hum Nutr, Appl Nutr* 39A:426–30, 1985.

Bowles, B, Stutte, P, and Hensley, J: Alternate massage in breastfeeding, *Genesis* 9:5–9, 1987/1988.

Bull, P, and Barger, J: Fingerfeeding with the SNS, *Rental Roundup* 4:2–3, 1987.

Caldeyro-Barcia, R: Milk ejection in women. In Reynolds, M, and Folley, S, eds.: *Lactogenesis, the initiation of milk secretion at parturition,* Philadelphia, 1969, University of Pennsylvania Press.

Cobo, E, et al.: Neurohypophyseal hormone release in the human. II. Experimental study during lactation, *Am J Obstet Gynecol* 97:519–29, 1967.

Costa, K: A comparison of colony counts of breast milk using two methods of breast cleansing, *JOGNN* 18:231–36, 1989.

de Sanctis, V, et al.: Comparison of prolactin response to

suckling and breast pump aspiration in lactating mothers, *La Ric Clin Lab* 11:81–85, 1981.

DeNicola, M: One case of nipple shield addiction, *J Hum Lact* 2:28–29, 1986.

Desmarais, L, and Browne, S: *Inadequate weight gain in breastfeeding infants: assessments and resolutions,* Lactation Consultant Series Unit 8, Garden City Park, N.Y., 1990, Avery Publishing Group, Inc.

Dodd, F, and Griffin, T: *Milking routines, machine milking,* National Institute of Research on Dairying, Reading, England, 1977, Shinfield, pp. 179–200.

Donowitz, L, et al.: Contaminated breast milk: a source of *Klebsiella* bacteremia in a newborn intensive care unit, *Rev Infec Dis* 3:716–20, 1981.

Drewett, R, Bowen-Jones, A, and Dogterom, J: Oxytocin levels during breastfeeding in established lactation, *Horm Behav* 16:245–48, 1982.

Edgehouse, L, and Radzyminski, S: A device for supplementing breast-feeding, *MCN* 15:34–35, 1990.

Egnell, E: The mechanics of different methods of emptying the female breast, *J Swe Med Assoc* 40:1–8, 1956.

Feher, S, et al.: Increased breastmilk production for premature infants with a relaxation/imagery audiotape, *Pediatrics* 83:57–60, 1989.

Fildes, V: *Breasts, bottles and babies,* Edinburgh, 1986, Edinburgh University Press, pp. 141–43.

Forte, A, Mayberry, L, and Ferketich, S: Breast milk collection and storage practices among mothers of hospitalized neonates, *J Perinatol* 7:35–39, 1987.

Goodman, G, and Grosvenor, C: Neuroendocrine control of the milk ejection reflex, *J Dairy Sci* 66:2226–35, 1983.

Gorewit, R, et al.: Current concepts on the role of oxytocin in milk ejection, *J Dairy Sci* 66:2236–50, 1983.

Grams, M: *Breastfeeding source book,* Sheridan, Wyo., 1988, Achievement Press, pp. 100–142.

Gransden, W, et al.: An outbreak of *Serratia marcescens* transmitted by contaminated breast pumps in a special care baby unit, *J Hosp Infec* 7:149–54, 1986.

Green, D, et al.: The relative efficacy of four methods of human milk expression, *Early Hum Dev* 6:153–59, 1982.

Howie, P, et al.: The relationship between suckling-induced prolactin response and lactogenesis, *J Clin Endocrinol Metab* 50:670–73, 1980.

Hughes, V, et al.: *Acute prolactin stimulation in breastfeeding women using three commercial breast pumps, manual expression and natural infant suckling,* Presented at the Congress for International Federation for Family Life Promotion, Nairobi, Kenya, 1989.

Jackson, D, et al.: The automatic sampling shield: a device for sampling suckled breast milk, *Early Hum Dev* 15:295–306, 1987.

Johnson, C: An evaluation of breast pumps currently available on the American market, *Clin Pediatr* 22:40–45, 1983.

Johnston, J, and Amico, J: A prospective longitudinal study of the release of oxytocin and prolactin in response to infant suckling in long-term lactation, *J Clin Endocrinol Metab* 62:653–57, 1986.

Kutner, L: Nipple shield consent form: a teaching aid, *J Hum Lact* 2:25–27, 1986.

Lawrence, R: *Breastfeeding: a guide for the medical profession,* St. Louis, 1989, The C.V. Mosby Co., pp. 183–85.

Leake, R, et al.: Oxytocin and prolactin response in long-term breast-feeding, *Obstet Gynecol* 62:565–68, 1983.

Marmet, C, and Shell, E: *Marmet technique of manual expression of breastmilk,* Encino, Calif., 1979, The Lactation Institute.

Maygrier, J: *Midwifery Illustrated,* Philadelphia, 1833, Carey & Hart, p. 173.

McNutley, et al.: Release of oxytocin and prolactin response to suckling, *Br Med J* 286:646–47, 1983.

Meier, P, and Wilks, S: The bacteria in expressed mothers' milk, *MCN* 12:420–23, 1987.

Merrill, W, et al.: Effects of premilking stimulation on complete lactation, milk yield and milking performance, *J Dairy Sci* 70:1676–84, 1987.

Minchin, M: *Breastfeeding matters,* Victoria, Australia, 1985, Alma Publications, pp. 142–45.

Moloney, A, et al.: A bacteriological examination of breast pumps, *J Hosp Infec* 9:169–74, 1987.

Morse, J, and Bottorff, J: The emotional experience of breast expression, *J Nurs-Midwif* 33:165–70, 1988.

Neifert, M, and Seacat, J: *Milk yield and prolactin rise with simultaneous breast pumping,* Presented at the Ambulatory Pediatric Association Meeting, Washington, D.C., May 7–10, 1985.

Neville, M: Regulation of mammary development and lactation. In Neville, M, and Neifert, M, eds.: *Lactation: Physiology, Nutrition and Breast-Feeding,* New York, 1983, Plenum Press, p. 118.

Newman, J: Breastfeeding problems associated with the early introduction of bottles and pacifiers, *J Hum Lact* 6:59–63, 1990.

Newton, M, and Newton, N: The let-down reflex in human lactation, *J Pediatr* 33:698–704, 1948.

Noel, G, Suh, H, and Frantz, A: Prolactin release during nursing and breast stimulation in postpartum and non-postpartum subjects, *J Clin Endocrinol Metab* 38:413–23, 1974.

Nwankwo, M, et al.: Bacterial growth in expressed breastmilk, *Ann Trop Paediatr* 8:92–95, 1988.

Petersen, W: *Dairy science: principles and practice,* Philadelphia, 1950, J. B. Lippincott Co., pp. 373–87.

Pittard, W, et al.: Bacterial contamination of human milk: container type and method of expression, *Am J Perinatol* 8:25–27, 1991.

Rees, D: Juice-jar breast pump, *Keep Abreast J* 2:225, 1977.

Rental Roundup: New product, SNS, 3:1–3, 1986a.

Rental Roundup: Warning: these devices can hurt a woman, 3:9–12, 1986b.

Sagi, R, Gorewit, R, and Zinn, S: Milk ejection in cows mechanically stimulated during late lactation, *J Dairy Sci* 63:1957–60, 1980.

Saint, L, Maggiore, P, and Hartmann, P: Yield and nutrient content of milk in eight women breast-feeding twins and one woman breast-feeding triplets, *Br J Nutr* 56:49–58, 1986.

Shrago, L: Product evaluation: nipple shields, *J Hum Lact* 4:169, 1988.

Sponsel, W: Simple and effective breast pump for nursing mothers, *Br Med J* 286:1676–84, 1983.

Stutte, P, Bowles, B, and Morman, G: The effects of breast massage on volume and fat content of human milk, *Genesis* 10:22–25, 1988.

Sutherland, A, and Auerbach, KG: *Relactation and induced lactation,* Lactation Consultant Series Unit 1, Garden City Park, N.Y., 1985, Avery Publishing Group, Inc.

Tyson, J: Nursing and prolactin secretion: principle determinants in the mediation of puerperal infertility. In Crosignani, P, and Robyn, C, eds.: *Prolactin and human reproduction,* New York, 1977, Academic Press, pp. 97–108.

Walker, M: How to evaluate breast pumps, *MCN* 12:270–76, 1987.

Weichert, C: Prolactin cycling and the management of breastfeeding failure, *Adv Pediatr* 27:391–407, 1980.

Wennergren, M, Wiqvist, N, and Wennergren, G: Manual breast pumps promote successful breastfeeding, *Acta Obstet Gynecol Scand* 64:673–75, 1985.

Whittlestone, W: The physiologic breastmilker, *NZ Fam Phy* 5:1–3, 1978.

Whitworth, N: Lactation in humans, *Psychoneuroendocrinology* 13:171–88, 1988.

Whitworth, N, et al.: The effect of fetal genotype on the human maternal PRL response to labor, delivery and breast stimulation, *Abst Proc Int Cong Prolactin* 4:60, 1984.

Wilks, S, and Meier, P: Helping mothers express milk suitable for preterm and high-risk infant feeding, *MCN* 13:121–23, 1988.

Williams, J, Auerbach, K, and Jacobi, A: Lateral epicondylitis (tennis elbow) in breastfeeding mothers, *Clin Pediatr* 28:42–43, 1989.

Woolford, M, and Phillips, D: *Evaluation studies of a milking system using an alternating vacuum level in a single chambered teatcup,* Proceedings of the International Symposium on Machine Milking, National Mastitis Council, 1978, pp. 125–49.

Woolridge, M, Baum, J, and Drewett, R: Effect of a traditional and of a new nipple shield on sucking patterns and milk flow, *Early Hum Dev* 4:357–64, 1980.

Zinaman, M: Breast pumps: ensuring mothers' success, *Contemp Obstet Gynecol* 32:55–62, 1988.

Zinaman, M, et al.: Acute prolactin, oxytocin response and milk yield to infant suckling and artificial methods of expression in lactating women, *Pediatrics* 89:437–40, 1992.

Appendix 11–1
Manufacturers/Distributors
of Breastfeeding Devices

Ameda/Egnell
765 Industrial Dr.
Cary, IL 60013
(Automatic electric breast pump,
battery pump, cylinder pump,
breast shells, nipple shields)

Bailey Medical Engineering
1820 Donna
Los Osos, CA 93402
(Nurture III small semiautomatic breast pump)

Cannon Babysafe Ltd.
Lower Rd.
Glemsford, Suffolk
England CO10 7QS
(Avent squeeze-handle breast pump,
silicone nipple shields)

CEA of Greater Philadelphia
127 Fayette St.
Conshohocken, PA 19428
(Comfi-Dri Milk Cups)

D.A. Kadan, Inc.
10100 Industrial Dr.
Pineville, NC 28134
(Kadan small semiautomatic electric pump)

Evenflo Products Co.
P.O.Box 1206
771 North Freedom St.
Ravenna, OH 44266–1206
(Cylinder pump, battery pump)

Gerber Products Co.
445 State St.
Fremont, MI 49412
(Cylinder pump, small semiautomatic electric pump)

Graham-Field, Inc.
400 Rabro Dr. East
Hauppauge, NY 11788
(Gentle Expressions battery pump,
The Rose automatic electric pump, breast shells)

International Design/Manufacturing, Inc.
305 Avenue G
Redondo Beach, CA 90277
(Happy Family cylinder pump)

Lact-Aid
P.O.Box 1066
Athens, TN 37303
(Tube feeding device)

Lopuco Ltd.
1615 Old Annapolis Rd.
Woodbine, MD 21797
(Loyd-B squeeze-handle pump)

Lunas Enterprises
Box 2400
Sitka, AK 99835
(Ora'lac pump)

Mada Medical Products, Inc.
60 Commerce Rd.
Carlstadt, NJ 07072
(Small semiautomatic pump)

Medela, Inc.
4610 Prime Parkway
P.O. Box 660
McHenry, IL 60051
(Automatic electric pump, manual pump, battery
pump, Lactina pump, breast shells, nipple shield,
Supplemental Nutrition System feeding tube
device)

Netsy Company
34 Sunrise Ave.
Mill Valley, CA 94941
(Breast shells)

Omron Marshall Products, Inc.
300 Lakeview Parkway
Vernon Hills, IL 60061
(Kaneson cylinder and Mag Mag battery
pumps)

Pharmics
1878 S Redwood Rd.
Salt Lake City, UT 84104
(Breast shells)

Ross Laboratories
585 Cleveland Ave.
Columbus, OH 43216
(Cylinder pump)

Sassy, Inc.
1534 College S.E.
Grand Rapids, MI 49507
(Infa cylinder pump)

Schuco, Inc.
P.O. Box 357
333 Westbury Ave.
Carle Place, NY 11514
(Small and large semiautomatic
electric pumps)

Sears, Roebuck and Co.
Chicago, IL 60684
(Cylinder pump)

Trigon Industries, Ltd.
12 Maidstone St.
CPO Box 3674
Auckland 2, New Zealand
(Whittlestone automatic electric pump)

White River-Natural Technologies
23010 Lake Forest Dr., Suite 310
Laguna Hills, CA 92653
(Cylinder pump, semiautomatic and
automatic electric pumps)

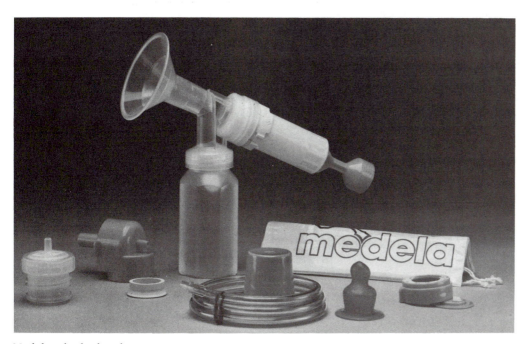

Medela cylinder hand pump
(Medela Inc., McHenry, Illinois).

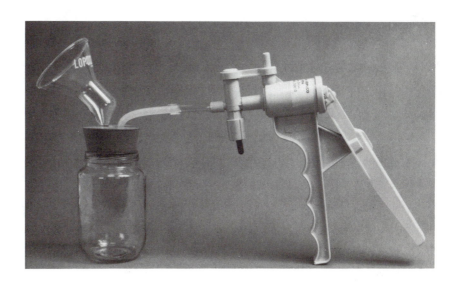

Loyd-B squeeze handle manual
pump (Lopuco Ltd., Woodbine,
Maryland).

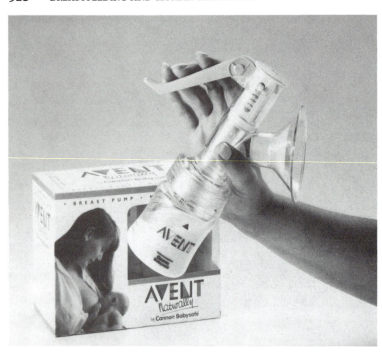

Avent squeeze handle manual pump (Cannon Babysafe Ltd., Suffolk, England).

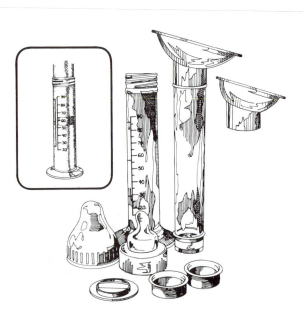

Happy Family cylinder hand pump (International Design/Manufacturing Inc., Redondo Beach, California).

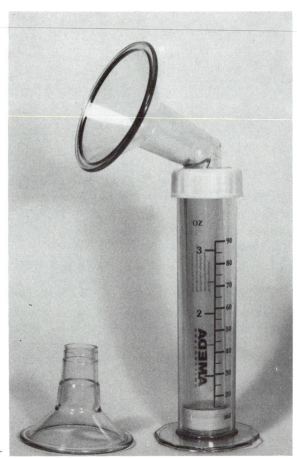

Hand pump (Ameda/Egnell, Cary, Illinois).

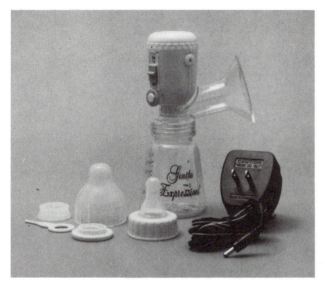

Gentle Expressions Battery Pump (Graham-Field, Hauppague, New York).

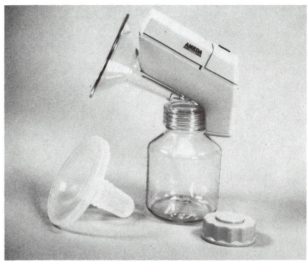

Lact-B battery operated pump (Ameda/Egnell, Cary, Illinois).

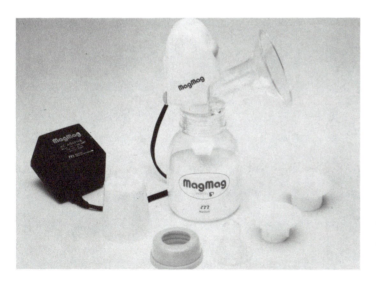

MagMag battery breast pump (Omron Marshall Products, Vernon Hills, Illinois).

Medela mini-electric battery pump (Medela Inc., McHenry, Illinois).

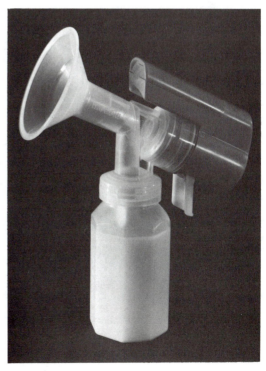

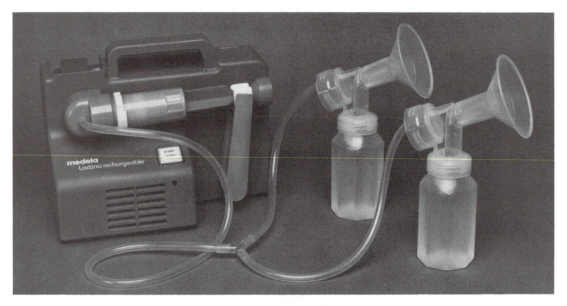

Lactina Rechargeable electric pump (Medela Inc., McHenry, Illinois).

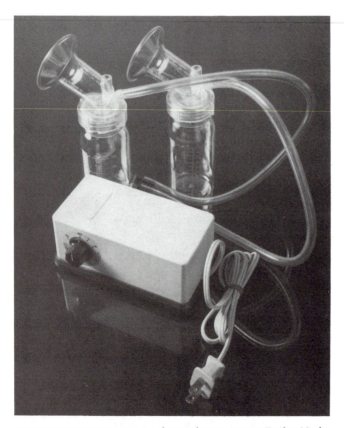

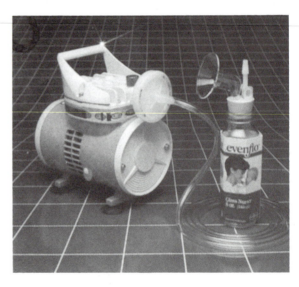

Schuco semi-automatic pump (Schuco Inc., Carle Place, New York).

Nurture III semi-automatic electric breast pump (Bailey Medical Engineering, Los Osos, California).

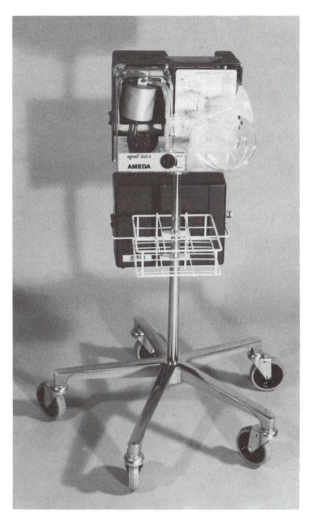

Automatic Electric Lact-E pump on trolley (Ameda/Egnell, Cary, Illinois).

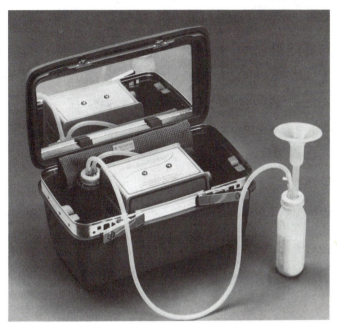

White River electric breast pump (White River-Natural Technologies, Laguna Hills, California).

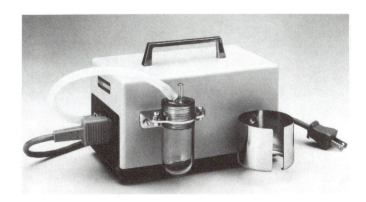

Mada semi-automatic electric breast pump (Mada Medical Product, Carlstadt, New Jersey).

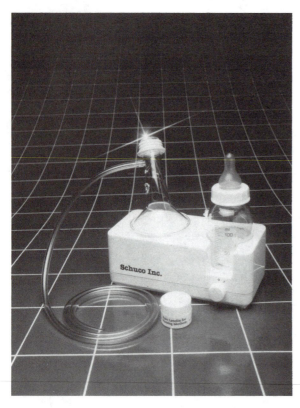

Schuco semi-automatic electric pump (Schuco Inc., Carle Place, New York).

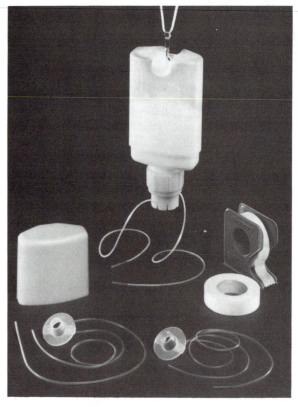

Supplemental Nutrition System (Medela Inc., McHenry, Illinois).

12

Jaundice and the Breastfeeding Baby

Few early experiences of the newborn are as apt to have a deterrent effect on breastfeeding as does the diagnosis of neonatal jaundice. This diagnosis causes more infants to be taken off the breast in the early newborn period than any other reason. In most cases, such intervention is unnecessary. It represents a failure of health-care workers to understand the normal physiology of the neonate and his adjustment to extrauterine life. Health-care workers must also understand the neonate's response to the routines that characterize many institutional birth sites in the early neonatal period. We begin this discussion with a review of the etiology of early-onset jaundice, followed by a discussion of late-onset jaundice, and the clinical implications of the normal infant's response to extrauterine life.

RICHARD A. GUTHRIE
KATHLEEN G. AUERBACH

EARLY-ONSET (NEONATAL) JAUNDICE

Following birth, the human neonate must initiate many activities which had previously been taken care of by the placenta. Instead of continuously feeding, as in the womb, the infant must learn to feed intermittently. Clearance of waste products is now taken over by the immature liver and kidneys. At the same time, these organs are confronted by a relatively concentrated load of bilirubin caused by the breakdown of red blood cells and the meconium that coats the intestines. Conjugated, water-soluble bilirubin is excreted by the kidneys in the urine; unconjugated, lipid-soluble bilirubin is excreted by the liver in the bile through the bowel. As the gut becomes coated and recoated with milk, recirculation of the unconjugated, lipid-carried bilirubin is re-duced, and more frequent stooling removes the unconjugated bilirubin.

Jaundice is caused by the accumulation of bilirubin in the tissue, particularly the skin, where it is visible as a yellow pigment. While the presence of jaundice in older children or adults is considered a pathologic condition, this is not true for the newborn. As a result of the relatively low level of maternal oxygen in placental blood, the fetus develops a relatively high red blood cell count with high hemoglobin; this increases the oxygen-carrying capacity of fetal blood. Fetal hemoglobin takes up oxygen poorly; thus there is need for more hemoglobin. When the baby is born, there is usually a relatively high level of red blood cells with a high level of fetal hemoglobin.

Fetal hemoglobin is well adapted to assist the fetus in the low-oxygen environment of the uterus. It has a low affinity for oxygen; therefore it picks up oxygen less well than does adult hemoglobin (which has more need for it). However it also releases the oxygen to peripheral tissue better, thus enabling the fetus to live and grow in a relatively low-oxygen environment.

Following birth, the low-affinity fetal hemoglobin becomes a liability in the high-oxygen environment of lung breathing, and the bone marrow switches to the production of adult hemoglobin (hemoglobin A). The red blood cells containing fetal hemoglobin can now be broken down and eliminated from the body. Hemoglobin is a complex molecule, consisting of heme, globin, and iron. When the hemoglobin molecule is broken down, iron returns to the bone marrow where it is used in hemoglobin synthesis. Globin returns to circulation in the blood. Heme is broken down into unconjugated bilirubin by the spleen.

Unconjugated or indirect bilirubin is a lipid-soluble compound and is transported from the spleen to the liver by attachment to transporting proteins such as albumin—in a fashion similar to the transport of cholesterol in the blood by opaproteins (lipid-transporting proteins which are synthesized by the liver). In the liver, the indirect bilirubin is detached from the carrier proteins and conjugated with other compounds, such as glucuronic acid. This results in conjugated or direct bilirubin, which is water soluble. Some conjugated bilirubin reenters the circulation and is excreted in the urine. Most, however, is excreted in the bile. Some unconjugated bilirubin is also excreted in the bile. High concentrations of direct bilirubin in serum usually indicate an obstruction of the biliary system, but otherwise this water-soluble bilirubin is not harmful.

It is the unconjugated or indirect, fat-soluble bilirubin that—in increasing concentrations—causes the baby to take on a yellowish cast to the skin and sclera (see Table 12–1). The concentration of indirect bilirubin can increase if its production exceeds the protein-carrying capacity of the blood, or if excretion is so slow that bilirubin accumulates faster than excretion and carrying capacity can handle (Gould et al., 1974; Chalmers, Campbell & Turnbull, 1975; Gale et al., 1990).

TABLE 12–1   RULE-OF-THUMB OBSERVATION AND ITS RELATIONSHIP TO BILIRUBIN LEVELS

Involvement of the Body	Serum Bilirubin Levels
Sclera	3 mg/dL
Face	5 mg/dL
Upper trunk	5–7 mg/dL
Complete trunk	7–10 mg/dL
Spread to extremities	10–12 mg/dL
Extremities yellow; palms and soles clear	12–15 mg/dL
Palms and soles yellow	>15 mg/dL

In the fetus, the gut is sterile; therefore, bilirubin excreted into the gut throughout fetal life accumulates in the meconium. Much of this bilirubin can be reabsorbed. If the body begins to feed, it can contribute to the bilirubin load which the newborn must excrete and thus contribute to the serum bilirubin level.

The large load of meconium bilirubin combined with the relatively slow functioning of the liver and the rapid breakdown of fetal hemoglobin may result in an early, temporary exaggeration of serum bilirubin concentration, which manifests itself in yellowing of the sclera and skin during the early neonatal period. This is a natural result of the normal physiologic process which every newborn experiences in the early extrauterine period (McDonagh, 1990). Generally, in African and Caucasian neonates a mean peak of 6 mg/dL occurs on the third or fourth day of life. Thereafter, serum bilirubin levels decline to about 2 to 3 mg/dL by the end of the first week of life and gradually reach the normal adult value (1 mg/dL) by the end of the second week (Gartner et al., 1977; Kivlahan & James, 1984). Higher values of 10 to 15 mg/dL will sometimes occur. There is no scientific evidence that bilirubin levels below 20 mg/dL in the first week of life and less than 25 mg/dL thereafter have any harmful effect on full-term, healthy infants (Newman & Maisels, 1990).

PATHOLOGIC JAUNDICE

Pathologic jaundice usually falls into three general categories: (1) disease which causes increased red cell hemolysis (such as Rh disease, ABO incompatibility, congenital spherocytosis, and other hemolytic processes); (2) a deficiency of carrier protein or binding sites (such as occurs with prematurity, sepsis, hypoxia, and the use of certain drugs); and (3) liver and metabolic disease (such as hepatitis, Crigler-Najjar syndrome, Rotor's syndrome, liver damage from cytomegalovirus, toxoplasmosis, rubella, syphilis, congenital biliary atresia, and metabolic problems such as galactosemia and hypothyroidism). Usually diseases causing a deficiency of carrier protein or binding occur after the first week of life and result in *late* onset of jaundice which can persist for several weeks.

FACTORS ASSOCIATED WITH EARLY-ONSET JAUNDICE

The medical and nursing literature is replete with discussions linking the presence or severity of neonatal jaundice to a wide range of variables, including mode of feeding (Newman & Gross, 1963) and hospital practices. Examination of the literature provides no clear picture of how these variables affect jaundice, because feeding groups are rarely defined in the same way and are rarely totally discrete. In addition, other factors (identified by different investigators as important) may have been allowed to vary without considering their potential influence as intervening variables.

INFANT CHARACTERISTICS

Race/ethnic group. Different racial groups appear to exhibit neonatal hyperbilirubinemia in varying degrees. Horiguchi and Bauer reported that Japanese neonates were more than three times as likely as Caucasian newborns to have jaundice—defined as a serum bilirubin level ≥10 mg/dL (Horiguchi & Bauer, 1975; Maisels et al., 1988). In their population sample, the groups were comparable with regard to maternal age, parity, intrapartum medication, type of delivery, and anesthesia received.

Fischer et al. (1988) compared Japanese and Caucasian neonates and found significantly higher serum bilirubin levels among the Japanese babies, regardless of feeding method. The authors suggest that genetic and/or environmental factors contributing to an increased rate of heme catabolism may explain the differences between the groups. Similar patterns have occurred when comparing other Asian neonates (for example, Chinese and Korean) with Caucasian infants.

Navajo Indian neonates also have been found to have substantially higher serum bilirubin levels than Caucasian infants at two days of age (Johnson et al., 1986). It was concluded that the higher bilirubin levels may be caused by differences in red cell metabolism and/or membrane structure. Saland, McNamara, and Cohen (1974) controlled for feeding method when they compared Navajo infants with Caucasian controls. They found that the Navajo infants exhibited higher serum bilirubin levels in all feeding groups and that the highest levels occurred when the Navajo infants were breastfed. Higher neonatal bilirubin levels in these groups may therefore be normal and should not precipitate intervention.

Birth weight. Osborn, Reiff, and Bolus (1985) noted that birthweight was related to the likelihood of hyperbilirubinemia. Specifically, lighter weight babies were more likely than heavier babies to become jaundiced.

Bracci et al. (1989) found that only birthweight and gestational age remained significantly associated with the likelihood of neonatal jaundice when they performed a linear regression analysis of numerous variables. They suggested that "most factors already reported in the literature play a minor role which may not merit attention from a preventive point of view" (Bracci et al., 1989).

Stool patterns. DeCarvalho, Robertson, and Klaus (1985) evaluated 24 exclusively breastfed and 13 exclusively formula-fed infants in the first three days after birth. Throughout the study period, the breastfed group was found to lose significantly more weight than the bottle-fed babies, but there was no correlation between weight loss and serum bilirubin concentrations. Stool frequency and volume also varied by feeding group, with the bottle-fed infants stooling more often and in greater volume than the breastfed babies. Examination of stool samples revealed that for the breastfed babies the amount of stool bilirubin increased as the volume of stools increased through the three-day study period. This was not the case for the bottle-fed babies. This may partially explain the greater frequency of jaundice in breastfed babies, so-called "breast*feeding* jaundice."

Frequent suckling has been found to shorten gut transit time and to promote stool output in both full-term (Cavell, 1981; Tomamasa et al., 1987; Weaver, Ewing & Taylor, 1988) and pre-term infants (Bernbaum et al., 1981). As breastfed babies increase their stool output, they excrete more stool bilirubin and have lower serum bilirubin concentrations, which suggests that early stimulation of intestinal motility may reduce the likelihood of hyperbilirubinemia (De Carvalho, Klaus & Merkatz, 1982). Thus, there is a need for early and frequent breastfeeding in newborn infants.

Weight loss. Among the numerous studies which have examined weight loss and its relationship to hyperbilirubinemia in neonates, Hall et al. (1983)

found that breastfeeding infants lost more weight during the first four days of life and remained lighter than bottle-fed infants during the same time period, but that there was no relationship between weight loss and bilirubin levels.

In their study of 588 consecutively born infants, Butler and MacMillan (1983) found that breastfed babies had a significantly higher incidence of elevated serum bilirubin than did the formula-fed infants—and that the breastfed infants lost the greatest amounts of weight. They concluded that weight loss may be a contributing factor in level of jaundice exhibited.

HOSPITAL ROUTINES

Routine care patterns have been implicated as influencing factors both in bilirubin levels and in breastfeeding patterns. For example, Osborn, Reiff, and Bolus (1985) reported that problems during labor and delivery, the use of general anesthetics, cesarean delivery, postnatal complications, blood group incompatibility, and bruising—as well as infant feeding method—were significantly correlated with jaundice in the neonate.

Anesthesia. Wood and colleagues (1979) found that when the mother received epidural anesthesia during labor, the infants of those mothers were more likely to exhibit hyperbilirubinemia than infants of mothers who did not. In addition, weight recovery was associated with hyperbilirubinemia. The authors did not speculate as to the reason for the association; however, it may be that infants with intrauterine exposure to such analgesics are slower to suckle, thereby placing themselves at greater risk for weight loss because they receive less milk, a finding supported by Matthews (1989).

Type of feeding. With few exceptions, neonatal jaundice is thought to occur with greater frequency and to rise to higher levels when the baby is breastfed than when he or she is artificially fed. In spite of the frequency of this finding, Maisels and Gifford (1983) reported that no cause was identified in more than one-half of the cases in which serum bilirubin concentrations exceeded 12 mg/dL in 264 term infants.

Dahms et al. (1973) studied 199 full-term infants, dividing them into four groups. Demand breastfeeders received no supplemental feedings and went to the breast by six hours after birth, nursing six to seven times every 24 hours. Demand formula feeders received no supplemental feedings, received their first formula feed by six hours after birth, and were fed six to seven times every 24 hours. Control breastfeeders did not go to breast until 20 hours or later after birth, and received four breastfeedings every 24 hours and two formula feedings in the nursery at night. The control bottle-feeders were not fed until 20 hours or later after birth and received six formula feedings every 24 hours. The two control groups also received one or two feedings of 5% dextrose. Bilirubin levels were not statistically different between the four groups. Perhaps the widely held belief that breastfed babies have a greater prevalence of hyperbilirubinemia is one of those things we all "know for sure that just aren't so"—even though the belief leads to many alterations of early feeding practices (the use of water supplements, for example) which may be deleterious to continued breastfeeding.

Frequency of feeding. De Carvalho, Klaus, and Merkatz (1982) evaluated the relationship between the frequency of breastfeeding and mean bilirubin levels on the third day of life. The infants in the two groups did not differ in length of feeds, weight loss during the first three days of life, or hematocrit readings. However, the 29 infants who comprised Group 1 had a mean feeding frequency of 6.8± 0.8/24 hours. Mean serum bilirubin levels on day three for this group was 9.3± 3.5. By contrast, the 26 infants who comprised Group 2 had a mean feeding frequency of 10.1± 1.6/24 hours and mean serum bilirubin levels of 6.5± 4.0, a statistically significant difference (<.01). De Carvalho, Klaus, and Merkatz (1982) concluded that "policies that reduce or limit the number of breastfeedings in the first days of life may interfere with normal mechanisms that eliminate bilirubin from newborn infants."

Supplemental feeds. Adams, Hey, and Hall (1985) examined the incidence of hyperbilirubinemia in 223 consecutively born full-term, healthy infants. In their analysis, breastfeeding was the best predictor of hyperbilirubinemia higher than 12 mg/dL. However, most babies received fewer than eight feedings in 24 hours. In addition, all of the breastfed infants in the study were complemented with water feedings after breastfeeding, and many received two or three formula feedings as well.

These factors raise questions about the degree to which reduced caloric intake (from water feeds) and infrequent feedings from the breast—as well as possible delay in establishing maternal milk supply because of infrequent stimulation—may have contributed to higher serum bilirubin concentrations.

Water supplementation. Nicoll, Ginsburg, and Tripp (1982) found that most full-term breastfed infants in their sample received supplementary feeds of water, dextrose, or formula during the first days of life. When they compared plasma bilirubin levels in babies grouped by supplemental feeding, they found that those infants having the highest bilirubin levels were those who had received water feeds in addition to breastfeeding. The group receiving dextrose had slightly lower bilirubin levels, while those babies who were exclusively breastfed had the lowest bilirubin levels. Although there was no relationship between weight loss and physiological jaundice, the amount of supplemental water or dextrose taken was reported to account for more than one-quarter of the infants' calculated daily fluid requirements—and raises the issue of the degree to which water and dextrose feeds reduce the total daily calories received. The authors speculate that since thirst is the primary drive of infant appetite (Taitz & Byers, 1972) supplementation which depresses the thirst response may reduce neonatal interest in breastfeeding, thereby interfering with lactation. In a recent study, Glover and Sandilands (1990) found that glucose water supplementation was not only associated with greater weight loss in the first week of life, but that length of hospital stay increased as the total volume of glucose water supplementation increased. One might ask if bottle-fed babies who develop hyperbilirubinemia may also be receiving more supplemental water feeds than is appropriate. Nicoll, Ginsburg, and Tripp (1982) suggest that the practice of supplementing breastfeeding babies should be discouraged. Furthermore, they speculated that not providing prepacked feeds, which have no redeeming benefits for their recipients, would result in a 70% savings in hospital costs for breastfeeding infants. Studies by De Carvalho, Hall, and Harvey (1981) and Clarkson, Cowan, and Herbison (1984) confirm these findings.

Stevenson et al. (1980) noted that breastfed neonates experience a temporary decline in the caloric intake, compared with that received continuously *in utero,* until the mother's milk supply begins to climb; thereafter, caloric intake is sufficient to sustain growth. Although bilirubin production appears to be the same in infants regardless of what they are fed, bilirubin clearance is slower in breastfed, compared with bottle-fed, infants. This slower bilirubin clearance may explain the higher serum bilirubin concentrations in breastfed neonates.

Laws (1981), in reply to the study by Stevenson et al., reported that while supplemented infants lost less weight than unsupplemented neonates, glucose supplementation appeared not to affect bilirubin levels or the likelihood of subsequent phototherapy for bilirubin concentrations exceeding 12 mg/dL. He suggests that instead of being concerned about the temporarily "calorically deprived" breastfed infant (a frequently used rationale for offering supplements), clinicians should direct their attention to the "'calorically supplemented' (overfed?)" bottle-fed baby, whose rapid bilirubin clearance may actually represent a deviation from the norm.

Kuhr and Paneth (1982) studied 135 consecutively born healthy newborns. Among the breastfed infants, jaundice (defined as a total serum bilirubin level > 10 mg/dL in the first four days of life) occurred with greater frequency than among the bottle-fed babies. In a subset of 44 breastfed infants, the investigators examined the effect of complemental glucose water feeds on likelihood and severity of jaundice. As the volume of glucose water intake increased, estimated breastmilk intake declined, prompting the authors to speculate that, because sugar water provides fewer calories for infants, it may contribute to impaired hepatic clearance of bilirubin. Their speculation suggests that breastfeeding may not have been the reason the infants were jaundiced; instead, glucose water supplementation may have been the culprit!

ROUTINE THERAPY FOR EARLY-ONSET JAUNDICE

Typically, therapy for early-onset jaundice has included interrupting breastfeeding, an action which in most cases is both unnecessary and introduces other negative consequences, including early breastfeeding termination (Elander & Lindberg, 1986; Kemper, Forsyth & McCarthy, 1989) and phototherapy. While exposing the infant's skin to light in the blue range of 460 to 480 nm wavelength appears to break down the bilirubin and render it water soluble, such therapy is not without risks. Because blue light can damage the cornea and possibly the retina, the baby's eyes must be covered during light therapy. Because the baby tends to sweat under the lights, dehydration can occur, particularly if the baby is left under the lights for long periods. Furthermore, in the absence of phototherapy, serum bilirubin levels drop of their own accord, thereby questioning the necessity of additional hospitalization in order to perform phototherapy. In the first week of life, in healthy full-term infants who are feeding well and voiding regularly, there is no scientific justification for instituting phototherapy for serum bilirubin levels under 15 mg/dL. Between levels of 15 and 20 mg/dL, careful assessment of the infant is warranted before using phototherapy. Lethargy, poor feeding, and infrequent stooling may contribute to a relatively rapid rise in serum bilirubin concentrations. Under such circumstances, phototherapy may slow the rise; however, improving the baby's feeding pattern is also necessary to increase the frequency of stooling and break the cycle of continued lethargy.

Until recently, little consideration has been given to the possible effects of routine treatment for jaundice other than its effect on the bilirubin concentrations. Kemper, Forsyth, and McCarthy (1989, 1990)

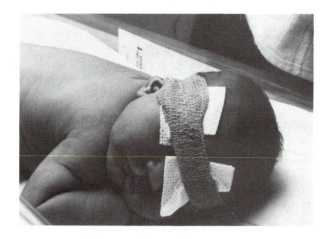

FIGURE 12–1   The baby's eyes must be covered during light therapy for jaundice.

ask if the benefits of such treatments may contribute to psychosocial and parenting risks previously ignored. In their matched sample of 124 control mothers and 85 mothers whose infants were diagnosed as jaundiced, they found that the mothers of the jaundiced babies were significantly more likely to consider the diagnosis of jaundice as moderately to very serious. This was especially true if the babies had received phototherapy to reduce the bilirubin levels. In addition, as late as one month after discharge, the mothers of the jaundiced babies were not sure that their babies had recovered. More than twice as many mothers of jaundiced infants had stopped breastfeeding, compared with the breastfeeding termination rate among the control group of mothers whose babies were not diagnosed as jaundiced.

Interruption of breastfeeding as a treatment for jaundice also played a role in breastfeeding rates at one month. Those who experienced an interruption of breastfeeding were only half as likely to be nursing one month postbirth if they also were diagnosed with jaundice. In those babies with no diagnosis of jaundice, breastfeeding interruption resulted in a 40% reduction in breastfeeding likelihood at one month.

In addition, the authors found differences between the groups in the frequency with which the mothers sought health care. More than twice as many mothers with jaundiced babies had more than two "well-child" visits within the first month and more than one "sick visit" in that same time period.

Summary of Characteristics of Early-Onset Jaundice

- Affects nearly all newborns
- Manifests itself after 24 hours of age
- Peaks on the third or fourth day of life
- Declines steadily through the first week to normal levels
- May be more obvious in all infants whose feeding is limited in frequency and/or duration, and with whom nonmilk complements or supplements are used
- Is self-limiting in a healthy, full-term infant
- Requires no intervention

Mothers of jaundiced babies were more than five times as likely as control mothers to have used an emergency room for a problem unrelated to jaundice in the baby's first month of life, and not to have left their babies in the care of someone else—even another adult family member.

By six months, the mothers of jaundiced babies were still more than twice as likely as control mothers to have used an emergency room for care for their baby, but they were also much more likely than the mothers in the control group to have left their babies for 48 hours (Kemper, Forsyth & McCarthy, 1990). The authors suggest that separating a mother from her baby and/or interrupting breastfeeding to treat a self-limiting condition must be considered a risk with potentially significant negative consequences. One can speculate that overconcern in the early neonatal period may result in an apparent reduction of concern in the postneonatal period—perhaps as a reaction to the stress of the diagnosis and the parental perceptions of vulnerability it engenders.

In addition to the psychosocial costs of a diagnosis of, and subsequent treatment for, jaundice, other investigators question whether routine evaluations and/or interventions may be appropriate, suggesting that they may be an unnecessary use of increasingly scarce health-care funds. Newman et al. (1990) examined the medical records of nearly 2,500 infants born at the University of California, San Francisco. They found that 447 (18%) of the babies born between 1980 and 1982 met the standard criteria for "nonphysiologic" hyperbilirubinemia; in 214 (48%) of these no cause of the jaundice was identified. On the basis of their examination, the investigators made five recommendations for determining when blood work for infants is necessary (see boxed checklist). The criteria recognize the effect of both feeding method and racial/ethnic heritage; they are aimed at avoiding the trauma of bleeding the infant unnecessarily and saving the high cost of testing infants who do not actually need these expensive tests, the results of which will yield no useful information.

LATE-ONSET JAUNDICE

Late-onset jaundice, as the name implies, cannot be distinguished from early-onset jaundice in the infant's first week. In an infant with late-onset jaun-

---

> **CONSIDERATIONS FOR DETERMINING THE NEED FOR LABORATORY EVALUATION OF HYPERBILIRUBINEMIA**[*]
>
> 1. If a newborn requires transfusion, search for evidence of hemolysis in the event that the infant shows signs of early-onset jaundice.
> 2. If a newborn is 24 hours of age or older and has a high bilirubin level, do follow-up tests, taking into account both racial origin and feeding experience. A high bilirubin level is defined as follows:
>
> | | If bottle-fed | If breastfed |
> |--------|---------------|--------------|
> | Black | 12 mg/dL | 14 mg/dL |
> | White | 14mg/dL | 16mg/dL |
> | Asian | 16mg/dL | 18mg/dL |
>
> 3. If an infant is not anemic and the Coombs test is negative, there is little justification for ordering additional tests.
> 4. If bilirubin levels continue to rise, it is important to attempt to identify the cause.
> 5. If an infant is seven days old or older, shows signs of illness, and the jaundice is prolonged, check a direct bilirubin to rule out cholestasis.

[*]Derived from Newman, TB, et al.: Laboratory evaluation of jaundice in newborns: frequency, cost, and yield, *Am J Dis Child* 144:364–68, 1990.

---

dice, serum bilirubin concentrations characteristically may begin to decline in the first week and then rise again, often climbing well above the level at which early-onset jaundice usually peaks. Late-onset jaundice is generally defined as a serum bilirubin concentration exceeding 10 mg/dL in the third week of life (Winfield & MacFaul, 1978; Clarkson, Cowan & Herbison, 1984). Approximately two to four percent of all full-term, healthy, breastfeeding non-Asian neonates will exhibit this condition, which is sometimes called breastmilk jaundice. Usually, breastfed infants with late-onset jaundice will have had earlier higher serum bilirubin levels than breastfeeding infants of the same age who do not exhibit late-onset jaundice. A recent study has shown that some normal, healthy, breastfeeding infants will have elevated bilirubin levels through the 16th day of life. The only difference between these babies and other breastfeeding infants in the study was the levels of bilirubin in the baby's blood and the mother's milk. The authors noted that the babies with high serum bilirubin levels into the third week of life (36% of the sample) did not differ from the babies with low serum bilirubin levels with regard to infant age, maternal age, or frequency of breastfeeding per day. The findings from this study may imply that elevated bilirubin levels are more likely to be a normal (though not yet completely understood) consequence of adjustment to extrauterine life, rather than an indication of a potentially serious pathology which requires intervention (Alonso et al., 1991).

Correctly identifying late-onset jaundice first requires that all other causes be ruled out. Obvious causes include organic and functional problems, such as intestinal obstruction, hemolytic disease, hypothyroidism, inherited hepatic glucuronyl transferase deficiencies, and transient familial neonatal hyperbilirubinemia (Gartner & Auerbach, 1987). In addition, the infant with late-onset jaundice is thriving, vigorous, and healthy—and is gaining weight appropriately. Thus, the diagnosis is often made after ruling out other explanations for late elevations of serum bilirubin.

Numerous explanations have been offered for this condition—including inhibited glucuronyl transferase, free fatty acid concentrations, increased enteric absorption of unconjugated bilirubin, and the high fat content of human milk, which becomes a factor after lactation has been established.

Arias et al. (1964) reported that a small group of mothers whose infants presented with late-onset jaundice appeared to have milk which inhibited the conjugation of bilirubin. Specifically, these mothers' milk *in vitro* inhibited the conjugation of bilirubin by more than 50% when compared with the conjugation of bilirubin by mothers' milk whose infants did not exhibit the syndrome. Verification of the conjugation-inhibiting factor was borne out when milk from the mothers of infants with the syndrome was given to two normal, full-term infants. Their serum bilirubin concentrations rose, but returned to normal when administration of the icterogenic milk was discontinued (Arias & Gartner, 1964). However, with the exception of Arthur, Bevan, and Holton (1966), other investigators were

unable to replicate the findings of Arias and colleagues (1964).

Based on studies in a rat model, inhibition of conjugation of bilirubin by the liver can result in late-onset jaundice. The exact cause of the inhibition of such conjugation of bilirubin remains a mystery. Gartner, Lee, and Moscioni (1983) found that inhibiting milk appears to exaggerate the absorption of bilirubin, in contrast to the effect of human milk samples from mothers of babies not exhibiting late-onset jaundice. Their milk, as with bovine milk samples, serves to prevent the absorption of bilirubin.

Investigators have also examined the variability of fat content in human milk. Bevan and Holton (1972) reported that the milk from mothers whose babies had late-onset jaundice inhibited conjugation by the liver and that this inhibition was caused by the free fatty acid concentrations in the milk after refrigeration. However, Odiévre and Luzeau (1978, 1982), Odiévre et al. (1973), and others (Bevan & Holton, 1972; Hargreaves, 1973) reported that when fresh unrefrigerated milk from mothers of jaundiced infants was examined, no concentrations in free fatty acids were evident.

Colostrum, the first milk available to the baby (Humenick, 1987) and most prominent in feedings through the first week of life, contains relatively more protein and less fat than mature milk. Within mature milk, foremilk has fewer calories and hindmilk more calories. As each feed progresses, the amount of hindmilk available to the infant increases (Woodward, Rees & Boon, 1989). Speculation has existed for some time that it is this increase in cream content which triggers the infant to stop suckling (Hall, 1975). The higher fat content in some mothers' milk may be a risk factor for late-onset jaundice, according to Amato, Howald, and von Muralt (1985). They found that the milk from mothers of babies with hyperbilirubinemia had significantly higher cream content than did the milk from mothers of babies without hyperbilirubinemia. Although evidence of continued elevated serum bilirubin concentrations may exist for several weeks, this finding is not sufficient to warrant the interruption of breastfeeding. In nearly all cases, serum bilirubin concentrations will continue to decline slowly over many weeks, eventually plateauing at the normal adult level of 1mg/dL. Generally, the likelihood is high that all children of the same mother will exhibit a similar pattern if breastfed.

CLINICAL IMPLICATIONS

Most infants will have elevated serum bilirubin levels in the first week of life. Although a wide variety of variables has been linked to the likelihood of elevated serum bilirubin, including some over which the clinician has no control, many hospital routines also have been implicated, particularly those governing frequency and duration of feeding. (See the accompanying boxed chart.)

It is appropriate for the clinician to examine those routines currently followed to determine which can be most easily altered or eliminated in order to reduce the likelihood that initiation of infant feeding *of any kind* in an institution contributes to early-onset jaundice. Whenever hyperbilirubinemia manifests itself in the first day of life, pathologic jaundice should be suspected, and steps should be taken to identify the cause in order to effect appropriate treatment while avoiding unnecessary overtreatment. The breastfeeding mother and baby should be observed carefully and assisted to begin breastfeeding so that frequent, effective feedings occur. If the baby is feeding poorly and/or exhibiting lethargy, supplementation at the breast may be used to break the cycle of lethargy, poor feeding, climbing serum bilirubin concentrations, more lethargy, which can result in symptoms of jaundice (Auerbach, 1986). For most breastfed babies, early-onset jaundice will peak on the fourth or fifth day, to be followed by a gradual decline in serum bilirubin levels as they approach the normal adult level of 1mg/dL.

The race of the infant and his parents should be noted in order to appropriately assess the baby's serum bilirubin levels. In the case of an American Indian infant or a baby of Mediterranean extraction, a test for glucose 6-phosphate dehydrogenase (G_6PD) should be requested.

Supplemental feedings of sterile water or glucose are neither indicated nor appropriate. If the baby is given phototherapy (which is rarely needed), the mother should be urged to offer feedings frequently, at least every two hours, to reduce the likelihood of dehydration. In situations in which mother and baby are still hospitalized, mobile phototherapy units placed in the mother's room will enable frequent feeding and more careful monitoring of the baby than occurs in busy nurseries, where crying babies tend to receive the most attention.

For the small percentage of infants who exhibit late-onset jaundice, organic or functional causes must first be ruled out. If the infant is thriving, frequent monitoring of serum bilirubin levels is recommended in order to discern whether the levels remain within an acceptable range. No known cases of kernicterus caused by breastmilk jaundice have been reported (Auerbach & Gartner, 1987); caution dictates that the risk of brain damage be minimized through careful monitoring and intervention in those situations in which serum bilirubin concentrations significantly exceed 20 mg/dL.

In most cases, the concentration of serum bilirubin will peak and then decline while the baby continues to breastfeed. Discreet observation of the infant and continued support and reassurance to the mother are all that is necessary. (See the boxed list of questions on p. 343.) In rare situations in which concentrations of serum bilirubin continue to climb, a brief period of breastfeeding supplementation may be helpful. Such supplementation can occur at the breast using a feeding tube device such as the Supplemental Nutrition System (SNS)™. The milk of another mother whose baby does not exhibit late-onset jaundice, or artificial formula made from bovine milk or a vegetable substitute, can be used in the feeding

HOSPITAL ROUTINES AND THEIR EFFECTS ON THE NEONATE

Hospital routines	Effect of routines on the neonate
Limited or infrequent feedings	Slowed gut motility
	Reduced stooling
	Greater frequency, volume of supplemental feeds
	Greater weight loss
	Higher bilirubin levels
Sterile water/glucose feedings	Caloric deprivation, contributory to "starvation-induced" jaundice
	Muting of thirst response
	Reduced neonatal interest in feeding
	Slowed weight gain
	Reduced breastmilk intake
	Slowed bilirubin clearance
	Higher bilirubin levels
Separation of mother and baby	Reduced satisfaction with hospital care
	Increased likelihood of supplementation
	Shorter breastfeeding duration
Phototherapy for jaundice	Increased risk of dehydration
	Separation of mother and baby
	Increased length of hospital stay
	Increased costs of hospitalization
	Shorter breastfeeding duration
	Abnormal care-giving patterns
	Enhanced likelihood of Incipient Vulnerable Child syndrome
	Greater frequency of use of expensive health-care facilities post hospitalization
	Questionable benefit in reducing bilirubin levels
	Shorter breastfeeding duration
Laboratory evaluations	Overall higher cost of hospital care
	More frequent use of additional laboratory tests
	Limited benefit for the majority of cases
	Increased parental anxiety

tube device. The addition of such milk will result in a decline in concentrations of serum bilirubin. When the mother prefers to give her baby only her own milk in the face of significant rises of concentrations of serum bilirubin which are suggestive of late-onset jaundice, her expressed milk should be heated to 56°C for 15 minutes and then cooled to body temperature prior to being offered to the baby in a bottle. Such heat treatment appears to alter the milk so that concentrations of serum bilirubin are reduced.

If the mother prefers to interrupt breastfeeding for 24 to 48 hours and give the baby some other milk from a bottle, this too will result in a decline in concentrations of serum bilirubin. After such a brief interruption, unsupplemented breastfeeding can continue. An initial small rebound response will occur, followed by gradually declining concentrations of bilirubin. Inter-

---

KEY QUESTIONS TO ASK WHEN ASSESSING THE RELATIONSHIP OF FEEDING TO JAUNDICE[*]

1. *How often is the infant being put to breast?* The total number of such episodes in each 24-hour period, as well as the duration of each episode should be noted.
2. *Is the baby suckling when put to breast?* Active suckling should be noted; in particular, the pattern and frequency of swallowing should be recorded.
3. *Has the baby begun stooling, and if so, how frequently is this continuing to occur?* Early stooling which does not continue may be an early indication of inadequate intake, particularly of a calorically dense fluid such as milk. If stooling is occurring, note the color and explain to the mother how she can verify through changes in stool color that the baby is obtaining milk from the breast.
4. *Is the baby receiving complementary or supplementary feedings?* Fluids offered after breastfeedings and fluids offered *in lieu* of breastfeedings may contribute to serious breastfeeding problems; they should be avoided. If additional fluid is deemed medically necessary, it should contain as many calories as human milk to avoid starvation-induced jaundice from insufficient caloric intake.
5. *Is the mother encouraged to nurse her infant at night?* In order to ensure frequent feedings, the lactating mother and her breastfeeding infant should have ample opportunities to breastfeed throughout the 24-hour day. In light of research which reveals that more appropriate neonatal and maternal sleep patterns occur when babies room-in (Keefe, 1987) and that more responsive care-giving ensues with such an arrangement (Keefe, 1988), the new family is well served when they have uninterrupted access to one another through the nighttime hours.

Derived from Auerbach, KG, and Gartner, LM: Breastfeeding and human milk: their association with jaundice in the neonate, *Clin Perinatol* 14:89–107, 1987.

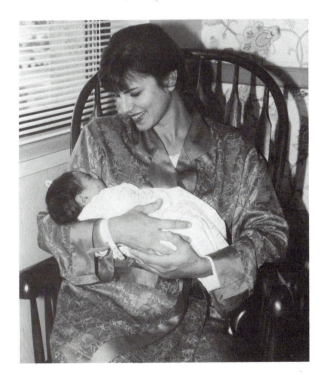

FIGURE 12–2 Neonatal jaundice rarely requires that breastfeeding be interrupted. (Courtesy Debi Leslie Bocar.)

rupting breastfeeding even for a few feedings is rarely needed and is discouraged since other methods of management will usually suffice. (See Table 12–2.)

SUMMARY

Jaundice in the newborn, in most cases, is an exaggeration of a normal physiologic process that can be managed conservatively and is not a contraindication of breastfeeding. If we understand the normal physiologic process and intervene only when absolutely necessary, there is no contraindication to the neonate's consumption of human milk, either by direct suckling at the breast or by tube-feeding for those who may be too small or too young to suckle.

Breastfeeding should never be interrupted because of a diagnosis of "physiologic" jaundice and should only rarely be interrupted for pathologic jaundice. Even in the presence of jaundice which is thought to be brought about by the breastmilk itself, there is no reason to wean the baby. Breastfeeding should be strongly encouraged for all mothers and all babies.

TABLE 12–2 CLINICAL CARE PLAN FOR PHYSIOLOGIC JAUNDICE

NURSING DIAGNOSIS: Deficit of maternal knowledge about physiologic jaundice

Case notes: A two-day-old Caucasian male neonate has a total bilirubin concentration of 8 mg/dL. At three days, the level is 13 mg/dL. The infant's skin about his head has a yellow cast when pressed above the nose and on the forehead; the rest of his body remains pink. The baby has been vigorous since birth and is breastfeeding effectively. The parents are concerned that "something might be wrong with our baby."

Assessment	Goals	Intervention	Rationale
Bilirubin rising 5 mg/day	Maintain lactation	Increase number of breastfeedings (q 3 hr at night; q 2 hr during day)	Milk intake stimulates bilirubin excretion
Yellowish cast confined to head	Reduce bilirubin levels	Discourage water/glucose feedings	Increase caloric intake
		Place infant near natural light	Natural light breaks down unconjugated bilirubin
Baby alert and vigorous	Prevent neuro complications	Obtain serum bilirubin q 24 hrs until levels decline	
		Observe for irritability and/or lethargy	
Sucking effectively	Maintain adequate hydration	Monitor number of wet diapers and stools (color, consistency)	
Breastfeeding *ad lib* until satiation 8–12 times/24 hrs		Observe for swallowing during feedings	
Parents express concern, confusion, anxiety about baby's status	Provide emotional support	Explain reason for jaundice and its benign nature	Teaching basic facts about jaundice fosters understanding and relieves unvoiced parental guilt feelings
		Reassure that lactation can and should continue	
		Encourage parents to express their concerns	Verbalization reduces anxiety
		Assure parents that baby's skin color will return to normal	
		Reassure parents that jaundice is not caused by anything they did or did not do; it is a normal occurrence of early neonatal life	

REFERENCES

Adams, JA, Hey, DJ, and Hall, RT: Incidence of hyperbilirubinemia in breast- vs. formula-fed infants, *Clin Pediatr* 24:69–73, 1985.

Alonso, EM, et al.: Enterohepatic circulation of nonconjugated bilirubin in rats fed with human milk, *J Pediatr* 118:425–30, 1991.

Amato, M, Howald, H, and von Muralt, G: Fat content of human milk and breast milk jaundice, *Acta Paediatr Scand* 74:805–6, 1985.

Arias, IM, and Gartner, LM: Production of unconjugated hyperbilirubinemia in full-term new-born infants following administration of pregnane-3(alpha), 20(beta)–diol, *Nature* 203:1292–93, 1964.

Arias, IM, et al.: Prolonged neonatal unconjugated hyperbilirubinemia associated with breast feeding and a steroid, pregnane-3(alpha), 20 (beta)-diol, in maternal milk that inhibits glucuronide formation in vitro, *J Clin Invest* 43:2037–47, 1964.

Arthur, LJH, Bevan, BR, and Holton, JB: Neonatal hyperbilirubinemia and breast feeding, *Dev Med Child Neurol* 8:279–84, 1966.

Auerbach, KG: Supportive management of the jaundiced breastfeeding infant, *Rental Roundup* 3:5–6, 1986.

Auerbach, KG, and Gartner, LM: Breastfeeding and human milk: their association with jaundice in the neonate, *Clin Perinatol* 14:89–107, 1987.

Bernbaum, JC, et al.: Enhanced growth and gastrointestinal function in premature infants given non-nutritive sucking, *Pediatr Res* 15:650, 1981.

Bevan, BR, and Holton, JB: Inhibition of bilirubin conjugation in rat liver slices by free fatty acids, with relevance to the problem of breast milk jaundice, *Clin Chim Acta* 41:101–7, 1972.

Bracci, R, et al.: Epidemiologic study of neonatal jaundice: a survey of contributing factors, *Acta Paediatr Scand* (suppl.) 360:87–92, 1989.

Butler, DA, and MacMillan, JP: Relationship of breast feeding and weight loss to jaundice in the newborn period: review of the literature and results of a study, *Cleve Clin Q* 50:263–66, 1983.

Cavell, B: Gastric emptying in infants fed human milk or infant formula, *Acta Paediatr Scand* 70:639–41, 1981.

Chalmers, I, Campbell, H, and Turnbull, AC: Use of oxytocin and incidence of neonatal jaundice, *Br Med J* 2:116–18, 1975.

Clarkson, JE, Cowan, JO, and Herbison, GP: Jaundice in full term healthy neonates—a population study, *Aust Paediatr J* 20:303–8, 1984.

Dahms, BB, et al.: Breast feeding and serum bilirubin values during the first 4 days of life, *J Pediatr* 83:1049–54, 1973.

De Carvalho, M, Hall, M, and Harvey, D: Effects of water supplementation on physiological jaundice in breastfed babies, *Arch Dis Child* 56:568–69, 1981.

De Carvalho, M, Klaus, MH, and Merkatz, RB: Frequency of breast-feeding and serum bilirubin concentration, *Am J Dis Child* 136:737–38, 1982.

De Carvalho, M, Robertson, S, and Klaus, M: Fecal bilirubin excretion and serum bilirubin concentrations in breast-fed and bottle-fed infants, *J Pediatr* 107:786–90, 1985.

Elander, G, and Lindberg, T: Hospital routines in infants with hyperbilirubinemia influence the duration of breast feeding, *Acta Paediatr Scand* 75:708–12, 1986.

Fischer, AF, et al.: Comparison of bilirubin production in Japanese and Caucasian infants, *J Pediatr Gastroenterol Nutr* 7:27–29, 1988.

Gale, R, et al.: Epidemiology of neonatal jaundice in the Jerusalem population, *J Pediatr Gastroenterol Nutr* 10:82–86, 1990.

Gartner, LM, and Auerbach, KG: Breast milk and breastfeeding jaundice, In Barness, LA, et al., eds.: *Advances in Pediatrics,* Volume 34, Chicago, 1987, Year Book Medical Publishers, Inc., pp. 249–74.

Gartner, LM, Lee, KS, and Moscioni, AD: Effect of milk feeding on intestinal bilirubin absorption in the rat, *J Pediatr* 103:464–71, 1983.

Gartner, LM, et al.: Development of bilirubin transport and metabolism in the newborn rhesus monkey, *J Pediatr* 90:513–31, 1977.

Glover, J, and Sandilands, M: Supplementation of breast-feeding infants and weight loss in hospital, *J Hum Lact* 6:163–66, 1990.

Gould, SR, et al.: Influence of previous oral contraception and maternal oxytocin infusion on neonatal jaundice, *Br Med J* 3:228–30, 1974.

Hall, B: Changing composition of human milk and early development of an appetite control, *Lancet* 1:779–81, 1975.

Hall, RT, et al.: Hyperbilirubinemia in breast- versus formula-fed infants in the first six weeks of life: relationship to weight gain, *Am J Perinatol* 1:47–51, 1983.

Hargreaves, T: Effect of fatty acids on bilirubin conjugation, *Arch Dis Child* 48:446–50, 1973.

Horiguchi, T, and Bauer, C: Ethnic differences in neonatal jaundice: comparison of Japanese and Caucasian newborn infants, *Am J Obstet Gynecol* 121:71–74, 1975.

Humenick, SS: The clinical significance of breastmilk maturation rates, *Birth* 14:174–79, 1987.

Johnson, JD, et al.: Exaggerated jaundice in Navajo neonates, *Am J Dis Child* 140:889–90, 1986.

Keefe, MR: Comparison of neonatal nighttime sleep-wake patterns in nursery versus rooming-in environments, *Nurs Res* 36:140–44, 1987.

Keefe, MR: The impact of infant rooming-in on maternal sleep at night, *JOGNN* 17:122–26, 1988.

Kemper, K, Forsyth, B, and McCarthy, P: Jaundice, terminating breast-feeding, and the vulnerable child, *Pediatrics* 84:773–78, 1989.

Kemper, KJ, Forsyth, BW, and McCarthy, PL: Persistent perceptions of vulnerability following neonatal jaundice, *Am J Dis Child* 144:238–41, 1990.

Kivlahan, C, and James, EJP: The natural history of neonatal jaundice, *Pediatrics* 74:364–70, 1984.

Kuhr, M, and Paneth, N: Feeding practices and early neonatal jaundice, *J Pediatr Gastroenterol Nutr* 1:485–88, 1982.

Laws, HF: Caloric deprivation questioned in breast milk jaundice (letter), *Pediatrics* 67:748–49, 1981.

Maisels, MJ, and Gifford, K: Neonatal jaundice in full-term infants: role of breast-feeding and other causes, *Am J Dis Child* 137:561–62, 1983.

Maisels, MJ, et al.: Jaundice in the healthy newborn infant: a new approach to an old problem, *Pediatrics* 81:505–11, 1988.

Matthews, MK: The relationship between maternal labour analgesia and delay in the initiation of breastfeeding in healthy neonates in the early neonatal period, *Midwifery* 5:3–10, 1989.

McDonagh, AF: Is bilirubin good for you? *Clin Perinatol* 17:359–69, 1990.

Newman, AJ, and Gross, S: Hyperbilirubinemia in breast-fed infants, *Pediatrics* 32:995–1001, 1963.

Newman, TB, and Maisels, MJ: Does hyperbilirubinemia damage the brain of healthy full-term infants? *Clin Perinatol* 17:331–58, 1990.

Newman, TB, et al.: Laboratory evaluation of jaundice in newborns: frequency, cost, and yield, *Am J Dis Child* 144:364–68, 1990.

Nicoll, A, Ginsburg, R, and Tripp, JH: Supplementary feeding and jaundice in newborns, *Acta Paediatr Scand* 71:759–61, 1982.

Odiévre, M, and Luzeau, R: Liplytic activity in milk from mothers of unjaundiced infants, *Acta Paediatr Scand* 67:49–52, 1978.

Odiévre, M, and Luzeau, R: More on breast-milk jaundice (letter), *J Pediatr* 100:671–72, 1982.

Odiévre, M, et al.: Effect of fatty acids on bilirubin conjugation, *Arch Dis Child* 48:984, 1973.

Osborn, LM, Reiff, MI, and Bolus, R: Jaundice in the full-term neonate, *Pediatrics* 73:520–25, 1985.

Saland, J, McNamara, H, and Cohen, MI: Navajo jaundice: a variant of neonatal hyperbilirubinemia associated with breastfeeding, *J Pediatr* 85:271–75, 1974.

Stevenson, DK, et al.: Pulmonary excretion of carbon monoxide in the human infant as an index of bilirubin production. IV: Effects of breast-feeding and caloric intake in the first postnatal week, *Pediatrics* 65:1170–72, 1980.

Taitz, LS, and Byers, HD: High calorie osmolar feeding and hypertonic dehydration, *Arch Dis Child* 57:257–60, 1972.

Tomamasa, T, et al.: Gastroduodenal motility in neonates: response to human milk compared with cow's milk formula, *Pediatrics* 80:434–38, 1987.

Weaver, LT, Ewing, G, and Taylor, LC: The bowel habit of milk-fed infants, *J Pediatr Gastroenterol Nutr* 7:568–71, 1988.

Winfield, CR, and MacFaul, R: Clinical study of prolonged jaundice in breast- and bottle-fed babies, *Arch Dis Child* 53:506–7, 1978.

Wood, B, et al.: Factors affecting neonatal jaundice, *Arch Dis Child* 54:111–15, 1979.

Woodward, DR, Rees, B, and Boon, JA: Human milk fat content: within-feed variation, *Early Hum Dev* 19:39–46, 1989.

SECTION
FOUR

Postnatal Period

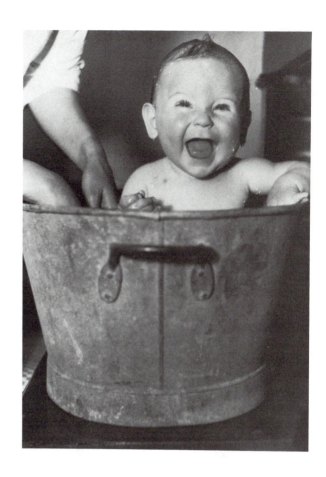

Most mothers are healthy when they give birth and begin breastfeeding. Some mothers are not. Other mothers encounter difficulties, many of which are preventable, and nearly all of which have solutions that will preserve the breastfeeding course. Nevertheless, other activities will influence whether and for how long the mother breastfeeds. Two such issues are her employment outside the home and concerns relating to control of her fertility and her resumption of sexual activity following the birth of her breastfeeding infant.

13

Maternal Health

Jan Riordan

Kathleen G. Auerbach

This section of the book continues with a discussion of acute and chronic maternal health problems that are considered to have an effect on lactation. The health of a mother directly affects her ability (both emotional and physical) to care for her infant. During their childbearing years, women, as a general rule, are healthy and fit. Illness is usually episodic: a head cold or a case of influenza. The nurse or LC, therefore, does not see many of the more serious health conditions described here. When she does, it is expected that she have a working knowledge of these conditions as well as the ability to develop a plan of care based on the wishes and needs of the breastfeeding mother who has a health problem.

MATERNAL NUTRITION: BASIC GUIDELINES

During the "hunger winter" in Holland in 1944–45, women were systematically undernourished as a result of wartime conditions. Dutch infants who were born during this period were found not to be affected by their mothers' inadequate nutritional intake. Slightly less maternal milk was produced than in previous years when the food supply was more ample, but neither duration of breastfeeding nor infant growth patterns were affected (Smith, 1947). Malnourished Brazilian women actually produce milk with a slightly higher fat content than well-nourished women (Spring et al., 1985); Nepalese women with milk protein malnutrition breastfed babies who were in the low-normal-range of weight and length for age yet appeared healthy; Bangladeshi women considered "marginally nourished" maintain an aver-

age daily milk production of 750 grams (Brown et al., 1986). These worldwide studies, taken together, support the theory that maternal nutrition has only a modest effect on milk production and on milk composition in the face of malnutrition.

While "mother nature" appears to protect maternal milk, maternal nutrition is an appropriate subject for discussion in relation to pregnancy and subsequent lactation. During pregnancy, many women are motivated to follow a more balanced and varied diet than they may have before they were pregnant. This motivation needs to be encouraged during lactation as well, although the emphasis on maintaining a "good" diet needs to be tempered by an understanding that caloric intake of *any* kind by the mother will assist in sustaining lactation. The lactating mother need not maintain a caloric intake that is markedly higher than she maintained prior to pregnancy: in most cases 200 to 500 calories in excess of that which is needed to maintain her own body weight will be sufficient.

Increased fluids also help, but should not be overemphasized. What the mother drinks will not markedly affect what she will provide to the baby through her breasts (whether this fluid is measured by quantity or assessed by color). If the mother drinks to meet her own thirst needs, she will be drinking enough to sustain lactation. The easiest way to assure this is to suggest that the mother have something to drink each time she sits down to breastfeed the baby. Additionally, she can check the color of her own urine as she voids throughout the day. With the exception of the first morning urination, if she is drinking enough liquids, her urine will be clear to light yellow. At the same time, she should not drink too many fluids as it may result in a reduction of milk production (Stumbo et al., 1985; Dusdieker et al., 1985, 1990; Illingworth & Kilpatrick, 1953).

A woman should be encouraged to follow a diet appropriate to her culture or subculture, eating foods with different colors, flavors, and textures—and in as natural state as possible. She should avoid processed foods as much as possible, particularly those using refined sugars. If the mother does not overeat and keeps her intake of animal fat low, she is unlikely to gain weight while she is breastfeeding, particularly in the early weeks when she is using more energy to make milk for her infant who is breastfeeding exclusively and nursing frequently.

The mother who chooses to diet while lactating should be encouraged to avoid crash or "fad" diets which promise large, quick weight loss, since fat-soluble environmental contaminants and toxins are released into the milk when caloric intake is severely restricted. Additionally, a marked reduction of caloric intake can result in fussiness in some babies. A safe maternal weight loss regimen includes careful analysis of the mother's own prepregnancy caloric needs, accompanied by a plan that enables her to maintain her own nutritional needs while the caloric content is gradually reduced. In most cases, a weight loss of no more than two pounds per week can be sustained during lactation without compromising the baby's milk supply or cream content. Butte and colleagues (1984a) found that mothers with less than 20% body fat did not produce less milk; rather, they ate more. These investigators also found that mothers who ate up to 2186 kcal/day not only produced ample milk but also experienced a gradual loss of maternal weight.

Numerous questions continue to be asked about the relationship between maternal nutritional intake and its effect on a mother's lactation course—as well as the effect of lactation on the mother's nutritional status. Following are nine frequently asked questions and answers:

1. *Aren't women at risk for loss of bone mineralization caused by calcium loss when they breastfeed?* No. While breastfeeding women's bone mineral content has been reported to be less than that of bottle-feeding mothers, other studies have found no reduction of bone density in women who

have breastfed up to four children (Hayslip et al., 1989; Koetting & Wardlaw, 1988).

2. *What about vitamin D? Can mothers provide enough of this vitamin to protect their breastfeeding babies against rickets?* Yes. Even in countries in the northern hemisphere where sunlight may be severely limited for several months of the year, there is no need to be concerned (Specker et al., 1987). One study found that among vegetarian women serum vitamin D concentrations were considerably higher among the lactating than among the nonlactating women (Ala-Houhala et al., 1988).

3. *Is it possible for teen-age mothers—who are still growing themselves—to make milk that will support appropriate infant growth?* Yes. Lipsman, Dewey, and Lonnerdal (1985) found only minimal differences between milk samples from teen-age mothers and older mothers; these differences probably had to do with when milk expression occurred. The mothers in their sample, regardless of age, were able to breastfeed successfully without compromising their infants' growth.

4. *What about folic acid? These are important to the growing infant.* Folate deficiency and resulting anemia is highly unlikely in the breastfeeding baby. One study found that folate levels in breastfeeding infants were two to three times higher than maternal levels and that nearly all of the comparison formula-fed babies had levels below the lowest concentrations in the breastfed infants. The authors raised concerns about the risk of folate deficiency in the formula-fed infants, not in their breastfed counterparts (Salmenpera, Perheentupa & Siimes, 1986).

5. *What about fatty acids? Does what the mother eats affect what is in the milk?* Yes. The dietary fatty acids consumed by the mother will be reflected in the milk the baby receives. Thus, if her diet is high in polyunsaturated fatty acids, these same fatty acids will predominate in the baby's milk (Vuori et al., 1982).

6. *What about vitamin B_6? If the mother's levels are low, will this affect her milk supply or her baby in any way?* Yes. Vitamin B_6 is an important water-soluble vitamin that is necessary for amino acid metabolism. A vitamin-B_6 deficiency in the mother's milk has recently been found to be related to lethargy in the baby and greater difficulty in consoling the infant when he became distressed (McCullough et al., 1990).

7. *What about iron in the mother's milk?* Several investigators have reported that breastfed infants use the iron available to them from their mothers' milk more efficiently than do babies being fed artifi-

cial milks (Woodruff, Latham & McDavid, 1977; Mc-Millan, Landaw & Oski, 1976). Duncan et al. (1985) found that the exclusively breastfed infant was not at risk for iron deficiency during the first six months of life. Pastel, Howanitz, and Oski (1981) found that exclusive breastfeeding through at least nine months met the iron requirements of full-term infants. In addition, investigators have reported that the gut flora and fecal specimens of infants fed artificial formula is closer to human milk patterns when they are not fed iron-fortified formulas (Mevissen-Verhage et al., 1985). In addition, it has been reported that breastfed infants who are fed solid foods early experience a drop in their iron absorption, thus suggesting a change in the bioavailability of iron to such infants (Oski & Landaw, 1980). Given these findings, the mother would be well advised to exclusively breastfeed her infant for as long as possible through the first six months of life without concern about the baby's iron stores. Thereafter, solid foods should be added slowly; if artificial formula is used, she might consider the low-iron varieties, rather than those that have been fortified with extra iron, until after her baby has completely weaned from the breast.

8. *Doesn't caffeine cause jitteriness in the baby and shouldn't the mother avoid such substances?* Caffeine, which is present in a wide variety of beverages and foods, appears to be present in very small to nondetectable levels in infant serum (Berlin et al., 1984; Ryu, 1985a, 1985b; Fulton, 1990). Nevertheless, the potential delay in elimination which has been observed in premature infants (LeGuennec & Billon, 1987) may be sufficient reason to avoid large quantities in the early postpartum period when its effect is most likely to be noticeable. Drinking an occasional beverage with caffeine is unlikely to have the same effect as continual doses.

9. *What are the nutritional consequences if the pregnant mother breastfeeds?* In many regions of the world, women breastfeed one child while they are pregnant with the next. Among rural Guatemalan women participating in a nutrition-supplementation study, lactation overlapped with pregnancy in one-half of the pregnancies. These pregnant mothers adjusted to the increased demands by eating more food supplements, and breastfeeding did not significantly affect the growth of their unborn babies (Merchant, Martorell & Hass, 1990).

Virtually everyone agrees that nutrition practices in the United States are poor; foods contain too much fat and processed sugars. One easy way for pregnant and breastfeeding mothers to improve their nutrition—and that of their family—is to eat more whole foods. About one-third of the calories that Americans take in come from "dismembered," not whole food. About two-thirds of our calories come from dismembered or partitioned foods such as purified sugar, fats and oils; they have been separated from whole foods, e.g., soybeans, milk, and milled grains (primarily white flour) which have had their nutrient-rich germ and bran removed. All of these dismembered foods supply calories, but little or none of the vitamins, minerals, and amino acids present in whole foods. Davis (1983) points out that "when individuals take half, two-thirds or even more of their calories in the form of dismembered foods, they automatically substantially reduce their intakes of all 45 nutrients across the board, and they significantly estrange themselves from our biological heritage of eating only the cells and tissues of plant and animal origin." Fig. 13–1 is a helpful eating guide, for

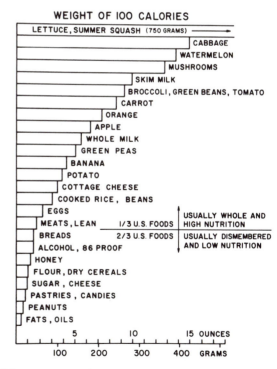

FIGURE 13–1 The weight of 100 calories of various foods. Small servings of dismembered foods supply the same number of calories as much larger servings of most whole foods. As a result, most people greatly overestimate the fraction of their diet which comes from whole foods. From Davis, DR: Nutrition in the United States: Much room for improvement, *J Appl Nutr* 356:17–29, 1983.

it graphically portrays caloric density by showing the weight of 100 calories of various foods.

FOODS THAT PASS THROUGH MILK

Most mothers can eat any food they wish without observing a problem in the baby. While milk is flavored by what the mother ingests, babies do not seem to mind. Some mothers, according to their culture, however, choose to avoid eating certain foods in order to avoid problems during pregnancy or lactation. In a study of Sudanese women, protein sources as well as salty, sour, and spicy foods were avoided during pregnancy on the grounds that these foods contributed to heartburn, diarrhea, colic, nausea, and vomiting (Osman, 1985). During lactation, these same women believed that prenatal restrictions of protein-rich foods should be removed and that energy-rich foods should be added to the diet as well. Drinking cow's milk was thought to increase their own milk production. The Sudanese culture values coming out of the postpartum period "fatter" than when the women had become pregnant. "It is considered a social prestige for her mother or the close relative who was nursing her, and indicates that she had been well looked after" (Osman, 1985).

Among women in Australia, a wide variety of foods are avoided by breastfeeding mothers, including (in order of frequency mentioned) cabbage, chocolates, spicy foods, peas, onions, cauliflower, and many other fruits or vegetables. The reasons given for avoiding these foods was their presumed association with problems for the breastfeeding baby—specifically colic and/or flatulence, diarrhea, and skin rashes, particularly on the face or diaper area. Cow's milk and dairy products were not among the proscribed foods, although they have been implicated in making symptoms of atopic disease worse in family members with a history of allergies (Eaton-Evans & Dugdale, 1986). Aside from cultural preferences, mothers can eat what they like, by and large, without any effects on their breastfeeding baby.

MATERNAL WEIGHT

The concerns lactating women have about their weight may be on either end of the weight spectrum: the mother is underweight and undernourished and concerned that undernourishment will reduce her milk production and/or the creamy portion of her milk. More commonly in developed countries, the mother is overweight and concerned that she will gain weight during her lactation course and/or be unable to diet.

The mother who breastfeeds can enjoy a diet that is higher in calories because she uses additional energy to make milk. At the same time her basal metabolic rate remains the same as the woman who is not lactating (Motil, Montandon & Garza, 1990). Many women lose unwanted weight during lactation without engaging in a weight loss program. Instead, they eat sufficiently to meet their own needs, yet lose weight through the energy their bodies use to make milk for their babies. Examination of the frequency of feedings, particularly in the first six months postpartum, reveals that women who breastfeed more frequently tend to lose weight more rapidly than women who breastfeed less frequently (Dugdale & Eaton-Evans, 1989). Furthermore, breastfeeding mothers tend to lose more weight in the first six months postpartum than bottle-feeding mothers (Bradshaw & Pfeiffer, 1988). However, if the new mother exercises, she will not diminish her milk production. Lovelady, Lonnerdal, and Dewey (1990) found that women who exercised gained less weight during their pregnancies; in addition, they made more milk, expended more energy, and were able to eat more than nonexercising women. Lactation was not adversely affected by exercise; in fact, overall breastmilk volume was higher when the women exercised.

Women who are undernourished face a different concern. They may worry that their milk is not good enough and thus they should not breastfeed. In the United States and other developed countries, too much emphasis has been placed on assuring a "good" diet *in order to breastfeed*. Yet, numerous studies have found that even women who have been undernourished their entire lives have provided ample breastmilk of a quality sufficient to enable their infants to grow and thrive for several months on breastmilk alone. The issue thus may not be *what* the mother eats, but rather that she receives food. If she does not obtain enough calories, her fat stores will be insufficient and depleted more rapidly. Where she obtains those calories may not always be optimal, but that she obtains them is critical. For the lactation consultant or other health-care worker who is providing information on nutrition, the primary message is that the mother should eat foods that will meet her needs for protein, carbohydrates, and fats. Ideally, she will choose foods which have a caloric content that is balanced with other foods that complement one another. In a situation where that is not possible, the priority is caloric intake rather than the "right" foods.

ALTERATIONS IN ENDOCRINE AND METABOLIC FUNCTIONING

Anything that affects the control of the endocrine system can also affect the production of breastmilk. The following discussion of diabetes mellitus, thyroid problems, and pituitary dysfunction explains uncommon conditions that may affect the breastfeeding mother's milk supply. Any woman with symptoms that suggest she might have an altered metabolic functioning should be referred to a physician for further testing.

DIABETES MELLITUS

Diabetes mellitus is a chronic disease of impaired carbohydrate metabolism caused by insufficient insulin or the inefficient use of insulin. Diabetes mellitus is classified into two main categories: insulin-dependent diabetes mellitus (IDDM) and noninsulin-dependent diabetes mellitus. Gestational diabetes is a glucose intolerance which manifests itself only during pregnancy. Most women with gestational diabetes will revert to normal and be reclassified as being impaired glucose tolerant following the birth of the baby. This discussion deals with insulin-dependent diabetes.

Any insulin-dependent pregnant woman is considered a high-risk obstetric patient (Summary and Recommendations of the Second International Workshop-Conference on Gestational Diabetes Mellitus, 1985). During pregnancy blood glucose levels should be kept below 130 mg/dL as much as possible. During labor, delivery, and for some time after delivery, blood glucose levels must be closely monitored. The mother receives insulin in intravenous dextrose and Ringer's solution, carefully regulated by an infusion pump or the Biostator. Cesarean deliveries are much more likely for the mother with diabetes.

The woman with insulin-dependent diabetes not only can breastfeed her infant but should be encouraged to do so despite the necessary technology required to bring the diabetic mother and her infant safely through childbirth (Engelking & Page-Lieberman, 1986). Colostrum helps to stabilize the infant's blood sugar and although breastfeeding should begin as soon after birth as possible, this usually does not occur. Babies of diabetic mothers are considered high-risk infants and are routinely placed in the special or intensive care unit immediately following delivery. Even if breastfeedings are delayed the mother should be encouraged to begin pumping as soon as she feels able. Delay in breastfeeding may be responsible for a lower volume of breastmilk in diabetic mothers following birth (Bitman et al., 1989; Miyake, 1989).

While studying 48 British women with IDDM, Whichelow and Doddridge (1983) described a change in hospital policy whereby the neonates of these mothers were no longer routinely separated from their mothers and taken to the special care unit. This change was accompanied by increases from 41 to 60% of infants who first suckled within 12 hours of delivery—and from 53 to 70% in the prevalence of mothers who were still breastfeeding at three months. Fewer mothers complained of difficulty in getting the infant to grasp the nipple and suckle well when breastfeeding was initiated early.

During the immediate postnatal period, sudden but normal hormonal changes cause drastic fluctuation in maternal blood glucose levels. Maternal hypoglycemia can be expected to occur from immediately postbirth to five to seven hours after delivery; insulin requirements usually decrease abruptly. In addition, lactose excretion in the urine drops to a low level two to five days after birth and then rises rapidly. These sudden metabolic shifts require close monitoring.

Lactose is reabsorbed from the breast and is normally excreted in the urine; therefore nurses and mothers should be aware that in testing the urine after delivery, the presence of lactose may result in a false-positive test if copper-reducing urine testing (Clinitest) is used. For this reason, Testape or Diastix, which measure only the glucose, is the preferred method. Once physiologically stable, the patient can return to subcutaneous injection insulin or to injection via a portable infusion pump. The pump is strapped to trunk, wrist, arm, or leg and automatically injects the correct insulin dosage throughout the day.

The Ames Glucometer or Dextrometer system is a

reliable, preferred method of testing blood glucose that can continue to be used by the mother at home. By keeping a daily record of blood glucose levels, the mother can self-monitor day-to-day changes. Once the blood glucose level stabilizes, it is generally lower during lactation. Ferris et al. (1988) compared 30 mothers with IDDM with 30 controls and found that fasting plasma glucose levels during the exclusive breastfeeding period were significantly lower than the glucose levels of the women with IDDM who had stopped breastfeeding, or who had never breastfed even in the face of markedly higher caloric intake by the breastfeeding mothers. Given the continuous conversion of glucose to galactose and lactose during milk synthesis, less insulin is required than if the mother were not breastfeeding. Davies et al. (1989) showed that diabetic women may need to reduce their insulin dose by about 27% of their prepregnancy dose to avoid hypoglycemic reactions.

Breastmilk nutrients vary slightly. Breastmilk fat content, especially the medium-chain fatty acids, appear to be slightly lower in diabetic women than in nondiabetic women (Bitman et al., 1989). Butte and colleagues (1987) studied five moderately controlled women with IDDM at three months postpartum. Milk concentrations of total nitrogen, lactose, fat, and energy were indistinguishable from concentrations in the milk of nondiabetic women; however, glucose concentrations in the milk of the diabetic women was higher and more variable, as was sodium.

In addition to the known physiological advantages of breastfeeding for both her infant and herself, breastfeeding helps fulfill the diabetic mother's need to feel normal. An advantage of working with diabetic women is their keen awareness of their body functions and the importance of diet. More than the average woman, they are knowledgeable about physiology and are quick to notice changes that forewarn problems.

Any sudden drop in blood glucose appears to affect milk production because of the secretion of epinephrine that accompanies hypoglycemia. For example, one mother's blood glucose level suddenly dropped to 19 mg/dL eight days following a cesarean birth. For the next 24 hours, which were spent in the hospital, she was unable to express any milk using an electric pump; but in the following days after returning home she began to rebuild her milk supply.

Diabetic mothers' breastfeeding experiences are like those of mothers who are not diabetic—except that there is some evidence that mothers with diabetes may be more susceptible to mastitis, especially if they are not well controlled (Ferris et al., 1988; Guthrie & Guthrie, 1982). Any infection will quickly raise the level of blood glucose. Self-care teaching should emphasize the importance of recognizing early symptoms of mastitis and seeking prompt treatment while continuing to breastfeed. Diabetic mothers also are at risk for candidiasis if blood glucose levels are elevated. Preventing this problem involves careful control of blood glucose, drying the nipple after breastfeeding, and being aware of the early symptoms (see Chapter 14 on Breast-Related Problems).

The mother with diabetes needs an additional 35 to 45 kcal/kg while breastfeeding (Ferris et al., 1988). As her child begins to wean, the mother will again need to make alterations in her diet and insulin intake to compensate for a decrease in milk production. If weaning is gradual, fewer problems and adjustments arise.

THYROID DISEASE

The thyroid gland controls the body's metabolism and promotes normal growth of central nervous system development. It produces three hormones: thyroxine (T_4), triiodothyronine (T_3), and calcitonin. T_3 and T_4, which are chemically similar, are known as thyroid hormones. Although the incidence of thyroid disease in pregnancy is rare (0.5–3%), it is important because of its potentially adverse effects on pregnancy and lactation.

Disorders of the thyroid gland have prompted some clinicians to recommend against breastfeeding for mothers with hypothyroidism or hyperthyroidism. While maternal hypothyroidism can be reflected in poor weight gain in the baby (see Chapter 19 on Slow Weight Gain), hyperthyroidism has no such effect.

Many thyroid tests are available for screening lactating women who are suspected of having thyroid disease. The once widely used basal metabolism test is generally inaccurate and is no longer used. The most cost effective, safe and sensitive test is the FT_4I test. If the results of the FT_4I test are high, an FT_3I test is ordered to confirm a diagnosis of hyperthyroidism. No special patient preparation is required for these laboratory tests; a peripheral venous blood sample is drawn. The radioactive iodine uptake test is not recommended during lactation because radioactive iodine transfers into the breastmilk and breastfeeding must be interrupted for at least 48 hours.

Hypothyroidism. Successful pregnancy is rare in women of childbearing age who suffer from untreated hypothyroidism; therefore, most breastfeeding women with a history of hypothyroidism are already receiving medical care.

For the untreated breastfeeding woman, hypothyroidism can result in a reduced milk supply. Other symptoms in the mother are thyroid swelling or nodules (goiter), intolerance to the cold, dry skin, thinning hair, poor appetite, extreme fatigue, and depression. When the thyroid deficiency is not known, these problems are often attributed to postpartum hormonal changes or changes in lifestyle (notably constant care of the baby) and the disease goes undiagnosed—at least for a time. When the infant of one mother suddenly and completely weaned, the mother, who was subsequently diagnosed with hypothyroidism, reported that she "never experienced any fullness in the breast—it was as though I'd dried up overnight" (LLLI, 1976).

These complaints, sometimes coupled with the infant's failure to gain weight satisfactorily on breastmilk alone, should alert the nurse or lactation consultant to the possibility of thyroid deficiency, and the mother should undergo further medical diagnostic evaluation. If replacement therapy of thyroid extract with synthetic T_4 (thyroxine, sodium levothyroxine, or Synthroid) or other thyroid preparation is adequate, the relief of symptoms, as well as an increase in the milk supply, can be quite dramatic. The daily replacement dose of thyroid is 0.1 to 0.3 mg of sodium levothyroxine or equivalent doses of other thyroid preparations. Women whose replacement therapy was determined before pregnancy should be reevaluated after the baby's birth to determine if adjustment is necessary.

Hyperthyroidism. An excess of thyroid hormone is characterized by loss of weight (despite an increased appetite), nervousness, heart palpitations, and a rapid pulse at rest. A well-developed case of hyperthyroidism with exophthalmos (bulging eyes) is called Graves' disease. Hyperthyroidism can develop for the first time postpartum. The ability to lactate does not appear to be affected, although the mother's nervousness may complicate her ability to cope with the daily care-giving of her infant.

Laboratory diagnosis of hyperthyroidism can be established by values from total thyroxine (TT_4), resin T_3 uptake, and FT_4I. According to Romney, Nickoloff, and Esser (1989) hyperthyroidism and thyroiditis can be reliably diagnosed with pertechnetate imaging in combination with clinical symptoms and plasma hormone levels. They claim that radioiodine studies should not be performed in women who wish to continue breastfeeding. Although radioiodine uptake may be considered necessary for establishing the treatment dose for hyperthyroidism, the uptake dose and agent then become irrelevant because breastfeeding must be discontinued when the woman is treated. When radionuclide evaluation of the thyroid is deemed essential, technetium-99m pertechnetate is the preferred agent. (See Table 13–3.)

Treatment usually involves giving an antithyroid drug to lower the maternal thyroid level. If needed, propylthiouracil (PTU) given orally (50 to 300 mg daily) is the treatment of choice for the lactating woman with hyperthyroidism. Although the infant may be monitored for thyroid function, PTU appears to have little effect on the thyroid functioning of the infant (Kampmann, 1980; McDougall & Bayer, 1986; Momotani et al., 1989). Another antithyroid drug, carbimazole, which is widely used in Great Britain, is converted by body metabolism to methimazole (Tapazole). In a case report of a mother who was being treated with carbimazole for hyperthyroidism (Rylance et al., 1987) neither of her breastfeeding twins showed any effects of the medication being administered to the mother; she continued breastfeeding.

PITUITARY DYSFUNCTION

Severe postpartum hemorrhage and hypotension may result in the pituitary gland's failure to produce gonadotropins, which leads to a condition known as panhypopituitarism or Sheehan's syndrome. Initial weight gain postpartum followed by weight loss, loss of pubic and axillary hair, intolerance to cold, breast tissue atrophy, low blood pressure, and vaginal tissue atrophy are symptoms of Sheehan's syndrome. Milder cases of pituitary disruption may occur with less severe symptoms and a delay in milk synthesis.

Prolactinomas (prolactin-secreting adenomas) are

pituitary tumors that stimulate the secretion of prolactin and produce secondary amenorrhea and galactorrhea. Women with this problem may breastfeed. In a study of 46 women with prolactinomas, Ikegami and colleagues (1987) reported the results of 51 pregnancies experienced by these women and their subsequent postpartum course. The women were in one of three treatment groups: surgery, surgery plus bromocriptine, and bromocriptine only. Although prolactin levels declined in all three groups after delivery in 87% of the patients, more women were breastfeeding from the group whose prolactinoma had been treated with bromocriptine. Moreover, no woman showed a sharp increase in prolactin levels during the postpartum period, and there were no symptoms of tumor enlargement. The authors suggested that breastfeeding should not be restricted in patients with prolactinomas. Holmgren et al. (1986) also studied women with prolactinoma. In the group of 35 women whom they followed, lactation did not appear to affect the secretory activity of the tumor and breastfeeding proceeded uneventfully.

CYSTIC FIBROSIS

Cystic fibrosis (CF) is a generalized hereditary disorder of infants, children, and young adults. It is associated with the widespread dysfunction of the exocrine glands and is marked by signs of chronic pulmonary disease, obstruction of the pancreatic ducts, and pancreatic enzyme deficiency. In the past, children with the disease rarely lived to adulthood. Early treatment has enabled young women with CF to marry and to give birth to children without evidence of the disease. About 50% of all patients with CF now live past 25 years of age, and more than one thousand women with this disease have become pregnant and given birth to healthy infants (Shiffman et al., 1989).

Generally, mothers with CF should be encouraged to breastfeed as much as any other mother, although Luder et al. (1990) report that most centers for cystic fibrosis treatment are less likely to report recommending breastfeeding when the mother has CF than when her infant has the condition. Concern about breastfeeding involves the possible risk to the mother's own health status while breastfeeding and caring for a young infant, not the quality of the breastmilk. Although there are some differences in lipid composition, the breastmilk of mothers with CF contains sufficient nutrients to supply the energy needs of the nursing infant (Bitman et al., 1987). Shiffman et al. (1989) reported two cases in which the mothers breastfed for one month and two months respectively, during which time the babies grew at appropriate rates. In both cases, the concentrations of milk sugar, electrolytes, sodium, potassium, and chloride were within normal values. At the same time, concentrations of milk proteins, fat, and IgA appeared to decrease during periods of pulmonary exacerbations.

While these women may breastfeed, they need close nutritional monitoring. Because the nutritional status of the person with CF is already compromised, the extra 500 kcal/day needed for breastmilk may cause excessive weight loss. One early case presentation discussed the breastfeeding course of a 20-year-old woman with CF. Her early breastfeeding course was normal, and the baby grew appropriately through the first 10 weeks postpartum. Thereafter, the mother continued to lose weight and her respiratory status began to worsen. She began antibiotic therapy and stopped breastfeeding. The baby remained free of illness even after being put on artificial formula (Welch, Phelps & Osher, 1981).

A later case report documented the normal growth of an infant through six weeks of exclusive breastfeeding by a 24-year-old mother with CF. These authors concluded that breastfeeding was an "acceptable option" for women with the disease, as long as the maternal diet was closely monitored and vitamin and caloric supplementation was offered when necessary (Golembeski & Emergy, 1989).

Breastfeeding has another advantage when the mother has CF. Since individuals with CF are chronic carriers of bacterial pathogens (such as *s aureus* and *Pseudomonas*), lymphocytes in breastmilk, sensitized to the bacterial pathogens carried by the mother, protect the infant against these infections (Welch, Phelps & Osher, 1981).

INFECTIONS

For most infections, the key word is "self-limiting." Usually infections are not life-threatening; furthermore, the infected mother provides antibody protection to her infant through continued breastfeeding, thereby decreasing her baby's exposure to infection or modifying the illness. When antibiotics are given to the mother, their use poses no danger to the infant and thus should not be used to justify an unnecessary interruption or cessation of breastfeeding.

In some cases, as with active tuberculosis, recommendations are contradictory. For example, Lawrence (1989) recommends discontinuing breastfeeding "if the infant has access to good alternative nutrition." However, this same author notes that "if it is safe for the mother to be in contact with her infant, it is safe for her to breastfeed" (Lawrence, 1989). In countries where tuberculosis is endemic, mothers continue to breastfeed without endangering their infants.

Another acute infectious disease, chicken pox, can result in severe illness in the adult. If the infant is born within the first five days of onset of the illness in the mother, varicella-zoster immune globulin (VZIB) will be given. Antibodies are produced and will appear in the milk. In one report of two different cases, the mother's milk was safe for the baby, although the presence of weeping lesions prevented one mother and baby from being housed together until somewhat later in the disease course (Frederick, White & Braddock, 1986).

DYSFUNCTIONAL UTERINE BLEEDING

Normal uterine bleeding (lochia) following birth ceases in about two to three weeks. In many primiparous mothers who are nursing frequently, such bleeding often stops within the first week to ten days. Abnormal bleeding can be caused by several factors. In the early weeks this may caused by placental fragments retained in the uterus; such fragments can also inhibit breastmilk production (Neifert, McDonough & Neville, 1981). Bleeding caused by a relaxed uterus occurs less often in the breastfeeding woman since the oxytocin released by the suckling infant causes the uterus to contract during each suckling episode. Later bleeding may be the result of miscarriage or the irregular onset of hormonal function. Treatment includes hormonal therapy or nonsteroidal, antiinflammatory drugs. If bleeding is excessive, prolonged, or unexplained, curettage of the uterine lining may be necessary.

For excessive postpartal bleeding, the physician usually orders several doses of methylergonovine maleate (Methergine), a derivative of an ergot alkaloid. Methergine can be given orally, intramuscularly, or intravenously. Unlike crude ergot preparations, there have been no adverse effects reported from the use of methylergonovine by nursing mothers. Methylergonovine does not suppress lactation. If the therapy is prolonged (beyond five days), the infant's pulse and blood pressure should be monitored (Lauwers & Woessner, 1990).

Anxiety always accompanies excessive bleeding. Nursing intervention should focus on relieving the mother's anxiety and assisting in determining the cause of the bleeding while maintaining breastfeeding. The mother should be referred to a physician for an immediate appointment or, if the bleeding is especially severe and a physician is not available, she should be taken to the hospital emergency room. Because leaving her alone only increases her fear, someone should stay with her until she can be medically evaluated. If a dilation and curettage (D & C) is necessary, it is usually done on an outpatient basis, which reduces both the likelihood and duration of mother-infant separation.

Occasionally hormone therapy, either estrogens or progesterone or a combination of both, may be necessary to control bleeding. If hormone therapy is advised, its risks and benefits must be considered in relation to continued breastfeeding. In this case, the mother may want to seek a second medical opinion for other options. The nurse can act as a sounding board in assisting her to make this decision.

RELACTATION

Relactation is the process of restimulating lactation. It can occur days, weeks, or months after prior lactation has ended (Waletzky & Herman, 1976). Brown (1977) notes that in the developing world, when war and other civil unrest have destroyed families, the key elements to successful relactation are a mother who is adequately nourished, a baby with a good sucking reflex, and a support system. At South African medical centers, relactation is routinely initiated as part of the rehydration therapy which is offered to ill, seriously malnourished infants whose nutritional difficulties start after weaning from the breast, when they develop diarrhea (Olango & Aboud, 1990) following the introduction of bottle-feedings. In these centers, the mothers are fed additional foods, the babies are put to breast frequently for long periods, and fed other foods only after suckling. The mothers live at the center with other mothers who are receiving the same assistance; they become a mutual support system along with the staff who strongly support the importance of reestablishing breastfeeding. In nearly all cases, the mothers successfully relactate and the babies' health status is improved.

In the developed world, the purpose of relactation and induced lactation is to enable breastfeeding after an untimely weaning, or to initiate breastfeeding which has been delayed by neonatal or maternal illness or prematurity (Auerbach, 1981; Auerbach & Avery, 1980). Relactation is also an option for a mother who bottle-feeds at first, but who has a change of mind and/or discovers that her infant cannot tolerate infant formula.

Generally, relactation is easier for the mother to accomplish the shorter the interval between the end of the pregnancy and the last day of previous breastfeeding (or pumping). A milk supply can be reestablished with sufficient, regular stimulation. Although metoclopramide has been used to assist mothers following a premature birth (Ehrenkranz & Ackerman, 1986), hormonal preparations are neither necessary nor appropriate in all cases. Furthermore, an important but often neglected consideration is the baby's willingness to return or go to the breast. In situations in which the baby has never been put to breast, the age of the infant at the time this is attempted makes a difference. The younger the baby, the greater the likelihood that he will be willing to suckle, particularly within the first three months of life. If the baby has previously breastfed the chances are greater, but in all cases promptly rewarding the baby when he first attempts to do so will increase the likelihood that the baby will continue to suckle.

The reason for relactation is important. If the baby has been found to be intolerant of all or most of the human milk substitutes that are available, the mother may be more committed to resuming breastfeeding or to increasing her milk supply sufficiently to meet her baby's needs. However, emphasis *only* on her milk as evidence of success can result in increasing her anxiety, thereby inhibiting her milk production and ejection reflex. Thus, the clinician needs to weigh carefully—with plenty of discussion with the mother—the benefits as well as the more problematic elements involved in relactation. The

clinician should encourage the mother both at the outset and throughout her relactation experience, but should also caution that reality may not follow her expectations.

Many health workers assume that if the mother has recently been lactating, all she needs to do is to return the baby to breast and her breasts will promptly respond to renewed stimulation by producing ample amounts of milk. This assumption must be tempered by knowledge of the reason for the termination of breastfeeding in the first place. If the mother was ill or injured, her own health status may influence how quickly her body responds to suckling stimulation. If the baby was ill or injured, his health status will determine how often, and how vigorously, he is able to suckle. Additionally, his age at the time he stopped breastfeeding and his age when it is resumed will determine how willing he is to do so. Generally, a baby under three months of age can usually be coaxed back to the breast. Between three and six months of age, individual infants may be more or less willing to do so; after six months of age, most babies cannot be convinced that the breast will provide either nutrition or nurturing. This poignantly points out that breastfeeding is a two-person activity; failure to keep this continuously in mind when assisting the mother to relactate is likely to result in disappointment and a sense of failure that is avoidable.

Realistic expectations are especially important with relactation, because so many unknowns characterize the situation. One mother, whose baby had been off the breast from six weeks of age through $3\frac{1}{2}$ months, desperately wanted to get her baby back to the breast after she returned home from emergency gallbladder surgery and a difficult recuperation. Her baby, however, had lost all recognition of the breast as a source of food or comfort. During her mother's absence, she had been fed by bottle, facing away from the body. When put to breast, the baby screamed inconsolably. The lactation consultant to whom the mother was referred cautioned the mother that the baby was rapidly developing a mind of her own and that she might not be coaxed back to the breast. The LC then suggested that the family begin finger-feeding the baby with a feeding tube device secured to the mother's largest finger under a rubber nipple shield, which felt like a bottle nipple. The mother began this method of feeding—holding the baby away from her body and gradually moving the infant closer to her chest as the baby relaxed and accepted this new way of feeding. After a few days, the mother was able to eliminate the rubber nipple shield. Several days later, she moved the feeding tube to her breast and provided the infant with additional fluid while her milk supply began to build. Three weeks after that she was able to eliminate the feeding tube device completely. Her infant continued to breastfeed exclusively until nine months of age, at which time she began to experiment with small amounts of solid food. The mother's final comment to the LC was, "If you had told me it would be easy, I would have been terribly disappointed. Your comment that it might or might not work kept me from feeling frustrated when Meghan occasionally took one step back after moving two steps forward the day before." (Personal communication to Kathleen Auerbach.)

INDUCED LACTATION

Preliterate peoples have long known that it is possible to induce lactation (Jelliffe & Jelliffe, 1972). Sutherland and Auerbach (1985) describe what they call "psuedo-induced lactation," to distinguish the mother who is still breastfeeding a birth-baby at the same time she attempts to breastfeed an adopted baby. They note that some of the features of relactation apply in such a situation, but that some of the same cautions relevant to other adoptive mothers are also relevant. A milk supply which is initially established by a birth-baby is not a guarantee of either the establishment of a complete milk supply or of a more rapid increase in any milk supply (Auerbach & Avery, 1981). This assumption is often misunderstood, particularly by those who have experienced unrestricted biological breastfeeding and who very much want to duplicate this experience with the adopted baby. Expecting that it will be easy to breastfeed another baby in addition to a birth-baby can result in frustration—plus an end to the induced lactation experience that is characterized more by anger directed at both oneself and at baby than by success.

Defining success as the presence of milk (Hormann, 1977) continues to influence care-givers and their clients as they prepare to breastfeed the adopted infant. Except in cases in which the adopted

infant is found to be completely intolerant of all artificial formulas, such an emphasis is usually misplaced. It can contribute more to a sense of failure than to the enhancement of the attachment process, which should be the primary consideration for breastfeeding an adopted infant.

In some cases, the adopted baby will switch from bottle to breast fairly easily. In preparation for adopting a Korean baby girl, one mother pumped her breasts for eight weeks, working up to four times a day by the time the baby arrived from Korea (Anderson, 1988).

> When we picked up Elissa I tried nursing her right away, but she wanted nothing to do with it. We had hoped she had been with a nursing foster mother but that had obviously not been the case, and she was very definite about preferring the bottle over the breast. The next night we persuaded Elissa to take the breast by using a rubber nipple shield with a nursing supplementer tube inside the shield. Since this seemed similar to her bottle nipple, she was willing to try it. The following day she decided the shield was too much trouble and willingly took my breast. We became a nursing couple with a minimum of problems. I had been expecting it to take about a month to switch from bottle to breast, and we did it in three days. I started to notice milk in my breasts after we had been nursing about four months, but the amount is minimal. I know the most important thing is the closeness of the nursing relationship. Breastmilk is an added luxury (Anderson, 1988).

Other mothers, however, have found that adopted babies will not go to breast. One mother who obtained an Asian baby from an overseas agency was told that her new daughter had been suckled by her birth mother. Although the baby was then housed for five months in an orphanage and bottle-fed before being placed with her adoptive family, her new mother offered the baby her breast. She reported that her baby reacted "in horror, as if she remembered having been nursed, but not by me!" (Personal communication to Kathleen Auerbach.) It became clear that breastfeeding would not work. This mother continued to offer as much body contact and touching as the baby would tolerate with bottle-feedings.

With a newborn or baby under one month of age,

the usual experience is that the baby will, with little encouragement, root at and accept the breast—especially if rewarded for such behavior. Most mothers find that avoiding bottles and using a tube feeding device which enables them to feed the baby at, if not from, the breast is all that is necessary to teach the baby to breastfeed. In many cases, a portion of the baby's total fluid nutritional needs will be obtained, particularly if the mother enhances opportunities for suckling stimulation with frequent breastfeedings—and does not become so concerned about milk production as an indicator of "success" that her own anxiety inhibits her milk-ejection reflex. Many such mothers often report mild-to-moderate changes in menstrual cycling, some breast changes (including a feeling of fullness, a change in breast shape, occasional leaking of milk), and other indicators of increasing milk production in the early adoptive nursing period when breastfeeding occurs very frequently. These changes are an indication of rises in prolactin and oxytocin hormone levels in response to infant suckling (Amico & Finley, 1986).

Another obvious indication of an increasing supply of breastmilk is the change in infant stools: less stool odor, a softening of the stool so that it more closely resembles the nearly liquid breastmilk stool, and a lightening of the color from dark brown to mustard yellow. Because these stool changes usually occur gradually, the health-care worker who is assisting the adoptive mother needs to remind her that they are an indication of an increase in the proportion of human milk vs. artificial formula that the baby is receiving.

In a few instances, mothers have reported a cessation of menstrual bleeding, although such a reaction is rare; it probably reflects a highly responsive mother and a baby whose suckling pattern is both vigorous and frequent. One mother laughingly reported, "If *your* baby sucked like a vacuum cleaner, you'd get milk in a week, too!" (Personal communication to Kathleen Auerbach.) Often the adoptive mother will find that as solid feedings increase in frequency and volume the amount of necessary supplemental fluid declines, thereby enabling her to be like many other breastfeeding mothers whose babies suckle with varying frequency yet who also enjoy solid foods and sips from a cup as they approach their first birthdays.

Even the highly motivated adoptive mother cannot be assured that she will produce milk. To do so without the benefit of a pregnancy that prepares her breasts for milk production, she is more obviously dependent on the suckling style of her baby—the frequency with which he is put to breast, the strength of his suckling, and the duration of each suckling episode.

The adoptive mother needs to be reminded that a recent birth and breastfeeding experience prior to the arrival of the adoptive baby is no guarantee that she will make sufficient milk to sustain the adoptive baby exclusively at the breast. The age of the birth-baby, the frequency of suckling, the use of solid food for either baby, and the age and frequency of suckling of the new baby—separately or in combination—are insufficient to explain why most women who attempt to tandem-breastfeed a birth-baby and an adopted baby are unable to develop a milk supply large enough to sustain the (usually younger) adopted baby (Auerbach & Avery, 1979). One explanation may involve the age of the baby for whom the milk was originally produced: the birth-baby. The mother's milk supply and its pattern of volume increase, plateauing and gradual decline over time, is a reflection of the older baby's physiological needs. In a situation in which an adopted baby is introduced and offered an opportunity to suckle, the milk continues to "age" in concert with the older birth-baby's maturation. Thus, if the mother is already at a stage where her milk volume has plateaued—which occurs at around the fourth month postpartum (Butte et al., 1984b)—or is declining, it may be increasingly difficult to markedly change that decrease in volume, even with the additional stimulation of a younger baby.

Keeping one's priorities clear from the outset can, however, provide the mother and baby with a unique relationship built on the special closeness that characterizes the breastfeeding experience. The clinician who assists a family with relactation or induced lactation is in a position to observe how mother and baby must truly work together to enjoy something which cannot be duplicated with any other method of feeding. The intimacy which mother and baby derive directly from induced lactation cannot be underestimated; often all family members benefit from the experience as they make this baby "their" baby in a way which cannot be ignored.

CONSIDERATIONS TO DISCUSS WITH THE MOTHER WHO IS CONTEMPLATING RELACTATION OR INDUCED LACTATION

1. What is the *primary* reason for relactation?
2. What is the baby's age at the time of relactation?
3. How much time has elapsed since the baby's birth (if never put to breast) or since the last breastfeeding/pumping?
4. How does the mother expect to judge whether she is "successful"?
5. If the mother obtains less than a full milk supply, how does she think she will feel? How will this influence her self-esteem and acceptance of herself as a good mother?
6. Are any immediate family members strongly opposed to her attempt to relactate? If so, how does she plan to get around such opposition?

7. How does she feel about using a device and/or artificial formula to preserve the baby's nutritional integrity while establishing her own milk supply?
8. How important to the mother is *any* increase in her milk supply?
9. If she is planning to induce lactation, does she feel that lack of a previous (successful) pregnancy/birth means she *must* breastfeed in order to feel like a normal mother? (This is a danger signal.)
10. If she is planning to induce lactation, how does she respond when it is suggested that she consider any milk she obtains "a bonus" rather than the primary reason for attempting to induce lactation?

IMPAIRED MOBILITY

Increasing numbers of women with disabilities are choosing to become pregnant and to breastfeed. For these women, breastfeeding is more than giving good nutrition; it helps to normalize this aspect of their life experience. According to one, "You feel a fierce determination, particularly if you have a permanent disability, to show the world that you can manage on your own and prove to everyone that you are a 'competent' mother" (NMAA, 1982). Breastfeeding builds the mother's confidence and self-esteem, proving that her body is capable of nourishing her baby even though she may be able to do little else quite so easily (Minami, 1990).

In some disorders involving impaired mobility, especially those which are immunologically mediated (such as rheumatoid arthritis, multiple sclerosis, myasthenia gravis), pregnancy may bring about a period of remission followed by postpartum relapse. Often, women suffering from such a disease feel so good during their pregnancy that they take it for granted that their condition has improved. When the condition worsens after birth, it is doubly difficult because additional energy is now required to care for a new baby.

MULTIPLE SCLEROSIS

Multiple sclerosis (MS) is a progressive degenerative neurologic disorder; its symptoms include weakness, fatigue, incoordination, paralysis, and speech and visual disturbances. It affects twice as many women as men, and the diagnosis is usually made during the reproductive years (20 to 40). The condition is known for its unpredictability and the variability of its prognosis and symptoms; the cause is unknown.

Pregnancy and the number of births a woman has experienced have no effect on long-term disability from MS (Poser & Poser, 1983). Studies (Korn-Lubetski et al., 1984; Poser & Poser, 1983; Nelson et al., 1988) consistently report remission of symptoms during pregnancy followed by substantially increased exacerbation (deterioration) in the postpartum period, especially in the first three months. The presence of an immuno-suppressive factor in the maternal serum during the pregnancy may be protective; the subsequent drop in serum hormonal levels after birth may provoke exacerbations.

Women with MS who breastfeed are no more likely than women who do not breastfeed to alter the risk or timing of the exacerbation in the postpartum period (Nelson et al., 1988). Fatigue and exhaustion from care of the infant is a particular problem in all cases, regardless of feeding method. According to one mother, "I was nursing every two-and-one-half hours around the clock; I was totally exhausted. Also I had insomnia and sometimes couldn't get back to sleep after nursing. . . . I had a bad exacerbation and my doctor prescribed a nurse that took care of both of us for two months. After that I used a babysitter, and now day care. I've recovered but I'm still more fatigued than before my pregnancy" (Kirshbaum, 1990). Disrupted sleep, compromised nutrition, excess weight, and lack of supportive household help—all risks during the postpartum period—are more likely to result in a worsening of the disease whether the mother is breastfeeding or formula feeding. These mothers, especially, need household support.

RHEUMATOID ARTHRITIS

Rheumatoid arthritis (RA) is a chronic inflammatory disease thought to be caused by a genetically influenced antigen-antibody response. Symptoms include pain and swelling of the joints, pain on movement, and fatigue. RA symptoms usually go into remission during pregnancy (75%) and relapse postpartum (95%). The mother may also be anemic because of blood loss resulting from salicylate therapy. Women with RA often feel overwhelmed with fatigue both during pregnancy and postpartum (Carty, Conine & Wood-Johnson, 1986). If the mother's hands and fingers are stiff, breastfeeding is simpler than artificial feeding, which requires more complex movements. Although this mother needs additional rest, she still needs to continue range-of-motion exercises. Periodic rest periods and wearing removable braces or splints to support joints will help reduce fatigue (Carty, Conine & Hall, 1990).

CLINICAL IMPLICATIONS

Disabled parents are adaptive and even ingenious in devising ways to carry out basic baby-care activities. Good parenting occurs even when the parent is severely disabled, as long as psychosocial functioning is not a problem. Generally, these parents find that breastfeeding is more convenient than bottle-feeding. Yet friends and relatives may react negatively, concerned that the mother should not breastfeed because of her limited energy and/or abilities. More than mothers with normal mobility, these women

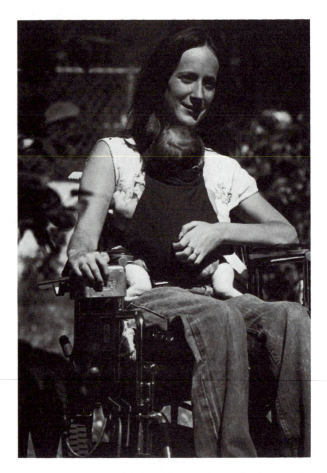

FIGURE 13–2   Disabled women are breastfeeding mothers, too.

need compassionate support and guidance. Suggestions for the physically disabled mother and her family on breastfeeding and baby care are listed in the box on p. 363.

The hospital birthing experience can be traumatic. Kopala (1989) interviewed seven mothers with mobility impairments including spina bifida, spinal cord injury, postpolio syndrome, and MS about their birth experience in the hospital. One mother, a paraplegic, felt that her knowledge about her body and its limitations was not respected by the staff. Less than 24 hours after undergoing a cesarean, she was told to get out of bed. She knew that without the use of both her arms—she had an intravenous line in one—she was "dead weight" and was afraid of being dropped or hurt (Kopala, 1989). Because the disabled mother is usually under continuing medical care and has so many needs, the health-professional working with the breastfeeding

---

BABY CARE GUIDELINES FOR MOTHERS WITH A PHYSICAL DISABILITY

- Mothers with some upper-body strength who are confined to wheelchairs can use a harness or a wide belt with a long strip of Velcro to lift and retrieve a crawling baby from the floor.
- Set up a special "place" for breastfeeding that is easily accessible and comfortable for the mother.
- If the baby is small, he can be laid diagonally across the mother's knees on a pillow to breastfeed. Arrange other pillows for support. The mother's feet should be supported.
- Changing tables and cribs can be adapted so that they are accessible to a wheelchair, and the room can be arranged so that moving about is minimized. A low-sided pram or baby stroller makes it easier to slide the baby out onto the mother's lap without requiring much lifting.
- A baby sling allows the mother's arms to be free while assuring that the baby is safe and supported during breastfeeding. This is also helpful when the mother has unilateral weakness or paralysis (e.g., from a stroke).
- A bell tied to the baby's shoes keeps track of where the mobile child is.
- A toddler will quickly learn to climb on his mother's knee for a ride and to sit still while the chair is moving.
- Give the baby extra cuddling, such as touching at night in bed, if there are barriers to physical contact during the day.

- Clothe the baby in overalls with crossed straps so it is easier to lean over and pick him up.
- Use a nursing bra that opens in the front, instead of the back—one with an easy-to-fasten clip or Velcro strap that can be fastened with one hand. Replace the usual clips for opening and closing the bra flap with Velcro.
- Alter (or have altered) maternity clothes with Velcro openings or large ring zippers. Antique buttonhooks are helpful for manipulating the small buttons found on many garments.
- Plan rest periods during the day: sit to work whenever possible.
- Sleep with the infant and/or have the father or someone bring the baby to the mother to nurse during the night.
- Use an intercom system that picks up the sound of the baby crying. If the mother is deaf, the sound can be transformed into flashing light signals.
- If the mother cannot lift both herself and the baby, she might spend the day on the floor (preferably carpeted)—feeding, changing, and playing with him. This enables her to roll the baby to her, instead of lifting him, when he needs attention. A bean bag will provide support for breastfeeding.

Derived from: Conine, TA, Carty, E, and Safarik, PM: *Aids and adaptations for parents with physical or sensory disabilities*, Vancouver, B.C., 1988, School of Rehabilitative Medicine, University of British Columbia, Canada, pp. 67–71; Nursing Mothers' Association of Australia: *Where there's a will, there's usually a way—breastfeeding when the mother has a disability*, Hawthorn, Victoria, Australia, 1982, The Association; Kirshbaum, M: The parent with a physical disability. In Auvenshine, JM, and Enriques, MG: *Comprehensive maternity nursing: perinatal and women's health*, Boston, 1990, Jones and Bartlett Publishers, Inc.; Minami, J: Helping mothers with chronic illness, *Leaven* 26:52–53, 1990.

---

disabled mother may find her role expanding to that of a case manager; she coordinates medical, family, and community support and services (Bowles, 1991). If the mother has someone to help her with the physical tasks, diplomatically arrange for that person to take over the household jobs and care for older children; let the mother take care of her baby. Everyone loves to take care of the new baby (rather than mopping the floor), but when others take over

care of the baby, the mother's role and her self-confidence diminishes.

Since many of these mothers are already on medication, the physician should be consulted about the safety of taking specific medication while breastfeeding. Most medications are compatible with breastfeeding (see Chapter 6 on Drugs and Breastfeeding). If the physician recommends weaning, the health-care provider should research the drug using up-to-date references, and if necessary, act as an advocate for the mother in her desire to continue to breastfeed.

For peer support, Carty, Conine, and Hall (1990) suggest setting up group sessions which might include any woman with a disability who has given birth in the last five years. The purpose of these sessions is to provide information on coping with the demands placed upon disabled women by pregnancy, birthing, and early infant care.

When first encountering a disabled mother who needs help with breastfeeding, it is easy for the caregiver to feel overwhelmed and inadequate. Having had the disability for a long time, the mother is usually more knowledgeable than anyone else about her problem (both her abilities and limitations); the health-care provider may not be. The reality of these feelings should be shared with the mother. The majority of disabled women do not require frequent hospitalizations; thus, nurses typically lack experience with these clients (Kopala, 1989). If they have experience in working with disabled individuals, it is usually in an institutional setting. Nurses and health-professionals can learn a great deal from the mother who has developed extraordinary survival skills to work around inconveniences. For example, a mother we know who has no left hand or lower left arm tends to breastfeed her baby on her left side, propping her baby against her upper left arm so that her free right hand is free. This mother also needs a battery or electric pump, not a hand-operated one.

Reinforcing the disabled mother's abilities, while supporting her against possible negative attitudes around her can make a positive difference. When the nurse assists this mother in the home, she, rather than the mother, is the guest. This requires a role change that may take some adjustment. Self-care presumes an optimal level of functioning as its goal. Functioning at an optimal level can occur for the physically disabled mother who desires to breastfeed her infant as much as it can for any mother.

Until recently, limited information was available on breastfeeding (and all other aspects of childbearing) among women with disabilities. Unfortunately society's general view is still that women with a physical disability are not capable of having or caring for a child. Even now there are only a few resources these families can seek for guidance. Two are La Leche League International and Nursing Mothers' Association of Australia (Minami, 1990; NMAA, 1982). Both organizations have educational materials, including cassette tapes and Braille, for the physically disabled mother who is breastfeeding. They will also refer the mother to another woman who has had a similar experience. The reader can find more information on childbearing among disabled women from an annotated bibliography developed by Kopala (1989).

SEIZURE DISORDERS

Seizure disorders are now classified into two major classes: partial and generalized. Partial or focal seizures begin in a specific area of the brain and produce symptoms ranging from simple repetitive movements to more complex abnormal movements and bizarre behavior. Generalized seizures have no specific point of origin in the brain. The most common type is a major motor seizure, formerly called grand mal epilepsy. Anticonvulsants appear in human milk in much reduced concentrations compared with maternal serum levels. Breastfeeding should be encouraged, keeping in mind that neonatal sedation can occur if the mother is receiving high doses of phenobarbitone, primidone, or one of the benzodiazepines. Brodie (1990) recommends that anticonvulsant therapy be tapered off prior to conception to avoid the higher risk of teratogenicity that such drugs pose.

Seizure disorders can be so well controlled by medications that seizures are rarely a problem for the lactating mother. However, nurses need to know about the effect of the medication on the breastfed infant. The physician will prescribe antiseizure medications based on diagnosis of the seizure and its pattern of occurrence, as well as on the tolerance and response of the mother to the prescribed drug. Common medications are phenytoin (Dilantin), carbamazepine (Tegretol), primidone (Mysoline), and phenobarbital. The American Academy of Pediatrics, Committee on Drugs classifies these and other antiseizure drugs (ethosuximide, thiopental and valporic acid) as being usually compatible with breastfeeding (see p. 156). Phenobarbital taken in higher than average amounts (50–100 mg two or three times/day), however, may cause drowsiness in infants or mothers; primidone may also cause sedation in the infant.

In the unusual case in which the mother has seizures, breastfeeding is in no way contraindicated. Dropping or harming the infant during a seizure is

---

**GUIDELINES FOR A BREASTFEEDING MOTHER
WITH A SEIZURE DISORDER**

1. Have a playpen available on each level of the house in which to quickly place the baby when a seizure seems imminent.
2. Pad the arms of the rocker or chair where the mother usually breastfeeds with extra pillows and cushions for protection.
3. Place guard rails padded with pillows around the mother's bed if she customarily takes her infant to bed to breastfeed.
4. Attach a tag stating that the mother has a seizure disorder, along with other pertinent information, to the baby, as well as the stroller or baby carrier, whenever she is away from home.

---

no more probable during breastfeeding than it is during bottle-feeding. Usually a prodromal warning (aura) alerts the mother of an impending seizure, and she is able to take safety precautions to protect her infant.

POSTPARTUM DEPRESSION

There are three types of depressive reactions following childbirth: (1) postpartum "blues"; (2) postpartum depression, a clinical depression; and (3) psychotic depression with delusions (Hopkins, Marcus & Campbell, 1984). About 70 to 80% of women experience a transient depression following birth, usually on the third postpartum day. The "blues" is usually temporary, accompanied by tearfulness and is more common in women having their first child.

In a critical review of the literature, Hopkins, Marcus, and Campbell (1984) estimate that as many as 20% of postpartum women have mild to moderate depression following childbirth. At the same time, the research on depression suffers from lack of a clear definition of clinical depression, especially for the postpartum mother. Every new mother experiences sleep disturbance, mood changes, and fatigue during normal postpartum that may be interpreted as clinical depression, so this percentage may be inflated.

New mothers with high levels of life stress and few supportive relationships, especially with a husband or partner, suffer more from postpartum depression (Hopkins, Marcus & Campbell, 1984). There is no consistent evidence that the mother's age, the number of children she has, or complications during the pregnancy and delivery are associated with the appearance of depression. Although mothers of preterm infants are more anxious and depressed than mothers of term infants in the first week following birth, this difference does not last beyond the first week (Gennaro, 1988).

Postpartum hormonal shifts play no clear role in depression; to ascribe depression to physical pathology is to miss the point that we ought to be looking at society's failure to give adequate social support to mothers. Maternal hormonal levels during lactation represent the *normal postpartum state;* thus, breastfeeding women should be at no greater risk for postpartum depression because their hormone levels are different from nonlactating women (Auerbach & Jacobi, 1990).

The few studies on postpartum depression and maternal hormones are conflicting. Harris et al. (1989) found that depression was associated with decreased prolactin concentrations in the early postpartum period. Since bottle-feeding mothers have low prolactin levels, they were also much more likely to exhibit symptoms of depression. Among breastfeeding mothers who became depressed, plasma prolactin levels were closer to the levels seen among the bottle-feeders than among their breastfeeding cohorts. On the other hand, Alder and Cox (1983) noted that mothers who totally breastfed their infants or who were on the pill had a higher incidence of postnatal depression than those who partially breastfed or who were not on the pill.

Psychotic depression or psychosis is rare, occurring in about one or two of every one thousand women who have a child (Lindstrom, 1984). The onset of the psychosis occurs within a few days to two weeks after delivery and symptoms peak at about six weeks postpartum. The mother with postpartum psychotic depression may have insomnia, irrational ideas, feelings of failure, self-accusatory thoughts, depression, fatigue, and hallucinations; sometimes she may threaten to commit suicide.

Hardly any problem is more distressing to all concerned than a mother suffering from postpartum depression psychosis. The family is in a state of severe crisis, disequilibrium, and suffers from lack of sleep. If the mother is breastfeeding, the consulting psychiatrist often insists upon weaning because of undue concern about a prescribed medication passing through the breastmilk. If she needs constant observation, there is the threat of hospitalization and separation, since most psychiatric facilities do not allow the infant to remain with the mother. The decision whether to hospitalize this mother and/or to wean the baby is agonizing. Care of the infant and possibly other children is an immediate concern. A severe maternal depression can also have a dramatic effect on the infant. Following a suicide attempt by his mother, a 12-month-old toddler suddenly refused any nourishment other than what he received from breastfeeding. All attempts to entice him into eating foods that he had formerly enjoyed were firmly refused for several months. He may have sensed that becoming totally dependent on his mother for food would ensure her continued presence.

CLINICAL IMPLICATIONS

Unfortunately, postpartum depression tends to occur when the maternal-infant bond is being formed. Every effort should be made to foster this crucial bond and breastfeeding as well. The mother with depression suffers a loss of maternal identity and self-esteem. When the infant stays with the mother, the mother recovers more quickly and has a lower relapse rate (Waletzky, 1981).

Mothers at risk for postpartum depression usually display emotional problems very soon after the birth of their child. In fact, experienced maternity nurses can usually identify the mothers who are likely to become depressed. Typically, this mother has difficulty bonding with her baby and will make self-accusatory remarks, such as "I am a terrible person" or "I have a lovely baby, a lovely house and a lovely husband, and I know I should be happy, yet I feel awful." Kitzinger (1989) reminds us that "few women are prepared for the resentment, the sense of inadequacy, the guilt, anger and murderous feelings we have as mothers. There is delight, discovery and joy, and sometimes sheer ecstasy too, and that makes it all worth while. But the trouble is that the image of motherhood is romanticized" (Kitzinger, 1989).

With early postpartum discharge, however, the hospital staff is only able to assess the problem; their most helpful intervention is to refer the family to a primary care physician or social worker for follow-up care. These providers need to be able to assess precipitating factors that increase the risk of postpartum depression, which include:

- a chronic history of maladjustment or inability to cope with stress
- lack of caring support from a partner/husband
- lack of a social network of support from relatives or close friends
- constant fatigue and lack of sleep
- mood swings, weepiness, anxiety.

If the mother is deeply depressed, she must be referred to a psychiatrist or psychologist who will probably initiate drug therapy. The risks and benefits of any particular agent must be carefully evaluated. Although most of these medications do not pass into the breastmilk in sufficient quantities to harm the infant, clearly the last word on prolonged high doses is not yet in. Medications commonly used to control symptoms of postpartum depression are phenothiazines such as perphenazine (Trilafon); antianxiety drugs such as alprazolam (Xanax); and tricyclic antidepressants such as imipramine (Tofranil) or nortriptyline (Pamelor). With the exception of phenelzine sulfate (Nardil), a MAO inhibitor, these medications appear to be relatively safe for short-term therapy. MAO inhibitors are generally not the drug of first choice to treat depression. The principle reasons for their more limited use are the dietary restrictions (i.e., avoiding tyramine-containing foods such as cheese and wine) the persons must observe while on these drugs (see Table 13–1).

The dosage of tricyclics is slowly increased over several days to minimize side effects. Sedation and other side effects may begin at once, but the antidepressant response occurs only after 10 to 21 days at full therapeutic dose. MAO inhibitors may produce a mild stimulation effect almost at once, but again, full therapeutic benefit may take two to six weeks. Antidepressants need not be continued indefinitely, and the drug will be discontinued after the mother has been asymptomatic for several weeks. Both tricyclics and MAOs are highly toxic in overdose. As a general rule, the physician will limit the prescription to a 7 to 10 day supply.

Chlorpromazine (Thorazine), a tranquilizer, has been

TABLE 13–1 DRUGS USED TO TREAT POSTPARTUM DEPRESSION

Drug Name	Usual Daily Oral Dosage (mg)	Use in Breastfeeding Mother and Safety Level
Antianxiety Drugs		
(Benzodiazepines)		
alprazolam (Xanax)	0.75–4	Use with caution; may accumulate in infant; do not use in first week.
diazepam (Valium)	5–40	Use with caution; may accumulate in infant; do not use in first week.
Tricyclics		
amitriptyline (Elavil)	50–300	Safe; no effects on infants reported; no apparent accumulation in nursing infant
desipramine (Norpramin)	50–300	Relatively safe
imipramine (Tofranil)	50–300	Relatively safe; infant would receive approximately .04 mg/kg/day; recommended initial therapeutic dosage for children is 1 mg/kg/day
nortriptyline (Pamelor)	25–100	Safe; not detected in serum of infant
MAO Inhibitors		
phenelzine (Nardil)	15–90	Contraindicated; inhibits lactation
tranylcypromine (Parnate)	10–30	Use with caution
Phenothiazines		
chlorpromazine (Thorazine)	30–1000	Relatively safe if average dosage; one report of infant drowsiness with high dosage; may increase mother's milk supply
mesoridazine (Serentil)	100–400	Relatively safe
perphenazine (Trilafon)	4–6	Safe; dose passed to child through milk is only 0.1% that given the mother
thioridazine (Mellaril)	150–800	Relatively safe

Data from: Riordan, J: Drugs excreted in breastmilk. In Pagliaro, L, and Pagliaro, AM: *Problems in pediatric drug therapy,* 2nd ed., Hamilton, Ill., 1987, Drug Intelligence Publications, Inc.; Lauwers, J, and Woessner, C: Chemical agents and breast milk, Garden City Park, N.Y., 1990, Avery Publishing Groups, Inc.; Lipkin, GB: Drug therapy in maternal care. In Spencer, RT, et al.: *Clinical pharmacology and nursing management,* 3rd ed., Philadelphia, 1989, J.B. Lippincott Co., pp. 1132–70.

prescribed for manic disorders in breastfeeding mothers. Chlorpromazine passes the milk in minute quantities and may actually increase milk production by blocking the prolactin-inhibitory factor. Lithium, sometimes prescribed for manic depressive states, may be used with caution if the mother's and infant's serum levels are closely monitored (Schou, 1990).

The mother with depression also needs help to build a supportive network; this is especially crucial for mothers of young infants who are relatively housebound and likely to be drained by the demands of child care. A friend of the mother, a neighbor, a La Leche League chapter, or a church group are all possibilities. Many countries already have supportive systems for these mothers built into their health care. For a clinical care plan for depression, see Table 13–2. Handford (1985) describes an effec-

tive Canadian system of self-help support programs for mothers suffering from postpartum depression. In Australia, this role is fulfilled by a domicilary nurse, an infant welfare sister, or a family aide (Scott, 1984). Not only do these support persons provide individual support but they also play a key role in facilitating the mother's peer relationship with other mothers. Reducing the social isolation of the depressed mother reinforces her identity and ability to cope. The quality of the marital relationship is of primary importance in the mother's postpartum adaptation, especially for first-time mothers. Since the father plays a key role, he should also be counseled and supported. If the mother and/or father are sleep-deprived, every effort should be made to devise a plan whereby they may sleep for at least six hours and thus benefit from the restoration of sleep.

TABLE 13–2 CLINICAL CARE PLAN

Nursing diagnosis: Coping, ineffective individual, related to stress or potential complications of perinatal period and to life changes

Assessment	Intervention	Rationale
Previous history of postpartum depression	Listen to mother describe her feelings	Postpartum depression is likely to recur with subsequent births
Beyond first week postpartum: Tearfulness Mood swings	Maintain a supportive and nonjudgmental attitude	Clinical depression occurs in about 20% of mothers
Feelings of failure Insomnia and fatigue Anxiety	Maintain her privacy and let her cry	Role changes and increased responsibilities cause stress
Suicidal thoughts	Assist in providing social support and physical help for mother and infant	
Possible disinterest in baby	Monitor baby's weight gain and general well-being	Infant may not be receiving adequate nurturing and care because of mother's depression
Depression worsens	Referral to psychologist or psychiatrist for counseling and evaluation for medication therapy	Antidepressant and/or antianxiety drugs are effective in treating depression
Mother taking medication for depression and wishes to continue breastfeeding	Research the effect of the medication upon the breastfeeding infant; recommend optional medications	Some medications are safe to take while breastfeeding

ASTHMA

About one percent of pregnant women have active asthma, which may improve, worsen, or remain unchanged during pregnancy (D'Alonzo, 1990). The course of asthma appears to be influenced by the gestational time: it is likely to worsen during the late second trimester, improve during the last four weeks of pregnancy, and revert back to the prepregnancy course within the first three months postpartum.

Lactation does appear to influence the course of asthma. The main concern is the effect of medications taken by the mother to control her asthma. Asthma therapy should be continued during lactation and generally does not have to be altered (D'Alonzo, 1990). The two central classes of antiasthmatic medications are corticosteroids and bronchodilators including beta-adrenergic agonists and theophyllines. Many of the new bronchodilators are available in metered aerosol form so that one inhalation delivers a given amount of a drug and the likelihood of overdose is small. Halogenated corticosteroids given by inhalation provide selective topical effects that lessen the amount of corticosteroids

transferred into breastmilk. Although theophylline is secreted in breastmilk, the infant receives only a small percentage (< 10%) of the maternal dose. Theophylline taken by the breastfeeding mother may occasionally result in infant irritability and insomnia, necessitating a decrease in the maternal dosage and/or temporary withdrawal (Yurchak & Jusko, 1976).

SMOKING

Smoking is a form of addiction; it affects the mother's general health, the milk she makes, her baby, and the breastfeeding course (Said, Patois & Lellouch, 1984). While nursing mothers tend to take fewer drugs of any kind than do nonbreastfeeding women, early weaning occurs more often when the mother is a smoker, usually exhibiting an inverse dose relationship (Woodward & Hand, 1988; Matheson, Kristensen & Lunde, 1990; Vio, Salazar & Infante, 1991). The dangers of nicotine exposure have only recently been identified. This may be because of the classification of nicotine as a "licit" (legal) drug (Fulton, 1990). Even the milk of nonsmokers has been found to include nicotine through passive exposure to the smoke of others (Trundle & Skellern, 1983). Nicotine concentrations—and those of its metabolite, cotinine—increase markedly in breast-milk immediately after smoking (Dahlström et al., 1990). The half-life of nicotine in milk is 97 ± 20 minutes (Luck & Nau, 1984). Steldinger and Luck (1988) report that levels of nicotine are higher in the mother's milk than in her serum; while both levels decline over time, the investigators recommend that breastfeeding mothers prolong the period between cigarette smoking and breastfeeding in order to reduce the amount of nicotine to which the baby is exposed.

The mother who smokes also exposes her infant to secondhand smoke, which raises inhaled carbon monoxide to unsafe levels, aggravates allergies and increases the risk of respiratory illnesses (Luck & Nau, 1985; Bonham & Wilson, 1981). Maternal cigarette smoking is associated with a 20 to 35% increase in respiratory illnesses and may have a deleterious effect on children's growth (Rona et al., 1981).

In many cases, women who have been moderate or heavy smokers will use their pregnancy as a motivation to reduce or stop smoking. The negative influence of smoking on breastfeeding needs to be shared with the mother; such knowledge may serve to strengthen her resolve to continue to reduce her use of nicotine or to stop altogether. Also, people who smoke are not always truthful about their smoking habits, and self-reports of nicotine use tend to correlate poorly with laboratory tests (Little et al., 1986). This may be important to consider when attempting to rule out factors which may contribute to inadequate milk production and/or compromised infant growth.

DIAGNOSTIC STUDIES USING RADIOISOTOPES

The degree of interference with lactation when radioactive drugs are used depends in part on the proposed dose and on the radioactive element to be used. Elements, such as iodide, are selectively concentrated in human milk; thus, their use may interrupt breastfeeding for a longer period (Romney, Nickoloff, and Esser, 1989). Studies using radioactive isotopes usually require that breastfeeding be interrupted until nearly all radioactivity is excreted in order to avoid its passage to the infant. Fortunately, most studies use an isotope such as technetium-99 which has a short half-life (4 hours). Iodine isotopes (123 and 131) have much longer half-lives, and breastfeeding has to be interrupted for a longer period. Gallium-67 requires two weeks before it is safe to resume nursing. In some cases, transmission can occur directly from the mother even when she cuddles the baby (Coakley & Mountford, 1985). Ways to reduce the effects of radiation therapy are seen in the boxed list of guidelines on this page. A list of radiopharmaceuticals and the approximate length of time they are present in human milk is given in Table 13–3.

DISCUSSION

Rehospitalization of a mother after she has gone home following delivery is a traumatic experience for all members of the family. A mother faced with separation from her infant, whether brief or prolonged, is a mother in crisis. For the breastfeeding woman and her infant it is essential that ongoing, intimate, and regular contact be maintained. During a postpartum illness, the baby should be allowed to room-in with the mother, or at least be brought to

---

REDUCING RADIATION EXPOSURE IN THE
BREASTFEEDING MOTHER AND HER INFANT

1. Make sure that the investigation is essential; avoid unnecessary tests.
2. Reduce the dose to the minimum required to obtain a diagnostic result.
3. Change the radiopharmaceutical to one with the least concentration in milk—or other more favorable dosimetric properties, including a shorter half-life.
4. Balance the inconvenience and disadvantage of interrupting breastfeeding against the potential risk of exposure to the infant.

From Coakley, AJ, and Mountford, PJ: Nuclear medicine and the nursing mother, *Br Med J* 291:160, 1985.

TABLE 13–3 SUMMARY OF ORIGINAL RESEARCH REPORTS AND REVIEWS, INCLUDING CLINICAL RECOMMENDATIONS AND AUTHOR COMMENTS

Radio-pharma-ceutical	Original (# cases) or Review*	Recommendation	Comment	Reference
^{99m}Tc04 (pertechnetate)	Review	Interrupt nursing and measure milk activity. Resume when activity <1mSv	Time to reduce to EDE <IMSv** is 36 hrs	3
	Original (1)	Discard milk during first 12 hrs after tracer administration	EDE to infant <1mSv	8
	Original (1)	Discard milk during first 12 hrs after tracer administration	Mean effective t1/2=3.2 hrs; total fraction of injected activity excreted into breast milk = 10.8×10^{-2}	1,2
	Original (2)	Discard milk during first 24 hrs after tracer administration	Recommendation made for doses up to 1.5 mCi*	9
	Original (1)	Discard milk during first 48 hrs after tracer administration		10
	Original (2)	Wait until breast milk activity is <6×10^{-3}uCi/mL	1/10 ICRP drinking water standard for ^{99m}Tc; level reached 20–32 hrs after tracer administration	6
	Original (1)	Discard milk during first 72 hrs after tracer administration levels	Waited until breast milk activity reached background	7
^{99m}Tc-MAA (macroaggregated albumin)	Review	Discard mild during first 6 hrs after tracer administration	EDE to infant <1mSv	3
	Original (6)	Discard milk during first 12 hrs after tracer administration	Mean effective t1/2=37 hrs; total fraction of injected activity excreted into breast milk = 3.2×10^{-2}	1,2
	Original (4)	Discard milk during first 24 hrs after tracer administration	Cumulative dose to infant=0.2mrad if nursing is resumed after 24 hrs	11
	Original (1)	Discard milk during first 24 hrs after tracer administration	Whole body dose to infant=<0.05mrem	12
	Original (1)	Discard milk during first 24 hrs after tracer administration	Also gave ^{99m}Tc-DTPA aerosol	13
	Original (1)	Discard milk during first 24 hrs after tracer administration	Estimated 24 hrs infant exposure if nursed=0.3mrad	14
	Original (1)	Interruption not essential		15
	Original (1)	Discard milk during first 24 hrs after tracer administration	Estimated dose to infant thyroid if nursed after 24 hr <1mrad	16
^{99m}Tc-RBC (erythrocytes)	Review	Interrupt nursing and measure milk activity.	Time to reduce to EDE <1mSv is approximately 13 hrs Resume when activity <1mSv	3
	Original (1)	Discard milk during first 24 hrs after tracer administration	Mean effective t1/2=7.7 hrs; fraction of injected activity excreted into breast milk = 6.1×10^{-5}	1,2
^{99m}Tc-DTPA (diethylene-thia-mine pentacetic acid)	Review	Interruption not essential.	EDE to infant, 1mSv	3

Reprinted with permission. Originally appeared in Fulton, B, and Moore, L: Radiopharmaceuticals and lactation, *J Hum Lact* 6:181–84, 1990.

(continue

Radiopharmaceutical	Original (# cases) or Review*	Recommendation	Comment	References
	Original (1)	Discard milk during first 4 hrs after tracer administration	Mean effective t1/2=3.7 hrs; total fraction of injected activity excreted into breast milk = 1.5×10^{-4}	1,2
	Original (1)	Discard milk during first 4 hrs after tracer administration	Total activity ingested was approximately 0.1% of ICRP annual limit for 6.6 kg infant nursing not interrupted	17
99mTc-DMSA	Review	Interruption not essential	EDE to infant <1mSv	3
99mTc glucoheptonate	Original (1)	Discard milk during first 4 hrs after tracer administration (although not essential)	EDE to infant <1mSv	3,8
99mTc-MDP (methylenediphosphonate)	Review	Interruption not essential	EDE to infant <1mSv	3
	Original (2)	Discard milk during first 4 hrs after tracer administration	Mean effective t1/2=4.2 hrs; total fraction of injected activity excreted into breast milk = 1.9×10^{-4}	1,2
99mTc-HDP	Review	Interruption not essential	EDE to infant <1mSv	3
123I-iodide	Review	Interrupt nursing and measure milk activity. Resume when activity <1mSv	Time to reduce to EDE <1mSv approximately 5 hrs	3
	Review	Avoid breastfeeding	Permissible milk concentration=1.9×10^{-6} uCi	18
	Review	Avoid breastfeeding	112 day delay following 100uCi dose	19
	Original (1)	Discard milk during first 36–72 hrs after tracer administration	Biologic t1/2=10.4 hrs	20
	Review	Discard milk during first 48–72 hrs after tracer administration	Based on extrapolated 131-I data	4
123I-IOH	Review	Interrupt nursing and measure milk activity. Resume when activity <1mSv	Time to reduce EDE to <1mSv approximately 8 hrs	3
125I-IOH	Review	Interrupt nursing and measure milk activity. Resume when activity <1mSv	Time to reduce EDE to <1mSv approximately 18 hrs	3
	Original (1)	Discard milk during first 12 hrs after tracer administration	Mean effective t1/2=4.3 hrs; total fraction of injected activity excreted into breast milk = 2.4×10^{-2}	1,2
125I-HSA	Review	Avoid breastfeeding	Time to reduce EDE to <1mSv approximately 206 hrs	3
	Original (2)	Discard milk during first 10 days after tracer administration		21

(continued)

Radio-pharma-ceutical	Original (# cases) Or Review*	Recommendation	Comment	Reference
[125]I-fibrinogen	Review	Avoid breastfeeding	Time to reduce EDE to <1mSv is 540 hrs	3
	Original (1)	Avoid breastfeeding	tl/2 in milk = 80 hrs	22
[131]I-iodide	Review	Avoid breastfeeding	Time to reduce EDE to <1mSv approximately 1727 hrs	3
	Review	Avoid breastfeeding	Biologic t1/2=21.9 days	19
	Review	Discard milk during first 8 weeks after tracer adminis-tration	Standard=1/10 yearly per-missible dose of ICRP. Dose=5uCi	4
	Original (2)	Discard milk during first 12 days after tracer administra-tion	ICRP drinking water stan-dard	6
	Original (1)	Discard milk during first 24 hrs after tracer administra-tion		23
	Original (2)	Avoid breastfeeding	Biologic t1/2 of radioiodine = 7 days in thyroid gland	24
^{131}I-IOH	Review	Interrupt nursing and mea-sure milk activity. Resume when activity <1mSv	Time to reduce EDE to <1mSv approximately 30 hrs	3
	Review	Discard milk during first 45 days after tracer administra-tion		4
	Original (6)	Discard milk during first 12 hrs after tracer administra-tion	Mean effective t1/2=4.5 hrs total fraction of injected ac-tivity excreted into breast milk=2.8×10^{-2}	1,2
[75]Semethionine	Review	Avoid breastfeeding	Time to reduce to <1mSv approximately 467 hrs	3
	Original (1)	Avoid breastfeeding		25
[67]Ga-citrate	Review	Avoid breastfeeding	Time to reduce to <1mSv approximately 427 hrs	3
	Review	Interrupt nursing for 4 weeks	Standard=1/10 of yearly per-missible dose by ICRP	4
	Original (1)	Avoid breastfeeding	Biologic t1/2 in milk = 9 days	26
[111]In-leukocytes	Original (1)	Interruption not essential	Maximum EDE to in-fant=1mSv	27
[51]Cr-EDTA	Review	Interruption not essential	Maximum EDE to in-fant=0.001mSv	3
	Original (2)	Discard milk after first 4 hrs after tracer administration	Mean effective t1/2=6 hrs; total fraction of injected ac-tivity excreted into breast milk=4.0×10^{-4}	1,2

*Indicates whether recommendation is based on original data or on a review of previously published/gathered data.
**mSv = milliSievart
uCi = microCurie
mCi = milliCurie
mrad = milirad
mrem = milirem

(continued)

1. Ahlgren L, et al: Excretion of radionuclides in human breast milk after the administration of radiopharmaceuticals. J Nucl Med 26:1085–90, 1985

2. Ahlgren L: Error in table (letter). J Nucl Med 27:151, 1986

3. Mountford PJ, Coakley AJ: A review of the secretion of radioactivity in human breast milk: data, quantitative analysis and recommendations. Nucl Med Comm 10:15–27, 1989

4. Romney BM, et al: Radionuclide administration to nursing mothers: mathematically derived guidelines. Radiology 160:549–554, 1986

5. Karjalainen P, Penttila IM, Pystynen P: The amount and form of radioactivity in human milk after lung scanning, renography, and placental localization by ^{131}I labelled tracer. Acta Obstet Gynecol Scand 50:357–61, 1971

6. Wyburn JR: Human breast milk excretion of radionuclides following administration of radiopharmaceuticals. J Nucl Med 14:115–17, 1973

7. Vagenakis AG, Abreau CM, Braverman LE: Duration of radioactivity in the milk of a nursing mother following Tc-99 administration. J Nucl Med 12:188, 1971

8. Mountford PJ, Coakley AJ: Breast milk radioactivity of ^{99m}Tc-pertechnetate and ^{99m}Tc-glucoheptonate. Nucl Med Commun 8:839–45, 1987

9. Ogunleye O: Assessment of radiation dose to infants from breast milk following the administration of Tc[99m]-pertechnetate to nursing mothers. Health phys 45:149–51, 1983

10. Pittard WB, III, Bill K, Fletcher BD: Excretion of technetium in human milk. J Pediatr 94:605–7, 1979

11. Cranage R, Palmer M: Breast milk radioactivity after [99m]TC-MAA lung studies. Eur J Nucl Med 11:257–59, 1985

12. Heaton B: The buildup of technetium in breast milk following the administration of [99]Tc[m]04 labelled macroaggregated albumin. Br J Radiol 52:149–50, 1979

13. Mountford PJ, et al: Breast milk radioactivity after a Tc-[99m] DTPA aerosal/Tc-[99m] MAA lung study. J Nucl Med 25:1108–10, 1984

14. Pittard WB, III, Merkatz R, Fletcher BD: Radioactivity excretion in human milk following administration of technetium Tc[99m] macro-aggregated albumin. Pediatrics 70:231–34, 1982

15. Tribukati B, Swedjemark GA: Secretion of [99]Tc[m] in breast milk after intravenous injection of marked macroaggregated albumin. Acta Radiol Oncol 17:379–82, 1978

16. Berke RA, et al: Radiation dose to breast-feeding child after mother has [99]Tc[m] MAA lung scan. J Nucl Med 14:51–52, 1973

17. Mountford PJ, Coakley AJ, Hall FM: Excretion of radioactivity in breast milk following injection of [99]Tc[m] DTPA. Nucl Med Commun 6:341–45, 1985

18. Romney B, Nickoloff EL, Esser PD: Excretion of radioiodine in breast milk. J Nucl Med 30:124–26, 1989

19. Dydek GJ, Blue PW: Human breast milk excretion of iodine-131 following diagnostic and therapeutic administration to a lactating patient with Graves' disease. J Nucl Med 29:407–10, 1988

20. Hedrick WR, DiSimone RN, Keen RL: Radiation dosimetry from breast milk excretion of radioiodine and pertechnetate. J Nucl Med 27:1569–71, 1986

21. Bland EP, et al: Radioactive iodine uptake by thyroid of breast-fed infants after maternal blood volume measurements. Lancet 1:1039–40, 1969

22. Palmer KE: Excretion of ^{125}I in breast milk following administration of labelled fibrinogen. Br J Radiol 52:672–73, 1979

23. Weaver JC, Kamm ML, Dobson RL: The excretion of radioiodine in human milk. J Am Med Assoc 173:872–75, 1960

24. Nurnberger CE, Lipscomb A: Transmission of radioiodine (I[131]) to infants through human maternal milk. J Am Med Assoc 150:1398–1400, 1952

25. Taylor DM, McCready VR, Cosgrove DO: The transfer of L-seleno-methionine-75SE to human milk and the potential radiation dose to a breast-fed infant. Nucl Med Commun 2:8083, 1981

26. Tobin RE, Schneider PB: Uptake of ^{67}Ga in the lactating breast and its persistence in milk. J Nucl Med 17:1055–56, 1976

27. Mountford PJ, Coakley AJ: Excretion of radioactivity in breast milk after an Indium-111 leukocyte scan. J Nucl Med 26:1096–97, 1985

her for breastfeeding at frequent intervals during her hospitalization. Nurses and LCs can be advocates for changing policies and for relaxing hospital restrictions which place an unnecessary additional hardship on families. For example, when the mother has a postpartum depression, denying the disturbed woman access to her infant imposes a justifiable paranoia—in addition to whatever thought disorder is already present.

Fortunately, a mother with an acute illness is now more likely to be treated as an outpatient rather than hospitalized. As a result, separation because of hospitalization is not as frequent a barrier to breastfeeding as it was a few years ago.

Chronic illnesses present a somewhat different potential dilemma for the breastfeeding mother and the clinician assisting her. In some cases, the nature of the chronic illness and its effect on the mother's functioning may interfere to a greater or lesser extent on her ability to breastfeed. In other cases, creative alternatives to "usual" solutions are all that is needed to give the mother the opportunity to experience the same infant feeding as other mothers who do not have a chronic illness. In addition, drug therapy, particularly because it is likely to be long-term, may pose risks to the breastfeeding infant which are not an issue if the mother has an acute, self-limiting illness. Thus, the clinician needs to look beyond the illness itself and examine how the condition is being managed, as well as what the mother wishes to do given complete information about the risks and benefits of breastfeeding for both herself and her baby—in light of her chronic illness. In many cases, the therapy of choice need not be changed, because it poses no dangers for the suckling infant. A case in point is the management of hypertension when the mother is lactating. According to White (1984), the drugs used for this condition appear to be safe for the breastfeeding baby.

Attention must be given to any situation which rarely receives notice. Care must be taken to accurately interpret the mother's desire to begin and/or to continue breastfeeding when faced with uncommon difficulties or situations. Occasionally when an illness or a breastfeeding problem occurs, health-professionals may be asked to give permission to wean to a woman who no longer wants to continue breastfeeding. Even if there is no reason to wean, a relatively minor difficulty can occasionally present a mother with a socially acceptable "out" from a situation which she is emotionally uncomfortable with, or finds inconvenient for her lifestyle. For the health-care worker who is enthusiastic about breastfeeding, personal feelings and the knowledge of the benefits of breastfeeding may conflict with the subtle response from the client which suggests she would rather wean. Typically, the comment that the physician, lactation consultant or nurse "told me to wean" because of a problem may partially reflect the mother's own wishes. Avoiding judgmental responses and encouraging her to air conflicting feelings may enable the mother to place her breastfeeding experience in context, so that she can focus on the positive aspects of her experience rather than upon its more problematic aspects.

SUMMARY

In this chapter we reviewed several health conditions which relate to the lactating mother and sug-

gested interventions that facilitate the lactation process. Admittedly, our discussion is far from inclusive of the full range of acute or chronic diseases the health-professional will find in practice. To find information on other health problems the mother may develop while she is lactating, we recommend several excellent gynecological and medical-surgical texts for physicians and nurses which more thoroughly discuss the conditions described here.

REFERENCES

Ala-Houhala, M, et al.: 25-hydroxyvitamin D and vitamin D in human milk: effects of supplementation and season, *Am J Clin Nutr* 48:1057–60, 1988.

Alder, EM, and Cox, JL: Breastfeeding and post-natal depression, *J Psychosom Res* 27:139–44, 1983.

Amico, JA, and Finley, BE: Breast stimulation in cycling women, pregnant women and a woman with induced lactation: Pattern of release of oxytocin, prolactin and luteinizing hormone, *Clin Endocrinol* 25:97–106, 1986.

Anderson, K: Nursing my adopted daughter, *New Beginnings* 4:108, 1988.

Auerbach, KG: Extraordinary breastfeeding: relactation/induced lactation, *J Trop Pediatr* 27:52–55, 1981.

Auerbach, KG, and Avery, JL: Induced lactation: a study of adoptive nursing by 24 women, *Am J Dis Child* 135:340–43, 1981.

Auerbach, KG, and Avery, JL: *Nursing the adopted infant: report from a survey, RHNI Monograph #5,* 1979.

Auerbach, KG, and Avery, JL: Relactation: a study of 366 cases, *Pediatrics* 65:236–42, 1980.

Auerbach, KG, and Jacobi, A: Postpartum depression in the breastfeeding mother: In *NAACOG Clinical Issues in Perinatal and Women's Health Nursing,* Philadelphia, 1990, J.B. Lippincott Co., pp. 375–84.

Berlin, CM, et al.: Disposition of dietary caffeine in milk, saliva, and plasma of lactating women, *Pediatrics* 73:59–63, 1984.

Bitman, J, et al.: Lipid composition of milk from mothers with cystic fibrosis, *Pediatrics* 80:927–32, 1987.

Bitman, J, et al.: Milk composition and volume during the onset of lactation in a diabetic mother, *Am J Clin Nutr* 50:1364–69, 1989.

Bonham, GS, and Wilson, RW: Children's health in families with cigarette smokers, *Am J Public Health* 71:290–93, 1981.

Bowles, BC; Breastfeeding consultation in sign language, *J Hum Lact* 7:21, 1991.

Bradshaw, MD, and Pfeiffer, S: Feeding mode and anthropometric changes in primiparas, *Hum Biol* 60:251–61, 1988.

Brodie, MJ: Management of epilepsy during pregnancy and lactation, *Lancet* 336:426–27, 1990.

Brown, KH, et al.: Lactational capacity of marginally nourished mothers: relationships between maternal nutritional status and quantity and proximate composition of milk, *Pediatrics* 78:909–19, 1986.

Brown, RE: Relactation: an overview, *Pediatrics* 60:116–20, 1977.

Butte, NF, et al.: Effect of maternal diet and body composition on lactational performance, *Am J Clin Nutr* 39:296–306, 1984a.

Butte, NF, et al.: Human milk intake and growth in exclusively breast-fed infants, *J Pediatr* 104:187–95, 1984b.

Butte, NF, et al.: Milk composition of insulin-dependent diabetic women, *J Pediatr Gastroenterol Nutr* 6:936–41, 1987.

Carty, E, Conine, TA, and Hall, L: Comprehensive health promotion for the pregnant woman who is disabled, *J Nurs-Midwif* 35:133–42, 1990.

Carty, E, Conine, TA, and Wood-Johnson, F: Rheumatoid arthritis and pregnancy: helping women to meet their needs, *Midwives Chron* 99:254–57, 1986.

Coakley, AJ, and Mountford, PJ: Nuclear medicine and the nursing mother, *Br Med J* 291:159–60, 1985.

Conine, TA, Carty, E, and Safarik, PM: *Aids and adaptations for parents with physical or sensory disabilities,* Vancouver, B.C., 1988, School of Rehabilitative Medicine, University of British Columbia, Canada.

Dahlström, A, et al.: Nicotine and cotinine concentrations in the nursing mother and her infant, *Acta Paediatr Scand* 79:142–47, 1990.

D'Alonzo, GE: The pregnant asthmatic patient, *Sem Perinatol* 14:119–29, 1990.

Davies, HA, et al.: Insulin requirements of diabetic women who breastfeed, *Br Med J* 298:1357–58, 1989.

Davis, DR: Nutrition in the United States: much room for improvement, *J Appl Nutr* 356:17–29, 1983.

Dugdale, AE, and Eaton-Evans, J: The effect of lactation and other factors on post-partum changes in body-weight and triceps skinfold thickness, *Br J Nutr* 61:149–53, 1989.

Duncan, B, et al.: Iron and the exclusively breast-fed infant from birth to six months, *J Pediatr Gastroenterol Nutr* 4:421–25, 1985.

Dusdieker, LB, et al.: Effect of supplemental fluids on human milk production, *J Pediatr* 106:207–11, 1985.

Dusdieker, LB, et al.: Prolonged maternal fluid supplementation in breast-feeding, *Pediatrics* 86:737–40, 1990.

Eaton-Evans, J, and Dugdale, AE: Food avoidance by breast-feeding mothers in southeast Queensland, *Ecol Food Nutr* 19:123–29, 1986.

Ehrenkranz, RA, and Ackerman, BA: Metoclopramide effect on faltering milk production by mothers of premature infants, *Pediatrics* 78:614–20, 1986.

Engelking, C, and Page-Lieberman, J: *Maternal diabetes and diabetes in young children: their relationship to breastfeeding,* Lactation Consultant Series (Unit 5), Garden City Park, N.Y., 1986, Avery Publishing Group, Inc.

Ferris, AM, et al.: Lactation outcome in insulin-dependent diabetic women, *J Am Diet Assoc* 88:317–22, 1988.

Frederick, IB, White, RJ, and Braddock, SW: Excretion of varicella-herpes zoster virus in breastmilk, *Am J Obstet Gynecol* 154:1116–17, 1986.

Fulton, B: Recreational drug use in the breastfeeding mother, Part 2: Licit drugs, *J Hum Lact* 6:15–17, 1990.

Gennaro, S: Postpartal anxiety and depression in mothers of term or preterm infants, *Nurs Res* 37:82–85, 1988.

Golembeski, DJ, and Emergy, MG: Lipid composition of milk from mothers with cystic fibrosis (letter), *Pediatrics* (suppl.) 31:631–32, 1989.

Guthrie, DW, and Guthrie, RA: *Nursing management of diabetes mellitus,* 2nd ed., St. Louis, 1982, The C.V. Mosby Co.

Handford, P: Postpartum depression: what is it, what helps? *Can Nurs* 81:(1):30–33, 1985.

Harris, B, et al.: The hormonal environment of post-natal depression, *Br J Psychiatry* 154:660–67, 1989.

Hayslip, CC, et al.: The effect of lactation on bone mineral content in healthy postpartum women, *Obstet Gynecol* 73:588–92, 1989.

Holmgren, U, et al.: Women with prolactinoma—effect of pregnancy and lactation on serum prolactin and on tumour growth, *Acta Endocrinologica* 111:452–59, 1986.

Hopkins, J, Marcus, M, and Campbell, SB: Postpartum depression: a critical review, *Psychol Bull* 95:498–515, 1984.

Hormann, E: Breast feeding the adopted baby, *Birth Fam J* 4:165–72, 1977.

Ikegami, H, et al.: Relationship between the methods of treatment of prolactinomas and the puerperal lactation, *Fertil Steril* 47:867–69, 1987.

Illingworth, RS, and Kilpatrick, B: Lactation and fluid intake, *Lancet* 2:1175–77, 1953.

Jelliffe, DB, and Jelliffe, EFP: Non-puerperal induced lactation (letter), *Pediatrics* 50:170–71, 1972.

Kampmann, JP: Proplythiouracil in human milk: revision of a dogma, *Lancet* 1:736–38, 1980.

Kirshbaum, M: The parent with a physical disability. In Auvenshine, JM, and Enriques, MG: *Comprehensive maternity nursing: perinatal and women's health,* Boston, 1990, Jones and Bartlett Publishers, Inc.

Kitzinger, S: *The crying baby,* New York, 1989, Penguin Books.

Koetting, CA, and Wardlaw, GM: Wrist, spine, and hip bone density in women with variable histories of lactation, *Am J Clin Nutr* 48:1479–81, 1988.

Kopala, B: Mothers with impaired mobility speak out, *MCN* 14:115–19, 1989.

Korn-Lubetski, I, et al.: Activity of multiple sclerosis during pregnancy and puerperium, *Ann Neurology* 16:229–31, 1984.

La Leche League International: *La Leche League News* 18:69, 1976, The League.

Lauwers, J, and Woessner, C: *Chemical agents and breast milk,* Garden City Park, N.Y., 1990, Avery Publishing Group, Inc., p. 41.

Lawrence, RA: Breastfeeding and medical disease, *Med Clin North Am* 73:583–603, 1989.

LeGuennec, J-C, and Billon, B: Delay in caffeine elimination in breast-fed infants, *Pediatrics* 79:264–68, 1987.

Lindstrom, LH: CSF and plasma β-Casomorphin-like opioid peptides in postpartum psychosis, *Am J Psychiatry* 141:1059–66, 1984.

Lipkin, GB: Drug therapy in maternal care. In Spencer, RT,

et al.: *Clinical Pharmacology and nursing management,* 3rd ed., Philadelphia, 1989, J. B. Lippincott Co., pp. 1132–70.

Lipsman, S, Dewey, KG, and Lonnerdal, B: Breast-feeding among teenage mothers: milk composition, infant growth, and maternal dietary intake, *J Pediatr Gastroenterol Nutr* 4:426–34, 1985.

Little, RE, et al.: Agreement between laboratory tests and self-reports of alcohol, tobacco, caffeine, marijuana and other drug use in post-partum women, *Soc Sci Med* 22:91–98, 1986.

Lovelady, CA, Lonnerdal, B, and Dewey, KG: Lactation performance of exercising women, *Am J Clin Nutr* 52:103–9, 1990.

Luck, W, and Nau, H: Nicotine and cotinine concentrations in serum and milk of nursing smokers, *Br J Clin Pharmacol* 18:9–15, 1984.

Luck, W, and Nau, H.: Nicotine and cotinine concentrations in serum and urine of infants exposed via passive smoking or milk from smoking mothers, *J Pediatr* 107:816–20, 1985.

Luder, E, et al.: Current recommendations for breast-feeding in cystic fibrosis centers, *Am J Dis Child* 144:1153–56, 1990.

Matheson, I, Kristensen, K, and Lunde, PKM: Drug utilization in breast-feeding women. A survey in Oslo, *Eur J Clin Pharmacol* 38:453–59, 1990.

McCullough, AL, et al.: Vitamin B_6 status of Egyptian mothers: relation to infant behavior and maternal-infant interactions, *Am J Clin Nutr* 51:1067–74, 1990.

McDougall, IR, and Bayer, MF: Should a woman taking propylthiouracil breast-feed? *Clin Nucl Med* 11:249–50, 1986.

McMillan, JA, Landaw, SA, and Oski, FA: Iron sufficiency in breast-fed infants and the availability of iron from human milk, *Pediatrics* 58:686–92, 1976.

Merchant, K, Martorell, R, and Hass, J: Maternal and fetal responses to the stresses of lactation concurrent with pregnancy and short recuperative intervals, *Am J Clin Nutr* 52:280–88, 1990.

Mevissen-Verhage, EAE, et al.: Effect of iron on neonatal gut flora during the first three months of life, *Eur J Clin Microbiol* 4:273–78, 1985.

Minami, J: Helping mothers with chronic illness, *Leaven* 26:52–53, 1990.

Miyake, A, et al.: Decrease in neonatal suckled milk volume in diabetic women, *Eur J Obstetr Gynecol Reprod Biol* 33:49–53, 1989.

Momotani, N, et al.: Recovery from foetal hypothyroidism: evidence for the safety of breast-feeding while taking propylthiouracil, *Clin Endocrinol* 31:591–95, 1989.

Motil, KJ, Montandon, CM, and Garza, C: Basal and postprandial metabolic rates in lactating and nonlactating women, *Am J Clin Nutr* 52:610–15, 1990.

Neifert, M, McDonough, S, and Neville, M: Failure of lactogenesis associated with placental retention, *Am J Obstet Gynecol* 140:477–78, 1981.

Nelson, LM, et al.: Risk of multiple sclerosis exacerbation during pregnancy and breast-feeding, *JAMA,* 259:3441–43, 1988.

Nursing Mothers' Association of Australia: *Where there's a will, there's usually a way—Breastfeeding when the mother has a disability,* Hawthorn, Victoria, Australia, 1982, The Association.

Olango, P, and Aboud, F: Determinants of mothers' treatment of diarrhea in rural Ethiopia, *Soc Sci Med* 31:1245–49, 1990.

Oski, FA, and Landaw, SA: Inhibition of iron absorption from human milk by baby food, *Am J Dis Child* 134:459–60, 1980.

Osman, AK: Dietary practices and aversions during pregnancy and lactation among Sudanese women, *J Trop Pediatr* 31:16–20, 1985.

Pastel, RA, Howanitz, PJ, and Oski, FA: Iron sufficiency with prolonged exclusive breast-feeding in Peruvian infants, *Clin Pediatr* 20:625–26, 1981.

Poser, S, and Poser, W: Multiple sclerosis and gestation, *Neurology* 33:1423–27, 1983.

Riordan, J: Drugs excreted in breastmilk. In Pagliaro, L, and Pagliaro, AM: *Problems in pediatric drug therapy,* 2nd ed., Hamilton, Ill., 1987, Drug Intelligence Publications, Inc.

Romney, BM, Nickoloff, EL, and Esser, PD: Excretion of radioiodine in breast milk, *J Nucl Med* 30:124–26, 1989.

Rona, RJ, et al.: Parental smoking at home and the height of children, *Br Med J* 283:1361, 1981.

Rylance, GW, et al.: Carbimazole and breastfeeding (letter), *Lancet* 1(8538):928, 1987.

Ryu, JE: Caffeine in human milk and in serum of breast-fed infants, *Dev Pharmacol Ther* 8:329–37, 1985a.

Ryu, JE: Effect of maternal caffeine consumption on heart rate and sleep time of breast-fed infants, *Dev Pharmacol Ther* 8:355–63, 1985b.

Said, G, Patois, E, and Lellouch, J: Infantile colic and parental smoking, *Br Med J* 289:660, 1984.

Salmenpera, L, Perheentupa, J, and Siimes, MA: Folate nutrition is optimal in exclusively breast-fed infants but inadequate in some of their mothers and in formula-fed infants, *J Pediatr Gastroenterol Nutr* 5:283–89, 1986.

Schou, M: Lithium treatment during pregnancy, delivery, and lactation: an update, *J Clin Psychiatry* 51(10):410–13, 1990.

Scott, D: Nursing the impaired mother-infant relationship in puerperal depression, *Aust J Adv Nurs* 1(4):50–56, 1984.

Shiffman, ML, et al.: Breast-milk composition in women with cystic fibrosis: report of two cases and a review of the literature, *Am J Clin Nutr* 49:612–17, 1989.

Smith, CA: Effects of maternal undernutrition upon the newborn infant in Holland (1944–45), *J Pediatr* 30:229–43, 1947.

Specker, BL, et al.: Effect of vegetarian diet on serum 1,25-dihydroxyvitamin D concentrations during lactation, *Obstet Gynecol* 70:870–74, 1987.

Spring, PCM, et al.: Fat and energy content of breast milk of malnourished and well nourished women, Brazil 1982, *Ann Trop Paediatr* 5:83–87, 1985.

Steldinger, R, and Luck, W: Half lives of nicotine in milk of smoking mothers: implications for nursing (letter), *J Perinat Med* 16:261–62, 1988.

Stumbo, PJ, et al.: Water intakes of lactating women, *Am J Dis Child* 142:870–76, 1985.

Summary and Recommendations of the Second International Workshop-Conference on Gestational Diabetes Mellitus, *Am J Clin Nutr* 85:1351–55, 1985.

Sutherland, A, and Auerbach, KG: *Relactation and induced lactation* (Unit 1), Lactation Consultant Series, Garden City Park, N.Y., 1985, Avery Publishing Group, Inc.

Tamminen, T: The impact of mother's depression on her breastfeeding attitudes and experiences, *J Psychosom Obstet Gynecol* (Suppl.)10:69–78, 1989.

Trundle, JI, and Skellern, GG: Gas chromatographic determination of nicotine in human breast milk, *J Clin Hosp Pharm* 8:289–93, 1983.

Vio, F, Salazar, G, and Infante, C: Smoking during pregnancy and lactation and its effects on breast-milk volume, *Am J Clin Nutr* 54:1011–16, 1991.

Vuori, E, et al.: Maternal diet and fatty acid pattern of breast milk, *Acta Paediatr Scand* 71:959–63, 1982.

Waletzky, L: Emotional illness in the postpartum period. In Ahmed, P, ed.: *Pregnancy, childbirth and parenthood,* New York, 1981, Elsevier North-Holland, Inc.

Waletzky, LR, and Herman, EC: Relactation, *Am Fam Phys* 14:69–74, 1976.

Welch, MJ, Phelps, DL, and Osher, AB: Breast-feeding by a mother with cystic fibrosis, *Pediatrics* 67:664–66, 1981.

Whichelow, MJ, and Doddridge, MC: Lactation in diabetic women, *Br Med J* 287:649–50, 1983.

White, WB: Management of hypertension during lactation, *Hypertension* 6:297–300, 1984.

Woodruff, CW, Latham, C, and McDavid, S: Iron nutrition in the breast-fed infant, *J Pediatr* 90:36–38, 1977.

Woodward, A, and Hand, K: Smoking and reduced duration of breast-feeding (letter), *Med J Aust* 148:477–78, 1988.

Yurchak, AM, and Jusko, WSJ: Theophylline secretion into breast milk, *Pediatrics* 57:518–20, 1976.

14

Breast-Related Problems

In nursing practice or lactation consultant counseling, as elsewhere, an ounce of prevention is worth a pound of intervention. Many difficulties women encounter while breastfeeding can be prevented by the self-care measures and breastfeeding education discussed in preceding chapters. When a woman fully understands how her body works, she is at less risk for frustration and failure when she encounters a barrier to breastfeeding. We turn now to specific breast problems, identifying how health-professionals can help.

Clinicians who work with breastfeeding women agree that breast and nipple problems can be common barriers to breastfeeding. During prenatal visits, women should be screened for unusual looking breasts, areola, or nipples, as well as lack of breast enlargement. Any of these conditions, coupled with previous breastfeeding difficulties, are high-risk indicators for breastfeeding problems (Livingstone, 1990).

Before discussing the more clinical aspects of breast-related problems, including surgery, the emotional significance of the female breasts deserves attention. Breasts are part of a woman's internalized body image which she develops around adolescence and carries with her for the rest of her life. They represent a woman's deepest sense of womanhood. Any change in her breasts—for instance, breast surgery—threatens this feminine internal view of self and creates a disequilibrium. When a woman's breasts are altered by illness or infection, this can be a double whammy: both her femininity and her ability to breastfeed can be threatened.

JAN RIORDAN

KATHLEEN G. AUERBACH

NIPPLE VARIATIONS

INVERTED OR FLAT NIPPLES

As pointed out in Chapter 4 the frequency of nipple inversion is unknown, although clinicians have reported that this condition sometimes is self-resolving from the beginning to the end of pregnancy. In many cases, the degree of inversion is such that it does not affect the ability of the baby to eventually grasp the areolar tissue and draw the nipple into the mouth, although this might take longer. Lactation consultants have observed that women who have markedly inverted nipples early in their first pregnancy and who go on to breastfeed have much less inversion with subsequent pregnancies. In some cases, these women have reported that the nipples which initially inverted between feedings with the first baby no longer do so with second and later infants.

The degree to which inverted nipples are an impediment to breastfeeding is partially caused by the belief that they prevent breastfeeding. How the nipple looks when it is not in the baby's mouth, however, does not always predict how well it will function. In most cases, as long as the mother positions the baby well back on the areola, so that the entire nipple is placed well back in the baby's mouth, there is no reason why a mother with inverted nipples should forgo breastfeeding. One hopes that soon careful ultrasound studies will be undertaken to observe how the inverted nipple responds to the negative pressure generated by suckling in the infant's mouth. Studies have already confirmed that during suckling the nipple elongates to double its "resting" length (Smith, Erenberg & Nowak, 1988). Such reactivity to infant suckling helps to explain why the degree of inversion appears to lessen after weeks or months of repeated suckling by the infant.

The clinician should examine the mother's breasts and nipples in the third trimester of pregnancy. At the time of this initial examination, discussion about breastfeeding can begin. If the mother has flat or inverted nipples, the following recommendations can be made.

Wear breast shells. Breast shells consist of two pieces of plastic, doughnut-shaped cups with inner and outer portions that snap together. By exerting a continuous, gentle pressure around the areola, the nipple is pushed through a central opening in the inner shell. Shells should be worn during the last trimester of pregnancy, initially for one to two hours each day. Gradually, the length of wearing time should be increased until they are worn all day.

Shells can also help to evert nipples after childbirth if they are worn one-half hour before a feeding. The mother may use the milk that collects in the cup if it is not more than one hour old; body warmth may foster bacterial growth. The cups are washed after each feeding and boiled once a day. Various trade names of these shells are Ameda/Egnell, Free and Dry, Hobbit Shields, Medela, Netsy, Nurse-Dri, and Woolwich. Shells with multiple airways (Ameda/Egnell and Medela) allow air to circulate to the nipple areola; if placed upwards, milk will not leak through the air holes. (See Chapter 11 on Breast Pumps and Technologies for a further discussion, photographs of shells, and addresses of manufacturers.)

Exercise the nipple/areola. As originally suggested by Hoffman (1953) and explained in Fig. 14–1, nipple exercises are used for separating adhesions which cause retraction or inversion. The nipple, which has tiny muscles that are highly elastic, is stretched forward and held outward several times a day. Based on extensive clinical experience in lactation, Chele Marmet and Ellen Shell, directors of The Lactation Clinic in Los Angeles,

believe that the Hoffman exercises are generally ineffective unless they are done numerous times each day (Marmet & Shell, personal communication, 1991).

Exercising the nipple just before latching-on a newborn, however, appears to effectively loosen the nipple tissue. The infant also stretches the nipples during feedings. Additionally, any change in the degree of eversion may result in greater confidence that breastfeeding will proceed without further difficulty. These exercises may also be helpful, insofar as the mothers who practice them become comfortable handling their breasts in a matter-of-fact manner.

Stimulate and shape the nipple just before the feeding. For a flat nipple (not inverted), massage the nipple or apply a cold cloth to help the nipple to evert outward. For an inverted nipple, instruct the mother to shape her nipple by placing her thumb about one-and-one-half to two inches behind the nipple (with her fingers beneath) and pulling back into her chest. This works best in a side-lying position (Huggins, 1986).

Apply suction by using a pump. Any pump can be used to help pull out the nipple immediately before the infant feeds.

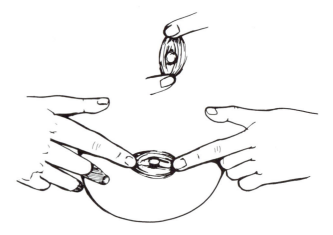

FIGURE 14–1 Hoffman's exercises. Mother places her thumbs opposite each other on either side of nipple, then gently draws thumbs distally or away from nipple. Repeat with thumbs above and below nipple. From Riordan, J: *A Practical Guide to Breastfeeding,* Boston, 1990, Jones and Bartlett Publishers, Inc., p. 118.

LARGE/ELONGATED NIPPLES

Nipples come in assorted sizes and shapes; like all anatomical structures they are genetically influenced. Boarman (personal communication, 1991) reports that a number of Asian mothers (Korean, Vietnamese, Filipino) in her practice have unusually long nipples. Generally, nipples which are larger or longer than normal are less likely to cause problems in breastfeeding than inverted or flat nipples. In fact, they are often viewed as an anatomical "gift" that will make breastfeeding easier. While this is true in many cases, exceptionally long or large nipples detract from breastfeeding, especially if the infant is small. Infants of mothers with extra-long nipples have been observed to gag after latch-on and "slide back" toward the nipple tip, which in some cases causes the mother to develop sore nipples. (See color photographs of extra-long nipples featured in the endpapers of this book.)

PLUGGED DUCTS

No one knows the specific cause of plugged ducts, but they are usually found in mothers who have an abundant milk supply and who do not adequately drain each breast (Livingstone, personal communication, 1991). Pathologic changes causing the "plug" within the breast are vaguely referred to in the literature as a stasis, clogging of milk, or "local accumulations of milk or dead cells that have been shed." A plugged duct is indicated by either of these two sets of symptoms: complaints of tenderness, heat, and possibly redness in one area of the breast; or, if the plug is located in a duct close to the skin, a palpable lump of well-defined margins which is not accompanied by generalized fever. Sometimes a tiny white plug can be seen at the opening of the duct on the nipple. One mother described it as "little bits of a hard white substance that is just beneath the surface of milk duct outlets." (See color photographs of plugged ducts featured in the endpapers of this book.)

Clinicians are aware of a higher frequency of plugged ducts during the winter season. The reason for this is not clear, although it may be related to the restricting effects of winter clothing or simply the cold weather. There is also some evidence that, whereas some women are predisposed to developing plugged ducts, others never do—even through multiple breastfeeding experiences. Plugged ducts can also lead to mastitis, especially if ignored or untreated. Self-care measures to recommend to a mother with a plugged duct are given in the boxed list below.

In an acute situation, stripping the breast effectively dislodges the blocked milk. If a mother has chronically recurring plugged ducts, some physicians elect to open the ducts with a sterile, needle-like instrument. After this is done, the milk may forcibly "shoot out" from the duct, and the mother feels relief. Incomplete drainage caused by a skipped feeding or a constricting bra, poor nutrition, and stress have all been implicated in the development of plugged ducts—but a cause and effect relationship has never been substantiated. Assessment should include a review of these possibilities with

---

SELF-CARE FOR TREATING A PLUGGED DUCT

- Continue to breastfeed often. Begin feeding on the affected breast to promote drainage.
- Apply moist heat to the area several times a day, generally before breastfeeding.
- Massage the affected breast before and during feeding to stimulate flow of milk. Support the breast with a cupped hand and use firm massage—starting at the periphery of the breast, using thumb to encourage flow of milk while baby suckles. Another option is to massage in a hot shower or bath. Outside of the shower try using an electric vibrator (on low setting).
- Soak the affected breast(s) by leaning over a basin of warm water, then gently massage.
- Change position of the infant during feedings to ensure drainage of all the sinuses and ductules in the breast. At least one position should result in the baby's nose being pointed toward the site of the plugged duct.
- Avoid any constricting clothing such as an underwire bra or straps on a baby carrier.

the mother and a review of events leading up to the plugged duct, especially if she has a repeated problem. There is no need for an antibiotic to treat a plugged duct, unless a fever and mastitis develop.

MASTITIS

Mastitis usually develops after the mother leaves the hospital. Nurses and LCs who practice in the community may be the first to speak with the mother whose symptoms suggest early indication of mastitis. The advice dispensed during this initial call can prevent the condition from advancing to an abscess, especially if the mother mistakenly thinks she should stop breastfeeding or has already done so.

The initial symptoms of puerperal mastitis may be fatigue, localized breast tenderness, and a flu-like, muscular aching. If a breastfeeding mother calls into the clinic or office complaining that she has the "flu," the first consideration is to rule out infectious mastitis (LLLI, 1991). Typically, fatigue, headache, and muscular aching are followed by fever, a rapid pulse, and the appearance of a hot, reddened, and tender area on the breast (see Table 14–1). The infection is usually unilateral and in one area (often in the upper outer breast quadrant), although it can occur in any area of the breast. Mastitis can occasionally occur bilaterally and may involve a large portion of the breast. The infection can also affect milk com-

position: an elevation of sodium and chloride in the milk from an infected breast has been noted in two reports (Conner, 1979; Thullen, 1988).

Among women who breastfeed long-term, mastitis is most likely to occur in the first several weeks after delivery. About one-third of the cases, however, occur after the infant is six months old. Another one-fourth of the cases were reported after 12 months of breastfeeding (Riordan & Nichols, 1990). Symptoms may last from two to four days followed by resolution. Early reports showed the incidence to be six percent or less (Waller, 1938; Leary, 1948; Marshall, Hepper & Zirbel, 1975); these studies, however, counted only those women who returned to the clinic or physician to treat their mastitis. The actual incidence is much higher; for long-term breastfeeders it may be as high as 33% (Riordan & Nichols, 1990). A number of factors are thought to predispose a woman to lactation mastitis. These include stress, fatigue, cracked or fissured nipples, plugged ducts, constriction caused by a tight bra or incorrect sleeping position, engorgement or milk stasis, and an abrupt change in frequency of feedings. When mothers who had mastitis were asked to list factors present before the breast infection, they rated fatigue, stress, and plugged ducts as most prevalent.

The best treatments for hastening recovery are continued breastfeeding, application of moist heat, increased fluids, bed rest, and the judicious use of antibiotics (Kimball, 1951; Marshall, Hepper & Zir-

TABLE 14–1 FACTORS ASSOCIATED WITH MASTITIS AS RATED BY PARTICIPANTS

Rank	Factor	Score	%
1	Fatigue	38	24
2	Stress	35	22
3	Plugged ducts	28	17
4	Change in number of feedings	24	15
5	Engorgement/stasis	17	10
6	Sore/cracked nipples	7	4
7	Family infection	6	4
8	Breast trauma	5	3
9	Poor diet	1	.6
10	Exercise	0	—
		161*	99.6

*Respondents mentioned more than one factor.
From Riordan, J, and Nichols, F: A descriptive study of lactation mastitis in long-term breastfeeding women, *J Hum Lact* 6:53–58, 1990.

TABLE 14–2 SELECTED ORAL ANTIBIOTICS FOR MASTITIS

Generic Name	Trade Name	Adult Dosage Ranges
Penicillinase-resistant penicillins		
Cloxacillin	Tegopen	PO 250–500 mg q 6hr
Dicloxacillin	Dynapen	PO/IM 125–250 mg q 6hr
Oxacillin	Prostaphlin	PO/IM 500 mg–1 g q 4–6hr
Cephalosporins		
Cephalexin	Keflex	PO 250–500 mg q 6hr
Cephradine	Anspor, Velosef	PO 250–500 mg q 6hr
Cefaclor	Ceclor	PO 250–500 mg q 8hr

bel, 1975; Thomsen et al., 1985; LLLI, 1991). It is well established in the medical literature (Marshall, Hepper & Zirbel, 1975; Newton & Newton, 1950) that mastitis is associated with the presence of staphylococci. Only rarely is a streptococcus involved; when it is, the mastitis may be bilateral (Schreiner et al., 1977). The standard antibiotic for lactation mastitis is a penicillinase-resistant penicillin or a cephalosporin that covers *Staphylococcus aureus* for 6 to 10 days (Thomsen et al., 1985). Dicloxacillin is often used as the most specific treatment for mastitis; however, as first-generation cephalosporins become available in their generic form at lesser cost, they will probably be used more (see Table 14–2). Both drugs are considered safe during lactation by most clinicians (Ogle & Davis, 1988).

For chronic mastitis, erythromycin at low doses (regular dosage 250–500 mg every 6 hours) or trimethoprim-sulfamethoxazole (Bactrim, Septra) over a longer period of time has been recommended (Cantlie, 1988). Trimethoprim-sulfamethoxazole and erythromycin are also options when the mother is allergic to penicillin. In a case report, trimethoprim-sulfamethoxazole (two tablets per day for ten days) was effective in preventing recurrence of mastitis in a patient with multiple incidences of mastitis who was allergic to penicillin (Hoffman & Auerbach, 1986).

These medications can be taken during breastfeeding without known untoward reactions in the infant.

A small percentage of breast infections develop into an abscess. An abscess, like a boil, is basically a collection of pus that must be drained. If the abscess is small, the pus may be aspirated with a needle. Livingstone (personal communication, 1991) reports some success with using fine-needle aspiration under ultrasound guidance to treat an abscess. For a larger abscess, the physician makes an incision and drains the area. According to Love (1990), "The surgeon will never sew up a drained abscess; that would lock the bacteria into the abscess, and almost insure the infection's return. I tell my patients to go home and rest; then, after 24 hours, begin taking daily showers; let the water run over the breast and wash away the bacteria, and then put a dressing over it to absorb oozing fluids from the incision." A tube is placed in the incision to promote drainage; in addition, manual expression helps eliminate pus and milk. The incision heals from the inside out within one to two weeks.

The major share of medical research on lactation mastitis has focused on pathology, biomedical analysis, and attempts to classify types of mastitis. Gibberd (1953), for instance, described two types of mastitis: cellulitis and adenitis. Cellulitis is thought to involve the interlobular connective tissue which has been infected by the introduction of bacteria through cracked nipples; it is treated with antibiotics. In adenitis, presumably, the breast ducts are blocked, and the clinical symptoms are less severe. Treatment involves getting the milk to flow with heat, expression, and pumping. Antibiotics are used only if the infection is not resolving (Livingstone, 1990). One newer therapy is breast stripping (Bertrand & Rosenblood, 1991).

Thomsen et al. (1985) proposes another classification based on leukocyte counts in milk taken from the infected breast:

- *Milk stasis:* Leukocyte count less than 10^6/mL of milk; symptoms lasting for an average of 2.1 days.
- *Noninfectious inflammation:* Leukocyte count more than 10^6/mL of milk; symptoms lasting about 5.3 days
- *Infectious mastitis:* Leukocyte count more than 10^6/mL and bacteria count more than 10^3/mL.

He recommends that antibiotic treatment be used only for infectious mastitis, the third classification. Although this taxonomy is helpful in theory, laboratory studies on mastitic milk are seldom done in practice. By the time the mother reports the problem to a physician, she has usually been ill for several hours, if not a day or two; the peak of the infectious process may already have passed, and she is getting well by the time she seeks medical treatment. Other drawbacks: the milk sample must be collected before any antibiotics are started; laboratory studies may take several days; and the testing expense may not be covered by health insurance.

SKIN RASHES AND LESIONS

Breast rashes and lesions on the nipple/areolar area are unusual and often difficult to diagnose. They are particularly distressing if they are painful. In one case (Brackett, 1988) a mother described a periodic burning sensation in the breast not related to actual breastfeeding. Most of the mother's areola was "itchy," flaky and red. The family lived without air conditioning during hot, humid weather. In addition, the mother swam in a chlorinated pool each day and often wore her bathing suit for some time after returning home. Thrush was ruled out as a possible cause of her problem. The mother stopped swimming and her rash resolved within two weeks.

A more severe breast skin problem is redness and itching accompanied by tiny ulcers on the nipple and areola that resemble chicken pox. Breastfeeding is extremely painful. As the ulcers heal they form scabs. The baby may or may not have similar perioral skin lesions. This condition requires referral to a physician, who should evaluate the mother for a possible staphylococcal or viral infection. Culture of the lesion should be taken during its early stages before it begins to dry and heal over.

Treatment will depend on laboratory results of a culture of the lesion and maternal serum antibody titers. If the lesions are herpes simplex, and the baby is under three weeks of age (Whitley et al., 1980), it is advisable for the mother to wean the infant, or to pump her milk until the lesions are healed. The mother will be treated with an antiviral ointment.

The breast lesions shown in the color photograph in the endpapers of this book were described by the lactation consultant who saw them (Zielinski, personal communication, 1987) as looking like chicken pox: the healing lesions were scabbing, the active lesions were oozing ulcerations, and the new lesions were tiny bright red flat areas. The mother complained of extreme, "razor blade-like" pain during feedings. She was evaluated by two physicians who offered differing diagnoses. Her pediatrician suggested it might be herpes virus, while her dermatologist felt that the mother had a staphylococcal infection. Neither physician obtained a culture or serum antibody titers. The woman was first treated for a staphylococcal infection, which worsened the problem, and then with an antiviral agent (Zovirax). The lesions began to resolve shortly after the mother applied Zovirax to her nipples and areola. The mother interrupted breastfeeding her 10-month-old baby for two weeks while the lesions healed; during this period she pumped and hand expressed her milk. She resumed full breastfeeding at the end of that time. The child had "fever blisters" every three or four months for some time after this episode, and the mother developed more breast lesions a few months after the first infection, which she again treated successfully with Zovirax. For more discussion on herpes virus, see Chapter 7.

CANDIDIASIS/THRUSH

When a mother has persistent sore nipples, candidiasis is likely. It is caused by a yeast, *Candida al-*

INTERVENTIONS FOR BREAST/NIPPLE
SKIN INFECTION

- Discontinue irritant
- Take frequent showers
- Wear all-cotton bras
- Expose breasts to sunlight (15 minutes) and to air
- Apply hydrocortisone cream (available over-the-counter) on the affected area twice a day; remove cream with clean cotton swab if used on nipple/areola
- Rinse nipple/areola area with warm water after each feeding; pat dry, then air dry with hair blower on the low setting

bicans, also called *Monilia* or thrush, when it occurs orally. Candida thrive in the warm moist areas of the infant's mouth and on the mother's nipples. Candidiasis should be suspected if the mother has been breastfeeding without discomfort and then rapidly develops extremely sore nipples, burning or itching, and possibly a shooting pain deep in the breast.

Although Candida is a naturally occurring yeast which lives in the mucous membranes of the gastrointestinal and genitourinary tract and on the skin, the use of antibiotics promotes overgrowth (Candidiasis); consequently, infants and women who have received antibiotic therapy are more susceptible to Candidiasis (Amir, 1991). Antibiotics are given routinely in a cesarean birth, making women who have had a C-section more susceptible to thrush. Moreover, chicken and beef eaters in the United States are exposed to antibiotics which are routinely given to poultry and livestock to ward off infections.

In checking for thrush, inspect the woman's breasts for inflammation of the nipples and areola. The inflammation is usually striking deep pink (see the color photograph in the endpapers of this book), sometimes with tiny blisters. The mother will complain of severe tenderness and discomfort, especially during and immediately after feedings.

The baby may have a diaper rash, with raised, red, sore-looking pustules and/or red scalded-looking buttocks. Also examine the child's mouth carefully for white patches surrounded by diffuse redness. The absence of symptoms in the child's mouth, however, does not rule out thrush, since the infant may be asymptomatic. On the other hand, thrush symptoms in the baby (temperament change, frequent suckling) can go unnoticed or be attributed to something else. Moreover, treatment may be needed even in the absence of positive cultures in the mother and the infant (Jennison, 1977). Whenever any woman has recurrent yeast infections, her sexual partner should be considered a potential reservoir of infection (Horowitz, Edelstein & Lippman, 1987). Pacifiers and bottle nipples are another source of recurrent thrush infection; they may harbor persistent oral *Candida* colonization (Manning, Coughlin & Poskitt, 1985) and should be replaced or boiled after each exposure to the infant's mouth.

Candidiasis is a "family" disease; it spreads quickly among family members, especially with intimate contact involving warm, moist areas of the body, as is the case with breastfeeding and sexual contact. Candidiasis which develops during breastfeeding can persist and recur unless all areas of possible infection in the baby, mother, and father are treated promptly and aggressively. The infant's mouth and anal area, as well as the mother's breasts (nipples and areola) and vagina are prime sites for candida infection; all should be treated simultaneously. Treatment for the infant includes placing an antifungal medication in the infant's mouth with a medicine dropper after feedings and swabbing it over the mucosa, gums, and tongue. This should be continued for two weeks.

The mother must also apply an antifungal topical cream or lotion to her nipples and breast before and after each feeding, as well as around the infant's entire diaper area if there is any redness. The mother may also have vaginal yeast infection and should simultaneously use an antifungal intravaginal preparation. Clotrimazole (Gyne-Lotrimin) has been approved as an over-the-counter drug in the United States and is available as a vaginal suppository or as a cream. The following are other recommendations to be considered on a case-by-case basis.

The mother can:

- expose her nipples directly to the sun for a few minutes twice a day
- dry her external genitalia with a blow dryer set on warm
- wear 100% cotton underpants and bras which can be boiled in plain water for 5 to 10 minutes to kill spores
- avoid baths with other members of the family
- use condoms during coitus since cross infection with her partner is possible (Clay et al., 1990).

Nystatin is the most commonly used medication for candidiasis. For a listing of recommended dosages of commonly used antifungal medications see Table 14–3. After taking an antifungal medication, mothers need encouragement and follow-up; they may not get immediate relief from pain because nystatin may not bring instant relief of symptoms (Zielinski, personal communication, 1990).

In the case of chronic candidiasis a restricted diet, along with prolonged nystatin treatment, is an option. A midwife (Clay et al., 1990) suggests a regimen for the mother that combines a strict yeast-free diet with oral nystatin (after consultation with a backup physician):

TABLE 14–3 SELECTED ANTIFUNGAL PREPARATIONS

Drug Name	Preparations	Usual Dosage
clotrimazole (Gyne-Lotrimin, Mycelex)	Creams, solutions, vaginal cream and vaginal tablets	Skin cream: apply twice a day Vaginal cream or tablet: 100 mg/day for 7 days or 200 mg/day for 3 days
gentian violet	Adults and children: 0.5%, 1% or 2% solution	Topical: Infant: 2–3 times over several days; use 1% solution; do not repeat
Ketoconazole (Nizoral)	Oral tablets	Oral: Adults: 200–400 mg/day, given in single dose Children weighing less than 20 kg: 50 mg/day Children weighing 20–40 kg: 100 mg/day
miconazole (Monistat)	Creams, lotions, vaginal cream and vaginal suppositories	Skin cream or lotion: apply 3–4 times/day Vaginal cream or suppository: 100 mg/day for 7 days
nystatin (Mycostatin)	Suspensions, cream, powders, ointment, and vaginal suppositories	Oral: Adults: 1,500,000 U–2,400,000 U/day divided into 3–4 doses Infants: 400,000–800,000 U/day, divided into 3–4 doses Topical: 1 million U applied 2 times/day Duration of therapy: at least 2 days after symptoms disappear Vaginal: 1–2 million units/day

- Nystatin (oral): 2 million units three times daily for four weeks; then 1 million units three times daily for the next four weeks; followed by 500,000 units three times daily for four weeks
- Restriction of all alcohol, cheese, bread, wheat products, sugar, honey and condiments
- Acidophilus (40 million to 1 billion viable units, approximately one tablet) daily

If nystatin does not clear the fungal infection, other antifungal medications such as miconazole (Monistat), clotrimazole (Gyne-Lotrimin), naftifine (Naftin), or oxiconazole (Oxistat), should be tried. Johnstone and Marcinak (1990) report a case in which nystatin oral suspension was applied to the infant's mouth lesions with a clean cotton swab four times a day for two weeks—and to the mother's nipples immediately after feedings. This treatment was ineffective. The mother then applied clotrimazole gel to her nipples and to the baby's oral lesions every three hours. After five applications, both mother and baby were symptom free. Ketoconazole (Nizoral) is now available orally and is used successfully by a family physician to treat candidiasis in the breast-feeding mother (Mathis, personal communication, 1991).

Gentian violet is an old-fashioned antifungal drug which is enjoying a comeback because it works well, is inexpensive, and does not require a prescription.

One drawback is that gentian violet stains anything it comes in contact with, although rubbing with alcohol helps remove the dye. In advising a mother who is using it, suggest that she keep her sense of humor and wear clothing she can throw away. She should use clean cotton swabs (Q-tips) to apply the gentian violet (0.25 or 0.5% solution) to the baby's mouth and diaper area, as well as to her nipples after feedings. When the purple stain disappears (about two days in the baby's mouth and within one day on his diaper area), it should be reapplied *only once or twice.* Prolonged use of gentian violet can cause irritation and ulceration of the infant's oral mucous membranes. In one case, a baby developed oral sores and swelling which were so painful that the infant refused to feed (Utter, 1990). One to two days after the gentian violet is applied, the epidermis on both the baby's diaper area and the mother's breasts may peel and become red. A & D ointment may then be applied to any red areas not thrush related.

Anything which comes in contact with the baby's mouth (pacifiers, rubber nipples, teethers, or toys), or the mothers's breasts (breast pump parts, bras, reusable breast pads) should be washed and then boiled daily, as the spores are heat resistant. Disposable breast pads should be thrown away after each feeding (Danforth, 1990).

In one case of thrush pictured in a color photograph in the endpapers of this book the infant remained symptom free for the entire four-month period, while the mother had repeated episodes of candidiasis. Because her baby's pediatrician would not prescribe treatment for the baby in the absence of a positive culture in his mouth, the mother limited treatment to her nipples. Within four days after resolving the painful blistering and redness, she experienced a new flare-up. After four such episodes within four months, she sought a second opinion and obtained medication for her infant as well as herself; after five days of treatments following *every* suckling episode, she was symptom free and remained so thereafter.

BREAST PAIN

When candidiasis infection is severe, it can involve the lower ducts and sinuses of the breast, in addition to the outer skin of the nipples and breast. When the ducts are infected, the mother is very likely to feel a burning sensation deep in the breast which is distinct from the burning sensation of the breast skin itself. Often the inner burning persists for several minutes after the baby has come off the breast. When the mother is treated with oral antifungal medication, the pain subsides (Johnstone & Marcinak, 1990). The more severe the candidiasis infection, the longer it takes for the treatment to work and for the pain to disappear.

Breast pain which may derive from any number of sources can be both disconcerting and discouraging (Lauwers & Woessner, 1987). In some cases, pressure on the brachial plexus can result in shooting pain in the breast. Identifying the cause of this pressure—a badly fitting bra or baby carrier straps which are pulled too tightly across the mother's back—is a key to alleviating such pain (Simkin, 1988).

Women have reported feeling shooting pain that coincides with powerful ejection of milk. Such episodes are most likely to occur in the first month of the breastfeeding course. When the milk-ejection reflex subsides, the pain often subsides as well. This temporary pain tends to occur more often in primiparous women; often the same mothers who have experienced it with a first breastfeeding baby do not experience a recurrence with later infants. This pain may reflect distension of the milk ducts, which is more obvious in the early first breastfeeding course than at later periods.

In cases in which the mother reports very intense pain coincidental with a vigorous milk-ejection response, the care-giver should encourage the mother to gently massage her breasts before putting the baby to breast—in order to enhance the likelihood of some initial leaking of milk before the baby's active suckling stimulates milk ejection. When the milk begins to drip freely, sprays, and then subsides, subsequent suckling is less likely to result in such intense discomfort. By the end of the first month, such pain is usually no longer present when the milk-ejection reflex is activated.

MILK BLISTER

Infrequently a whitish, tender area—or milk blister—develops on the upper areola. This blister is thought to be caused by nipple-pore milk which has been sealed over by the epidermis and has triggered an inflammatory response. Persistent and very painful during feeding, it can remain for several days or weeks and then spontaneously heal by a peeling away of the epithelium over the affected area. In some cases, a sterile needle aspiration may be necessary to draw out the fluid. With ice packs, an analgesic to relieve discomfort, and a topical antibiotic, breastfeeding can continue and healing is rapid.

In addition to the larger blister, tiny blisters may appear on nipples which appear to have a whitish fluid within, possibly milk. These blisters are sore and painful. Vitamin E ointment, applied sparingly and wiped off before feedings, and breast shells, which take pressure off the nipples, relieve discomfort and possibly aid healing.

MAMMAPLASTY

Breast augmentation and reduction are increasingly common surgical procedures. Since 1960, two million women have had breast implants; during 1988 alone, 70,000 breast augmentations were performed in the United States. While augmentation is for cosmetic effect, reduction of very large breasts is often performed to reduce discomfort from neck and back pain.

Sooner or later the clinician will see a client who has had breast augmentation or reduction—and who wants to know if she will be able to breastfeed her baby. The ability to breastfeed following these surgical procedures depends on the type of surgery, the specific technique used, whether neural pathways were severed, and the amount of breast tissue removed. Generally speaking, breastfeeding is possible following augmentation surgery, but usually not after reduction surgery unless feedings are supplemented; however, exceptions occur in both instances. An explanation of the differences in the operative procedures is crucial to understanding the subsequent effect on lactation.

BREAST REDUCTION

The two techniques used for breast reduction are the *pedicle* technique and the *free-nipple* technique. With the pedicle technique, the nipple and areola remain attached to the breast gland on a pedicle, while the excess tissue is "reduced": a wedge is removed from the sides and underside of the breast (see Fig. 14–2). Since the breast, its ducts, blood supply, and some nerves remain intact, breastfeeding has been possible after this operation but no data is available on the number of successes. The ability to breastfeed is dependent on whether the surgeon deliberately tries to leave nerve pathways and blood supply intact or whether he removes the tissue without regard for these structures.

The free-nipple technique (autotransplantation of nipple) involves removing the nipple/areola entirely from the breast and preserving it in saline (much like a graft) while the breast glandular tissue is removed. Then the nipple/areola is stitched back in place. This technique is used for women with extremely large breasts and is designed to reduce risks and compli-

cations. Breastfeeding may be possible with the pedicle technique but it is rarely possible with the free-nipple technique since the blood supply of nipple/areola is completely severed (Barnett, 1990), and damage to the nerves occurs. Several cases of spontaneous galactorrhea in women following reduction mammaplasty are reported in the literature; none of these women had breastfed for several months before the surgery (Menendez-Graino et al., 1990; Song & Hunter, 1989).

MASTOPEXY

Mastopexy is a "breastlift" in which sagging breasts are uplifted and made firmer (see Fig. 14–3). The operation involves removing excess skin and breast tissue and elevating the nipple. It may be done either in the hospital or in the physician's office. While there may be a very slight loss of sensation in the nipple or areola, the operation should not affect the ability to breastfeed (Love, 1990).

AUGMENTATION

Because augmentation surgery is most often performed on women during their childbearing years, LCs are likely to be asked about it by their clients (see Fig. 14–4). Four techniques are used to enlarge the breasts.

Infra-submammary. An incision is made under the breast and the implant is placed under the breast tissue. One disadvantage is that the scar is very visible and is easily irritated by a bra.

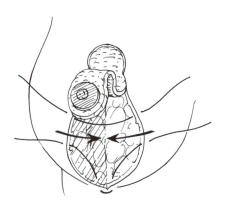

A. Wedge of breast tissue removed, areola pulled up, gap closed

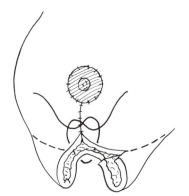

B. Excess tissue removed, skin closed with stitches

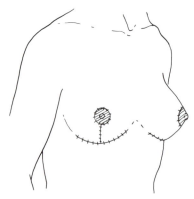

C. Post–operative appearance

FIGURE 14–2.   Breast reduction.

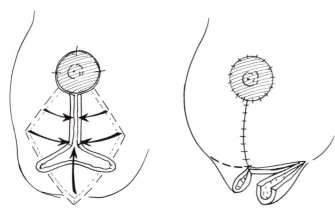
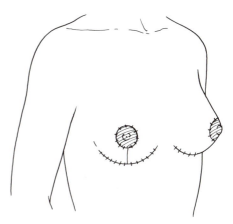

A. Skin edges pulled together   B. Excess tissue removed   C. Post–operative appearance

FIGURE 14–3.   Breast "lift" or mastopexy.

Periareolar technique. An incision is made around the areola/nipple. While the scar is less visible, there often is a loss of sensation.

Transareolar. An incision is made across the areola/nipple area. This technique is preferred by Asian women because they are less likely to have severe scarring, which is common among them. Bar-

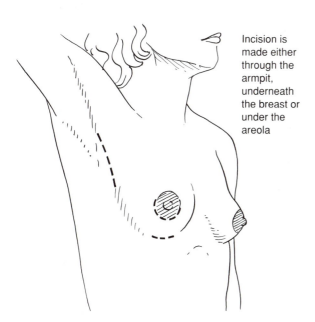

Incision is made either through the armpit, underneath the breast or under the areola

FIGURE 14–4.   Breast augmentation. Incision is made either through the armpit, underneath the breast, or around the areola.

nett (1990) describes this technique as "unphysiological" and advises against its use. Full lactation is almost always impossible after this procedure because the glandular tissue, nerves, and blood supply are extensively disrupted. This should be made clear to any woman who contemplates having this procedure.

Axillary. An incision is made underneath the arm and the implant is placed below the gland. While there are few scars and no interference with breast tissue and lactation, this type of implant makes breast cancer harder to detect, and there is a possibility of contractures. If the implant is placed below the muscle, it interferes less with mammograms.

The implant itself is either silicone gel, saline water, or silicone gel surrounded by a polyurethane bag. If the woman intends to breastfeed, Barnett (1990) recommends using a saline water implant. Silicone is a highly inert substance, but charges have been made that it may "bleed" into body tissues and fluids (including breastmilk), thereby affecting the immune system and causing toxic reactions in the mother ("Face-to-face," Chung, 1990). Plastic surgeons countercharge that most women are satisfied with their implants and that virtually everyone has some silicone in their bodies. Silicone is a major ingredient in drugs such as Di-Gel and is added to processed foods, hand lotion, hair spray, and other common products.

Only one prospective study on the effect of

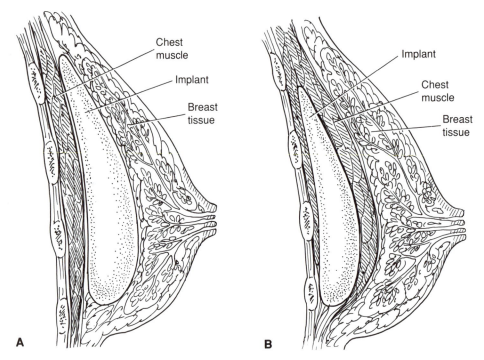

FIGURE 14–5.   Location of breast implant. **A**, Implant placed between breast and muscles. **B**, Implant placed under muscles.

mammaplasty on breastfeeding outcomes is reported. Neifert et al. (1990) conducted a study on 319 primiparous women who were breastfeeding healthy, full-term infants. Women who had previous breast surgery had greater than a threefold risk of lactation insufficiency compared with women who had not had surgery. The mothers with periareolar incisions were almost five times more likely to have insufficient milk than were those with no breast surgery. Women with breast incisions in other locations had no statistically significant increase in risk of lactation insufficiency compared with those who never had breast surgery.

BREAST LUMPS AND SURGERY

What if a breastfeeding mother develops a lump or nodule in her breast? Warnings by the American Cancer Society have made American women keenly aware of breast lumps, and the woman discovering one is usually anxious and perhaps frightened. However, a breast lump in a lactating woman is most often a galactocele or a milk-filled lacteal cyst caused by plugged milk in the ducts. A galactocele is usually tender and will atrophy rather rapidly and disappear in a matter of days.

If it does not resolve or reduce in size, the LC should refer the mother to a physician or surgeon for an examination. If it appears to be a cystic mass, a needle aspiration is done to determine whether it is fluid filled. To aspirate a cyst, the physician first cleans and anesthetizes the skin, immobilizes the mass with his hand, and inserts a 20-to-22-gauge needle to draw out fluid. This procedure collapses the cyst and solves the problem. Cysts are almost never malignant. If a biopsy is necessary, one of four methods may be used (Love, 1990):

- fine-needle biopsy which draws out a few cells
- larger-needle ("tru-cut") biopsy which cuts out a small piece of tissue without an incision
- incisional biopsy which takes a much larger piece
- excisional biopsy in which an entire lump is removed.

A known breast mass (by palpation) can be evaluated further, usually by biopsy or ultrasound, to determine whether it is fluid filled (cystic or benign) or solid (possibly malignant). Because of the tissue density of the lactating breast, mammography is often inconclusive. Most diagnostic procedures are performed on an out-patient basis, either in a freestanding ambulatory clinic or minor operating room. Using the lowest dosage possible of local anesthetic minimizes the amount of anesthetic the infant might ingest with the next breastfeeding (Love, 1990). When the mother resumes breastfeeding depends on her comfort level and the type of procedure used, but she should certainly be able to resume within 12 hours. Although the area will be tender, resuming feedings needs to be weighed against the discomfort of engorgement and/or listening to the cries of an unhappy child. If breastfeeding is not resumed within 12 hours, have the mother pump her breasts to relieve the pressure. Too much milk pressure and stasis could lead to undue stress on the surgical site and infection.

Day (1986) describes a case in which a woman underwent biopsy of her right breast after suspicious calcifications were found by xeromammography. Biopsy was accomplished with a wedge-shaped resection at the nine o'clock position through a circumareolar skin incision with excellent cosmetic results. The pathology report indicated a benign "fibrocystic" condition. Following the delivery of her next baby, the woman's breasts became engorged symmetrically. By the fourth postpartum day she noted that her right breast remained engorged after breastfeeding, although her left breast seemed relieved of its milk supply. The client subsequently used warm packs, oxytocin nasal spray (on the right side only), plus an electric breast pump in efforts to build up her milk supply in the treated breast. At no time was more than two mL of milk obtained from the right breast using the electric pump—despite having successfully breastfed her first child on both breasts. Day suggests that the surgeon must weigh cosmetic considerations of breast surgery against the need for an adequate biopsy and the threat to future milk ejection.

FIBROCYSTIC DISEASE

Fibrocystic breast disease (benign breast disorder) is a general term that describes a number of benign breast conditions. It should not be assumed that fibrocystic disease refers only to those breasts with cysts or nodules; the term is also used to include breasts with evidence of hyperplasia, metaplasia, and atypia, among other conditions (Brucker & Scharbo-DeHaan, 1991). The American Cancer Society recommends that clinicians use the term "fibrocystic changes"; nevertheless, the diagnosis of fibrocystic disease is commonly used because it guarantees reimbursement by health-care insurers.

About one-half of all women of childbearing age will develop one of these conditions at some point. Years of menstrual cycling will eventually produce dense or fibrous breast tissue. Women usually develop cysts in their thirties. Because of its occurrence rate, the condition is sometimes referred to as a non-disease.

From 50 to 75% of all breast biopsies are done because of clinical diagnoses of fibrocystic disease (Norwood, 1989). About one-fourth of women with fibrocystic disease develop gross evidence of a cyst or a fibroadenoma, a smooth, round lump which moves around easily when palpated. Fibroadenomas can vary from the size of a pea to the size of a lemon. A needle aspiration helps to confirm the diagnosis. If no fluid can be aspirated, a fibroadenoma is likely. Tissue is sent to the lab to confirm the diagnosis. Fibroadenomas are harmless in themselves and, if the woman is lactating, most surgeons choose to delay surgery at least until lactation ceases and the child is completely weaned. In middle-aged or older women, fibroadenomas are usually removed at the time they are diagnosed.

A mother with persistent benign breast disease is commonly advised to reduce or eliminate caffeine (coffee, tea, cola, chocolate) and to take vitamin E supplements. There are as many studies (Minton, 1979; Cheek, 1979; Gonzalez, 1980) substantiating these recommendations as there are those negating it (Allen & Froberg, 1987; Lubin et al., 1985; London et al., 1985).

BLEEDING FROM THE BREAST

Red-tinged, pink, or rusty breastmilk is relatively rare, but it does occur and causes concern as it signals the presence of blood. There are several possible antecedent factors which lead to bleeding in the milk ducts. For example, one mother with severely retracted nipples had painless bleeding from her breasts after wearing breast shells late in pregnancy. After reducing the wearing time of the shells, the bleeding ceased.

In other cases, the etiology of the bleeding is not so clear. Chele Marmet (1990) has worked with several mothers whose milk appears brown or "rusty"—like rusty water emitted from pipes which haven't been used for a long while. Hence she calls it the "rusty-pipe" syndrome. This syndrome appears to occur more often in primiparous mothers during early stages of lactogenesis and is not associated with any discomfort. O'Callaghan (1981) reported 37 cases of this syndrome involving 32 Australian women. Most of these women reported that their breast discharge was either red or brown. Its earliest appearance was during the fourth month of pregnancy, and it was associated with antenatal breast expression in a little over one-half of the mothers. Dairy farmers report similar "rusty milk" from cows calfing for the first time—and suggest that the reason is slight internal bleeding from edema during the cow's first engorgement.

Bright red bleeding from the breast in the absence of nipple soreness or cracking indicates that the mother should be assessed for the possibility of an intraductal papilloma. This is a small, benign, wartlike growth on the lining of the duct that bleeds as it erodes. Usually no mass or tumor is palpable, and there may or may not be moderate pain and discomfort. Often the bleeding stops spontaneously without any treatment, but if bleeding continues the woman should be medically evaluated. The physician will probably remove it surgically to make sure that it is an intraductal papilloma and not something more serious. In any case, reassure the mother that the infant is not harmed by the intake of small amounts of serosanguinous discharge.

BREAST CANCER

Breast cancer diagnosed during pregnancy or lactation is rare—occuring in about 0.03% of pregnancies. Only one to two percent of breast cancer overall is diagnosed during pregnancy or lactation (Hoover, 1990). However remote, there is a possibility of a tumor or nodule being malignant. Breastfeeding does *not* prevent breast cancer, although some studies conclude that it provides a protective function. For a woman who is at risk for breast cancer, prolonged breastfeeding may at least delay its occurrence. The longer a woman breastfeeds, the less likely she is to develop breast cancer before menopause. Following menopause there is no difference in the rate of breast cancer among women based on the length of time the mother breastfed. Several studies support this statement.

Ing, Ho, and Petrakis (1977) reported that women in fishing villages near Hong Kong customarily breastfeed only with the right breast. Among these women, they reported a four-fold, highly significant increased risk of cancer in the unsuckled breast after menopause.

Byers et al. (1985), in a study of premenopausal women in New York state, identified a negative association between duration of breastfeeding and risk of breast cancer. The protective effect of lactation held after Byers controlled for such factors as age, parity, age at first pregnancy, age at menarche, and education. Byers concludes that a woman's risk of developing premenopausal breast cancer decreases steadily for every 12 months she breastfeeds (Byers et al., 1985).

McTiernan and Thomas (1986) conducted a case-control study of women in Washington state. Premenopausal women who had lactated had less than one-half the risk of developing breast cancer than did the control group, which had never lactated. A dose-response was noted, with the risk of breast cancer declining as the duration of breastfeeding in-

---

BREAST RESEARCH LACKING

Ignorance about female biology still impedes the treatment of breast cancer and other diseases of women, a panel of scientists said Thursday. "There's no research on the normal breast," said Susan Love, an author and professor of surgery at Harvard. "Therefore, we don't have a clue when carcinogens are acting." Yet breast cancer will strike one woman in 10 in her lifetime, and will kill 44,000 this year, she said.

The Wichita Eagle, Monday, December 10, 1990

creased; this was particularly strong among premenopausal women. The protective effect of breastfeeding persisted even after controlling for maternal age, parity, and age at first full-term pregnancy.

The length of time that the mother breastfeeds may also play a role in breast cancer. Kvåle and Heuch (1987) reported a curvilinear relationship between the duration of breastfeeding and the risk of breast cancer. The highest risk existed among women who had breastfed four to ten months. Women who breastfed for less than four months or longer than ten months had lower risks for breast cancer. For all nongenital cancers, the duration of breastfeeding appeared to reduce risk in linear fashion.

Layde et al. (1989) also found that risk of breast cancer declined in inverse proportion to the length of breastfeeding. In their analysis of the experiences of 4,599 women, the mother's age at first full-term pregnancy exerted the strongest influence on reducing the risk of breast cancer. Thereafter, the number of births (parity) and the duration of breastfeeding became important elements. Women whose breastfeeding career exceeded 25 months had the lowest risk for breast carcinoma.

Other studies show that breastfeeding/lactation neither prevents nor delays breast cancer. Siskind et al. (1989) found that Australian women who had breastfed were only slightly less likely to develop breast cancer than women who had not breastfed. The greatest protective effect occurred if the first child was breastfed. There were no differences in the risk ratio after breastfeeding when comparing premenopausal and postmenopausal women. Likewise, London et al. (1990) found no independent association between lactation and risk of cancer; however, only six percent of the women in the study had breastfed for at least 24 months.

Patients diagnosed with breast cancer during pregnancy and lactation are largely in their thirties and forties. They have had multiple pregnancies and relatively few deliveries; usually there has been a long interval since a previous pregnancy or childbirth (Deemarksy & Semiglazov, 1987). Unlike women who are past menopause (Dunne, 1988), premenopausal women are more likely to have breast cancer that is not hormone dependent.

Most studies in the past 30 years have convincingly shown that the poor prognosis for patients with breast cancer discovered during pregnancy is attrib-utable more to delay in diagnosis and reluctance to treat patients aggressively, rather than to any detrimental effect of pregnancy or lactation itself (Donegan & Spratt, 1988; Hoover, 1990; Ribeiro & Palmer, 1977). The delay is due to: denial (by both the physician and the mother) that the disease occurs in pregnant women, breast tenderness, and lobular hyperplasia, which hides a tumor and hinders its detection, giving it time to grow and spread. Lactating breasts are very dense (see Fig. 4–9), making mammography or thermography of little value in diagnosis.

Contrary to this view, Tretli et al. (1988) studied 20 breast cancer patients diagnosed during pregnancy and 15 patients diagnosed during lactation. Taking the stage of the disease, age and calendar year into account, the pregnancy group showed a significantly poorer prognosis compared with the control group. The lactating group did not have a poorer prognosis than the control group, although there was a tendency in this direction.

Approximately seven percent of fertile women treated for mammary carcinoma subsequently become pregnant, usually within the first five years. Their survival rate has been the same as for women who have never been pregnant (Donegan & Spratt, 1988; Deemarsky & Semiglazov, 1987). Previously, it was widely taught that subsequent pregnancy and lactation aggravated the course of mammary cancer; however, outcome and survival rates are similar for both pregnant and nonpregnant women who are of similar age and disease stage at the time of diagnosis (Peters & Meaken, 1965; Cooper & Butterfield, 1970; Schweppe, Mohlen & Beller, 1979).

As long as the woman remains clinically free of cancer, there is no therapeutic benefit in interrupting the pregnancy. If advanced cancer is diagnosed in the first or second trimester, however, treatment often requires that the pregnancy be terminated—since chemotherapy, radiation or hormone therapy place the fetus at risk (Deemarsky & Semiglazov, 1987). Some women who have had a unilateral mastectomy breastfeed after a subsequent pregnancy. The mother should be encouraged to alter her baby's position frequently to provide optimal stimulation to all portions of the breast.

One of the myths about breastfeeding and cancer is that a baby can receive cancer-causing viral particles in human milk. This is not true—there is no increased incidence of breast cancer in breastfed daughters of women who have had breast cancer (Morgan, Vakil & Chipman, 1974; Miller & Fraumenti, 1972). There is, however, some evidence (Goldsmith, 1974) that following an experience of the infant rejecting the breast without apparent reason, a woman may be more likely to develop breast cancer in the rejected breast. In such cases close surveillance is probably needed.

Pregnant women diagnosed with early breast cancer are treated medically like nonpregnant women. Hornstein, Skornick, and Rozin (1982) have outlined a protocol for breastfeeding following a diagnosis of breast cancer.

1. If breast cancer is diagnosed toward the end of pregnancy, the woman will undergo immediate surgery. If chemotherapy follows, the mother should not breastfeed.
2. If the diagnosis is made during lactation, lactation should be immediately suppressed by medications other than estrogen. Other standard treatments for carcinoma are then started.
3. Following the diagnosis of breast cancer, subsequent pregnancies should be delayed until the period of greatest risk is over (three to five years). After this time the patient/mother may breastfeed.

EFFECT OF RADIATION AND CHEMOTHERAPY

Green (1989) reported that a woman who received breast radiation treatment for an infiltrating ductal carcinoma became pregnant 19 months after the irradiation treatment. After giving birth to a healthy infant, she began breastfeeding. The irradiated breast neither enlarged nor produced colostrum. Two days after the untreated breast began leaking milk, the treated breast did so; however, it never produced the same volume of milk as the untreated breast, even though the baby suckled from both breasts. Approximately four weeks after lactation began, it ceased in the treated breast; however, lactation continued on the untreated side. Laboratory analysis of a milk sample from the treated breast revealed a much higher than expected level of sodium, probably because the breast was undergoing involution (Alpert & Cormier, 1983; Thullen, 1988). In addition, triglyceride levels were approximately one-third the level in the milk from the untreated breast, while alkaline phosphatase levels were 43% higher than those found in the milk from the untreated breast.

David (1985) also reports the lactation experience of a woman with a history of fibrocystic disease who was treated with radiation therapy for a small mass in the right breast. Following an uneventful pregnancy one year after completion of the radiation therapy, she gave birth to a healthy infant, who suckled well from both breasts. The right breast enlarged during pregnancy, but not as much as the left breast. Following the baby's birth, she experienced near-normal lactation from the treated breast.

Women receiving chemotherapy for breast cancer—or for any other cancer—should not breastfeed. All chemotherapeutic drugs cross into the milk. While the milk levels are low, these toxic compounds are potent antimetabolites. They are potentially toxic to the infant.

CLINICAL IMPLICATIONS

MASTITIS

A mother with mastitis feels ill. Often she is discouraged. She asks, "Why does this have to happen to me?" She may even contemplate weaning. This is a time when she needs mothering herself—a role that the LC can assume as she reassures the mother that the infection will resolve and that to stop breastfeeding will only increase the risk of infection and/or recurrence. Tender loving care goes a long way in helping the mother through this difficult time. She also needs specific advice and a plan for care (see Table 14–4). A long-term plan for self-care of mastitis should also be provided. A considerable number of mothers develop mastitis more than once during the course of lactation (Riordan & Nichols, 1990). Therefore certain women may be prone to the condition, and prevention is important. Review with the mother all the possible factors that preceded and may have contributed to mastitis.

Fatigue and stress. Mothers rate stress and fatigue as major factors leading to mastitis. The effect of stress on the individual's immune defense system has been substantiated. Recounting events leading up to mastitis, a mother explained, "My husband took a new job which meant moving out of state. I also was planning a christening party in order to fit it

TABLE 14–4   MASTITIS TEACHING PLAN

Content/Goal	Teaching
Prevention	
To reduce stress and fatigue related to childbearing responsibilities	
Management of work	Prioritize tasks from most important to least important.
	Encourage other family members to assist in routine household tasks.
	Delay return to job as long as possible.
Management of socializing	Hold one informal open house for all friends/relatives to see new baby.
	Install telephone answering machine and keep on "answer."
	Turn down social invitations.
Adequate rest and sleep	Take day naps when infant sleeps.
Avoid plugged ducts	Breastfeed often: 8–12 times/day.
	Massage any reddened area of breast, especially while breastfeeding.
Avoid change in number of feedings	Pump or express milk if a feeding is skipped.
Engorgement/stasis	Pump or express milk if breasts become overfull/distended.
	Wear bras without support underwires.
Care if mastitis occurs	
To prevent breast abscess and hasten recovery	
Self-care and relief of discomfort	Recognize early signs and symptoms: redness, fatigue, fever, chills.
	Rest with infant and fluids at bedside.
	Continue frequent breastfeedings.
	Monitor oral temperature.
	Place moist warm packs at site of infection and over nipple.
Medical care	Take antibiotics as prescribed.
	Take antipyretic to reduce fever.

From Riordan, J, and Nichols, F: *J Hum Lact* 6:53–58, 1990.

in before moving away. Everything happened very rapidly and my baby was only two weeks old." Typically mothers who develop mastitis are stressed from overwork and/or lack of sleep; they describe themselves as exhausted as a result of circumstances above and beyond the normal stresses of taking care of the infant. A mother wrote, "I was doing too much—just starting to get out with my first baby and trying to get ready for our first Christmas."

Plugged Duct. As discussed earlier, some women repeatedly develop plugged ducts, some of which lead to a full-blown infection. It is not uncommon to be able to see this "plug" as a white "head" and feel pressure and tenderness around the plug. Gentle massage above the area of tenderness may

help while the baby is breastfeeding from that breast, particularly if the plug is newly formed (Marmet & Shell, personal communication, 1991).

Decrease in number of feedings. A sudden drop in the number of feedings usually leads to breast distention. If the number is reduced for any reason, milk collects in the ducts and stasis may occur; one mother reported, "We were on vacation 1,000 miles from home. After driving for two days and exclusively breastfeeding, we arrived at our destination and the feedings were cut back quite a bit. The infection started a few days after this."

Engorgement/stasis. A decrease in the frequency of feedings presents the potential for engorgement or milk stasis. In one case a mother whose infant was sleeping 10 hours at night was plagued with repeated mastitis. When she awakened in the morning, her breasts were always hard and sore. As soon as she began waking up her baby for a night feeding she had no more problems.

Sore/cracked nipple. A breakdown in the epidermis provides an avenue of entry into the breast tissue; however breakdown is not a prerequisite for a breast infection. Mastitis from sore, cracked nipples usually occurs in the first few weeks postpartum.

Other factors. Other conditions, such as breast trauma, poor maternal nutrition and vigorous exercise (particularly of the upper arms and chest) have been mentioned anecdotally as factors leading up to mastitis. These should also be noted in the patient's assessment and history, in the event that they predispose the mother to mastitis.

Finally, the LC should encourage the mother to seek medical help early if and when symptoms recur. Some mothers, especially if they are experienced long-term breastfeeders (Riordan & Nichols, 1990) do not consult their physicians even though their mastitis warrants medical attention.

BREAST SURGERY AND ABSCESS

With abscess drainage, lump removal, or biopsy, there is usually no reason the mother should stop breastfeeding. The exception is the case in which a perioareolar cut interferes with the nerve supply to the nipple, severs milk ducts, and leads to lactation failure (Day, 1986; Neifert et al., 1990). Even in such an instance, breastfeeding may still be possible if the other breast is unaffected. After a biopsy, the baby usually feeds only from the unaffected breast. While waiting for the affected breast to heal, the mother hand expresses or pumps milk from the affected side. Protocol at the Lactation Clinic in Los Angeles, however, calls for continued feeding on the affected breast as long as the incision/stitches are dorsal to the nipple and areola, and the mother does not find this objectionable (Marmet & Shell, personal communication, 1991).

If the wound is left open to drain, breastfeeding can be "messy," as milk and other body fluids may leak from the ducts. The mother should be prepared to replace soiled dressings with clean pads. Milk leaking from the wound may slow healing. As a result, the mother is at risk for a breast infection or a milk cyst; a low-dose prophylactic antibiotic is sometimes used to avoid infection. If the problem persists, gradual weaning from the affected side might be necessary while the baby feeds from the unaffected side. Usually the mother resumes breastfeeding on the affected breast when the drain and/or stitches are removed—and when she can tolerate it. A child's reaction to being prevented from feeding from the affected breast (sometimes his "favorite" breast) varies. Some cooperate without a fuss; others are distraught and actively fight to breastfeed there.

If breast cancer is diagnosed during lactation, breastfeeding is always terminated. Subsequent surgery, possible radiation, and chemotherapy make continued lactation impossible. Whether a woman should become pregnant again and breastfeed after she has had breast cancer is a medical decision. While it is not generally encouraged, there are no studies which demonstrate that a subsequent pregnancy accelerates cancer. However, many physicians are reluctant to advise breastfeeding because of limited data on the outcomes.

Many mothers have shared their breastfeeding experiences after breast surgery in La Leche League's *New Beginnings* (formerly La Leche League News), a rich source of clinical information. One mother (Hart, 1980) had a lump removed as an outpatient. The following day her breast started swelling with stored milk because her baby had not nursed from that breast. After expressing by hand for 12 days, she began feeding her infant again on the affected breast. Her milk supply in the affected breast returned; however for two to three days, nursing was uncomfortable.

Another woman (Paster, 1986) underwent a breast biopsy under general anesthesia for a lump which was deep within her breast. Within 12 hours of the procedure, she was able to nurse on the affected side. Although painful at first, by the second or third day breastfeeding was quite tolerable. The mother found that putting pressure (splinting) on the dressing helped allay the feeling that the baby would pull the incision apart. At first, there was some lessening of milk production, since about 25% of the ducts had been disturbed. Subsequently, the mother nursed another baby without noticing any difference in milk production in the affected breast.

In a third case (Resico, 1990), the nipple was cut

from top to bottom during a surgical procedure— and lifted to remove a lump the size of a golfball. The surgeon suggested that the mother not attempt to breastfeed when she became pregnant because he felt he had severed milk ducts during surgery. Surprisingly, the mother was able to breastfeed from that breast. This suggests one of two possibilities: either some of the ducts were not actually severed, or it is possible for milk ducts to recanalize with one another after having been severed.

Any woman contemplating breast surgery needs to be fully informed about the procedure and the different techniques which are available. A chart that shows the anatomy and lactational functions of the breast is indispensable for explaining the possible effects of surgery. If the patient is highly motivated to breastfeed, it is the clinician's responsibility to counsel her and suggest techniques which are less disruptive to breastfeeding than others. If the surgery is very likely to disrupt breastfeeding, that information should be made clear to the woman before the operation. At the same time, it is almost impossible to predict whether or not breastfeeding will be successful.

There are few studies on breastfeeding outcomes following breast surgery to guide us. Hatton and Keleher (1983) presented two cases of women who breastfed after reduction mammaplasty in which the surgical procedure used was nipple transposition. In the first case, the mother prenatally prepared her breasts for breastfeeding and expressed colostrum, which was very reassuring to her. During her postpartum stay she breastfed frequently and for long periods. Her follow-up care consisted of frequent phone calls by the nurse-midwives as well as several office and home visits. At two-and-one-half weeks of age, the baby weighed two ounces less than at birth, even though he was being breastfed every two hours during the day and every six hours at night. At seven weeks of age the infant was at the 20th percentile for weight, and the mother started formula supplements. She continued to breastfeed with supplements for several months. Prolactin levels were obtained from this mother before and after breastfeeding her six-week-old infant. Her prebreastfeeding prolactin level was 80 ng/mL; after breastfeeding it was 245ng/mL, indicating a normal prolactin response to suckling and an intact neuroendocrine pathway.

The second case report concerned a mother who likewise massaged and prepared her breasts during pregnancy. She was able to express a small amount of colostrum which greatly encouraged her. Her breasts became fully engorged on the second day after delivery. During the first month the baby gained weight slowly but he continued to nurse frequently. At one month the baby was just above the 10th percentile for weight and was increasingly fussy. By eight weeks he had dropped to the fifth percentile, and he was breastfeeding very frequently. The baby was started on formula supplements when he was three months of age. In retrospect, the client remembered feeling guilty for delaying formula supplements, even though she thought that supplements would further decrease her milk production. The authors concluded that for these mothers the possible necessity of supplements for their babies should be discussed antepartally. If supplements become necessary, a Lact-aid device could be used so that the milk production is stimulated by allowing the infant to suckle at the breast while receiving a supplement.

Following the publication of these cases in the *Journal of Nurse-Midwifery,* Schoch (1985) responded with a report of a similar outcome in another woman. This mother also started off well, with both breasts becoming full of milk after delivery. As the breastfeeding course progressed, however, the untreated breast was noticeably larger and produced more milk than the treated breast. An occasional bottle of formula was started in the third week. During the fourth week, mastitis set in on the untreated breast, and the mother decided to slowly stop breastfeeding—because of the low milk supply of the treated breast and her reluctance to breastfeed with only one breast. This mother did not regret her actions and felt that the baby benefited from breastfeeding in the first critical weeks; if she has another baby, she will again attempt to breastfeed.

If a woman has already had breast surgery and wants to know if she can breastfeed, it is vital that the care-giver ask about the specific details of the surgery and assess the scarring in order to determine the surgical technique which was used. Following breast surgery, the ability to breastfeed depends on the location of the incision, the techniques employed, and the extent of damage to the tissue, especially to blood and neural pathways. Before any biopsy or breast surgery is performed on any woman of childbearing age, *informed consent dictates that she know the probable effect of the surgery on her ability to breastfeed. The client's motivation to breastfeed is critical to the outcome.*

If the client is able to express colostrum during pregnancy, she may feel optimistic about being able to breastfeed. At the same time, her inability to express colostrum does not necessarily mean that she cannot breastfeed (Hatton & Keleher, 1983). However, not every woman who has milk after birth will be able to fully lactate. Breastfeeding may go along well for days or weeks, with the infant gaining weight—until the rapidly growing baby's demand for milk exceeds the mother's ability to produce the amount needed (Petok, personal communication, 1990).

Breast reduction surgery and transareolar augmentation surgery are particularly damaging to breastfeeding. The mother who has had one of these procedures needs to consult a health-professional experienced with such cases. The health-professional should provide a forthright discussion about the likelihood of successful lactation and options for supplemental feedings (especially in later months). There are very few individuals who have the expertise to do this. Plastic surgeons, while they may be sympathetic to breastfeeding, are more interested in the surgical technique and the cosmetic results; they are generally uninformed about breastfeeding. The risks of such surgery are high. One of the consequences is loss of sensation. Courtiss and Goldwyn (1976) found that two years following augmentation mammaplasty 15% of the patients still had decreased sensation in the nipple and areola. In other cases, LCs have been told by their clients that their nipples are "hypersensitive"; none, however, describe an improved sensation (Marmet & Shell, personal communication, 1991).

An experienced lactation consultant, Petok (personal communication, 1990) has worked with many mothers who have had mammaplasty surgery. If the mother has had reduction surgery, Petok reports that the mother often gratefully accepts whatever ability she still has to breastfeed, without regretting that she had the surgery. If breastfeeding is not at all possible, and she had it to do all over again, she would still choose to have the reduction. Marmet and Shell (personal communication, 1991) believe this percentage is much lower, about 25%, that "most women go into reduction surgery uninformed about the consequences of surgery on breastfeeding and their sex lives and later they are angry about this."

Likewise, some women who have had augmentation surgery become angry that their surgeons did not discuss with them the procedure's negative impact on breastfeeding. These women are also angry with themselves for proceeding with the surgery without having been completely informed. Some of these women say that if they had it to do over again, they would not have the surgery. Some made the decision at a time in their lives when they were not feeling good about themselves. They feel guilty about having the implant and are reluctant to tell their pediatrician about their surgery, especially if their baby fails to adequately gain weight because their breasts are not producing enough milk.

Most of what we do for our clients is to give of ourselves—the therapeutic self. So when a mother faces surgery or other procedures on her breasts that are painful—and that might also potentially alter and/or scar her breasts—encourage her to openly express her feelings. Tell her it's all right to cry or to scream if she feels like it. The nurse or lactation consultant is there to listen and to give her support.

SUMMARY

Breast-related problems constitute a substantial proportion of clinical breastfeeding counseling. The overuse of antibiotics which leads to candidiasis and the surge in the popularity of cosmetic breast surgery are "man-made" barriers to breastfeeding; they are peculiar to affluent countries. Breast cancer is quite likely another disease of the developed world.

Women have the right to be fully informed about any medical procedure, especially a surgical one, because the outcome is apt to be irreversible. Part of the health-professional's responsibility is to act as a client advocate. The client should know all options available to her (including the right to refuse surgery) and all probable outcomes before consenting to a medical procedure.

A study of the effects of breast surgery (especially breast augmentation which is popular among the childbearing age group) is a research priority. Such a study could be done nationwide by collectively pooling data on these cases.

REFERENCES

Allen, SS, and Froberg, DG: The effect of decreased caffeine consumption on benign proliferative breast disease: A randomized clinical trial, *Surgery* 101: 720–30, 1987.

Alpert, SE, and Cormier, AD: Normal electrolyte and protein content in milk from mothers with cystic fibrosis: an explanation for the initial report of elevated milk sodium concentration, *J Pediatr* 102: 77–80, 1983.

Amir, LH: Candida and the lactating breast: predisposing factors, *J Hum Lact* 7: 177–81, 1991.

Barnett, A: *Breast surgery and breast feeding,* International Lactation Consultant Association Conference, July 13–15, 1990, Scottsdale, Ariz.

Bertrand, H, and Rosenblood, LK: Stripping out pus in lactational mastitis: a means of preventing breast abscess, *CMAJ* 145: 299–306, 1991.

Brackett, VH: Eczema of the nipple/areola area, *J Hum Lact* 4: 167–68, 1988.

Brucker, MC, and Scharbo-DeHaan, M: Breast disease: The role of the nurse-midwife, *J Nurs-Midwif* 36: 63–73, 1991.

Byers, T, et al.: Lactation and breast cancer: evidence for a negative association in premenopausal women, *Am J Epidemiol* 121: 664–74, 1985.

Cantlie, HB: Treatment of acute puerperal mastitis and breast abscess, *Can Fam Phys* 34: 2221–26, 1988.

Cheek, W: Benign breast lumps may regress with diet, *JAMA* 241: 1221, 1979.

Clay, LS, et al.: Chronic moniliasis, *J Nurs-Midwif* 35: 377–84, 1990.

Conner, AE: Elevated levels of sodium and chloride in milk from mastitic breast, *Pediatrics* 63: 910–11, 1979.

Cooper, DR, and Butterfield, J: Pregnancy subsequent to mastectomy for cancer of the breast, *Ann Surg* 171: 429–33, 1970.

Courtiss, EH, and Goldwyn, RM: Breast sensation before and after plastic surgery, *Plast Reconstr Surg* 58(1): 1–12, 1976.

Danforth, D: Could it be thrush? *Leaven* 26: 56, 1990.

David, FC: Lactation following primary radiation therapy for carcinoma of the breast (letter), *Int J Radiat Oncol Biol Phys* 11: 1425, 1985.

Day, TW: Unilateral failure of lactation after breast biopsy, *J Fam Pract* 23: 161–62, 1986.

Deemarsky, LJ, and Semiglazov, VF: Cancer of the breast and pregnancy. In Ariel, IM, and Cleary, JB: *Breast cancer: diagnosis and treatment,* New York, 1987, McGraw-Hill Book Co., pp. 475–88.

Donegan, WL, and Spratt, JS: *Cancer of the breast,* Philadelphia, 1988, W.B. Saunders Co., pp. 685–87.

Dunne, CR: Hormonal therapy for breast cancer, *Canc Nurs* 11: 288–94, 1988.

"Face-to-face with Connie Chung": Breast Implants, CBS, December 10, 1990.

Gibberd, GF: Sporadic and epidemic puerperal breast infections, *Am J Obstet Gynecol* 65: 1038–41, 1953.

Goldsmith, HS: Milk rejection sign of breast cancer, *Am J Surg* 127: 280–81, 1974.

Gonzalez, ER: Vitamin E relieves most cystic breast disease, may alter lipids, hormones, *JAMA* 244: 1077–78, 1980.

Green, JP: Post-irradiation lactation (letter), *Int J Radiat Oncol Biol Phys* 17: 244, 1989.

Hart, J: Nursing after breast surgery, *La Leche League News* 22: 10, 1980.

Hatton, M, and Keleher, KC: Breastfeeding after breast reduction mammaplasty, *J Nurs-Midwif* 28(4): 19–22, 1983.

Hoffman, JB: A suggested treatment for inverted nipples, *Am J Obstet Gynecol* 66: 346, 1953.

Hoffman, KL, and Auerbach, KG: Long-term antibiotic prophylaxis for recurrent mastitis, *J Hum Lact* 1: 72–75, 1986.

Hoover, HC: Breast cancer during pregnancy and lactation, *Surg Clin North Am* 70: 1151–63, 1990.

Hornstein, E, Skornick, Y, and Rozin, R: The management of breast carcinoma in pregnancy and lactation, *J Surg Oncol* 21: 179–82, 1982.

Horowitz, BJ, Edelstein, SW, and Lippman, L: Sexual transmission of candida, *Obstet Gynecol* 69: 883–86, 1987.

Huggins, K: *The nursing mother's companion,* Boston, 1986, The Harvard Common Press, pp. 46–47.

Ing, R, Ho, JHC, and Petrakis, NL: Unilateral breast-feeding and breast cancer, *Lancet* 2: 124–27, 1977.

Jennison, RF: Thrush in infancy, *Arch Dis Child* 52: 747–49, 1977.

Johnstone, HA, and Marcinak, JF: Candidiasis in the breastfeeding mother and infant, *JOGNN* 19: 171–73, 1990.

Kimball, ER: Breastfeeding in private practice, *Northwestern University Medical School Bulletin* 25: 257–60, 1951.

Kvåle, G, and Heuch, I: Lactation and cancer risk: Is there a relation specific to breast cancer? *J Epidemiol Commun Health* 42: 30–37, 1987.

La Leche League International: *The womanly art of breastfeeding* (5th ed.), Franklin Park, Ill., 1991, The League, pp. 139–41.

Lauwers, J, and Woessner, C: Pain—more than discomfort to breastfeeding women, *Int J Child Educ* 2: 30–32, 1987.

Layde, PM, et al.: The independent associations of parity, age at first full term pregnancy, and duration of breastfeeding with the risk of breast cancer, *J Clin Epidemiology* 42: 963–73, 1989.

Leary, WG: Acute puerperal mastitis: a review, *Calif Med Soc* 68: 147–49, 1948.

Livingstone, V: Problem-solving formula for failure to thrive in breast-fed infants, *Can Fam Phys* 36:1541–45, 1990.

London, RS, et al.: The effect of vitamin E on mammary dysplasia: a double-blind study, *Obstet Gynecol* 65: 104, 1985.

London, SJ, et al.: Lactation and risk of breast cancer in a cohort of US women, *Am J Epidemiol* 132: 17–26, 1990.

Love, SM: *Dr. Susan Love's breast book,* Reading, Mass., 1990, Addison-Wesley Publishing Co., Inc., pp. 32–121.

Lubin, F, et al.: Coffee and methylxanthines and breast cancer: A case-control study, *Jr Nat Can Inst* 74: 569–73, 1985.

Manning, DJ, Coughlin, RP, and Poskitt, EME: Candida in mouth or on dummy? *Arch Dis Child* 60: 381–82, 1985.

Marmet, C: *Breast assessment: A model for evaluating breast structure and function,* La Leche League International, Annual Seminar for Physicians, Boston, July 11–13, 1990.

Marshall, BR, Hepper, JK, and Zirbel, CC: Sporadic puerperal mastitis: an infection that need not interrupt lactation, *JAMA* 233: 1377–79, 1975.

McTiernan, A, and Thomas, DB: Evidence for a protective effect of lactation on risk of breast cancer in young women, *Am J Epidemiol* 124: 353–58, 1986.

Menendez-Graino, F, et al.: Galactorrhea after reduction mammaplasty, *Plast Reconstr Surg* 85: 645–46, 1990.

Miller, R, and Fraumenti, J: Does breastfeeding increase the child's risk of breast cancer? *Pediatrics* 49: 645–46, 1972.

Minton, JP: Response of fibrocystic disease to caffeine withdrawal and correlation of cyclic nucleotides with breast disease, *Am J Obstet Gynecol* 135: 157, 1979.

Morgan, RW, Vakil, DV, and Chipman, ML: Breastfeeding family history and breast disease, *Am J Epidemiol* 99: 117–22, 1974.

Neifert, M, et al.: The influence of breast surgery, breast appearance, and pregnancy-induced breast changes on lactation sufficiency as measured by infant weight gain, *Birth* 17: 31–38, 1990.

Newton, M, and Newton, N: Breast abscess as a result of lactation failure, *Surg Gynecol Obstet* 91: 651–55, 1950.

Norwood, SL: Fibrocystic breast disease, *JOGNN* 19: 116–19, 1989.

O'Callaghan, MA: Atypical discharge from the breast during pregnancy and/or lactation, *Aust NZ Obstet Gynaecol* 21: 214–16, 1981.

Ogle, KS, and Davis, S: Mastitis in lactating women, *J Fam Pract* 26: 139–144, 1988.

Paster, BA: Surgery on the nursing breast, La Leche League, *New Beginnings* 2: 92, 1986.

Peters, MV, and Meaken, JW: The influence of pregnancy on carcinoma of the breast, *Prog Clin Cancer* 1: 471, 1965.

Resico, S: Nursing after breast surgery, La Leche League, *New Beginnings* 6: 118, 1990.

Ribeiro, GG, and Palmer, MK: Breast carcinoma associated with pregnancy: a clinician's dilemma, *Br Med J* 2: 1524–27, 1977.

Riordan, J, and Nichols, F: A descriptive study of lactation mastitis in long-term breastfeeding women, *J Hum Lact* 6: 53–58, 1990.

Schoch, RN: Letters to the editor, *J Nurs-Midwif* 30: 240, 1985.

Schreiner, RL, et al.: Possible breast milk transmission group B streptococcal infection, *J Pediatr* 91: 159, 1977.

Schweppe, K-W, Mohlen, KH, and Beller, FK: Mamma-karzinom und schwangerschaft, *Geburtshilfe Frauenheilkd* 39: 1083–90, 1979.

Simkin, P: Intermittent brachial plexus neuropathy secondary to breast engorgement, *Birth* 15: 102–4, 1988.

Siskind, V, et al.: Breast cancer and breastfeeding: results from an Australian case-control study, *Am J Epidemiol* 130: 229–36, 1989.

Smith, WL, Erenberg, A, and Nowak, A: Imaging evaluation of the human nipple during breast-feeding, *Am J Dis Child* 142: 76–78, 1988.

Song, IC, and Hunter, JG: Galactorrhea after reduction mammaplasty, *Plast Reconstr Surg* 84: 857, 1989.

Thomsen, AD, et al.: Course and treatment of milk stasis, noninfectious inflammation of the breast, and infectious mastitis in nursing women, *Am J Obstet Gynecol* 149: 492–95, 1985.

Thullen, JD: Management of hypernatremic dehydration due to insufficient lactation, *Clin Pediatr* 27: 370–72, 1988.

Tretli, A, et al.: Survival of breast cancer patients diagnosed during pregnancy or lactation, *Br J Cancer* 58: 382–84, 1988.

Utter, AR: Gentian violet treatment for thrush: can its use cause breastfeeding problems? *J Hum Lact* 6: 178–80, 1990.

Waller, HK: *Clinical Studies in Lactation,* London, 1938, Heinemann, Medical Books, pp. 115–135.

Whitley, RJ, et al.: The natural history of herpes simplex virus infection of mother and newborn, *Pediatrics* 66: 489–94, 1980.

SUGGESTED ADDITIONAL READINGS

Biggs, TM, and Humphreys, DH: Augmentation mammaplasty. In Smith, JW, and Aston, SJ: *Grabb and Smith's plastic surgery* (4th ed.), Boston, 1991, Little, Brown & Co.

Fisher, JC, and Rudolph, R: Augmentation mammaplasty. In Fisher, JC, Guerrerosantos, J, and Gleason, M: *Manual of aesthetic surgery,* New York, 1985, Springer-Verlag.

Lewis, CM, and Fisher, JC: Breast reduction/elevation. In Fisher, JC, Guerrerosantos, J, and Gleason, M: *Manual of asthetic surgery,* New York, 1985, Springer-Verlag.

Woessner, C, Lauwers, J, and Bernard B: *Breastfeeding today,* Garden City Park, N.Y., 1987, Avery Publishing Group, Inc., pp. 183–86.

15

Maternal Employment and Breastfeeding*

KATHLEEN G. AUERBACH

The decision to continue breastfeeding following return to employment, be it part-time or full-time, may represent a significant departure from the decisions of a woman's mother and grandmother. She may be the *first* mother in her family to return to work before her child is in school; she may also be the *first* mother to have chosen to breastfeed, and she is very likely to be the *first* mother to have chosen to combine both roles. As such, she is a pioneer; like the pioneers who preceded her across the plains, she may feel that she is facing innumerable unknowns for which she is woefully unprepared.

How many women work outside the home? This question is difficult to answer, because what one chooses to count influences the answer. U.S. Census data reveals that more than one-half of all women with children under the age of three are in the labor force, and that most of these work full-time (Facts on Working Women, 1989). Working wives and mothers are the rule rather than the exception, and many of these women will return to work during the period when they are most likely to be breastfeeding.

Three factors influence whether breastfeeding can be combined with maternal employment: (1) the nature of the mother's work (is it physically demanding or potentially hazardous; can she arrange breaks for feeding or pumping?); (2) the baby's age; and (3) the amount and type of support the mother has from family, child-care people, and others whose opinions are important to her (Shepherd & Yarrow, 1982).

Being employed, particularly more than 20 hours

per week, does have a significant negative influence on breastfeeding duration (Gielen et al., 1991; see also Auerbach & Guss, 1984). Hence many women, when faced with the need to consider both, choose not to breastfeed at all (Livingstone & Grams, 1985), or to wean the baby in advance of returning to paid employment outside the home. While breastfeeding is possible after the mother returns to work, surveys conclude that the employed mother is less likely to continue to breastfeed than is the woman who chooses to stay at home during her baby's early infancy. Ryan and Martinez (1989) found that initiation of breastfeeding was as likely among women planning to return to work as among those who were planning to stay home; however, only 10% of the employed mothers were breastfeeding six months later, compared with 24% of unemployed women who were breastfeeding their six-month-olds.

Most worldwide studies, particularly those conducted in developing countries, report that working negatively affects breastfeeding (Thimmayamma, Vidyavati & Bhavani, 1980; Al-Sekait, 1988; Marshall, 1988). On the other hand, an Israeli study found that women who worked outside the home during their pregnancy are more likely than nonworking pregnant women to breastfeed (Birenbaum, Fuchs & Reichman, 1989). This chapter examines these and other issues and offers specific guidelines for the health-care worker who is asked to counsel or to provide information to women anticipating a return to work outside the home when their babies are breastfeeding.

---

*Sections of this chapter are derived from Auerbach, KG: Assisting the employed breastfeeding mother, *J Nurs-Midwif* 35:26–34, 1990.

This chapter is divided into two parts. The reader interested in the "how-to's" of assisting an employed breastfeeding mother may wish to read only Part 1, which offers such advice. Part 1 focuses on how the health-care provider can assist the employed breastfeeding mother from pregnancy onward, highlighting those elements which have been found to work for others. Part 2 discusses some of the contextual issues surrounding breastfeeding and employment, including legal issues, the pull between home and work, and the experiences of health-care workers.

WHY WOMEN WORK

Most women work because they need the money. Many more women today are the sole support of their families than in previous years: some are married to men who are underemployed; others are "putting hubby through" trade school, college, or graduate school. When the paycheck arrives, they receive tangible evidence that what they do counts for something. More important, the paycheck enables them to keep a roof overhead and food on the table. Many women also work because they gain self-esteem by being valued for their marketable skills. In addition, the social rewards of the time they spend with other adults on the job makes them feel good about themselves—that they are improving the skills for which they sought higher education (of whatever level) and that they as individuals (and their skills) are not going to "stagnate" and become outdated from lack of use. Why then do women work? For the same reasons that most men work.

However, in a society in which many people still hold fast to the myth of the family with only one income-earner (male), a full-time homemaker/mother (female), and two to four children (preferably both sons and daughters), accepting that women work for the same reasons as men creates discomfort.

PRENATAL PLANNING/PREPARATION

Just as pregnancy is a time of planning that focuses on caring for the baby and breastfeeding, pregnancy is the best time to plan for one's return to the employment scene. Most women already have decided how they will feed the baby, often prior to the onset of the pregnancy. However, many need to use the pregnancy as a time when they learn specifics about how to do so. Because so many myths exist about breastfeeding and so many different individuals may take the view that combining breastfeeding (a home activity) with employment (a work and nonhome activity) is inappropriate, the health-care worker who has contact with the employed pregnant woman does her a great service simply by asking how she plans to combine the two tasks after the baby's arrival. In many cases, the mother's reply to such a question will identify fallacies that need to be debunked and areas of information that need to be shared.

First, encourage the mother to *learn* as much as she can *about breastfeeding*. Discussing the changes in the breasts which most mothers observe during pregnancy is a good way to help the mother see that such physical changes require consideration of other kinds of changes that are going to occur. Primary among them is the baby's need for the mother and how this need can be met—even if they must be separated for many hours on a regular basis. Encouraging the mother to attend breastfeeding classes or a group, such as La Leche League, whose support of breastfeeding is unquestioned, will go a long way toward providing her with people from whom she can receive ongoing support and assistance.

Next, help her to *begin making plans* for her baby and for breastfeeding both after the baby arrives and when she returns to work. The employed mother who is breastfeeding will want to determine whether she can use her work breaks to nurse her baby and whether lunchtime breastfeeding will be permitted in the center or at the day-care worker's home. If she is entitled to two small "coffee" breaks a day, can they be combined into a single longer period that will enable her to see her baby, and breastfeed, or take a more leisurely period for expressing her milk? In some settings, "baby breaks" at the job site are a possibility. In situations in which the father works nearby, a family lunch break may be enjoyed: both parents and baby can meet for some quiet midday contact. Another question to ask is whether the day-care provider is familiar with human milk and how to warm it, if it can be refrigerated or frozen at the day-care center, and—if provided—whether it will be used. Additionally, the mother needs to ask how babies are fed at the day-care center; specifically, are they given a bottle to hold while lying alone in a crib or on a pad on the floor, or are they held? Women who have bottle-fed other infants may be unaware that most breastfeeding babies under three months of age have no idea how to hold a bottle; they expect to be held when fed. The mother should insist that her baby be held in arms when fed if this is important to her.

THE PUERPERIUM

When women choose to return to work is influenced by a number of factors. In most cases, the duration of paid or unpaid maternity leave plays a major role. In the case of the birth of a premature baby, the additional and unexpected costs of extended hospital care may also contribute to the decision. Youngblut, Loveland-Cherry, and Horan (1990) found that women who had already planned to return to work were very apt to do so after the birth of a premature infant. The employed women were less satisfied with their situation than the unemployed women, suggesting that the decision to return to work in the face of increased financial need did not totally redirect their concerns away from the baby during this period.

If she expects to express milk after her return to work the new mother may bring a breastpump to the hospital. Assisting her in its use at this time can reduce future difficulties. If she wishes to learn how to express milk, the hospital stay is a good time to introduce hand-expression techniques. However, neither breast pumping nor expression should be stressed at this time as a necessary daily activity. Simply knowing that she can do it and that the time for more active involvement in perfecting these skills will come a bit later is all that is necessary during the hospital stay. Placing too much emphasis on practicing them before the mother's milk supply is well established is self-defeating—unless her baby is ill or born prematurely, and she must use these techniques as a substitute for regular breastfeeding. With a healthy, term infant, the mother's best preparation for an ample milk supply when she returns to work is frequent, unlimited breastfeeding and getting to know her baby before they must be separated.

As with other breastfeeding mothers, assistance with the early breastfeedings that will occur in the hospital can help her to focus first on her baby and on learning new skills. Often the questions which are answered about breastfeeding and the baby's behavior at this time will set the stage for how the mother views later breastfeedings. When does she feel most capable of learning new skills? How has her baby indicated that he is learning, too? Is she identifying changes that indicate each is getting more comfortable with the other? Each of these issues, when supported positively, can give the mother a sense of accomplishment.

Caring for a neonate with a wobbly head and subtle, easily missed cues can be a frightening experience for the new mother. Furthermore, her relationship with other people may have changed. No longer is she simply a wife, if married. Now she is a wife and mother. If she has never been a mother before, her often unvoiced worries about whether she will be a "good" mother can be overwhelming. Skilled observation of early breastfeeding encounters enables the health-care worker to point out ways in which both mother and baby are learning from one another and working well together. Raising issues that other mothers have voiced, but which she may not have expressed, can aid greatly in the mother's growing sense of competence as a parent.

Most striking in the early weeks postbirth is the mother's own physical and emotional adjustment to motherhood: learning to read her baby's cues and remaking her family to include the new little person who represents such a responsibility. The early breastfeeding period is sometimes fraught with difficulties. How they are defined and how the mother copes with them can determine whether she sees herself as a successful breastfeeding mother—or as one who is continuing to struggle in the face of evidence that bottle-feeding seems easier.

When the mother compares learning to be a mother with returning to paid employment (a role with which she may be far more comfortable), she may be influenced by the expectation of others that "of course, she will be going back to work"—as if her work at home counts for nothing. It is no wonder that so many young women today look to a return to a known role as wage earner as a way of guaranteeing that they are still functioning, capable, successful adults. Unlike their grandmothers and greatgrandmothers, who looked on motherhood as a rewarding role for which they received plaudits and recognition, young women today too often view mother-hood as a not-always-sought-after experience with myriad pitfalls. Not the least of which is how to interact with a nonverbal creature who seems only to want to nurse insatiably, but who never sleeps very long and insists on being cared for constantly—even when the mother herself feels inadequate to the daily, to say nothing of the hourly, tasks of nurturing.

How, then, does the new mother cope? If she has a job, she returns to it. If she can arrange it, a relative takes over the care of her baby, for several hours a day. If no relative is available, she hires a stranger to do so—in her own home, in the stranger's home, or in a day-care center where other infants, toddlers, and/or young children are brought each day.

RETURNING TO WORK

The first day a mother returns to work, even when she has prepared for it throughout her time at home after the baby's birth, is often one characterized by the emotional and physical tugs she feels, the tears that slide unbidden down her cheeks, and the many times she pulls out pictures of the baby to share with her co-workers. Rarely is this day one in which she is as productive as she was prior to the baby's birth.

Informing the mother that her first day back is one for showing off the baby photos and straightening her desk so that her infant's picture is prominently displayed is one way to let her know that things will not be the same and that—however prepared she thinks she is—it may be one of the most difficult days she has experienced. The depth of her attachment to the baby means that regardless of the baby's age, this day simply will be one to "get through." "It was no easier with my second than it was with my first. The only reason I was not a basket-case with my third," reported one employed mother, "was that I brought her with me. Believe it or not, I got just as much work done as before—precious little!"

The timing of return to work, particularly if it is full-time, will influence the breastfeeding-specific problems that the mother encounters and how long she may have to deal with them (Auerbach & Guss, 1984; Kearney & Cronenwett, 1991). In one study, breastfeeding difficulties tended to cluster in the first four months of the baby's life (Auerbach, 1984). The sooner the mother returned to work, the longer

she had to deal with one or more of these hurdles, which included:

* concern about an inadequate or fluctuating milk supply
* engorgment
* leaking
* emotional lability
* the need to express or pump milk (its frequency, duration, and likelihood over time)
* the baby's need for frequent feedings, particularly if he was very young when she returned to work
* the baby's frequently changing feeding patterns, including appetite spurts and nighttime nursings.

Added to these difficulties is her low reserve of energy, a problem endemic to all new mothers. The mother needs to be informed that each of these difficulties will resolve over time and that the longer she is home with the baby, the less likelihood there is that any of these issues will prove insurmountable. Remind her that none of these issues are major obstacles after the baby is older than four months; this may encourage her to see that the difficulties need not reduce breastfeeding duration when the mother returns to work very soon after her baby's birth. Such information may assist her in making decisions about the length of her leave from work, if she has an opportunity to extend it beyond the usual four to six weeks (Frederick & Auerbach, 1985).

Helping the mother to harbor realistic expectations about her first days on the job will enable her to see that most of the problems she encounters will not be specific to breastfeeding; rather, they are specific to the overworked woman with a family. However, *how* she plans to breastfeed can make a difference. For example, Morse, Bottorff, and Boman (1989) interviewed 61 mothers who intended to continue breastfeeding after they returned to work. The strategies the mothers selected for breastfeeding influenced how long they did so. Those women who practiced "demand breastfeeding" were more likely to breastfeed longer, even though they tended to return to work sooner. Strategies least likely to result in longer duration of breastfeeding included using formula routinely or going from demand feedings to minimal (one or two per day) breastfeeding. These investigators also noted that the proximity of the baby to the work site significantly influenced the likelihood of breastfeeding duration. Those mothers whose babies were nearby had a mean breastfeeding duration of 21.6 weeks, compared with those whose babies were not nearby; their breastfeeding duration averaged only 17 weeks.

There are many ways in which breastfeeding can be continued after the mother returns to work—including the use of hand expression, breast pumping, having the baby brought to the mother during meal breaks, or using formula for those feedings which occur during the mother's work day (Broome, 1981). Each of these alternatives represents an option that deserves discussion. In those cases in which a family history of allergies has been identified, formula use should be avoided for as long as possible. Setting up the right care situation for the baby may actually solve many of the problems that the mother feels certain will negatively affect her baby's growth and development. For example, several women in one international study reported resenting deeply the time the sitter had with the baby (Auerbach, 1984). The opportunity to see the baby during the day resolved this difficulty for some of these mothers.

BREAST PUMPING/EXPRESSING

Prior to the mother's return to work, the lactation consultant or other health worker who is counseling her will want to discuss the need to express milk when she is away from her baby. The older the baby and the fewer number of times per day that he nurses, the less the likelihood that the mother will be required to do so. Thus, a mother who plans to work a shift when her baby usually sleeps may not need to express milk while she is at work.

According to Auerbach and Guss (1985), a week to 10 days before the mother returns to work is a good time to begin practising expression and pumping and to begin building a stockpile of milk in order to:

- learn how to relieve physical discomfort from overfull breasts
- obtain milk for the baby's other feedings
- maintain her milk supply at an optimal level

As a general rule, the earlier in the postpartum period that the mother returns to full-time work, the more frequently she will need to express or pump her breasts. Expressing or pumping milk at work in order to give the baby human milk feedings in her absence is only one reason for doing so. The mother is also protecting her baby from infections and allergies, which have been discussed earlier. In addition, the mother who is comfortable on the job is a more efficient worker. If she feels, as one mother put it, "that I am going to explode and *gallons* would flood the room," she cannot concentrate on her work. Furthermore, painful engorgement contributes to embarrassing leaking, an increased risk of mastitis from milk stasis, and reduction of her milk supply from overfullness of the ducts. (See the following boxed questions.)

For a baby who is less than two months old, one to two ounces for each feeding will be sufficient. When

---

QUESTIONS TO ASK A MOTHER WHO IS PLANNING TO USE A BREAST PUMP*

1. Are the instructions accompanying the pump understandable, accurate, and easy to follow?
2. Is the pump physically comfortable to use?
3. How available are parts for the pump?
4. What is the cost (daily, weekly, monthly) of using the pump?
5. What pumping options are available in her community or worksite?
6. What is the experience of other women who have used breastpumps in her community or worksite?
7. Does the mother feel emotionally/psychologically comfortable pumping her milk? If she does not, has she considered expressing her milk by hand or breastfeeding without expressing her milk for the periods when she is separated from her baby?

*Derived in part from Auerbach, KG: Assisting the employed breastfeeding mother, *J Nurs-Midwif* 35:26–34, 1990.

she begins expressing milk, the mother may be dismayed that she obtains so little (sometimes barely enough to cover the bottom of a small four-ounce bottle). Remind the mother that each time she expresses milk, or uses an efficient pump which does not cause pain, she will probably get more milk. Just as she had to learn to breastfeed, her body needs to learn to respond to the stimulation of hand expression or breast pumping in order to trigger milk ejection. (See Chapter 11 for techniques for maximizing milk ejection.) One lactation consultant tells each mother who is planning to return to work to expect no more than one-half ounce with the first several pumping/expression sessions. Since most mothers will obtain more than this, especially after several sessions, such a comment results in a sense of success for the mother, who may view how much milk she obtains as an indicator of the adequacy of her supply. If she exceeds what "the expert" has told her to expect, surely she will succeed!

During practice sessions, she should express or pump in the morning, when she is more likely to feel rested, rather than later in the afternoon or evening. Usually two practice sessions, timed about one hour after two consecutive morning nursings, are sufficient to develop her milk expression skills. Mothers

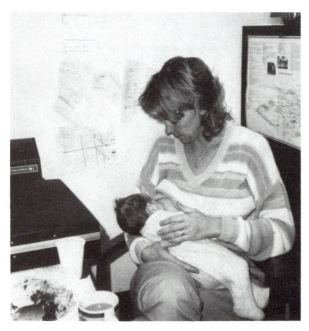

FIGURE 15–1   Breastfeeding in the workplace.

who feel particularly full late in the evening have also found that expressing at this time helps to build up a sizable stockpile of milk. Remind a mother that the milk she obtains in this way is "excess," not an indication of the amount of milk the baby obtains. Furthermore, residual milk is present after all breastfeedings, regardless of the rate at which the baby is growing (Dewey et al., 1991).

When planning pumping sessions, ask the employed mother to practice the 5–15–5 rule. The first and last "fives" refer to two very short, "pump for comfort" sessions in the midmorning and midafternoon. Rarely do such periods last longer than five minutes. Some mothers will choose simply to excuse themselves to the women's room, where they express briefly into the sink until the breast fullness they are feeling has subsided; they then return to their work station. At a meal break, the mother then expresses or pumps her breasts for 15 to 20 minutes and saves this milk for later use. As the mother becomes adept at expressing/pumping, and as her baby gets older, she may find that she can reduce the number of pumpings to two/day and then to one/day. Some women have combined the midmorning and midafternoon coffee breaks into a single longer period more conducive to breast expression.

When babies are cared for near the worksite, mothers often use this time, as well as lunchtime, to go to the baby for a relaxed midday nursing; sometimes they have the baby brought to them. In either case, breastfeeding stimulates the breasts more effectively than the best electric pumps or the accomplished mother who is comfortable hand expressing her milk. Furthermore, both parties enjoy their time together; more than one mother has commented on how much easier it was to return to work after having "touched base" with the baby, while grabbing a quick sandwich at the sitter's or the day-care center.

If the mother is more comfortable using a breast pump than hand expressing, she will need to purchase a breast pump. The breast pump market has expanded rapidly in recent years. As usual, one gets what one pays for. Questions the mother should ask when selecting a pump include:

- Is the pump easy to clean?
- Is the pump comfortable to use?
- Is the pump easy to use?
- Is the pump effective in obtaining milk quickly?

- Are the instructions for pump use clear and easy to understand?
- Are extra/replacement parts available without having to purchase an entire kit?
- What is the overall cost of using the pump (not just the initial purchase price)?
- Are both single and double pumping options available if desired?
- What have other mothers reported about using the pump in question?

The first important consideration is that the pump must be easy to clean. If the user cannot be assured that cleaning is possible at home, with or without a dishwasher, the pump should not be purchased. Generally, any pump with a bulb syringe attachment is difficult to clean and should be avoided.

The pump should be easy and comfortable to use. No single pump works optimally for every mother. This may relate to the closeness of fit of the pump flange on the mother's breast, to the angle of "pull" of cylinder-style pumps, and other factors as yet undiscovered. The angle of the flange varies from one pump to another, as do the shape, size, and degree of fullness of each mother's breasts. Optimally, the mother should try using several pumps before purchasing one. The next best alternative is to talk with other mothers who are successfully pumping and compare the efficiency and reported comfort of different pumps. However, it is important to keep in mind that what works for one mother may not always work for another.

The *length* of pumping experience may be more important than *duration* of a given pumping session in obtaining breastmilk. One mother who used a hospital "Lactation Station" obtained 15 ounces in 20 minutes, during which time she had to empty the collection bottles at least once to avoid their overfilling! Another mother, who used the same mechanical equipment, obtained six ounces in 20 minutes. Other mothers averaged seven to nine ounces after 15 minutes of pumping. Still another mother sometimes obtained as much as 10 ounces and other times as little as five. All mothers obtained less milk at the end of the work week than they did at the beginning.

The lesson learned from these mothers is that efficiency needs to be gauged by whether the mother is comfortable with the pump during its use, whether her breasts feel softer after using the pump, and

whether—over time—the amount of milk she obtains tends to increase. When she begins offering solid foods, breastfeedings become less frequent and/or shorter. When this occurs, the amount obtained by pumping also usually declines. If answers to these questions are in the affirmative, the pump can be considered efficient. The least effective pumps obtain less milk over time and the mother's discomfort increases.

The health-care worker who assists the mother should be familiar with instructions for all pumps in order to clarify instructions that are incomplete, unclear, or written in an unfamiliar language. Additionally, pump instructions should be reviewed to determine whether pictures demonstrating use of the equipment are accurate. In one study, the instructions of several hand-operated pumps included illustrations and recommendations that resulted in Tennis Elbow (Williams, Auerbach & Jacobi, 1989).

If the mother cannot obtain replacement parts or extra pieces without purchasing an entirely new kit, the cost of using the pump may become prohibitive. The same is true if she plans to use a battery-operated pump with cost-effective batteries and/or a rechargeable battery pack. (See Chapter 11 on Breast Pumps.) The least expensive breast pumps tend not to have replacement parts. Since double pumping is more effective in obtaining milk quickly than pumping each breast separately, electric pumps without this option should be carefully considered (Auerbach, 1990b).

STORAGE

Research supports the notion that human milk is a dynamic substance that kills bacteria. This ability is highest in the first several hours after expression, even when it is unrefrigerated (Pittard et al., 1985; Barger & Bull, 1987; Nwankwo et al., 1988), and some investigators have reported that colony counts remain low in such milk for at least 48 hours (Larson et al., 1984). For this reason, when women use clean containers, in which their own fresh milk is stored for less than six to eight hours prior to refrigeration, they are not endangering their healthy babies. (See the list of guidelines on p. 408.) Other mothers who prefer to refrigerate their milk should do so in a clean, capped container and use the milk within two days after it has been refrigerated. Mothers who express milk on a Friday to use the following Monday often freeze their milk. Milk stored in the freezer compartment of a refrigerator (top, bottom, or side models) should be placed as far away from the door as possible; most mothers use frozen milk within one month of the date when it was expressed. If a deep-freezer is used to store the milk, it can be used up to six months after the date of expression. The mother should be reminded that human milk is a substance whose "age" matches that of the baby. Milk obtained when the baby was three months old will not as completely meet that same baby's needs when he is six months old.

Once the milk has been refrigerated or frozen, it should be thawed and warmed to body temperature by placing it under the faucet in a sink and running gradually warmer water over the container. It is inappropriate to thaw milk overnight, this practice enables bacteria in the milk to multiply. Neither should it be heated very quickly on a stove or in a microwave oven. Vitamin C and other properties, including IgA (Sigman et al., 1989) are easily destroyed when milk is heated too hot; the protein is altered as well. Additionally, microwave heating nearly always results in uneven distribution of the heat, which usually goes unnoticed because the container rarely feels as warm as the center portion of the fluid (Hibbard & Blevins, 1988; Nemethy & Clore, 1990). Thus, the milk can be too hot in some spots and substantially cooler in others. Even water-warmed milk should be mixed well and tested on the inside of the caregiver's wrist before offering it to the baby. Mixing should be done not only for heat distribution, but also to assure that the creamy portion of the milk is resuspended. The fat content of milk is altered with refrigeration, as well as when the milk is frozen and then thawed for reuse (Silprasert et al., 1986). Loss can be minimized when the container is shaken well before offering its contents to the baby.

GENERAL GUIDLINES FOR STORING HUMAN MILK

- Always use a clean container.
- Label each container with date and time of the earliest contribution to the container, particularly if "layering" different expressions into the same container.
- Store milk in the approximate quantities that the baby is likely to need for one feeding.
- If refrigerated within six hours, store in a clean, tightly capped container for the unrefrigerated interim period.
- If refrigerated, use within two to five days.*
- If frozen in a refrigerator freezer section, use within one month.*
- If frozen in a deep-freezer, use within six months.*
- Discard any remaining milk which was not used at the feeding for which it was thawed and warmed.
- Remind the mother that the "age" of the milk should be matched as closely as possible to the baby's age in order to optimize the degree of "fit" between the baby's needs and the properties of the milk.

*Shake while thawing to remix the creamy portion which separates during storage.

AT WORK AND AT HOME

After the mother has returned to work most concerns tend to focus on the baby: in particular, is he getting enough milk to continue to grow well? Weighing the baby helps the mother to see that the baby's growth is not being compromised because she has returned to work. So is a reminder that many babies take less human milk from a bottle than the mother—or the care-giver—expects. Many women working part-time have found that their three-month-old babies—or even older infants—prefer to wait until the mother returns home, rather than to accept a bottle, even if it contains her own heated milk. Still other babies who refuse a bottle will happily accept a cup or a spoon of milk, particularly when it is offered matter-of-factly.

Breastfeeding at home during nonworking days helps to maintain a milk supply when the mother may be most concerned about providing for her young baby. The LC who counsels the breastfeeding mother needs to assure her that reducing fluids on Monday, when she returns to work and is concerned that her abundance will show by inadvertent leaking—and increasing them on Friday evening—will help to increase milk production if she is fearful that it is inadequate and/or not sufficient to meet her baby's needs.

FEEDING OPTIONS

Bottle-feeding. Most people think that a baby must be bottle-fed when he or she is not breastfed. Many a working mother worries that her baby will reject a bottle in her absence. To avoid this, some women have been told to begin bottle-feeding once a day immediately after the baby's birth. The clinical experiences of many lactation consultants who have worked with breastfeeding mothers suggest that this works only rarely. First, early introduction of a bottle is more likely to result in nipple confusion; even when this problem does not arise, the baby may still reject the bottle, particularly when he reaches two-and-one-half to three months of age. If the baby is over four weeks old when the bottle is introduced, the risk of nipple confusion is reduced and the likelihood of rejection is low—provided that someone else introduces the bottle and patiently helps the baby to learn how to use it. If the baby is nearing three months when the mother returns to work she may wish to forgo using a bottle entirely and have the baby's father teach the baby how to use a cup. Because adults use cups and babies are inveterate imitators of the actions of their parents, most babies will eagerly use a cup.

A week or 10 days before the mother returns to work is plenty of time to reassure her that her baby will not starve in her absence, and that her baby will learn how to use a bottle without difficulty. If her husband is the designated teacher of bottle-feeding, it is important to pick a time when the mother is not around. Ask the father to prepare the bottle about one-half hour before the baby is likely to indicate that he wants to feed, since a bottle is apt to be rejected if the baby is famished. He then places the baby in his arms, sitting in a place other then where the mother usually nurses the baby. The father should keep the baby's head somewhat higher than the rest of his body and present the bottle so that the teat is well into his mouth—centered on the tongue but not so steeply held as to cause choking. The father should talk or sing to the baby as he patiently waits for him to accept this new feeding method. Very often, the baby will, after a few tentative sucks, begin to empty the bottle.

Because bottle-feeding is more likely to cause the baby to swallow air, frequent burping (often after each ounce that is ingested) will be necessary. By stopping and starting the baby on the bottle, feedings last somewhat longer and are more likely to include the socializing behavior which is such a natural part of breastfeeding.

Caution the bottle-feeding care-giver to use a towel or other absorbent cloth under the baby to catch spills. Remind the mother or care-giver that nonhuman milk will stain and smell to a greater degree than human milk. Finally, reassure the father that it is acceptable if the baby takes only a small amount of milk—there is no need to "empty" the bottle. On the other hand, if the baby drains the bottle in very short order, this is not necessarily an indication that the baby needs more. Rather, the hole in the rubber teat may be too large, or the steepness of the bottle is such that the baby has no choice but to drain the container to avoid choking.

Some babies will express clear preferences for particular rubber nipples/teats. If one is rejected, try others. Teats that have been warmed under hot tap water are more likely to be accepted.

Cup feeding. The father or care-giver sits the baby up in his or her arms, supporting the head and neck. Lean the baby forward slightly and tip the cup into his mouth so that a small amount of fluid is presented. Because sipping is different from suckling, nipple confusion is unlikely to occur. After the first sip, the baby who has sufficient coordination and hand control usually reaches forward and grasps the cup on either side, an indication that he is interested in continuing the activity! Any cup will serve the purpose. Parents who prefer spouted ones often do so because of less spillage. Dropper-like containers which have contained liquid baby medicines are a good beginning "cup." Small plastic specimen cups, shot glasses, and all manner of small cups have been used and have been reported to work well. Premature babies have been taught to cup-feed prior to beginning to breastfeed (Armstrong, 1987); parents should be reassured that their baby can learn to cup-feed early, even before he is able to sit.

Spoon-feeding. Spoon-feeding proceeds much like cup-feeding, except that the fluid is poured into the spoon—or the spoon is dipped into the liquid—and offered to the baby. It involves a sipping action and thus eliminates nipple confusion. Very small infants have been taught to spoon-feed. It takes a bit longer than cup- or bottle-feeding, but is well accepted by infants.

LOSS OF SLEEP

Fatigue is an issue for all parents of infants. Other issues are no time (for the mother), feeling unhappy and/or guilty about leaving the baby to go to work, and loss of nighttime sleep (Auerbach, 1984).

Sleep deprivation is a fact of life for nearly all parents of very young infants. Many employed breastfeeding mothers who work during the day find that their baby's sleep pattern changes after they return to work. Instead of taking short naps during the day and sleeping longer at night, the baby begins to sleep for very long periods during the day and to remain awake later into the evening. This may be a coping behavior that enables the baby to tolerate many hours away from his mother. This behavior leads to "reverse cycle breastfeeding." Often, the baby's waking time with his mother is spent engaging in many short breastfeeding episodes and other time nestled in her arms. Such behavior need not mean that the mother loses still more sleep. In fact, what better built-in "excuse" does the mother have for lying down on the couch when she gets home than breastfeeding? "Sleep saving" techniques that families have found work well include keeping the baby's cradle or crib in the parents' room; creating an extension on the parents' bed; "graduating" from a double to a queen- or even king-size mattress; and placing a spare mattress on the floor of the baby's room for late-night cuddling and nursing away from other family members. This last option works best for those near-toddlers and larger babies who tend to "sing" when they eat—sometimes loudly enough to waken nearby sleepers.

THE TRIPLE BREEDER-FEEDER-PRODUCER

Boulding (1976) has noted that women's productivity is rarely considered until they leave the home. Only recently has women's contribution as a homemaker been a topic of discussion taking into consideration its economic value and worth. The result, however, is rarely a decision to pay housewives to stay at home in order to continue their role full time. Instead, women have been sold the notion that they can "have it all, all at the same time" (Gilbert,

Holahan & Manning, 1981). That most women have discovered the inherent falsity of such a premise only adds emphasis to Boulding's (1976) conclusion:

> When women have too heavy a work burden with the triple breeder-feeder-producer role, the whole society suffers. Women suffer role strain, men suffer role deprivation, and children suffer from inadequate experiences of relating to the human community.

Given an acceptance of the notion that we expect too much of women when we ask them to be full-time mothers and full-time workers at the same time, is part-time employment during their children's early years the answer? Perhaps. In more than one study, part-time workers, male or female, blue-collar or white-collar, expressed greater satisfaction with their situation and more interest in their jobs than did full-time employees (Ferree, 1976). Increasingly, women are choosing to return to paid work on a part-time basis before resuming full-time employment. Factory workers have reported being able to arrange additional break time to rest when they could not delay their return to work. Sometimes this break was used to express milk; in other cases, women took catnaps. Often such part-time white-collar work begins at home, particularly where electronic linking to the job via computer modems and fax machines is possible. Such an option means that the mother can practice resuming a very organized way of life while she is still learning that a freer form to the day, the norm when a baby's needs come into play, has its own rewards.

Still another option is job-sharing. Advantages to the employer include greater productivity, greater worker satisfaction, and lower turnover. Such sharing of responsibilities is well suited to factory work, as well as white-collar and executive slots.

Job-sharing is an alternative to full-time work that seems especially viable for nurses. At least one pair of lactation consultants made such an arrangement with their hospital employer. According to Lindeke and Iverson (1986), the advantages of job-sharing include the following:

- one full-time position, for which all duties and responsibilities are assumed
- each of the partners is an integral part of the work group

- each receives fringe benefits based on the time they work
- both partners can remain fully involved in work-related activities
- both partners can be considered for promotion and career development, just as they would if working full-time.

Where job-sharing works best, each partner fills in the other regarding work issues before the first partner leaves for home. In most cases, each is more rested than a full-time worker and thus is more efficient during her four-hour workday than either would be for half of a full workday. The flexibility of job-sharing may be just the ticket for an employee who wishes to maintain work skills while avoiding stress and burn-out which may occur with having young children.

Breastfeeding is easier when the mother works less than a full day. Both Auerbach and Guss (1984) and Gielen et al. (1991) found that the length of the mother's work day shortened the length of time the mother breastfed. Women who ease back into a work setting, through a delay in their return, more flexible hours, or a flexible work site (beginning at home and going to a more distant site somewhat later), have reported being happier with themselves and their employment situation than women who felt forced into making decisions they were not sure were right for them.

MATERNITY LEAVE

Eighty-five percent of American female workers will become pregnant at some time during their working lives (Kamerman, Kahn & Kingston, 1983). Most of these women will continue to work through much of the pregnancy; in fact, the majority will take so little time off following the birth of the baby that they are considered not to have left the labor force at all! American legislation has taken a protective posture toward the pregnant worker in the past—with mixed results (Gardin & Richwald, 1986). On the one hand, some argue that the pregnant woman and the fetus she carries are a "protected class" deserving of special dispensation. However, feminists and others argue that to grant pregnant women such a status begins the slide down the slippery slope of discrimination against all women—under the guise of "protecting" women from themselves (Erickson, 1979). One result is that most employers ignore the preg-

nancy for as long as possible, offering no special consideration for women during this period and hoping that no special needs arise. Some employment is indeed restricted during the perinatal period in certain occupational settings; additionally, there is little legal protection of income, benefits, seniority status, or reinstatement of employment after the pregnancy.

Barriers to breastfeeding while the mother is employed outside the home are many and include role overload and multiple demands on the working mother's time (Auerbach, 1984); sexual discrimination and harassment on the job (*New York Times,* 1984); lack of child care at or near the work site (Morse, Bottorff & Boman, 1989); lack of appropriate support systems, such as paid maternity leave and flexible work arrangements after the baby is born (Koop & Brannon, 1984); lack of opportunities to express and/or store milk for later use (Katcher & Lanese, 1985); lack of awareness of the importance of breastfeeding to the mother and baby; and an expectation that maternal employment is a legitimate reason for weaning the baby (Lawrence, 1982).

These barriers raise issues about the impact of women's work on breastfeeding and the legitimacy of promoting breastfeeding among working women (Barber-Madden, Petschek & Pakter, 1987)—and, conversely, about the impact of breastfeeding on women's abilities, inclination, and/or motivation to work outside the home! Removing the barriers that exist, as seen in Table 15–1, requires both short-term and long-term strategies, and involves the concerted efforts of individuals at specific work sites, as well as at the state and federal levels, particularly where policy decisions may influence future actions (U.S. Department of Health and Human Services, 1984). When such strategies are implemented, support for breastfeeding also benefits other family responsibilities and concerns. Breastfeeding may simply be more visible evidence that the worker comes to the job from a family and will return to that unit when the work day is over. Thus, linking breastfeeding promotion and support policies to the general needs of all family members may enable what could be seen as legislation for the minority to be sought under the legitimate guise of legislation which supports the health and well-being of all members of society.

Kurinij et al. (1989) note that most employers in the United States do not follow a general maternal leave policy, thereby forcing many women to return to paid employment during the very period which is

TABLE 15–1   BARRIERS TO BREASTFEEDING WHILE EMPLOYED AND SUGGESTED STRATEGIES*

Barriers	Short-term Strategies	Long-term Strategies
Lack of child care at/near workplace	Information about child care located near the worksite Child-care information and referral system	Government policies enabling most employers to subsidize child care
Conditions of work environment	Provide breastfeeding breaks for mothers Provide a place for mothers to express/pump their milk and store for later use	Options for flex-time, job-sharing, part-time work at the worksite Options to work from home, either part-time or full-time Options to bring a nonmobile infant to the worksite with mother
Employer policies: inadequate maternity insurance programs	Encourage legislation for disability insurance in states in which it does not yet exist	Establish a national maternity policy with job-protected maternity leave featuring full or partial wage replacement, plus health coverage
Society-wide attitudes about breastfeeding	Develop public education programs for school-age children	Develop educational attitudes and programs about breastfeeding
Mother's lack of information about breastfeeding	Establish worksite prenatal programs about working, maternity leave and breastfeeding	Integrate material knowledge with information about employer policies and options
Lack of understanding and knowledge of health-professionals about breastfeeding and employment	Develop professional education programs for health-care workers, at all levels	Integrate material on lactation into curricula in professional training programs at undergraduate and graduate levels

*Derived in part from Barber-Madden, R, Petschek, MA, and Pakter, J: Breastfeeding and the working mother: barriers and intervention strategies, *J Public Health Pol* 8:531–41, 1987.

most likely to interfere with breastfeeding and the baby's need for a great deal of care-giving by the mother. She suggests the "need for the development and implementation of a maternal leave policy, particularly for women who choose to breastfeed" (Kurinij et al., 1989). Morse, Bottorff, and Boman (1989) recommend that "day-care facilities should be constructed near the workplace, rather than in the suburbs, and that lactating mothers should be provided with adequate time to nurse their infants as well as to eat their own lunch during the workday." This conclusion is based on their finding that convenience of the baby to the worksite increased the breastfeeding duration among their Canadian subjects. Some large corporations do provide such a service. For example, Apple, a giant in the computer industry, provides an on-site day-care center which gradually reduces costs as the age of the child increases. The monthly charge for a child under age two was reported to be $575/month in 1989, i.e., less than $4.00/hour. Both the DuPont corporation and Merck subsidize off-site centers for the children of their employees. Most of these opportunities sound good; however, Gielen et al. (1991) found that the opportunity to leave work to breastfeed the baby during the day, or to express and store milk during the work day (evidence that the worksite was "accommodating" to breastfeeding), did not result in an increase in breastfeeding duration. The *opportunity* to take advantage of an option is not the same as the *option* itself! Gardin and Richwald (1986) suggest that the protection of the pregnant worker in the future must derive from the restructuring of the employment system so that it includes worksite day-care, affordable and available temporary employment options, parental leave opportunities, and flexible job-sharing arrangements. Maternity leave policies need to accommodate the mother's minimum goal of breastfeeding for four to six months, rather than the far more common pattern of requiring her to return to work by six weeks postbirth or earlier. Additionally, opportunities should be provided for mothers to return to work part-time, perhaps engaging in job-sharing or flexible time arrangements, particularly when they first return to paid employment (Gielen et al., 1991). Few studies examining the effects of mother-child separation and substitute care on attachment behavior have included information related to infant feeding at the time the mother went back to work. One study that took into account how the infants and young children were fed found that breastfeeding was most likely to be discontinued when the child was placed in day-care (Weile et al., 1990).

The political waffling which has occurred in the last two decades reflects, at least in part, the wide range of opinions regarding the need for women to stop work during their pregnancy in order to protect the health of the mother and her growing fetus. A survey of members of the American College of Obstetricians and Gynecologists (Barman, 1984) revealed that most physicians think that the pregnant woman should stop working about two weeks before her expected date of confinement. However, some physicians suggested doing so as early as four months before delivery, while others recommended no cessation of work at all! Controlling the type of work done (sedentary, standing and walking, or physically strenuous) had little effect on the range of responses, except that slightly more physicians felt that women in physically strenuous jobs should cease such activity one month (or earlier) before the baby's expected due date. What is most surprising about this finding is that the same publication also discusses a federally funded study which found that birthweight drops the longer women remain on the job past 28 weeks of gestation. Of all working mothers who participated in the collaborative perinatal project, only white women with sedentary jobs—and no other children at home—gave birth to normally grown babies if they continued to work. Particularly among black women, working past 28 weeks of gestation resulted in a plummeting of infant birthweights (Barman, 1984). A recent study found that pre-term birth was significantly more likely to occur when working women had jobs requiring prolonged standing rather than sedentary or active jobs. Low birthweight, however, was only slightly more

likely in the women with jobs requiring prolonged standing (Teitelman et al., 1990).

The obstetricians offered no specific time frames for optimal time to return to work after the baby's birth. Even women who had a cesarean birth were thought to be ready to return to work after 35 to 48 days. At least in the United States, the strong work ethic adhered to by most physicians (male and female) may influence them to choose not to view pregnancy as a disability and to encourage women—as a result of the physician's own expectations—to return to paid work as soon as possible. In the military, for example, the duration of maternity leave is only four weeks. Thereafter, the military woman on active duty, whether she is enlisted or an officer, is expected to put in a full day's work. The fact that few women in the United States receive any kind of mandated paid maternity leave may also contribute to this point of view. In countries where paid leaves are longer, the pattern of a mother's return to work outside the home is later. In Russia, for example, the period of time off is 18 months.

Phelan (1991) reports that maternity leave policies in Boston-area hospitals vary markedly. Most of the responding hospitals reported having written policies about maternity leave; however, most were plagued by unclear definitions of coverage. Another finding was a general lack of acceptance of pregnant residents in these hospitals. In the absence of a maternity leave policy, women residents tended to hide their pregnancy for as long as possible and attempted to create maternity leave by combining personal leave, sick time, and vacation benefits.

A recent study compared the attitudes of pediatricians with pediatric residents regarding motherhood during residency (Balk, Christoffel & Bijur, 1990). Both groups felt that a medical residency was more deleterious than other work in which women might engage and had a negative effect on the fetus. More than one-half thought that the infant also suffered emotionally, and 80% or more felt that maternal employment had a deleterious effect on breastfeeding.

The U.S. Family and Medical Leave Act (FMLA), which if passed would guarantee job protection for a woman choosing to stay home with a new baby or a sick family member for up to 12 weeks, has generated vehement discussion. Those in favor of the bill argue that women are the only ones who can have babies and that they should not be penalized for doing so. Opponents cite the cost to business of such a long period of time away from the job and suggest that such a requirement would result in reticence to hire women during their childbearing years.

In spite of the women's movement and the presence of women in the work force, parenting and household responsibilities continue to fall on the mother (Zambrana, Hurst & Hite, 1979; Hochschild & Machung, 1989). This pattern has not changed since the time when the percentage of employed mothers began to climb rapidly. In 1973, for example, working wives averaged four to eight hours per day of household work; nonemployed housewives averaged six to 12 hours daily. Husbands of employed and unemployed wives contributed an average of 11 hours weekly, or less than two hours daily—regardless of their wives' employment status (Walker, 1973).

THE "WAR" BETWEEN WORK AND HOME

Perhaps this discomfort with what "today's" woman has chosen has created the lack of understanding and empathy that exists between employed women and at-home women. On the one hand, the mother at home feels ignored and devalued. She is right to feel this way, for our society rarely values that which has no price. Precisely because she is not paid, what she does is economically invisible. In fact, most social scientists remain at a loss when it comes to classifying "housewives/homemakers." Thus, social analysts tend to maintain them in a separate category and ignore them in most analyses, especially those relating to economic contributions.

On the other hand, the employed mother, who is struggling to maintain her equilibrium while she simultaneously attempts to be all things to all people, feels ignored and devalued. She, too, is right to feel this way. Although she brings home a paycheck for the work she does at the office or factory, her at-home work does not go away. Rarely is it shared by more than a minuscule amount with her spouse if she is married. In spite of the fact that the majority of the married households in the country include two workers, it is the wife who schedules a plumber to fix a broken pipe or an electrician to see about a faulty wire; one quickly gains a sense of the degree to which working women feel continually pulled in different directions!

The mother at home may both envy and resent her employed counterpart. After all, *she* gets paid for what she does. *She* wears silk blouses and has power lunches with the corporate leaders. *She* may be one of those corporate leaders. They do not recognize that she also has children to care for, worry about, and fret over—plus feel guilty about because there is never enough time.

To the woman at work, the mother at home has it made. *She* doesn't have to work; *she* has someone to take care of her. *She* has time for her children. *She* can watch soap operas! They do not recognize that the woman at home often feels that she too is pulled in different directions as she attempts to make time for each person's needs and schedules, as well as the household chores which are neverending and for which she receives neither pay nor societal recognition.

Each wants to think that she is managing her life the "right" way, even though she may feel that the "other" alternative has many benefits. The mother at home is attempting to live the myth of the intact American family that never really existed for the majority of women, but which is still touted as the ideal on television shows, in radio dramas, and in books. Remember the *Dick and Jane* series? It wasn't the father who wore the apron; nor was it the mother who opened the gate of the white picket fence and left for work every morning. The woman at work is also attempting to live out a new myth that came to life in the 1960s after *The Feminine Mystique* exposed the *Dick and Jane* myth for what it was—and discussed the realities of the at-home woman whose children no longer need her and whose husband is bored with her. In addition, today's working woman is attempting to live out yet another myth which suggests that women can and should be able to have it all: marriage, career, and children. This myth sounded good, even great, to some who had seen how stultified their own mothers had become by living only for others and not for themselves. But the fallacy of this myth was that it was touted by women who weren't raising infants.

What we have here is a lack of recognition that each group is operating under the unreality of an unattainable myth. Neither woman is fully right or fully wrong; each woman is doing the best for her family and each struggles with what oftentimes seem to be insoluble problems and unresolvable situations. Each needs the support of the other; each shares far more similarities with the other than differences. Most important about those shared similarities, both groups of women are caring for children and wanting to do the best for them in an environment that

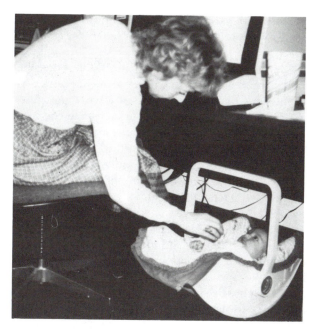

FIGURE 15–2 Baby goes to work with mom.

values women far less than they are worth—and children even less. The at-home woman deserves to be valued for her truly priceless (not valueless) activity: rearing and caring for children. The working woman needs to be valued sufficiently so that her special procreative and nurturing capabilities are not ignored simply because she goes out of the house to earn a living.

What has this to do with breastfeeding—particularly when the mother returns to paid work? The relative invisibility of breastfeeding in today's world is symptomatic of the relative invisibility of most women's accomplishments. Women must value one another and recognize how each affirms female existence and their contribution to life. Only through such valuation will the barriers eventually be gathered together and burned on the bonfire of enlightened self-interest.

THE IMPORTANCE OF SOCIAL SUPPORT

The employed breastfeeding mother is a pioneer insofar as there is no precedent for it. She is walking the edge of a life experience where none of her older female relatives have ever trod. She may be the first among her circle of friends to have a baby, to breastfeed, and to return to work, full-time or part-

time. If she is married, her husband probably has never seen his female relatives practicing this kind of mothering. Thus, they are setting out on an adventure that places their family at the cutting edge of social change.

Such a position is likely to be unsettling, precisely because there are few established rules governing action. Until they find peers who have done the same thing—and lived to laugh about the inevitable "potholes of life" that will surely trip them up—the employed breastfeeding mother and her spouse will need the support of other family members, friends, and colleagues whose opinions matter to them. Who these key support people will be varies by ethnic group. Baranowski et al. (1983) report that the male partner is the most important person for the Anglo mother. However, among black women, a close friend was most influential, while Mexican-American mothers sought the support of their own mothers.

When combining breastfeeding and employment, the mother needs several types of social support, specifically:

- a person who cares about her and what she wants for her baby
- a role model
- a knowledgeable advisor
- a person who obviously values breastfeeding
- a person on whose shoulder she can lean or cry

A person who cares about her and what she wants for her baby. This is most often the baby's father, but not all fathers are supportive of breastfeeding. Most Caucasian mothers, however, will look first to the baby's father for support.

A role model. This person has breastfed her own baby while employed, has enjoyed her experience, and focuses more on the positive aspects of breastfeeding, while helping the mother to work through the difficult situations that inevitably arise from time to time. The friend who has breastfed can be a particularly powerful ally for Hispanic women or women from low-income groups (Barron et al., 1988).

A knowledgeable advisor. A lactation consultant is a natural in this role. So is another health-care provider who has counseled other successful breastfeeding and working mothers. Least likely to be an appropriate choice here is a health-care worker whose personal experience combining breastfeeding and working was more negative than positive.

A person who obviously values breastfeeding. The La Leche League leader or Nursing Mothers counselor fits this role beautifully. She is both enthusiastic and knowledgeable about breastfeeding. Her support and information can be critical to the working mother, when she chooses to nurture her baby in a manner that is not supported by all family members or friends.

A person on whose shoulder she can lean or cry. Husbands are rarely the best choice here. Too often, when the mother complains that things are not going well, the husband—in a sincere desire to give his wife permission to make her life easier—may suggest that she stop breastfeeding "if it is causing so much hassle." He may not want her to do so, but he may feel that this is the only suggestion he can provide which gives them some control. The role model or knowledgeable advisor may provide that shoulder to lean on which the mother needs. So also may the person who values breastfeeding. In some cases, however, this person may be a sister or a dear friend whose familiar voice over the long-distance phone lines may be just the tonic the new mother needs as she struggles with one more new experience and feels alone as she does so. Whoever this person is, simply knowing that the shoulder is available may give the mother sufficient strength of purpose to persevere. Most often, it is this person who can help her distinguish between baby-related and sitter-related problems.

The more people who support the mother's actions, the more likely she is to feel that she can maintain her equilibrium during the rough spots in her journey through motherhood (Lancaster, 1975; Saunders & Carroll, 1988). While commitment is clearly necessary whenever a person takes on a new role (Coreil & Murphy, 1988), the support of others cannot be underestimated, particularly when there is little shared past experience.

HEALTH-CARE WORKERS: A SPECIAL CASE?
Because health-care workers, particularly physicians, midwives, and nurses, are often asked for their assistance when a breastfeeding mother is planning to return to the work force, it is important to examine their experiences, which often form the basis of professional recommendations (Reifsnider & Myers, 1985).

Auerbach and Guss (1985) found differences between three health-care worker groups: physicians, technicians, and nurses. Nurses were significantly less likely ($p<.001$) to work a full day after the birth of a baby whom they were breastfeeding. Perhaps because they chose not to return to full-time work, more nurses gave their babies only human milk for missed feedings. And they were more likely to have positive contact with local breastfeeding support groups.

Such contact influenced when these health-care workers introduced solid foods to their babies, and the timing of introduction of solid foods was predictive of the age of the infant at weaning from the breast. Eighty-five percent of the health workers who introduced solids when the baby was less than four months old had weaned the baby from the breast before the baby's twelfth month.

In contrast, the majority of physicians in this study introduced solid foods very early; and they were more likely than nurses to routinely, sometimes exclusively, use artificial baby milk rather than expressed human milk for missed feedings. This helps to explain why early weaning occurred more often among the physicians, most of whom felt that their work was an impediment to breastfeeding, even when they did not return to full-time employment. They also reported being unable to arrange regular breaks for pumping or expressing, or for nursing the baby. Such "time poverty" is most likely when job demands are determined by the often unpredictable needs of others.

The degree to which physicians may be frustrated by the feeling that breastfeeding is easier for others to schedule, is reflected in Balk and Yellin's (1982) letter decrying the lack of support and encouragement from colleagues when pediatric residents choose to breastfeed. A more recent examination (Balk, Christoffel & Bijur, 1990) of the perceived effect of residency workload on pregnancy—on the mother and her baby, as well as on breastfeeding—makes clear that the earlier concerns of Balk and Yellin have not abated.

Yet, the difficulties identified by health-care workers can be resolved. Katcher and Lanese (1985) reported that the availability of an electric breast pump in an accessible location in a hospital, along with supportive professional advice, resulted in longer breastfeeding duration and a slightly earlier return to work.

Nurses are more likely than other married women to be in the work force when they have young children at home (Greenlear, 1983; Hardin & Skerret, 1981). Many nurses continue to breastfeed after they return to work. The nature of their employment includes the opportunity to select work shifts–which may mean that the baby never misses a regular feeding and/or that the father is the sole care-giver during the mother's work hours (Sandroff, 1980). Employers often prefer to hire nurses part-time because fringe benefits do not have to be paid for part-time workers. And for nurses in the United States, 12-hour shifts three days a week, an increasingly common option, may make breastfeeding easier simply because these mothers are away from home fewer days of the week. While a 12-hour day may be no "picnic," such an arrangement is more feasible than that which exists for women who are in jobs such as sales, or positions that require a great deal of travel. Yet, in all these situations, women have breastfed for many months or years. And, at least one airline guarantees flight attendants a job after a six-month maternity leave when they breastfeed. Flight attendants who bottle-feed are expected to return to work after six weeks.

Said one nurse: "It makes a difference where you work when pumping your breasts. As a nurse, no one makes a big deal of it when I pump and put my milk in the refrigerator. But my friends in business jobs tell me that they wouldn't do that—pumping milk on the job makes them less a businesswoman." At least one group of attorneys would disagree. In their office supply closet next to a stack of legal pads is a pile of breast pads! Such an image suggests that breastfeeding has become one more experience which working mothers can share.

THE DAY-CARE DILEMMA

Whether to use a day-care facility, *where* such care will be provided, *when* the baby will be enrolled, and for *how many hours* and days, plus *its effects* on both the child and her or his parents: all of these issues figure in decision-making of the early postpartum period. The mother who knows she will return to full-time or part-time paid work outside the home

often agonizes about how best to care for her child when she must be absent from the home (Zambrana, Hurst & Hite, 1979). In some cases, the father may take on such care, particularly when the parents' work hours differ, or when the father's work is flexible and he can rearrange his schedule to accommodate his spouse's work requirements. In some families, the wife/mother is the only employed parent and her husband's lack of employment or student status may be such that child care is more easily managed.

In other families, however, the mother may not have a spouse who is available; or she may be a single parent. Other relatives may not be potential care-givers—because of geographic distance, disinclination to provide such assistance, physical or psychological incapacity, and many other reasons. When a relative is not available or is not considered appropriate, the parents must decide what kind of care the child will receive and where he or she will receive it.

Early discussions of the effect of maternal employment on the infant or young child focused on the psychological effects of separation. Perhaps because so many investigators were themselves mothers using substitute care for their own children, many studies focused not on separation effects on the child, but rather whether the mother was "happy" or "satisfied" as a working or nonworking mother (Caldwell et al., 1970; Wallston, 1973; Smith, 1981; Boswell, 1981; Hock, 1978, 1980; Hardin & Skerret, 1981). Their conclusions may have reduced the guilt of the investigators and the other professionals reading their findings, for most could then say without difficulty *they* were happy in their careers; therefore, *their children* were protected from the potential ill effects of substitute care. Although occasional evidence of attachment deficits crept into the literature, usually in the form of the mother's interpretation of fussy behavior as a rejection of her mothering or some other kind of personal affront (Hock, Christmas & Hock, 1980), most findings of this kind were viewed as aberrant and were dismissed as unimportant.

Among the first investigators to suggest that day-care contributed to altered attachment behavior was Blehar (1974), who found that children who began attending day-care before two years of age showed avoidance behavior when they were reunited with the mother; children who began day-care at three years of age were more likely to show anxious, ambivalent behavior. As a result of this and later studies, the attachment process is again being evaluated. Schwartz (1983) examined attachment behavior in 50 infants who were 18 months of age. Seventeen of the children attended day-care all day; 16 did so for part of the day in a home with a single substitute care-giver and one to eight other children; a control group of 17 children had no day-care experience. The children in the first two groups began day-care prior to nine months of age. When compared, the children in full-time day-care, but not those in part-time day-care, were significantly more likely to avoid the mother on reunion, thus suggesting alteration in expected attachment behavior in children of this age group.

Barglow, Vaughn, and Molitor (1987) compared 54 middle-class children who were cared for *in their own homes,* beginning at least four months before their first birthday, with 56 children of the same age whose mothers remained in the home through the child's first year. The investigators identified less secure attachment behavior, particularly in firstborn children, in the day-care group.

Infants who received more than 20 hours of day-care per week were more likely to avoid their mothers when they were reunited than were children who were in day-care less than 20 hours per week, according to Belsky and Rovine (1988), as well as Belsky, Steinberg, and Walker (1982). The mothers of babies who were classified as insecure in their attachments also expressed greater career motivation for working, implying not only that they had returned to work earlier, but that their orientation toward work may have contributed to how they viewed their babies.

Alternatives to infant day-care need to be developed and government-supported. One such alternative is a system that enables—perhaps even encourages—parents to remain with their infants during the first few months of life. This could be accomplished with paid infant-care leaves, not to be confused with maternity leaves, which are often viewed as a form of disability. The People's Republic of China, which has a long history of group child rearing, does not allow infants to be placed in such group care during the first four months of life. In Sweden, a mother may receive up to one year of paid leave—and take another six months of unpaid leave—without fear of losing her job. In Denmark, women receive paid maternity leave for the first six months after birth. Most babies enter day-care in their seventh

month of life, when their mothers return to full-time employment. The mean age when breastfeeding was stopped for the Danish babies who were placed in day-care was six months (Weile et al., 1990).

Brazelton and Als (1979) have speculated that four months of close mother-baby interaction is essential for the maternal-infant bond to be cemented and for optimal infant development to be achieved. It is difficult to see how such development can be attained when mothers and babies are separated for long hours many days a week, beginning just a few weeks after the baby's birth.

In addition to attachment issues, the likelihood of childhood illness as a result of out-of-home care during the early years is also being raised. Fleming et al. (1987) found that among those children attending day-care full-time, 31% of upper respiratory tract infections and 66% of ear infections were attributable to day-care attendance.

Bell et al. (1989) reported that children in day-care were 4.5 times more likely to be hospitalized than children cared for in other settings. This was usually the result of an increased rate of placement of tympanostomy tubes for recurrent ear infections. They also noted that childhood illness accounted for 40% of parental absenteeism from work. Parents whose children went to day-care settings outside the home required more than one-half day per month at home because of illness, compared with one-third day at home because of illness for children cared for in other ways. In the study by Bell et al. (1989) most of the children under 12 months of age who were being breastfed were also being cared for in their own homes when the mothers were employed. Hospitalization occurred for 1.7% of those children who were cared for in their own homes, but for more than three times as many (5.7%) of those who were cared for at a day-care center.

Wald et al. (1988) also compared types of child-care arrangements in assessing the frequency and severity of infections among children in day-care. Children in group care (two to six children) or day-care (seven or more children) were significantly more likely than children cared for at home to experience at least six respiratory infections, more than 60 days of illness, and more than four severe illnesses in an 18-month period. Children cared for at home had far fewer episodes of infection than did children in day-care. Hospitalization for myringotomy and tube placement occurred in 21% of the children in day-care compared with only 3% of those who received care at home. Other health problems associated with day-care attendance include streptococcal infections (Rauch et al., 1990); otitis media (Wald et al., 1988; Fosarelli, 1990); respiratory disease (Anderson et al., 1988); diarrhea (Bartlett et al., 1985a, 1985b); and hepatitis A (Hadler & McFarland, 1986).

When group day-care is used, whether it provides quality care depends in large part on the size of the group, the ratio of staff members to children, and staff training. Day-care that is viewed as psychologically healthy tends to occur in the same centers where the spread of infectious disease is minimal. Quality day-care is possible but costly, often averaging between $3,000 and $5,000 per year (1986 figures) per child. Most of this cost is for staff, the majority of whom are notoriously underpaid (Zigler & Muenchow, 1986; Wong, 1986). Parents must determine whether it is economically feasible to plow such a substantial portion of a mother's after-tax income into day-care. In a recent survey of more than 2,500 women throughout the United States and Canada, including U.S. military personnel stationed overseas, the cost of day-care, regardless of the site, ranged from $50 to $500 per week. Average weekly day-care costs were more than $200. How many women make enough money to be able to afford to pay a day-care worker what her time and expertise are worth remains an open question—and may explain why so many young children are inadequately cared for when their mothers must be away from them.

CLINICAL IMPLICATIONS

When providing information about breastfeeding and employment, it is best to sprinkle such information throughout several different discussions of breastfeeding, maintaining a matter-of-fact attitude and establishing a positive expectation that this combination of roles is possible. Discuss breastfeeding with the mother well in advance of her return to work. The lactation consultant may suggest that options exist about which her client may be unaware. Is she the first person with her job to continue breastfeeding? Is there a place at work where she can go to express milk and store it for later use at home or at the sitter's? Who will be a support system for her? Have some of her breastfeeding co-workers returned to work later than she may have thought was re-

quired? Have some them chosen not to return to work, or found ways to rearrange their work so that they could do it at home? More women are starting their own businesses and/or are joining the increasing numbers of workers whose offices are "at home." In many white-collar jobs, home computers, modems, electronic mail, telephone answering machines, and fax machines make home offices a viable option for many. One reason for this exodus from the traditional work setting is the increasing recognition by parents of the importance of being with their children when they are young.

The role overload ("Superwoman") of the full-time employed mother necessitates that she learn how to organize her time for maximum efficiency (Vaughn & Wittig, 1980). In breastfeeding, she has found an ideal combination for meeting the physical and psychic needs of her young child. At the same time, she need not feel that she must shorten the period of lactation that she had planned.

A frank discussion of the different ways in which women have chosen to structure their breastfeeding is necessary. There is no *one* way to do things. For example, some women will choose to give their babies only human milk during their absence. Such a decision requires that the mother begin to obtain additional milk before her return to work; additionally, she may need to arrange to pump or express her milk more than once a day in order to maintain a supply that meets her baby's needs as completely as possible. (See the boxed review of decisions on pp. 421–423.)

Other mothers may choose not to express their milk at all. These women will need to know that expressing "for comfort," at least during the first week or two, may be necessary if they are to avoid unpredictable, potentially embarrassing "leak spots" while their body is adjusting to no breast stimulation during the work day. Additionally, encourage them to have someone introduce a bottle or cup of artificial formula to the baby well in advance of the mother's first day at work in order to make other plans if the baby develops an allergic reaction.

Some mothers will choose to return to work as soon as possible, often because they are financially unable to do otherwise; other women will make every effort to delay returning to work. The type of job the woman has, the degree of involvement of co-workers and bosses, as well as her relationship with them, her seniority, and a wide array of other factors will influence these decisions. The health worker can provide information about maternal employment and breastfeeding, but only the woman herself can implement them.

Share with the mother how other women have coped with similar situations, answer her questions based on study findings, whenever possible. (See Table 15–2.) Decisions relating to day-care are those most likely to be fraught with high emotion. Babies *do* know when a mother is not available and adapt to her absence by altering sleep patterns. Changes in wakeful and sleepy periods are typical in families in which the mother works at times when the baby has previously been awake a great deal. Increased breastfeeding frequency when the mother is home ("reverse cycle nursing") is a common reaction, particularly in very young babies who breastfeed often. Such a pattern needs to be pointed out to the sitter; ask that she not wake the baby for feedings. Instead, let the baby tell her when he should be fed during the day. These "reverse cycle nursing" episodes do not always increase during the mother's nighttime sleeping hours; rather, they tend to be more frequent during the early daytime hours when she is preparing to leave for work and during the evening hours after she has returned home. Many mothers

find that setting the alarm an hour earlier than they plan to be "up" reminds them to offer the baby the breast while they snooze before heading for the shower or the kitchen to start the day. If she is encouraged to see this as the baby's touching and social time, the mother is more likely to view such behavior as a sign of the baby's attachment to her.

There is no "magic bullet" that will resolve day-care issues. Unlike other countries where government subsidies enable many mothers to stay home for a substantial period following the birth of their babies, the United States has no federal policy supporting maternity leave. At the same time, increasing numbers of families make economic choices that mandate a two-worker household. (See the boxed review of day-care options on p. 421.) And day-care workers, often because they are so poorly paid, represent a workforce that has a high turnover, inadequate training, and lack of job commitment.

Finally, just as with other breastfeeding women, the health-care worker needs to place each mother's experience in context of the total picture. (See the boxed review of decisions on pp. 421–423.) The LC needs to identify first what the mother wants for herself and her baby; after that, supporting the mother's goals for herself and her family is relatively easy.

TABLE 15–2   STUDY FINDINGS AND RECOMMENDATIONS TO OFFER THE EMPLOYED BREASTFEEDING MOTHER*

Study Findings	Recommendations to Share
Successful, employed breastfeeding mothers . . .	
. . . were most anxious about the baby and breastfeeding in the first week of employment.	Arrange to return to work late in the week in order to look forward to a weekend that is only a day or two away.
. . . waited until the baby was four months old or older before returning to work.	Stay home as long as possible.
. . . used part-time/flex-time options when they first returned to work.	Return on less than a full-time schedule in the beginning.

. . . expressed milk during their absences:
  (a) especially in the first month
  (b) to remain physically comfortable
  (c) to reduce the likelihood of leaking
  (d) to collect milk for later use.
	Learn how to express/pump milk.

. . . obtained less milk at the end of the work week than at the beginning.	Increase fluids near the end of the work week; to avoid overfullness on Mondays, restrict fluids slightly.
. . . complained most often about exhaustion.	Use breastfeeding as a "break" from home chores.
. . . viewed breastfeeding as the key to continued "connection" with the baby in spite of separations.	Only the mother can enjoy the closeness that breastfeeding represents.

*Derived from Table 2 in Auerbach, KG: Assisting the employed breastfeeding mother, *J Nurs-Midwif* 35:28, 1990.

DAY-CARE OPTIONS

Center day-care: It usually includes a large number of children who are often segregated into smaller groups by age. Such facilities

- have long hours (some open as early as 6 A.M. and remain open as late as midnight)
- are licensed
- often offer a variety of formal learning experiences, particularly for three-year-olds and older preschoolers
- may provide "after-school" programs for school-age children of working parents
- may or may not take children under the age of two months.

Family day-care: The child is cared for in another home; this is the largest system of out-of-home care in the United States. It includes three different types of homes:

- *Unregulated:* These are neither licensed nor registered with a municipal or state agency.
- *Regulated:* These are licensed, usually by a municipal or state governmental body. This

means that they are limited in the number of children who can be cared for and they must conform to basic health and safety measures, such as the number of beds available for rest periods and proper, safe play equipment.

- *Sponsored or supervised homes:* These are usually part of a network or organization of child-care providers. In some cases, worksites will sponsor certain homes that provide day-care for their workers' children. Such homes are also licensed.

In-home care: Such facilities are less likely to be studied by investigators; these homes are less visible in that the care-giver comes to the child. Usually, the number of children cared for in the home is limited to those living there, although occasionally the care-giver may bring her own children to the site. Care-givers may be relatives of the child(ren) or a nonrelative. The major disadvantage is the high expense.

DECISIONS OF THE EMPLOYED BREASTFEEDING MOTHER

When to Return to Work

1. *Never!* This situation is occurring more often with mothers who have three children rather than two, and more often with mothers who have two children rather than one. Often the mother feels that she lost or missed something by returning to work after the birth of her first baby; this results in making different decisions with later-born offspring. Thus a woman who remains in the workforce, or who returns very soon after her first child's birth, will reduce the time she spends working outside the home after the birth of her second or third child. This is particularly true if the woman is married and her husband earns a salary sufficient to fully sustain the family.

2. *Later than six months.* This situation occurs very rarely, usually in situations in which the woman is a private practitioner or entrepreneur and chooses to be a full-time mother rather than a paid worker for this period of time.

3. *Between four and six months.* Some women workers are looking on this as "earned" time off, during which they can concentrate on enjoying their new and exciting mothering role without having to worry about planning for a "immediate" return to work. In the United States, most such leaves are unpaid; thus, their likelihood of occurrence is low, unless the woman exercises a great deal of control at work and/or is highly placed in the company—or is an owner.

(Box continues)

4. *Between six weeks and three months.* Often such a planned return can be arranged, particularly if the mother is a highly valued employee and a replacement would be more expensive to train than the cost of simply waiting for the original employee to return. Many mothers who have negotiated a return at three months or later have done so by offering to begin to work at home ahead of that time.

5. *As soon as maternity leave is over or when the employer asks/insists.* In some cases, the employer will ask the mother to return as early as three weeks postpartum. In other cases, often out of fear of loss of employment, the woman will return even earlier. This is inappropriate. As a countertactic, learn when employees (female and male) who have had abdominal surgery are expected to return to full-time employment.

How Long to Breastfeed

1. *Until her baby shows no more interest in breastfeeding.* Cues to lack of interest need to be identified so that the mother does not assume weaning is occurring when the baby is cutting teeth or engaging in a nursing strike.

2. *Until her baby gets teeth or reaches a certain age.* The significance of developmental milestones varies by ethnic and social group as well as by the expectations of immediate family members. Many mothers who had decided to breastfeed for a very short period may select later milestones after their baby has "captured" them in the early breastfeeding period.

3. *Until she returns to work.* Many uninformed women begin at this point, and change their minds after they learn something about how to combine breastfeeding with employment.

To Express or Pump Milk

1. *Regularly, often more than once/day, for as long as the mother chooses to supply this milk to her baby.* These mothers are most likely to find that their employment has minimal effect on the duration of their breastfeeding experience.

2. *Once per day.* Many of these mothers often find that the first week or so following their return to work is the most difficult to manage—because one pumping or expression session per day is not sufficient to prevent painful overfilling of the ducts and spontaneous leaking which draws attention to them as breastfeeding mothers. Thereafter, fullness usually does not continue, but they also find that their milk supply declines more rapidly than they had anticipated. Often, they regret their decision not to pump or express milk more often; however, by the time they realize what has happened, the baby is no longer interested in breastfeeding, and an untimely weaning—one which occurs before the mother wished—has occurred.

3. *For only a brief period after returning to work, until the body adjusts and breast fullness no longer occurs.* Many mothers often assume that "their" jobsite will not permit them an opportunity to express milk or to pump their breasts—without having determined whether this is actually true. However, it is the rare situation where employees are not allowed to go the restroom throughout the workday. Explaining that pumping need not be time consuming may help them to see that such activity can be incorporated into their workday with minimal disruption.

4. *Never!* Many mothers are initially uncomfortable with handling their breasts and may express this in reticence to learn how to express milk (Morse & Bottorff, 1988) or to pump their breasts.

When to Use Artificial Baby Milk for Missed Feedings.

1. *For no feeding that the baby needs in the mother's absence.* Many mothers who are aware of the risks of artificial feeding and the unique benefits of breastfeeding are in this group. In many cases in which the mother expresses milk more than once throughout her working day, the period of exclusively human milk feedings—even in her absence—can extend past the period

when the baby is introduced to solid foods. As the baby's needs begin to outstrip her ability to meet them, other nonhuman milk feedings may need to be introduced.

2. *For those feedings for which her own expressed milk is not available or has been used up earlier.* Many women with babies older than four months are in this category. Often the mother's milk supply is beginning to decline at about the time the baby has another appetite spurt and a rapid growth period. Although most missed feedings use her previously obtained milk, the care-giver may be required to use formula for other feedings if the supply of human milk is depleted. One option these mothers often use is the substitution of some solid foods for milk feedings—in order to extend the period of time when the baby receives only human milk as fluid nourishment.

3. *For all feedings as soon as the mother returns to work.* These women are also the least likely to express or pump their breasts. Often, they view human milk as a more convenient way of feeding when they are home, but see no real benefit in providing their milk if the baby cannot breastfeed directly. In addition, they often perceive that their work environment is not conducive to expressing or pumping and storing their milk for later use. Many physicians fall in this group.

Where the Baby Will Be Cared For

1. *In the mother's own home.* This is the most expensive form of care and therefore the least likely to occur. The mother who contemplates such care needs to be aware of IRS regulations governing employment of a person on the employer's premises, which also dramatically increase the cost of such care.

2. *In the home of a neighbor or friend.* Such care is often arranged informally, "over the back fence." It can work well if the arrangement is maintained in a businesslike manner. Problems tend to arise when differences of opinion regarding discipline and other aspects of child care occur. However, such care may also be beneficial to the child, who is not removed from his own neighborhood and who has access to playmates with whom he will share many experiences.

3. *In the home of a stranger who provides day-care services.* Many such homes are unlicensed; others are licensed by the city or state in which they operate. Care needs to be taken that the home provides what the mother wants for her child, including a minimum number of children of the same age. However, when the child being cared for is less than one year of age, expecting one person to also care for more than two older babies is less than optimal. Older children can be a blessing or a curse, depending on their behavior toward the little one.

4. *In a day-care center.* This is the most visible portion of day-care in the United States. While media coverage of such centers has focused on the nightmares of alleged (and actual) abuse and neglect, a center needs to be carefully evaluated before placing a child, particularly an infant, there. The staff-member-to-child ratio, the cleanliness and safety features of the facility, and opportunities for structured and unstructured learning all need to be assessed. The opinions of previous users of the center should be sought. If a center operator cannot provide the names of several previous clients, the parents considering such a center should run rapidly out the door!

SUMMARY

The role of the health-care worker is to inform the mother that she is not alone and that what she is likely to encounter has, in most cases, been faced by other women. In some cases, they found partial solutions; in other cases, their solutions enabled them—and now her—to proceed with breastfeeding with minimal interruption. Whatever the mother's individual situation, the person providing information needs to do so from a perspective of what has worked for others, recognizing that each mother's situation has its own unique strengths and pitfalls.

In settings where institutionalized day-care is well organized and carefully supervised, many families' concerns can be set aside. In other day-care situations, the increased illness rates and other questions related to meeting the infant's and child's many needs bear considerable concern. At-home care is both more expensive and more difficult to obtain; at the same time, it provides no guarantee that some of the problems which have surfaced in group settings, including child neglect and/or abuse, will not also occur.

ISSUES RELATING TO MATERNAL EMPLOYMENT AND BREASTFEEDING: SAMPLE CASE STUDIES

These cases may be used in a class exploring issues relating to maternal employment and breastfeeding, or in leading a discussion on how to assist the breastfeeding employed mother. They represent actual situations. Questions that are appended are designed to provoke discussion.

A. Mary Smith delivered her third child yesterday. She wonders aloud whether she should breastfeed. She says she will be returning to her part-time job (four hours/day; five days a week) when the baby is six weeks old. Her two other children, now ages four and seven, respectively, were bottle-fed. She said in her childbirth class that she wanted to nurse this, her last, baby.

B. Sharnelle Johnson is returning to work full-time when her firstborn is four weeks old. She just got her job last month and needs to return to it soon. She works eight hours per day, 5 days a week; her travel time to and from work is 30 minutes. Her mother, who bottle-fed all nine of her children, has agreed to watch Sharnelle's daughter for her. Sharnelle's job involves warehouse and packing duties. She operates a folklift and does some manual lifting as well. All her co-workers are men.

C. Debbie Andersen is going back to finish her junior year in high school three months after giving birth. She says she wants to breastfeed; it is now her third day postpartum and she and the baby are doing well.

D. Joan Gilbert has taken a 10-week leave from her private pediatric practice after the birth of her second baby. Her husband is completing law school this year. Joan nursed her first baby for eight weeks before discovering that her patients' needs were more intrusive than she had expected.

For each of the above case studies, answer the following questions:

1. What additional information do you need?
2. What will you tell her about (a) breastfeeding; (b) being a new parent; (c) continuing to breastfeed after she returns to work/school; (d) child behavior in the first year?
3. What, specifically, does she need to know about combining breastfeeding and working/going to school?
4. How might others (grandparents, spouse, friends) help her?
5. If this is not her first breastfeeding experience, how might she be more successful this time than she was the first time?
6. If she has never breastfed before, what does she need to know about how breastfeeding and breastfed babies are different from bottle-feeding and bottle-fed babies?
7. What particular elements about her work/school situation are apt to be most troublesome regarding her baby's needs and her breastfeeding experience?
8. Should she even bother to breastfeed?
9. How can you help her to have a positive breastfeeding experience?

The length of time children breastfeed (even for two years) represents a very small amount of the total time that child will live in the parents' home. The time of the mother's employment is likely to last far longer than the child's infancy. The longer the mother is home during the baby's early weeks and months, the shorter the time when breastfeeding is most likely to be negatively affected by that employment.

REFERENCES

Al-Sekait, MA: A study of the factors influencing breastfeeding patterns in Saudi Arabia, *Saudi Med J* 9:596–601, 1988.

Anderson, LJ, et al.: Day-care center attendance and hospitalization for lower respiratory tract illness, *Pediatrics* 82:300–308, 1988.

Armstrong, H: Breastfeeding low birthweight babies: advances in Kenya, *J Hum Lact* 3:34–37, 1987.

Auerbach, KG: Assisting the employed breastfeeding mother, *J Nurs-Midwif* 35:26–34, 1990a.

Auerbach, KG: Employed breastfeeding mothers: problems they encounter, *Birth* 11:17–20, 1984.

Auerbach, KG: Sequential and simultaneous breast pumping: a comparison, *Int J Nurs Stud* 27:257–65, 1990b.

Auerbach, KG, and Guss, E: Health care workers who breastfeed: implications for patient management, *J Am Med Women's Assoc* 40:111–15, 1985.

Auerbach, KG, and Guss, E: Maternal employment and breastfeeding: a study of 567 women's experiences, *Am J Dis Child* 138:958–60, 1984.

Balk, SJ, and Yellin, TG: Breast-feeding during pediatric residency: is 'breast-fed is best fed' only for others? (letter), *Pediatrics* 70:654, 1982.

Balk, SJ, Christoffel, KK, and Bijur, PE: Pediatricians' attitudes concerning motherhood during residency, *Am J Dis Child* 144:770–77, 1990.

Baranowski, T, et al.: Social support, social influence, ethnicity and the breastfeeding decision, *Soc Sci Med* 17:1599–1611, 1983.

Barber-Madden, R, Petschek, MA, and Pakter, J: Breastfeeding and the working mother: barriers and intervention strategies, *J Public Health Pol* 8:531–41, 1987.

Barger, J, and Bull, P: A comparison of bacterial composition of breast milk stored at room temperature and stored in the refrigerator, *Int J Child Educ* 2:29–30, 1987.

Barglow, P, Vaughn, BE, and Molitor, N: Effects of maternal absence due to employment on the quality of infant-mother attachment in a low-risk sample, *Child Dev* 58:945–54, 1987.

Barman, MR: Guidelines on time off from work, *Contemp Ob-Gyn* 23:81–127, 1984.

Barron, SP, et al.: Factors influencing duration of breast

feeding among low-income women, *J Am Diet Assoc* 88:1557–61, 1988.

Bartlett, AV, et al.: Diarrheal illness among infants and toddlers in day care centers. I. Epidemiology and pathogens, *J Pediatr* 107:495–502, 1985a.

Bartlett, AV, et al.: Diarrheal illness among infants and toddlers in day care centers. II. Comparison with day care homes and households, *J Pediatr* 107:503–9, 1985b.

Bell, DM, et al.: Illness associated with child day care: a study of incidence and cost, *Am J Public Health* 79:479–84, 1989.

Belsky, J, and Rovine, MJ: Nonmaternal care in the first year of life and the security of infant-parent attachment, *Child Dev* 59:157–67, 1988.

Belsky, J, Steinberg, LD, and Walker, A: The ecology of day care. In Lamb, ME, ed.: *Nontraditional Families: Parenting and Child Development,* Princeton, N.J., 1982, Lawrence Erlbaum Associates, pp. 71–115.

Birenbaum, E, Fuchs, C, and Reichman, B: Demographic factors influencing the initiation of breast-feeding in an Israeli urban population, *Pediatrics* 83:519–23, 1989.

Blehar, MC: Anxious attachment and defensive reactions associated with day care, *Child Dev* 45:683–92, 1974.

Boswell, J: The dual-career family: a model for egalitarian family politics, *Elem School Guid Counsel* 15:262–68, 1981.

Boulding, E: Familial constraints on women's work roles, *Signs* 1:95–117, 1976.

Brazelton, TB, and Als, H: Four early stages in the development of mother-infant interaction, *Psychoanal Study Child* 34:349–69, 1979.

Broome, M: Breastfeeding and the working mother, *JOGN Nurs* 10:201–2, 1981.

Caldwell, BM, et al.: Infant day care and attachment, *Am J Orthopsychiatry* 40:397–412, 1970.

Coreil, J, and Murphy, JE: Maternal commitment, lactation practices and breastfeeding duration, *JOGNN* 17:273–78, 1988.

Dewey, KG, et al.: Maternal versus infant factors related to breast milk intake and residual milk volume: the DARLING study, *Pediatrics* 87:829–37, 1991.

Erickson, N: Pregnancy discrimination: an analytical approach, *Wom Rights Rep* 5:83–105, 1979.

Facts on Working Women; 1989: No. 89-3, U.S. Bureau of Labor Statistics, Washington, D.C., 1989, U.S. Government Printing Office.

Ferree, MM: Working-class jobs: housework and paid work as sources of satisfaction, *Soc Prob* 23:431–44, 1976.

Fleming, DW, et al.: Childhood upper respiratory tract infections: to what degree is incidence affected by day care attendance? *Pediatrics* 79:55–60, 1987.

Fosarelli, P: Infectious conditions in day care: there is more than enteritis and rhinitis, *Am J Dis Child* 144:955–56, 1990.

Frederick, IB, and Auerbach, KG: Maternal-infant separation and breast-feeding: the return to work or school, *J Reprod Med* 30:523–26, 1985.

Gardin, SK, and Richwald, GA: Pregnancy and employment leave: legal precedents and future policy, *J Public Health Pol* 7:458–69, 1986.

Gielen, AC, et al.: Maternal employment during the early postpartum period: effects on initiation and continuation of breast-feeding, *Pediatrics* 87:298–305, 1991.

Gilbert, LA, Holahan, CK, and Manning, L: Coping with conflict between professional and maternal roles, *Fam Rel* 30:419–26, 1981.

Greenleaf, NP: Labor force participation among registered nurses and women in comparable occupations, *Nurs Res* 32:306–11, 1983.

Hadler, SC, and McFarland, L: Hepatitis in day care centers: epidemiology and prevention, *Rev Infec Dis* 8:548–57, 1986.

Hardin, SB, and Skerret, K: Counseling working mothers, *J Nurs-Midwif* 26:19–25, 1981.

Hibbard, R, and Blevins, R: Palatal burn due to bottle warming in a microwave oven, *Pediatrics* 82:382–84, 1988.

Hochschild, A, and Machung, A: *The Second Shift: Working Parents and the Revolution at Home*, New York, 1989, Viking Penguin.

Hock, E: Working and non-working mothers and their infants: a comparative study of maternal caregiving characteristics and infant social behavior, *Merrill Palmer Q* 26:79–101, 1980.

Hock, E: Working and non-working mothers with infants: perceptions of their careers, their infants' needs and satisfaction with mothering, *Dev Psychol* 14:37–43, 1978.

Hock, E, Christmas, K, and Hock, M: Career-related decisions of mothers of infants, *Fam Rel* 29:325–30, 1980.

Kamerman, SB, Kahn, AJ, and Kingston, P: *Maternity Policies and Working Women,* New York, 1983, Columbia University Press.

Katcher, A, and Lanese, MG: Breastfeeding by employed mothers: a reasonable accommodation in the workplace, *Pediatrics* 25:644–47, 1985.

Kearney, MH, and Cronenwett, L: Breastfeeding and employment, *JOGNN* 20:471–80, 1991.

Koop, CE, and Brannon, L: Breastfeeding—the community norm: report of a workshop, *Public Health Rep* 99:549–58, 1984.

Kurinij, N, et al.: Does maternal employment affect breastfeeding? *Am J Public Health* 79:1247–50, 1989.

Lancaster, J: Coping mechanisms for the working mother, *AJN* 75:1322–23, 1975.

Larson, E, et al.: Storage of human breast milk, *Infec Control* 5:127–30, 1984.

Lawrence, RA: Practice and attitudes toward breast-feeding among medical professionals, *Pediatrics* 70:912–20, 1982.

Lindeke, LL, and Iverson, SL: Job sharing: an employment alternative for nurse practitioners, *Pediatr Nurs* 12:101–4, 1986.

Livingstone, VH, and Grams, GD: Breast-feeding and the working mother, *Can Fam Phys* 31:1685–93, 1985.

Marshall, L: Breastfeeding and its alternatives among Papua New Guinea career women—an issue in economic development, *Ecol Food Nutr* 20:311–22, 1988.

Morse, JM, and Bottorff, JL: The emotional experience of breast expression, *J Nurs-Midwif* 33:165–70, 1988.

Morse, JM, Bottorff, JL, and Boman, J: Patterns of breastfeeding and work: the Canadian experience, *Can J Public Health* 80:182–88, 1989.

Nemethy, M, and Clore, ER: Microwave heating of infant formula and breast milk, *J Pediatr Health Care* 4:131–35, 1990.

New York Times: Chief denies Iowa firemen were sexist, January 25, 1984, p. C–8.

Nwankwo, MU, et al.: Bacterial growth in expressed breast-milk, *Ann Trop Paediatr* 8:92–95, 1988.

Phelan, EA: A survey of maternity leave policies in Boston area hospitals, *J Am Med Wom Assoc* 46:55–58, 1991.

Pittard, WB, et al.: Bacteriostatic qualities of human milk, *J Pediatr* 107:240–43, 1985.

Rauch AM, et al.: Invasive disease due to multiply resistant *Streptococcus pneumoniae* in a Houston, Tex., day-care center, *Am J Dis Child* 144:923–27, 1990.

Reifsnider, E and Myers, ST: Employed mothers can breastfeed, too! *MCN* 10:256–59, 1985.

Ryan, AS, and Martinez, GA: Breast-feeding and the working mother: a profile, *Pediatrics* 83:524–31, 1989.

Sandroff, R: Nurse/mother: how to cope with a double career, *RN* 43:52–57, 1980.

Saunders, SE, and Carroll, J: Post-partum breast feeding support: impact on duration, *J Am Diet Assoc* 88:213–15, 1988.

Schwartz, P: Length of day-care attendance and attachment behavior in eighteen-month-old infants, *Child Dev* 54:1073–78, 1983.

Shepherd, SC, and Yarrow, RE: Breastfeeding and the working mother, *J Nurs-Midwif* 27:16–20, 1982.

Sigman, M, et al.: Effects of microwaving human milk: changes in IgA content and bacterial count, *J Am Diet Assoc* 89:690–92, 1989.

Silprasert, A, et al.: Effect of storage on the creamatocrit and total energy content of human milk, *Hum Nutr, Clin Nutr* 40C:31–36, 1986.

Smith, EJ: The working mother: a critique of the research, *J Voc Behav* 19:191–211, 1981.

Teitelman, AM, et al.: Effect of maternal work activity on preterm birth and low birth weight, *Am J Epidemiol* 131:104–13, 1990.

Thimmayamma, B, Vidyavati, M, and Bhavani, B: Infant feeding practices in working mothers in an urban area, *Ind J Med Res* 72:834–39, 1980.

U.S. Department of Health and Human Services, USPHS: *The Surgeon General's Workshop on Breastfeeding and Human Lactation*, DHHS Publication No. HRS-D-MC 84-2, 1984, p. 64.

Vaughn, LS, and Wittig, MA: Occupation, competence, and role overload as evaluation determinants of successful women, *J Appl Soc Psychol* 10:398–415, 1980.

Wald, ER, et al.: Frequency and severity of infections in day care, *J Pediatr* 112:540–46, 1988.

Walker, KE: Household work time: its implications for family decisions, *J Home Econ* 65:7–11, 1973.

Wallston, B: The effects of maternal employment on children, *J Child Psychol Psychiatry* 14:81–95, 1973.

Weile, B, et al.: Infant feeding patterns during the first year of life in Denmark: factors associated with the discontinuation of breast-feeding, *J Clin Epidemiology* 43:1305–11, 1990.

Williams, JM, Auerbach, KG, and Jacobi, A: Lateral epicondylitis (Tennis Elbow) in breastfeeding mothers, *Clin Pediatr* 28:42–43, 1989.

Wong, DL: Helping parents select day-care centers, *Pediatr Nurs* 12:181–87, 1986.

Youngblut, JM, Loveland-Cherry, CJ, and Horan, M: Factors related to maternal employment status following the premature birth of an infant, *Nurs Res* 39:237–40, 1990.

Zambrana, RE, Hurst, M, and Hite, RL: The working mother in contemporary perspective: a review of the literature, *Pediatrics* 64:862–70, 1979.

Zigler, E, and Muenchow, S: Infectious diseases in day care: parallels between psychologically and physically healthy care, *Rev Infec Dis* 8:514–20, 1986.

16

Fertility, Sexuality and Contraception During Lactation

Fertility, sexuality, and contraception are interrelated areas in nonpregnant, nonlactating women. Breastfeeding acts, and is acted, upon by each of these entities; thus, the reproductive aspects of women's lives are more complex during lactation than during the nonlactating state (see Fig. 16–1). Al-

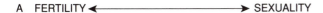

A FERTILITY ⟷ SEXUALITY

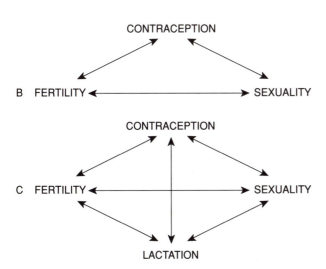

FIGURE 16–1 The interrelationships among fertility, sexuality, contraception and lactation. **A,** In the absence of a family-planning intention, the phenomena of reproduction and sexual behavior (fertility and sexuality) are related in the most simple and direct manner. **B,** When a family-planning method is used for spacing or limiting pregnancies, it clearly affects fertility, and sometimes also sexual behavior (e.g., coitus-dependent methods). **C,** Lactation can have independent effects on fertility, sexual behavior, and contraceptive decisions and patterns of use.

KATHY I. KENNEDY

though breastfeeding clearly has a fertility-reducing effect on the nursing mother, the nature of this effect is not fully understood. In general, the child's suckling initiates a cycle of neuroendocrinologic events which result in the inhibition of ovulation. One result of this inhibition is the creation of the hypoestrogenic state in the woman. Consequently, the dry, sometimes atrophic vaginal mucosa may result in painful intercourse for many breastfeeding women. Because of this and other circumstances, some investigators conclude that breastfeeding women have sexual relationships infrequently and are thus at reduced risk of pregnancy for behavioral reasons. Emotions related to motherhood, such as intensive (albeit normal) involvement with the infant, and feelings of undesirability on the part of a woman who has not recovered her prepregnancy body may affect her sexual behavior as well. Fear of subsequent pregnancy may also play a role in coital behavior and therefore risk of pregnancy. Not all contraceptives are appropriate during breastfeeding, but since some may actually relieve the vaginal symptoms of hypoestrogenicity as well as lessen the fear of pregnancy, coital frequency may also be related to family-planning choice. These are but a few examples of the interrelationships among fertility, sexuality, contraception, and lactation, so it is fitting that they should be explored together.

This chapter reviews current research on fertility and contraception and critiques the conventional wisdom as well as those few insights from research on sexuality during breastfeeding. There are three sections covering lactation as it relates to (1) fertility, (2) sexuality, and (3) contraception.

FERTILITY

THE DEMOGRAPHIC IMPACT OF BREASTFEEDING

The natural birth-spacing effect of breastfeeding has been recognized for many years. In the past few decades, demographers have been able to quantify, in various ways, the degree of contraceptive protection that results from breastfeeding. In the early 1970s it was determined that, in the developing world, nearly universal breastfeeding provided more woman-months of contraceptive protection than all other modern family planning methods combined (Rosa, 1975). It is not clear whether this situation still holds in the 1990s. Two more decades of expanding contraceptive choices to women in the developing world have reduced birth rates in countries as diverse as Bangladesh, Thailand, and Kenya (Mauldin & Segal, 1988; United Nations, 1989).

More sophisticated analyses in the early 1980s revealed that, in populations without access to modern methods of family planning, birth spacing is the major determinant of total fertility (the total number of children a woman will bear) and that the birth interval is dependent for the most part on breastfeeding (Bongaarts & Menken, 1983; Bongaarts & Potter, 1983).

One of the newest approaches taken by demographers to express the fertility-suppressing effect of breastfeeding is to determine the extent to which contraceptive prevalence would need to increase in order to offset a projected decline in breastfeeding—with its concomitant decrease in natural contraceptive protection (Bongaarts & Potter, 1983). For example, in a country like Senegal, where contraceptive prevalence is low and breastfeeding prevalence is high, Thapa, Short, and Potts (1988) have estimated that an erosion in breastfeeding duration of only 25% would require nearly a threefold increase in contraceptive prevalence in order to prevent an increase in the existing, already high fertility in the country. The authors estimate that total fertility would rise by nearly 12% if such a decline in breastfeeding occurred without a simultaneous increase in contraceptive use.

In general, those more developed settings in which the erosion of breastfeeding practices has been profound are the very countries in which contraceptive prevalence is high. Thus, in the United States and the United Kingdom the contraceptive effects of breastfeeding are demographically insignificant.

Scientific interest in the profound and irreproducible benefits of breastfeeding to the *child* has been expanded to a research interest in the effects of lactation on the *woman,* including new and interesting research on the contraceptive effects of lactation.

MECHANISMS OF ACTION

During the normal menstrual cycle in the nonlactating woman, the hypothalamus secretes gonadotropin-releasing hormone (GnRH) in a pulsatile fashion, which in turn triggers a pulsatile release of luteinizing hormone (LH) from the anterior pituitary. LH pulses play a major role in follicular growth and estrogen secretion. In the first days of the cycle, the growing ovarian follicles produce increasing amounts of estrogen, which in turn appear to increase the frequency of LH pulses. When estrogens reach a critical level, there is a surge of LH followed by ovulation in about 17 hours. After ovulation a corpus luteum is formed that produces estrogens and progesterone. During the luteal phase GnRH pulsatility is decreased in association with an increase in the hypothalamic opioid activity.

By about four weeks postpartum, plasma levels of LH return to a level below normal in lactating women, while normal levels are observed in non-breastfeeding, postpartum women by this time (Glasier, McNeilly & Howie, 1983). In fully breastfeeding women, LH remains at a baseline below normal even in the presence of follicular development (Glasier, McNeilly & Howie, 1984). Presumably suckling reduces the secretion of GnRH by the hypothalamus, which results in a dampening of LH pulsatile secretion (see Fig. 16–2). An experiment to test this presumption involved the administration of pulsatile GnRH to breastfeeding women, after which follicular development, ovulation, and luteinization were observed (Glasier, McNeilly & Baird, 1986).

It is accepted by some scientists that suckling stimulates the hypothalamic secretion of beta-endorphin, which in turn inhibits the so-called hypothalamic-LH pulse generator. A study of lactating

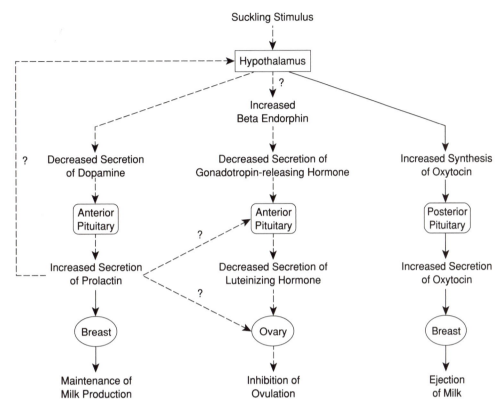

FIGURE 16–2   Physiological mechanisms involved in lactational infertility. Adapted with permission from Short, RV: Breast feeding, *Scient Am* 250(4):38, 1984.

ewes shows an increase in the release of beta-endorphin into the hypophyseal portal vessels in response to suckling (Gordon et al., 1987). Plasma beta-endorphin levels were seen to increase significantly during suckling in women (Franceschini et al., 1989), leading the authors to suggest an extrahypophyseal source of beta-endorphin, although there is debate over whether the opioid crosses the blood/brain barrier—and thus what this peripheral beta-endorphin finding means (Tay, 1991).

Increased levels of prolactin are clearly associated with breastfeeding patterns (Gross & Eastman, 1985). Inhibitory effects of prolactin on gonadotropin secretion and/or ovarian function have been postulated. However, the role of prolactin is uncertain since some lactating women show normal ovulatory cycles despite high levels of prolactin (Díaz et al., 1989) and because pulsatile GnRH infusion can induce follicular development and ovulation in hyperprolactinemic breastfeeding women (Glasier, McNeilly & Baird, 1986). Possibly the decline in

suckling causes both the decrease in prolactin and the improvement in LH pulsation, while the relationship between prolactin and hypothalamic inhibition is only coincidental (McNeilly, 1988; Tay, 1991).

The current understanding of the neuroendocrinologic mechanisms relative to lactational infertility is by no means complete. The complexity of the process is appreciated, as is the irony that the baby is in charge of it all.

LACTATIONAL AMENORRHEA

Lactational amenorrhea is rightly regarded as a period of natural infertility. In fact, it is quite clear that it is the period of "lactational amenorrhea" rather than the period of "breastfeeding" that should be considered the phase of natural infertility (Kennedy, 1986; Short et al., 1991). Reviews of the international literature have shown that between 3 and 10% of women conceive during lactational amenorrhea if they are not otherwise practicing contraception (Van

Ginnekin, 1974; Rolland, 1976; Badroui & Hefnawi, 1979; Simpson-Hebert & Huffman, 1981). These percentages are crude indices of the contraceptive efficacy of lactational amenorrhea, and are not directly comparable to Pearl pregnancy rates or life-table rates. Also, these percentages are uncontrolled for the time postpartum when the mothers conceived. (Some women may have become pregnant soon after delivery, but others may have remained amenorrheic for two or more years before they conceived.)

Studies are currently underway to calculate the lifetable pregnancy rates during lactational amenorrhea so that this natural contraceptive can be more easily evaluated in the context of all family planning methods. Current studies suggest that the expected protection afforded by amenorrhea is quite high—and competitive with reversible methods of fertility regulation such as pills or IUDs. In several breast-feeding studies, the researchers retrospectively calculated rates of ovulation or pregnancy during lactational amenorrhea. One recent analysis of 236 urban women in Chile found only a 0.9 probability of pregnancy at six months among amenorrheic women who did not feed their babies any breastmilk substitutes. In contrast, menstruating, breastfeeding mothers who gave milk supplements had cumulative probabilities of pregnancy of 35.6 and 54.7 at six and 12 months respectively (Diaz et al., 1991). In a study of 101 Australian women, an estimated cumulative probability of conception during lactational amenorrhea was calculated based on an observed rate of the recovery of ovulation. The estimated probabilities of pregnancy were 1.7 at six months and 7.0 at one year postpartum (Short et al., 1991; Lewis et al., 1991). An analysis of data on 346 amenorrheic women who were not practicing contraception was pooled from nine studies in eight countries; it yielded a 12-month cumulative lifetable pregnancy rate of 5.9% (Kennedy & Visness, 1992). This study reflects the combined effects of many different breastfeeding patterns and styles or timings of weaning. These three analyses support the assumptions about earlier, more crude estimates of 3 to 10% pregnancy rates during lactational amenorrhea, which did not control for time postpartum.

A small number of women experience their first normal postpartum ovulation and conceive during the period of lactational amenorrhea. To the best of our knowledge, a woman will have no more than one ovulation during amenorrhea. If she does ovulate during amenorrhea, it will usually occur shortly (0–3 weeks) before the first postpartum menses.

Some women repeatedly experience "inadequate" menstrual cycles—i.e., cycles in which too little progesterone is produced to sustain a fertilized ovum after the end of lactational amenorrhea. Indeed some women who wish to conceive are unable to do so until after the breastfeeding child has been totally weaned, as even token breastfeeding may provide enough inhibitory stimulus to prevent ovulation or to allow adequate progesterone production.

Generally, the earlier in the postpartum period that a woman experiences her first menses, the less likely it is that this first bleeding episode will be preceded by ovulation (Howie et al., 1981; Perez et al., 1972; Howie et al., 1982b). The earlier in the postpartum period that the first ovulation occurs, the less likely it is to be characterized by a luteal phase of adequate duration and progesterone production (Howie et al., 1982a).

SILENT OVULATION

Some researchers who have measured ovarian hormone production throughout the period of amenorrhea have suspected a phenomenon called "silent ovulation," or the occurrence of ovulation which is not followed by either menses or pregnancy. This suspicion grew from observations of elevated estrogen secretion followed by progesterone production in the same or similar sequence—and at levels one would expect to observe in connection with ovulation (Shaaban, Sayed & Ghaneimah, 1987). Further studies involving prospective ultrasonographic observation as well as hormone measurement suggest that in such cases a leading follicle develops but is luteinized without ever having ruptured. The luteinization of an unruptured follicle and/or the generation of ovarian cysts (which may or may not secrete estrogen at levels compatible with ovulation) are phenomena which may be more common during lactation than has been appreciated previously (Flynn et al., 1991).

THE SUCKLING STIMULUS

The suckling child is the stimulus that controls the negative feedback inhibition of the normal cycling of the hypothalamic-pituitary-ovarian axis, yet accurate measurement or quantification of the suckling stimulus is difficult. In general, researchers have relied on measures such as the *frequency* of breastfeeding episodes, the *duration* of each episode, *total minutes of suckling,* and *intervals between suckling episodes,* as well as each of these measures classified by day and by night. All of these approaches result in indices of how often suckling occurred but not of other suckling characteristics, such as the strength of the stimulus and/or the volume of milk obtained. Various creative approaches to measuring suckling strength and milk volume have been attempted, such as breastmilk expression, test-weighing mothers and babies before and after a breastfeed, isotope dilution, and Moire topography (Arthur et al., 1989). Unfortunately, the methodology required to measure, for example, pounds of pressure per square inch on the nipple, or minuscule changes in the baby's weight before and after a feeding, have rendered measurement of these variables on a large scale virtually impossible.

A simpler approach was taken in a study of the recovery of ovulation during lactation in Manila (the Philippines) and Baltimore, Maryland. Researchers determined that breastfeeds as a proportion of all feeds (a reflection of the *relative* frequency of breastfeeds) was the best correlate of the risk of ovulation during breastfeeding. Women whose first ovulation occurred before six months had a significantly lower percentage of breastfeeds to total feeds in the first six months (84%) than did women whose first ovulation occurred later (88%) (Gray et al., 1990; Eslami et al., 1990). Even this simple measure, however, may be impractical for mothers to calculate each day (i.e., whether she is giving more or less than 85% of the baby's feedings as breastfeeds).

The Manila study is one of a number which sought to develop simple guidelines for the optimum time for breastfeeding women to start using a modern contraceptive and/or to take full advantage of the natural protection from pregnancy that is provided by breastfeeding. Such guidelines usually involve some simple sign or behavior, such as a number of breastfeedings per day needed to prevent ovulation. The guideline must be based on phenomena easily observed or recorded by the woman in order to have widespread applicability.

Studies in Scotland and Denmark showed that no woman ovulated if she breastfed her baby at least six times in 24 hours for a total of at least 65 minutes (McNeilly, Glasier & Howie, 1985; McNeilly et al., 1983; Andersen & Schioler, 1982). A study in central Africa found that six suckling episodes per day were effective in maintaining levels of prolactin consistent with anovulation (Delvoye et al., 1977). However, subsequent prospective studies on the return of ovulation during lactation found no such minimum value of breastfeeding frequency that could be relied upon to suppress ovarian activity (Rivera et al., 1988; Israngkura et al., 1989; Shaaban et al., 1990; Elias et al., 1986). In these studies, some women ovulated despite up to 15 breastfeeding episodes per day (Israngkura et al., 1989), and a case of conception in the face of 12 breastfeeds per 24 hours has been reported (Khan et al., 1989). Some of the wide range of minimal feeding frequency required to prevent ovulation is because of problems of reliability of measurement across studies and between individual women. Additionally, the nature of a breastfeed changes from setting to setting and from woman to woman. For example, for some women, a breastfeed is a highly ritualized affair that takes some time to accomplish. It involves changing the baby's diaper; preparing a beverage for the mother to consume during the feed; taking the phone off the hook; settling into a particular rocking chair; suckling for 20 minutes or so; and putting the baby (who may have slipped off to sleep) back into his or her crib. These breastfeeds occur, for example, five to six times a day and one to two times per night, perhaps with the baby nursing in the parents' bed. By contrast, another woman may identify her baby's cue to feed before the first whimper. She puts the baby to her breast for three to four minutes until he/she regains serenity, as often as 15 to 20 times day and night. It is not surprising, then, that a "magic number" of breastfeeds has not been identified which will keep all women ovulation free.

Having concluded that there is no universally reliable breastfeeding frequency associated with anovulation, it is important to note that the frequency of breastfeeding remains an important determinant of lactational infertility (Jones, 1988, 1989). Indeed, the frequency of breastfeeding during both day and night, as well as the number of minutes of suckling per feed or per day, are all related to the duration of infertility; these relationships are shown most clearly in studies with large numbers of subjects. Nevertheless, these study results are difficult to apply to any given breastfeeding woman with adequate certainty due to the normal variation in end-organ response to the (same) suckling stimulus.

SUPPLEMENTAL FEEDING

The role supplementation plays in the return of fertility is anything but straightforward. A prevailing assumption is that anything which decreases the child's suckling behavior or the need to suckle will be a secondary cause of the recovery of fertility. Supplementation may have the effect of decreasing hunger, thirst, and possibly the emotional need for comfort, thereby reducing suckling at the breast.

The pioneering work of the Medical Research Council in Edinburgh found this to be the case (Howie et al., 1981). In a sample of Scottish women, the initiation of supplements to the infant occurred very shortly before the first ovulation. Supplementation was thought to be almost causally related to the recovery of ovulation because of the close temporal relationship between the two events. By contrast, in studies in developing countries, instances have been observed in which supplements are introduced to the baby without an impact on the underlying maternal ovarian hormone profile. (See Fig. 16–3,A.) In such cases, however, the supplements are usually gradual *additions* to the baby's diet, and, like the maternal ovarian hormone levels, the breastfeeding behaviors remain essentially unchanged. By contrast, in the Scottish studies, a supplement was generally a milk-substitute which was given as a *replacement* for a breastfeed, and the suckling stimulus was indeed decreased. A study of well-nourished Australian women who breastfed for an extended period of time also did not find supplementation to be associated with returning fertility (Lewis et al., 1991), perhaps because the introduction of supplements was gradual and quantities small.

Supplementation has also been shown to have an effect on the duration of lactational amenorrhea independent of breastfeeding frequency and duration (Jones, 1989; Benitez et al., 1992). It is possible that supplementation changes some of the more elusive characteristics of breastfeeding, such as suckling strength, rather than just frequency and duration.

The relationship between daily suckling frequency and the total number of minutes of suckling is difficult to generalize across mother-baby pairs. Many investigators assume that since frequent suckling produces higher milk yields than occasional suckling, mothers who feed frequently will also feed for a longer total duration. The more milk there is, the longer it will take for the baby to obtain it. Howie et al. (1981) found this relationship to be so strong that one characteristic could be ostensibly substituted for the other.

Like every other aspect of breastfeeding (and fertility), this generalization needs to be tempered by recognition of normal individual variations. For example, the personal need of the baby to suckle for comfort may affect both breastfeeding frequency and duration. Some babies are efficient sucklers and obtain milk quickly while others are more methodical and unhurried, just as children and adults vary in their speed of food consumption at the dinner table.

While the Edinburgh study reported a very high positive association between suckling frequency and duration, this has not been reported in all studies. In an investigation of breastfeeding mothers in Manila (Benitez et al., 1992), the association between suckling frequency and duration at one month postpartum (0.52) was not significant. This finding suggests that if such an association exists, it does not hold for all women. Fig. 16–4 displays the breastfeeding frequency and minutes of suckling for four women in this study, including their individual correlation coefficients. Across the four panels, the gamut of possibilities can be seen: high-positive, low-positive, high-negative, and low-negative associations.

One of the most promising correlates of the duration of lactational infertility is actually a measure of *not* breastfeeding. The interval between breastfeedings is an inverse expression of both frequency and duration because the number of intervals will be high if frequency is high, and the size of the average interval will be low if the duration or the frequency of breastfeeds is high. Measuring average intervals between feedings yields no new information or advantage over measuring frequency and duration of feedings. However, the *longest interval* between feedings reflects a different characteristic from all others mentioned thus far.

The strength and the nature of the relationship between infant feeding characteristics (such as breastfeeding frequency and time until supplementation) and the return of fertility changes with the duration of lactation. For example, if the duration of lactation is short, supplementation is probably more strongly associated with the return of fertility than if lactation extends over a long period.

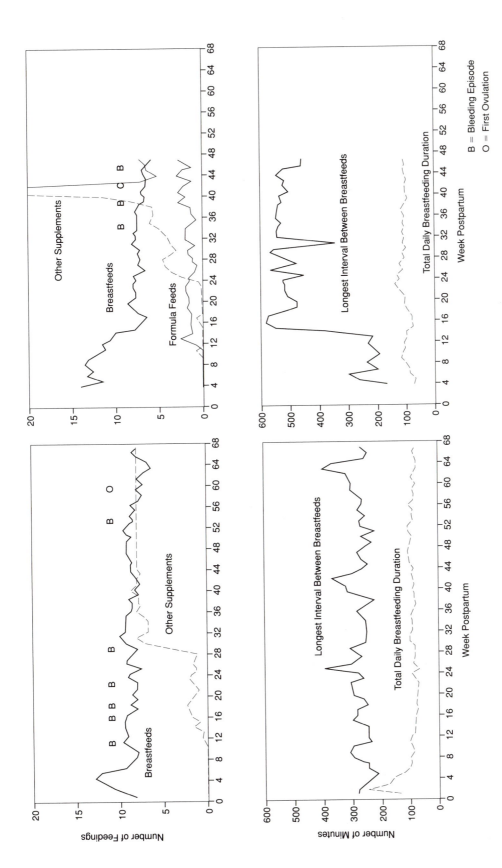

FIGURE 16–3 The effect of supplementation on breastfeeding. **A,** In one example the introduction of supplements at postpartum week 20 had absolutely no effect on breastfeeding frequency, duration, or the interval between feedings. **B,** In another example the introduction of supplements at about week nine coincided with a decrease in breastfeeding frequency and an increase in the longest interval between breastfeeds. Ovulation was still postponed for about 10 months, probably because breastfeeding frequency and duration were high enough. In-house data from Family Health International; Roberto Rivera, Durango II Study, 1991.

435

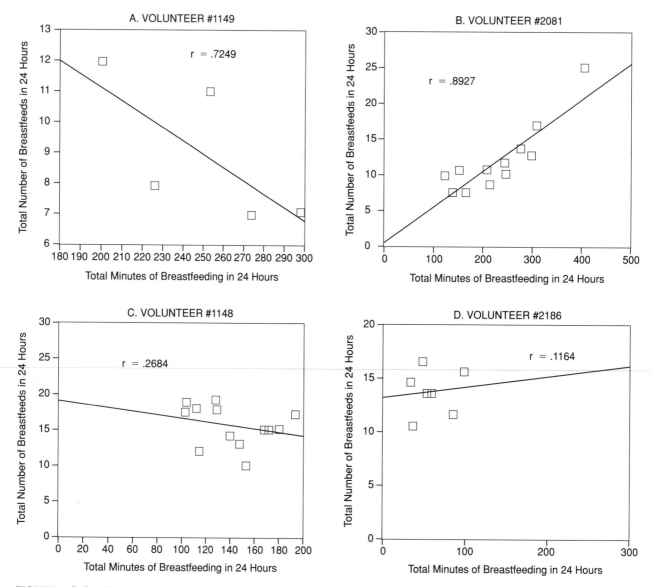

FIGURE 16–4 The association between the frequency of breastfeedings and the number of minutes of suckling within the same woman is sometimes strong (**A** and **B**), sometimes weak (**C** and **D**), sometimes negative (**A** and **C**) and sometimes positive (**B** and **D**). Unpublished data derived from Benitez et al. (1992).

THE REPETITIVE NATURE OF THE RECOVERY OF FERTILITY

In an unpublished study of two consecutive pregnancies in 160 women in France, Ecochard (personal communication, 1990) determined that the recovery of ovulation was likely to occur at the same time postpartum relative to menses—as long as the duration of breastfeeding was similar from child to child of the same mother. Women with parity 2 or higher who used the so-called natural family-plan-

ning method kept daily prospective infant feeding charts, as well as records of basal body temperature (BBT) and other natural fertility symptoms. The first ovulation was said to have occurred at the time of the first BBT shift that was followed by menses. (BBT shift occurs in response to a rise in progesterone production by the ovaries. The ovary does not normally secrete progesterone except as a consequence of ovulation.) In 119 of the women studied, roughly the same breastfeeding pattern was repeated from one child to the next of the same woman. (Twenty-six did not breastfeed either baby; 51 breastfed both babies for less than three months; and 42 breastfed both babies for more than three months. The total length of breastfeeding ranged from zero to 23 months.) Among the 119, the first breastfeeding experience was compared with the second to determine if ovulation occurred before or after the first menses. When the investigators controlled for the category of breastfeeding duration mentioned above, a highly significant association between the first and second experiences was seen. (Mantel-Haenszel Chi-square = 10.2, p <.002.) Further, the association between the first and second durations of amenorrhea was strong (R^2 = .538) and the relationship significant (analysis of covariance F = 2.92, p <.0001 for short durations of breastfeeding and F = 5.13, p < .0001 for long durations).

Gross, Ecochard, and Parenteau-Carreau (personal communication, 1990) analyzed data from four studies which suggest that past experience has a highly significant predictive effect on the subsequent duration of lactational amenorrhea. The four studies included that of Ecochard in France, described above, as well as data on 89 women in Australia, 97 women in the Philippines, and 16 women in Canada. In each of these studies, the association between the durations of lactational amenorrhea for consecutive postpartum experiences was statistically significant; correlation coefficients ranged from .62 to .92.

From a large prospective study of Bangladeshi women, 418 women were observed through two consecutive breastfeeding intervals. The first length of amenorrhea had significant predictive value for the subsequent length of amenorrhea. The author concluded that information on previous experience with lactational amenorrhea should be incorporated into guidelines for the introduction of family planning during lactation (Ford, 1991).

The analyses by Ecochard, Gross, and Parenteau-Carreau (personal communication, 1990), as well as by Ford (1992) suggest that women can expect a similar pattern of recovery of fertility from one birth to the next, provided that the breastfeeding pattern does not change dramatically.

THE BELLAGIO CONSENSUS

By the late 1980s, researchers on five continents had completed prospective studies of breastfeeding women, measuring their ovarian hormone levels and sometimes other objective physiologic parameters in order to learn about the recovery of fertility during lactation. Many of these researchers were brought together by Family Health International at the Bellagio Conference and Study Center in Italy (with support from the Rockefeller Foundation, the World Health Organization and the United States Agency for International Development). The purpose of this assembly was to determine whether the researchers' findings about women with vastly different patterns of breastfeeding behavior could be synthesized into a statement about how breastfeeding women might predict their recovery of fertility. The conclusions of the group are listed in the box below.

The basis for the consensus in 1988 was a body of published and unpublished studies of the pregnancy rates (three studies in two countries), as well as data on the probability of a recognizable pregnancy from prospective studies of the recovery of ovulation during lactation (10 studies in seven countries). Among these studies, the highest pregnancy rate reported in fully breastfeeding amenorrheic women during the first six months postpartum was lower than 2% (Family Health International, 1988; Kennedy, Rivera & McNeilly, 1989).

THE CONCLUSIONS OF THE BELLAGIO CONSENSUS

Breastfeeding should be regarded as a potential family planning method in all maternal and child health programs in developing and developed countries.

Postpartum women should be offered a choice of using breastfeeding as a means of family planning, either to help achieve optimal birth spacing of at least two years, or as a way of delaying the introduction of other contraceptives. They should be informed how to maximize the antifertility effects of breastfeeding to prevent pregnancy.

Breastfeeding provides more than 98 percent protection from pregnancy during the first six months postpartum if the mother is "fully" or nearly fully breastfeeding and has not experienced vaginal bleeding after the 56th day postpartum.

From *Lancet* ii(8621):1204–5, 1988; *Contraception* 39 (5):477–96, 1989.

The Bellagio consensus is important because it reflects principles that are believed to be applicable cross culturally. Yet this aspect of the consensus is also one of its weaknesses: by making generalizations that apply to a range of breastfeeding patterns and practices, some possible situations could not be accommodated. For example, in societies in which a child is breastfed for two years or more, or among La Leche League mothers in industrialized countries who choose to breastfeed for these longer periods, lactational amenorrhea alone may be a viable marker of returning fertility. Cognizant of this, Kennedy, Rivera, and McNeilly (1989) cautioned:

> Guidelines specific to a particular country or population for using breastfeeding as a postpartum family planning method can be developed based on this consensus. Local infant feeding practices, the average duration of amenorrhea and the ongoing changes in women's status and health practices should be considered in adapting these general guidelines.

The consensus is also important because it represents the framework for the actual use of lactational amenorrhea as a method of contraception. Guidelines on how to integrate the Lactational Amenorrhea Method (or LAM) into family planning and breastfeeding support programs have been developed based on the Bellagio consensus (Labbok et al., 1990b). A prospective study of LAM used by 422 middle-class women in Santiago, Chile, found a cumulative six-month life table pregnancy rate of 0.45% (Perez, Labbok & Queenan, 1992). Additional research is also underway on the potential effectiveness of LAM beyond six months and on whether women can understand the guidelines.

SEXUALITY

Human sexuality in the 1990s promises to be no less complex than in previous decades. The variety of living arrangements in combination with various sexual orientations makes for new circumstances in which sexuality is expressed. Although the following discussion will presuppose a marriage or stable union between a breastfeeding woman and her male partner, this presupposition is simply for convenience. It seems safe to assume that the majority of lactating mothers are heterosexual; there is virtually no information in the scientific literature about the sexuality of breastfeeding single and lesbian women. Nevertheless, it is likely that much of the following discussion will apply to these women also.

This discussion is also based on the assumption that libido or sexual desire is the main driving force or motivation for sexual expression (although the desire to please one's partner is also recognized as a motivation). Yet we acknowledge that many women have intercourse against their will and/or without sexual desire. This chapter does not consider the role of breastfeeding in coercive or indifferent sexual relationships.

LIBIDO

There are at least five categories of factors that may influence sexual drive or desire during lactation, namely:

- common situational factors unrelated to breastfeeding
- libido-inhibiting influences related to parturition
- libido-inhibiting influences of lactation
- libido-enhancing factors related to pregnancy, birth and lactation
- factors related to the breastfeeding woman's partner.

Common situational factors unrelated to breastfeeding. Many preexisting factors which either facilitated or inhibited sexual arousal before pregnancy or birth will remain a part of one's living experience, family routine, or personal preference after the birth of the child. Preexisting factors that inhibit libido—such as the chronic illness of one of the partners, fear of pregnancy, or lack of privacy—persist and are unrelated to breastfeeding. If a couple has a dysfunctional or unsatisfying sexual rapport, this is no more likely to be spontaneously remedied by lactation than a faltering marriage is to be "saved" by adding a child to the family chemistry.

Conversely, there is no reason to assume that individualized stimuli *per se,* such as a preferred cologne, a special song, or candlelight, should lose their excitatory effects because a baby joins the family. Opportunity to attend to the old stimuli, however, is another matter. Some of the preexisting sexual stimuli or circumstances associated with sexual opportunity may be decreased due to having a young baby in the home. For example, the couple may find that they now lack time alone and that they endure constant interruptions—especially, it seems, at night. The quiet evening at home may seem gone forever.

Libido-inhibiting influences related to parturition.   The natural process of physical recovery from childbirth takes about six weeks, and postpartum abstinence is sensible until the time of the postpartum checkup. This medical visit can occur earlier, and if the woman decides that she wants to be sexually active before six weeks postpartum, she should insist on receiving medical attention earlier.

The tenderness from episiotomy or vulvo-vaginal or perineal damage following vaginal delivery usually lasts for several months. Although the mother's stitches may have healed, she may still experience discomfort upon intercourse. In a study of 93 parturients in New South Wales, Australia, the median time required to achieve comfort during intercourse was three months, with a range of from one to more than 12 months. Whether or not the women had episiotomies (58 yes, 35 no) did not affect the time until painfree intercourse was experienced, but this may be because of the commonness of tearing (69%) of the vulval tissues, which required sutures in the women who did not have an episiotomy (Abraham et al., 1990). In a longitudinal study of 119 primiparous women attended at a London teaching hospital, 40% complained of soreness and occasionally painful intercourse at three months postpartum (Robson, Brant & Kumar, 1981). Another study of British women reported dyspareunia during the first postpartum intercourse in 40% of mothers; of these, 64% refrained from further coitus after the initial distressing event (Grudzinskas & Atkinson, 1984). The anticipation of pain during intercourse may cause the woman to avoid sexual suggestion. A clear understanding of her feelings and communication with her partner may help the couple to defer intercourse until some future time and free them to express their love and caring—or perhaps to use other means of mutual sexual expression and gratification.

Soon after delivery, women experience a precipitous decline in ovarian steroid levels. This drastic change is sometimes associated with noticeable mood changes. The immediate effect is usually temporary and probably overlaps with the period of recommended postpartum abstinence. In some women,

postpartum depression can follow delivery immediately or occur after a few days or weeks. Although the etiology of postpartum depression is not well understood, this depression probably has both endogenous and exogenous sources. Some women experience emotional vulnerability when their progesterone levels are low, such as during the postpartum period. (By way of analogy, the symptoms of premenstrual syndrome in the nonpregnant woman are often relieved by progesterone administration.) The overwhelming needs of the new baby plus other familial and extrafamilial responsibilities seem enough to make a normal person weary; exogenous sources of postpartum depression should not be underestimated (see Fig. 16–5). Depression is commonly characterized by a lack of sexual drive, and the "postpartum blues" is no exception.

Even if the mother does not experience postpartum depression, she will probably be spending most of her emotional energy caring for and bonding with her newborn. This process is sometimes likened to a love affair in which infatuation with one's beloved is like an obsession. It is difficult to refrain from thinking about and doing things for the person who is the object of one's affection. Between mother and child, this bonding serves exceedingly important functions by creating an enduring parental talent and commitment in the mother and a sense of trust and security in the infant. However, this process can interfere with the mother's emotional availability for her partner.

Psychological factors unrelated to hormones or to attachment can also be strong inhibitors of libido. Fear of pregnancy can be an important inhibitor of sexual drive. If the new baby was unplanned, especially if a contraceptive failure occurred, sexual inhibition could understandably be great. Parents of a firstborn sometimes have trouble synthesizing the roles of "lover" and "mother" or "father," because the parental role was previously understood subconsciously to be asexual. Colic or minor or major problems with the infant can decrease sexual interest by either partner, and if a difficult parenting challenge is faced by a mother who has no previous parenting experience, she may be even less emotionally available to her partner. Preexisting marital difficulties may manifest themselves in an exclusive emphasis on the child and neglect of the adult love relationship. One mother suggested that the factors contributing to a decrease in the frequency of sexual relations were not very complex or deeply rooted and

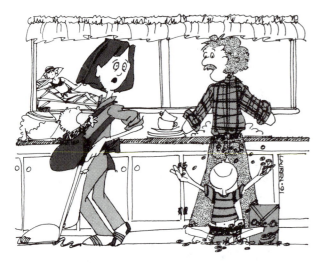

FIGURE 16–5   The overwhelming needs of the new baby plus other familial and extrafamilial responsibilities seem enough to make a normal person weary. When you have kids, there are lots of other things to do.

were probably unrelated to any particular psychological construct. She declared simply: "Our priorities changed! When you have kids, there are lots of other things to do, and your values change."

Libido-inhibiting influences of lactation.   Libido is thought to be elevated during the middle of the menstrual cycle in normal, nonlactating women. The midcycle is the period during which peaks in follicle stimulating hormone (FSH), LH, and estrogen are observed. Accordingly, libido in the breastfeeding woman may be linked to one or more of these substances, or to a drop in prolactin which, during breastfeeding, is elevated above the levels in normally cycling women. The study of parturients in New South Wales showed that breastfeeding duration longer than five months was associated with longer duration of discomfort during intercourse, as well as longer periods of lactational amenorrhea (Abraham, 1990). This finding supports an association between the hormonal milieu during breastfeeding and sexual activity. Alder and Bancroft (1988) found that women who bottle-fed tended to resume coitus earlier and had intercourse more frequently than breastfeeders, which similarly supports a hormone-libido association. However, these same researchers had earlier found no relationship between basal prolactin levels, estrogen levels, or even the return of follicular development with measures of sexuality in breastfeeding women (Alder et al., 1986). Some design problems could account for these results, namely the retrospective nature of the data collected, the small number of women under study, and the infrequent intervals of data collection. A possible explanation is that hormones may in fact exert some influence over sexual desire, but that there are other factors with greater influence over sexual behavior than the hormonal milieu.

Nonbreastfeeding, postpartum women produce low levels of estrogen until they begin to recover fertility at one to two months postpartum. Among breastfeeding women, this period of hypoestrogenemia can endure for the entire lactation course.

As in menopause, lactation-related hypoestrogenemia can cause the vaginal epithelium to be very thin and to secrete little fluid during arousal. Dryness and pain are experienced during intercourse and vaginal tears are possible. Atrophy of the vaginal mucosa can be relieved quickly and easily by the use of inert, water-based lubricants. Estrogen cream is sometimes prescribed for vaginal application and yields satisfactory results in many cases. However, the vagina is so efficiently absorptive that users should be alert to the possible consequences of estrogen administration, such as the recovery of ovulation and a decrease in breastmilk production.

As if the emotional demands of parenthood are not enough, breastfeeding adds another dimension of complexity. Exhaustion may be the most pervasive inhibitor of sexual desire (see Fig. 16–6). The London study of primiparous women mentioned earlier reported that 25% of mothers indicated that tiredness reduced their libido and/or enjoyment of sex (Robson, Brant & Kumar, 1981). Of course, the nonbreastfeeding woman with a new infant is also vulnerable to exhaustion, especially if she has other small children to care for. Yet breastfeeding women may be more vulnerable if frequent night feeding disturbs their sleep. If the breastfeeding child sleeps in the parents' bed, this may afford the mother a better night's sleep. Conversely, the presence of the child could inhibit sexual expression.

Emotional attachment between the mother and child is thought to be more intense if the dyad is breastfeeding rather than bottle-feeding (Bottorff, 1990; Virden, 1988; Wrigley & Hutchinson, 1990). Emotional availability of the mother for her sexual partner may be correspondingly reduced. Describing her feelings during lactation, one mother reported:

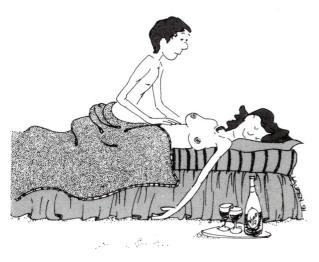

FIGURE 16-6   Exhaustion may be the most pervasive inhibitor of sexual desire.

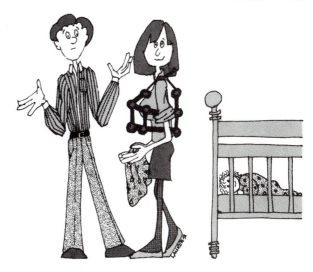

FIGURE 16-7   If the breasts are "off limits," sexual expression may be negatively affected.

When you are home and you touch, hold, hug, and nurse all day, you're not so interested in it when your husband walks through the door. But then his day has been all talk all day and no touch, and he's ready. It creates a problem (Riordan, 1983).

Some men may feel that they are in competition with the baby, not only for the breastfeeding woman's attention but for her breasts. The woman's breasts are often an important aspect of eroticism for the couple. If either or both partners feel that the breasts are "off limits" for sexual play because the woman is producing milk, then the couple's sexual expression may be negatively affected. Even if the couple feels no taboo about the woman's breasts, there may be a dislike of milk leakage and thereafter a fear of eliciting it. The breasts may be tender, and the new mother may be tired of having her breasts "handled" (see Fig. 16-7). Conversely, there is little harm in breast stimulation and even suckling by the woman's partner, especially after the baby has had his fill. The partner may actually help to prevent or relieve engorgement by periodically stimulating the breast leakage.

Libido-enhancing factors related to pregnancy, birth and lactation.   Especially in the context of a planned pregnancy, the birth can be a positive and fulfilling experience, and many couples express this mutual happiness in lovemaking. Childbirth is a major life event, and when this occurs under emo-

tionally and physically healthy conditions, sexual expression can be particularly joyful and rewarding.

In contrast to the possible inhibitors mentioned above, pregnancy, childbirth, and breastfeeding can also have the effect of magnifying an appreciation of the womanliness of the mother by her partner. For example, to some men and women, the shape or fullness of the lactating breasts is particularly arousing.

The breastfeeding woman may feel more interested in sexual relations after a few months postpartum because of the interaction of some of the factors mentioned. Her perineum is less tender, she may be experiencing some ovarian activity, she no longer has the body shape of a pregnant woman and she feels more normal. One mother described it this way:

To me, sex is best of all during the later breastfeeding period because (1) I feel physically better than at any other time (2) no fear of pregnancy and no contraceptives needed because for me breastfeeding is a 100% effective contraceptive for at least one year after the birth of a baby, and (3) there is something about nursing a little baby that gives you an "all's right with the world" kind of feeling. I feel so happy and loving toward my whole family, husband, and other children as well as the baby. Sex just seems to be a nice, natural expression of this good feeling (Kenny, 1973).

Human sexual expression can be a creative activity in addition to being procreative. It is also obviously a personal endeavor for the lovers as individuals and as a couple. For this reason, some potentially inhibiting factors may actually be arousing factors which add to the likelihood that the couple will have sexual intercourse. For example, one couple may make love more frequently in times of stress, while another couple may experience a paucity of emotional reserve for lovemaking under the same circumstances. The former pattern may be quite functional because orgasm helps to release tension and promotes relaxation and a feeling of well-being, thus providing one or both partners with more psychic energy with which to cope with the causes of stress. For some couples, pregnancy itself often stimulates erotic responses. Therefore to some people, having given birth and becoming nonpregnant again may be less sexually stimulating than being "great with child." Because each person and each couple is unique, any discussion of sexuality during lactation must be couched in generalities, recognizing that individual expression varies widely.

Factors related to the breastfeeding woman's partner. The possibility of role conflict has already been mentioned and is a reminder that men also experience psychological adjustments to accommodate the major life event of birth. No doubt the experience is most profound the first time that a man becomes a father. While the male partner is often assumed ever ready, willing, and wanting sex, this is an overgeneralization, possibly reflecting the relative lack of a cycle in the male capacity to fertilize. Men are subject to libidinal influences in everyday life, and, analogous to the female perspective discussed at the beginning of this section, these facilitators and inhibitors do not disappear with the birth of his child or during the lactation course of his partner.

When the man has witnessed his pregnant partner's metamorphosis into lactating mother, this may affect his perception of her as a sex partner, either because of her body's obvious changes or because of the meaning he ascribes to her maternity. Motherhood may make her more or less sexually appealing to him.

Fear of hurting a postpartum woman during vaginal intercourse may inhibit male sexual expression. A man may feel guilty for desiring his breastfeeding partner if he perceives that she has "more important" maternal matters. Identifying and talking about their sexual feelings, desires, and inhibitions, while earnestly caring for the welfare of each other, can help the couple through this sometimes awkward period.

SEXUAL BEHAVIOR DURING LACTATION

In order to measure a level of sexual functioning or behavior in breastfeeding women, researchers have studied the resumption of postpartum intercourse and coital frequency. First intercourse and coital frequency are relatively easy variables to quantify, although they certainly do not yield a complete understanding of sexual functioning during lactation. Unfortunately, little qualitative information about sexual behavior during lactation is reported in the scientific literature. Few studies of sexual behavior during lactation contain large numbers of subjects, and the results of the studies are sometimes contradictory.

First postpartum intercourse. In one study in the postnatal hospital clinic of a city in England, 328 women were interviewed. By the time of the postnatal visit, 51% had already resumed intercourse, most frequently (the mode) during the fifth week postpartum (Grudzinskas & Atkinson, 1984). An intensive study of 25 breastfeeding women in Edinburgh, Scotland, found that six to seven weeks was the mean time preceding initial postpartum intercourse. In a prospective study of 130 breastfeeding women in Santiago, Chile, the participants had "usually" resumed sexual relations by the beginning of the second month (Diaz et al., 1982). In a probability sample of U.S. women taken from 1979 to 1982, only 4.3% of lactating women reported that they were not yet sexually active at three months postpartum (Ford & Labbok, 1987).

A population-based survey of 3,080 parturients was conducted in Cebu, the Philippines, where breastfeeding is the norm. The study included all identified pregnancies in 27 administrative districts in and around metropolitan Cebu. The period of time with the highest probability of return to coitus was six weeks postpartum, although about 80 women (2.7%) had still not resumed coitus by two years. A multivariate analysis sought to identify factors that could predict the return to coitus. A woman was more likely to become sexually active postpartum if her husband was present, if she was not breastfeeding, and if she was menstruating (i.e., not amenorrheic). The likelihood of postpartum inter-

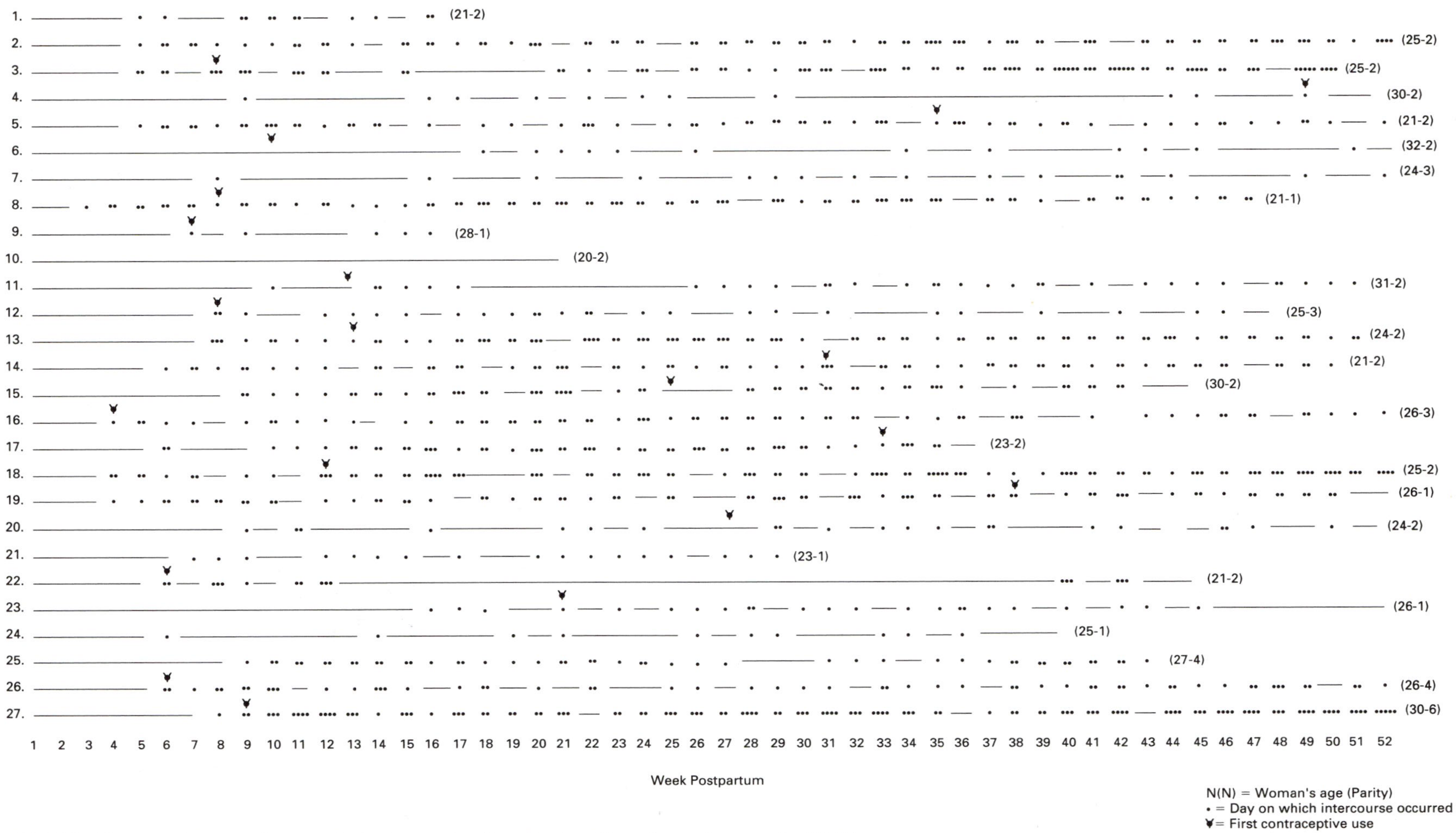

FIGURE 16–8 Incidence of coitus during breastfeeding. Derived from Israngkura et al. (1989).

N(N) = Woman's age (Parity)
• = Day on which intercourse occurred
▶ = First contraceptive use

Week Postpartum

443

course also increased if the woman was younger; was better educated; had other young children (less than seven years of age) in the home; had a less crowded home; lived in a nuclear household; was from an urban area; and/or had been attended by a trained health worker (Udry & Deang, in press).

In a study involving 27 breastfeeding women in Bangkok, Thailand, the mean time until the first postpartum coitus was 7.8 weeks (Israngkura et al., 1989). However, although an arithmetic mean can be calculated, average time does not tell the whole story. In this sample, the range of time until the first coitus was from three weeks to more than 21 weeks postpartum (Fig. 16–8).

Postpartum coital frequency.   An analysis of retrospective and prospective data on coital frequency was performed using information provided by 91 nonpregnant, nonlactating women in North Caro-

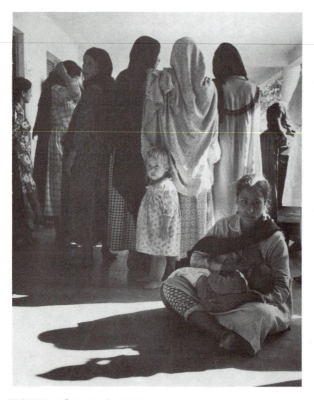

FIGURE 16–9   In the WHO perspective, family planning is concerned with the quality of life. It is a way of thinking and living that promotes the health and welfare of the family group and thus contributes to economic and social development. In an Egyptian health centre, family planning care is included within maternal and child health services.

lina who were married or living with a male partner as if married. First the women reported from memory their "usual" weekly frequency of sexual intercourse. Then they recorded each morning, for one to three months, whether they had intercourse during the previous 24 hours. The women reported a significantly higher frequency of coitus for the period prior to the first interview (2.5 times per week) compared with their later prospective recordings (1.7 times per week)—an average of 0.8 episodes per week. This overestimate occurred uniformly in subgroups of women and was thought to be caused by the women's tendency to report a frequency that would exist in the absence of travel, illness, menses, and other influencing factors. The prospective data showed trends toward decreased coital frequency with increasing age, education, income, and duration of relationship. Also, women currently using an intrauterine device (IUD) or who had had a tubal ligation had intercourse twice as often (2.0 times per week) as women with "no" contraceptive use (1.1 times per week) (Hornsby & Wilcox, 1989). Although the North Carolina analysis is a study of the methodology for obtaining information about coital frequency, it offers a clear example of the potential bias incurred with the use of retrospective data. Although it is a study of normally cycling women, it provides a good context in which to view studies of coital frequency during lactation (see Fig. 16–9).

Fig. 16–8 indicates the frequency of coitus for breastfeeding women in the Thai study for up to a year postpartum (Israngkura et al., 1989). After the first intercourse, average weekly frequency (data collected prospectively) was about once per week. However, again there were differences among women. One woman (number 27) reported intercourse on an average of three times per week, and her frequency tended to increase over time. Another (number 11) had intercourse about once a week, while woman number 24 had her first postpartum intercourse at six weeks postpartum, but not again until 14 weeks postpartum—and only sporadically thereafter. This variation in coital behavior may be similar to the variation which would be expected among normally cycling, nonbreastfeeding women in stable relationships.

A nonrandom, nonrepresentative sample of breastfeeding women using the symptothermal method associated with natural family planning (NFP) centers in three countries was studied prospectively. The occurrence of intercourse and other variables was recorded in a daily diary. The average weekly frequency of intercourse ranged from zero to about four in the first six months postpartum during lactation (see Table 16–1). The women from the Canadian center reported relatively low mean frequencies (always less than once per week) compared with the others, while those from the English center reported relatively higher mean frequencies (always once or more per week). These group differences could be the result of subtle differences in the NFP rules taught by each center for determining the number of "safe days" (days judged not fertile) for intercourse. In all three groups, coital frequency decreased somewhat over time; this was most pronounced in the Canadian group, particularly in the first six months postpartum. The number of recommended days of abstinence can be expected to increase during the recovery of fertility, and this could account for the small decrease in coital frequency noted. The information from these 75 women in developed countries cannot be generalized to other populations; these women serve as examples within particular cohorts of a moderate range of coital frequency (Kennedy et al., 1990, unpublished, in-house data from Family Health International).

In the aforementioned study in Santiago, Chile,

the reported coital frequency ranged from one to six times per week in the first six months postpartum among breastfeeding women (Diaz et al., 1982). Conversely, the Cebu study found a remarkable lack of variance in coital frequency in the first six months postpartum. The women were asked every two months about the frequency of intercourse in the previous week. After controlling for a large number of potentially influential factors, coital frequency of 0.5 to 0.6 times per week did not vary meaningfully with any of the demographic or situational factors observed (Udry & Deang, in press). This finding has led the researchers to conclude that just because a woman has returned to coitus does not mean that she's having (much) sex!

The variability in coital frequency in the Cebu study could not be well explained by factors such as age and education. Other factors, such as fear of pregnancy, may be a stronger correlate of sexual behavior, as may psychological factors, such as perceived locus of control (the perception that one is in control of one's life and fate rather than the victim of forces outside oneself).

On an individual basis, coital frequency may only be important to know so that it may be compared with frequency before the pregnancy and/or the birth. The Edinburgh study mentioned above prospectively measured coital frequency during weeks

TABLE 16–1 AVERAGE WEEKLY FREQUENCY OF INTERCOURSE AMONG BREASTFEEDING USERS OF NFP IN THREE CENTERS BY MONTH POSTPARTUM

Month Postpartum	Montreal (N)	Mean	Sydney (N)	Mean	Birmingham (N)	Mean	Total (N)	Mean	Min	Max*
2	(25)	.80	(25)	.88	(24)	.99	(74)	.89	0	3.68
3	(25)	.71	(25)	.79	(25)	1.15	(75)	.88	0	2.93
4	(24)	.54	(24)	.80	(25)	1.37	(73)	.91	0	3.97
5	(24)	.55	(24)	.78	(23)	1.45	(71)	.92	0	4.20
6	(23)	.59	(22)	.78	(21)	1.15	(66)	.83	0	3.16
7	(22)	.54	(20)	.81	(18)	1.06	(60)	.80	0	2.33
8	(21)	.41	(17)	.78	(14)	1.32	(52)	.80	0	4.67
9	(17)	.33	(14)	.81	(12)	.99	(43)	.70	0	2.10
10	(16)	.36	(13)	.99	(10)	1.13	(39)	.81	0	2.10
11	(13)	.46	(12)	1.04	(5)	.89	(30)	.78	0	3.50
12	(10)	.49	(10)	.88	(3)	1.01	(23)	.73	0	2.06

*Greatest mean observed during the month
Gross et al., personal communication, 1990.

12 to 24 postpartum and found a mean frequency of 1.2 times per week. The recalled prepregnancy frequency was 2.6 times per week (p < .01) (Alder et al., 1986). In light of the findings of Hornsby and Wilcox (1989), it is possible that the retrospectively generated prepregnancy frequency was an overestimate. Also, it is not clear whether the prepregnancy period being recalled is a time in which pregnancy was actively sought, which could inflate sexual frequency above previous or later levels for the couple.

Does breastfeeding affect the resumption of sexual activity or coital frequency? The earliest research concluded that breastfeeding enhances these overt measures of sexuality; more recent papers suggest that breastfeeding reduces coital sexual expression; other reports in the literature say that there is no difference. Alder and Bancroft (1988) reported that, when compared with bottle-feeders, breastfeeding women showed a lower preferred frequency of intercourse; delayed the resumption of coitus for a longer period; had a greater reduction in sexual interest and enjoyment compared with prepregnancy levels; experienced more pain during intercourse; and were slightly more depressed at three months postpartum. All of these differences disappeared by six months except for dyspareunia.

By contrast, works by Masters and Johnson (1966) and by Kenny (1973) reported a more prompt return of sexual desire, plus a return to higher levels of sexual functioning, among breastfeeding women than among bottle-feeders. These earlier works were conducted during a time and at locations in which breastfeeding was not popular. It is unknown whether women who were less sexually inhibited were the ones who breastfed.

In 1981, Robson, Brant, and Kumar reported that breastfeeding showed no influence over several indices of maternal sexuality in 119 primiparas in London. Grudzinskas and Atkinson (1984) reported that breastfeeding was not related to the resumption of coitus in their sample of 328 women.

What do these conflicting results mean? Does breastfeeding stifle sexual experience, accelerate it, or neither? Some methodologic explanations have been offered; they should be considered carefully. In addition, psychologically, behaviorally and biologically based hypotheses are needed. Can breastfeeding have *either* an inhibiting or a stimulating effect? Perhaps breastfeeding is a swing factor, sometimes enhancing sexual feelings and sometimes acting as the obstacle to their expression. Studies on the return of ovulation during breastfeeding have shown that the physiologic response to ostensibly the same suckling stimulus can be greater or lesser for different women.

The small studies of coital resumption and frequency have been more detailed and provide an appreciation of the range of possibilities regarding these two variables. The results of the large Cebu study, with its representative sample, provide a reminder that people in the same population behave in a way that can be generalized—e.g., these Filipinas generally resumed coitus after one month postpartum and had intercourse about once every two weeks, at least until the sixth month postpartum. Both the variety of individual behaviors and the conclusions from the large dataset are credible in light of the previous section on sexuality during lactation.

CONTRACEPTION

The "vital complementarity" between breastfeeding and family planning for the health of both mother and child has been eloquently expressed (Labbok, 1989). During lactation, the choice of whether to practice contraception, and if so how, requires different considerations compared with the same choice during the nonlactating state. The array of available family-planning methods has been put into a hierarchy according to their general advisability for use during breastfeeding (Labbok et al., 1990a). The hierarchy of family planning options (see Table 16–2) places nonhormonal methods as the first choice, progestin-only methods as the second choice, and methods containing estrogen as a distant third to be used only when other methods are unavailable. At least three parameters must be considered when evaluating the appropriateness of a contraceptive for use during lactation: the hormonal content of the method, the family-planning intention (whether contraception is used for spacing or for limiting pregnancies), and the timing of introduction of the method.

TABLE 16–2 FAMILY-PLANNING OPTIONS AS THEY RELATE TO THE SPECIFIC CONCERNS OF BREASTFEEDING WOMEN

Method	Advantages	Disadvantages	Comments
FIRST CHOICE: NONHORMONAL METHODS			
CONDOMS	No effect on breastfeeding. Can be very effective if used correctly	May be irritating to vagina and may require additional lubrication.	Offers some protection against sexually transmitted diseases. No risks to mother or child.
DIAPHRAGMS	No effect on breastfeeding. Can be very effective if used correctly.	Diaphragm must be refitted postpartum after the uterus has returned to the prepregnancy size.	May not be widely available. Effectiveness depends on use with a spermicide.
SPERMICIDES	No effect on breastfeeding. Can be very effective if used correctly	May be irritating to the genital area. May be irritating to the male partner.	Small amounts may be absorbed into maternal blood and there may be some passage into milk; there is no known effect on the infant.
INTRAUTERINE DEVICES (Nonhormonal IUDs)	No effect of IUD itself, or of the copper in some IUDs, on breastfeeding. Very effective.	Possible risk of expulsion and uterine perforation if not properly placed, or if inserted prior to six weeks postpartum.	Insertion may need to be delayed until after six weeks postpartum to reduce the possibility of expulsion and/or perforation of the uterus.
NATURAL FAMILY PLANNING (Periodic abstinence)	No effect on breastfeeding. Can be very effective if used correctly.	May require extended periods of abstinence. May be difficult to interpret fertility signs during breastfeeding.	Additional training of method users may be necessary to accurately interpret signs and symptoms of fertility during breastfeeding. Calendar rhythm method alone has limited value prior to first ovulation.
VASECTOMY (Male voluntary surgical sterilization)	No effect on breastfeeding. Nearly 100% effective.	Minor surgery with chance of side effects for father. It is irreversible.	A recommended method if no more children are desired. Counseling necessary for couples. No risk to mother or child.
TUBAL LIGATION (Female voluntary sterilization)	No direct effect on breastfeeding. Nearly 100% effective.	May involve short-term mother/infant separation. Anesthesia can pass into breastmilk and sedate the infant. Surgery, in general, has risks. It is irreversible.	A recommended method if no more children are desired. General anesthesia is not recommended. Counseling necessary for couples.
SECOND CHOICE: PROGESTIN-ONLY METHODS			
PROGESTIN-ONLY METHODS (Mini-pill, injectables, implants)	Can be very effective. May increase milk volume. Effectiveness during breastfeeding approaches that of combined pill.	Some hormone may pass into breastmilk.	There is no evidence of adverse effects on the infant from the very small amount of hormone which passes into the milk.
THIRD CHOICE: METHODS CONTAINING ESTROGEN			
COMBINED ORAL CONTRACEPTIVES (Estrogen and progestin)	Very effective.	Estrogens may reduce milk supply. Some hormone may pass into breastmilk.	There is no evidence of a direct negative effect on infants; however, in some women, suppression of milk supply appears to lead to earlier cessation of breastfeeding. If these methods cannot be avoided, **breastfeeding can and should continue,** as it continues to offer important health and nutritional benefits for the infant or toddler.

Adapted with permission of the Institute of International Studies in Natural Family Planning, Washington, D.C., 1990.

TIMING THE COMMENCEMENT
OF A FAMILY-PLANNING METHOD:
THE DOUBLE-PROTECTION DILEMMA

The question of when a postpartum woman should begin practicing contraception has no easy answer. A family-planning provider may be tempted to give a safe response and advise that family planning is needed immediately after the baby's birth. Indeed, several authorities advocate this practice. Certainly, for methods that do not depend on correct use by the woman or couple for long durations, such as IUDs or tubal ligation, there is no need to postpone the service; but for methods such as oral contraception, which depend on consistent and correct application by the user, immediate use postpartum may not always be the best approach.

Fig. 16–10 graphically demonstrates how the natural protection from breastfeeding, which is characterized by lactational amenorrhea, overlaps the protection from contraception—from the time that family planning begins until the time that amenorrhea ends. This overlap can be considered a period of double protection. A recent analysis of demographic data from Zimbabwe in 1988 showed that 30% of total contraception use in the country overlapped with lactational amenorrhea (Adamchak & Mbizvo, 1990).

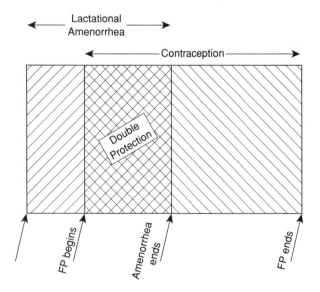

FIGURE 16–10 Double protection from pregnancy. The period between the time that family planning begins and amenorrhea ends is mostly a period of double protection from pregnancy.

When the duration of natural infertility resulting from lactation is brief, e.g., three to six months, there may be some benefit to double protection. For example, it may help the couple to establish good family-planning habits as soon as they resume sexual relations; this could be of great value when the return of fertility is expected sooner rather than later. Additionally, there is no guesswork involved in deciding when to start practicing contraception.

Even if the couple knows how to identify the return of fertility—as in the case of a couple who understands the Bellagio guidelines—the couple may not act on their knowledge. Having been out of the practice of using contraceptives, a couple may simply not believe that one day they are free of risk and the next day they are not. Being out of practice, they may simply forget to use condoms or take the pill. Concern that postpartum couples will not begin a method when they become at risk, or will not resume their method, consistently jibes with the hesitation found in the current medical literature about when to start contraception during lactation. For example, in the same short document, the medical advisory panel of the International Planned Parenthood Federation (IPPF, 1990) gives two somewhat contradictory recommendations:

> Contraceptive measures should be used as soon as any of the risk factors mentioned [the first postpartum menses, the introduction of supplementary milk or food to the infant, and six months postpartum] is present.
>
> . . .
>
> Couples should not take the risk of unprotected intercourse assuming wrongly that they can rely on lactational infertility.

Since the family-planning movement was established, professionals in the field have believed and advocated that there is no condition under which breastfeeding alone should be relied upon for its contraceptive benefits. Although family-planning professionals do not deny the current research to the contrary, the previous position has long been practiced and preached. A certain degree of skepticism, however, is healthy at this time, as the body of research literature is still growing.

Contraceptive Technology, an important clinical reference for family planning in the United States, suggests:

If a woman intends to breastfeed on demand and during the night, not introducing supplementary food, she may be able to postpone the introduction of an additional contraceptive method for 6 months, provided she continues breastfeeding fully both day and night and has not resumed menses. (We stress, however, that the majority of U.S. women do not fulfill these conditions.) Thus, U.S. clinicians should caution patients against relying on breastfeeding alone for contraception (Hatcher et al., 1990).

In Zimbabwe, the average duration of lactational amenorrhea in 1988 was $12\frac{1}{2}$ months (Adamchak & Mbizvo, 1990). By contrast, women in the United States breastfeed and experience amenorrhea for much shorter periods. Between 1987 and 1988 only 56% of all U.S. mothers ever breastfed (Ryan et al., 1991), with only a small proportion still breastfeeding (at least once a day) after six months. Supplementation occurs early too, which suggests that the pool of U.S. mothers eligible to adhere to the Bellagio guidelines is smaller than in other cultures.

When the durations of breastfeeding and amenorrhea are short, the potential for double protection is small. It is among successful breastfeeders who are amenorrheic for long periods that double protection *may* be problematic if temporary family-planning methods are discontinued after brief periods or are used unreliably. Double protection is a dilemma when people do not practice contraception consistently and correctly for long periods of time. People get tired of using contraceptives: they run out of supplies, and access to methods—especially those available only by prescription—is not always easy, inexpensive, or timely. Users are often not taught properly, so they do not understand how their method works. An analysis of data on contraceptive use in the Philippines revealed that in common use, oral contraceptive pills were no more effective than the rhythm method used with withdrawal (Laing, 1985). The low level of actual effectiveness of the pill has been attributed to high discontinuation of the method and poor compliance with instructions for its use. Although the theoretical efficacy of the pill is extremely high, in actual use, as many as 16 to 20% of users have had unplanned pregnancies while on it. One of the primary causes appears to be its incorrect use (Potter & Williams-Deane, 1990). In addition, the percentages of women continuing to use reversible methods for one year are not impressive. For example, use of the pill, IUDs, condoms, diaphragms, and spermicides in the United States are continued for one year by only 75%, 74%, 73%, 69%, and 55% of users, respectively (Trussell & Kost, 1987; Trussell et al., 1990). Roughly 63% of those who discontinue their previous method of contraception do not replace it with another (Grady, Hayward & Florey, 1988).

It is important to clarify that if method continuation is very good, then double protection is not a serious problem. Some methods, like tubal ligation, are not susceptible to continuation problems. If a woman wants to use a method that has a predetermined duration of effectiveness which is significantly longer than the duration of amenorrhea, then that method should be considered, even during amenorrhea. If a permanent method is the woman's informed choice, then double protection is not at issue.

At least two more factors must be considered. Women who are breastfeeding may be more interested in spacing their pregnancies rather than in limiting them. Women who desire another pregnancy after optimal spacing (for example, two years) may not want a long-acting method, such as tubal ligation, Norplant (subdermal implants which deliver contraceptive hormones into the blood), or possibly even IUDs. Some temporary methods well suited to spacers are also methods which are unforgiving of incorrect use. By contrast, a factor that weighs in favor of encouraging double protection is that accidental pregnancies early in the postpartum period are the ones which are most important to avoid, because of their adverse health consequences to the mother, her breastfeeding child, and developing fetus. This situation is far more serious in developing country settings.

It is easier to speak with certainty about the double-protection dilemma on a demographic level than on a clinical one for individual women because the personal manifestations of double protection have not been studied. If the lessons learned on a population level are applicable to individuals, then the use of lactational amenorrhea as a family-planning method under the Bellagio guidelines should be recommended in the United States only for mothers with a history of breastfeeding of at least 9 to 12 months who have experienced amenorrhea for six months or longer. Special care should be taken to teach and counsel primiparas about sound breast-feeding skills if they intend to breastfeed for at least several months—and especially if they wish to benefit from the natural contraceptive protection associated with lactational amenorrhea. The caution of the IPPF and others about advocating the informed use of lactational amenorrhea is fully understandable given the lamentable practice of limited breastfeeding in the United States and some other developed countries.

THE CONTRACEPTIVE METHODS

The following discussion describes the advantages and disadvantages of various contraceptive methods used during the postpartum period and/or during lactation. It is not intended to be an exhaustive exposition of the methods. Instead it emphasizes the implications of the use of the methods for the breastfeeding mother and baby. A fully detailed discussion of instructions for use, as well as the contraindications of each method unrelated to breastfeeding, can be found in the most recent edition of *Contraceptive Technology* (Hatcher et al., 1990).

The array of existing methods of family planning is theoretically impressive, although even in the most industrialized countries women's first choices are not always available, sometimes because of regulatory agency restrictions. For example, although the injectable contraceptive Depo-provera (a progestin injection with contraceptive efficacy of three months' duration) is currently available as a contraceptive in many other countries, it is not yet approved for contraceptive use in the United States.

Nonhormonal methods. The permanent methods of family planning—now the most popular category of methods in the United States—all fall under the nonhormonal method category. They are highly appropriate methods provided that a couple wishes to prevent any future pregnancy, has been properly counseled, fully appreciates the irreversibility of the procedure, and is fully satisfied with the decision to use a permanent method.

When a permanent method is indicated, vasectomy is one of the most appropriate alternatives available, because it is safe, effective, and should have no effect whatsoever on lactation. After the vasectomy, the male reproductive tract continues to clear itself of sperm during about 20 ejaculations. If

the woman is not pregnant, the couple needs to use a second method of contraception for a period of time in order to be fully protected. The couple may feel that the vasectomy is ideally timed either during the pregnancy itself or in the first few months postpartum, especially if the current pregnancy was unplanned. In an era of only one or two children per family, however, the presumed final pregnancy often is highly planned. If so, couples may feel more comfortable postponing vasectomy until after the pregnancy, in case a miscarriage should occur, or even until after the infancy period of the child.

Female sterilization carries several advantages. It is safe, effective, and relatively convenient since it can be performed in hospital—even on the delivery table. There is a potential negative effect of the sterilization *procedure* on lactation, in that general anesthesia used may synergistically interfere with the early breastfeeding pattern. The mother needs time to recover from the anesthesia, and during this period she is not breastfeeding. By the time she begins to breastfeed, the anesthetic agent has passed into her milk, contributing to the baby's drowsiness and making it difficult to feed effectively. In addition, the pain she feels may temporarily reduce her ability or desire to breastfeed, and it may limit her options for comfortably positioning herself or her infant for breastfeeding. If the mother is experienced and/or well counseled, and if hospital staff does not interfere by bottle-feeding the baby, this interruption of early breastfeeding should not have serious consequences for lactation.

Studies reviewed in the early 1980s have reported that up to 7% of women express regret about tubal sterilizations (Divers, 1984; Grubb et al., 1985). In general, regret over the procedure and/or desire for reversal has been associated with younger age (e.g., under 30) or low parity at the time of the procedure, as well as remarriage, the death of a child after the procedure, and having the procedure with a concurrent cesarean section or during the puerperal or postabortion period. Occasionally, lower socioeconomic class and lack of having a child of a specific gender have also been associated with regret over having the procedure. It is possible that regret is intensified when pre-, post- and intraprocedural factors interact, such as when a young woman with few children is sterilized immediately postpartum, and she later remarries.

Of more than 5,000 women in the Collaborative

Review of Sterilization, a U.S. multicenter prospective observational study, 2.0% and 2.7% reported that they regretted their sterilization one and two years after the procedure, respectively. The preoperative risk factors for experiencing regret after two years were identified as an age of less than 30 and (for whites) concurrent cesarean section (Grubb et al., 1985). Chi et al. (1989c) also reported that women whose tubal ligations were combined with the cesarean procedure were more likely to have characteristics associated with later regret.

Counseling is crucially important when helping women or couples to select the best family-planning approach for them. When a permanent method is a serious consideration, counseling must begin long before the procedure and be repetitive. This may be especially important when younger women of low parity express an interest in the procedure during the puerperium, as well as when young men under the same conditions consider vasectomy.

Nonhormonal intrauterine devices (IUDs) have been shown to have either no effect or a positive effect on lactation (Koetsawang, 1987). One study found Copper T-380A IUD insertion easier and less painful during lactation, with possibly higher continuation rates than in nonlactating women (Chi et al., 1989a; Chi et al., 1989b). IUDs inserted during the postpartum period tend to be expelled more frequently than IUDs inserted at other times. However, insertion immediately after delivery of the placenta (within 10 minutes) by an experienced person who places the device high in the fundus significantly reduces the chance of expulsion (Chi & Farr, 1989). Breastfeeding has not been found to increase the risk of expulsion when the device is inserted at this time or after the postpartum period (Chi et al., 1989a; Cole et al., 1983).

A study of U.S. women found the risk of uterine perforation to be significantly elevated in women who were breastfeeding at the time of insertion (Heartwell & Schlesselman, 1983), although large studies have been unable to confirm this (Chi, Feldblum & Rogers, 1984; Farr & Rivera, in press). Insertion by an experienced person is thought to minimize the risk of perforation.

Because of the advantages of immediate postplacental insertion, contraceptive counseling and informed consent to IUD insertion should occur long before labor and delivery. Counseling on postinsertion care is also important. Women should be encouraged to have early postpartum checkups and to return if the IUD thread is missing, because expulsion, if it occurs, often does so soon after insertion.

Little research has been conducted on the effectiveness of barrier methods used during lactation. Clinical trials of contraceptive efficacy have deliberately excluded breastfeeding women because their naturally subfertile state may influence pregnancy rates. The relative effectiveness of the various barrier methods vis-à-vis each other is probably maintained during lactation.

Barrier and/or spermicidal methods are the most widely used contraceptives among lactating U.S. women (Ford & Labbok, 1987). Several characteristics of these methods make them particularly attractive during the breastfeeding period. Condoms, diaphragms, sponges, and spermicides are all coitus-dependent methods. Even if couples prefer other methods, they may find these methods useful if they are having intercourse less frequently than before the pregnancy. The lubricative effect of the spermicide can be welcome if the woman experiences vaginal symptoms from estrogen suppression. The contraceptive sponge, the diaphragm, and the cervical cap should not be used in the first six weeks postpartum in order to avoid postpartum endometritis, a serious complication of the puerperium. This leaves the condom as the barrier method of choice during the early postpartum period. Condoms can be purchased with or without a lubricant coating and/or a spermicide in the reservoir. A condom used with a spermicide, whether applied by the user or as part of the condom itself, should have better contraceptive efficacy than the condom alone.

The diaphragm that a woman used prior to her pregnancy is apt to be unsuitable in size after childbirth. A new diaphragm can be fitted at the postpartum checkup. With the gain or loss of every 10 pounds, a new diaphragm may need to be sized in order to achieve effective protection, and a clinical gynecologic visit should be sought for this purpose. The diaphragm should always be used with a spermicidal cream or jelly.

The vaginal contraceptive sponge is a safe and convenient barrier method. It can be purchased over the counter and is perceived to be less messy to use because the sponge comes with spermicide already in it. The contraceptive efficacy of the sponge used by parous women has been found to be significantly lower than among women who have never had a child, with up to 28 pregnancies per 100 parous women in the first year of use (McIntyre & Higgins, 1986).

Spermicidal cream, jelly, foam, or foaming tablets used alone are not as effective in preventing pregnancy as a spermicide used with a barrier, such as a sponge, diaphragm, or condom. Yet they represent a significant improvement over unprotected intercourse; they also have the advantage of being widely available and can be purchased over the counter.

Hormonal methods. Hormonal contraceptive methods are not the category of first choice for breastfeeding women. The main reason is that all steroid hormones, natural or synthetic, are detectable in milk to some degree (Johansson & Odlind, 1987). The effect of the infant's exposure to exogenous hormones is presumed to be minor because very small amounts of hormone are excreted in the milk or absorbed by the infant. Since the fetus is exposed to very high levels of progesterone *in utero,* exposure to small quantities of progesterone in milk may be of no consequence. Nevertheless, the long-term effects of consumption of exogenous steroid hormones on development are as yet unknown. Several ongoing studies are addressing this important question (Rivera, personal communication, 1991).

Hormone formulations containing estrogen have been observed to decrease the milk supply in several studies (Koetsawang, 1987; WHO, 1988). Therefore, combined estrogen-progesterone methods (usually in the form of combined oral contraceptive pills) are contraindicated unless there is no other alternative. If combined pills (including low-dose formulations) are the only choice, they should begin no earlier than six weeks postpartum in order for the mother and baby to achieve a reasonable level of milk production, although it is recommended that they be avoided for at least six months.

Progesterone metabolism by the baby appears to vary across formulations of progestin-only methods; little is known about the degree to which the child absorbs the progesterone it consumes. Progestin-only pills, injections, and subdermal implants usually have not been associated with reduced milk volume or impaired infant growth (McCann et al., 1989; Koetsawang, 1987). Although one large study found no adverse effects of progestin-only pill initiation at one week postpartum, progestin-only methods are most commonly begun only after breastfeeding has been well established—and then at the lowest practical effective dose. Progestin-only pills are marginally less effective than combined estrogen-progesterone formulations, but still highly effective when taken consistently and correctly. Progestin-only pills, however, are somewhat unforgiving of incorrect use—e.g., missing a pill. One study of 200 breastfeeding women using the progestin-only oral contraceptive norgestrel (0.075 mg) reported discontinuation and method failure rates of 32.5 and 3.4, per 100 respectively, at 12 months (Canto et al., 1989).

Norplant subdermal implants were approved for contraceptive use by the U.S. Food and Drug Administration in December, 1990. Some family-planning programs in other countries have advocated the implant of the levonorgestrel-containing silastic rods in breastfeeding women as early as six weeks postpartum, while others advocate beginning the method at six months postpartum—in order to initiate progestin-only contraception after the milk supply has been well established. The implants maintain a level of serum levonorgestrel which is lower than the levels achieved with progestin-only pills; thus Norplant should have no effect on milk production or infant growth. The currently available progestin-only injectable contraceptives create much higher circulating levels of steroid than either the oral pills or implants.

The quality and composition of breastmilk during hormonal contraceptive use has been given a modest amount of attention. Different studies of progestin-only injectables and progestin-only pills have reported conflicting results regarding the protein and fat content of milk—finding it increased, decreased, or unchanged. Lactose concentrations, however, appear to be unaffected (Koetsawang, 1987).

Natural methods. The Billings' Ovulation Method and the Symptothermal Method are considered to be modern natural family-planning (NFP) methods because they are based on sound scientific research. The methods require abstinence from intercourse during the fertile period, which is identified by observing the woman's physical signs and symptoms—e.g., cervical mucus volume, color, stretchiness, sensation, and clarity; basal body temperature; cervical position; and breast tenderness. The modern natural methods are highly effective when used correctly, but most studies observe a great deal of incorrect use. Incorrect use is usually the failure to abstain from intercourse during the fertile period rather than a misunderstanding of the method or how to use it.

Modern NFP methods have been adapted for use during lactation, but their effectiveness during this time has seldom been systematically evaluated (Labbok et al., 1991; Perez et al., 1988). As is the case with the study of barrier contraceptives, previous efficacy of research has excluded all but ostensibly normally cycling women. One study observed a poor association between estrogen metabolite excretion and women's reports of the cervical mucus symptom which is regulated by estrogen (Brown, Harrison & Smith, 1985). Basal body temperature is unknowable unless the woman has at least six hours of uninterrupted sleep; this requirement excludes many fully breastfeeding women, particularly in the early months of lactation. Although the methods can be taught and learned in simple terms (and illiterate women in many countries have learned to use the modern NFP methods), it seems logical that learning is easier during normal cycles compared with the hypoestrogenic period of lactation. Therefore, couples who wish to use natural methods to space or limit pregnancies during lactation are at an advantage if they have learned how to use their NFP method of choice prior to conception and subsequent lactation. Knowledge of the fertile period is also useful for achieving pregnancy.

The Lactational Amenorrhea Method (LAM) is the deliberate nonuse of a contraceptive method, despite the intention to prevent pregnancy during the period of lactational amenorrhea, under very specific circumstances: (1) the woman is breastfeeding her child exclusively (or nearly exclusively), i.e., no supplemental feedings[*]; (2) the woman has experienced no vaginal bleeding or spotting after lochia ends (all bleeding, spotting, or bloody vaginal discharge before postpartum day 56 can be ignored); and (3) the child is less than six months of age. LAM is based on the Bellagio consensus (FHI, 1988; Kennedy, Rivera & McNeilly, 1989). It can be considered a natural family-planning method or a way to time

[*]LAM includes the condition that the child is receiving no supplements. Given enthusiastic breastfeeding, at least one study has shown that the presence or absence of supplements does not matter (Short et al., 1991)

the commencement of use of another contraceptive (Gross, 1991).

CLINICAL IMPLICATIONS

When a woman or couple makes a legitimate family-planning decision and/or chooses a method for achieving their family-planning ideal based on full and accurate information and reflection, that person or couple has maximized the likelihood of being satisfied with the decision or choice and of using the chosen method correctly and effectively.

Informed choice has been defined as follows:

> effective access to information on reproductive choices and to the necessary counseling, services and supplies to help individuals choose and use an appropriate method of family planning, if desired (Piotrow, 1989).

Informed choice should be viewed as a continuing process which parallels changing procreative desire and phase of life, as well as personal changes over time. It is naive to think that family-planning intentions will remain fixed throughout life, and equally naive to suggest that one type of contraceptive is appropriate for the same person throughout all the reproductive years. An appropriate range of available methods includes both male and female methods—and permanent methods as well as long- and short-acting temporary ones. If only a limited range of methods is available to the health-care provider, he or she should be prepared to offer referrals to help meet the patient's needs.

Information can be shared with patients in different ways, using the written word through pamphlets, books, and posters, or the spoken word through videos, audio-visual presentations, or "class-style" (part lecture, part participatory) discussions. Providing information, however, is not sufficient. An interpersonal exchange is necessary to ensure that effective communication of information has been achieved and also to provide clarification and counseling. The desired result of counseling is a patient or couple who has made a choice based on full understanding of the alternatives—and who has made that choice freely, unaffected by the counselor. Information should flow freely between the provider/counselor and the woman/couple. This circum-

---

ISSUES TO CONSIDER WHEN DISCUSSING FAMILY PLANNING WITH THE LACTATING MOTHER

Questions

1. Does the mother wish to limit or space any future pregnancies? If so, what method(s) of family planning does she prefer?

2. If she has breastfed a previous child, how long did she remain amenorrheic? What factors may have influenced the duration of her lactational amenorrhea?

3. If she has not breastfed before, how does she plan to do so? Is she familiar with the factors that can reduce the duration of lactational amenorrhea?

4. If she wishes to have no more children, how will her family be affected if a temporary method of contraception fails and she becomes pregnant before she had planned, or in the face of a desire to have no more children?

Information to Share

1. Discuss the effectiveness of the mother's preferred method(s) and offer additional information about other contraceptives as well. Include information about the effect of each method on lactation and on the suckling child.

2. This information may predict the degree of double protection she may experience by using both a contraceptive and breastfeeding to reduce the risk of an unplanned pregnancy.

3. Review the factors that reduce the duration of lactational amenorrhea and increase the early resumption of fertility. Pay particular attention to what is meant by exclusive or nearly exclusive breastfeeding, the impact of pacifier use, regular use of solid foods in the infant's diet, and supplementary bottle-feedings.

4. When the reproductive intention is to prevent any future pregnancies, it is especially important that a highly effective contraceptive method be chosen. Double protection is not an issue under this circumstance.

---

stance exists, ideally, between the lactation consultant and the breastfeeding woman. The lactation consultant needs to be well versed in available family planning services and alternatives in her community; perhaps most important, the health-care provider should be aware of the possible interaction of various contraceptives with breastfeeding as discussed in this chapter. Counseling is needed *before* delivery, especially for the immediate postpartum insertion of an IUD or for postpartum sterilization.

Accurate information is an essential tool for the lactation consultant, and posing the questions in the boxed copy above will help her ascertain some essential information. Additionally, such accurate information will influence the ability of the woman or couple to make a decision without undue influence from the consultant. When the couple freely makes informed choices, the lactation consultant is better able to support the woman and her family in their choices.

SUMMARY

Fertility, sexuality, and contraception are normally related, but each of these aspects of reproduction also affects or is affected by lactation. A clear understanding of the interrelationships of these elements is essential if the health-care provider is to discuss issues and concerns of the lactating mother as she seeks to determine her fertility in concert with her sexual self. The health-care provider will benefit from an understanding of the relationship between physiological responses to suckling stimulation and the resumption of fertility. Additionally, the breastfeeding woman needs to be prepared for the ways in which her own breastfeeding experience may alter her sexual feelings as well as her fertility—in the early weeks postbirth as well as when her breastfeeding child is weaning.

Double protection from pregnancy may occur when a fully breastfeeding woman is practicing contraception prior to the resumption of menses during the first six months postpartum, and possibly even later. Information about different methods of family planning will be received with varying degrees of acceptance and compliance, depending on how well a given method or combination of methods can be incorporated into each sex partner's short- and long-term plans for family life. The degree to which double protection is unnecessary will vary from one family to the next, depending upon the degree to which an unplanned pregnancy is a serious disruption of that family's plans for its individual members.

The health-care provider who is assisting the lactating mother should be thoroughly familiar with how lactation, fertility, sexuality, and contraception are intertwined threads in the cord of life experience in order to best serve the breastfeeding family.

ACKNOWLEDGMENTS

Cynthia Visness and Theresa Burton assisted in preparing the figures and text of this chapter. Their contributions are sincerely appreciated, as are the valuable reviews by Nancy Williamson, Ph.D.; Roberto Rivera, M.D.; Gary Grubb, M.D.; Barbara Gross, Ph.D.; and Soledad Diaz, M.D. The personal communications of the scientists noted within are important in shaping the current thinking about fertility, contraception, and sexuality during breastfeeding, and each researcher is thanked and appreciated most sincerely. Partial support for this work was provided by the U.S. Agency for International Development through a cooperative agreement with Family Health International, Research Triangle Park, North Carolina. The views expressed here are those of the authors and do not necessarily reflect those of USAID or FHI.

REFERENCES

Abraham, S: Recovery after childbirth, *Med J Aust* 152:387, 1990.

Abraham, S, et al.: Recovery after childbirth: a preliminary prospective study, *Med J Aust* 152:9–12, 1990.

Adamchak, DJ, and Mbizvo, MT: The relationship between fertility and contraceptive prevalence in Zimbabwe, *Int Fam Plann Persp* 16:103–6, 1990.

Alder, E, and Bancroft, J: The relationship between breastfeeding persistence, sexuality, and mood in postpartum women, *Psychol Med* 18:389–96, 1988.

Alder, EM, et al.: Hormones, mood and sexuality in lactating women, *Br J Psychiatry* 148:74–79, 1986.

Andersen, AN, and Schioler, V: Influence of breastfeeding pattern on pituitary-ovarian axis of women in an industrialized community, *Am J Obstet Gynecol* 143:673–77, 1982.

Arthur, PG, et al.: Measuring short-term rates of milk synthesis in breastfeeding mothers, *Quart J Exp Phys* 74:419–28, 1989.

Badroui, MHH, and Hefnawi, F: Ovarian function during lactation. In Hafez, ESE, ed.: *Human Ovulation*, Amsterdam, 1979, Elsevier-North Holland Biomedical Press, pp. 233–41.

Benitez, I, et al.: Extending lactational amenorrhea in Manila: a successful breast-feeding education program, *J Biosoc Sci* 24:211–31, 1992.

Bongaarts, J, and Menken, J: *Determinants of fertility in developing countries*, New York, 1983, Academic Press, Inc., pp. 27–60.

Bongaarts, J, and Potter, RG: *Fertility, biology and behavior*, New York, 1983, Academic Press, Inc.

Bottorff, JL: Persistence in breastfeeding: a phenomenologic investigation, *J Adv Nurs* 15:201–9, 1990.

Brown, JB, Harrison, P, and Smith, MA: A study of returning fertility after childbirth and during lactation by measurement of urinary estrogen and pregnanediol excretion and cervical mucus production, *J Biosoc Sci* 9(suppl.):5–23, 1985.

Canto, TE, et al.: Mini pill in lactating women, *Contraception* 39:589–601, 1989.

Chi, IC, and Farr, G: Postpartum IUD contraception—a review of an international experience, *Adv Contraception* 5:127–46, 1989.

Chi, IC, Feldblum, PJ, and Rogers, SM: IUD-related uterine perforation: an epidemiologic analysis of a rare event using an international dataset, *Contracept Deliv Syst* 5:123–30, 1984.

Chi, IC, et al.: Performance of the Copper T-380A intrauterine device in breastfeeding women, *Contraception* 39:603–18, 1989a.

Chi, IC, et al.: Insertional pain and other IUD insertion-related rare events for breastfeeding and non-breastfeeding women—a decade's experience in developing countries, *Adv Contraception* 5:101–19, 1989b.

Chi, IC, et al.: Tubal ligation at cesarean delivery in five Asian centers: a comparison with tubal ligation soon after vaginal delivery, *Int J Gynecol Obstet* 30:257–65, 1989c.

Cole, LP, et al.: Effects of breastfeeding on IUD performance, *Am J Public Health* 73:384–88, 1983.

Delvoye, P, et al.: The influence of the frequency of nursing and of previous lactation experience on serum prolactin in lactating mothers, *J Biosoc Sci* 9:447–51, 1977.

Diaz, S, et al.: Contraceptive efficacy of lactational amenorrhea in urban Chilean women, *Contraception* 43:335–52, 1991.

Diaz, S, et al.: Fertility regulation in nursing women: I. The probability of conception in full nursing women living in an urban setting, *J Biosoc Sci* 14:329–41, 1982.

Diaz, S, et al.: Circadian variation of basal plasma prolactin,

prolactin response to suckling and length of amenorrhea in nursing women, *J Clin Endocrinol Metab* 68:946–55, 1989.

Divers, WA: Characteristics of women requesting reversal of sterilization, *Fertil Steril* 41:233–36, 1984.

Elias, MF, et al.: Nursing practices and lactational amenorrhea, *J Biosoc Sci* 18:1–10, 1986.

Eslami, SS, et al.: The reliability of menses to indicate the return of ovulation in breastfeeding women in Manila, The Philippines, *Stud Fam Plann* 21:243–50, 1990.

Family Health International: Breastfeeding as a family planning method, *Lancet* ii:(8621):1204–5, 1988.

Farr, G, and Rivera, R: Interactions between IUD and breast-feeding status at time of IUD insertion: analysis of PCU 380A acceptors in developing countries, *Am J Obstet Gynecol* (in press).

Flynn, AM, et al.: Ultrasonic patterns of ovarian activity during breastfeeding, *Am J Obstet Gynecol* 165:2027–31, 1991.

Ford, K: Correlation between subsequent lengths of postpartum amenorrhea in a prospective study of breastfeeding women in rural Bangladesh, *J Biosoc Sci,* 24:89–95, 1992.

Ford, K, and Labbok, M: Contraceptive usage during lactation in the United States: an update, *Am J Public Health* 77:79–81, 1987.

Franceschini, R, et al.: Plasma beta-endorphin concentrations during suckling in lactating women, *Br J Obstet Gynaecol* 96:711–13, 1989.

Glasier, A, McNeilly, AS, and Baird, DT: Induction of ovarian activity by pulsatile infusion of LHRH in women with lactational amenorrhea, *Clin Endocrinol* 24:243–52, 1986.

Glasier, A, McNeilly, AS, and Howie, PW: Fertility after childbirth: changes in serum gonadotrophin levels in breast and bottle feeding women, *Clin Endocrinol* 19:493–501, 1983.

Glasier, A, McNeilly, AS, and Howie, PW: Pulsatile secretion of LH in relation to the resumption of ovarian activity postpartum, *Clin Endocrinol* 20:415–26, 1984.

Gordon, K, et al.: Hypothalamo-pituitary portal blood concentrations of B-endorphin during suckling in the ewe, *Reprod Fertil* 79:397–408, 1987.

Grady, WR, Hayward, MD, and Florey, FA: Contraceptive discontinuation among married women in the United States, *Stud Fam Plann* 19:227–35, 1988.

Gray, RH, et al.: Risk of ovulation during lactation, *Lancet* 335:25–29, 1990.

Gross, B: Is the lactational amenorrhea method a part of natural family planning? Biology and policy, *Am J Obstet Gynecol* 165:2014–19, 1991.

Gross, BA, and Eastman, CJ: Prolactin and the return of ovulation in breastfeeding women, *J Biosoc Sci Suppl.* 9:25–42, 1985.

Grubb, GS, et al.: Regret after decision to have a tubal sterilization, *Fertil Steril* 44:248–53, 1985.

Grudzinskas, JG, and Atkinson, L: Sexual function during the puerperium, *Arch Sex Behav* 13:85–91, 1984.

Hatcher, RA, et al.: *Contraceptive Technology,* New York, 1990, Irvington Publishers, Inc., pp. 461–74.

Heartwell, SF, and Schlesselman, S: Risk of uterine perforation among users of intrauterine devices, *Obstet Gynecol* 61:31–36, 1983.

Hornsby, PP, and Wilcox, AJ: Validity of questionnaire information on frequency of coitus, *Am J Epidemiol* 130:94–99, 1989.

Howie, PW, et al.: Effect of supplementary food on suckling patterns and ovarian activity during lactation, *Br Med J* 283:757–59, 1981.

Howie, PW, et al.: Fertility after childbirth: adequacy of postpartum luteal phases, *Clin Endocrinol* 17:609–15, 1982a.

Howie, PW, et al.: Fertility after childbirth: postpartum ovulation and menstruation in bottle and breastfeeding mothers, *Clin Endocrinol* 17:323–32, 1982b.

International Planned Parenthood Federation: *IPPF Med Bull* 24:2–4, 1990.

Israngkura, B, et al.: Breastfeeding and return to ovulation in Bangkok, *Int J Gynaecol Obstet* 30:335–42, 1989.

Johansson, E, and Odlind, V: The passage of exogenous hormones into breastmilk: possible effects, *Int J Gynaecol Obstet* 25(suppl.):111–14, 1987.

Jones, RE: Breastfeeding and postpartum amenorrhea in Indonesia, *J Biosoc Sci* 21:83–100, 1989.

Jones, RE: A hazards model analysis of breastfeeding variables and maternal age on return to menses postpartum in rural Indonesian women, *Hum Biol* 60:853–71, 1988.

Kennedy, KI: *Breastfeeding as a child-spacing mechanism,* Abstracts of papers presented at the IVth Congress of the International Federation for Family Life Promotion, Ottawa, June 29, 30, and July 1, 1986, pp. 51–52.

Kennedy, KI, and Visness, CV: Contraceptive efficacy of lactational amenorrhoea, *Lancet* 339(8787):227–30, 1992.

Kennedy, KI, Rivera, R, and McNeilly, AS: Consensus statement on the use of breastfeeding as a family planning method, *Contraception* 39:477–96, 1989.

Kennedy, KI, et al.: The NFP-LAM interface: observations from a prospective study of breastfeeding NFP users, *Am J Obstet Gynecol* 165:2020–26, 1991.

Kenny, JA: Sexuality of pregnant and breastfeeding women, *Arch Sex Behav* 2:215–29, 1973.

Khan, T, et al.: A study of breastfeeding and the return of menses and pregnancy in Karachi, Pakistan, *Contraception* 40:365–76, 1989.

Koetsawang, S: The effects of contraceptive methods on the quality and quantity of breastmilk, *Int J Gynaecol Obstet* 25(suppl.):115–28, 1987.

Labbok, MH: Breastfeeding and family planning programs: a vital complementarity. In Baumslag, N, ed.: *Breastfeeding: the passport to life,* New York, 1989, NGO Committee for UNICEF.

Labbok, M, et al.: *Guidelines for breastfeeding in family planning and child survival programs,* Washington, D.C., 1990a, Institute for International Studies in Natural Family Planning.

Labbok, M, et al.: The lactational amenorrhea method: examples of a teaching unit. In Rodriguez-Garcia, R, Schaeffer, LA, and Yunes, J, eds.: *Lactation Education for Health Professionals,* Washington, D.C., 1990b, Pan American Health Organization, pp. 70–96.

Labbok, MH, et al.: Ovulation method use during breastfeeding: is there increased risk of unplanned pregnancy? *Am J Obstet Gynecol* 165:2031–36, 1991.

Laing, JE: Continuation and effectiveness practice: a cross-sectional approach, *Stud Fam Plann* 16:138–53, 1985.

Lewis, PR, et al.: The resumption of ovulation and menstruation in a well-nourished population of women breastfeeding for an extended period of time, *Fertil Steril* 55:529–36, 1991.

Masters, WH, and Johnson, VE: *Human sexual response,* Boston, 1966, Little, Brown & Co.

Mauldin, WP, and Segal, SJ: Prevalence of contraceptive use: trends and issues, *Stud Fam Plann* 19:335–53, 1988.

McCann, MF, et al.: The effects of a progestin-only oral contraceptive (levenorgestrel 0.03 mg) on breastfeeding, *Contraception* 40:635–48, 1989.

McIntyre, SL, and Higgins, JE: Parity and use-effectiveness with the contraceptive sponge, *Am J Obstet Gynecol* 155:796–801, 1986.

McNeilly, AS: Suckling and the control of gonadotropin secretion. In Knobil, E, and Neill, J, et al., eds.: *The Physiology of reproduction,* New York, 1988, Raven Press, pp. 2336–49.

McNeilly, AS, Glasier, A, and Howie, PW: Endocrine control of lactational infertility-I. In Dobbing, J, ed.: *Maternal nutrition and lactational infertility,* New York, 1985, Raven Press, pp. 1–24.

McNeilly, AS, et al.: Fertility after childbirth: pregnancy associated with breastfeeding, *Clin Endocrinol* 18:167–73, 1983.

Perez, A, Labbok, MH, and Queenan, JT: Clinical study of the lactational amenorrhoea method for family planning, *Lancet* 339:968–70, 1992.

Perez, A, et al.: Use-effectiveness of the ovulation method initiated during postpartum breastfeeding, *Contraception* 38:499–508, 1988.

Perez, A, et al.: First ovulation after childbirth: the effect of breastfeeding, *Am J Obstet Gynecol* 114:1014–47, 1972.

Piotrow, PT: *Informed choice: report of the Cooperating Agencies Task Force,* Baltimore, 1989, The Johns Hopkins University, Center for Communication Programs, pp. i, 2–68.

Potter, L, and Williams-Deane, M: The importance of oral contraceptive compliance, *IPPF Med Bull* 24:2–3, 1990.

Riordan, J: *A practical guide to breastfeeding,* St. Louis, 1983, The C.V. Mosby Co., p. 339.

Rivera, R, et al.: Breastfeeding and the return to ovulation in Durango, Mexico, *Fertil Steril* 49:780–87, 1988.

Robson, KM, Brant, HA, and Kumar, R: Maternal sexuality during first pregnancy and after childbirth, *Br J Obstet Gynaecol* 88:882–89, 1981.

Rolland, R: Bibliography (with review) on contraceptive effects of breastfeeding, *Biblio Reprod* 28:1–4, 93, 1976.

Rosa, FW: The role of breastfeeding in family planning, *WHO Protein Advisory Group Bull* 5:5–10, 1975.

Ryan, AS, et al.: A comparison of breastfeeding data from the National Surveys of Family Growth and the Ross Laboratories Mothers Surveys, *Am J Public Health* 81:1049–52, 1991.

Shaaban, MM, Sayed, GH, and Ghaneimah, SA: The recovery of ovarian function during breast-feeding, *J Steroid Biochem* 27:1043–52, 1987.

Shaaban, MM, et al.: The recovery of fertility during breastfeeding in Assiut, Egypt, *J Biosoc Sci* 22:19–32, 1990.

Short, RV: Breast feeding, *Scient Am* 250(4):3541, 1984.

Short, RV, et al.: Contraceptive effects of extended lactational amenorrhea: beyond the Bellagio consensus, *Lancet* 337:715–17, 1991.

Simpson-Hebert, M, and Huffman, SL: The contraceptive effect of breastfeeding, *Stud Fam Plann* 12:125–33, 1981.

Tay, CCK: Mechanisms controlling lactational infertility, *J Hum Lact* 7, 15–18, 1991.

Thapa, S, Short, RV, and Potts, M: Breastfeeding, birthspacing and their effects on child survival, *Nature* 335 (6192):679–82, 1988.

Trussell, J, and Kost, K: Contraceptive failure in the United States: a critical review of the literature, *Stud Fam Plann* 18:237–83, 1987.

Trussell, J, et al.: Contraceptive failure in the U.S.: an update, *Stud Fam Plann* 21:51–54, 1990.

Udry, JR, and Deang, L: Determinants of coitus after childbirth, *J Biosoc Sci,* in press.

United Nations: *Levels and trends of contraceptive use as assessed in 1988,* New York, 1989 United Nations, pp. 17–28.

Van Ginnekin, JK: Prolonged breastfeeding as a birth spacing method, *Stud Fam Plann* 5:201–6, 1974.

Virden, SF: The relationship between infant feeding method and maternal role adjustment, *J Nurs-Midwif* 33:31–35, 1988.

World Health Organization: Effects of hormonal contraceptives on breast milk composition and infant growth, *Stud Fam Plann* 19:361–69, 1988.

Wrigley, EA, and Hutchinson, SA: Long-term breastfeeding: the secret bond, *J Nurs-Midwif* 35:35–41, 1990.

17

Child Health

JAN RIORDAN

Breastfeeding has long been considered health promotion, and the positive effect of breastfeeding on protecting the health of the baby has been the subject of extensive study and review. Attention has focused on breastfeeding as a means of reducing infections; other aspects of breastfeeding on child development are not as recognized. This chapter provides the reader with an overview of child-health issues. Discussion begins with the fundamentals of normal growth and development of infants and children and then moves on to review prominent theories of child development. The rich textures of mother-infant social interaction, woven from sophisticated sensory abilities of the newborn, creates a lifelong bond. In infancy this bond creates distress and protest (on the part of both mother and infant) when the mother and infant are separated. Next, the topic turns to such children's health issues as immunization and dental health to answer questions that care providers are frequently called upon to provide. This is followed by practical considerations of introducing solids. The chapter concludes with a discussion of weaning.

Before addressing specific elements of growth and development, it is useful to consider a handful of studies which compare developmental outcomes between breastfed and bottle-fed babies. A few studies (Broad, 1972; Hoefer & Hardy, 1929; Rogerson & Rogerson, 1939) have found that the developmental status of children who were breastfed was higher than those who were fed with other milks. The methods used in these studies have been criticized, however, because the authors failed to control for socioeconomic and educational factors—e.g., the education of the mother. Later studies which did control for these factors confirm that breastfeeding

appears to have a small but significantly positive effect on development.

Rodgers (1978) analysed U.K. National Survey of Health and Development data and showed a small but significant advantage for the children who were breastfed. Fergusson, Beautrais, and Silva (1982) looked at the relationship between breastfeeding and childhood intelligence and development in New Zealand children. Even when the mother's intelligence and education, the family's socioeconomic status, and the baby's birth weight and gestational age were taken into account, breastfed children had slightly higher intelligence test scores than bottle-fed infants. Two years later, Taylor and Wadsworth (1984) found a positive correlation between duration of breastfeeding and children's performance in vocabulary and visual-motor coordination tests.

Finally, Morrow-Tlucak, Haude, and Ernhart (1988) compared the cognitive development in breastfed and bottle-fed children living in Ohio. The investigators used rigorous covariate control, including controlling for the home environment (HOME scale), in order to determine if the previously discerned advantage to breastfed children was evident early in development. They found that breastfed infants scored higher on the Mental Development Index of the Bayley Scales at one and two years of age. At six months of age, the breastfed babies scored higher than the bottle-fed infants but the difference did not reach significance.

These results raise questions. What specific elements of breastfeeding play a role in promoting development? Is it nutritional or immunological aspects of breastmilk? Or is it the interactions between the mother and infant during breastfeeding? Although clear-cut evidence regarding the causation of an apparent relationship between breastfeeding and increases in cognitive and developmental abilities cannot be made, these studies indicate that further benefits accrue from breastfeeding. Additionally, researchers in infant development may wish to incorporate breastfeeding status in future studies.

GROWTH AND DEVELOPMENT

PHYSICAL GROWTH

Infant and child growth is affected by genetic makeup, general health, and nutrition. Infants and children vary in their tempo of growth and development, which tends to be marked by spurts of growth separated by plateaus. Still, there are universal patterns of growth for all children. These universal patterns include *cephalocaudal* growth (growth that proceeds from head to foot), *proximaldistal growth* (growth that occurs from the center outward), and *general-to-specific* movements. The fact that the infant's head accounts for about one-fourth of the infant's length at birth illustrates cephalocaudal direction of growth. Maturation of motor skills also follows the cephalocaudal pattern: an infant masters control of his head before he masters arm and trunk control; this is followed by leg control. (See Fig. 17–1A.)

Proximaldistal and general-to-specific development is illustrated by the sequence of muscle control: infants control large muscles before they control small muscles. For example, the child is able to wave "bye-bye" before he is able to grasp with his whole hand—and before he is able to hold a small object with his thumb and forefinger (pincer grasp).

WEIGHT AND LENGTH

Change, rather than stability is the hallmark of infancy; weight progresses faster in infancy than at any other time of life. The average neonate weighs about 3000 to 4000 grams ($6\frac{1}{2}$ to $8\frac{1}{2}$ pounds). Because full-term infants are born with excess fluid, they lose five to ten percent of their birthweight following birth and then stabilize within a few days. Generally speaking, infants double their birth weight by about five months of age, triple it by one year of age, and quadruple it by two years of age.

As discussed in various chapters in this book, weight patterns of formula-fed infants differ from infants who are fed exclusively at the breast. Their weights are similar for the first several months; then at three to four months formula-fed infants begin to weigh more than their breastfed counterparts. Breastfed babies gain an average of 35 grams (approximately one ounce) per day at one month and 19 grams (0.6 ounce) per day at four months. Formula-fed infants gain an average of 34.4 grams per day at one month and 23 grams per day at four months (Butte et al., 1990).

Length at birth is about 50 to 53 centimeters (20 to 21 inches) and, on the average, male infants tend to be five ounces heavier and one-half inch longer than females. A baby grows about one inch each month for the first six months and about one-half inch per month for the next six months. By the infant's first birthday, his length has increased by 50%. Length and head circumference growth for both breastfed and formula-fed infants are similar (Butte et al., 1990). The weight of the baby's brain increases most rapidly during infancy as nerve cells enlarge, become longer and branched, and gain myelin sheathing. By 18 months of age, the infant's brain is 75% of its adult weight. If the infant becomes malnourished, the first growth factor to be affected is weight. Only when malnourishment is severe and long-standing are the infant's length or head circumference compromised.

SENSES

Neonates and young infants have remarkably well-developed sensory capabilities. At birth the infant's auditory nerve tracts have sufficient myelin sheathing to allow them to hear well; they can differentiate various tastes and smells. As long as two months before birth, hearing develops in the womb. The fetus is already responding to internal sounds from the mother as well as to noises outside the mother. Some young infants, for instance, appear to recognize their mother's favorite soap opera when it comes on television. Neonates discriminate between differences in pitch and can detect the direction of the source of sound (Levanthal & Lipsitt, 1964; Weir, 1976).

Shrill, low sounds are likely to disturb and alarm the infant while soft, high-pitched sounds have a calming effect; therefore, the higher-range tones of the female voice tend to quiet and focus the baby's attention. In a nursery when one baby starts crying, others will do the same. Newborns respond to sound by differentiating the care-giver's voice from strangers' voices. They also sense heat, cold, pressure, and pain.

The neonate's vision is less developed because retinal structures and the optic nerve are not yet complete. A neonate focuses mainly on large objects close to his face and sees best at a range of 8 to 12 inches, with 9 inches as the optimum—just about the distance between the baby's face and the mother's face while the baby is being held at the breast level. Neonates are able to follow and track a moving object with their eyes and prefer moving objects to stationary ones (Kessen, Haith & Salapatek, 1970).

Babies seem to have an innate visual preference. They prefer more complex stimuli, such as the human face, to a plain surface and will look at a face longer than at other visual patterns (Fantz, 1965; Kagan, 1966; Lewis, 1969). Infants have dark, smoky eyes at birth. Their lids are puffy and the tear ducts do not function. Eye muscles may occasionally drift to a crossed position.

REFLEXES

The fragile appearance of neonates belies the sophistication of their reflexes, which are designed to enhance survival. Reflexes protect the infant and give the central nervous system and brain time to mature and begin to take over the coordinated behaviors (Table 17–1).

Reflexes directly applicable to breastfeeding are the rooting, suckling, swallowing, and gag reflexes. The rooting reflex initiates the act of suckling milk from the mother's breast and is considered vital to life. Although the sucking reflex is less intense during the first three to four days of life, it can be elicited by stroking the infant's lips. Normally present at 32 weeks of gestation, the suckling reflex is developed at 34 weeks of gestation; however, synchronized coordination of suckling and swallowing with breathing appears to be achieved consistently only by infants of more than 37 weeks postconception age (Bu'Lock, Woolridge & Baum, 1990). By three to four months after birth, the rooting reflex begins to diminish. In Chapter 4, Anatomy and Psychophysiology, we describe the infant's oral/suckling capabilities as the cockpit of the nervous system. The presence of rooting, sucking, swallowing, and gag reflexes are barometers that indicate an intact, functioning central nervous system.

LEVELS OF AROUSAL

Young infant behavior can be described by several levels of arousal states (Gill et al., 1988; Prechtl & Beintema, 1975). The Anderson Behavioral State Scale (1988) is a 12-category scale with states ranging from very quiet sleep to hard crying (see the boxed list on p. 462 of 12 behavioral states). The infant's most complex interaction with his environment is made in the quiet awake state; in this state,

TABLE 17–1   REFLEXES OF THE NEONATE

Reflex	Stimulus/description	Appears/disappears
Rooting	Stroke infant's cheek/head will turn toward stimulus	Birth/disappears by 3–4 mo when awake and by 7–8 mo when asleep
Sucking	Stroke infant's lips; place clean finger in infant's mouth/elicits strong sucking movement	Birth/12 mo
Swallowing	Place liquid on posterior tongue/swallow follows	Persists throughout life
Gag	Stimulate posterior pharynx with object	Persists throughout life
Extrusion	Touch infant's tongue/tongue thrusts outward	Birth/2–4 mo
Moro (startle)	Loud noise; jarring/lowering infant's head	Birth/1–4 mo
Tonic neck	Rotate infant's head to one side while infant lies on back/arm and leg extend on the side the infant faces; opposite arm and leg are flexed	Birth to 2 mo/4–6 mo
Babinski	Gentle stroking on the sole of the foot/produces fanning and extension of the toes	Birth/about 18 mo

---

ANDERSON BEHAVIORAL STATE SCALE: BEHAVIORAL STATES

Sleep

Very quiet sleep
Quiet sleep
Restless sleep
Very restless sleep

Awake

Drowsy
Alert inactivity
Quiet awake

Restless

Restless awake
Very restless awake
Fussing
Crying
Hard crying

Derived from Gill, NE, et al.: Effect of nonnutritive sucking on behavioral state in preterm infants before feeding, *Nurs Res* 37: 347–50, 1988.

---

the neonate fixates on and follows objects and turns his head toward any sound. The neonate becomes more alert when he senses a new stimulus; when it is a repetitive stimulus, the infant responds less or *habituates* to the stimuli (Als & Brazelton, 1981). This decrement in response allows the neonate to control his behavioral state. Overactive infants are said to lack this ability to habituate or respond less to repeated stimuli.

THEORIES OF DEVELOPMENT

NATURE VS. NURTURE

Which is most important in a child's development—nature (genes, heredity) or nurture (environment)? At one end of the spectrum the way a child develops is thought to be determined at conception; at the other end, it is seen as a product of the environment. While we can demonstrate by studies cited at the beginning of this chapter that breastfeeding appears to maximize development, the issue is still complex. For example, are the overall parenting patterns of a woman who chooses to breastfeed different from those of a woman who chooses to bottle-feed? We cannot say that any one aspect of child development is determined exclusively by either nature or nurture—clearly each plays a role. The extent of influences from nature vs. nurture differ among developmental theorists. How these two issues interact are

addressed in two popular theories about child development.

ERIKSON'S PSYCHOSOCIAL THEORY

Eric Erikson (1963, 1968) identified eight stages of development which center about conflicts. These conflicts are central issues of crucial importance to the personality at each stage of life. Characteristics of the first two stages (infant and toddler) of Erikson's theory are shown in Table 17–2. Each stage requires resolution of its particular conflict, and each stage widens the social radius of the infant's influence. The first conflict is trust vs. mistrust. According to Erikson, the first year is when confidence in having one's needs met and feeling physically safe results in the infant's either trusting or mistrusting his environment.

Once trust, as opposed to mistrust, is established, the toddler moves into the next stage, in which autonomy must be mastered over shame and doubt. By then ($1\frac{1}{2}$ to 3 years of age), he walks, runs, and expresses himself verbally, eagerly exploring his exciting new world, but still needing reassurance and returning to his mother for "emotional refueling." If an infant is lovingly fed and his biological needs are cared for, he develops a sense of trust in the world. Being left hungry or crying for long periods results in a sense of mistrust of the world. Breastfeeding for nourishment becomes breastfeeding for reassurance and comfort in this stage. The process of individua-

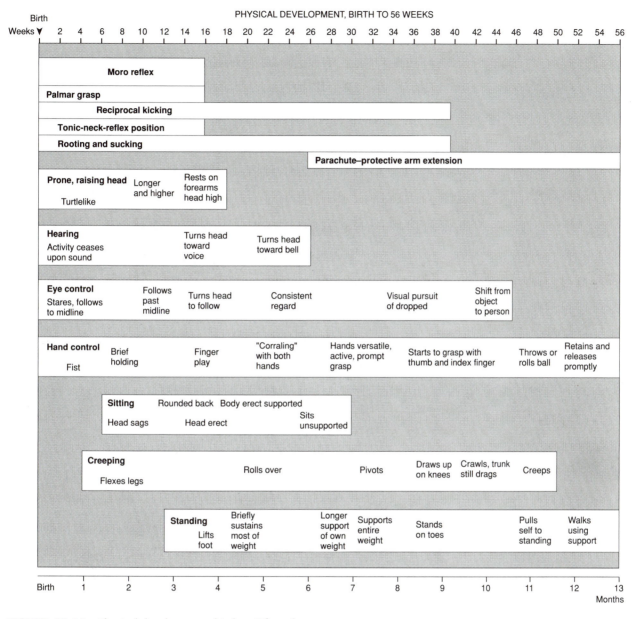

PHYSICAL DEVELOPMENT, BIRTH TO 56 WEEKS

FIGURE 17–1A   Physical development, birth to 56 weeks

tion, a realization that he is a separate individual, un-folds gradually as the child begins to assert control over his life.

PIAGET'S COGNITIVE THEORY

Piaget (1952) stresses the major periods through which humans pass in the course of intellectual maturation. The first is the sensorimotor stage, in which

an infant's knowledge of the world comes primarily through his sensory experiences and motor activities. This period begins with the reflex stage and lasts until the child is two-years old; its main features are seen in Table 17–2.

As infants experience sensory and motor activities, they construct *schemas* (concepts or models) for dealing with information and experiences. These schemas are put into play through complementary

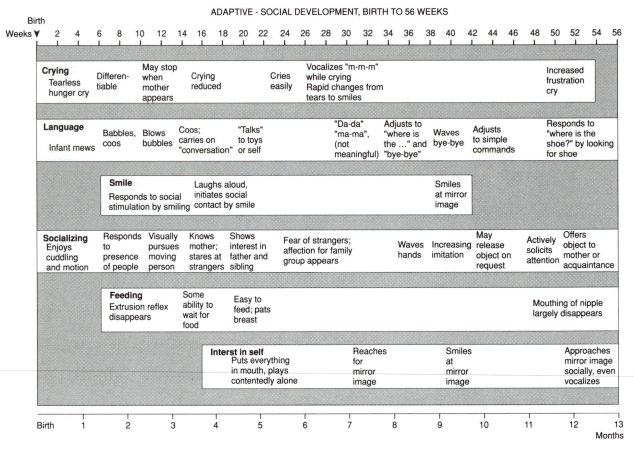

FIGURE 17–1B Adaptive-social development, birth to 56 weeks

processes of assimilation and accommodation. *Assimilation* refers to the process of absorbing new information from the environment and using current structures to deal with the information. *Accommodation* refers to the process whereby the infant alters his or her behavior and adjusts existing schemas to the requirements of objects or events in order to integrate new learning with old—and thus adapt to their ever expanding environments.

Hayes (1987) gives the following example:

> If a child is breastfed, and a pacifier is given to him for the first time, the pacifier nipple may be sufficiently different so that the old sucking patterns do not work well. When this happens, disequilibrium occurs, and the child must restructure the existing view of suckling so it fits with the new information or experience. This process is accommodation. Through these processes, schemas are developed and refined.

The concept of *object permanence* is a feature of the sensorimotor period. Piaget suggests that the infant younger than six to nine months of age lacks the ability for mental representation of the unseen. For instance, when an object such as a toy is out of sight, it ceases to exist and the infant does not search for it. With the ability for mental representation, the infant realizes that an object or person continues to exist when out of sight and he searches for a hidden object. It is now quite certain that person permanency precedes object permanency: an infant does recognize his mother, father, or caretaker long before eight months, and thus experiences loss or anxiety of an all-important person when he or she is not present. Later, as the child broadens the ability to recognize a separate existence from his mother, he begins to tolerate brief periods of separation from different caretakers. The ability roughly coincides with diminishing separation anxiety and with Erikson's estab-

TABLE 17–2   THEORIES OF DEVELOPMENT

Theorist	Infant	Toddler
Erikson (psychosexual)	Trust vs. mistrust (birth to 1 yr)	Autonomy vs. shame and doubt (1 to 3 yrs)
	Requires basic needs (food, comfort, warmth) to be met	Increasing independence in eating, dressing, toileting, and bathing
	Learns to trust self (and environment)	Father becomes important
	Mutual giving and getting between self and caregivers	Limits (firm and consistent) lead to security
	Mistrust results if needs not met consistently or inadequately	Acquires "will"; feeling of self-control, bias for self-esteem
Piaget (cognitive)		Excessive criticism and expectation of perfection leads to shame and doubt about ability to control self and world
	Sensorimotor (birth to 2 yrs); uses senses, motor skills, reflexes to explore	Proconceptual (2 to 7 yrs)
		Self-centered; other centeredness begins
	Object performance	Perception from own point of view
	Trial and error	Use of symbols, especially language
	"Insight" problem solving	Literal interpretation of works and action
	Able to think before they act (18–24 mo)	Judges thing for outcome, consequence to self
		Transductive reasoning

Derived from Erickson, E: *Childhood and society,* New York, 1963, W.W. Norton & Co., Inc.; Piaget, J, and Inhelder, B: *Psychology of the child,* New York, 1969, Basic Books, Inc.

lishment of trust progressing to the beginnings of autonomy.

Piaget's *preoperational period* characterizes toddlers and children from about two to seven years of age. During this period, children develop new abilities to think about situations rather than to just behave in them. The acquisition of expressive language marks the beginning of the preoperational stage of intellectual development. Children in this age group view everything in relation to themselves and are unable to take the role of another: this is called *egocentrism.* This egocentricity leads them to believe that their thoughts and actions are shared by others.

SOCIAL DEVELOPMENT

As infants grow, their periods of waking and socializing lengthen. By six to eight weeks of age, a baby smiles spontaneously to pleasurable stimuli, particularly at human faces. Babies coo and babble to their parents and other fascinated adults who coo and babble back.

By three months the infant is interested in his environment and playfully reaches out to grasp objects, including breasts, nipples, noses, and hair. By six months of age, the infant reaches out to be picked up, squeals with pleasure at recognition of his mother, and enjoys games such as peek-a-boo (Table 17–3).

LANGUAGE/COMMUNICATION
Because infants hear well from birth, they are soon able to discriminate between different intonations, as well as between vowels and consonant sounds. This ability to understand the spoken word is called passive or *receptive language.* The ability to produce meaningful utterances is called *expressive language.* The speech center in the brain borders on the areas of the motor cortex which control both mouth-tongue movement and hand movement. This proximity explains why we tend to express ourselves with our hands as well as our mouths. Infants, as well, use many gestures in association with sounds and expressive language. Children consistently acquire language communication in the following sequence:

TABLE 17–3   CHARACTERISTICS OF INFANTS' THINKING: SENSORIMOTOR STAGE

Major Task

Conquest of object

Throughout this stage, infants are unable to think. Intelligence proceeds from directly acting, as a whole, on the environment to more goal-directed attending to and action on particular objects to make specific events occur. All the senses and motor skills are actively used to define and interpret objects and events.

Perception

Birth to 3 months: View of world and self undifferentiated; unconscious of self.

4 to 6 months: View of world centered around body: self-centered.

After 6 months: View of world as centered around objects.

6 to 12 months: Self seen as separated from objects.

12 to 18 months: Objects seen to have constancy and permanence.

18 to 24 months: Represents spatial relationships between objects and between objects and self (e.g., knows smaller things fit inside larger things.)

Thought

Birth to 3 months: Not present. Uses inborn reflexes and senses.

4 to 6 months: Questions presence of thought. Uses combination of reflexes and senses purposively. Develops habits.

6 to 12 months: Knows objects by how he or she uses them. Knows objects have constant size before knows objects have same form; serially acts out two previously separate behaviors in goal-directed sequences.

12 to 24 months: Object permanence stimulates purposive, intentional use of behaviors to find hidden objects and to cause event via trial and error—problem solve via "insight": can now see effect when given the cause (e.g., knows where train will come out when goes into tunnel). Symbolism and memory begin—uses deferred imitation to discover new ways of acting (e.g., when "pretends" sleep means "know" symbolic sleeping).

Reasoning

Birth to 6 months: Not present.

6 to 24 months: Syncretism: (1) perceives "whole"—impression without analysis of parts or synthesis of relations, (2) lacks systematic exploratory behavior until end of stage, (3) begins to connect series of ideas together into a confused whole.

Language

Birth to 3 months: Undifferentiated cry. Use of different intensities, patterns, and pitches of cry for different feelings (e.g., pain, hunger, fatigue).

6 to 8 weeks: Cooing: contented and happy sounds.

3 to 6 months Babbling: repeated various sounds for sensation of pleasure. *Laughing:* when happy or excited.

6 to 12 months: Spontaneous vocalization: imperfect imitation. *Echolalia:* conscious imitation of sounds.

12 to 18 months: Expressive jargon: use for information, rhythms, and pauses to imitate sentence sounds. *Holophrases:* use of one word to convey meaning. *Gestures:* substitute for or add meaning to speech.

18 to 24 months: Telegraphic speech: use of noun and verb to convey many meanings.

Play

Birth to 6 months: Exercise play: repetition of actions and sounds for pleasure (e.g., rolling over, babbling)

6 to 12 months: Exploratory play: pleasure from causing effect and reconfirming skill (e.g., "peek-a-boo," "drop and retrieve," "pat-a-cake"").

12 to 24 months: Deferred imitation: imitates previously observed actions (not reasons for or purposes of actions) from memory (e.g., pretends to be "Daddy" and goes through getting dressed, shaving, then walks outside, and gets in the "car").

From Servonsky, J, and Opas, SR: *Nursing management of children,* Boston, 1987, Jones and Bartlett Publishers Inc., p. 22.

- Crying—from birth; different rhythms signify emotions and needs (hunger, anger, pain)
- Cooing and gooing—after two weeks; a wide variety of meaningless speech sounds (see Fig. 17–1B)
- Babbling—3 to 12 months; "mama-mama," "dada-dada"
- Holophrasing—12 months; one word sentences
- Telegraphic speech—18 months; subject-verb-object
- Complete sentences—two years.

A baby's duration of crying during the early months of life typically increases until about six weeks of age, followed by a gradual decrease until four months of age (Brazelton, 1962; Bernal, 1972; Wessel et al., 1954; Rebelsky & Black, 1972). Infants cry more and are more wakeful during the late afternoon and evening (Emde, Gaensbauer & Harmon, 1976; Rebelsky & Black, 1972). If the infant is carried during fussy periods, crying and fussing decrease but the number of the infant feedings and the dura-

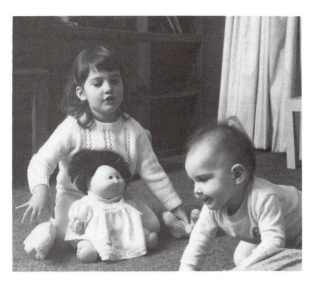

FIGURE 17–2 Developing motor skills by exploring the environment.

tion of his sleep does not change (Hunziker & Barr, 1986).

Although infants differ individually in the number of hours of sleep, *each baby gets as much sleep as he needs.* Newborns sleep an average of 16.5 hours per day; some sleep a total of about 10 hours, others sleep up to 23 hours. Generally infants fuss and cry before falling asleep. The sleeping pattern of breastfed infants differs from formula-fed infants. Breastfed infants wake more often during the night and have shortened sleep patterns (Elias et al., 1986; Carey, 1974). The expression, "he sleeps just like a baby," simply isn't true during the first few months of life for any infant. The typical pattern is one of frequent, short periods of sleep interrupted by crying and fussing. This occurs night and day. The so-called infant "sleep disorders" being diagnosed today are not disorders at all but are normal sleep patterns.

Babies coo, goo, and babble whenever they are alert and content. These sounds change from week to week and are elicited by the smiling faces of adults, by voices, or by touch. Any mother who has breastfed knows that feeding at the breast is a prime time for her baby to communicate actively with coos, babbling, and speech sounds as he looks directly into the eyes of his mother. These exquisite sensory interchanges further bond the mother and baby.

Mothers speak to their infants in a universal dialogue that Sears (1987) calls "motherese." According to Sears:

they instinctively use exaggerated upbeat tones and facial gestures to talk to babies. Mothers use slowly rising crescendo and decrescendo allowing the baby time to process each short vocal package before the next communication arrives. How a mother talks to her baby is more important than what she says.

This sing-song quality of the mother's speech is tailored to the baby's listening abilities. Smiling, grasping, and talking all play important roles in the attachment process, i.e., the reciprocal development of an affectional tie between the mother or care-giver and the baby.

During these interactions the mother not only gives care to her infant but the newborn gives care back to his mother. For this reason, Anderson (1977) calls the mother and infant "mutual care-givers":

As the mother holds her infant to her breast, assumes the *en face* position, and talks to her newborn, her eyes are the optimal distance away and her head, mouth and eyes move slowly and within a closely circumscribed range. Her newborn will also be sending stimuli, such as changes in facial expression, vocalizations, and eye-to-eye contact. The mother's response to such stimuli is immediate.

In a review of the theoretical framework for studying factors which affect the maternal role, Mercer (1981) emphasized the role of the infant in his mother's maternal role-taking process. The newborn's ability to see, hear, and track the human face shows socialization capabilities at birth which allow the infant to be an active partner with the mother in the attachment process.

The infant uses play as a part of the communication process. During the earliest (sensorimotor) stage of life, infants begin with exercise play, such as repeating newly learned actions for pleasure. Stick out your tongue at a young infant and he will stick out his tongue at you. Next, they play using exploration of their skills—crawling backwards down the stairs, for example, or pushing their finger into mother's mouth while breastfeeding and then squealing with glee when she pretends to bite the finger. Table 17–4 shows infant psychosocial and breastfeeding behaviors at certain points of development. The older baby's playful activities as he breastfeeds are a part of communication and attachment with his mother. Deferred imitation play be-

TABLE 17–4 INFANT PSYCHOSOCIAL AND BREASTFEEDING BEHAVIORS BY AGE

Age	Psychosocial behavior	Breastfeeding behavior
First day postpartum	Quiet alert state following birth followed by long sleep.	May or may not feed following delivery. Sleepy, learning how to suckle.
1 mo	Follows objects with eyes; reacts to noise by stopping behavior or crying.	Becoming efficient at suckling; feedings last approximately 17 minutes. Feedings now 8 to 16 times per day.
2 mo	Smiles; vocalizes in response to interactions.	Easily pacified by frequent breastfeedings.
3 mo	Shows increased interest in surroundings. Voluntarily grasps objects. Vocalizes when spoken to. Turns head as well as eyes in response to moving object.	Will interrupt feeding to turn to look at father or other familiar person coming into room and to smile at mother.
4–5 mo	Shows interest in strange settings. Smiles at mirror image.	Continues to enjoy frequent feedings at the breast.
6 mo	Laughs aloud. Shows increased awareness of care-givers vs. strangers. May become distressed if mother or care-giver leaves.	Solids offered. Fewer feedings. Feeds longer before sleep for the night. May begin waking to nurse more often at night.
7–8 mo	Imitates actions and noises. Responds to name. Responds to "no." Enjoys peek-a-boo games. Reaches for toys that are out of reach.	Will breastfeed anytime, anywhere. Actively attempts to get to breast, i.e., will try to unbutton mother's blouse.
9–10 mo	Distressed by new situations or people. Waves bye-bye. Reaches for toys that are out of reach.	Easily distracted by surroundings and interrupts feedings frequently. May hold breast with one or both hands while feeding.
11–12 mo	Drops objects deliberately to be picked up by other people. Rolls ball to another person. Speaks a few words. Appears interested in picture books. Shakes head for "no."	Tries "acrobatic" breastfeeding, i.e., assumes different positions while keeping nipple in mouth.
12–15 mo	Fears unfamiliar situations but will leave mother's side to explore familiar surroundings. Shows emotions, e.g., love, anger, fear. Speaks several words. Understands meaning of many words.	Uses top hand to play while feeding: forces finger into mother's mouth, plays with her hair, and pinches her other nipple. Pats mother's chest when wants to breastfeed. Hums or vocalizes while feeding. Verbalizes need to breastfeed—may use "code" word.
16–20 mo	Has frequent temper tantrums. Increasingly imitates parents. Enjoys solitary play or observing others. Speaks 6 to 10 words.	Verbalizes delight with breastfeeding. Takes mother by the hand and leads her to favorite nursing chair.

TABLE 17–4 INFANT PSYCHOSOCIAL AND BREASTFEEDING BEHAVIORS BY AGE

Age	Psychosocial behavior	Breastfeeding behavior
20–24 mo	Helps with simple tasks. Has fewer temper tantrums. Engages in parallel play. Combines 2 or 3 words. Speaks 15 to 20 words.	Stands up while nursing at times. Nursing mostly for comfort. Feeding before bedtime is usually last feeding before weaning. Willing to wait for feeding until later when asked to do so by mother.

gins at around 18 months of age when toddlers begin to imitate the behavior and language they see and hear. For example, little girls, who are already adopting the gender role of their mothers, will very seriously and readily "nurse" their dolls at their "breasts." (See Fig. 17–3.)

ATTACHMENT/BONDING

This exquisite dance of reciprocal reinforcement between the mother-infant dyad leads to the mother "taking-in" her maternal role, cementing the mother-infant bond. Early theorists paved the way for understanding the processes of bonding and attachment. Konrad Lorenz (1935) noted the behavior and imitation of the mother animal by the young which is necessary for survival and labeled it *imprinting*. It is believed that attachment and bonding are the human equivalent of imprinting.

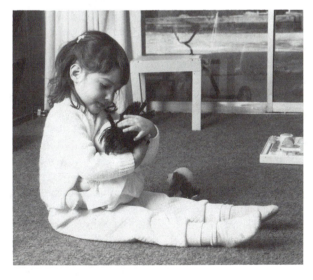

FIGURE 17–3 Child "nursing" doll.

In the early 1950s Bowlby (1951) emphasized the importance of an infant's developing a primary attachment to a caring, responsible adult. A decade later, Harlow and Harlow (1965) demonstrated the importance of contact comfort for the attachment and emotional well-being of the newborn rhesus monkey. When presented with "surrogate" mothers—one formed out of unpadded chicken wire and equipped with milk-filled bottles, the other made out of padded terry cloth but without bottles—the baby monkeys spent much more time with the warm, cloth-covered mothers, only going briefly to the bottles for food.

Rubin (1967) showed a progressive attachment which results from touching: a mother first explores her newborn's extremities with her fingertips, rapidly moves to the baby's arms and legs, and finally caresses the trunk with the palm of her hand. Rubin (1977) prefers the term "binding-in" to bonding because it more accurately describes the formative stages of the maternal-child relationship as a process, not a state:

A conceptual model for the binding-in processes might well be like the weaving of a tapestry. Not a cord, nor a bond, nor a welding job, rather a large creative work, framed between the child and the mother's own significant social world, systematically and progressively developed for durability against time and stress to form the substance of her own personal identity and the fabric of her relationship with this particular child.

Ainsworth and colleagues (1978) studied brief infant separation from mothers in a laboratory situation to measure the degree of attachment. Mothers defined by the researchers as "securely attached" to their infants were most sensitive to their baby's needs, whereas mothers identified as "insecurely attached" to their infants were less emotionally expressive, felt more aversion to close body contact with the babies, and were more frequently irritated, resentful, and angry (Ainsworth, 1982).

A multitude of circumstances affect the mother-child relationship, which begins before the child is born; even unseen, the mother imagines or fantasizes about her child. According to Ann Clark (1976):

> Her perceptions of the "dream child" and, subsequently, her relationship with that child will not only be influenced by her self-concept but also by her total life experience. Her culture, social relationship, economic status, and state of health can all add to or detract from her relationship with her unborn child. If she experiences social isolation and economic deprivation during her pregnancy, her emotional reserves will be lowered. If she experiences physical discomfort and ill health, her physical stamina may be depleted. Thus, the support she receives during pregnancy and from her total environment will affect her acceptance and readiness for mothering.

The infant's birth forces the mother to compare her real-life baby with her dreams, fantasies, and expectations. If reality and expectations are congruent, attachment begins soon after birth; if they are divergent, the mothers must first work through the loss of the "dream child" and strive to fall in love with this stranger who bears little resemblance to the child of her fantasies.

Klaus and Kennell (1975) moved the concept of attachment one step further by popularizing the existence of a sensitive period for attachment shortly after birth. Barring excessive medication of the mother during delivery, a newborn will normally be in an alert state for at least one hour following birth. During this period, the mother will spend a significant amount of time gazing *en face* into her infant's eyes, touching, and stroking. The neonate is born in a state of readiness for this human interaction. The infant's remarkable perceptual and sensory abilities (hearing, seeing, smelling, and tasting) at birth facilitate the attachment process. As attachment becomes established, the newborn is observed to move his arms and legs in rhythm to the cadences of the mother's voice—in a synchronic pattern which may be the foundation for later speech (Condon &

Sander, 1974). Such interaction is commonly known as entrainment, and its effects carry over into later life.

An active partner in the attachment process, the infant initiates about one-half of parent-infant interaction. Through predictable and clear-cut transmission of *cues* or nonverbal signals, neonates are capable of producing the desired behavior in the parent and selectively reinforcing parent behavior. In many ways the infant is as competent as the parents, "perhaps even more so than young, inexperienced parents" (Anderson, 1981; Bell, 1974).

The baby's cry (impossible to ignore for very long) is his cue for attention, and his mother responds by picking up, feeding, or carrying him. The perceptive mother is attuned to her baby's cues and reacts to them appropriately. If he coos and smiles, she reacts happily to his pleasure. The infant's contentment or irritability signal the mother to increase or decrease stimulation. If parents are aware of these cues as a method of communication for their infant, they respond by viewing their infants as individuals. Informing mothers about the behavioral characteristics of their babies is an effective means of enhancing the interaction between a mother and her infant (Anderson, 1981; Clark, 1976). Breastfeeding, with its frequent touching, holding, and eye-to-eye contact, offers enhanced opportunities for attachment and responding to infant cues. Certainly the frequency of subjective verbal responses by mothers who state they "feel closer" to the breastfed child merits serious consideration. By breastfeeding the infant may exert more control: for example, the decision to end the feeding is a shared decision between the mother and baby when the mother "reads" and responds to her baby's behaviors. In bottle-feeding, on the other hand, the mother is chiefly responsible for ending the feeding.

The 1970s social movement to incorporate rooming-in and mother-baby care into hospital maternity care spawned many studies on maternal-infant attachment and bonding. Most of these studies demonstrated that increased mother-baby contact was associated with stronger attachment (Anisfeld & Lipper, 1983; Klaus et al., 1970; Kontos, 1978; Thomson, Hartsock & Larson, 1979; Anisfeld et al., 1990). It was also shown that children who have minimal separation from their mother after birth have higher levels of parental interaction and personal health in later years (deChateau & Wiberg, 1977; O'Connor et al., 1979). This proliferation of

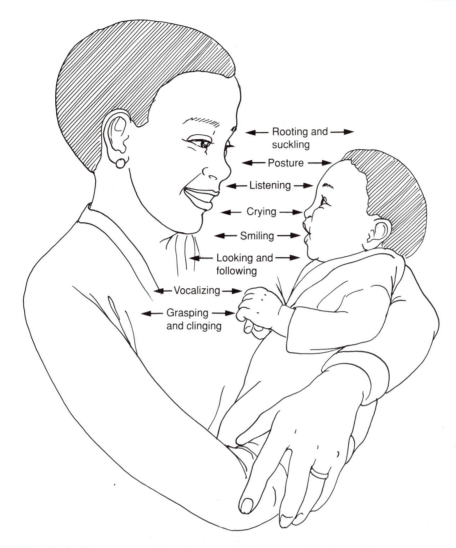

FIGURE 17–4 Components of attachment and their interaction in specific areas. From Mott, S, Fazekas, NF, and James, SR: *Nursing care of children and families,* Menlo Park, Calif., 1985, Addison-Wesley Publishing Co., Inc., p. 206.

research on attachment and the benefits of rooming-in ceased in the 1980s because rooming-in and mother-baby care was incorporated by most hospitals and because of criticisms that other maternal factors—such as age, education, and socioeconomic status—explained more of the variance in maternal attachment than did early contact (Campbell & Taylor, 1979; Lamb, 1983; Siegel et al., 1980; Svejda & Campos, 1980).

As a result, the current view of attachment and bonding is that while immediate postpartum mother-child contact is desirable, it is not critical. Almost all parents are attached to their babies, even if they experience marked disruption of the early par-

ent-child contact which most healthy mothers and babies now take for granted (see Chapter 9). Parents should be assured that not having the opportunity to interact and bond with their baby soon after birth does not cause irreparable damage to their child (Klaus & Kennell, 1982; Wolff, 1970).

TEMPERAMENT

During the past two decades researchers have studied the temperament of the infant and how it influences parenting. The longitudinal work of Thomas and Chess (1977) and Thomas et al. (1963) suggests that every child exhibits a particular temperament from birth and that (1) infants have individual characteristics even as newborns; (2) these characteristics differentiate infants one from another; and (3) they remain constant over time. Categories of response which influence a child's temperament include: activity level; regularity of body functions; adaptability; response to new situations; sensory threshold; intensity of reaction; quality of mood; distractibility; and attention span and persistence. These characteristics were rated for three temperaments: the easy child, the difficult child, and the slow-to-warm-up child (Thomas & Chess, 1977). Characteristic temperament styles of each are seen in Table 17–5.

Sears (1987) reduced these three temperament characteristics into two categories, which he terms "high-need" and "low-need" babies, and popularized the concept for parents to understand and use. High-need babies are fussy, seem to breastfeed "all the time," and cry if put down; low-need babies are content, cuddly and do not need constant carrying or attention. Two questionnaires or tools for assessing the temperament of an infant or child are the Infant Temperament Questionnaire (ITQ) for infants four to 12 months of age (Carey & McDevitt, 1978) and the Toddler Temperament Scale for children one to three years of age (Hegvik, McDevitt & Carey, 1982). The ITQ scores identify a child's temperamental style; the results may be used as an opportunity for making parents aware of their child's temperament and for suggesting appropriate parenting skills.

TABLE 17–5   CHARACTERISTICS OF TEMPERAMENT STYLES IN CHILDREN

Factor	Easy child	Slow-to-warm-up child	Difficult child
Activity level—amount of physical activity during sleep, feeding, play, dressing	High	Medium	Low
Regularity—of body functions in sleep, hunger, bowel movements	Fairly regular	Variable	Fairly irregular
Adaptability to change in routine—ease or difficulty with which initial response can be modified in socially desirable way	Generally adaptable	Variable	Generally slow to adapt
Response to new situations—initial reaction to new stimuli, foods, people, places, toys, or procedures	Approach	Variable	Withdrawal
Level of sensory threshold—amount of external stimulation, such as sounds or changes in food or people, necessary to produce a response	High threshold (much stimulation needed)	Medium threshold	Low threshold (little stimulation needed)
Intensity of response—energy content of responses regardless of their quality	Generally intense	Variable	Generally mild
Positive or negative mood—energy content of responses regardless of their quality	Generally positive	Variable	Generally negative
Distractibility—effectiveness of external stimuli (sounds, toys, people) in interfering with ongoing behavior	Easily distractible	Variable	Nondistractible
Persistence and attention span—duration of maintaining specific activities with or without external obstacles	Persistent	Variable	Nonpersistent
Percentage of all children	40%	15%	10%

Source: Carey, WB, and McDevitt, SC: Revision of the Infant Temperament Questionnaire, *Pediatrics,* 61:735–39, 1978.
From Servonsky, J, and Opas, SR: *Nursing management for children,* Boston, 1987, Jones and Bartlett Publishers, Inc., p. 180.

STRANGER DISTRESS

As the infant grows older the significance of his major care-giver is recognized, and during the second half of the first year of life another developmental phenomenon appears: stranger distress. The infant, who up to that time has been curious about everything in his environment including strangers, suddenly frowns, cries, and may even attempt physical escape when a stranger approaches. Stranger distress appears quite suddenly as early as six months but more commonly at eight months. It is more pronounced when the mother or primary caretaker is not present. As a consequence, exposure to a variety of strangers is disruptive to an infant at this age. Although stranger distress occurs at about the same period of development as separation anxiety, it is a separate phenomenon.

SEPARATION

As mother or father leave the room, anxious eyes follow. Almost instantly the child's face is contorted by rage; he cries loudly and may throw himself wildly about, kicking and screaming. No action brings solace at this point. This behavior is the first phase of separation anxiety, a phenomenon which emerges toward the middle of the first year of life, peaks from 13 to 20 months, and decreases after the second birthday. Separation anxiety, according to psychoanalytic theory, is the painful effect of anxiety engendered by the threat of actual separation from a loved one. Bowlby (1973) and Robertson (1958) delineated three phases of separation anxiety in young children: protest, despair, and denial.

Protest.   In an angry and yearning attempt to recover his mother or primary caretaker, the child violently cries and throws himself about, kicking and screaming. He is angry at the world and at his mother for leaving him. He feels that she must be angry with him also, since she left him. The protest phase can last from a few hours to several days depending on the energy of the child, his age, relationship with his mother, and the quality of the new environment.

Despair.   Gradually the child moves into quiet grieving and mourning as he begins to accept his fate. He shows little interest in his environment but suffers intensely; his expression is one of great sadness. Regressive behavior, such as thumb-sucking, occurs as the child turns inward for solace.

Detachment or denial.   The child develops a defense mechanism to deal with his loss by detaching himself from the importance of his mother's love. He gradually begins to interact with others, approaching anyone and even appearing cheerful. This stage is often misinterpreted as adapting or "settling in." Actually, he is coping with his loss by indiscriminately attaching to caretakers. When he is reunited with his mother at this point, he may appear uninterested and not seem to recognize her.

IMPLICATIONS FOR PRACTICE

Deviations from these normal patterns of attachment signal that a problem may be present; hence assessing the infant's or child's growth and developmental level—and being able to apply a working knowledge of developmental patterns—is as important as knowing the specifics of a child's health problem. If a baby is being examined, for example, the close proximity of his mother helps to reduce stranger distress. Although "friendly" (nonwhite) appearing clothing helps to ameliorate the baby's distress, by no means does it prevent his crying and avoidance behavior as the examiner approaches him—especially for the first time.

How can health-care workers who are strangers to the child minimize this fear? First, take advantage of his attachment to his mother by relating to the mother first in the presence of the child. During this interaction with his mother, the child is carefully observing her response to and acceptance of the "stranger" and will take cues from her. Even body position is important: turning slightly sideways away from the child to avoid *en face* contact while talking with the mother is less threatening to the child. Renee Spitz (1946) demonstrates in one of his films that when a stranger approaches with his back to the child, the child instead of crying, becomes curious and will even reach out after a bit and tug at the stranger. Using a soft, low voice instead of a loud or high-pitched one is more pleasing to the child and facilitates his acceptance of this new person in his life.

Nursing and medicine have made great progress in recognizing and applying development theories into practice. Since a comprehensive listing and discussion of developmental assessment and screening tools is not within the scope of this book, we refer the reader to the many excellent references that discuss child development in detail. In addition, we remind the reader about the use of assessment tools, such as the Bayley Scale of Infant Development, the Denver Development Screening Test, and the Brazelton Neonatal Behavior Assessment Scale.

IMMUNIZATIONS

Immunizations have greatly reduced the incidence of childhood diseases worldwide. Many infections which contributed to high infant mortality in the past can now be prevented through a series of immunizations. Smallpox, for example, has been virtually eliminated and poliomyelitis, rubella, and rubeola have decreased markedly since the rigorous enforcement of a series of immunizations. In the United States, the Federal Immunization Initiative of 1977 provides access to immunization for everyone, regardless of ability to pay (Richmond & Filner, 1979).

In the United States the usual schedule is for three immunizations for DPT-OPV (diphtheria, pertussis or whooping cough, tetanus, and oral polio vaccine) in the first year of life and one each for measles, mumps, and rubella, plus another for *H. influenzae* type b in the second year of life. The *H. influenzae* type b vaccine has been approved by the FDA for use at two, four, and six months of age, with a booster at 15 to 18 months of age. Children aged six to 12 months are at highest risk of *H. influenzae* type b infection. The exact timing of the immunizations is not nearly as important as the fact that the child eventually receives all of the immunization doses. Primary immunization of infants and children as currently recommended by the Committee of Infectious Diseases of the American Academy of Pediatrics is given in Table 17–6.

Hepatitis B is a major public health problem in the western Pacific and in central southern Africa. Of the estimated 300 million chronic carriers of hepatitis B virus in the world, about 80% live in Asia and Oceania. Many countries and areas in the western Pacific region, including China, have started routine hepatitis B immunization of newborns.

Generally, vaccines which contain attenuated "live" organisms are more effective than inactivated

TABLE 17–6 SCHEDULE OF IMMUNIZATIONS FOR INFANTS AND CHILDREN (American Academy of Pediatrics, 1991)

Age	Type of vaccine
2 months	DTP, TVOPV, HbOC or PRP-OMP
4 months	DTP, TVOPV, HbOC or PRP-OMP
6 months	DTP, HbOC (TVOPV optional)
12 months	PRP-OMP
15 months	MMR, HbOC[a]
18 months	DTP, TPOPV[b]
4–6 years	DTP, TVOPV
11–12 years	MMR
14–16 years	Td, TVOPV
Thereafter	Td every 10 years

DTP = diptheria, tetanus toxoid and pertussis

TVOPV = trivalent live oral polio vaccine

HbOC = Haemophilus influenzae b congugate, Hib-TITER™ by Praxis

PRP-OMP = Haemophilus influenzae b (Hib) conjugate, PedvaxHIP™ by Merck, Sharp and Dome

MMR = live attenuated measles, mumps and rubella viruses

Td = adult tetanus toxoid and adult diptheria toxoid

[a]Tuburculin testing may be done at the same visit
[b]May be given simultaneously with MMR at 15 months
Note: A child should receive either HbOC or PRP-OMP, not both. Each vaccine is equally effective using the appropriate schedule. Once a dose of one type of Hib vaccine is given, the vaccinated child should continue to receive that same type of vaccine.
American Academy of Pediatrics: *Report of the committee on infectious diseases,* Elk Grove, Ill., 1991.

or "killed" vaccines. Live vaccines induce long-lasting immunity but they are also likely to cause adverse reactions, such as that seen in the vaccine for pertussis. Although killed vaccines are noninfectious and can be prepared in a purified form, they usually induce a shorter period of protection; therefore booster injections may be needed (Bellanti, 1990). Most vaccines are given parenterally; an exception is the live oral polio vaccine.

Live-virus vaccines do multiply within the mother's body, but most are not secreted in breast milk. The exception is rubella (Losonsky et al., 1982), which can be transmitted through breastmilk; however, the infection is well tolerated by the infant (Wolfe, 1990). Earlier concerns about the possibility that breastmilk antibodies may neutralize the virus after vaccination have not been substantiated. Krogh et al. (1989) compared breastfed and formula-fed infants of a group of mothers who had been immunized with the rubella vaccine postpartum with a second group of naturally immune women who were seropositive for rubella and did not receive immunization after childbirth. Subsequent immunization with rubella vaccine of breastfed infants whose mothers had received postpartum immunization resulted in a serum antibody response that was similar to the response observed in the formula-fed infants or the infants of naturally immune mothers who had not received immunization. Thus, early neonatal exposure to the rubella virus in breastmilk does not enhance or suppress subsequent responses to rubella vaccination in early childhood.

Breastfed infants are also successfully immunized with oral poliovirus vaccine while receiving breastmilk, and it is *not* necessary to withhold breastfeeding after administration of OPV. In a retrospective study of 52 breastfed infants and 53 bottle-fed infants, Deforest et al. (1973) reported that serum antibody responses after oral polio vaccine administered at two, four, and six months of age—without withholding breastfeeding for any period of time—were comparable with those of bottle-fed in-

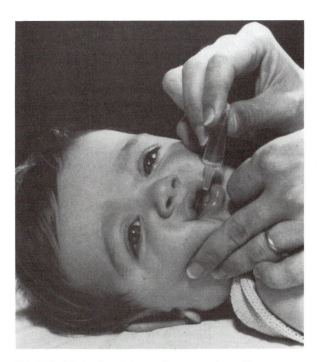

FIGURE 17–5 Receiving polio protection. (Courtesy WHO/PAHO/C. Gaggero.)

fants who were similarly vaccinated. John and colleagues (1976) later confirmed these results in a study of 300 American Indian infants.

In fact, breastfeeding may enhance immunity in some cases. Pabst et al. (1989) found that infants who were breastfeeding had enhanced cell-mediated immune response to Bacille Calmette Guerin (BCG) vaccine given at birth. In another study, by the same group of investigators, breastfed infants immunized with *H. influenza* type b vaccine had higher antibody levels at seven months and at 12 months of age—strong evidence that breastfeeding enhances the active immune response in the first year of life.

Considerable controversy surrounds the pertussis (whooping cough) vaccination. Some parents fear having their child vaccinated for whooping cough because the vaccine has been associated with encephalopathy following its administration. Symptoms, usually convulsions and coma, develop within a few days. Risk of damage to the infant's central nervous system from the vaccine varies depending on the source: from one out of 62,000 vaccinations (Children at Risk, 1987; Coulter & Fisher, 1985) to one out of 310,000 vaccinations (Fulginiti, 1984). If a child develops a high fever, drowsiness, or a convulsion after an initial DPT injection, pertussis should be omitted for all subsequent injections and DT used. Some physicians give partial doses, particularly when parents report that the baby has developed reactions to previous doses.

During 1989 and 1990, the federal vaccine injury compensation system set up by the National Childhood Vaccine Injury Compensation Act of 1986 paid nearly 27 million dollars to families of children injured or killed by vaccines (DPT, 1990). It is hoped that an improved acellular pertussis vaccine that has much less risk will soon be available. Of an estimated 3.5 million children born each year, 90% receive five doses of pertussis vaccine in the first five years of life.

DENTAL HEALTH

The first primary (deciduous) teeth to erupt are the lower central incisors, which appear at about six to eight months of age. By $2\frac{1}{2}$ years of age, children have a full set of primary teeth which will be replaced by permanent teeth. While breastfeeding helps to protect the teeth, healthy dental practices should in no way be neglected because the child is breastfeeding. Teaching and guidance to parents should encourage:

- optimal prenatal nutrition and restriction of refined carbohydrates in the child's diet (including fluids the older infant drinks from a cup)
- use of fluorides when the amount in the water supply is inadequate (parents can check with the local health department); human milk contains only trace amounts, even if the mother is drinking fluorinated water
- regular brushing as soon as the primary teeth erupt
- no coating of pacifiers with sweeteners or the use of hard-candy pacifiers
- dental visits after about two years of age.

Nursing-bottle caries is a term applied to progressive dental caries aggravated by sucking on a bottle while sleeping. Decay usually starts with the maxillary (upper) incisors and often spares the mandibular (lower) incisors. Overall, breastfed children have less dental decay than those who are fed otherwise (Tank & Storvick, 1965). The probable reasons for this include the mechanical differences between breastfeeding and bottle-feeding. Drawn deep into the child's mouth, the human nipple rests at the junction of the hard and soft palate during breastfeeding, posterior to the child's teeth. A suckle is automatically followed by a swallow, thus preventing the teeth from being bathed in pooled milk. By contrast, the milk from a bottle flows out spontaneously with only the slightest pressure into the anterior part of the mouth, permitting stagnation of the milk on and around the teeth (Abbey, 1979).

Brams and Maloney (1983), Gardner, Norwood, and Eisensen (1977) and Kotlow (1977) have reported a condition similar to nursing-bottle caries which occurred in breastfed children, especially those who breastfed for two to three years and spent long, uninterrupted periods at the breast. Their experience probably represents a very small percentage of all the young children who breastfeed for long periods at night through the millenia.

As the numbers of breastfeeding toddlers increase, however, it is reasonable to expect that some of them will develop dental disease, especially after the introduction of solids which often contain sugar. Dental caries is also thought to be an inherited trait;

therefore, these children probably represent a group who are more susceptible, and prolonged nocturnal exposure to human milk becomes a risk factor. It could be argued that some breastfed children develop caries not because they were breastfed, but in spite of it. Unfortunately, the susceptibility of the child's teeth to decay cannot be clinically predicted, and caries may be extensive before they become evident.

Oral-facial development is a health issue in which breastfeeding has a measurable impact. The oral-facial development of a child is affected by feeding methods, swallowing patterns, and finger sucking (Sanger & Bystrom, 1982). There are several mechanisms by which bottle-feeding might contribute to the development of malocclusion, such as a forward thrusting of the tongue, which in turn leads to underdevelopment of the masseter and buccinator muscles (Stanley & Lundeen, 1980; Straub, 1960), abnormal swallowing patterns, and increased prevalence of nonnutritive sucking. Two studies suggest that breastfeeding prevents malocclusion.

While some researchers have shown minimal (Myers & Hertzberg, 1988) or no (Humphreys & Leighton, 1950) differences in the frequency of malocclusion based on the method of feeding, a retrospective study by Adamiak (1981) in Czechoslovakia found that the longer the duration of breastfeeding, the lower the incidence of malocclusion anomalies. Among those breastfed for less than three months or not at all, 36% had anomalies, whereas 24% of those breastfed for longer than six months had anomalies. Labbok and Hendershot (1987) analyzed data from the Child Health Supplement of the 1981 National Health Interview Survey and also found that increased duration of breastfeeding was associated with a decline in the proportion of children with malocclusion. This trend was constant for all variables tested and remained even when adjusted for age and maternal educational level as a proxy of socioeconomic status.

SOLID FOODS

For every breastfed infant a point is reached when breastmilk alone no longer fulfills the baby's nutritional needs. If breastfeeding is continued exclusively, the baby will eventually become malnourished (Mata, 1990). How long exclusive breastfeeding can satisfy the nutrient needs of babies is a crucial public-health issue, especially in areas with an unsafe water supply and poor sanitation, where early supplements are likely to be associated with infections (Naing & Co, 1991).

WHEN SHOULD THEY BE INTRODUCED?

Solid foods are not necessary, nor are they recommended, before the baby is four to six months of age (AAP, 1980; AAP, 1981). Developmental cues for introducing solid foods to the infant are the fading of his tongue-extrusion reflex, eruption of teeth, the ability to sit, and purposeful movement of the baby's hands and fingers, all of which normally occur during the middle months of the first year of life. Also, in the full-term baby, the prenatal storage of iron acquired during the last trimester of pregnancy gradually begins to diminish by four to five months of age. This approach suggests developmental readiness for solids.

Most infants will at first actively resist the advances of even the most enterprising mother in her attempts to spoon-feed him during the early months of life. Before six months of age, a baby has an extrusion-tongue reflex and is unable to push food to the back of his mouth. The newspaper cartoons of a triple-bibbed infant propped in a high chair and surrounded by a wide circumference of newspapers and spit-out food reflects an unpleasant reality. Developmentally speaking, the ability to tolerate solids offers no evidence that their early introduction is advantageous. In fact, the practice may initiate a chain of disadvantages that include allergies and obesity (Guthrie & Riordan, 1977).

Early introduction of solids is still a common practice in the United States, even though the American Academy of Pediatrics' Committee on Nutrition has consistently held that no nutritional advantage results from the introduction of supplemental foods prior to four to six months of age (AAP, 1981). In fact, mothers sometimes competitively seek to outdo one another in initiating solid food, as if how soon an infant eats adult food is a measure of his maturity (Parrago et al., 1988). A few far-seeing and alert pediatricians have warned against the early introduction of solid foods (Gyorgy, 1957). They argued that the practice was not substantiated by sound nutritional principles but was rather the result of both commercial marketing and maternal competition.

Despite official recommendations and a concerted effort to teach parents to delay solids, many infants still receive solid foods during their first few months of life. The first solid food is usually cereal, which is given in the evening because some parents wrongly believe that feeding solids to the baby will help him sleep through the night. However, feeding infants solids prior to bedtime is not related to evening sleep patterns; according to well-controlled studies, babies who receive solids before bedtime have the same sleep patterns as babies who are not given solids (Keane et al., 1988; Macknin, Medendorp & Maier, 1989).

WHAT SHOULD BE OFFERED?

If solids are started after six months of age the sequence of foods is not critical. If solids are introduced earlier, then the following order is suggested: fruits, meats and cereals, yellow vegetables, and lastly legumes. For cereal which requires mixing with a liquid, breastmilk (instead of cow's milk) avoids any potential allergic reaction. Egg yolk, if carefully separated from the white (which is highly allergenic), is high in protein and iron, hypoallergenic, and therefore safe.

Infants need additional water when solids are started because of their added osmolar load. Juices, which are good sources of vitamin C, can be introduced when the child can drink from a cup. Using one with a tight-fitting lid or a straw prevents excessive spilling at first.

A basic rule is to feed the infant foods in as close to a natural state as possible: pieces of raw, peeled apples, slices of banana, toasted whole wheat bread, orange sections, and a chicken leg with the skin removed are all good choices. They can be picked up and held and are tasty, nutritious, and satisfying to chew. Giving small amounts at first and gradually increasing the amount (along with continued breast-feeding) avoids constipation. Mothers should be prepared for changes in consistency, odor, and frequency of stool when solids are begun. To test for allergy, each new food should be fed for at least one week before a new one is added. Generally all foods which are eaten by the family can be given to the infant in a consistency that he can handle. The beginning eater enjoys foods of all kinds and relishes the tactile pleasures of squeezing, smearing, and crushing his food—an activity he should be allowed with impunity since it is also a learning experience. General guidelines for initiating solid foods are in Table 17-7.

The optimal way to introduce solid foods to the

TABLE 17–7 INTRODUCING SOLID FOODS INTO A BREASTFED INFANT'S DIET

When to introduce	Approximate total daily intake of solids*	Description of foods and hints about giving them
6–7 mo if infant is breastfed	Dry cereal. Start with ½ tsp (dry measurement), gradually increase to 2–3 Tbsp. Vegetables: Start with 1 tsp. gradually increase to 2 Tbsp. Fruit: Start with 1 tsp. gradually increase to 2 Tbsp. Divide food among 4 feedings per day (if possible).	Cereal: Offer iron-enriched baby cereal. Begin with single grains. Mix cereal with an equal amount of breastmilk Vegetables: Try a mild-tasting vegetable first (carrots, squash, peas, green beans). Stronger-flavored vegetables (spinach, sweet potatoes) may be tried after the infant accepts some mild-tasting ones. Fruits: Mashed ripe banana and unsweetened, cooked, bland fruits (apples, peaches, pears) are usually well liked. Apple juice and grape juice (unsweetened) may be introduced. Initially, dilute juice with an equal amount of water. Introduce one new food at a time and offer it several times before trying another new food. Give a new food once a day for a day or two; increase to twice a day as the infant begins to enjoy the food. Watch for signs of intolerance. Include some foods that are good sources of vitamin C (other than orange juice).
6–7 mo if infant is breastfed	Dry cereal. Gradually increase up to 4 Tbsp. Fruits and vegetables: Gradually increase up to 3 Tbsp of each Meat: Start with 1 tsp and gradually increase to 2 Tbsp. Divide food among 4 feedings per day (if possible).	Meat: Offer pureed or milled poultry (chicken or turkey) followed by lean meat (veal, beef); lamb has a stronger flavor and may not be as well liked initially. Liver is a good source of iron; it may be accepted at the beginning of a meal with a familiar vegetable. Continue introducing new cereals, fruits, and vegetables as the infant indicates he is ready to accept them, but always one at a time; introduce legumes last.
7–9 mo if infant is breastfed	Dry cereal: Up to ½ c. Fruits and vegetables: Up to ¼ to ½ c of each. Meats: Up to 3 Tbsp. Divide food among 4 feedings per day (if possible).	Soft table foods may be introduced; for example, mashed potatoes and squash and small pieces of soft, peeled fruits. Toasted whole grain or enriched bread may be added when the infant begins chewing. If introduction of solids is delayed until now, it is not necessary to use strained fruits and vegetables. Continue using *iron-fortified* baby cereals.
8–12 mo	Dry cereal: Up to ½ c. Bread: About 1 slice. Fruits and vegetables: Up to ½ c of each. Divide food among 4 feedings per day (if possible).	Table foods may be added gradually. Cut table foods into small pieces. Start with ones that do not require too much chewing (cooked, cut green beans and carrots, noodles, ground meats, tuna fish, soft cheese, plain yogurt). If fish is offered, check closely to be sure there are no bones in the serving. Mashed, cooked egg yolk and orange juice may be added at about 9 months of age. Sometimes offer peanut butter or thoroughly cooked dried peas and beans in place of meat.

Modified from Suitor, CW, and Hunter, MF: Nutrition principles and applications in health promotion. Philadelphia, 1980, J.B. Lippincott Co.
*Some infants do not need or want these amounts of food; some may need a little more food.

baby is to offer tastes from the mother's or father's plate at mealtime. If the baby has teeth and is ready for them, mashing with a fork is all that is necessary. Over the next few weeks, the baby begins to take so much from the mother's plate that it becomes necessary to prepare his own plate of food from the family meal (NMAA, 1979).

If additional baby food needs to be mashed or blended, foods prepared at home are not only more wholesome and nutritious but also cost less than commercially prepared baby foods. Carrots and apple sauce, for example, cost about one-half the store price when prepared at home. Beef and chicken blended in the kitchen provide more nutrients by weight than their commercial counterparts, chiefly because they contain less water. With the aid of an electric blender, food mill, or grinder, preparing baby food is easily accomplished. The foods should be selected from high-quality fresh or frozen fruits, vegetables, or meats, with special attention to hygienic preparation and storage. For convenience, small individualized portions can be stored safely in the refrigerator or freezer for reasonable periods of time.

Some parents prefer to buy commercial baby food rather than to make their own. Commercial baby food is generally produced by pulverizing fruit, grain, vegetable, and meat ingredients with water and adding filler ingredients. In the typical selection of strained foods purchased by the average mother, about 80% of the calories are carbohydrates in the form of modified starch and sucrose. Since 1977, leading manufacturers of baby food have stopped adding salt and sugar to their products.

WHERE SHOULD SOLID FOODS BE GIVEN?

The best place to feed a baby is at the family table at mealtime—in a high chair or on someone's knee. Young children love to be considered one of the family and sit at the same height as the rest of the family. Even before the infant is ready to take solids, he enjoys being nearby during meals and can "join in" by chewing on food like bread crust or a carrot.

WHY SHOULD SOLIDS BE DELAYED?

Babies who are started on solid food early (before five to six months) and who have a family history of allergy are more likely to develop atopic disease (allergic asthma, allergic rhinitis, atopic dermatitis, food allergy) according to a Finnish study (Kajosaari

& Saarinen, 1983) of 135 exclusively breastfed infants of allergic families. Total solid food elimination for the first six months of life, in addition to exclusive breastmilk feeding, appears to reduce atopic disease in children who are at hereditary risk. The protective effect against eczema afforded by solid food postponement lasts up to one year of age.

IgE, which is associated with allergy, rises in direct time sequence to the introduction of solid foods. IgE is also associated with allergy verified by a positive skin-test later in life. Before the age of six months, the infant's intestine lacks the necessary digestive enzymes to completely digest complex proteins and starches down to amino acid and simple sugars. At the same time, the infant's intestinal mucosa is permeable to some intact proteins and starches. These incompletely digested peptides and starches can be absorbed and serve as sensitizing agents to the infant's immune system. IgE is then produced and allergy results in some, perhaps many, infants. When solids, especially wheat, egg whites, pork, and legumes, are withheld from the potentially allergic child until the immature immunity period has passed, the symptoms are minimized or even prevented (Glaser, 1973). At age six months, the infant produces sufficient IgA antibody to prevent absorption of food antigens through the intestinal wall, thus reducing food allergy (Saarinen et al., 1979).

Because there is a tendency for mothers to force food on the baby by encouraging him to finish the jar of baby food without taking cues of satiation from the baby, it was thought that the potential for obesity increases with the giving of early solids. More recent research, however, has not shown a relationship between obesity during infancy and the time when solid foods were introduced (Davies et al., 1977; Kramer, 1981; Read & Boling, 1982; Yeung et at., 1981). Nevertheless, teaching the young child to eat beyond satiation may contribute to later food problems and should be avoided.

OBESITY

Obesity affects between 11 and 19% of American children (Wishon & Kinnick, 1986). Whether obesity stems from excessive adipose cells laid down during the first year of life ("fat-cell" theory), or from hypothalmic or behavioral factors is still unclear. There is evidence of a genetic component: children of obese parents are more likely to be overweight themselves. (Copeland & Baucon-Copeland, 1981; Dietz, 1983; Taitz, 1977). On the other hand, it is possible that overweight mothers are likely to be more anxious about food and push their children into eating more, thereby creating a persistent food-reward system which can lead to overeating for the rest of the individual's life.

Is an obese infant likely to become an obese adult? It depends upon who is asked. Several investigators claim that fat babies have an increased risk of obesity during adulthood (Brook et al., 1975; Fisch et al., 1975; Kramer, 1981; Shulka et al., 1972), while others deny that infant obesity usually leads to adult obesity (Roche, 1981; Zack et al., 1979).

The same conflict surrounds measuring the effect of feeding method (breast or bottle) on adult obesity. A major obstacle in studies has been confounding factors, e.g., the mother's nutritional awareness, and methodological problems, e.g., operational definitions of obesity, the distinction between a "breastfed" infant vs. a "bottle-fed" infant, and the timing of feedings. Kramer (1981) attempted to prevent these biases in a case-control study of 639 young patients 12 to 18 years of age living in Montreal. He sought to control bias by (1) classifying each subject as either obese, overweight, or nonobese based both on relative weight and skinfold criteria; (2) obtaining feeding and family history as well as demographic data "blindly" by telephone; (3) operationalizing the definition of breastfed to mean having received no more than one bottle-feeding per day; and (4) statistically controlling for confounding effects of family history.

Study results suggested that breastfeeding provides a significant protective effect against subsequent obesity which persists at least through adolescence. The protection appears to rise slightly with increased duration of breastfeeding. Delayed introduction of solid food, on the other hand, had little if any additional benefit. Breastfeeding had a far weaker effect on obesity, however, than did genetic, racial, socioeconomic, and behavioral factors. All factors being equal, breastfeeding appears to afford a two- to fourfold benefit which lasts at least until adolescence.

WEANING

In the United States, weaning usually takes place in the first year of life. Women who breastfeed longer than this have difficulty with acceptance by relatives, peers, and health professionals (Morse & Harrison,

1987). If "baby-led weaning" is practiced, weaning usually takes place between the child's second and fourth birthday. To counteract social pressures for early weaning, women with breastfeeding toddlers find peer support for each other, sometimes changing their circle of friends. In a study by Wrigley and Hutchinson (1990) of 12 mothers who practiced long-term breastfeeding, one mother reported that "her obstetrician told her anyone who breastfed an infant past six months of age was 'perverted.' Another said that her father thought she was 'strange.'" Many health-care workers, who wholeheartedly support breastfeeding and would never advocate taking a security blanket away from a baby, reel in horror when a mother breastfeeds a walking child.

Ideally, the time for weaning is a joint decision, in which both the mother and baby reach a state of readiness to begin weaning around the same time; however, this is not always the case. The child may be ready before his mother; more often, the mother is ready before her child. Sometimes the decision is made to wean quickly. Although the literature offers considerable advice about gradual weaning, there is little information for the anxious mother in a situation in which weaning must be rapid and will necessarily be traumatic. Rago (1991) reported that the following nondrug therapies may make deliberate weaning easier and at the same time avert plugged ducts and/or mastitis:

- shower and allow the warm water to run over the breasts, or soak the breasts by lying down in the tub
- use a breast pump or manual expression to relieve breast fullness
- wear a supportive, comfortable bra
- observe for signs of plugged ducts or a breast infection
- expect to feel very emotional during this time and seek support from people who will listen sympathetically
- give the baby extra cuddling and holding.

It may take several days before the mother finds it is no longer necessary to express breastmilk for comfort. A standard Australian method for reducing engorged breasts is to wear cool raw cabbage leaves in the bra and change them every two hours (Rosier, 1988). Doing so has been reported to quickly relieve engorgement, thereby increasing the mother's comfort.

QUICK, EASY-TO-PREPARE INFANT FOODS

- Yogurt (low-fat)
- Fresh fruit—cut-up apples, pears, oranges, bananas, grapes, or any fruit in season
- Cheese—cut into chewable pieces
- Toast of whole grain bread—cut into strips
- Chicken—leg, wing, or cut-up pieces
- Egg—soft-boiled; hard-boiled as finger food
- Vegetables—mashed; whole (peas); in strips or pieces as finger food
- Crackers—whole grain; with peanut butter or cheese spread
- Custard
- Cottage cheese
- Dried fruit—apples, dates, figs, prunes (pitted)
- Liver—sautéed and cut into strips
- Tuna—drained; with grated cheese

IMPLICATIONS FOR PRACTICE

Care providers assume responsibility for educating families in optimal infant feeding practices and for providing rationale and support when they are needed. It was pointed out in Chapter 2 in the first section of this book that the introduction of foods other than breastmilk is culturally influenced and common worldwide. In a study of the feeding patterns of urban black infants, in Cleveland, Ohio, Parrago et al. (1988) found that 20% of three-week-old infants were receiving baby foods. Their mothers encouraged the babies to eat as much as possible, believing that a plump baby represents the picture of health. Competition among mothers also leads to the early introduction of baby foods (Guthrie & Riordan, 1977). Mothers, feeling pressure to give their babies solids, may misinterpret the baby's cries as hunger, when the baby merely needs stimulation by holding and interacting. Important points to share with new parents are:

- continue frequent breastfeedings with lots of cuddling and holding

- remember that crying is not always a sign of hunger—it can mean that the infant needs to be held, rocked, and soothed
- delay the introduction of solid foods until around the middle of the first year of life when the baby indicates that he is ready for them
- prepare foods for the infant in as close to a natural state as possible
- have easy-to-prepare foods available for quick meals for the infant (see the boxed list on this page)
- bring the baby to the family meal table whenever possible
- introduce one new food at a time, and offer it several times before trying another new food, observing for signs of intolerance or allergy.

It is not unusual for children, usually from about two years of age, to become very fussy about food and refuse to eat certain items; they may especially dislike vegetables. Children will go through periods of eating very little for periods lasting as short as a week to as long as a few months and then gradually start eating more again. The mother should be reassured that "this too shall pass" and that the child will start eating again. Meanwhile, she should make the food he does like easily available and neither force the child to eat nor mask his natural appetite by offering sugary foods (NMAA, 1979).

Choices about weaning should be based on the mother's own wishes rather than on expectations of others and should call for active listening to her feelings. If the mother enjoys meeting her baby's needs by breastfeeding but feels great pressure to wean, pointing out the advantages of continued breastfeeding and the cultural differences in weaning practices may be all the reinforcement she needs. On the other hand, if she expresses resentment each time her baby breastfeeds and is impatient for each feeding to end, she is entitled to know options for safe and comfortable weaning techniques.

SUMMARY

Imperative to assisting a breastfeeding family is recognition and knowledge of a wide array of areas of child health. Taking the holistic view, breastfeeding is not an isolated activity but one aspect of the child's overall health and welfare. This chapter offers readers basic information derived from research findings and clinical experiences. Parent teaching and incorporating research findings into the daily lives of families are the linchpins of effective practice.

REFERENCES

Abbey, LM: Is breastfeeding a likely cause of dental caries in young children? *J Am Dent Assoc* 98:21, 1979.

Adamiak, E: Occlusion anomalies in preschool children in rural areas in relation to certain individual features, *Czas Stomat* 34:551–55, 1981.

Ainsworth, MDS: Early caregiving and later patterns of attachment. In Klaus, MH, and Robertson, MO, eds.: *Birth, interaction and attachment: Pediatric round table series 6*, Skillman, N.J., 1982, Johnson & Johnson Baby Products Co.

Ainsworth, MDS, et al.: *Patterns of attachment*, Hillsdale, N.J., 1978, Lawrence Erlbaum Associates, Inc.

Als, H, and Brazelton, TB: A new model of assessing the behavioral organization in preterm and full term infants, *J Am Acad Child Psychol* 20:239, 1981.

American Academy of Pediatrics, Committee on Nutrition: Nutritional aspects of obesity in infancy and childhood, *Pediatrics* 68:880–83, 1981.

American Academy of Pediatrics, Committee on Nutrition: On the feeding of supplemental foods to infants, *Pediatrics* 65:1178, 1980.

American Academy of Pediatrics: *Report of the committee on infectious diseases*, Elk Grove, Ill., 1991.

Anderson, CJ: Enhancing reciprocity between mother and neonate, *Nurs Res* 30:89–93, 1981.

Anderson, GC: The mother and her newborn: mutual caregivers, *JOGN Nurs* 6:50–55, 1977.

Anisfeld, E, and Lipper, E: Early contact, social support, and mother-infant bonding, *Pediatrics* 72:79–83, 1983.

Anisfeld, E, et al.: Does infant carrying promote attachment? An experimental study of the effects of increased physical contact on the development of attachment, *Child Dev* 61:1617–27, 1990.

Bellanti, JA: Pediatric vaccinations: Update 1990, *Pediatr Clin North Am* 37:513–30, 1990.

Bell, RQ: Contributions of human infants to caregiving and social interaction. In Lewis, M, and Rosenblum, LA, eds.: *The effect of the infant on its caregiver*, New York, 1974, John Wiley & Sons, Inc., pp. 1–19.

Bernal, J: Crying during the first ten days of life, *Dev Med Child Neurol* 14:362–72, 1972.

Bowlby, J: *Attachment and loss: Vol. 2, Separation*, New York, 1973, Basic Books, Inc.

Bowlby, J: *Maternal care and mental health*, Geneva, 1951, World Health Organization.

Brams, M, and Maloney, J: "Nursing bottle caries" in breast-fed children, *J Pediatr* 103:415–16, 1983.

Brazelton, TB: Crying in infancy, *Pediatrics* 29:579–88, 1962.

Broad, B: The effects of infant feeding on speech quality, *NZ Med J* 76:28–31, 1972.

Brook, CG, et al.: Influence of heredity and environment in determination of skinfold thickness in children, *Br Med J* 2:719–21, 1975.

Bu'Lock, F, Woolridge, MW, and Baum, JD: Development of co-ordination of sucking, swallowing and breathing: ultrasound study of term and preterm infants, *Dev Med Child Neurol* 32:669–78, 1990.

Butte, NF, et al.: Energy utilization of breast-fed and formula-fed infants, *Am J Clin Nutr* 51:350–58, 1990.

Campbell, SBG and Taylor, PM: Bonding and attachment: theoretical issues, *Sem Perinatol* 3:3–13, 1979.

Carey, WB: Night waking and temperament in infancy, *J Pediatr* 84:756–58, 1974.

Carey, WB, and McDevitt, SC: Revision of the Infant Temperament Questionnaire, *Pediatrics* 61:735–39, 1978.

Children At Risk: *DPT dilemma*, Rochester N.Y., April 1987, *Democrat and Chronicle* Special Report, p. 5.

Clark, AL: Mother-child relationships, *MCN* 2:94–99, 1976.

Condon, WS, and Sander, LW: Neonate movement is synchronized with adult speech: interaction participation and language acquisition, *Science* 183:99, 1974.

Copeland, ET, and Baucon-Copeland, S: Child obesity: a family systems view, *Am Fam Phys* 24:153–57, 1981.

Coulter, HL, and Fisher, BL: *DPT: A shot in the dark*, New York, 1985, Warner Books, Inc. pp. 371–75.

Davies, DP, et al.: Effects of solid foods on growth of bottle-fed infants in the first three months of life, *Br Med J* 2:7–8, 1977.

deChateau, P, and Wiberg, B: Long term effect on mother-infant behavior of extra contact during the first hour postpartum, *Acta Paediatr Scand* 66:137, 1977.

Deforest, A, et al.: The effect of breast-feeding on the antibody response in infants to trivalent oral poliovirus vaccine, *J Pediatr* 83:94–95, 1973.

Dietz, WH: Childhood obesity: susceptibility, cause, and management, *J Pediatr* 103:676–86, 1983.

Dissatisfied Parents Together (DPT): Compensation system begins to pay out awards, National Vaccine Information Center, *Vaccine News* 5(1):2,6, 1990.

Elias, F, et al.: Sleep/wake patterns of breast-fed infants in the first 2 years of life, *Pediatrics* 77:322–29, 1986.

Emde, RN, Gaensbauer, TJ, and Harmon, RJ: *Emotional expression in infancy: a biobehavioral study*, Psychological Issues, Monograph 10(#37), New York, 1976, International Universities Press, Inc.

Erikson, EH: *Childhood and society* (2nd ed.), New York, 1963, W.W. Norton & Co., Inc.

Erikson, EH: *Identity, youth and crisis*, New York, 1968, W.W. Norton & Co., Inc.

Fantz, RL: Visual perception from birth, as shown by pattern sensitivity, *Ann NY Acad Sci* 118:739–814, 1965.

Fergusson, DM, Beautrais, AL, and Silva, PA: Breastfeeding and cognitive development in the first seven years of life, *Soc Sci Med* 16:1705–8, 1982.

Fisch, RO, et al.: Obesity and leanness at birth and their relationship to body habitus in later childhood, *Pediatrics* 56:521–28, 1975.

Fulginiti, VA: Immunization. In Kempe, CH, Silver, HK, and O'Brien, D, eds.: *Current pediatric diagnosis and treatment*, 8th ed., Los Altos, Calif., 1984, Lange.

Gardner, DE, Norwood, JR, and Eisensen, JE: At-will breastfeeding and dental caries: four case reports, *J Dent Child* 44:186–91, 1977.

Gill, NE, et al.: Effect of nonnutritive sucking on behavioral state in preterm infants before feeding, *Nurs Res* 37:347–50, 1988.

Glaser, J: *Prophylaxis and allergic disease in infancy and childhood: allergy and immunology in children,* Springfield, Ill., 1973, Charles C Thomas, Publisher.

Guthrie, RA, and Riordan, J: Fact and fantasy: solids and infant nutrition, *J Kansas Med Soc* 78:388–92, 1977.

Gyorgy, P: Trends and advances in infant nutrition, *W Va Med J* 53:121, 1957.

Harlow, HF, and Harlow, M: The affectional systems. In Schrier, A, Harlow, H, and Stollnitz, F, eds.: *Behavior of nonhuman primates,* Vol II, New York, 1965, Academic Press, Inc.

Hayes, JS: Theories of child development. In Servonsky, J, and Opas, SR: *Nursing management of children,* Boston, 1987, Jones and Bartlett Publishers, Inc., pp. 230–61.

Hegvik, R, McDevitt, SC, and Carey, W: The Middle Childhood Temperament Questionnaire, *J Dev Behav Pediatr* 3:197–200, 1982.

Hoefer, C, and Hardy, MC: Later development of breast-fed and artificially fed infants, *JAMA* 92:615–19, 1929.

Humphreys, HG, and Leighton, BC: A survey of antero-posterior abnormalities of the jaws in children between the age of two and five and a half years of age, *Br Dent J* 88:3–15, 1950.

Hunziker, UA, and Barr, RG: Increased carrying reduces infant crying: a randomized controlled trial, *Pediatrics* 77:641–48, 1986.

John, TJ, et al.: Effect of breast-feeding on seroresponse of infants to oral poliovirus vaccination, *Pediatrics* 57:47, 1976.

Kagan, J: Infant's differential reactions to familiar and distorted faces, *Child Dev* 36:519–32, 1966.

Kajosaari, M, and Saarinen, UM: Prophylaxis of atopic disease by six months' total solid food elimination, *Acta Paediatr Scand* 72:411–14, 1983.

Keane, V, et al.: Do solids help baby sleep through the night? *Am J Dis Child* 142:404–5, 1988.

Kessen, W, Haith, MM, and Salapatek, PH: Human infancy: a bibliography and guide. In Mussen, PH, ed.: *Carmichael's manual to child psychology,* New York, 1970, John Wiley & Sons, Inc.

Klaus, M, et al.: Human maternal behavior at first contact with her young, *Pediatrics* 46:187–92, 1970.

Klaus, MH, and Kennell, JH: *Maternal-infant bonding: the impact of early separation and loss on family development,* St. Louis, 1975, The C.V. Mosby Co.

Klaus, MH, and Kennell, JH: *Parent-infant bonding,* 2nd ed., St. Louis, 1982, The C.V. Mosby Co.

Kontos, D: A study of the effects of extended mother-infant contact on maternal behavior at one and three months, *Birth Fam J* 5:133–40, 1978.

Kotlow, LA: Breast-feeding: a cause of dental caries in children, *J Dent Child* 44:192–93, 1977.

Kramer, MS: Do breast-feeding and delayed introduction of solid foods protect against subsequent obesity? *J Pediatr* 98:883–87, 1981.

Krogh, V, et al.: Postpartum immunization with rubella virus vaccine and antibody response in breast-feeding infants, *J Lab Clin Med* 113:695–99, 1989.

Labbok, MH, and Hendershot, GE: Does breast-feeding protect against malocclusion? An analysis of the 1981 Child Health Supplement to the National Health Interview Survey, *Am J Prev Med* 3:227–32, 1987.

Lamb, M: The bonding phenomenon: misinterpretations and their implications, *J Pediatr* 102:249–50, 1983.

Levanthal, AS, and Lipsitt, LP: Adaptation, pitch discrimination and sound localization in the neonate, *Child Dev* 35:759–67, 1964.

Lewis, M: Infant's responses to facial stimuli during the first year of life, *Dev Psychol* 1:75–86, 1969.

Lorenz, KZ: The companion in the environment of the bird, *J Ornithol* 83:137–215, 289–413, 1935.

Losonsky, GA, et al.: Effect of immunization against rubella on lactation products. II. Maternal-neonatal interaction, *J Infec Dis* 145:661, 1982.

Macknin, ML, Medendorp, SV, and Maier, MC: Infant sleep and bedtime cereal, *Am J Dis Child* 143:1066–68, 1989.

Mata, L: Breast-feeding, infections and infant outcomes: An international perspective. In Atkinson, SA, Hanson, LA, and Chandra, RK: *Breastfeeding, nutrition, infection and infant growth in developed and emerging countries,* St. John's Newfoundland, Canada, 1990, ARTS Biomedical Publisher.

Mercer, R: A theoretical framework for studying factors that impact on the maternal role, *Nurs Res* 30:73–77, 1981.

Morrow-Tlucak, M, Haude, RH, and Ernhart, CB: Breastfeeding and cognitive development in the first 2 years of life, *Soc Sci Med* 26:635–39, 1988.

Morse, JM, and Harrison, M: Social coercion for weaning, *J Nurs-Midwif* 32:205–10, 1987.

Mott, S, Fazekas, NF, and James, SR: *Nursing care of children and families,* Menlo Park, Calif., 1985, Addison-Wesley Publishing Co., Inc., pp. 182–83, 206.

Myers, A, and Hertzberg, J: Bottle-feeding and malocclusion: Is there an association? *Am J Orthod Dentrofac Orthodont* 93:149–52, 1988.

Naing, K-M, and Co, T-T: Growth and milk intake of exclusively breast-fed Myanmar infants, *Eur J Clin Nutr* 45:203–7, 1991.

Nursing Mothers Association of Australia: Introduction of solid foods to baby's diet, *NMAA News* 15(4):1–5, 1979.

O'Connor, S, et al.: How does rooming-in enhance the mother-infant bond? *Soc Pediatr Res* 13:336, 1979.

Pabst, HF, et al.: Effect of breast-feeding on immune response to BCG vaccination, *Lancet* 1(Feb 11):295–96, 1989.

Parrago, IM, et al.: Feeding patterns of urban black infants, *J Am Diet Assoc* 88:796–800, 1988.

Piaget, J: *The origins of intelligence in children* (Cook, M, trans.), New York, 1952, International Universities Press.

Piaget, J, and Inhelder, B: *Psychology of the child,* New York, 1969, Basic Books, Inc.

Prechtl, J, and Beintema, D: *The neurological examination of the full term infant,* Child development medical series, 12, Philadelphia, 1975, J.B. Lippincott Co.

Rago, JL: Helping a mother wean with the electric breast pump, *Rental Roundup* 8(3):8–9, 1991.

Read, MH, and Boling, MA: Effect of feeding practices on the incidence of iron deficiency anemia and obesity in a native American population, *Nutr Rep Int* 26:689–702, 1982.

Rebelsky, F, and Black, R: Crying in infancy, *J Genetic Psychol* 121:49–57, 1972.

Richmond, J, and Filner, F: Infant and child health needs and strategies. In: *Healthy People: The Surgeon General's Report of Health Promotion and Disease Prevention,* USDHHS, PHS Publication No. 79–55071A, Washington, D.C., 1979, U.S. Government Printing Office.

Robertson, J: *Young children in hospital,* New York, 1958, Basic Books, Inc.

Roche, AF: The adipocyte-number hypothesis, *Child Dev* 52:31–43, 1981.

Rodgers, B: Feeding in infancy and later ability and attainment: a longitudinal study, *Dev Med Child Neurol* 20:421–26, 1978.

Rogerson, BFC, and Rogerson, CH: Feeding in infancy and subsequent psychological difficulties, *J Ment Sci* 85:1163–82, 1939.

Rosier, W: Cool cabbage compresses, *Breastfeed Rev* 12:28–31, 1988.

Rubin, R: Attainment of the maternal role, I. Processes. II. Models and referrants, *Nurs Res* 16:237, 342, 1967.

Rubin, R: Binding-in in the postpartum period, *MCN* 6:67–75, 1977.

Saarinen, UM, et al.: Prolonged breast-feeding a prophylaxis for atopic disease, *Lancet* (8135):163–66, 1979.

Sanger, R, and Bystrom, E: Breastfeeding: does it affect oral facial growth? *Dent Hygiene* 56:44–47, 1982.

Sears, W: *Growing together,* Franklin Park, Ill., 1987, La Leche League International, pp. 30, 71.

Servonsky, J, and Opes, SR: *Nursing management of children,* Boston, 1987, Jones and Bartlett Publishers, Inc., pp. 22, 180.

Shulka, A, et al.: Infantile overnutrition in the first year of life, *Br Med J* 4:507, 1972.

Siegel, E, et al.: Hospital and home support during infancy: impact on maternal attachment, child abuse and neglect and health care utilization, *Pediatrics* 66:183–90, 1980.

Spitz, R: Anaclitic depression, *Psychoanal Study Child* 2:313–42, 1946.

Stanley, E, and Lundeen, D: Tongue thrust in breast-fed and bottle-fed school children: a cross-cultural investigation, *Int J Oral Myol* 6:6–16, 1980.

Straub, W: Malfunction of the tongue, *Am J Orthodont* 46:404–24, 1960.

Suitor, CW, and Hunter, MF: *Nutrition principles and applications in health promotion,* Philadelphia, 1980, J.B. Lippincott Co.

Svejda, MJ, and Campos, J: Mother-infant "bonding": failure to generalize, *Child Dev* 51:779, 1980.

Taitz, LS: Obesity in pediatric practice: symposium on nutrition in pediatrics, *Pediatr Clin North Am* 24:107, 1977.

Tank, G, and Storvick, CA: Caries experience of children of one to six years old in two Oregon communities, *J Am Dent Assoc* 70:101, 1965.

Taylor, B, and Wadsworth, J: Breastfeeding and child development at 5 years, *Dev Med Child Neurol* 26:73–80, 1984.

Thomas, A, and Chess, S: *Temperament and development,* New York, 1977, Brunner/Mazel, Inc.

Thomas, A, et al.: Behavioral individuality in early childhood, New York, 1963, New York University Press.

Thomson, M, Hartsock, T, and Larson, C: The importance of immediate postnatal contact: its effect on breastfeeding, *Con Fam Phys* 25:1374–78, 1979.

Weir, L: Auditory frequency sensitivity in the neonate: a signal detection analysis, *J Exp Child Psychol* 21:219–25, 1976.

Wessel, MA, et al.: Paroxysmal fussing in infancy, *Pediatrics* 14:421–34. 1954.

Wishon, PM, and Kinnick, VG: Helping infants overcome the problem of obesity, *MCN* 11:118–21, 1986.

Wolfe, MS: Vaccine for foreign travel, *Pediatr Clin North Am* 37:757–69, 1990.

Wolff, PH: "Critical periods" in human cognitive development, *Hosp Pract* 11:77–87, 1970.

Wrigley, EA, and Hutchinson, SA: Long-term breastfeeding: The secret bond, *J Nurs-Midwif* 35:35–41, 1990.

Yeung, DL, et al.: Infant fatness and feeding practices: a longitudinal assessment, *J Am Diet Assoc* 79:531–35, 1981.

Zack, PM, et al.: A longitudinal study of body fatness in childhood and adolescence, *J Pediatr* 95:126–30, 1979.

18

The Ill Breastfeeding Child

JAN RIORDAN

Why devote an entire chapter to health problems of infants and children relating to breastfeeding when details of these problems can easily be found in other books? Because the care of a breastfeeding infant differs from that of an artificially fed one, and these differences in the breastfeeding child and his family require special consideration when the breastfeeding baby or young child is ill. Also, the crucial role of nursing in direct primary care of a child with a health problem often makes the difference between unnecessary weaning and continued breastfeeding. Despite its many advantages, it is often assumed that breastfeeding must be terminated when a serious illness strikes. Even when breastfeeding continues, a disruption of the established patterns is inevitable. Nurses and health-care workers must know when and how to intervene effectively to improve a child's health status without unnecessarily disrupting the breastfeeding course.

The purpose of this chapter is to provide specific information on selected health problems that affect breastfeeding. There are obviously far more pediatric health problems than those presented here. Pumps and other lactation technologies described in Chapter 11 will be an integral part of nursing interventions.

INFECTIONS

The infant is exposed to a variety of pathogens in his environment. Breastfeeding enhances the infant's immune system and helps to protect the baby from infections. During the past two decades, numerous research studies have documented the protection breastfeeding affords against many infections during infancy and childhood. For example, investigators have discovered that breastfed infants are less likely to develop urinary tract infections (Piscane, Graziano & Zona, 1990). This protective effect appears to be more striking and easier to demonstrate in settings where poverty, malnutrition, and poor hygiene are prevalent (Kramer, 1988).

A study by Chen, Yu, and Li (1988) which reports the effect of artificial feeding on hospitalization rates in China, the world's most populous country, is of special interest for further testing the protectiveness of breastfeeding. After controlling for potentially confounding factors (infant gender, infant weight, parent education, smoking), Chen, Yu, and Li established that artificially fed infants were twice as likely to be hospitalized for respiratory infections and about one-third more likely to be hospitalized for gastroenteritis or other infections during the first 18 months of life (Tables 18–1 and 18–2).

Two years later, Howie et al. (1990) reported a prospective study on breastfeeding and infant illness in Dundee, U.K.; like Chen, Yu, and Li, they also controlled for confounding variables. In the study by Howie and colleagues, however, the data was collected prospectively by the health visitors as they made home visits. Their results were similar to those of Chen, Yu, and Li: babies who were breastfed for 13 weeks or more had less gastrointestinal illness than those who were bottle-fed from birth for the first 13 weeks of life. While breastfeeding is protective, this protection is not always complete, especially if the baby is partially breastfed and nurses are

TABLE 18–1 HOSPITAL ADMISSION RATE PER 100 INFANTS FOR THE FIRST 18 MONTHS OF LIFE BY DIAGNOSIS AND FEEDING TYPE

	Feeding Type		
Diagnosis	**Breast (n = 670)**	**Artificial (n = 388)**	**Total (N = 1,058)**
Respiratory infections	7.0	13.7	9.5
Gastroenteritis	3.6	5.2	4.2
Other infections	1.5	2.1	1.7
Other diseases	3.4	4.1	3.7

From Chen, Y, Yu, S, and Li, W: Artificial feeding and hospitalization in the first 18 months of life, *Pediatrics* 81:58–62, 1988.

sometimes called on to care for a breastfeeding child with an infection.

GASTROINTESTINAL

The infant may have diarrhea with the flu; however, since the breastfed infant's stools are normally loose, what is thought to be "diarrhea" by an uninformed individual may be a normal stool pattern. Vomiting and diarrhea are common in children, but far less common in breastfed children, particularly during the period of exclusive breastfeeding (Huffman & Combest, 1990; Haffejee, 1990; Popkin et al., 1990). While the primary cause is viral or bacterial invasion

of the GI tract, vomiting and diarrhea also occur as a result of infections and disorders of other body systems. All infants "spit up" occasionally; this does not necessarily mean that the infant is ill. An infant with persistent vomiting, however, should be examined for other problems if an infection is ruled out.

Water is lost from the body through urine, feces, and evaporation from the skin and lungs. Because the infant has a relatively greater body surface area compared to body mass, larger amounts of fluid are lost through the skin. If the baby is nauseated, he will take less fluid, and vomiting will cause direct fluid loss. If he also has diarrhea the loss of fluid may be profound, and dehydration is a real threat. Excessive

TABLE 18–2 HOSPITAL ADMISSION RATE FOR RESPIRATORY INFECTIONS PER 100 INFANTS FOR THE FIRST 18 MONTHS OF LIFE BY FEEDING TYPE AND CONFOUNDING VARIABLES*

	Feeding type		OR_{M-H}	X^2_{M-H} Test *P* Value
	Breast	**Artificial**		
Sex				
Boys	7.1 (22/322)	14.4 (33/299)	2.08	<.01
Girls	6.9 (24/348)	12.6 (20/159)		
Birth wt (g)				
<2,500	10.5 (2/19)	23.8 (5/21)	2.07	<.01
≥2,500	6.9 (45/651)	12.8 (48/367)		
Father's education				
University	4.8 (4/84)	8.6 (6/70)	2.16	<0.1
Secondary or primary	7.3 (43/586)	14.8 (47/318)		
Smoking status				
Smoking	7.7 (38/491)	15.4 (42/273)	2.18	<.01
Nonsmoking	5.0 (9/179)	9.6 (11/115)		

*Numbers in parentheses are numbers of infants/total number of infants.

From Chen, Y, Yu, S, and Li, W: Artificial feeding and hospitalization in the first 18 months of life, *Pediatrics* 81:58–62, 1988.

gastrointestinal losses, particularly diarrhea, involve losses of sodium and potassium along with water. The risk of dehydration and acidosis occurs if losses are extensive; prompt fluid replacement may be necessary.

Following birth, newborns have an excess amount of body fluids which gradually disappear in two or three days. After that time, infants are vulnerable to rapid and extreme disturbances in hydration because they have such a small extracellular fluid reserve. Until the infant is about two years of age, he has a relatively larger percentage of extracellular fluid and a greater fluid intake and output than the adult. The daily exchange of fluid volume for an infant is about 40%. For example, an infant who weighs seven kilograms has an extracellular fluid volume of 1750 mL. This baby will drink about 700 mL and excrete about 700 mL daily. An adult, on the other hand, will exchange only about 14% of extracellular fluid daily. Thus, following the newborn period (when the baby has excess fluid), fluid loss in an infant who does not eat or drink for a day is more critical than in an adult who does not eat or drink in the same period.

Hydration can be assessed by observing the infant's general responsiveness and skin turgor. Dehydrated babies are listless and look and act sick. The degree of dehydration is best determined by the extent of rapid body weight loss. If a baby was 10 kg and is now 9 kg, then he has had a 10% loss, which is considered moderate dehydration. Other evidence of dehydration includes:

- depressed anterior fontanel
- dry mucous membranes
- small urinary output—few wet diapers
- cool, clammy extremities—especially the fingers and toes.

Normally, six to eight cloth diapers wet with urine in a 24-hour period is an indication of adequate hydration; however, frequent stools confuse estimates of urine output. With dehydration, the specific gravity of the urine (normal is 1.010–1.020) will be high, indicating a diminished water intake.

Treatment for dehydration requires replacement of fluid and electrolyte losses. At home, extra fluids can be given with a spoon or dropper if the infant is too young to drink from a cup. The parents should also place the infant on his abdomen with his face to one side to prevent aspiration if he is regurgitating.

If the baby is willing to take anything by mouth, it should be breastmilk (Ruuska, 1992). Even partial breastfeeding reduces the severity and duration of diarrhea episodes—and the likelihood of mortality from diarrhea (Sachdev, et al., 1991). Although many health professionals advise that even breastfed infants should be taken off milk products in the event of vomiting and diarrhea, this is seldom necessary. Human milk should not be classified as part of, or identical to, cow's milk and other dairy products. Because breastmilk digests so rapidly, even the infant who is vomiting regularly will absorb some of the nutrient and fluids of the milk before it is regurgitated. The most appropriate management includes continued breastfeeding with or without solids, as determined by the child's willingness to eat. Only a fully-formula fed infant requires a reduction or elimination of milk feedings if the diarrhea persists or worsens (Brown, 1991). Sodas or jello water offer little in the way of nourishment and none of the immunities of breastmilk. After being told to interrupt breastfeeding because her infant was vomiting and had a mild fever, a mother who is also a nurse reported:

> He needed to breastfeed and refusing him for 24 hours would have been devastating. I walked him around to quiet him, waiting as long as I could between feedings. The breastmilk stayed down about 20 minutes before he vomited it up, but at least I felt like he was getting something.

Acute diarrhea continues to be a cause of hospitalization in young children, and deaths still occur. Ruuska and Vesikari (1991) followed 336 Finnish children from birth to $2\frac{1}{2}$ years of age to determine the incidence of acute diarrhea. More than half of the children had no diarrhea, 26% had one episode, and 19% had two or more episodes of diarrhea. Rotavirus was by far the most common pathogen. About two-thirds of the infants were breastfed over six months; breastfeeding for less than six months was associated with a higher incidence of rotavirus diarrhea between 7 and 12 months of age, but not thereafter.

If a severe gastroenteritis develops during weaning, a time when this is a likely occurrence, the baby may be brought into a clinic or hospital for intravenous replacement of fluids. Usually a five percent dextrose-containing solution (D_5W) with added so-

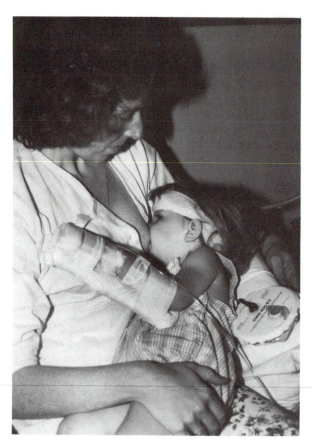

FIGURE 18–1 Comfort at breast while receiving an IV infusion. (Courtesy Debi Leslie Bocar.)

dium (Na) and potassium (K) is given for 24 to 48 hours. Before potassium is added, however, it must be determined that the infant's renal system is functioning, since accumulation of potassium in the system is life-threatening.

RESPIRATORY

Infection of the respiratory tract, the most common cause of illness in infancy and childhood, is usually caused by a virus. Infants with few outside contacts develop fewer respiratory infections than children in day-care settings. If a child is breastfed, he is less likely to develop a serious respiratory infection, even when exposed to others who are ill or contagious. Although newborns may have an infection without a fever, children from six months to three years of age will readily develop a fever—sometimes before any other sign of a respiratory problem is apparent. If the fever is 104° F (40° C), the child is at risk for febrile

convulsion with tonic-clonic characteristics. Other symptoms of a respiratory infection include wheezing, hoarseness, cough, and the presence of abnormal respiratory chest sounds, such as rhonchi, rales, and hyperresonance, as well as the absence of normal lung sounds.

If a breastfeeding infant does develop a respiratory infection, it is usually an upper-respiratory infection, and he is less likely to be hospitalized (Cunningham, Jelliffe & Jelliffe, 1991). Care is given at home unless the child's symptoms worsen. In helping the family of a breastfed child with a respiratory infection, several points should be emphasized.

First, instead of the usual response of wanting to breastfeed more when sick, *the infant may be less interested in feedings* and may even refuse the mother. Such infants are nose breathers, blocked airway passages pose the risk of compromising oxygen intake during feeding. To make it easier for the infant to breathe, the mother should feed him sitting up, holding him in an upright position as much as possible. For older infants and children, decongestant nose drops can be administered 15 to 20 minutes before breastfeeding. A less satisfactory way to clear nasal secretions is to gently suction them out by using a nasal infant aspirator or rubber ear syringe. Saline nose drops also help clear nasal passages and promote feeding. To prepare saline drops at home, simply dissolve one teaspoon of salt in one pint of warm water. For older infants and children who tolerate nose drops, a vasoconstrictor such as phenylephrine will shrink the mucous membranes. Two to three drops are gently placed into each of the child's nostrils for three to five days until breathing is easier.

Second, the infant *may not be as hungry as before.* Anorexia (loss of appetite) and vomiting is often a result of respiratory infections in a toddler or small child, especially if he is coughing. If hydration is not a problem, he should be allowed to determine his own need for food. Once the acute symptoms have passed, his appetite returns, usually in a day or two. Until then, the mother should pump or hand express her breastmilk. Acetaminophen will reduce the fever and make the child more comfortable. If the infant or child has laryngeal involvement, with hoarseness or a croupy cough, a cool-mist vaporizer in the room or area where he sleeps is still thought to soothe and moisten mucous membranes, despite lack of evidence that vaporizers are effective (Colombo, Hopkins & Waring, 1981). An inexpensive, time-honored, and effective method for creating concentrated steam and temporarily relieving croup is for the parent, while safely holding the child, to turn on hot water in an empty shower stall with the bathroom door closed. Fifteen minutes may be all that is necessary for relief. Wrapping the infant with a dry blanket or towel will be needed afterwards to prevent the child from becoming chilled.

Bronchiolitis.   Acute bronchiolitis is a respiratory infection that may follow an upper respiratory tract infection (URI). It is most common during the winter months, affects young infants, and lasts about two weeks. Breastfeeding has a protective effect against respiratory syncytial virus (RSV), the primary causative pathogen (Pullan et al., 1980). These viruses cause extensive inflammation which leads to necrosis of bronchiole cells, edema, and increased secretions. The baby can inhale easily because the bronchioles dilate on inspiration and air goes around the obstruction; exhalation, however, is difficult because the airway narrows, trapping air distal to the obstruction. Because bronchiolitis is a viral illness, antibiotics are used only if a secondary bacterial infection develops. Most cases of bronchiolitis are self-limiting and hospitalization is not necessary. The baby is given supportive treatment at home and continues to breastfeed.

Pneumonia.   Pneumonia is almost always viral, not bacterial. Respiratory syncytial virus (RSV) is responsible for most viral pneumonias in young children. Antibiotic therapy is usually given until it is determined that the pneumonia is not bacterial. Hospitalization may be necessary, and the child may be placed in a Croupette to aid breathing.

Bacterial pneumonia, while uncommon, is a serious disease and is seen more often in infants than in children. The *pneumococcus* is the most common (90%) organism in bacterial pneumonia. Infants with bacterial pneumonia become acutely ill and rapidly develop a high temperature which may be accompanied by seizures. In most cases, these infants are hospitalized and given intravenous antibiotics and other measures to reduce their fever. Antimicrobial therapy has significantly reduced morbidity and mortality from bacterial pneumonia.

A Croupette or mist tent imposes a necessary, albeit therapeutic, isolation of the child from the parent, but there is no reason for it to interfere with breastfeeding if the child is interested. Taking him out of the tent for brief periods of holding and feeding has more benefits than risks. Another alternative is for the mother to climb into the tent and have the side of the tent zipped to prevent loss of cool mist and oxygen. Many mothers have done it as shown in Fig. 18–2. Other than being nontraditional, it has no disadvantages, and the mother's presence quickly quiets a crying, unhappy infant who has little energy to spare.

MENINGITIS

Meningitis is an acute inflammation of the meninges caused by a viral or bacterial pathogen. When meningitis occurs in the breastfed infant it is usually, but not always, aseptic or viral in origin. Meningitis is also associated with other viral diseases, such as enteroviruses, measles, mumps, or herpes. The range of clinical symptoms and their severity varies widely and may be sudden or gradual in onset. Signs of meningeal irritation include nausea and vomiting, as well as a tense anterior fontanel. Other neurological signs are pain when the baby's head is moved and a positive Brudzinski's sign (lower limbs flex spontaneously when his neck is flexed).

One mother whose breastfeeding child developed meningitis on a family vacation reported, "We had no idea of just how sick he was, but I had a strong feeling that if we did not get him to a doctor he would die. He didn't have much fever, but he had

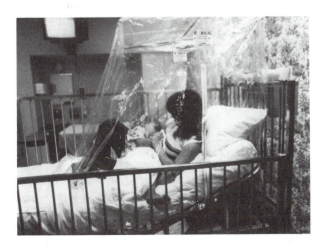

FIGURE 18–2   Breastfeeding in a Croupette. (Courtesy La Leche League International.)

stopped nursing and he no longer seemed to recognize his older brother and sister. Every time I moved him he would cry."

The child with meningitis is hospitalized, and a lumbar puncture is done in order to culture cerebrospinal fluid. Intravenous antibiotics are usually administered, and the child is isolated until bacterial meningitis can be ruled out. The mother will need help in careful handling of the IV site (usually in the child's arm) when moving her child to her breast. Infants are sometimes uninterested in breastfeeding for a day or two during the acute phase but then resume breastfeeding as eagerly as before.

Bacterial meningitis is a serious disease that requires hospitalization, sometimes in intensive care. In neonates the causative organisms are *Escherichia coli* and group-B streptococci; in infants *Meningococcus* or *Hemophilus influenzae*. Meningitis from *Hemophilus influenzae* is now preventable by immunization. Breastfeeding is associated with significant reductions in bacterial meningitis; formula-fed infants have a four- to sixteen-fold risk of developing *H. influenzae* bacteremia and meningitis (Cochi et al., 1986; Istre et al., 1985).

OTITIS MEDIA

Inflammation of the middle ear is the most prevalent childhood disease after respiratory tract infections. It occurs most often in male children from six months to three years of age. Bottle-feeding increases both the risk of otitis media and the duration of the illness (Saarinen, 1982; Teele, Klein & Rosner, 1989). It generally occurs following a respiratory infection when the child suddenly develops a fever and sharp, constant pain in one or both ears. Infants become very irritable, frequently pulling or tugging at the affected ear; a child verbalizes pain. Most middle-ear infections are caused by *H. influenzae* and are treated with a penicillinase-resistant antibiotic such as amoxicillin. An analgesic such as acetaminophen may be given to relieve pain and fever. An infant with a middle-ear infection will breastfeed more often for solace and will hold his head carefully in an attempt to protect against pressure on the painful ear during breastfeeding. If episodes of acute otitis media occur frequently, it may be wise to keep the child on maintenance antibiotic therapy.

ALTERATION IN NEUROLOGIC FUNCTIONING

The suck-swallow reflexes in a full-term, healthy infant are usually neurologically mature at birth, and the infant usually has little difficulty in establishing a pattern of satisfactory suckling. This is not true for the neurologically damaged child, however. Any neurologic deficit which affects neuromuscular function carries the risk that the child will have feeding difficulties. Suckling and swallowing, as well as breathing, are integrated under medullary (brainstem) control. When this control is impaired, the normal muscle tension involved in these functions becomes dystonic and flaccid. As a result, feeding, either by breast or by bottle, can be difficult and frustrating. As pointed out in Chapter 10 on high-risk infants, breastfeeding requires *less energy* than bottle-feeding—just the opposite of what had been previously believed. Despite these problems, a number of determined women, with the help of their physicians, nurses and others, have breastfed these children, developing techniques through trial and error that overcome these initial problems.

DOWN SYNDROME

The risk of Down syndrome increases with maternal age, which is the only clearly defined factor known to increase the likelihood of faulty chromosome distribution and Down syndrome. A chromosome study can be done early in pregnancy by obtaining amniotic fluid by amniocentesis. Common characteristics include epicanthal folds, broad hands with shortened fingers, a simian crease (single crease across the upper palm), flattened forehead, a small mouth, and hypotonicity. In about one-third of these infants, heart development is incomplete (most commonly septal defects), and surgery may be required; incomplete development of the intestine is also common.

In addition to requiring special assistance with feedings (especially when young), these infants need extra stimulation through frequent touching, exercising of extremities in a patterned sequence, carrying, and being spoken to in a varied voice pitch and intonation. In short, the parents should be encouraged to play, laugh, and have fun with the baby. Since the infant with Down syndrome has increased respiratory secretions, the same activities that stimulate the infant's sensory system also help postural drainage, thus preventing the pooling of mucus.

MYELOMENINGOCELE

Abnormalities along the neural axis occur often enough to warrant their discussion in relation to breastfeeding. With successful surgical interventions many of these infants are able to function and fully participate in life—including being able to breastfeed. In myelomeningocele, a segment of the spinal cord and meninges protrudes though a defect in the bony spine, usually in the lumbosacral region. The infant may have some weakness or complete flaccid paralysis of the legs, as well as bladder and bowel control dysfunction later on. The important aim of early care is to prevent infection of the sac and to preserve muscular and neurologic functions. Surgical correction to close the opening is done as early as possible, preferably in the first 24 to 48 hours of life. If the defect is extensive, one or more surgical procedures will be done later using skin flaps.

Since the infant is in the intensive care unit during the critical period, the parents should be encouraged to be with their baby and to help in care-taking whenever possible. If the mother is able to feed the infant by breast, the nurse should stay with her during the first several feedings, especially helping her to carefully pick up the infant and position him on the breast while protecting the sac or the surgical site from any pressure. A typical feeding position can be used if the mother's elbow is rotated around a protective device (see Fig. 18–3) to avoid pressure on his back. The infant can also be fed with the mother lying next to him on a bed. Feedings should be brief at first to conserve the infant's energy. Since the infant cannot be burped or bubbled in the normal way, gently rubbing him between his shoulders or rocking on a firm surface helps to release any ingestion of air. If brainstem impairment is involved, the baby may not be able to breastfeed for a long time, if ever. Yet stimulating lactation so that the mother's milk can be given to the infant is immensely rewarding to her.

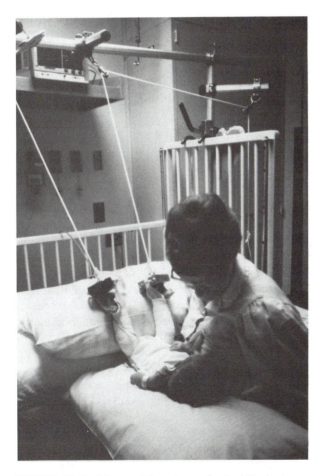

FIGURE 18–3   It's possible to breastfeed while the infant remains in traction.

HYDROCEPHALUS

Hydrocephalus, which sometimes occurs with myelomeningocele, is an accumulation of fluid in the intracranial cavity caused by an interference in the flow or absorption of cerebrospinal fluid. In communicating hydrocephalus, the infant has normal communication between the ventricles and the subarachnoid space; in the noncommunicating type, the infant's brain has a partial or complete blockage between these two areas. Circulation of the cerebrospinal fluid is blocked at some point within the ventricular system, preventing its flow to the subarachnoid spaces.

As the fluid distends the ventricles, the infant's head enlarges, and the sutures begin to separate with bulging fontanels. The "setting sun" (the white-of-the-eye shows above the iris and below the upper lid) sign of the eyes from the intracranial pressure, a high-pitched cry, muscle weakness, and severe neurologic defects occur if the hydrocephalus is already advanced at birth or is allowed to progress.

Surgery should be performed as soon as the diagnosis is made. The surgical treatment is by means of a shunt to bypass the obstruction point and to drain the cerebrospinal fluid to another area, usually the peritoneum, where it is absorbed and finally excreted.

The infant with hydrocephalus requires careful nursing care, and the parents need emotional support. Breastfeeding is often possible; with early treatment many children can lead normal lives. Care must be taken when positioning and supporting the infant's head; feeding while lying down with his head supported by a pillow is probably the most comfortable position for the infant with advanced hydrocephalus. To prevent regurgitation, feedings should be frequent and on demand. When there is severe brain damage and breastfeeding is not possible, some mothers of hydrocephalic infants pump their milk, deriving satisfaction from still being able to give their baby their milk in a gavage tube or bottle.

CLINICAL IMPLICATIONS

When an infant is ill, nothing should be assumed without actually putting the baby to breast to see if he is interested in suckling. Even when a child has a known neurological condition with hypotonia, such as Down syndrome, he may be able to feed effectively. In a study of 59 breastfed infants with Down syndrome, one-half of the infants had no difficulty in establishing suckling; four were slow in doing so for less than one week; eight took one week in establishing suckling; and 16 took longer than one week in doing so (Aumonier & Cunningham, 1983).

McBride and Danner (1987) describe suckling disorders in neurologically impaired infants and suggest helpful techniques to improve suckling abilities. Many of the following suggestions for breastfeeding these special babies derive from this discussion:

1. Arrange a comfortable and quiet environment (with soft lighting and pillows) for feedings.
2. Encourage the mother to find a completely comfortable position for herself and to try different positions for her infant.
3. Teach the mother to use the "dancer hand" position to help stabilize the infant's lower jaw (see Fig. 18–4). While the breast is supported with the last three fingers, the thumb and index

finger surround the infant's jaw and rest against his cheeks, applying gentle pressure. The infant is in an upright position, and his chin rests in the web between the thumb and index finger. Swallowing is easier going with the force of gravity rather than against it; plus, body alignment in a sitting position facilitates the passage of food.
4. Hold the breast so that it angles slightly upward. This prevents the infant from getting too much milk at once.
5. Hand express a few drops of milk into his mouth to arouse his interest or brush the nipple on the center of his lower lip to stimulate his rooting reflex. Placing a thumb under the baby's bottom lip or chin encourages bilabial closure and suction.
6. Teach the mother to pump her breasts following the feeding. The hind milk obtained from pumping after feeding has a higher fat content and may be useful for supplementary feedings.
7. Feed the infant frequently.
8. Consider providing the mother with a feeding tube device so that the infant obtains additional milk, thus getting more milk for less effort.

CONGENITAL DEFECTS

CONGENITAL HEART DEFECTS

Infants with congenital heart defects include those who are free of symptoms and those with such severe defects that any exertion, including feeding, can cause cyanosis and early signs of a congestive heart failure. For many infants, congenital heart defects are not severe enough to interfere with breastfeeding; nurses should encourage breastfeeding for these infants as they would for any other.

Frequently, there are so few symptoms that the problem is not recognized until later in life. A serious problem, however, can cause the infant to suckle poorly and to tire easily at the breast. He may begin with vigorous suckling, pulling away after a few minutes to rest. Typically the hungry infant will again grasp the breast, and the cycle is repeated (Shor, 1978). After a time, an inadequate intake of breastmilk leads to failure to gain weight. Medical interventions with drug therapy such as digitalis can alleviate lack of oxygenation and increase cardiac

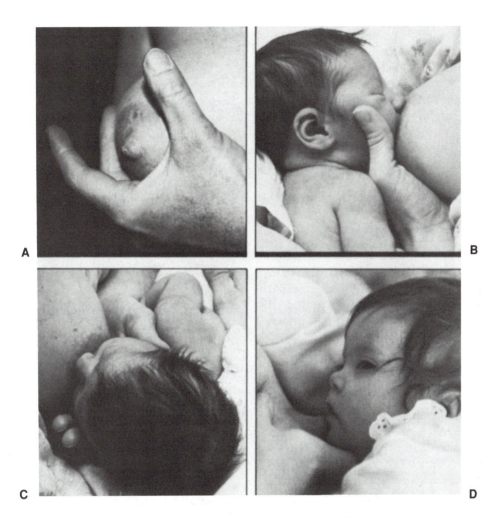

FIGURE 18–4 Mother breastfeeding using the "dancer hand" position. **A,** The mother's hand that supports the breast slides forward so that the breast is supported by three fingers rather than four. The index finger is bent slightly so that the thumb and index finger form a U. **B,** This position helps the baby suckle effectively without using energy to stabilize his jaw. **C,** The breast is supported with the last three fingers; the thumb and index finger surround the infant's jaw and rest against his cheeks, applying gentle pressure. **D,** Using a modified "dancer hand" position to provide chin support only. From Danner, SC, and Cerutti, ER: *Nursing your baby with Down's Syndrome,* Rochester, N.Y., 1984, Childbirth Graphics, Ltd., p. 9.

output. Often corrective surgery is indicated in one or several stages.

With a severe defect, the infant can show early signs of heart failure, becoming cyanotic with fast respirations (tachypnea) and pulse rate (tachycardia). While she is holding her infant, the baby's heartbeat may be so prominent that the mother is aware of it. Any of the symptoms described, along with auscultation of abnormal heart sounds or palpa-

tion of a thrill or unequal femoral pulses, should lead the health worker to suspect a cardiac defect. The child should be immediately referred to a pediatrician for subsequent diagnostic testing to determine whether a defect is present and what type it is.

There are several points to remember in helping the breastfeeding mother. First, encourage her to feed frequently in an upright position for short periods of time to avoid distending the infant's stomach and impeding his breathing capacity. If the infant is distressed during feeding, pumping some of the milk and feeding it through a feeding tube device to him at the same time he is feeding at the breast will reduce his exertion. Corrective or palliative surgery such as pulmonary banding can dramatically improve the infant's condition.

When surgery is performed, feeding at the breast as soon as oral feedings can be resumed reduces the trauma of the surgery and hospitalization. If the child is too ill to hold to feed, arrange for the mother to stay close to her baby so she can see him and reach out and touch him.

ORAL AND GASTROINTESTINAL DEFECTS

Esophageal reflux (chalasia).   Rarely, a breastfeeding infant will develop persistent, nonprojectile vomiting because of laxity of the lower esophageal muscles, which causes frequent return of stomach content into the esophagus. This problem is much more pronounced in formula-fed infants, presumably because the stomach digests formula or cow's milk more slowly and less completely than breastmilk (Heacock et al., 1992).

Frequent vomiting starts within one week after birth, especially when the infant is lying down. A barium swallow x-ray examination can confirm the diagnosis of esophageal reflux. The condition tends to be self-limiting after several weeks and is minimized if the mother breastfeeds the infant in an upright position. Medications can be given which promote gastric emptying, such as metaclopramide (dopamine blocker) and bethanechol (cholinergic drug).

Pyloric stenosis.   Pyloric stenosis, a hypertrophy of the pyloric sphincter, develops a few weeks after birth with vomiting that becomes progressively more severe and projectile. Rapid dehydration and electrolyte imbalance become a threat. During and following a feeding, it is possible with side lighting to see peristaltic waves that pass from left to right; an olive-shaped tumor (the hypertrophic pylorus) can be palpated in the right upper quadrant of the abdomen.

Surgery can be delayed until the infant is rehydrated and the electrolyte imbalance restored. All feedings have to be temporarily interrupted for a day or so after surgery. The mother should be advised to feed with only one breast and for a short time at first to prevent overfilling. The infant must be handled very carefully, "as if he were made of crystal." Using an infant seat for a few days may help to stabilize his position during feeding.

This problem is usually not seen in a breastfed infant; where breastfeeding rates have risen there has been a decrease in the incidence of pyloric stenosis. Habbick (1989) conducted a case-control study of the hospital charts of 91 infants with pyloric stenosis and matched these infants with a control group. Bottle-feeding was 2.9 times more prevalent among the infants with pyloric stenosis than among the control subjects.

Tracheoesophageal fistula (T-E fistula).   In the most common form of esophageal anomaly, tracheoesophageal fistula (T-E fistula), the upper end of the esophagus ends in a blind pouch with a fistula connecting the lower segment of the esophagus to the trachea. An infant who has unexplained episodes of coughing, choking, and cyanosis while feeding, as well as increased mucus secretion may be suspected of having T-E fistula. Feeding at the breast is the optimal way to check for this problem because colostrum is secreted in only small amounts at first; therefore if a fistula is present, no great amount of fluid can be aspirated, and this fluid is not an irritant.

T-E fistula, a rare defect (1:3,000 live births), is suspected when the baby has extreme difficulty feeding. A catheter is passed into the esophagus to see if gastric secretions can be aspirated; it is a practice that should *not* be done routinely. If gastric content cannot be determined and other symptoms are present, medical attention should be obtained at once. If the diagnosis is confirmed by x-ray examination and sonography, surgery is performed to connect the esophagus by end-to-end anastomosis.

Postoperatively, the infant is placed in an isolette with his head elevated. He should have continuous low suction in the esophageal pouch and intermittent low suction to the gastrostomy tube. Until the infant can take oral feedings, the mother can maintain lactation by pumping or by hand expressing milk. Her milk should be saved and frozen according to the storage guidelines in Chapter 15. If temporary bottle-feeding is required to test for feeding tolerance, breastmilk should be used, since human milk is a physiologic fluid and less irritating than glucose water.

As soon as the suture line begins to heal, the mother can breastfeed while simultaneously feeding her baby milk through the gastrostomy tube. Oral stimulation, either by feedings or pacifier, are extremely important. To meet the oral needs of the infant, a pacifier may be necessary until breastfeedings can be resumed. Usually it takes a few days before the baby begins to breastfeed enthusiastically.

Imperforate anus.   This anomaly ranges from no opening at all to a normal appearing rectum that ends in a blind rectal pouch just above the opening; it is only confirmed by careful examination and a diagnostic x-ray examination. Treatment requires reconstruction of the anal opening with surgery. In postoperative nursing care, the area around the surgical repair site should be kept clean and dry to promote healing. As soon as peristalsis returns, the infant can be fed from his mother's breast. The normally loose stools of the breastfed infant lessen the risk of constipation with subsequent breakdown of the surgical area and local infection.

Following her infant's surgery for high, imperforate, anal defect that included a temporary colostomy, one mother was encouraged by her physician to resume breastfeeding two days later. When the infant suddenly developed Ritter's disease (toxic epidermal necrolysis) and had to be rehospitalized, she continued to breastfeed and alternately pump her milk for tube feedings. A few months after recovering, the baby underwent pull-through surgery to bring the colon back down to the anal opening with anoplasty. Solids were deliberately delayed to avoid any undue pressure until the colostomy was completely closed at eight months of age. The child continued to breastfeed until he weaned himself at 18 months.

Cleft lip and palate.   Cleft lip and palate are congenital malformations characterized by incomplete fusing of the central processes around the upper jaw and lip. The clefting may involve only the lip, may extend into the hard and soft palate, and may be unilateral or bilateral. The general classifications include:

- CL: Lip only
- CLP: Both the lip and palate
- CP: Hard and soft palate only

Cleft lip and cleft palate each account for 25% of the malformations; clefting of both of these structures is found in 50% of all cases; therefore, the nurse or lactation consultant will work most frequently with cases involving both the lip and palate.

Surgical repair of the lip is done before the palate. Early surgery (during the first three weeks of life) enhances bonding attachment to a more "normal" infant whose appearance is closer to the ideal baby that the parents expected; it appears to have no greater risks than later surgery (Weatherley-White et al., 1987). Surgical closure of the palate between six months and three years of age takes advantage of normal palatal changes in development.

If the infant has unilateral cleft lip with only minor alveolar ridge deficiency and no palate involvement, he will probably be able to breastfeed before surgery is performed. He must, however, find a way to form a satisfactory seal with his mouth and nose defect. Mothers of these infants have found that by holding their infant inward, pressing the cleft as tightly to the breast as possible, and placing a thumb or index finger over the cleft, enough suction is created for the infant to effectively milk the breast. When necessity demands, the infant is amazingly adaptive and the breast is far more flexible than a rigid bottle teat. Radiographic observation of an infant with a bilateral cleft lip showed that during suckling the tongue is grooved longitudinally, and a peristaltic wave moves backward and obliterates the groove, presses on the nipple, and expresses the milk from it (Jenkins, 1978).

Following surgical repair of the lip, the baby may breastfeed. Weatherley-White and colleagues (1987) at Children's Hospital, Denver, Colorado, offered mothers of 60 infants undergoing surgery for cleft lip the option to breastfeed immediately after surgery. The breastfed infants attained adequate oral intake in a shorter time than babies fed with a cup. The only surgical complication occurring was a partial separating of the lip on the third post-operative day—in a baby fed by cup. No breastfed infant sustained any gross clinical changes attributable to nursing. At the same time, of the 15 babies with complete cleft lip and palate who attempted breastfeeding, only one continued to breastfeed, while the other 14 were switched to a bottle by their mothers. The authors failed to mention if any of these infants wore an artificial palate (see Table 18–3).

When the hard and/or soft palate are also involved in the cleft (CP and CLP), feeding at the breast is more difficult. Since there is a direct space into the nasal cavity, the infant must quickly gulp his food between breaths to prevent regurgitation through his

TABLE 18–3   CLEFT LIP SURGERY: WEIGHT GAIN AND COST DIFFERENCES BETWEEN GROUPS

Category	1-Month Gain	3-Month Gain	Hospital Stay	Cost
Breastfeeders*	28%	67%	2.1 days	$2,552
Cup-feeders	16%	50%	3.3 days	$3,178

*Cleft lip only babies
From Weatherly-White, RCA, et al.: Early repair and breastfeeding for infants with cleft lip, *Plast Reconstr Surg* 79:879–85, 1987.

nostrils. This is not possible unless the milk flows easily and quickly into the back of the oral cavity where it can be swallowed rapidly. One mother started breastfeeding her twins without realizing that one of them had a cleft of the soft palate. The

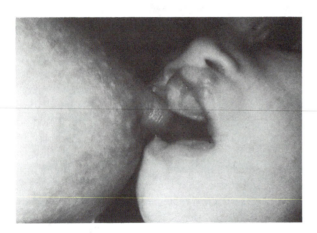

A

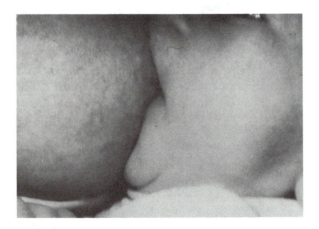

B

FIGURE 18–5   **A,** Infant with cleft lip and complete cleft of hard and soft palates. Palatal obturator in place. **B,** Same infant at breast (**A** and **B** courtesy David Barnes, D.D.S.)

infant cried constantly from hunger and could only drink the milk already let-down in the breast. After discovering the cleft, the mother noticed that by milking the breast with her gums and tongue, the child could suckle effectively when the breasts were full and hard. "Then we discovered that the only purpose of the suction was to draw in and keep the nipple in her mouth. I found that by placing my index finger on the top edge of my areola and my middle finger on the bottom, I could press my nipple out between these fingers; it would protrude as if it were full of milk. I held the nipple in her mouth during the whole feeding as much as I would a bottle and its nipple" (Grady, 1977). After four months of using this technique, supplementation was no longer necessary, and the baby was able to breastfeed without additional assistance. Even when this technique is used successfully, the infant must develop strong muscles and jaw capabilities to withdraw the milk.

A palatal obturator, a plastic dental appliance made by a dentist from impressions of the infant's mouth, covers the cleft in the palate and improves the infant's ability to suckle. With early breastfeeds with this artificial palate, the baby does not tire as easily when the feed is finished or "topped-off" with expressed breastmilk using a supplementation device. Sometimes denture powder helps to hold the dental palate firmly in place.

In another case from the author's practice, a determined mother successfully breastfed her infant who had bilateral cleft lip and complete clefts running through the entire hard and soft palate. By first stimulating her milk supply by hand expression and electric pump, this mother found that she was able to breastfeed using the following techniques:

1. Hold the infant sitting up directly facing the mother, with infant's legs spread on each side, and his head slightly tilted backward.
2. Push the breast into the baby's mouth as far as

possible. In this way, the breast helps to seal the cleft.

3. Massage the breast before the feeding to let-down the milk. The mother reported, "When it did, he thought he had done it!"
4. Stimulate suckling motions by placing fingers under his jaw and firmly pushing up and down. The infant soon catches on and initiates the suckling movements himself, which become stronger.

In the interval between experimentation with different methods of feeding, breast pumping helps to maintain lactation. Unless the mother is very efficient in hand expression, an electric pump is recommended, particularly one with a double kit for simultaneous pumping of both breasts to save time and energy. Meanwhile, the infant can be fed breastmilk by using various methods. Some parents find that a small spouted cup works well. Others favor an eye-dropper, a rubber-tipped syringe, or a pipette. Feeding tube devices (see Chapter 11) have been used successfully for infants with cleft palates. The Beniflex Nurser is another alternative for feeding breastmilk.

Choanal atresia. Choanal atresia is a narrowing of the posterior nares which prevents an infant from drawing air through his nose and breathing normally. A rare congenital anomaly, it is a life-threatening emergency in the neonate who develops respiratory distress following birth. Surgery is usually attempted after the second or third week of life, depending on the condition of the infant and his ability to breath through his mouth. The reconstructive surgery for choanal atresia is highly specialized, and the family will probably have to travel to a regional medical center for the surgery. Surgical placement of nasal stents relieves the baby's respiratory distress.

Following the insertion of an oral airway, if the mother desires, she should be encouraged to breast-feed or pump her milk for bottle-feeding. The mother will need to be alert for choking during suckling because the infant is unable to breathe through his nose. Feedings need to be interrupted between swallows to allow the infant time to breathe through his mouth (Ledonne, 1986). If the baby is unable to feed from the breast or bottle, breastmilk may be given through a naso-gastric tube, but the infant will be expected to take oral feedings before he is released from the medical center.

Ledonne (1986) describes a case in which the mother of a child with choanal atresia gradually switched the baby from formula to breastmilk and continued nursing until he was nine months of age. The mother's desire to breastfeed necessitated cutting down the stents so that they would not be occluded by the breast. In addition, the mother held the baby as upright as possible while feeding to reduce the amount of milk that remained in the rear portion of the nasal stents. The infant needed to be suctioned after every feeding because the stents became plugged, causing difficulty in nasal breathing.

The baby with choanal atresia may resist taking any type of oral feeding at first—breast or bottle—and he will curl up his tongue to protect himself against the possibility of choking. After desperately trying every "trick the doctors and nurses knew," a mother tearfully pleaded with her baby that she had tried everything possible to get him to eat and that now it was his turn to do his part. The mother reported: "Then I laid down on the couch with him and for the first time he took my breast and started feeding. It was like he was saying to me, 'OK mom, I didn't know it was this bad'" (Smith, personal communication, 1991).

CLINICAL IMPLICATIONS

One out of 50 newborns is born with a significant congenital defect, many of which are genetically determined. When the child has myelomeningocele, a cleft palate, or any other abnormality that requires special care over a long period of time, the parents must adjust psychologically after the birth to the discrepancy between the ideal child wished for during pregnancy and the real child they have. For the mother who intended to breastfeed, the loss of a perfect infant is compounded by the possible loss of being able to feed her infant at her breast; sensitivity to these legitimate feelings is essential. The potential for breastfeeding depends on several variables: the extent of the problem and its short- and long-term implications for feeding; the mother's degree of motivation; and the help she receives.

Surgery has made it possible to correct congenital defects, enhance the quality of life, and to prolong life. Preparing the breastfeeding child who is to have surgery depends on his developmental level and his ability to comprehend and reason. Toddlers and pre-schoolers have vivid imaginations and a strong negative reaction to any procedure in which skin is broken; they may interpret syringes to be knives or daggers. Play interviews encourage children to express their fears and feelings about hospitalization and surgery through play.

Preparing the breastfeeding infant or child for surgery is similar to preparing the nonbreastfeeding child. One or both of the parents is encouraged to stay with the child as much as possible. Many surgical procedures are now conducted on an out-patient basis, with the family coming to the hospital in the morning and returning home later that day. If the surgery is major and if the baby will be anesthetized, the mother and father accompany the child to the doors of the surgery suite and then wait in a family waiting area on the pediatric unit for their child to return.

Some hospitals allow breastfeeding up to two hours prior to the induction of anesthesia. In a study (Schreiner, Triebwasser & Keon, 1990) which compared gastric fluid volume and pH levels in two groups of children, one group was permitted clear liquids (apple juice, water, jello, or soda) until two hours before surgery. The other group fasted after 8:00 P.M. on the previous evening. The authors concluded that drinking clear liquids up to two hours prior to anesthesia induction added no additional risk for aspiration of gastric contents. While breastmilk was not specifically listed as a "clear liquid" in this study, it is a physiologic fluid that is digested very rapidly and completely.

In some cases, the infant is so ill that the parents are told he may not survive. In such instances should health workers encourage the mother to establish and maintain a milk supply when she may not have the infant for very long? Experience leads us to believe that she should; doing so makes her feel that she has done everything possible for her infant. Moreover, if the infant does die, grieving occurs more normally when the mother has attached herself emotionally to the infant when he is alive. Giving herself through her milk enhances attachment and bonding as much as looking at and touching her baby.

With the medical technology now available, most infants with congenital abnormalities survive and go on to live relatively normal lives. During the first months after birth, if hospitalization, surgery, or the infant's weakness interfere with normal breastfeeding, the mother must depend on other means to stimulate her milk supply and remove her milk. To do this, she needs specific information on what

pumps or lactation aids are available, and how she can obtain the one most suitable for her.

It is best *not* to offer a rubber nipple of any kind to a breastfeeding neonate or young infant in order to prevent the baby from becoming nipple-confused. But the question arises: If a rubber nipple *is* used, what kind is best? There is no "special" kind of nipple that effectively simulates actual suckling at the breast and thereby prevents nipple confusion. If the infant is under four weeks of age, any oral fluids that are given *temporarily* may be given using one or more of the following:

- a feeding tube device such as those described in Chapter 11
- small medicine cup
- spouted cup
- syringe attached to tube
- syringe-like device used to give medicine to infants
- periodontal syringe (dental supply store).

In working with a mother whose self-esteem has already been undermined by the loss of the expected "perfect child," the nurse or lactation consultant must make every effort to avoid stimulating any further feelings of failure. Therefore, all words and actions should be carefully chosen. One such mother was devastated after being told, "We've never seen anything like this before," when she was unable to express any milk using an electric pump. Already having a child that was different from the one she had expected, she could not tolerate being thought of as different again, although for another mother the remark might have gone unnoticed. For this mother, maintaining her milk supply until she could breastfeed directly was a way of retaining normalcy in her relationship with her infant. Ironically, the pump was later found to be faulty. This suggests that, unless proven otherwise, the pump should always be suspected *first* when a mother has problems using it.

METABOLIC DYSFUNCTION

INBORN ERRORS OF METABOLISM

More than 100 metabolic diseases can be detected in infancy. Of these, only a few cause a health problem, and only a few are suitable for routine screening. Neonatal screening is determined by state law, and

TABLE 18–4   COMPARISON OF SERUM PHENYLALANINE CONCENTRATIONS BY MONTH FOR BREASTFED AND FORMULA-FED INFANTS WITH PHENYLKETONURIA*

| Month | Serum Phenylalanine (μmol/L) X ± SD(n) | |
	Breastfed	Formula-fed
1	993 ± 285 (16)	1084 ± 395 (10)
2	478 ± 145 (17)	454 ± 139 (10)
3	472 ± 194 (16)	478 ± 206 (10)
4	617 ± 176 (13)	630 ± 218 (10)
5	599 ± 151 (12)	593 ± 218 (10)
6	557 ± 157 (11)	684 ± 254 (9)

*No significant differences between groups

From McCabe, L, et al.: The management of breast feeding among infants with phenylketonuria, *J Inher Metab Dis* 12:467–74, 1989.

there is no national policy in the United States for routine metabolic screening. All states, however, require screening for phenylketonuria (PKU) and hypothyroidism. Other metabolic disorders for which screening is often done are galactosemia, maple syrup urine disease, and homocystinuria (Tiwary, 1987). In the United States, where most infants are born in a hospital or clinic, the hospital staff is responsible for obtaining the samples. With early discharge, this is sometimes done after the mother and baby go home. With a home delivery, the responsibility is with the attending physician or midwife.

Two rare disorders, phenylketonuria and galactosemia are briefly discussed here because of their effect on breastfeeding. PKU is an inherited metabolic disorder associated with mental retardation. Because of liver enzyme deficiency, the affected child is unable to metabolize the essential amino acid phenylalanine, one of the 20 amino acids necessary for growth. Accumulation of high levels of phenylalanine in the infant appears to prevent normal development of the brain and central nervous system (see Table 18–4).

Almost all infants in the United States are screened for PKU at birth. After two days of feedings, the infant's heel is pricked with a lancet and a few drops of blood are allowed to fall onto a specially prepared filter paper (the Guthrie test). The first test may be false-negative before higher levels of phenylalanine have had a chance to develop and be detected; therefore, the test should be repeated later. Even

then, there are problems with reliable testing. False-positive tests have caused extreme concern and resulted in (in the past) immediate weaning—only to be found to be inaccurate.

Breastfeeding an infant with PKU is not contraindicated as was previously believed. Human milk has relatively low levels of phenylalanine; breastfed infants who receive a daily amount of 362 mL (first month) to 464 mL (fourth month) of breastmilk each day have a lower phenylalanine intake than infants who are fed exclusively on low-phenylalanine formula during their first six months of life (McCabe et al., 1989). Total or partial breastfeeding can therefore be encouraged if the infant's phenylalanine levels are closely monitored (Miller & Chopra, 1984). Supplemental formula should be Lofenalac, a casein-free hydrolysate from which 95% of the phenylalanine has been removed.

Another hereditary metabolic condition, galactosemia, occurs once in about every 85,000 births. A rare disorder of the metabolism of galactose-1-phosphate, galactosemia is an enzyme deficiency that is transmitted as an autosomal recessive trait. With galactosemia, the liver enzyme that changes galactose to glucose is absent; as a result the infant is unable to metabolize lactose. Any intake of galactose results in liver dysfunction and disease.

These infants appear normal at birth but soon start having feeding difficulties. Vomiting and poor weight gain follow. Without treatment, cerebral impairment and lethargy appear at first, followed by mental retardation. Galactosemia is one of the few cases that demands immediate and total weaning, since breastmilk has a high lactose content. All milk and galactose-containing foods must be eliminated from the diet and the infant placed on special galactose-free formula such as Nutramigen. Reassure the mother that by holding and stroking during bottle-feedings she can meet the emotional-social needs of her infant.

CONGENITAL HYPOTHYROIDISM

Congenital hypothyroidism is caused by a lack of thyroid secretion—either because the thyroid gland is absent or because there is an inborn enzymatic deficiency in the synthesis of thyroxine. A transient (noncongenital) form of hypothyroidism develops from transfer in utero of antithyroid drugs or use of povidone-iodine on the mother at the time of deliv-

TABLE 18–5 MEAN (± SEM) THYROXINE (T$_4$ AND TRIIODOTHYRONINE (T$_3$) LEVELS OF BREASTFED (BF) AND FORMULA-FED (FF) CHILDREN WITH CONGENITAL HYPOTHYROIDISM

Age, Mo	T$_4$, nmol/L		T$_3$, nmol/L	
	BF	FF	BF	FF
1	161.4 ± 9.4	110.7 ± 9.4*	2.7 ± 0.2	30. ± 0.2
2	169.6 ± 7.8	128.4 ± 8.0*	2.6 ± 0.2	3.1 ± 0.2
3	173.4 ± 7.5	154.5 ± 7.7	3.0 ± 0.1	3.2 ± 0.3
4	176.6 ± 7.6	172.8 ± 8.2	3.2 ± 0.2	3.0 ± 0.2
6	174.2 ± 13.3	169.0 ± 6.3	3.0 ± 0.1	3.0 ± 0.1
9	163.2 ± 9.8	153.9 ± 6.3	2.8 ± 0.1	3.1 ± 0.2
12	161.5 ± 5.2	121.7 ± 4.5	2.4 ± 0.2	2.8 ± 0.1

*p <.001.
From Rovet, JF: Does breast-feeding protect the hypothyroid infant whose condition is diagnosed by newborn screening? *Am J Dis Child* 144:319–23, 1990.

ery (Delange et al., 1988). Routine screening results show that congenital hypothyroidism occurs in only one of every 4,000 to 5,000 births.

In the early weeks, parents of an untreated infant may praise their "good baby" because he cries so little. Unless treated, the symptoms of hypothyroidism become noticeable in three to six months. After three months, classic symptoms of myxedema appear: coarse, brittle hair; anemia; a large, protruding tongue; a wide forehead; and lack of skeletal growth. Impairment of the baby's nervous system can lead to severe mental retardation.

Does breastfeeding protect the infant with congenital hypothyroidism? For breastfeeding infants, T$_4$ levels appear to normalize (i.e., >130nmol/L) by one month of age as seen in Table 18–5 (Hahn et al., 1986; Rovet, 1990). Thus, because breastmilk contains small quantities of thyroid hormones not found in commercial formula preparations, breastfeeding may provide minimal protection to the infant with congenital hypothyroidism before treatment can be given (Bode, Vanjonack & Crawford, 1978; Hahn et al., 1983; Varma et al., 1978). At the same time, the presence of these hormones does not alter the accuracy of the screening program for congenital hypothyroidism (Hahn et al., 1986). Any child with congenital hypothyroidism will need lifelong thyroid replacement therapy regardless of how he is fed. A synthetic levothyroxine sodium (Synthroid or Levothroid) is usually given.

CELIAC DISEASE

Often called malabsorption syndrome or gluten enteropathy, celiac disease is characterized by changes in the intestinal mucosa or villi that prevent the absorption of foods, mainly fat. The mucosal damage appears to be from a sensitivity to the gluten factor of protein found in wheat, rye, oats, and barley. Formula-feeding and the early introduction of solids accelerates the development of celiac disease (Greco et al., 1988), which explains why the incidence of celiac disease has declined in the United States as breastfeeding rates have risen (Dossetor, Gibson & McNeish, 1981). Celiac disease is thought to be either an inborn error of metabolism or an immune system disorder. It is only recently that a link has been made between the mammary tissues and other secretory mucosal sites as part of the immune system (Slade & Schwartz, 1987).

The infant with this disorder will gain adequate weight and show no symptoms until solids containing gluten are introduced into his diet. Then the clinical symptoms are insidious and chronic. Because fat is not absorbed, the child's stools become frothy in appearance, foul smelling, and excessive. Deficiencies of the fat-soluble vitamins (A,D,K, and E) appear. If the disease progresses without treatment, abdominal distension and general wasting are evident.

Primary prevention is family teaching and encouraging women with a family history of this disease to breastfeed for a long period and to delay giving their baby solids. The affected child's diet must be modified and vigorously maintained to exclude gluten, thus improving food absorption and preventing malnutrition.

CYSTIC FIBROSIS

Cystic fibrosis (CF), a congenital disease manifesting itself as a chronic generalized dysfunction of the exocrine (mucus-producing) glands, occurs once in every 1,500 to 2,000 live births. The glands of the affected child produce abnormally thick and sticky secretions that block the flow of pancreatic digestive enzymes, clog hepatic ducts, and impede the movement of cilia in the lungs. The increased sodium chloride in the child's sweat provides an important diagnostic clue: the family reports that the child tastes salty when kissed.

Another early manifestation of cystic fibrosis is intestinal obstruction or *ileus*. The newborn's meconium blocks the small intestine and gives rise to signs of intestinal obstruction, including abdominal distention, vomiting, and failure to pass stools. In spite of a voracious appetite, the infant fails to gain weight. When he begins to eat cereals and solids, the stools become bulky, more frequent, foul smelling, and frothy. Pulmonary complications are almost always present, and the child suffers persistent, severe respiratory infections because of retained mucus.

Care primarily involves protection from respiratory infection by postural drainage, aerosol therapy, and medications such as expectorants and antibiotics. To replace pancreatic enzymes which the child is not producing, pancreatic enzyme replacement (Pancrease) is given mixed in soft foods such as applesauce.

There is no need to interrupt breastfeeding. In fact, breastfeeding is recommended. Babies with CF produce normal levels of gastric lipase, which is a major digestive enzyme. This enzyme, together with milk lipase in breastmilk, may help the infant with CF to absorb fat efficiently, according to Dr. Margit Hamosh, Professor of Pediatrics, Georgetown University Medical Center (personal communication, 1991). Human milk contains appreciably greater amounts of lipase than cow's milk. Pasteurization destroys milk lipase and rapid loss of activity occurs at room temperature (Ross & Sammons, 1955).

Dodge (1985), diSant'Agnese and Hubbard (1984), and Rooney (1988) suggest that some breastfed infants with CF will develop symptoms only *after* breastfeeding stops. Moreover, it appears that solely breastfed infants are taller and heavier than solely formula-fed infants (Holliday et al., 1991). Since the infant with CF is prone to severe respiratory infections, he needs the additional immunological protection conferred by breastmilk. In a recent survey (Luder et al., 1990) of U.S. cystic fibrosis centers, most centers recommended breastfeeding alone— or with pancreatic enzyme supplement and/or hydrolyzed formula. This is a reversal from previous reports in which breastfeeding was contraindicated.

ALLERGIES AND FOOD INTOLERANCE

It is widely recognized that breastfed infants and children are less susceptible to food allergies (Cunningham, Jelliffe, & Jelliffe, 1991). During the past several decades, numerous studies have been published on the relationships between infant feeding and allergies (see Chapter 5). In the majority of these studies, the findings suggest that the mode of feeding during the first few months of life affects the incidence of allergies and the risk of allergic disease in subsequent years. This association arises both from the protective effect of breastmilk and from the adverse effect of cow's milk (and to a lesser extent, other foods).

Nurses, especially those in pediatric settings, know that this advantage of breastfeeding is not to be taken lightly. The unhappy sequence of intolerance to formula starts when the infant becomes fussy, colicky, and has diarrhea. Next, the baby develops eczema while the parents and the physician frantically search for a formula he can tolerate. This experience is an unnecessary emotional and economic burden to the family and a health risk to the infant that may have lifelong consequences.

Food allergy is generally defined as an altered adverse reaction to a foreign substance or antibody accompanied by immunologic changes, notably a rise in IgE. The most common offending foods that tend to produce allergic responses in Western cultures are cow's milk, peanuts, eggs, seafood, and egg whites (see Table 18–6). Infants with food allergies are more likely to have families with atopic disease and mothers who were nauseated during pregnancy (Baylis, Leeds & Challacombe, 1983). *Food intolerance,* on the other hand, is a broad term that includes any adverse response to food and is not limited to a rise in IgE. This term includes *food sensitivity.* Sensitivities include lactose intolerance, celiac disease, and any condition in which the infant cannot tolerate certain foods (McCarty & Frick, 1983). The initial exposure is *sensitization,* which does not usually result in allergic symptoms. With a subsequent exposure, however, allergic symptoms become evident within days. This distinction helps to make it clear why a baby given a routine cow's milk formula in the hospital may not experience a reaction until the next exposure several days or weeks later. If the mother is not informed of the routine supplement given in her absence when the baby was in the nursery, she may not recognize that the sensitizing event occurred in the hospital.

Cow's milk allergy is the most common nutritional allergy during infancy. Some infants who are exclusively breastfed develop allergic symptoms following their first exposure to cow's milk because they have been previously sensitized to it transplacentally, through their mother's milk, or in the hospital nursery (Host, Husby & Osterballe, 1988).

In cow's milk allergy, vomiting may be accompanied by chronic diarrhea, colic, colitis, excessive crying, a reluctance to feed, and poor sleep patterns. Eczema, urticaria (itching), a severe diaper rash, and excessive pallor may also be present. Infants tend to have an individual way of responding to allergies. For instance, from the same food, one infant will develop diarrhea, colic, or gastrointestinal problems; another responds through his central nervous system and becomes irritable or hyperactive; and a third may have dermatologic symptoms such as urticaria or eczema.

The list of allergy symptoms is long: an allergic child may have rhinitis, otitis media, coughing, asthma, conjunctivitis, nausea, vomiting, anorexia, and frequent respiratory infections. Dark circles under the eyes ("allergic shiners") are a common indicator of allergy in the older child. Because foods belonging to the same botanical group have similar antigens, they can trigger a similar allergic response in the same child. Onions, for instance, along with garlic, leeks, and asparagus all belong to the same botanical family; allergy to one may mean allergy to the others (Suitor & Hunter, 1980).

ALLERGIES WHILE BREASTFEEDING

A few completely breastfed infants receiving no other foods react to foods passed from the mother to the baby via her breastmilk. The main offender is cow's milk (Jakobsson & Lindberg, 1978; Host, Husby & Osterballe, 1988; Machtinger & Moss, 1986). Other foods implicated in allergies to breastmilk are eggs (Matsu-

TABLE 18–6 TYPES OF FOODS COMMONLY ASSOCIATED WITH ALLERGIC REACTIONS

Food	Sources
Cow's milk in any form	Butter, bread, pudding, yogurt, cheese, baked goods, sherbet, ice cream, creamed soups, powdered milk drinks, gravies
Eggs, especially egg whites	Cakes, cookies, custard, baked goods, pancakes, French toast, root beer, mayonnaise, breaded foods, some cake icing, meatloaf, noodles
Wheat	Baked goods, pasta, wieners, bologna, some canned soups, some pudding and gravies, pudding, some textured vegetable protein
Peanuts, legumes	Peanut butter, beans, peas, lentils, and foods containing soy protein, soy flour, or oil
Nuts and Kola nuts	Candy, granola, baked goods, chocolate, cocoa, cola beverages
Fish or shellfish	Any fish or food fried in same oil as fish, cod liver oil, pizza with anchovies
Corn	Corn cereals, corn chips, Cracker Jacks, corn tortillas and other Mexican foods, popcorn, cornstarch, cornmeal
Citrus fruits	Orange, lemon, lime, grapefruit, fruit desserts, fruit punch
Tomatoes	Juice, meatloaf, stew or other mixed dishes, spaghetti, pizza, catsup
Spices	Cinnamon, catsup, chili, pepper, vinegar

mara et al., 1975), chocolate, fish, citrus (fruits), and peanuts (Cant, Marsden & Kilshaw, 1985; Chandra et al., 1986; Hattevig et al., 1989). Symptoms in the infants include eczema, diarrhea with foul-smelling stools, vomiting, colic (Host, Husby & Osterballe, 1988), excessive sleep, screaming (Sutin, 1988), and blood-streaked stools (Klein, Shvartzman & Weizman, 1990; Perisic, Filipovic & Kokai, 1988; Wilson, Self & Hamburger, 1990).

Eliminating foods in the mother's diet, especially cow's milk, usually solves the problem. If the elimination diet is to be of any value, however, it has to be carefully followed and clearly spelled out—written instructions are the most helpful, while scrupulous reading of labels on packaged foods helps avoid inadvertent consumption of foods that should be eliminated. It is necessary in some cases to remove all dairy foods. The extent of this elimination is described by a mother whose son developed eczema while she was exclusively breastfeeding:

> I stopped drinking milk and expected instant miracles, but nothing changed. I cut cheese and yogurt out of my diet and still saw no improvement. Eventually, I had to eliminate all dairy products as well as products containing even trace amounts of milk. Then I could see the improvement (Sutin, 1988).

If the mother does not eat dairy products, she must take sufficient calcium in other foods and from calcium supplements.

The most effective prevention of allergies in infants involves exclusive breastfeeding for the first several months and gradual introduction of solid foods, one at a time, observing for any symptoms of allergy. Kajosaari and Saarinen (1983) evaluated the prophylactic effect of six months' total solid food elimination in exclusively breastfed Finnish infants—compared to infants similarly breastfed who started solid food at about three months of age. At one year the children who had not received solids until six months of age had atopic eczema and food allergy less frequently than the early solid groups (Kajosaari & Saarinen, 1983).

Delaying solids for somewhat longer in infants who are highly allergic to a variety of foods is safe, provided the hemoglobin level is monitored at intervals. Usually the hemoglobin remains within the normal range because of the efficient absorption of the iron in breastmilk; however, the mother must be prepared to breastfeed often to provide the necessary calories that otherwise would have been provided by solids.

HYPOGLYCEMIA

During the last trimester of pregnancy, the fetus builds up his supply of glycogen reserves. After birth these reserves sustain the full-term infant during the birth process and for the first two or three days—until he receives sufficient amounts of breastmilk from his mother. Symptoms of hypoglycemia (low blood sugar) are vague and similar to those caused by many other conditions, such as tremors, jitteriness, lethargy, and a weak or high-pitched cry. About one-half of infants with low blood sugar will not show any of these symptoms.

Infants considered at risk are screened for hypoglycemia within the first hour after birth with a Dextrostix or Chemstrip-BG, which are read manually after placing blood on the reagent strip or by a glucose reflectance meter. Two specimens of blood should be analyzed because of possible error when conducting these sensitive tests. For instance, the blood must remain on the Dextrostix for exactly one minute and then be compared to the color chart. Delayed reading may result in an inaccurate measurement. Other factors that affect the reliability of the Dextrostix are overwashing and improper storage of the reagent strips. Color changes that indicate a blood glucose level of less than 45 mg/dL should be confirmed by a laboratory analysis of whole blood.

In the full-term, healthy newborn, hypoglycemia is traditionally defined as a blood glucose level below 30 mg/dL in the first day of life, or less than 40 mg/dL in the second day of life (Cornblath, 1976; Heck & Erenberg, 1987). The blood glucose reaches its lowest level between one and two hours after birth and then it gradually rises. If the infant is not started on feedings until three hours of age, blood glucose levels still rise and at three hours are significantly higher than one-hour values (Srinivasan et al., 1986). See Table 18–7 for glucose values.

The level of acceptable serum glucose concentrations is being revised upward in some hospitals to 40 and 45 mg/dL, with the result that breastfeeding neonates, who ingest only 25 to 30% of the amount of milk ingested by bottle-fed infants (Heck & Erenberg, 1987), are commonly diagnosed as hypoglycemic and given supplements. The medical com-

TABLE 18–7 PLASMA GLUCOSE VALUES DURING FIRST WEEK OF LIFE (ALL GROUPS) REGARDLESS OF TYPE OF FEEDINGS

	Plasma Glucose			
Age (hr)	Number of Samples	Mean	SD*	Range
0	52	107	35	55–265
1	52	56	19	17–119
2	51	60	11	39–96
3	51	70	13	39–97
4	49	68	14	40–112
6	69	65	13	40–101
12–24	40	67	14	46–117
25–48	55	71	10	48–98
49–72	55	73	13	50–114
73–96	35	83	12	56–116
97–168	26	80	12	54–192

*Standard deviation.
From Srinivasan, G, et al.: Plasma glucose values in normal neonate, *J Pediatr* 109:114–17, 1986.

munity is debating the definition of "normal" blood values of neonates. Some of the controversy is because the definition of hypoglycemia used today was derived from early studies which examined whole blood glucose levels of infant groups by birth weight and which were adjusted upward to approximate plasma levels. Since then, recognition of gestational age and the common administration of dextrose solution during labor and delivery has led some physicians to recommend that glucose levels should be maintained at above 40 mg/dL.

Using the classic definition of hypoglycemia (below 30%) of Cornblath (1976), incidence rates have ranged from four percent (Gutberlet & Cornblath, 1976) to a high of 11.4% (Lubchenco & Bard, 1971). But when the 40 mg/dL criterion is used, about 20% or *one fifth* of newborns, regardless of how they are fed, would be diagnosed as hypoglycemic (Sexon, 1984), which seems unreasonably high. In this same study, Sexson measured neonatal hypoglycemia in infants with hypoglycemia in a level-one nursery. Of the 232 babies, 168 (72%) had one or more so-called "risk" factors for hypoglycemia! This extraordinary incidence probably points to the nonspecific nature of many of the risk factors. Of

those infants with a known risk factor, 120 did not have hypoglycemia when the definition of a glucose value of less than 40 mg/dL was applied.

Whether infants with glucose values between 30 and 40 mg/dL are at risk for problems to the same degree as infants with lower glucose values is not known. Clearly, using high glucose values as the definition of hypoglycemia for both breastfed and formula-fed infants is questionable, particularly since formula and glucose supplements compromise breastfeeding. Weaning to formula can lead to allergies and many other health problems discussed throughout this book.

Hypoglycemia can be prevented in most cases by putting the baby to breast early and often after delivery. If breastfeedings are poorly tolerated and low serum glucose levels continue, intravenous glucose or formula should be given, but not oral glucose water. In addition to its low caloric content, glucose water is stressful to the infant's pancreas and carries the risk of rebound hypoglycemic problems; thus it is a poor nutritional substitute.

SUDDEN INFANT DEATH SYNDROME (SIDS)

Two of about every 1,000 live-born infants die suddenly, usually in their sleep without apparent cause. Put to bed without any indication that something was wrong, save perhaps a minor upper respiratory infection, the child later is found lifeless. Most of the deaths from SIDS, a major cause of infant death, occur between two and six months of age, with a peak at about 10 weeks of age. The incidence is greater during winter months and in lower socioeconomic groups.

Lack of breastfeeding has been shown to be a risk factor for SIDS (Biering-Sørensen, Jorgensen & Jørgen, 1978; Damus et al., 1988; Froggat, Lynas & MacKenzie, 1971; Hoffman et al., 1988; Mitchell, Stewart & Becroft, 1991). Results of the National Institute of Child Health and Human Development SIDS Cooperative Epidemiological Study conducted in six U.S. cities showed that only 9.8% of SIDS cases were mostly or only breastfed infants, compared to 27.7% and 22.3% of the two nonbreastfed control groups (Hoffman et al., 1988).

Also known as "crib death" or "cot death," there are many theories about the cause of SIDS. At autopsy, total closure of the upper airway seems to be the cause of death; findings include pulmonary congestion, lung hemorrhage, and respiratory inflammation. SIDS is now diagnosed only for an infant who was previously healthy, and the diagnosis is not confirmed until autopsy. Current theories of cause include fulminating infection, laryngospasm, anaphylactic reaction to cow's milk protein (Coombs & McLaughlan, 1982), sleep disorders, apnea (Gould, 1983), and botulism (Arnon, 1986).

Bernshaw (1991) suggests that breastfed infants are at lower risk for SIDS because they: (1) have shorter periods of uninterrupted sleep; (2) are more likely to sleep with the mother, who responds to breathing changes in her baby; (3) receive greater immunological protection; and (4) are less likely to be exposed to agents that cause an anaphylactic reaction.

In so-called "near misses" for SIDS, parents report finding the infant apneic, pale, or cyanotic and requiring vigorous stimulation or resuscitation. The infant may be placed on an apnea monitor because a second apneic episode is not uncommon. It must be pointed out, however, that only a minority of SIDS victims have had documented life-threatening apnea; conversely, most infants with episodes of apnea do not die.

Community-based health personnel, specially trained to work with families who have lost a child through SIDS, are an invaluable resource for helping parents. The breastfeeding mother, in addition to her emotional anguish, has painful, engorged breasts, full of milk for the child who is no longer there. One of the many therapeutic actions at this critical time is helping her with physical relief of her engorgement. She should be taught to express as much milk as is necessary for comfort until the milk reabsorbs. A slight fever during the period of milk reabsorption may be expected in some cases.

While counseling the parents, make them aware that nothing they could have done would have prevented the events from happening. Often, parents are overwhelmed with guilt; any comments that suggest shirked responsibility—such as "Did you check on your baby?"—should be avoided. Pamphlets that have helpful information for parents are available from the National Foundation for Sudden Infant Death, Inc.[*]

[*]National Foundation for Sudden Infant Death, Inc., 2 Metro Plaza, Suite 205, 8240 Professional Place, Landover, MA 20785.

HOSPITALIZATION

Like any crisis, hospitalization can be a time for learning and growth. Chances for a positive experience increase when the mother stays with her child, who finds security and comfort in breastfeeding. Helping has less to do with using specific techniques than with being sensitive to human beings.

The goal of self-care for the hospitalized infant or child is to minimize the discrepancy between care provided at home and the care given in the hospital setting, as well as to maintain and strengthen family unity. Thus, for the child who is breastfed, feeding and nurturing patterns should approximate as closely as possible the normal, home situation. Obviously, this is not always possible. Surgery, diagnostic tests, and other therapeutic interventions may represent obstacles, but the goal is still the same.

A complete data base and assessment help achieve the goal of minimizing the discrepancy of care, and thus trauma, to the child. Through the assessment phase, collection of both subjective and objective data occurs through interviewing and observation. Only by acquiring information can personalized and individualized care be given to families. One method for gaining a data base on normal activity of daily living patterns before hospitalization is to have the mother or father complete a detailed questionnaire. If the child is breastfeeding, some appropriate questions that should be asked during the history-taking include:

- How often does he breastfeed at home?
- How do you usually feed him—sitting up or lying down?
- Does he take any solids or supplements?
- Is he accustomed to his own bed or does he come in bed with you at night for feedings?
- What is his favorite word for breastfeeding?

If the breastfeeding child is old enough to talk, the family may use a "code" word for breastfeeding, such as "nummies," "yum-yum," "nursie," "snugglies," "night-night," or "side." A family who called breastfeeding "night-night" enjoyed the reaction of relatives and friends when the "good" little girl asked to "night-night" all by herself (Bumgarner, 1980). Keep these code words in mind the next time a breastfeeding toddler keeps demanding a "nursie"—he may not mean the nurse. Acceptance of the normalcy of a walking and talking child who breastfeeds is discussed further in Chapter 2.

PARENTAL STRESSES

Driving to and from the hospital from their home 100 or more miles away to alternate staying with their sick infant, a breastfeeding mother and her husband try to cope. With three other children at home, they can snatch only a few hours of sleep at a time. It is the third surgical procedure for their infant, who was born with a congenital defect. Although their physician encourages them that the prognosis is good, the worry and strain seem endless. The mother expresses her milk with a pump when necessary, and her baby is able to breastfeed part of the time. Lately she can express only a few drops at a time, and she can hardly feel a let-down. She wonders how long she will be able to continue lactating.

All parents of ill children are under stress, but consider the effects of chronic stress on a parent who must deal with it over many months and perhaps years, such as the family described here. When it becomes apparent that the ill child may have to be hospitalized, one of the first concerns of the mother is whether she will be able to continue breastfeeding. She has already recognized the unique healing effect of putting an irritable, fussy child to breast when he is hurt or ill. Continuing to breastfeed, unless the child refuses, preserves a sense of normalcy in an otherwise highly stressful time. The mother needs reassurance that breastfeeding can continue and that assistance is available if breastfeeding must be temporarily interrupted. Many hospitals now have breast pumps available for the mother to use to alleviate any discomfort from engorgement. When the child must undergo a surgical procedure or other intervention, particularly if it will be painful, encourage the mother to breastfeed as soon as possible afterward. It is hard to say who benefits more, the mother or the baby, when the sobbing child settles into his mother's lap for the comfort of her breast. What is readily apparent is the relief from stress for them both. A careful explanation of the procedure beforehand will also relieve the mother's anxiety; this relief is in turn transmitted to the child. Parents can handle nearly any treatment if they know what it will be. Of all nursing interventions, anticipatory guidance is one of the most effective.

What about the father? During the stress of the child's illness, attention is often focused on the mother and the ill child. Because his wife is breastfeeding, she will be the one spending most of the time at the bedside. While his child is in the hospital, the father is expected to be the Rock of Gibraltar, an anchor in a sea of distress. In addition to carrying on job responsibilities, he has the responsibility of keeping things running at home, nurturing and caring for the other children, and spending as much time as possible at the hospital. Fathers are people, too, and the stresses they feel are enormous.

These stresses affect the marriage bond. The divorce rate in families with a child born with a neural tube defect was nine times greater than the divorce rate for the normal population (Tew et al., 1977). When a sick child becomes the focus of a mother's attention, other relationships and responsibilities become secondary. Some husbands, sensing this, withdraw emotionally until the crisis is over. Yet, for other couples, their mutual concern causes them to grow closer and draw emotional support from one another. Some parents feel guilty about making love while their child lies ill. If it seems appropriate, point out that sexual enjoyment reinforces their bond with one another—a bond that strengthens them during this difficult period.

The family's response to the chronic illness involves not so much the event itself as it does a particular family's definition or perception of the event, as well as the family's resources to help them deal with the stress. A family with no health insurance and little or no savings perceives their child's chronic illness as more stressful than a family with health insurance, a sufficient income, and savings on which to draw if necessary.

Unreasonable as such feelings may be, both parents may harbor feelings of guilt for bringing on the illness—or for not recognizing how sick the child was in early stages. Questions like "What have I done?" or "What should I have done?" torment them. It is easier for the breastfeeding mother, who continues to be in close contact with her child as she participates in his recovery, to deal with these feelings than it is for the father. Picking up cues about his feelings and encouraging him to talk about them helps; it also provides the opportunity to reassure him that his feelings are normal. The therapeutic value of "talking it out" is significant enough to produce physiologic changes associated with stress reduction (Foster, 1974). Hearing their own statements aloud releases the parents' tension and speeds resolution of their inner conflicts.

Hospitalization brings about a disruption of lifestyle and environment to the family that is tantamount to culture shock. A barrage of unfamiliar stimuli is thrust on them: infusion pumps that periodically sound an alarm, mist tents, and a constantly rotating staff of new faces all place tremendous stresses on the family. Normally affable parents can be demanding and even hostile when anger becomes a by-product of their stress and guilt. These defensive behaviors are part of the parents' coping strategies for managing their feelings. Defense mechanisms, such as denial and rationalization, help protect families from painful realities and are not necessarily evidence of maladaptive behaviors. Although it can be difficult and even painful to deal with such parents, I would far rather work with these concerned parents than with those who are unconcerned or passive. Sympathetic listening and simple, understanding statements—such as, "I can see you are upset," or "This is such a difficult time"—can help parents through this trying time. If hospital nurses rationally assess parents' behaviors and use of defenses, their interactions with parents will be more therapeutic.

The first response of parents whose children are diagnosed with a chronic illness is shock. Their lives resemble an emotional rollercoaster. This initial disorganization and upheaval does not last long, however. As early as a few months after the diagnosis, the family begins to pull together their resources and develop a support system. Although for many parents their child's diagnosis is the worst problem they have ever faced, they are able to make many adjustments in a short period of time. The family gradually recovers and begins to cope.

Some parents, who are many miles from home during their child's hospitalization, must arrange for sleeping accommodations in the area if both are not allowed to stay overnight at the hospital. One father of a child in my unit rode the bus for six hours one-way and back each weekend to visit his wife and baby in the hospital. If the stresses are severe and lengthy, the marital relationship may suffer. Hospital social workers are valuable for helping parents deal with stress when their child is hospitalized.

Parents of hospitalized babies form new friendships that serve self-care groups. The mothers of breastfeeding babies sharing the same hospital room can form a self-care group.

> I was nervous and upset when Meghan and I arrived at the hospital but the staff made me feel right at home. I soon found out there were many other mothers staying with their children and we would get together in the parent's lounge after our children were sleeping to share our thoughts and try to unwind (LLLI, 1978).

Support groups of other parents experiencing a similar life crisis are effective because each person in the group understands the day-to-day issues and problems of caring for an ill child or rearing one with a chronic disease. Nevertheless, support groups are not for all parents—some are so overwhelmed by their own problems that they are not able to reach out and support others. Asking these individuals to participate helps neither them nor the other group members.

COPING WITH SIBLINGS

Siblings are often the forgotten members of the family when attention and concern is focused on the sick child. In nursing, the concept of family-centered care extends to every person in the family, including the children at home, who frequently react to their brother's or sister's illness with anger, resentment, jealousy, and guilt. The situation is especially difficult when an older child is hospitalized and a younger breastfeeding baby or toddler is at home. The mother is emotionally torn between being with her sick child and attending her breastfeeding baby, who so obviously needs her. If the baby is one of breastfeeding twins or if the mother is breastfeeding both a walking child and a baby, the problem is further compounded. Most hospitals encourage siblings (who are not infectious) to visit their brother or sister in the hospital. Institutions that do not do so may add to the family's stress by enforcing isolation when contact would be most beneficial to all parties. When the ill child is at home, siblings may bear additional responsibilities of child care or helping with household tasks.

EMERGENCY ADMISSION

Staff nursing in emergency situations takes split-second reactions and demands a thorough background of a wide range of nursing knowledge. No one nurse, of course, can be expected to know everything. In addition, patients come and go quickly; they are transferred to other units of the hospital or dismissed without being seen again.

Unless the nurse has had personal experience

with a breastfeeding infant or child, she is unlikely to understand all the needs of the family who comes into the emergency unit with a child who is being breastfed. An example is a situation in which the mother, not the child, became very ill. She overheard the harried nurse say, "If she had given that baby a bottle, we wouldn't be in this mess," when the infant first refused and later vomited bottle-feedings. Because emergencies distort perceptions and magnify emotions, criticism is not always a fair analysis of the situation, but there is a lesson for us here. The RN reacted defensively to a life need. The parent may then have mistrusted that their medical needs would be handled well. How do we avoid insensitivity in care when we are faced with a situation beyond our experience or understanding? The best way is to look at the family's needs through the eyes of each family member and actively attempt to support their wishes when an emergency threatens the symbiosis of a breastfeeding relationship.

HOME, THE REBOUND EFFECT

The child's reactions following hospitalization depend on the extent of trauma he has undergone and his defenses for protecting himself. Almost all hospitals now encourage a parent to stay with the child during hospitalization. Fagin (1966) clearly indicates that when parents room-in with the child, very little behavior changes occur upon returning home. If the young child has experienced a painful separation, he may at first refuse the breast and show little interest in his mother or family, using withdrawal as a means of coping. Or he may cry a great deal and want to be held and breastfed exceptionally often, vigorously protesting having his mother out of sight for even a moment. Emotional upheaval, including nightmares and insomnia, are common during the first few weeks following hospitalization, and all members of the family must also adjust.

Short separations during hospitalizations are usually inevitable; however, if a child feels safe and secure in his parent's love, trauma from the illness and temporary separations give way to restoration of trust after being reunited with his family. Helping parents to recognize this is vital to nursing care of the hospitalized child. Inherent in any crisis is the potential for bringing families closer together with new awareness and appreciation of one another.

CHRONIC GRIEF AND LOSS

When the breastfeeding child is chronically ill or has a disabling defect, the disappointment, sorrow, and frustration of parents can be overwhelming. Instead of the perfect child expected during the pregnancy, there is an intense feeling of loss. If the child requires indefinite special care and attention, there is a persistent effect described by Olshansky (1962) as chronic sorrow. Unlike acute grief, which is limited in time, chronic sorrow is prolonged and recurrent. Through grieving, coping processes evolve, and parents can find satisfaction and even joy from their child: "The shock and numbness linger for days, even months. . . . It is only after you have gotten over that first crisis that you begin to realize a life and soul have been given into your care." (Good, 1980). The onset of chronic sorrow is variable among families and sometimes difficult to identify; most important, however, is the recognition that this condition is a natural outgrowth of parenting and is an adaptive response (Lemons & Weaver, 1986).

Breastfeeding has an ameliorating effect for both the child and the parents when chronic illness is involved. The baby receives added protection from his higher risk of infection and also benefits from close contact and stimulation. Engendered in the parents, especially the mother, is the satisfaction of giving something special to her child which helps her deal with her feelings of loss. As one mother (Good, 1980) of a baby with Down syndrome said: "As I looked back at Chad's first year, I'm sure that breastfeeding and that closeness that comes with it helped me to love and accept him just as he was. There were still lots of tears sometimes falling on my special baby as we rocked along and I had many anxieties about the future."

THE MAGIC-MILK SYNDROME

In the process of grieving, parents move through several stages of adjustment. After the initial shock and emotional numbness they reach a stage characterized by rationalization, denial, and sometimes a search for a magic cure. If the baby is not being breastfed, a few frightened parents will desperately search for donated breastmilk in hopes that it will cure their child. The unique properties of breastmilk are so well known that it is sometimes perceived by parents to contain magic properties. The health-care provider needs to validate the value of human milk but at the same time help the parents to recognize that their baby may need more than breastmilk can offer at this moment.

There, are, of course, cases in which breastmilk can help—children with allergies and metabolic disorders may respond well to breastmilk. Chapter 22 (on milk banks) discusses some situations in which it is life-saving. In these situations in which the need is real and substantiated by medical opinion, the child should receive breastmilk from a milk bank if at all possible.

EMPTY CRADLE

The tremendous task of coping and somehow continuing with life must be faced by parents when their child dies. The first reactions of shock, disbelief, and denial are all the more intense when the death is unexpected, as with sudden infant death syndrome. Parents need to be able to express their feelings by crying, screaming, or just quietly talking about how they feel.

Compassionate care assists closure after death. Giving the parents the opportunity to hold their child and to say good-bye helps this process. Afraid at first, one family changed their minds and cradled their dead baby in their arms. "Holding him is what helped us most to accept the death of our baby; it made us feel he was really our own. He smelled sweet and felt soft, and we just stroked him and talked with him for awhile."

The focus of concern is often on the mother. The father, who has had a significant, loving relationship with his child, is sometimes forgotten. The cultural stereotype of male stoicism belies his feelings of shock, grief, and pain. Fathers also need to grieve but sometimes require different kinds of outlets to express it.

As the shock subsides, acute mourning and bereavement are followed by a developing awareness of the full impact of their loss. Guilt, silent or expressed, is an almost universal emotion during this period, and the parents examine their past misdeeds. Questioning the nurse about the possible effects of heredity on the disease is likely as their grief turns inward in the form of self-blame. Explanations of hereditary factors must be honest and factual, tempered with an understanding of what the parents are able to accept.

Physical symptoms such as sleeplessness or a lack of appetite often accompany the parents' feelings of loss and pain. Some parents describe feeling "dead inside" or having a "hole inside that nothing can fill." The breastfeeding mother may have to cope with the physical discomfort of breast fullness and leaking for awhile and should be advised to express her milk once or twice for relief. Occasionally, a mother will continue to pump her milk for several weeks, donating it to a milk bank so that other children may benefit from it. Doing so is her way of coping by maintaining visible evidence of the existence of the lost child. When she offers to do so, the best approach is to put her in touch with a milk bank whose staff members can assist her.

CLINICAL IMPLICATIONS

Families differ in their response to the birth of a child with a defect or a chronic illness, and they will need support from health-care professionals to help them adjust. Therefore, it is important for the professional to have a working knowledge of grief and crisis theories and the skills to implement them. While it is not within the scope of this chapter to review all such theories, the nurse or lactation consultant who works with these families will find additional education and study on parental grief helpful. Following are basic principles of care for any breastfeeding child who is ill. Since these are general principles, they may not be applicable to every situation:

1. Breastfeed the baby in an upright position (generally speaking), since this position facilitates swallowing which may be impaired. Additionally, the mother is able to closely observe her baby during the feeding.
2. Teach the mother alternative feeding methods, such as using a tube feeding device, small cup, or medicine dropper to supplement with breastmilk. Provide her with a breast pump, if needed.
3. Minimize the child's separation from the family. Infants and children should be cared for in their own home with the care provider's assistance and monitoring of the family's capabilities.
4. Help the family to mobilize and supplement their resources. Provide them with some of the excellent books available for parents with hand-

icapped children. Refer them to appropriate specialized health professionals and parent support groups, which can provide them with information in writing.

5. Remind the mother that breastfeeding is *less* (not more) strenuous than bottle-feeding.

6. Accentuate the child's positive attributes and strengths by making such comments as "What a beautiful child" or "He's so strong!"

7. Praise *any* progress in breastfeeding, no matter how small.

8. Read the mother's cues which tell you if she wants to continue to lactate/breastfeed. Give permission and assistance to wean if this is her wish.

9. Maintain the family's hope that tomorrow will be better.

When an infant dies, in the process of detachment, memories that tie the mother to the child must be painfully relived before they are slowly put aside. Especially important to her is the acknowledgement that *her* child was special: she should never be denied the right to her sorrow. Remarks such as "It just wasn't meant to be"—or "You can always have another baby"—are hurtful. They provide no consolation whatsoever regarding her loss of *this* baby. Statements such as "I'm sorry about your baby"—or "If you want to talk, call me"—are consoling and show sensitivity. Following are suggestions based on the author's experiences (as well as those of other health-care professionals) which have been found to help parents and families through the grief process:

1. Call the baby by his name. Having a baby is such a joyful experience; some of that is still there, even though the baby might be stillborn.

2. Acknowledge the parent's loss by sending cards or calling. If the person does not know the parents well, anything more may be too much.

3. Feel your way through the conversation, getting feedback from the parent; wait for him or her to lead the way. Make sure they know you are available to talk whenever needed.

4. If the mother was lactating, help her to remain comfortable. Mothers who lose a baby after 20 weeks of gestation may become engorged—which sometimes comes as a complete shock. The physician may order a lactation suppressant. Often, women are reluctant to relieve their discomfort by expressing milk for fear of stimulating more milk; encourage the mother to express some milk for comfort. Rarely will the discomfort last long (LLLI, 1987).

5. Help the parents to verbalize feelings of anger, fear, guilt, and anxiety by validating them.

Prolonged or abnormal grief is more often seen in the mother than in the father. This is more likely to happen if she has lost another significant person in her life and never resolved that loss, or if she has emotional problems. If her late child was chronically ill, a mother can miss the special mothering role that made her feel useful, important, and needed.

For many parents, the peer support system that previously helped them in parenting and breastfeeding changes in significance; seeing other breastfeeding mothers and their babies may be a painful ordeal. The mother may assiduously avoid them, choosing only one or two especially close peers with whom she can privately talk about her feelings and emotional pain. One of the community support systems available for parents during this difficult period is Aiding Mothers Experiencing Neonatal Death (AMEND). This group has trained counselors to individually help parents work through their grief.

SUMMARY

There are unique considerations for helping the breastfeeding mother and her family when her infant or young child is ill. These special needs can be met by recognizing the developmental stage, assessing family lifestyle, reducing parental stress, involving the parents in direct care of their child, and, most of all, minimizing separation between family members. Discontinuing breastfeeding is rarely necessary for the child with a health problem, although feeding patterns may have to be modified. Too often, however, weaning is automatically assumed, and once the infant is weaned a new cycle of health problems, especially allergies, can appear.

Each family is unique. The experience of one situation can never be duplicated: therefore, care providers helping families with an ill breastfeeding child must use versatility and a firm knowledge of the nature of the health problem. Just as important is recognition of the psychologic needs of the breastfeeding child and his family, especially the mother.

Interventions also require awareness of devices that aid lactation and how they can be obtained. The reader is referred to Chapter 11, Breast Pumps and Technologies, for detailed information. Support must come from the health-care team, not just one or two of its members; therefore, communication among the staff is essential for continuity of care. Ideally, one individual serves as the case manager and coordinates the entire spectrum of the health care in all its settings, whether in the hospital or out in the community. As needs arise, the nurse not only gives customary hands-on care but also acts as a family advocate and broker of additional services (Rogers, Riordan & Swindle, 1991). This health-care worker also informs the parents about every aspect of the health problem and includes them in decision-making, creating mutual respect and a working relationship between health-care workers and the family.

If the child dies, comprehending the impact of the parents' grief and their stage of adaptive coping requires special sensitivity and crisis-intervention skills to help the bereaved parents in their journey through pain toward an adaptive resolution of their loss, which comes only after a long, slow process of working through their grief. As preoccupation with memories lessen, they are able to establish new interests and develop new goals. "Time heals all wounds" is true in the sense that healing occurs with time, but the emotional scars and the times of feeling empty and lonely will endure as long as they live.

REFERENCES

Arnon, SS: Infant botulism: anticipating the second decade, *J Infec Dis* 154:201–6, 1986.

Aumonier, ME, and Cunningham, CC: Breastfeeding in infants with Down's syndrome, *Child Care Health Develop* 9:247–55, 1983.

Baylis, JM, Leeds, AR, and Challacombe, DN: Persistent nausea and food aversions in pregnancy, *Clin Allergy* 13:263–69, 1983.

Bernshaw, NJ: Does breastfeeding protect against sudden infant death syndrome? *J Hum Lact* 7:73–79, 1991.

Biering-Sørenssen, E, Jorgensen, T, and Jørgen, H: Sudden infant death in Copenhagen, 1956–1971, I. Infant feeding, *Acta Paediatr Scand* 67:129–37, 1978.

Bode, HH, Vanjonack, WJ, and Crawford, JD: Mitigation of cretinism by breastfeeding, *Pediatrics* 62:13–16, 1978.

Brown, KH: Dietary management of acute childhood diarrhea: optimal timing of feeding and appropriate use of milks and mixed diets, *J Pediatr* 118:S92–98, 1991.

Bumgarner, NJ: *Mothering your nursing toddler*, Franklin Park, Ill., 1980, La Leche League International.

Cant, AJ, Marsden, RA, and Kilshaw, PJ: Egg and cow's milk hypersensitivity in exclusively breastfed infants with eczema, and the detection of egg protein in breastmilk, *Br Med J,* 291:932–35, 1985.

Chandra, RK, et al.: Influence of maternal food antigen avoidance during pregnancy and lactation on incidence of atopic eczema in infants, *Clin Allergy* 16:563–69, 1986.

Chen, Y, Yu, S, and Li, W: Artificial feeding and hospitalization in the first 18 months of life, *Pediatrics* 81:58–62, 1988.

Cochi, SL, et al.: Primary invasive *Hemophilus influenzae* type b disease: a population-based assessment of risk factors, *J Pediatr* 108:887–96, 1986.

Colombo, JL, Hopkins, RL, and Waring, WW: Steam vaporizer injuries, *Pediatrics* 67:661–63, 1981.

Coombs, RRA, and McLaughlan, P: The enigma of cot death: Is the modified-anaphylaxis hypothesis an explanation for some cases? *Lancet* 1:1388–89, 1982.

Cornblath, M: Diagnosing and treating neonatal hypoglycemia, *Contemp Ob-Gyn* 8:95, 1976.

Cunningham, AS, Jelliffe, BD, and Jelliffe, EF: Breast-feeding and health in the 1980s: A global epidemiologic review, *J Pediatr* 188:659–66, 1991.

Damus, K, et al.: Postnatal medical and epidemiological risk factors for the sudden infant death syndrome. In Harper, RM, and Hoffman, HJ, eds.: *Sudden infant death syndrome: risk factors and basic mechanisms,* New York, 1988, PMA Publishing Co., pp. 187–201.

Danner, SC, and Cerutti, ER: *Nursing your baby with Down's syndrome,* Rochester, N.Y., 1984, Childbirth Graphics, p. 9.

Delange, F, et al.: Topical iodine, breastfeeding, and neonatal hypothyroidism, *Arch Dis Child* 63:106–7, 1988.

diSant'Agnese, PA, and Hubbard, VS: The pancreas. In Taussig, LM, ed.: *Cystic fibrosis,* New York, 1984, Thieme-Stratton Inc., pp. 278–79.

Dodge, JA: The nutritional state and nutrition, *Acta Paediatr Scand* 317(supp.):31–37, 1985.

Dossetor, JFB, Gibson, AAM, and McNeish, AS: Childhood coeliac disease is disappearing, *Lancet* 1(8215):3322–23, 1981.

Fagin, C: *The effects of maternal attendance during hospitalization on the post hospital behavior of young children,* Philadelphia, 1966, F.A. Davis Co.

Foster, SB: An adrenal measure for evaluating nursing effectiveness, *Nurs Res* 23:118, 1974.

Froggatt, P, Lynas, MA, and MacKenzie, G: Epidemiology of sudden unexpected death of infants (cot death) in Northern Ireland, *Br J Prev Soc Med* 25:119–34, 1971.

Good, J: *Breastfeeding the Down's syndrome baby*, La Leche League International, Franklin Park, Ill., 1980, The League.

Gould, JBL: SIDS—A sleep hypotheses. In: *Sudden infant death syndrome,* New York, 1983, Academic Press, Inc., pp. 443–52.

Grady, E: Breastfeeding the baby with a cleft of the soft palate, *Clin Pediatr* 16:978–81, 1977.

Greco, L, et al.: Case-control study on nutritional risk factors in celiac disease, *J Pediatr Gastroenterol Nutr* 7:395–99, 1988.

Gutberlet, RL, and Cornblath, M: Neonatal hypoglycemia revisited 1975, *Pediatrics* 58(1):10–17, 1976.

Habbick, BF: Infantile hypertrophic pyloric stenosis: a study of feeding practices and other possible causes, *Clin Comm Stud* 140:401–4, 1989.

Haffejee, IE: Cow's milk-based formula, human milk, and soya feeds in acute infantile diarrhea: a therapeutic trial, *J Pediatr Gastroenterol Nutr* 10:193–98, 1990.

Hahn, HB, et al.: Breastfeeding and neonatal screening for congenital hypothyroidism, *Tex Med* 82:46–47, 1986.

Hahn, HB, et al.: Thyroid function tests in neonates fed human milk, *Am J Dis Child* 137:220–22, 1983.

Hattevig, G, et al.: Effect of maternal avoidance of eggs, cow's milk and fish during lactation upon allergic manifestations in infants, *Clin Exp Allergy* 19:27–32, 1989.

Heacock, HJ, et al.: Influence of breast versus formula milk on physiological gastroesophageal reflux in healthy, newborn infants, *J Pediatr Gastroenterol Nutr* 14:41–46, 1992.

Heck, LJ, and Erenberg, A: Serum glucose levels in term neonates during the first 48 hours of life, *J Pediatr* 110:119–22, 1987.

Hoffman, HJ, et al.: Risk factors for SIDS: Results of the National Institute of Child Health and Human Development SIDS cooperative epidemiological study. In Schwarz, PJ, Sauhall, DP, and Valdes-Dapnea, M: *The sudden infant death syndrome*, New York, 1988, New York Academy of Sciences.

Holliday, KE, et al.: Growth of human milk-fed and formula-fed infants with cystic fibrosis, *J Pediatr* 118:77–79, 1991.

Host, A, Husby, S, and Osterballe, O: A prospective study of cow's milk allergy in exclusively breast-fed infants, *Acta Paediatr Scand* 77:663–70, 1988.

Howie, PW, et al.: Protective effect of breastfeeding against infection, *Br Med J* 300:11–16, 1990.

Huffman, SL, and Combest, C: Role of breast-feeding in the prevention and treatment of diarrhea, *J Diarrhoel Dis Res* 8:68–81, 1990.

Istre, GR, et al.: Risk factors for primary *Hemophilus influenzae* disease: increased risk from day care attendance and school-aged household members, *J Pediatr* 106:190–95, 1985.

Jakobsson, I, and Lindberg, T: Cow's milk as a cause of infantile colic in breast fed infants, *Lancet* 2:437–39, 1978.

Jenkins, GN: *The physiology and biochemistry of the mouth* (ed. 4), London, 1978, Blackwell Scientific Publications.

Kojosaari, M., and Saarinen, UM: Prophylaxis of atopic disease by six months' total solid food elimination, *Acta Paediatr Scand* 72:411–14, 1983.

Klein, E, Shvartzman, P, and Weizman, Z: Blood-streaked stools in two breast-fed siblings, *J Fam Pract* 30:713–14, 1990.

Kramer, M: Infant feeding, infection and public health, *Pediatrics* 81:164–66, 1988.

La Leche League International: *La Leche League News* 20:6, 1978.

La Leche League International: *The womanly art of breastfeeding* (4th ed.), Franklin Park, Ill., 1987, The League.

Ledonne, C: Hospital and home care of the infant with congenital bilateral choanal atresia, *JOGNN* 15:244–48, 1986.

Lemons, P, and Weaver, DD: Beyond the birth of a defective child, *Neonatal Netw* 5:13–19, 1986.

Lubchenco, L, and Bard, H: Incidence of hypoglycemia in newborn infants classified by birth weight and gestational age, *Pediatrics* 47:831–38, 1971.

Luder, E, et al.: Current recommendations for breast-feeding in cystic fibrosis centers, *Am J Dis Child* 144:1153–56, 1990.

Machtinger, S, and Moss, R: Cow's milk allergy in breast-fed infants; the role of allergen and maternal secretory IgA antibody, *J Allergy Clin Immunol* 77:341–47, 1986.

Matsumara, T, et al.: Egg sensitivity and eczematous manifestations in breast-fed newborns with particular reference to intrauterine sensitization, *Ann Allergy* 35:221–29, 1975.

McBride, MC, and Danner, SC: Sucking disorders in neurologically impaired infants, *Clin Perinatol* 14:109–30, 1987.

McCabe, L, et al.: The management of breastfeeding among infants with phenylketonuria, *J Inher Met Dis* 12:467–74, 1989.

McCarty, EP, and Frick, OL: Food sensitivity: keys to diagnosis, *J Pediatr* 102:645–52, 1983.

Miller, SA and Chopra, JG: Problems with human milk and infant formulas, *Pediatrics* 74(supp.):639–47, 1984.

Mitchell, EA, Stewart, AW, and Becroft, DMO: Results from the first year of the New Zealand cot death study, *NZ Med J* 104:71–75, 1991.

Olshansky, S: Chronic sorrow: a response to having a mentally defective child, *Soc Casework* 43:190–93, 1962.

Perisic, VN, Fillpovic, D, and Kokai, G: Allergic colitis with rectal bleeding in an exclusively breast-fed neonate, *Acta Paediatr Scand* 77:163–64, 1988.

Piscane, A, Graziano, L, and Zona, G: Breastfeeding and urinary tract infection, *Lancet* 336(8706):50, 1990.

Popkin, BM, et al.: Breast-feeding and diarrheal morbidity, *Pediatrics* 86:874–82, 1990.

Pullan, CR, et al.: Breastfeeding and respiratory syncytial virus infection, *Br Med J* 281:1034–36, 1980.

Rogers, M, Riordan, J, and Swindle, D: Community-based nursing case management pays off, *Nurs Man* 22:30–34, 1991.

Rooney, K: Breastfeeding a baby with cystic fibrosis, *New Beginnings,* 4:43–44, 1988.

Ross, CA, and Sammons, HG: Non-pancreatic lipase in children with pancreatic fibrosis, *Arch Dis Child* 30:428–31, 1955.

Rovet, JF: Does breast-feeding protect the hypothyroid infant whose condition is diagnosed by newborn screening? *Am J Dis Child* 144:319–23, 1990.

Ruuska, T: Occurrence of acute diarrhea in atopic and non-atopic infants: the role of prolonged breast-feeding, *J Pediatr Gastroenterol Nutr* 14:27–33, 1992.

Ruuska, T, and Vesilkari, T: A prospective study of acute diarrhoea in Finnish children from birth to 2-1/2 years of age, *Acta Paediatr Scand* 80:500–507, 1991.

Saarinen, UM: Prolonged breastfeeding as a prophylaxis for recurrent otitis media, *Acta Paediatr Scand* 71:567–71, 1982.

Sachdev, HPS, et al.: Does breastfeeding influence mortality in children hospitalized with diarrhoea? *J Trop Pediatr* 37:275–79, 1991.

Schreiner, Ms, Triebwasser, A, and Keon, TP: Ingestion of liquids compared with preoperative fasting in pediatric outpatients, *Anesthesiology* 72:593–97, 1990.

Sexson, WR: Incidence of neonatal hypoglycemia: a matter of definition, *J Pediatr* 105:149–50, 1984.

Shor, VZ: Congenital cardiac defects: assessment and case finding, *AJN* 78:256, 1978.

Slade, HB, and Schwarz, SA: Mucosal immunity: the immunology of breast milk, *J Allergy Clin Immunol* 80: 348–58, 1987.

Srinivasan, G, et al.: Plasma glucose values in normal neonates; a new look, *J Pediatr* 109:114–17, 1986.

Suitor, CW, and Hunter, MF: Nutrition; principles and practice, Philadelphia, 1980, J.B. Lippincott Co.

Sutin, R: Eliminating foods worked wonders, *New Beginnings* 4:145, 1988.

Teele, DW, Klein, JO, and Rosner, B: Epidemiology of otitis media during the first seven years of life in children in greater Boston: a prospective cohort study, *J Infec Dis* 160:83–94, 1989.

Tew, BJ, et al.: Marital stability following the birth of a child with spina bifida, *Br J Psychiatry* 131:79–82, 1977.

Tiwary, CM: Neonatal screening for metabolic and endocrine diseases, *Nurse Pract* 12:28–41, 1987.

Varma, SK, et al.: Thyroxine, tri-iodothyronine, and reverse tri-iodothyronine concentrations in human milk, *J Pediatr* 93:803, 1978.

Weatherley-White, RCA, et al.: Early repair and breast-feeding for infants with cleft lip, *Plast Reconstr Surg* 79:879–85, 1987.

Wilson, NW, Self, TW, and Hamburger, RN: Severe cow's milk induced colitis, *Clin Pediatr* 29:77–80, 1990.

SUGGESTED READINGS

Servonsky, J, and Opas, SR: *Nursing management of children,* Boston, 1987, Jones and Bartlett Publishers, Inc.

Whaley, LF, and Wong, DL: *Nursing care of infants and children,* (ed. 3), St. Louis, 1987, The C.V. Mosby Co.

19

Slow Weight Gain and Failure to Thrive

KATHLEEN G. AUERBACH

JAN RIORDAN

One of the most distressing clinical situations is a breastfeeding baby who is gaining weight poorly or not at all. Because the breastfeeding mother and baby operate as a team, when one partner fails to do his "job," it affects the other partner as well. In some cases, the baby's inability to effectively stimulate the maternal milk supply will result in a gradual reduction of that supply of needed nutrients. In other cases, the baby is unable to suckle appropriately as a result of neurological impairment or other reasons. In rarer situations, the mother's ability to make milk in sufficient quantity to totally nourish her baby at the breast is impaired. Both short- and long-term intervention may be needed to resolve the situation satisfactorily, while preserving the important breastfeeding relationship, as well as infant access to those elements in human milk that cannot be provided in artificial form.

This chapter discusses clinical situations involving poor weight gain and distinguishes between slow weight gain and failure to thrive. Because there are many reasons for inadequate weight gain, we identify the circumstances that may precede or contribute to the problem, noting whether they are management problems or whether they are infant- or mother-related. In all instances, the nutritional integrity of the baby is the paramount concern.

NORMAL GROWTH

Weight norms collected in the last century show that following birth in the hospital, most neonates lose approximately 5 to 10% of their birth weight. Breastfed infants usually regain their birth weight by the second week. Generally, babies—regardless of how they are fed—double their birth weight at about five to six months of age and triple their birth weight by one year of age. In some cases, these milestones may be reached earlier without implying infantile obesity.

Weight gain is not the only criterion to evaluate in normal growth patterns—body length and head circumference are also important parameters of growth. An infant who is 20 inches long at birth can be expected to be approximately 30 inches high at one year of age, or $1\frac{1}{2}$ times his birth length. Brain growth is rapid, and in the first year an infant's head circumference will increase approximately 7.6 cm (3 inches); it will increase another 7.6 cm in the next 16 years of life.

Although breastfed and formula-fed infants grow at about the same rate for the first few months, after this time babies fed formula begin to exceed their breastfed counterparts. Butte, Smith, and Garza (1990) found that breastfeeding infants gain about 34.5 gm/day at one month of age, while formula-fed infants gain 34.4 gm/day. By four months of age there is a substantial difference between them—18.7 gm/day for breastfed babies and 23 gm/day for formula-fed babies. Also, by four months of age, the breastfed baby's total daily energy expenditure is less than his formula-fed counterpart; he takes less milk, and he uses it more efficiently.

Normal growth reflects heredity for the individual

infant. Often, mothers (and fathers!) of slow-gaining infants, after asking their parents or finding their infant growth records, learn that they too gained weight slowly as infants. Frequently, the pattern of growth of the first baby will be observed in later babies, even if the method of feeding differs. In some families, *when* the baby gains is also governed by heredity. For example, although most babies gain more weight in the first year than in the second year of life, in some families all the infants tend to gain weight far more rapidly in the second year than in the first—regardless of the timing of supplementary foods and/or the frequency of breastfeeding. Although our culture tends to equate plumpness with well-being, obesity is not a sign of health. Thus, method of feeding—although an obvious element when considering nutritional intake—is not the only determinant of growth. Assessment of factors which may contribute to the pattern of growth of a young infant or child must, therefore, include consideration of the contribution of genetic heritage.

GROWTH CHARTS

Growth charts are intended to be used to record the growth of the individual child. They are standards based on *percentiles,* sometimes called percentile rank. In a growth chart based on percentiles, such as the ones shown in Fig. 19–1 and Fig. 19–2, all the measurements of a large sample of children are ranked in size, from the smallest to the largest, and are assigned percentiles which correspond to their position in the rank order. For example, the middle measurement, or *median,* is called the 50th percentile; a percentile of 90 indicates a measurement that is as great or greater than that of 90% of the children in the sample. One-half the children in a normal distribution can be expected to fall between the 25th and 75th percentiles, which are equidistant from the median; 80% of the children can be expected to fall between the 10th and 90th percentiles.

Growth can also be expressed in terms of *standard deviation.* The standard deviation (SD) is a statistical measure of variability, or the extent to which measurements deviate from the mean, or norm, of all the measurements in the sample. It is expressed as a distance in either direction from the mean, along the baseline of a normal distribution. About 68% of growth measurements of children can be expected to fall between +1 and –1 standard deviations from the mean; 95% fall between +2 and –2 SD, and 99% between +3 and –3 SD.

The most commonly used charts in the United States are from the National Center for Health Statistics (NCHS, 1977), which maintain separate charts for girls and for boys. The charts for children from birth to 36 months of age include measurements of head circumference, body weight by age, recumbent length by age, and weight by length. Currently, no charts reflect the normal growth of the breastfed infant. The sample of babies used to create growth charts were predominantly bottle-fed and often included infants who were introduced to supplementary solid foods very early in life (Tanis, 1985).

THE SLOW-GAINING INFANT

The term "slow-gaining infant" has been used to characterize infants whose weight

- shows slow but steady growth and, when charted on a standardized growth chart, remains between the same two percentiles over time
- exhibits growth for height, length, and weight that is proportional
- reaches developmental milestones within the normal time periods

Although such infants appear to weigh less than many of their age-mates, they are healthy and happy. In short, they are at the low end of the normal range of growth for healthy infants. Often intervention is not necessary, although mismanagement of breastfeeding should be ruled out as a factor contributing to such slow but steady weight gain.

Familial weight and stature are important criteria to consider when evaluating an infant who appears to gain weight slowly (Christian et al., 1989). The child of parents who are of small stature should not be expected to be in the 95th percentile for height, for example. Normal growth parameters of Asian families are not the same as those of northern Europeans, whose adult stature and weight is considerably different from that of the adult Asian. When the average growth rates of American and Chinese children are compared on the standard NCHS growth chart, the mean height and weight for Chinese children fall into the 10th percentile, as compared to the mean growth measurements for white American

BOYS: BIRTH TO AGE 36 MONTHS—PHYSICAL GROWTH (LENGTH, WEIGHT), NCHS PERCENTILES

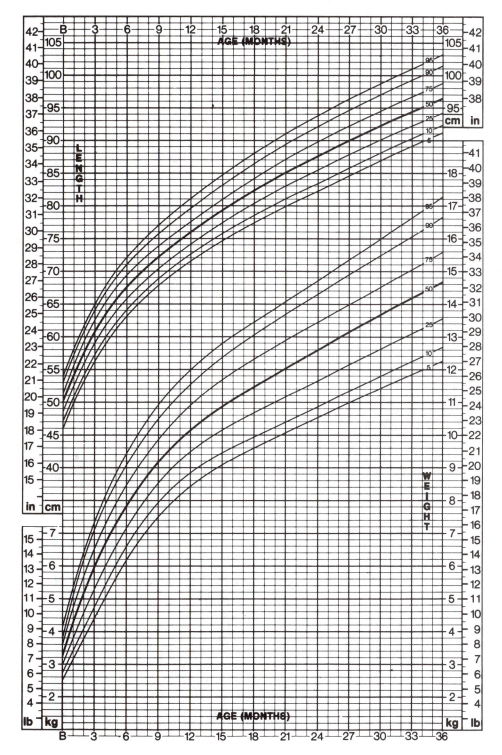

FIGURE 19–1   Standardized height-and-weight chart for boys (from birth to 36 months of age). Modified from Hamill, PVV, and others: Physical growth: National Center for Health Statistics percentiles, *Am J Clin Nutr* 32:607–629, 1979. (Data from the Fels Research Institute, Wright State University School of Medicine, Yellow Springs, Ohio.)

GIRLS: BIRTH TO AGE 36 MONTHS—PHYSICAL GROWTH (LENGTH, WEIGHT), NCHS PERCENTILES

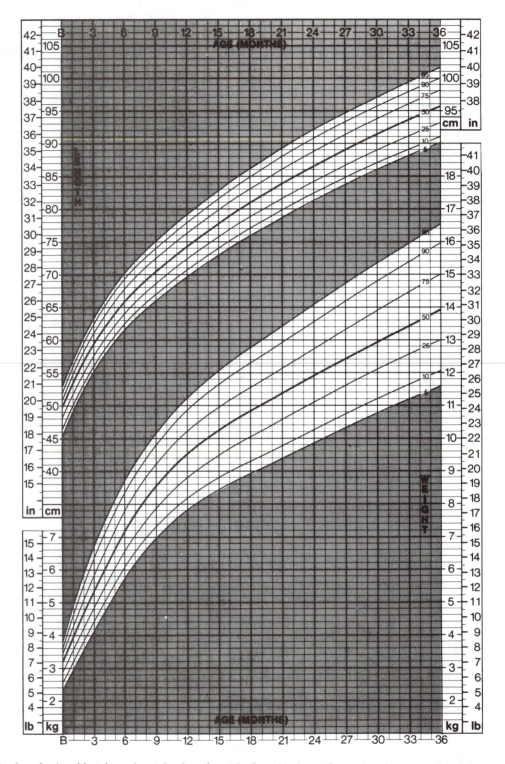

FIGURE 19–2 Standardized height-and-weight chart for girls (from birth to 36 months of age). Modified from Hamill, PVV, and others: Physical growth: National Center for Health Statistics percentiles, *Am J Clin Nutr* 32:607–629, 1979. (Data from the Fels Research Institute, Wright State University School of Medicine, Yellow Springs, Ohio.)

children, which comprise the 50th percentile (Whaley & Wong, 1989, p. 1094).

In addition to genetic heritage, numerous factors—including organic disease—can contribute to slow weight gain. (See the following boxed list.) Thus, any slow-gaining or poorly feeding infant should be evaluated to rule out an underlying illness or some organic problem before feeding method is considered a cause (Lukefahr, 1990).

FAILURE TO THRIVE (FTT)

There is no universally accepted definition for failure to thrive (FTT). Infants are generally considered failing to thrive, however, when their weight drops below the third percentile, or is two standard deviations below the mean on a standard growth chart. Indications of poor weight gain in the breastfed baby which may lead to failure to thrive include either or both of the following: the baby has not regained its birth weight within the first three weeks of life and/or the baby is gaining less than four ounces per week.

Failure to thrive accounts for two to five percent of pediatric hospital admissions. FTT is neither a medical nor a nursing diagnosis, but rather a cluster of symptoms occurring concurrently. FTT is classified into three categories:

1. *Organic FTT* is caused by physical factors such as renal disease, congenital defects, and other conditions given in the following boxed list.
2. *Nonorganic FTT* is the absence of physical evidence indicating that organic disease is a cause of weight loss; it points to environmental factors, such as insufficient caloric intake or a disturbance in the mother-baby relationship.
3. *Mixed FTT* is a combination of organic and nonorganic factors. For example, if the baby is unable to suckle adequately because of an undiagnosed neuromuscular problem, the mother may feel that her baby's inability to feed well is her fault. This may block the interplay of positive interaction and reciprocal play often associated with feedings.

Most cases of FTT are not caused by a physical problem. Of 38 breastfed infants with FTT seen in one pediatric practice, only seven (18%) were associated with an underlying physical illness (Lukefahr,

---

> **CONDITIONS THAT MAY CAUSE INFANT FAILURE TO GAIN WEIGHT**
>
> Biliary atresia
> Central nervous system insult
> Cleft palate
> Congenital cardiac anomalies
> Cystic fibrosis
> Galactosemia
> Glycogen storage disease
> Hyperthyroidism—inherited or acquired
> Hypoadrenalism
> Hypocalcemia
> Hypothyroidism (maternal)
> Intestinal malabsorption syndrome
> Megacolon
> Narcotic addiction (maternal)
> Obstruction of gastrointestinal tract
> Parasitic infection
> Renal insufficiency
> Urinary tract infection

1990). One-half of the babies diagnosed as failing to thrive because of organic illness were taken to the pediatrician between one and six months of age. About 40% of the cases were attributed to maternal misinformation or mismanagement, and 16% were thought to be caused by insufficient milk production (primary lactation failure). This study is congruent with an earlier study which reports organic FTT in 18% of the study cases, whether the babies were bottle-fed or breastfed (Sills, 1978).

Feeding styles of breastfed infants with weight loss tend to fall into two categories: the fretful, underfed baby and the contented, underfed baby (Davies, 1979). The fretful baby is characterized by constant crying; irritability associated with frequent, short feedings; and colic. The mother, who is under stress and worried about the baby, has a poor let-down reflex, which results in a vicious cycle of ineffective feedings and anxious interactions between mother and infant. The contented baby, on the other hand, is placid and gives the impression of being satisfied after feedings. This infant allows long intervals between feedings and sleeps long hours through the night. If the mother is feeding on demand, she doesn't realize that she needs to initiate more feedings. In general, mothers try to meet the norms of their society and/or family; thus, she will heed the common admonition not to pick up the baby so much—"you might spoil him."

It is uncommon to find maternal deprivation as a factor when the breastfed baby fails to thrive. Probably the reason for this is that deciding to breastfeed involves self-selection; the mother who chooses breastfeeding is more likely to be committed to her baby, a commitment which is incompatible with maternal deprivation. Moreover, the holding and skin-to-skin touching which occur with feeding at the breast in most cases preclude the possibility that the baby will be touch-deprived. Because of the intimate interaction required with breastfeeding, these infants usually function within normal developmental limits until their malnutrition becomes extreme, unlike many failure-to-thrive infants who are not breastfed. Lack of a support system for parents, however, is a significant factor in FTT. Breastfeeding mothers of infants for whom inadequate weight gain becomes a severe problem seldom have family or close friends whom they see frequently and/or who are available to give them emotional support.

When a baby fails to thrive, he must be referred to the direct care of a physician who will conduct a thorough assessment, including a complete physical examination and laboratory studies. The assessment is usually made by a multidisciplinary team, including the nurse, LC, physician, social worker, dietitian, and psychologist. The first approach is to feed the baby supplementary foods without changing any other aspects of care-giving. If weight gain occurs, the cause is considered to be nonorganic and the result of insufficient caloric intake.

FACTORS ASSOCIATED WITH INADEQUATE CALORIC INTAKE

Inadequate intake of breastmilk may be caused by a number of factors that may center around the baby, the mother, or breastfeeding management. (See Table 19–1.)

MANAGEMENT FACTORS

Limited length of feedings. Inadequate frequency and duration of feedings is a major factor leading to FTT in breastfed babies. Asking how long each feeding usually lasts and who stops it can indicate how advice has influenced the mother's breastfeeding pattern. Howie et al. (1981) found that five-to-seven day-old infants averaged 17 minutes of suckling per feeding period, with a range of seven to 30 minutes. It is reasonable to assume that newborns will suckle as long as they need to suckle and that some feedings will be shorter, while others will be longer. In both cases, encouraging the mother to look to the baby for cues regarding when to end the feeding is more appropriate than suggesting an arbitrary time limit.

When a mother restricts breastfeeding time—often because she has been told that her breasts contain a finite amount of milk or that the baby gets it within a particular time period—and then supplements her infant, she unwittingly begins the process of weaning. The breasts receive less stimulation, and the milk supply begins to decrease (Frantz, 1980).

McNeilly and colleagues (1983) have substantiated multiple let-down responses through successive bursts of oxytocin release during the same breastfeeding episode. Although the infant of an experienced breastfeeding woman with a very active let-down response may consume his total feeding quite rapidly—for example, within five to 10 minutes—and still gain weight well, this is the exception rather than the rule. The volume of milk received depends on the length of the feeding and the strength of the infant's suckling.

Many mothers report that their babies happily breastfed from just one breast and never have problems, but it should be kept in mind that infants who are *not* gaining weight adequately may begin to gain weight when both breasts are used at each feeding (Frantz, Fleiss & Lawrence, 1978). Feeding from both breasts has been reported (Woolridge, Ingram & Baum, 1990) to stimulate the breasts to produce more milk (782 mL) than does feeding from just one breast (713 mL). Although the average daily fat content of ingested milk is somewhat lower (44.3g/L) when the baby feeds from two breasts than when the baby feeds from one breast (52.7g/L), the baby's total fat intake is about the same (Woolridge, Ingram & Baum, 1990).

Insufficient number of feedings. When the baby is "content to starve" (Davies, 1979), the mother may conclude that lack of interest by the baby, or his willingness to go long periods between feedings, is an

TABLE 19–1 SUMMARY OF PROBLEMS AND INTERVENTIONS WITH SLOW WEIGHT GAIN WHEN ORGANIC CAUSES HAVE BEEN RULED OUT

	Assessment	Intervention	Rationale
Mismanagement	Mother removes baby before he finishes feeding.	Encourage mother to let infant self-limit feed by monitoring swallows. Teach her the swallow sounds.	Breastfed newborns need some long feeds. Length of feed is proportional to quality of suckle.
		Explain to mother who overdresses her infant that the baby may need to be awakened to finish the feeding.	Overheated infants decrease their suckling; swaddled newborns assume a sleep state.
	Long interval between feedings (4 hrs or more).	Suggest baby be allowed to feed often.	Breastfed newborns feed every 2 to 3 hrs. Some newborns "cluster" feed, i.e., many feeds after a longer sleep.
		Discourage pacifier use in the beginning weeks of breastfeeding.	Baby's desire to suckle is a survival mechanism and indicates need to feed. Keeping all suckling at the breast helps establish good maternal milk supply.
	Infant sleeping longer than a 4 hr-stretch at night before 8 to 12 weeks. Mother promotes long sleep at night.	Teach parents not to expect a young infant to "sleep through the night."	Sleeping 6 hrs usually occurs after six weeks
		Suggest additional waking if infant sleeps a long period.	Prolactin levels are highest from 10 P.M. to 2 A.M., and infants feed best at night.
	Mother offering water to reduce jaundice.	Discontinue water in favor of more frequent breastmilk feeding.	Milk feeds lower bilirubin levels faster than water feeds.
Disorganized suck	Infant feeds with eyes closed.	Feed lightly clothed.	Infants often find mother's arms "womb-like" and assume a state of near sleep.
	Suckles and swallows audibly only during let-downs—rest of feeding is a nonnutritive suckling pattern.	Have mother monitor nutritive suck-swallow pattern and have her switch breasts when swallows cease.	Fast milk flow improves suckle.
	Infant feeds frequently (q 1 hr) or continuously.	Explain that if infant feeds more effectively, he won't feed as often. However, very infrequent feeds will not improve nursing behavior.	Smaller intake results in more frequent feedings. Small bursts of nutritive suckling may not have completed the feeding, and the baby is still hungry.

(continued)

TABLE 19–1 SUMMARY OF PROBLEMS AND INTERVENTIONS WITH SLOW WEIGHT GAIN WHEN ORGANIC CAUSES HAVE BEEN RULED OUT (*cont'd*)

	Assessment	Intervention	Rationale
	Infant fusses when laid down.	Encourage nutritive suckling throughout entire feeding to avoid long periods between bursts of suckling.	
	Infant sleeps long stretches at night.	Waken infant at least q 4 hrs at night.	Establish more efficient daytime feeds.
Immature CNS or neuromuscular disorder	Poor suckling caused by poor coordination and/or muscle tone (hypotonia/hypertonia).	Realign infant for postural control. Baby should have chin near chest and flexion of arms, legs, hips, and feet.	Flexion helps organize oral motor function and normalizes tone.
	Breastfeeds continuously and when put on a 2-hr schedule loses weight. Mother states she hears swallows only for the first 5 minutes into the feeding.	Teach "switch" nursing; if not effective, use feeding tube device.	Tube device organizes a suckle, changes the pattern at the swallow phase, and initiates a sustained coordination. "Switch" nursing may not produce enough flow to sustain a nutritive suckle.
	Use of feeding tube device causes infant to gain weight and causes a noticeable increase in mother's milk supply within 48 hrs.	Assist in developing an optimal feeding plan. Evaluate the feeding tube size. It may be too large.	A fast milk flow may overwhelm the infant.
	Need for supplement increases or remains the same	Point out his progress. Explain CNS development in infants.	Most infants gradually develop organized CNS and neuromuscular abilities on their own by the third month.
	Baby continues to have diminished muscle tone and skill in suckling.	Refer for comprehensive pediatric evaluation. Pediatrician may refer to neurologist.	Degenerative neuromuscular disease often becomes more evident with time.

Derived from Frantz, K: Slow Weight Gain. In Riordan, J: *A practical guide to breastfeeding*, St. Louis, 1983, The C. V. Mosby Co.

indication that he is satiated. Usually, the number of feedings declines gradually over several days in the first few weeks postpartum, until the baby is nursing five or fewer times in a 24-hour period. In some cases, an infrequent number of breastfeedings will be combined with overly long periods of what the mother perceives to be suckling, but which may do little more than keep the nipple and areola wet with the baby's saliva. In other cases, infrequent nursings may dwindle into sleep shortly after the baby has received some milk, particularly if the baby has become progressively weaker as his nutritional intake declines.

In the absence of a neurological problem with the baby, a marked increase in breastfeedings, usually in combination with a feeding tube device which provides extra calories with little effort on the part of the baby, will change the baby's breastfeeding pattern dramatically. Instead of very long, inefficient feedings separated by more than four hours, the baby becomes more obviously wakeful at the breast, obtains more milk in a shorter period, and begins to spontaneously express a desire to nurse. In some cases, after the mother has insisted that the baby nurse more frequently, she will report a feeling of fullness in her breasts just prior to a breastfeeding as a "new" experience—or one that has not occurred since the first week postpartum. This feeling is an indication of increased milk production in response to increased stimulation through breastfeeding.

Improper positioning. As already noted in Chapter 9, positioning is an obvious, often overlooked, element in maternal breastfeeding behavior. However, the baby's position at the breast and the mother's own body position and her comfort when holding her baby are important preliminaries to effective breastfeeding.

Positioning errors that most often contribute to poor breastfeeding do not provide the baby with an opportunity to suckle comfortably. Usually, his body is turned away from the mother's, which results in an attempt to suckle "over his shoulder," or in a manner that forces his head to tilt away from the breast. (The baby then slips on and off as he attempts to make and retain contact.) Or he is pressed too closely to the top of the breast and not close enough to that portion under the areola. (His receding chin is not in contact with the mother's breast, and his nose is buried in her soft breast tissue, which requires him to suckle briefly and then pull away in order to breathe.) In any case, the baby expends a great deal of energy attempting to remain comfortable, failing to do so, and coming on and off the breast.

If the mother has breastfed before, often she will assume a body position relative to the baby which replicates how her previous child suckled when he was weaning or near the end of the breastfeeding course. While an older baby can suckle in a wide variety of positions as a result of more well-developed musculature and maturity, the newborn is unable to control his body as easily. Thus, when held too low, he either cannot reach the breast, can do so barely, or has to hang on by clamping his jaws onto the nipple, much as a climber who is slipping attempts to maintain his position. The result is a mother who reports sore nipples and a baby who gains weight poorly, who fusses at the breast, falling off frequently, and who eventually begins to refuse to have to fight in order to eat.

Very often, simply helping the mother to correctly position the baby for breastfeeding quickly changes the dynamics between mother and baby so that each is more comfortable: the baby is better able to suckle without causing the mother discomfort and without

having to struggle to obtain milk. In a situation in which the mother's milk supply is reduced because of poor feedings by a baby who has been poorly positioned for several weeks, the mother will need careful, written instructions to help her unlearn what she has been practicing for so long. The removal of pain is a strong incentive for her to correct herself when she inadvertently slips into old routines. By the same token, the baby who is finally positioned comfortably for several feedings is more inclined to protest when placed inappropriately at the breast.

The Maternal-Infant History Form appearing in Appendix 19–1 of this chapter is a helpful tool for gathering important information about the mother and the baby when the infant has trouble gaining weight. It is important for the clinician to incorporate issues relating to both the baby and the mother and to identify necessary referrals to other health-care disciplines as part of a team approach.

INFANT FACTORS

While lactation-related difficulties are probably responsible for the majority of failure-to-thrive cases in a breastfed baby, illness, which accounts for almost one case in five (Lukefahr, 1990), must be ruled out. Careful history-taking, laboratory studies, and observation will establish whether an organic disease has resulted in the infant taking in insufficient calories.

Even when the baby does have an underlying health problem, breastfeeding may ameliorate, rather than worsen, the condition. For example, poor weight gain has been associated with cystic fibrosis. Some infants with cystic fibrosis, however, have shown a slow but steady weight gain and may even remain asymptomatic throughout the breastfeeding course. In other cases, they have shown only minimal evidence of the disease while being breastfed. One author of this chapter has worked with families whose infants were diagnosed with cystic fibrosis early in infancy. They continued to breastfeed while receiving oral enzyme therapy in addition to milk through a feeding tube device. This approach controlled symptoms of the disease, improved weight gain, and provided the babies with the all-important immunological protections available only by receiving human milk. The opportunity to continue to provide human milk to infants with cystic fibrosis has only recently been considered in the standard therapy offered these children (Holliday et al., 1991; Luder et al., 1990).

Hypothyroidism in the infant also needs to be ruled out when poor weight gain occurs. Some studies indicate that human milk may contain sufficient thyroid hormone to temporarily mask, but not prevent, hypothyroidism (Sack, Amado & Lunenfeld, 1977; Rovet, 1990). Initial symptoms of hypothyroidism include poor suckling, slow weight gain, and infrequent stooling. Mandatory screening in most states usually identifies this problem before it becomes severe enough to cause mental retardation.

Disorganized suckling.   If the infant's suckling is impaired, it will affect how much and what kind of milk he gets. When the infant's pattern of suckling improves, the mother's milk supply increases. The strength of the suckle in facilitating the let-down reflex and obtaining adequate volume and fat concentrations for the infant is as important as the frequency or duration of the feedings (Auerbach & Eggert, 1987). Thus, the management of his feeds will need to be different from that of a baby who gains weight normally.

A careful history of the mother's birth experience and early breastfeeding may reveal mismanagement of early lactation in the hospital—combined with lack of sufficient skilled help to identify that her baby's suck is disorganized and needs assistance (Klaus, 1987; Livingstone, 1990). However, babies born at home, where none of the hospital routines that can interfere with early breastfeeding are present, may also exhibit a disorganized suck pattern. Thus, while it is important to rule out mismanagement issues which may be contributing to the problem, one must not be fooled into thinking that their elimination alone will resolve the issue.

Disorganization of suckling, a temporary condition, is most often seen in infants under one month of age, particularly if the baby was born prematurely or to mothers who received obstetric medications. Time and appropriate assistance are needed to help the baby to organize what is primarily a reflex action at this time. In most situations, one or more of the following elements is present:

1. The baby frequently suckles with his eyes closed throughout the feeding. The baby is not asleep, although he may appear to be. When removed from the breast, he may fuss and cry, prompting the mother to put him back for another round of extended suckling with minimal swallowing.

2. The baby may suck and swallow rhythmically one to three times at the beginning of a feeding, when the mother's body is responding to the baby's grasp of the breast with an initial spurt of milk; however, when lesser milk volumes provide a less obvious stimulus, the baby appears to flutter his tongue. Often the chin can be observed moving rapidly in very brief excursions, which place only minimal pressure on the lactiferous sinuses.

3. The mother reports that the baby's suck is difficult to feel, or "doesn't feel very strong," or is "very soft." If the mother has previously breastfed an infant who gained weight appropriately, she may compare the relative strength of her first baby's suck with that of this infant. If this is the first baby the mother has breastfed, she may comment either that "it hurts when he nurses," or that "it is hard to tell if he is doing anything."

4. The mother is unable to identify a swallow, or reports that the baby swallows for a very brief period and then falls asleep.

Over time, the mother's milk supply, which may have been adequate to copious early in the lactation course, will decline as a result of lack of sufficient stimulation. Often the mother has been told that she doesn't have enough milk without also being informed that her baby's lack of consistent or effective stimulation is the primary cause of her inadequate production. If the mother has successfully breastfed a previous baby, she may ask if the baby is doing something wrong. If she is a mother who is breastfeeding for the first time, she very often blames herself for attempting breastfeeding, particularly if other relatives, friends, or health care-givers are questioning the adequacy of her milk—its quality or quantity.

As noted in Chapter 4, suckling during milk flow occurs at the rate of about one suckle per second; a swallow follows each suckle. Although this is the general rule, toward the end of the feed nutritive suckling can slow down to one swallow for every three suckles and still be within the normal range (Bowen-Jones, Thompson & Drewett, 1982).

Nonnutritive suckles have often been described by mothers as "very soft" and observed by lactation consultants as a "quiver" or "fluttering" action on the chin. Milk is usually available to the infants with this suckling pattern only when it leaks out of the breast, when the milk let-down reflex occurs spontaneously, or when the baby momentarily suckles well at the beginning of the feed. Many slow-gaining breastfed infants engage in a pattern of suckling without swallowing, often when the nipple is not drawn well into the mouth.

Whenever an infant is not gaining weight well, it is important to observe breastfeeding to determine how the infant suckles and what the mother is doing, as well as what she reports she is feeling when the baby is at the breast. Begin by asking the mother for permission to watch her baby feeding at the breast. The mother often feels that *she* has done something wrong if her infant is a slow weight-gainer. The mother's positioning of her own body and her baby should be noted, as well as the baby's action during the breastfeeding (Escott, 1989). Infant swallows sound like soft exhales. Their frequency and pattern of occurrence, as well as when they cease, should be noted.

Changing the conditions surrounding suckling will elicit the baby's maximum potential for appropriate behavior. For example, flexing the baby's body places his head in a position that brings the infant's tongue forward, which is an added advantage for the breastfeeding baby. Adding a liquid flow will organize suckling action by triggering a swallow (K. Frantz, personal communication, 1991).

While assessment of the suckling reflex is part of the neurological portion of the normal examination of newborns, a digital suckling assessment may also be indicated if a breastfeeding problem is identified.

Neurologic dysfunction. In some cases, the baby's suckle is not disorganized, but rather exhibits a pattern suggestive of dysfunction. Unlike a disorganized suck, which is a temporary condition most apt to occur for a relatively brief period after birth and which usually resolves spontaneously, a dysfunctional suckle may be a sign of a mild to severe neurologic problem.

Persistent poor suckling, particularly if it is associated with a delay in reaching developmental milestones, suggests neurologic dysfunction. Because the tongue, jaws, and lips are operated by muscles which are innervated by the central nervous system, a neurologic dysfunction often manifests itself first in a feeding problem (McBride & Danner, 1987).

In some cases, the neurologic problem is transi-

tory and caused by central nervous system immaturity. As the infant matures, feeding problems disappear spontaneously. A baby who displays hypertonia as a result of immaturity usually responds to postural control measures, such as flexion and calming, while rapidly maturing.

Those infants with hypotonia build their muscle tone more gradually than babies with hypertonia and usually need a feeding tube device at the breast for an extended period of time. Examples of how such specialized therapy has been used to assist the slow-gaining breastfeeding infant can be found in Desmarais and Browne (1990).

Referral to a physical therapist who has had specialized training in assessing and treating feeding problems can improve the efficiency of the infant's suckling. The physical therapist (PT) or occupational therapist (OT) who prove most helpful for infants with suckling problems have additional neurodevelopmental treatment training and certification (NDT*) based on the research of Morris and Klein (1987), Bobath (1971), and Mueller (1972). Such a therapist assesses and works with the baby's entire body musculature and movements which affect his oral motor function (K. Frantz, personal communication, 1991).

A feeding tube device may be used with these infants while the mother's milk supply is increasing, simultaneously enhancing the milk let-down response while the baby is learning to suckle more effectively. A physical therapist can further assist the family to maintain flexion during bathing and diaper changes, as well as in holding the baby and in other daily activities, so that the infant can more easily control his own actions.

Infants with a disorganized suck rarely need a feeding tube device for their entire breastfeeding course, unless other problems exist. In most cases, the timing of elimination of the feeding tube device is dictated by the baby's need for less than a few ounces of milk per day. Often, the mother is the first to recognize that the baby's suckle is consistently stronger—from first grasp to last suck into satiated drowsiness. At that time, it is appropriate for the care-giver to encourage the mother to cease using the "coaxer" because it is clear that neither the baby nor she need it any longer.

*Contact: Neurodevelopmental Treatment Association, P.O. Box 70, Oak Park, IL 60303.

In some cases, a mother whose self-confidence has been severely shaken by the baby's previous failure to gain weight appropriately may be hesitant to eliminate the visible message that her baby is receiving milk. After all, she can see what the baby gets from the feeding tube device. The use of a chart, which shows how the volumes obtained from supplementation have declined as the baby continued to gain weight well, can be an important tool in demonstrating to the mother that her own milk supply is now adequate to continue to meet the baby's needs.

Ankyloglossia (Tongue-tie). An infant with a short frenulum may or may not be able to suckle efficiently at the breast (Berg, 1990; Marmet, Shell & Marmet, 1990; Nicholson, 1991b; Notestine, 1990; Ward, 1990; Wilton, 1990). In situations in which the condition prevents the infant from moving his tongue forward sufficiently to support and cup the elongated nipple and areola in order to form it into a teat, maternal nipple soreness is often the first sign that the infant is suckling inappropriately. This sign is followed by poor weight gain in spite of frequent breastfeeding and obvious interest in suckling. (See Fig. 19–3.)

When the lingual frenulum is clipped, relief from nipple pain and a markedly changed "feel" of the infant's suckling pattern in noted by the mother. In nearly all cases, the baby whose previous weight gain was minimal improves. In some cases, a short frenu-

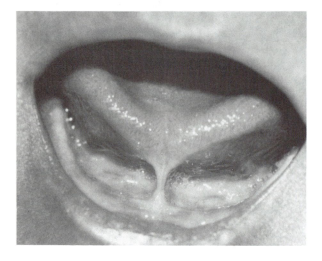

FIGURE 19–3 A severe tongue-tie. (Courtesy Gregory E. Notestine, D.D.S.)

lum will, over time, be stretched by the baby's suckling action and other movements of the tongue, so that clipping is not necessary. Obviously, the degree of severity of both mother's and infant's conditions will determine whether poor weight gain secondary to ankyloglossia is an issue which requires intervention rather than the patient application of "tincture of time."

MATERNAL FACTORS

The mother's rigid adherence to a "demand-feeding" philosophy, coupled with the baby's failure to express a need to be fed or to protest when too much time has elapsed between feedings, are significant factors in failure to thrive (Pfeifer & Ayoub, 1978). If the mother has no previous experience in mothering or breastfeeding, she may not realize that feedings at the breast should occur frequently, particularly in the early weeks. The problem is compounded if the baby has a passive temperament and/or a pattern of infrequent feeding is established which fails to meet the baby's nutritional needs. Often the mother describes her slow-gaining baby as a "good" baby who responds with quiet smiles and is often active and alert. Pfeifer and Ayoub (1978) note that these mothers often have dependent personalities and spend a great deal of time meeting the needs of their families at the expense of their own needs; often the father's emotional support is limited.

Physical problems deriving from the mother are less common than problems on the baby's side of the breastfeeding equation; however, they can include maternal hypothyroidism, drug use, and insufficient glandular tissue, among others.

Hypothyroidism. Thyroid-deficient mothers may not produce enough milk; this lack of adequate milk can be one of the diagnostic signs of maternal hypothyroidism. Correcting the mother's dose of thyroid medication will often result in an adequate weight in the infant as a result of a more copious milk supply (Neville & Berga, 1983). If the mother reports a history of thyroid deficiency, she should be reevaluated. The physician will probably order a T_4 test to measure her thyroid level.

Drug use. Drugs taken by a woman, particularly estrogen-containing birth control pills, may decrease her milk supply. Other drugs that are sometimes suspect include antihistamines and sedatives. A detailed discussion of the effect on medications on the breastfeeding mother and baby is found in Chapter 6.

Insufficient glandular tissue.   Neifert and Seacat (1987) have described women with a congenital lack of glandular breast tissue which led to failure to thrive in their infants. This is a *rare* phenomenon. Reduction mammoplasty can have a similar effect (Nicholson, 1991a) because such a surgical procedure often results in cutting milk ducts or altering nerve stimulation of the nipple area. Breastfeeding need not be halted because of this problem. A feeding tube device can be used to make up the difference in milk volume, while providing the baby with whatever volume of milk his mother is producing.

Poor let-down reflex.   Factors reported to interfere with the milk let-down reflex include maternal hormonal problems, fatigue, excessive amounts of caffeine (Berlin et al., 1984), smoking (Dahlstrom et al., 1990; Steldinger & Luck, 1988), and the effects of certain drugs (Atkinson & Biggs, 1988; Batagol, 1989; Berlin, 1989; Riordan & Riordan, 1984). Although many mothers may not be affected by any of the above, each element is important to consider when attempting to assess factors contributing to poor weight gain in the breastfeeding infant.

CLINICAL IMPLICATIONS

A prenatal history, perinatal information, and a feeding history should be obtained. When collecting this information, it is necessary to note how the mother talks about her baby, as well as the parent-infant emotional relationship. A thorough history may elicit enough information so that laboratory testing is not necessary. The health-care worker should be empathetic and kind during this interview, avoiding any hint that the parents are to blame. In the authors' experience, most parents of slow-gaining breastfed babies are already distraught—they feel helpless, guilty, and already blame themselves, usually unjustly. Following taking the history, ask the mother to breastfeed her baby using both breasts, so that a complete assessment of a feeding can be made. In addition to suckling, note the mother's level of com-

fort, body positions, eye contact, and verbalizations with the infant.

If the baby is severely malnourished or dehydrated, he may have to be hospitalized; in most cases, however, the slow-gaining breastfeeding baby can be treated on an out-patient basis. If the infant is hospitalized, caloric intake is closely monitored and recorded, and the baby is weighed at the same time each day, under similar conditions. An accurate record of intake and output is kept, including weighing the diapers. The nurse records the number, character, color, and consistency of the stools. Serum samples will be drawn from the infant for laboratory testing to rule out organic disease, and the stool will be tested for occult blood as well as for reducing substances. A Denver Developmental Screening Test may be administered to determine the baby's level of developmental maturity and whether a program of structured stimulation is needed to foster his development.

Treatment will depend upon the results of assessment and testing. Organic disease, if found, will be treated. In cases in which the mother is simply uninformed about basic breastfeeding, supplementation to preserve the baby's nutritional integrity until the mother's milk supply is adequate, teaching, and close supervision will suffice. In other rare cases, the mother (and possibly other family members) will require the assistance of a psychologist or social worker. In almost all circumstances, the mother may continue to breastfeed; feedings may be augmented by formula, expressed breastmilk, or solid foods. Optimally, the mother is given a feeding tube or some other device for supplementing the baby at the breast (Weichert, 1979).

DEVICES FOR SUPPLEMENTATION

The use of a cup or spoon or a feeding tube device that cues the baby when to swallow—and requires him to do so when his oral cavity is filled with milk— usually results in a steady, and sometimes rapid, resolution of the problem. Feeding tube devices are described in Chapter 11 and are discussed here only in terms of slow weight gain. Fig. 19–4 shows a commonly used device, the Supplemental Nutrition System™ (SNS).

The use of such a device almost always prompts maternal questions about how much milk the baby needs to ingest in order to grow and how she can tell

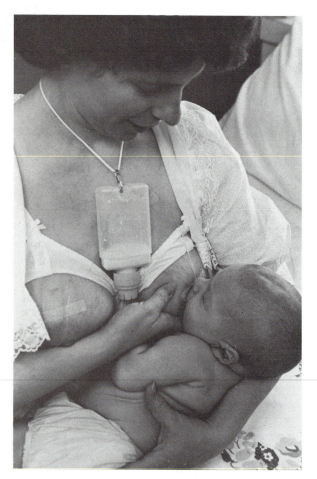

FIGURE 19–4 The Supplemental Nutrition System™ (SNS) feeding tube device. (Courtesy, Medela, Inc., McHenry, Ill.)

whether her own milk supply will increase when the baby is obviously deriving nutrients from the feeding tube device. Particularly in the first several days or week of use, the amount of supplemental fluid taken from the feeding tube device will climb, sometimes rapidly, for the mother should be told not to limit the amount the baby receives.

Any mother who is contemplating use of a feeding tube device should be reminded of the following four points:

1. A general rule of thumb is to begin with two to three ounces in the feeding tube device and to add one-half ounce more than the baby took the previous feeding—until he is leaving about one-half ounce in the feeding tube device for at least three feedings. At this point, the mother need

not continue to add fluid to the amount the baby has been taking.

2. After a period of time, which varies from one baby to the next, the amount of milk the baby takes from the feeding tube device will begin to decline. When this occurs consistently over several feedings, the mother can be instructed to reduce the amount in the feeding tube device to about one-half ounce more than the baby usually takes. This extra one-half ounce assures that the baby will receive milk rather than air from the tube.

3. Usually the reduced amount of milk taken from the feeding tube device declines in stages, with plateaus in between. In some cases, these plateau periods coincide with temporary appetite spurts of the baby which are age-appropriate.

4. Remind the mother—usually at each visit and often during phone follow-ups which occur between visits—that the baby is gaining weight during the course of the use of the feeding tube device, even as the amount being taken from that container declines. The boxed guidelines on p. 529 show the approximate amount of milk the baby should receive in the feeding tube device to support growth.

A baby whose suckling pattern is assisted in becoming more organized simultaneously begins to stimulate the mother's breasts more appropriately while using a feeding tube device. Such stimulation, in the absence of maternal breast tissue deficits, usually results in an increase in milk production. Often a first sign that the mother reports, usually within days of using the feeding tube device, is a feeling of breast fullness on waking. Thereafter, she may note spontaneous milk leakage from the contralateral breast when the baby is suckling. If she has never noted this before, it is time for congratulations! At the same time, the mother, who has been instructed in how to identify swallows, reports that the baby is more consistently and rhythmically swallowing. Usually, when a rhythmical suck-swallow pattern is established, the baby keeps his eyes open through most of the feeding.

Often, a previously fussy baby is noticeably more relaxed in demeanor and behavior. Note that the first photograph on p. 530 (Fig. 19–5) shows a two-month-old infant who looked and acted passive. When he went to breast, he immediately closed his eyes and appeared to be asleep; however, he could

GUIDELINES FOR USING A FEEDING TUBE DEVICE

1. Ask the mother to begin using the device when she and the baby are most rested, usually in the morning or at a time when other household/family activities are unlikely to require her attention.

2. Prepare the feeding *before* the baby becomes hungry or fussy. If the baby is frantic, the mother will become anxious.

3. Fill the device and position the tubing so that it extends slightly past the end of the mother's nipple. Use any kind of hypoallergenic tape to hold the tubing in place. If the baby appears to be sucking only on the end of the tubing, pull it back so that it is flush with the end of the mother's nipple.

4. Most babies will take most of the fluid in the device within the first 30 minutes. If the baby is actively suckling, but the device is flowing very slowly or not at all, test it by filling it with water and holding it upside down. Then, test it again by squeezing gently on the container to activate the flow. If the device is working properly, there should be a steady drip from the end of the tubing. In some cases, rapidity of flow can be increased by allowing the unused tubing (that which might be attached to the contralateral breast) to remain "open." By taping the tubing end-up along the side of the container it will not drip milk, but it will allow air intake into the bottle portion, thereby increasing milk flow from the other tubing. However, rapidity of flow ideally should be determined by the baby and his suckling pattern. In most cases, increasing the rapidity of flow by opening the other tubing will not be necessary.

Amount of Supplement to Use

If a feeding tube device is used to assist the baby to gain weight, both the care-giver and the mother need to know how much supplement the baby needs in order to grow. In the table below, find the weight of the baby and identify in the second or third column the approximate amount of milk required per day for that weight. Subtract the amount of milk the baby took from the feeding tube per day. The figure remaining is a rough estimate of breastmilk the baby received.

Infant weight	Approximate daily milk requirement	
lb	**oz**	**mL**
5	13	371
6	16	457
7	19	542
8	21	600
9	24	685
10	27	771
11	29	828
12	32	914

Example:
(a) Infant weight: 7 lb, 2 oz, which means that approximately 19 oz or 542 mL of milk is needed per day
(b) Amount taken from tube device/day = 9 oz of supplemental milk
(c) 19 oz − 9 oz = approximately 10 oz of breastmilk was taken
2. Another method of figuring required intake is to take the baby's weight in pounds and convert it into ounces. Divide that number by 6; the result is the total number of ounces of milk the baby needs in 24 hours to secure a 4 to 6 oz gain per week (Petok, personal communication, 1991).
Example:
(a) Infant weight: 7 lb, 2 oz = 114 oz
(b) 114 oz ÷ 6 = 19 oz per day
(c) 19 oz per day divided into 8 feedings (approximately every 3 hours) suggests that about 2-1/3 oz should be placed in the feeding tube device for each feeding.

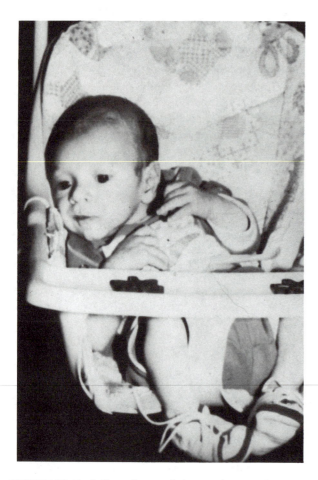

FIGURE 19–5   Infant who was failing to thrive at two months of age due to disorganized suckling.

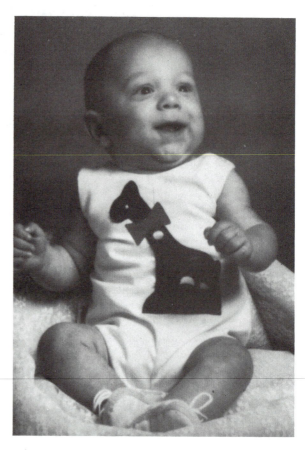

FIGURE 19–6   Same infant who was previously failing to thrive at four months of age, following correction of suckling pattern.

not be put down without continually fussing and crying. Bottle-feedings after breastfeeding brought his weight up temporarily, but because the mother's two previous children had stopped breastfeeding soon after being given bottles because of poor weight gain, she was reluctant to continue artificial feeding. At two months of age, this baby was two ounces below his birth weight; he had gained two pounds on bottle-feedings and then lost them again before being seen for breastfeeding evaluation and assistance. Two months later (Fig. 19–6), he was in the 75th percentile for weight and a happy, smiling baby, who, according to his mother, "almost never cries." In the first week of supplementation using the feeding tube device at the breast, he gained two pounds—such a pattern of very rapid gaining early in the supplementation period is nearly always catch-up growth. Thereafter, the rate of gain approaches that which one would expect in a baby who is breastfeeding effectively.

This infant started out getting 20 oz of supplement in the SNS per day (in addition to milk at the breast). He peaked at 32 oz of supplement in the SNS per day during the week when he gained two pounds. Thereafter, his daily supplementation amount came down steadily with two-to-four day plateaus between declines that usually lasted approximately one week each. It took him four months to come off the SNS. It usually takes twice as long as the age of the baby at the time of first visit, but every baby is different. One four-week-old baby (seen by the same LC) who exhibited an identical suckling pattern was off the same feeding tube device in 19 days. Fig. 19–7 illustrates the usual pattern of intake of supplemental fluid—the mother's own expressed milk, donated human milk, or artificial baby milk—that is

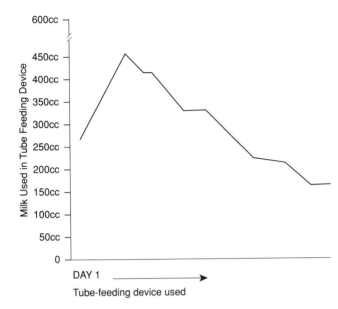

FIGURE 19–7   Characteristic pattern of supplemental milk intake when a baby's disorganized suckling pattern is being improved.

placed in the feeding tube device and thus can be measured.

OTHER METHODS

Sometimes drugs may be given to the mother to increase her milk supply. Chlorpromazine (Thorazine) is known to increase milk production by raising the prolactin level. Metoclopramide (Reglan) has also been found to increase prolactin levels and subsequent milk production in mothers (Gupta & Gupta, 1985; Ehrenkranz & Ackerman, 1986). Breast pumping may also be helpful, particularly if low milk supply is secondary to poor infant suckling. However, the degree of emphasis on breast pumping needs to be determined within the context of daily living. A mother with several other children, or one very busy toddler, who has no household assistance may find that being asked to pump her breasts—in addition to the time she is already spending with each feeding episode—may discourage her from continuing with the care plan. Unless a family history of allergies is identified, the judicious use of formula in the feeding tube device may assist continued breastfeeding.

SUMMARY

Breastfeeding is a normal physiologic process; however, problems such as poor weight gain occasionally occur. A first step in helping the mother of a baby who is gaining weight poorly is to identify aspects of her experience which differ from the normal breastfeeding course. Identification and treatment of any underlying illness—and managing the problem while preserving breastfeeding—should be the ultimate goal.

The majority of cases resulting in nutritional failure to thrive derive from nonorganic or environmental barriers which lead to inadequate weight gain. Therefore, in assessing the infant who is failing to thrive, mother and baby, as interacting individuals working as a team, must be evaluated together. Assessment and treatment is most effective when it includes evaluation of mother and baby during several breastfeeding sessions.

Often, the mother's knowledge of breastfeeding is assumed to be greater than it is, particularly if she has breastfed more than one baby. Assessing the mother's understanding of the underlying factors contributing to her baby's difficulties with breastfeeding is the first step in helping her to see where her behavior fits into the picture and how her own knowledge of her baby is essential as a care plan is developed to improve the infant's weight gain.

Many mothers have breastfed successfully in the most daunting situations, positions, and surroundings—and their infants thrive. However, when an infant fails to do so, consideration must be given to *all* the possible factors which may be contributing to the problem. At the same time, support should be offered for continued breastfeeding by avoiding any treatment option that separates the baby from the mother.

Every mother and infant are unique. Close and continuing follow-up care, by telephone and face-to-face visits, not only supports the mother during a stressful, fearful time but also informs the health-care provider by enabling her to evaluate the results of her care plan.

REFERENCES

Atkinson, HC, and Biggs, EJ: The binding of drugs to major human milk whey proteins, *Br J Clin Pharmacol* 26: 107–9, 1988.

Auerbach, KG, and Eggert, LD: The importance of infant suckling patterns when a breast-fed baby fails to thrive, *J Trop Pediatr* 33:156–57, 1987.

Batagol, R: Drugs and breastfeeding, *Breastfeed Rev* 14: 13–20, 1989.

Berg, KL: Two cases of tongue-tie and breastfeeding, *J Hum Lact* 6:124–26, 1990.

Berlin, CM: Drugs and chemicals: exposure of the nursing mother, *Pediatr Clin North Am* 36:1089–97, 1989.

Berlin, CM, et al.: Disposition of dietary caffeine in milk, saliva, and plasma of lactating women, *Pediatrics* 73: 59–63, 1984.

Bobath, B: *Abnormal postural reflex activity caused by brain lesions,* 2nd ed., London, 1971, Heinemann, Medical Books.

Bowen-Jones, A, Thompson, C, and Drewett, R: Milk flow and sucking rates during breastfeeding, *Dev Med Child Neurol* 24:626–33, 1982.

Butte, NF, Smith, EO, and Garza, C: Energy utilization of breast-fed and formula-fed infants, *Am J Clin Nutr* 51: 350–58, 1990.

Christian, PS, et al.: Relationship between maternal and infant nutritional status, *J Trop Pediatr* 35:71–76, 1989.

Dahlstrom, A, et al.: Nicotine and cotinine concentrations in the nursing mother and her infant, *Acta Paediatr Scand* 79:142–47, 1990.

Davies, DP: Is inadequate breast-feeding an important cause of failure to thrive? *Lancet* 1:541–42, 1979.

Desmarais, L, and Browne, S: *Inadequate weight gain in breastfeeding infants: assessments and resolutions* (Unit 8), Lactation Consultant Series, Garden City Park, N.Y., 1990, Avery Publishing Group, Inc.

Ehrenkranz, RA, and Ackerman, BA: Metroclopramide effect on faltering milk production by mothers of premature infants, *Pediatrics* 78:614–20, 1986.

Escott, R: Positioning, attachment and milk transfer, *Breastfeed Rev* 14:31–37, 1989.

Frantz, K: Slow weight gain. In Riordan, J: *A practical guide to breastfeeding,* St. Louis, 1983, The C. V. Mosby Co.

Frantz, K: Techniques for successfully managing nipple problems and the reluctant nurser in the early postpartum period. In Freier, S, ed.: *Human milk: its biological and social value,* Amsterdam, 1980, Exerpta Medica, pp. 314–17.

Frantz, KB, Fleiss, PM, and Lawrence, RA: Management of

the slow-gaining breastfed baby, *Keep Abreast J* 3:287–308, 1978.

Gupta, A, and Gupta, P: Metaclopramide as a lactagogue, *Clin Pediatr* 24:269–72, 1985.

Holliday, KE, et al.: Growth of human milk-fed and formula-fed infants with cystic fibrosis, *J Pediatr* 118:77–79, 1991.

Howie, PW, et al.: How long should a breast feed last? *Early Hum Dev* 5:71–77, 1981.

Klaus, MH: The frequency of suckling: a neglected but essential ingredient of breast feeding, *Obstet Gynecol Clin North Am* 14:623–33, 1987.

Livingstone, VH: Problem-solving formula for failure to thrive in breast-fed infants, *Can Fam Phys* 36:1541–45, 1990.

Luder, E, et al.: Current recommendations for breast-feeding in cystic fibrosis centers, *Am J Dis Child* 14:1153–56, 1990.

Lukefahr, JL: Underlying illness associated with failure to thrive in breastfed infants, *Clin Pediatr* 29:468–70, 1990.

Marmet, C, Shell, E, and Marmet, R: Neonatal frenotomy may be necessary to correct breastfeeding problems, *J Hum Lact* 6:117–21, 1990.

McBride, MC, and Danner, SC: Sucking disorders in neurologically impaired infants: Assessment and facilitation of breastfeeding, *Clin Perinatol* 14:109–30, 1987.

McNeilly, A, et al.: Release of oxytocin and prolactin in response to suckling, *Br Med J* 286:257–59, 1983.

Morris, S, and Klein, M: *Pre-feeding skills,* Tuscon, Ariz., 1987, Therapy Skill Builder.

Mueller, H: Facilitating feeding and pre-speech. In Pearson, PH, and Williams, CE, eds.: *Physical therapy services in the developmental disabilities,* Springfield, Ill., 1972, Charles C Thomas, Publisher.

National Center for Health Statistics: *NCHS growth curves for children: Birth–18 years,* PHS Publication No. 78-1650, Washington, D.C., 1977, U.S. Department of Health, Education and Welfare.

Neifert, M, and Seacat, J: Lactation insufficiency: A rational approach, *Birth* 14:182–88, 1987.

Neville, MC, and Berga, SE: Cellular and molecular aspects of the hormonal control of mammary function. In Neville, MC, and Neifert, M, eds.: *Lactation: physiology, nutrition and breast-feeding,* New York, 1983, Plenum Press, pp. 162–63.

Nicholson, WL: Breastfeeding after breast reduction: guidelines for mothers, *Breastfeed Rev* 2:174–77, 1991a.

Nicholson, WL: Tongue-tie (ankyloglossia) associated with breastfeeding problems, *J Hum Lact* 7:82–84, 1991b.

Notestine, GE: The importance of the identification of ankyloglossia (short lingual frenulum) as a cause of breastfeeding problems, *J Hum Lact* 6:113–15, 1990.

Pfeifer, DR, and Ayoub, C: Nonorganic failure to thrive in the breastfeeding dyad, *Keep Abreast J* 3:283–86, 1978.

Riordan, J, and Riordan, M: Drugs in breastmilk, *AJN* 84:328–32, 1984.

Rovet, JF: Does breast-feeding protect the hypothyroid infant whose condition is diagnosed by newborn screening? *Am J Dis Child* 144:319–23, 1990.

Sack, J, Amado, O, and Lunenfeld, B: Thyroxine concentration in human milk, *J Clin Endocrinol Metab* 45:171–73, 1977.

Sills, R: Failure to thrive, *Am J Dis Child* 132:967–69, 1978.

Steldinger, R, and Luck, W: Half lives of nicotine in milk of smoking mothers: implications for nursing (letter), *J Perinat Med* 16:261–62, 1988.

Tanis, AL: Growth in breastfed babies, *Breastfeeding Abstr* 4:13, 1985.

Ward, N: Ankyloglossia: a case study in which clipping was not necessary, *J Hum Lact* 6: 126–27, 1990.

Weichert, CE: Lactational reflex recovery in breast feeding failure, *Pediatrics* 63:799–803, 1979.

Whaley, LF, and Wong, DL: *Essentials of pediatric nursing* (3rd ed.), St. Louis, 1989, The C.V. Mosby Co., p. 1094.

Wilton, JM: Sore nipples and slow weight gain related to a short frenulum, *J Hum Lact* 6:122–23, 1990.

Woolridge, MW, Ingram, JC, and Baum, JD: Do changes in patterns of breast usage alter the baby's nutritional intake? *Lancet* 336(8712):395–97, 1990.

Appendix 19–1

From Desmarais, L, and Browne, S: *Inadequate weight gain in breastfeeding infants: assessments and resolutions* (Unit 8), Lactation Consultant Series, Garden City, N.Y., 1990, Avery Publishing Group, Inc. Reprinted with permission.

MATERNAL-INFANT HISTORY FORM*

Infant's Name: _____

Mother's Name: _____

Consultation For: _____

Office Tel.: (   )
Or call   -   from
(hours/A.M., P.M.) Weekdays and
(hours A.M., P.M.) Weekends

Date: _____

Phone Number: _____

PART I. PATIENT HISTORY

Please describe in your own words why you have sought this breastfeeding consultation. _____

_____

_____

_____

_____

_____

_____

Past Maternal Medical History

Yes No   Are you in good health? If not, describe any medical problems.

_____

_____

Are you taking:

Yes No   Birth control pills?
Yes No   Prescription medications?
Yes No   Non-prescription (over-the-counter) medications?
Yes No   Have you had any thyroid problems at any time in your life?
Yes No   Are you taking any thyroid medications *now*? If so, what kind; dosage?

Yes No   Do you have any endocrine ("glandular") problems?
Yes No   Have you had any previous surgery?
Yes No   Have you ever had breast surgery? If so, specify when, what, and for what reason.

_____

_____

Yes No   Do you have any allergies?
Yes No   Did you observe any breast changes during pregnancy? Describe.

Yes No   Did you take any medications during pregnancy? If so, which one(s); what dosage?

_____

Yes No   For this baby and any other breastfed infants, did your milk "come in" on or before the third postpartum day?

Maternal Family History

Has anyone in your family had a history of any of the following problems? If so, specify below.

Yes No   Breastfeeding problems?
Yes No   Eczema or allergy to food, pollen, or other substances?
Yes No   An infant who had difficulty gaining weight?
Yes No   Metabolic or malabsorption disease?
Yes No   Cardiac or neurologic problems?

_____

_____

_____

_____

_____

Maternal Habits

Yes No   Do you smoke? If so, specify brand and number per day.

_____

Yes No   Do you drink coffee or tea? If so, specify number of cups per day.

_____

Caffeinated?   Yes _____ No _____

Decaffeinated?   Yes _____ No _____

Herbal?   Yes _____ No _____

Type of herbal tea: _____

Yes No   Do you drink caffeinated sodas? If so, specify number per day; ounces per day.

_____

* Special acknowledgement for the technical assistance of
Janet Repucci, BS, MT (ASCP), IBCLC.

Yes No   Do you drink alcohol? If so, specify what type, and how much per day/week/month.

_____

Yes No   Do you use recreational drugs? If so, specify kind and frequency.

_____

Maternal Diet

Yes No   Do you eat regular meals?
How would you rate the food you eat?
Excellent   Good   Poor

Yes No   Do you currently take prenatal vitamins? If so, specify brand and type.

_____

Yes No   Do you take any other vitamins? If so, specify brand(s) and type(s).

_____

Yes No   Are you on a restricted diet of any kind (e.g., vegetarian, low sodium)? If so, specify type of restriction and purpose. _____

_____

Yes No   Are you currently on a weight loss diet?
Yes No   Are you drinking more fluids now that you are nursing?

Maternal Social History

Are you: single ____ married (how long?) ____ divorced (how long?) ____

Do you: own _____ rent _____ live with relatives _____

How long have you lived there? _____

Who lives in your household? (list all) _____

_____

Please supply the following information about each of your children?

	Age	Breastfed?	How long?
1st (oldest) child	_____	_____	_____
2nd child	_____	_____	_____
3rd child	_____	_____	_____
4th child	_____	_____	_____
5th child	_____	_____	_____
6th child	_____	_____	_____

How would you describe your relationship with the baby's father?

Good _____   Fair _____   Poor _____

Yes No   Do you have a busy lifestyle? If so, describe.

_____

Yes No   Do you have any source(s) of anxiety or tension? If so, describe.

_____

Yes No   Do you have any friends or relatives who have breastfed their babies? If so, describe. _____

_____

Yes No   Are any of your relatives or close friends opposed to/nonsupportive of breastfeeding? If so, describe.

_____

Breastfeeding Preparation

When did you decide to breastfeed this baby?

_____ before pregnancy

_____ early pregnancy (in the first 4 months)

_____ late pregnancy (in the last 3 months)

_____ after the baby's birth. When was that? Why? Specify reason.

_____

Who most influenced your decision to breastfeed? _____
How long do you want to breastfeed?

_____ up to 6 weeks

_____ up to 3 months

_____ up to 6 months

_____ up to 1 year

_____ until the baby weans

_____ other (specify) _____

Yes No   Have you read anything about breastfeeding? If so, specify.

_____

Yes No   Have you attended any classes or support groups for breastfeeding? If so, when, and by whom? _____

Yes No   During your pregnancy, were your breasts examined? If so, provide name of care provider.

_____

Infant's Birth History

Type of delivery:
Vaginal: _____ augmented   _____ forceps   _____ suction

Cesarean; why? _____

Yes No   Labor experienced? Length? _____
Yes No   Were medications given during labor or delivery? If so, what kind?

_____

Yes No   Was it a difficult birth? If so, describe.

_____

Yes　No　Were medications taken after birth? If so, what kind? For what reason?

_____

Place of birth:　　　　home ___　birth center ___　hospital ___

If not at home, where was baby kept?　in nursery ___　rooming in ___

If rooming in, what kind of plan? (How many hours with mother?) _____

Yes　No　Were you separated from infant for any length of time? If so, why?

_____

Maternal Feeding Experience

When infant nurses, do you feel: tingling _____　warmth _____

burning _____　filling _____

leaking on other side _____　nothing _____　other _____

If other, describe. _____

Yes　No　Do you have a quiet place for nursing? If not, where do you usually nurse?

_____

Yes　No　Do you use a rocking chair for nursing?

Have you ever experienced any of the following?
Yes　No　Sore nipples.
Yes　No　Plugged duct.
Yes　No　Breast infection.
Yes　No　Severe engorgement.
Yes　No　A feeling of being ''softer'' after a feeding.
Yes　No　Discomfort from fullness in the breasts.

Infant Feeding History

First time infant was put to breast was _____ hours after birth.
Yes　No　Did infant take to nursing easily?
Yes　No　Has your baby received any bottle-feedings? If so, when and why? _____

_____

What was in the bottle(s)?　Human milk only _____

Other(?) _____
Yes　No　Does your baby feed at each breast at each feeding?

How long on each breast at each feeding? _____
How many times on each breast at each feeding?

_____

How long is each feeding, on average? _____
Yes　No　Does the infant pause often during a feeding?
Yes　No　Do you hear the baby swallowing?
Yes　No　Does the baby make clicking or popping sounds while nursing?
Yes　No　Does the baby initiate the end of each feeding?
Yes　No　Does the baby appear to be satisfied at the end of a feeding? How would you rate his sucking?
poor ___　weak ___　average ___　strong ___
Yes　No　Does he burp easily?
When is he burped? _____

What technique is used? _____

Yes　No　Does the baby spit up or vomit after a feeding? If so, how often does this occur?

_____

Number of wet diapers per day? _____
Yes　No　Are paper diapers used?
Number of stools per day? _____　Consistency _____　Color _____

Is infant　　placid ___　average ___　active ___　fussy ___

When during the day/night is the baby awake? _____

What is your baby's longest sleep period? _____

When? _____

At what time is baby put to bed for the night? _____
Yes　No　Is this bedtime regular?

Circle the time when feedings begin on a typical day.

Midnight　1　2　3　4　5　6　7　8　9　10　11AM
Noon　　 1　2　3　4　5　6　7　8　9　10　11PM

Yes　No　Is a pacifier used? If so, what kind? _____
How often? _____
Yes　No　Does the baby suck his thumb or fingers?
Yes　No　Does the baby have ''colic?''
Yes　No　Has the baby begun receiving solid foods? If so, what are they? How often?

_____

Infant Medical History

Infant's Expected Date of Birth: _____

Infant's Actual Date of Birth: _____

Infant's Birth Weight: _____　Infant's Current Weight: _____

Infant's APGAR Scores: _____ 1 minute _____ 5 minutes

Yes　No　Were there any problems with the infant immediately after birth? If so, describe. _____
Yes　No　Has the infant had any problems since birth? If so, describe. ___

_____

Yes　No　Was the infant jaundiced? If so, peak bilirubin level? _____
On what day? _____
Yes　No　Is the infant receiving any medications? If so, what kind? What dosage? Why? _____

_____

Yes　No　Is the infant receiving any vitamins? If so, what kind? What dosage? Why? _____

_____

Yes　No　Has the infant had any other tests performed (especially for slow weight gain)? If so, what kind? When? Where? _____

_____

Yes　No　Does the infant have a milk allergy? If so, to what kind of milk? When did it first appear? _____

_____

Yes　No　Does the infant have cystic fibrosis?

PART II: PHYSICAL EXAMINATION

For each structure being examined, assign one of the two following codes: **0** (within normal range), **X** (abnormal). If abnormal, specify problem.

Maternal Examination

Right   Left

Nipple size: _____   _____

Protractility: _____   _____

Other: _____   _____

Notes: _____

_____

_____

Infant Examination

1. Infant behavior at time of exam: _____

_____

2. Measurements:

	Date	Weight	Length	Head Circumference
At birth:	_____	_____	_____	_____
Discharge date:	_____	_____	_____	_____
Today:	_____	_____	_____	_____

Notes: _____

_____

3. Muscle Tone _____

Positions (supine, prone, other) _____

_____

Notes: _____

_____

4. Oral exam:

Notes

Mouth _____ _____

Jaw _____ _____

Tongue: _____ _____

Frenulum: _____ _____

Palate: _____ _____

Digital suck exam: _____

_____

_____

Clinical Data

Enter all data (test, date, results) pertaining to creamatocrit, prolactin, triple prolactin, maternal thyroid, etc. _____

_____

_____

_____

ASSESSMENT SUMMARY

Summarize problems in order of impact upon breastfeeding:

1. _____
2. _____
3. _____
4. _____
5. _____

MANAGEMENT PLAN

Key to above numbers:

1. _____
2. _____
3. _____
4. _____
5. _____

PHYSICIAN FOLLOW-UP

Date _____

Notes _____

_____

PATIENT FOLLOW-UP

Date _____

Notes _____

_____

SECTION

FIVE

Contemporary Issues

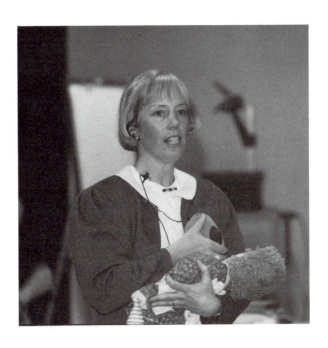

Out of need new methods of coping are developed. The development and expansion of lactation consulting as a new member of the allied health field highlights—by its very existence—the degree to which other health-care providers have tended to ignore the needs of breastfeeding babies and their lactating mothers. At the same time that these needs have been reemphasized, the market of products designed for lactating mothers has exploded, particularly in developed countries. Yet, as with other products, all are not what they seem or have been purported to be. Milk banks represent a means of obtaining a scarce resource yet they may disappear entirely in light of often unwarranted fears about the spread of AIDS through breastmilk. The political implications of continued use of human milk from banks is an ongoing story that continues to unfold. At the same time, we need more research in order to expand our knowledge of the lactation process and the variations in breastfeeding behavior. Only with such research will myths about breastfeeding be put to rest, and clinical care-giving begin to provide the help that lactating mothers deserve for themselves and their babies.

20

Work Strategies and the Lactation Consultant

KATHLEEN G. AUERBACH

JAN RIORDAN

A lactation consultant (LC) is a specialist trained to focus on the needs and concerns of the breastfeeding mother-baby pair and to prevent, recognize, and solve breastfeeding difficulties. The lactation consultant's services do not replace those of the physician, nurse, or any other health-care worker; instead the LC is an extender of maternal-child services. Today's lactation consultants work with the public in many settings: hospitals, clinics, private medical practice, community health departments, and home health agencies. Almost all LCs are women, and many have educational and clinical backgrounds in the health professions.

The lactation consultant is a new occupational category under the broad umbrella of allied health workers. Prior to recognition of the LC as a specific paid position in 1985, individuals serving breastfeeding women did so as volunteers and/or as unrecognized private practitioners. The lack of standardization of skills and minimal competencies led to formal development of the occupation. This occurred, in part, through a certification examination, as well as through the establishment of an international organization, International Lactation Consultant Association (ILCA), which publishes a journal on issues relating to human lactation and breastfeeding. This chapter traces the historical roots of lactation consultants and discusses work-related issues.

HISTORY

In a cultural setting in which nearly all mothers breastfed, help with breastfeeding was available through the shared knowledge of other family members, neighbors, and friends. As childbirth came to be managed by health professionals in hospital settings, however, knowledge of lactation, which a mother formerly shared with her daughters or a sister with her younger siblings, was set aside.

Thus, during the 1960s at the nadir of breastfeeding in the United States, and shortly thereafter in other countries, including Australia, volunteer breastfeeding support groups became a major source of assistance and information about how to breastfeed (Phillips, 1990b). As the numbers of breastfeeding mothers increased, health-care providers at first denounced these groups; later they came to appreciate them for the important role they played in helping mothers and in forcing the medical profession to consider lactation as an integral part of prenatal and postpartum care (Gerrard, 1974, 1975; Jelliffe & Jelliffe, 1977). In a salute to La Leche League International, Lee Forest Hill, the editor of the *Journal of Pediatrics,* praised: "A dedicated women's organization has taken on the task of attempting to restore what is called by some, 'the lost art of breastfeeding.' Certainly, their efforts deserve the commendation of the medical and nursing professions" (Hill, 1968).

As these volunteers relearned the art of breastfeeding, they also sought more knowledge of the science of lactation. La Leche League responded by providing scientific research information to their group leaders, who serve as mother-to-mother helpers, and by publishing a quarterly newsletter, *Breastfeeding Abstracts,* which focuses exclusively on the scientific literature. La Leche League also has a professional liaison department whose members seek to cultivate and maintain communication links to health providers in local communities.

Out of this context, some experienced breastfeeding support group members began to look beyond what they would accomplish as volunteers. Many of these women sought to apply in a paid work setting what they had learned from many years of helping breastfeeding mothers. From this small beginning grew the notion of the need for a new health-care worker.

CERTIFICATION

In 1981, an experienced La Leche League leader from Virginia, JoAnne Scott, was asked to develop a certification and training program for lactation consultants. This need derived from (1) an awareness that many health-care providers discredited the accomplishments of the volunteer because she was unpaid and (2) a need to establish minimum standards for individuals who were already providing lactation consultant services for a fee. A certification program was viewed as a way to recognize the important role of the volunteer and to provide a recognized credential that identified a certain level of competence (Scott, 1990).

Scott contacted a small group of other women who had come to the field of lactation through voluntary mother-to-mother service, mostly through La Leche League. In 1984, these women gathered and concluded that legitimacy of the field would be heightened if minimal standards of knowledge and skills were recognized through a certification examination.

The first examination was administered in July, 1985, under the International Board of Lactation Consultant Examiners, Inc. (IBLCE).* Since 1985, a certification examination has been given annually in three languages (English, Spanish, and German) in 11 countries on seven continents, including North America, Europe, the Pacific basin, and Africa. So far over 2,500 candidates have been certified, approxi-

*The International Board of Lactation Consultant Examiners, Inc., can be reached at 2315 Wickersham Cove, Germantown, TN 38139; (901) 755–6233.

mately 80% of whom live in the United States and Canada (Tanis, Coleman & Gross, 1990). Periodic recertification as an LC is required through the acquisition of continuing education credits and by reexamination. This dual recertification option increases the likelihood that the LC will remain current in a rapidly changing field.

Early candidates for the certification examination had a baccalaureate degree and were originally trained through La Leche League leadership accreditation. After the first year, affiliation with La Leche League declined, while affiliation with a hospital or clinical setting increased. Although there was no correlation between educational attainment and test scores in the first year of the examination, in subsequent years a baccalaureate (or higher) degree was significantly related to higher test scores. Among non-nurses, however, an inverse relationship exists between education and test performance. Persons with a master's degree (or greater) do not obtain higher scores than those with a lower level of educational attainment (Riordan, 1990). The authors of the first evaluation of certification candidates (Riordan & Auerbach, 1987) speculated that the pass rate would decline as the backgrounds of the candidates broadened to include individuals with fewer years of clinical experience prior to their taking the examination. As can be seen in Table 20–1, this speculation appears to have been borne out.

In the United States certification is respected and popular in the health professions. Over 40 specialty certifications exist in the field of nursing alone, despite the fact that certification is a voluntary credential. Some state laws limit clinical service in hospitals to licensed medical or nursing staff only, often for legal reasons. However, awarding credentials by certification evidence of their competency to practice enables LCs with other educational prerequisites to see clients under medical supervision. Such credentials afford opportunity for practice to clinical psychologists, physical therapists, and others who may not be licensed, but who have passed certification examinations.

DEVELOPING A LACTATION PROGRAM

In-hospital breastfeeding programs or clinics are developing throughout the United States. According to Anderson and Geden (1991), of 293 surveys returned from hospital-based nurses, 12% report having a lactation consultant in their institution, and

TABLE 20–1   IBLCE EXAMINATION SUMMARY DATA, 1985–1991

Year of Examination	Number of Candidates	Mean Passing %	Pass-Fail Score	Pass Rate
1985	259	72.8	61.8	94.6
1986	222	72.6	62.9	93.2
1987	281	72.5	63.8	90.7
1988	281	74.0	64.6	91.1
1989	306	76.1	67.5	92.5
1990	428	72.0	65.0	89.0
1991	683	72.9	64.0	91.1

Adapted from Riordan, J: A statistical overview of IBLCE certification exams, *J Hum Lact* 6:90–92, 1990; reprinted with permission.

about 80% had a breastfeeding protocol. Most nurses learned about breastfeeding on the job rather than as part of their educational experience (89% vs. 28%, respectively), and only a minority received in-service programs on breastfeeding, relying instead on journals or books to stay current.

In New York state, a 1984 law mandated that any institution providing care for new mothers and babies had to have at least one person on staff who was designated to serve as a resource for other staff and to provide breastfeeding assistance to patients. Initially, many hospitals met the letter of the law by assigning someone already on staff, most often a nurse, to be the lactation person. Often, these individuals were no more prepared than other staff members to provide assistance to breastfeeding mothers or to serve as a resource for their colleagues. However, since the law was enacted, many of these individuals have taken it upon themselves to become more informed about breastfeeding. Still others have sought certification as lactation consultants (Roseanne Orlando, personal communication, 1991).

Although only a small number of hospitals in the United States have a lactation program, most that do have several elements in common. The following boxed list identifies the elements most often found in hospital-based programs.

A lactation program may take many guises. A breast pump rental depot, because it is so likely to generate revenue, may serve as a first kind of service for breastfeeding women (Rago, 1987). A lactation service may be part of a community health program already in place, but which is funded for a breast-feeding clinic and/or promotion program (Dublin, 1989). Such programs often require that the LC become cognizant of the political as well as the social climate, not only of the particular agency for whom she works, but the larger community which it serves. For example, in a community where the health-care workers are already well versed in assisting breastfeeding mothers and babies, the presence of a lactation clinic may simply be part of an environ-

---

HOSPITAL-BASED LACTATION
PROGRAMS/SERVICES

- Telephone hotline and/or "warmline" (which may serve as a referral source, in addition to offering assistance without requiring an office visit)
- Prenatal education about breastfeeding (breastfeeding classes)
- In-hospital postbirth assistance with breastfeeding (one-on-one)
- At-home postbirth assistance with breast-feeding
- Pump rental and sales
- Breastfeeding problem-solving clinic (often both in-patient and out-patient service)
- Education: seminars, classes, clinical experience
- Preceptorship (less often offered; sometimes limited only to those individuals with a medical or nursing license)
- Research on lactation/breastfeeding issues (most often at a tertiary-care medical center)
- Evaluation of lactation products/devices and services

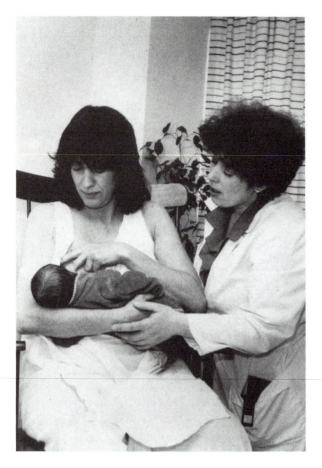

FIGURE 20–1   Assistance early promotes maternal confidence.

ment supportive of lactation. In another community, where breastfeeding is not seen as part of the regular health care, establishing such a clinic may represent a departure from previous care patterns.

A lactation program may also develop out of a patient-education program that began with childbirth preparation and other classes designed to meet the many needs of pregnant and postpartum women and their families. From such a base of clients who have already developed rapport with the patient educator, additional classes may be provided, including prenatal breastfeeding classes, as well as follow-up services after the babies are born and the mothers' questions become more frequent.

Other programs are the outcome of patient surveys, often pertaining to satisfaction with care they received as new mothers. In one case, a survey included questions relating to the mothers' interest in using the services of a lactation clinic, a phone hotline, and a prenatal or postpartum breastfeeding class (Wilton, 1989). Still others have developed from an identified need of a hospital to "keep up with the medical Joneses"; that is, when a competing hospital provides and then publicizes its lactation consultant services, other hospitals compete by providing similar services.

How those services are structured will vary by the institution. In some programs, the LC sees all new mothers who indicate that they plan to breastfeed. In other cases, she sees all new mothers, identifying her clients when they tell her how they are feeding their babies. A few LCs counsel both breastfeeding and bottle-feeding mothers. Other institutions restrict the LC's contact only to those breastfeeding mothers for whom the referring obstetrician or pediatrician have asked for a consultation and follow-up care.

Whatever system is used, estimate the anticipated workload prior to the start of the lactation service. Predicting the actual number of work hours will be based upon the number of births in the institution and the percentage of mothers who are breastfeeding. Thus, daily rounds may be appropriate in a hospital where the LC sees fewer than 10 patients per day; it may not be appropriate if more than 10 breastfeeding mothers are housed in the maternity unit on a given day—unless there is more than one lactation consultant in the service. A hospital with 3,000 deliveries each year should have at least three full-time LC positions in order to avoid burnout and get the job done. In addition, the service—to be effective—should be available seven days a week, on all shifts. Most hospital lactation programs, based on the 1:1000 ratio, are woefully understaffed and only provide part-time service as a result of partial shift coverage or coverage for less than seven days a week.

One of the newer programs is at Georgetown University (Washington, D.C.). It began with a "hotline" service for mothers, prenatal breastfeeding classes, and breastfeeding classes on the maternity unit. A grant from the March of Dimes established a Community Human Milk Bank at the hospital in 1976. Later, a LC training program was developed which provides both class lectures (40 hours) and a clinical site for hands-on training.

The Beth Israel Medical Center Lactation Program (New York City) was developed by its first director, pediatrician Marvin Eiger. A nurse-lactation consultant and a non-nurse lactation consultant provide prenatal and postpartum teaching to breastfeeding mothers. They are an integral part of the education of prospective LCs and other health-care workers through regularly sponsored seminars, grand rounds, and other teaching courses. Additionally, hands-on training opportunities are offered which enable the prospective LC to gain valuable experience under supervision. The Lactation Institute in Encino, California, is now affiliated with Pacific Oaks College and offers a specialization in lactation as part of a degree program. (See Chapter 8 for more information.)

PLAYING POLITICS

When proposing a lactation program, it is essential to realize that such a service will overlap with the interests of several ongoing departments or programs. As a result, it is both politic and appropriate to involve all such departments in the early stages of the proposal process. "Touching base" and developing a working relationship with hospital decision-makers is critical. Without it, any hope of establishing a program is seriously undermined, and the likelihood of the program becoming an integral part of the institution remains low.

Any new program will stand a good chance of *not* being implemented without someone with power pushing it. A powerful figure in the institution who is committed to pushing the program keeps up the momentum even when efforts might wane. A sponsor with "clout" is needed to give the major push beyond the actions of the innovators and to commit resources from the institutional budget. This person can be a high-level administrator, chief of staff, or chairman of a department. Kantor (1983) calls this individual the "prime mover" or an "idea sponsor": "prime movers push in part by repetition by mentioning the new idea or practice on every possible occasion in every speech and at every meeting."

Department heads particularly critical to securing support for the new program include the supervisor of maternity nursing (who may oversee labor and delivery, postpartum and nursery units, and sometimes the intensive care nursery); the supervisor of the pediatric unit; as well as the chairman or medical director for obstetrics/gynecology, pediatrics, and in some cases, family medicine. If the institution has a midwifery service, the support of its director should also be sought. Usually, department heads meet as a committee to review requests and attempt to solve problems. These committees should be approached when proposing a new lactation service (Bachman, 1987).

If the institution has an employee health department or a women's health clinic, their supervisors should be informed of the proposal and asked for their support. Any documents which highlight how the new program will assist and support the services that are already being provided helps build their acceptance. For example, the supervisor of employee health may be particularly interested in learning that the lactation program will include services to employees, such as a special place where newly returning employees can express or pump their breasts or nurse their babies during work hours. The women's health service may want to know how to refer clients to the lactation service and/or how they can take advantage of the resources of the lactation service as it relates to information pertaining to the use of medication during lactation.

Experienced lactation consultants who have started a lactation service point out the importance of not taking for granted that everyone knows about the service and/or what it offers (Williams, 1986). Being as visible as possible around the hospital helps to get the word out. The lactation consultant is a member of the staff and thus able to attend staff meetings for the departments (nursing service, family practice, pediatrics, obstetrics) in which the lactation service will have the greatest impact. In all cases, each contact and presentation must focus on the ways in which the department and institution will benefit from the service. While improved patient care is an obvious item to mention, most hospitals expect that *any new service will generate income for the institution or at least pay for itself.*

What priority do lactation services have for hospital administrators? Keep in mind that hospital administrators choose new programs from dozens of new possibilities for hospital investment—another magnetic resonance imager vs. a new diabetes center. Before deciding, administration first looks at two "bottom-line" factors: revenue and marketing potential. When it comes to any new health program, money speaks loudest. For example, while it appears obvious that premature infants should receive follow-up home care, it was not taken seriously by health officials until Brooten and colleagues (1986) at the University of Pennsylvania School of Nursing showed that postdischarge home visits for very low-birth-weight infants could save as much as 334 million dollars annually in the United States.

While lactation services will bring minimal revenue to the hospital compared to "high-tech" machines, such services are an effective marketing tool for the hospital. Women, after all, make most of the decisions about choosing health-care services for all family members. Thus, health strategists claim that if the mother uses a certain hospital for having her baby and she liked the service she received there, she will probably use that same hospital again for the family's future health-care needs. It is well established in the United States and many other countries that women who are most likely to breastfeed are educated and in the middle-to-higher income brackets; thus, a lactation service increases the hospital's visibility and credibility with young, educated families who have a high earning potential. The income-generating nature of patient care makes such a service attractive, particularly in settings where local hospitals are competing for the same patient dollars. The new trend in hospitals is product-line management, an approach which markets a product-line of services: lactation services are a new "product" that medical centers can offer to their "customers" (Sonstegard, 1988).

Support for a lactation program must come from different areas, including nursing services, medical services (particularly family practice, internal medicine, obstetrics/gynecology, and pediatrics), and ancillary services, such as those pertaining to billing and supplies. If the health professionals running the lactation service are part of a major teaching medical center, they should have a faculty status, particularly if they will have responsibility for teaching medical and/or nursing students (Best, 1987).

Just as the lack of physicians' support can prevent a program from being added to the array of services already offered, physicians' support can pave the way for the addition of a lactation program. Such support is most likely to be obtained if the key physicians—often chiefs of service or department heads—see that a lactation program will meet needs that they feel are important. In some cases, the need for such a service is highlighted through a physician's (or his spouse's) own experiences with breastfeeding. In other cases, the comments of patients often highlight a need and generate the physician's initial interest in such a service.

Physicians are powerful figures in the hospital; therefore, maintaining positive relations with physicians, both staff and attending, is critical. The physician as "gatekeeper" plays a major role in the fiscal health of a hospital. If the physician's patients do not want to go to a particular hospital because it lacks certain amenities—such as a lactation service—the hospital administrator, with the backing of several physicians, may choose to back such a program rather than lose patients to a competing institution in an adjoining community or even within the same city. Physicians have the influence to make or break the program, and physician support should be encouraged and nurtured. Supportive physicians are more likely to be:

- young mothers who breastfed
- fathers of breastfed children
- physicians building a new practice, particularly in an area of the city where breastfeeding is valued by young parents
- physicians from countries where breastfeeding is the norm.

Mothers who are satisfied with the help they received with infant feeding are very likely to stay with the physician for other aspects of care. It is advisable to get input on all important plans from the physicians most influential to your program. For example, before putting forth a breastfeeding protocol for your unit or agency, distribute it to the appropriate physicians with a note asking for their input.

There will always be a few physicians who are not supportive of lactation services and who feel that their turf has been invaded. The best way to handle the situation is to "hang tough"—be courteous but make it clear that you intend to continue with your plans with or without their help. It has been noted that physicians who are consistently antagonistic to the program usually have had a personal (negative) family experience with breastfeeding. If the resistive physician is male, chances are that his wife chose not to breastfeed or had an unhappy experience with breastfeeding.

The first several months of existence of a lactation service, as with any new service, are usually characterized by generalized good will. The team approach, which involves several different areas within the institution, becomes important in providing continued support for the lactation service. This is particularly true if the lactation service has neither a medical director on a daily basis nor one whose reputation within the medical community is well established. Potential antagonists usually hold their tongues and bide their time; they are willing to allow the lactation service personnel to "make a mistake." During this "honeymoon" period, the LC often finds her enthusiasm carries her further than she imagined. This experience encourages confidence that many short-term goals will be met.

Nine to 18 months into the existence of the lactation service, problems that have not been resolved become more noticeable. For example, if in-service programs have been provided for all areas of the hospital except the emergency room and the intensive care nursery, this lack of coverage may become an issue. It is at this time that antagonists to the service begin to make their opinions known to their peers. Sometimes this takes the form of a direct challenge to the lactation service personnel to "prove their worth"—monetarily, as well as in terms of quality of service. Failure to support the service may take the guise of structuring the service in such a way that it cannot develop a financial base sufficient to support itself, or removing its financial or administrative underpinnings and thereby "killing" it (Eiger, 1991). This is particularly likely if physicians must write an order for lactation services to be provided—and the physicians remain unconvinced that such a service is necessary.

Changing well-established routines is a major source of conflict between other health-care workers and the lactation service personnel, even when the change is supported by research. Since few people like to do things differently and most health professionals tend to provide service as they were taught in medical or nursing school (Auerbach & Walburn, 1987a, 1987b), recommendations from the LC can cause resentment and irritation among the nursing and medical staff.

When any change in protocols or routines—however small—is contemplated, the wise LC will enlist the assistance of those most likely to be affected by such change. Such preplanning can go a long way toward defusing potential antagonism and/or reducing resistance to change. Nearly always, this means consulting with the physicians who write the orders and the nurses who are expected to carry them out. Even something so apparently insignificant as the removal of supplemental water bottles from the cribs of neonates will require meetings and discussions—often with a committee mandated to initiate the change.

Additionally, in-service programs are needed to explain the change. When a team approach is used, change is more likely to be accomplished, and compliance is more likely to occur. After change is instituted, additional in-servicing is often necessary—to assure that all staff members are following the new

protocol and to iron out any difficulties that may arise as the new protocol is put into effect.

THE UNIQUE CHARACTERISTICS OF BREASTFEEDING COUNSELING

There are unique aspects of working with breastfeeding women that differ from other areas of health care. First, breastfeeding is a very emotional subject—it is an integral part of human sexuality, not just an infant feeding method. It touches deep-seated feelings which people have about themselves and their bodies that reach back to childhood. This makes breastfeeding counseling, like sex counseling or childbirth education, unusually sensitive. The health-care workers assisting breastfeeding families must be especially intuitive, caring listeners and advisors. It was probably because of these necessary traits that the term lactation "counselor" was chosen.

The second unique characteristic of breastfeeding counseling is that working with new mothers and babies is a popular and thus, competitive, activity. *Everyone* loves taking care of babies. Not only are newborns adorable, but the mothers and fathers are healthy and (generally) happy. By working on the hospital maternity unit or in a birth center, the nurse gets to play a paid, starring, ongoing role in the usually joyous family dramas of birthing. As a result, nurses compete to work there, and the maternity unit/nursery area has a low rate of staff turnover. In fact, one reason why introducing change in maternal care nursing has been difficult is because nurses continue work in the same maternity area for so many years. Gardner (1978) has described competition to "play the mother" as an unconscious conflict between nurses and new mothers.

The third characteristic is that breastfeeding counseling is done almost exclusively by women who must daily interact and work with other women: mothers and other female health workers. It is now recognized that women interact in the work place differently than men. Awareness and understanding of the typical ways that women interact with women and compete with each other gives the nurse or LC who comes onto the unit or into the community agency as a "new kid on the block" an advantage (Gilligan, 1982). The following elements outline the differences between women working together and men working together and the reasons for these differences.

1. *Women tend to suppress anger and express it covertly behind their co-workers' backs instead of openly and confrontationally.* Women learn, early on, ways of dealing with one another that are different from the ways men deal with one another. For example, boys learn at an early age that it is alright to openly fight with one another; even knocking each other down is often praised as "manly" (Melia, 1986). Girls, on the other hand, learn that they should be "nice" to everyone, not to fight, and especially not to hit anyone. These are called "Mommy's Rules" (Davidson-Crews, 1989), and they are deeply imbedded female behaviors, especially in white, middle-class, American women.

2. *Women are afraid to be criticized and take criticism personally.* As young children, women have been socialized to derive their self-worth from external, rather than internal sources; therefore, they tend to react excessively to others' opinions, whether positive or negative. If criticized, women are more likely to hold grudges for long periods; men are more likely to confront, disagree, and then forget. Remember: If you're afraid of criticism, don't give birth!

3. *Women do not work as well in teams as men.* Women have not used the give-and-take team concept of "you help me and I'll help you and we'll both get ahead." Instead, women operate on a higher utopian level: what is RIGHT and JUST is more important than any other consideration. Women act as policemen of one another, making sure that what their co-worker does is right and correct, and "trashing" them to keep them in their place.

4. *Women tend to become "over friendly," one-on-one.* Women who work together become fast friends with another female co-worker and tell each other their deepest secrets, which are sometimes used against each other when the friendship dissolves. Women give away power by giving away too much of themselves. Men rarely develop intimate, "tell-all" friendships with their co-workers. Women are more likely to work for social rewards; men work for money.

These three characteristics—the emotional quality of breastfeeding, the popularity of caring for babies, and the dysfunctional, covert games that women use in the work environment—set the stage for potential difficulties between the LC and the nurse, the nurse and the breastfeeding mother, the volunteer counselor and the LC, and the female physician and the LC.

The standards of behavior in the workplace are set according to men's rules, but that does not negate feminine qualities. Feminine, nurturing qualities are positive qualities that help us in working with breastfeeding families. Our best qualities have to do with becoming attached—developing close relationships and friendships with others. These attributes are critical for nurses and LCs if they are to empathize with breastfeeding women. However, when women personalize the business or professional setting, it is counterproductive to professional or business goals.

Survival requires that we learn to work within two concurrent cultures: the culture of nurturing and caring, and the culture of the profession's business. Business is not about friendship or family; it's about accomplishing tasks efficiently. Virginia Woolf noted that the values of women differ from the values of men; yet, she added, "it is the masculine values that prevail" (Woolf, 1929). Women are apt to succeed in the workplace when they use their womanly strengths of compassion and intuitiveness in their work, while playing by men's rules, using the suggestions in the following boxed list.

While harsh, a primer entitled *How to Swim with Sharks* (see the accompanying excerpt on pp. 551–552) is for the benefit of those who, by virtue of their occupation, find that they *must* swim *and* that the water is infested with sharks.

TIPS FOR WORKING WITH WOMEN CO-WORKERS
IN WORK SETTING

- Be friendly, but do not strive to be close friends.
- Be overt, not covert.
- If there's a problem, confront, forget, and move on.
- Communicate.
- Do not make scenes or public outbursts.
- Accept and love yourself.
- Accept (and appreciate) that some people are not your friends, now or ever.

HOW TO SWIM WITH SHARKS*

Swimming with sharks is like any other skill; it cannot be learned from books alone; the novice must practice in order to develop the skill. The following rules simply set forth the fundamental principles which, if followed, will make it possible to survive while becoming expert through practice.

Rule 1. *Assume unidentified fish are sharks.* Not all sharks look like sharks, and some fish which are not sharks sometimes act like sharks. Unless you have witnessed docile behavior in the presence of shed blood on more than one occasion, it is best to assume an unknown species is a shark.

Rule 2. *Do not bleed.* It is a cardinal principle that if you are injured, either by accident or by intent, you must not bleed. Experience shows that bleeding prompts an even more aggressive attack.

The control of bleeding has a positive protective element for the swimmer. The shark will be confused as to whether or not his attack has injured you, and confusion is to the swimmer's advantage. On the other hand, the shark may know he has injured you and be puzzled as to why you do not bleed or show distress. This also has a profound effect on sharks. They begin questioning their own potency or, alternatively, believe the swimmer to have supernatural powers.

Rule 3. *Counter any aggression promptly.* Sharks rarely attack a swimmer without warning. Usually there is some tentative, exploratory aggressive action. It is important that the swimmer recognizes that this behavior is a prelude to an attack and takes prompt and vigorous remedial action. The appropriate countermove is a sharp blow to the nose. Almost invariably this will prevent a full-scale attack, for it makes it clear that you understand the shark's intentions and are prepared to use whatever force is necessary to repel his aggressive actions.

Some swimmers mistakenly believe that an ingratiating attitude will dispel an attack under these circumstances. Those who hold this erroneous view can usually be identified by their missing limb.

Rule 4. *Get out if someone is bleeding.* If a swimmer (or shark) has been injured and is bleeding, get out of the water promptly. The presence of blood and the thrashing of water will elicit aggressive behavior even in the most docile of sharks. No useful purpose is served in attempting to rescue the injured swimmer. He either will or will not survive the attack, and your intervention cannot protect him once blood has been shed.

Rule 5. *Use anticipatory retaliation.* A constant danger to the skilled swimmer is that the sharks will forget that he is skilled and may attack in error. Some sharks have notoriously poor memories in this regard. This memory loss can be prevented by a program of anticipatory retaliation. The skilled swimmer should engage in these activities periodically, and the periods should be less than the memory span of the shark. Thus, it is not possible to state fixed intervals. The procedure may need to be repeated frequently with forgetful sharks and need be done only once for sharks with total recall.

The procedure is essentially the same as described under Rule 3—a sharp blow to the nose. Here, however, the blow is unexpected and serves to remind the shark that you are both alert and unafraid. Swimmers should take care not to injure the shark and draw blood during this exercise for two reasons: First, sharks often bleed profusely, and this leads to the chaotic situation described under Rule 4. Second, if swimmers act in this fashion it may not be possible to distinguish swimmers from sharks.

Rule 6. *Disorganize an organized attack.* Usually sharks are sufficiently self-centered that they do not act in concert against a swimmer. This

Continued

*The author, Voltaire Cousteau, died in 1812. He is thought to be a descendant of Francois Voltaire and an ancestor of Jacques Cousteau. The essay was originally written for sponge divers, but may have broader implications. It was translated from the French by Richard J. Johns, a French scholar and Massey Professor and Director of the Department of Biomedical Engineers, The Johns Hopkins University and Hospital, 720 Rutland Avenue, Baltimore MD 21205.

lack of organization greatly reduces the risk of swimming among sharks. However, upon occasion the sharks may launch a coordinated attack upon a swimmer or even upon one of their number.

The proper strategy is diversion. Sharks can be diverted from their organized attack in one of two ways. First, sharks as a group are especially prone to internal dissension. An experienced swimmer can divert an organized attack by introducing something, often something minor or trivial, which sets the sharks to fighting among themselves. Usually by the time the internal conflict is settled the sharks cannot even recall what they were setting about to do, much less get organized to do it.

A second mechanism of diversion is to introduce something which so enrages the members of the group that they begin to lash out in all directions, even attacking inanimate objects in their fury.

What should be introduced? Unfortunately, different things prompt internal dissension or blind fury in different groups of sharks. Here one must be experienced in dealing with a given group of sharks, for what enrages one group will pass unnoted by another.

It is unethical for a swimmer under attack by a group of sharks to counter the attack by diverting them to another swimmer. It is, however, common to see this done by novice swimmers and by sharks when they fall under a concerted attack.

ASSERTIVENESS

To be assertive is to be self-confident and to feel comfortable when presenting oneself and one's views to another (Clark, 1984). When women act assertively, they may be accused of being "aggressive," an attack on their use of actions that would not be viewed as negative were the same tactics employed by men. Women who have been taught that it is appropriate for men to be aggressive and women to be passive are hesitant to act assertively. The assertive person:

- takes an active rather than a passive orientation toward work
- works constructively and collaboratively
- is able to give and take criticism and assistance
- deals with anxiety and fear in order to continue to function effectively.

Assertiveness and aggressiveness are not the same thing, although many people think they are. The goal of aggressive behavior is to win. Unfortunately, the price of winning is not only negative feelings, such as humiliation and resentment, but a consequent sense of loss by all parties. This is particularly true when the original loser in an encounter attempts to get back at the aggressor through sarcasm, defiance, passive resistance, and other behavior which does not deal with the original behavior in a straightforward manner. Aggressive behavior is reactive; assertive behavior is initiating and enables the person to participate in active learning experiences. Ultimately, such active learning supports continued assertive behavior.

Assertiveness is neither manipulative, nor does it imply an uncaring attitude to people. When challenged, an assertive person is able to identify the strengths and limitations of that which she has proposed. She is able to say "I don't know" if she doesn't have an answer to a question. She does not become defensive or give up in the face of such a challenge. The dialogue shown in the following boxed scenario is an example of a situation in which all parties acted assertively. In this scenario, the positive elements included:

- avoiding personal attacks
- providing factual information
- asking for assistance and support in a straightforward manner.

In addition, each person displayed a willingness to work around other responsibilities in order to produce a solution (additional in-services). The discussion focused on the need for consistent information without accusing or humiliating any one staff member. The LC was not defensive when the nursing manager (NM) laughingly implied that she was

Problem to be Solved: Postpartum patients are becoming confused about breastfeeding because different staff members are providing conflicting information. The LC has asked for a meeting with the postpartum nursing manager (NM) to discuss the issue.

LC: I have observed some problems that are contributing to patient confusion about breastfeeding. [Factual statement.]

NM: What is that? [Asking for information.]

LC: Mrs. A, Mrs. B, and Ms. D were all told to give water instead of breastfeeding during the night shift, to nurse every two hours on the morning shift, and every three to four hours on the P.M. shift. [Additional information.]

NM: Do you know who gave them that information?

LC: The charts were signed by. . . . [Additional information; no accusations.]

NM: Do you want me to talk with them?

LC: That might be helpful. I was also wondering if we should schedule another group of in-services and go over the basic information all the patients need to hear. [Offers suggestion.]

NM: Will you take responsibility for setting it up?

LC: If you can tell me what the best times would be.

NM: (*Laughter*) Pushy, pushy. OK. Thursday is good.

LC (*Checking her calendar*): That's not good for me. I have several meetings that day. Can we schedule it next week?

NM (*Shutting her calendar forcefully*): That's not good. We'll have to put it off 'til next month.

LC: I'd really prefer that we get at this problem sooner. How about next week? [Focuses on the effect of the problem for them as a group.]

NM (*Opens her calendar again*): Wednesday looks good—if you can come in a bit early to get the night shift before they leave? I'll tell their unit leader to start reports earlier than usual.

LC (*Writes in times in her calendar*): Sure. Thanks so much. I knew you would help solve this problem.

"pushy." Had she done so, the discussion could have degenerated into a match of one-up-personship, which would have solved nothing. Assertive communication avoided antagonism, accusations, or a passive refusal. This encounter was a "win-win" situation for both the NM and the LC; they came to a joint agreement about the legitimacy of the problem and how best to attempt to resolve it.

ROLES AND RESPONSIBILITIES

The lactation consultant is responsible to the mothers she sees to provide up-to-date and accurate information and appropriate assistance (Marmet & Shell, 1990). In a medical center setting, however, such service will be molded by the other services also provided there.

Said one hospital-based lactation consultant:

When I started this [job], I went through culture shock. I had been a childbirth educator and had no experience on the postpartum floor. My impression was that I'd walk in the patient's room and help with breastfeeding. I didn't expect to walk in and find babies being fed with glucose water, supplemental formula and babies being discharged without weights. I expected to learn from the nursing staff, but they either did not know about breastfeeding or did not keep up. Somehow, I thought the staff nurses would already have the theory behind the practice, but they didn't, so I had to start from square one. I have in my mind ideas of how it should be up there on the floor; I need to know more about how to validate what I do.

This LC's shock is not an uncommon experience and reinforces the importance of in-servicing healthcare workers in the maternal-child area of the hospital. From such an experience, as well, come the seeds of burnout, if the lactation consultant does not have a support network of individuals who, like herself, are knowledgeable about lactation but who may work with many people who are not.

Staff in-services on breastfeeding increase the likelihood that the staff will give breastfeeding mothers consistent breastfeeding information. According to Cohen (1987), "the patient usually takes for granted that the person they spoke to knows exactly what should be done. If confusion or controversy is found among the staff, we cannot expect the patient to become knowledgeable and comfortable with learning mother-infant tasks."

While in-servicing is an important, perhaps even essential, role of the lactation consultant, like the proverbial horse brought to a watering hole, one can offer but not impel other health-care workers to drink from the pool of knowledge. One cause of the reluctance of others to avail themselves of formal or informal in-service opportunities is the dependence of other staff members on the LC to "take care of" all the breastfeeding issues. Those issues may involve highly complex problems requiring the teamwork of many individuals from an array of disciplines, or they may involve simply providing basic assistance in putting the baby on the breast and teaching basic breastfeeding information. Moreover, in a situation in which a lactation consultant is not available on all shifts or all days, this person cannot possibly always "be there." Rather than expecting her to "do it all," it is more effective for her to reach the staff so that all health-care workers are operating from the same frame of reference in how they assist breastfeeding mothers and when they will intervene to resolve a difficulty.

Another function of the lactation consultant—whether she is located in a hospital or has her own private practice—is to evaluate products related to lactation and to share her evaluations with others (Shrago, 1988). Evaluation of pumps and other technologies sometimes result in other benefits: assessment forms identify special needs of the new mother or her baby (Dodgson, 1989); and consent forms enable the breastfeeding mother to make a clear, informed choice (Kutner, 1986; Bull, 1986).

LCS AND VOLUNTARY COUNSELORS

The relationship between LCs and voluntary breastfeeding counselors has been discussed and debated. Gardiner et al. (1986) note that the client is apt to obtain more complete services when lactation consultants maintain a congenial, reciprocal relationship with volunteer counselors, as well as other health-care professionals in their community.

When the volunteer counselor and the LC work together, each contributes valuable skills toward the same end: a mother's positive breastfeeding experience and her baby's optimal start in life. (See Table 20–2.)

TABLE 20–2   WAYS IN WHICH THE VOLUNTEER COUNSELOR AND THE LC SUPPORT THE BREASTFEEDING MOTHER

	Volunteer Counselor	Lactation Consultant
Setting	Her home	Health-care clinic
	Mother's home	Hospital
		Doctor's office
		LC's office
		Mother's home
Communication	Telephone	Face-to-face
Timing of contact	Prenatally	Prenatally
	After hospital discharge	In hospital and after hospital discharge
Type of assistance	Lifestyle oriented	Problem-oriented
	Mother-to-mother	In-patient assistance
	Ongoing follow-up	Short-term
	Preventive	Episodic
Referral	To LC, M.D., other specialists	To volunteer, M.D., other specialists, including other LCs

Because the role of the lactation consultant is new, many other health providers are unclear about what to expect of this new allied health-care worker. If their experience has been with community-based voluntary breastfeeding counselors, they may assume that "lactation consultant" is simply a new title for a resource with which they may be familiar. To clarify areas of expertise which can be expected of such an individual, the International Lactation Consultant Association has developed a set of recommendations and related competencies for LC practice. (See Appendix F.)

In many ways, the volunteer counselor and the lactation consultant provide similar services. They most often differ about where such service is provided, the nature of clinical assistance, and the degree of follow-up care. For example, volunteer breastfeeding counselors are an excellent source of preventive health-care information pertaining to breastfeeding and lactation. They also spend more time giving long-term assistance than the lactation consultant, particularly if the latter sees clients in a clinic or hospital setting. It is not uncommon for a mother to continue to receive assistance and caring concern from a volunteer breastfeeding counselor through the entire lactation course; only rarely will a lactation consultant meet with a client regularly through that entire period. Instead, she is more apt to have sporadic contact, initiated by the client when a specific question or concern arises. However, the LC is more apt to have the experience to assist a mother when specific clinical skills are needed to assess or to resolve a problem. One recent report of mothers who sought assistance at a lactation clinic identified several factors, many related to breastfeeding initiation in hospital or early feeding practices, that may have contributed to the mothers' difficulties. Such findings can be highlighted in in-service presentations when hospital staff seek feedback regarding the recommendations they are offering or the practices they know to be routine (Mukasa, 1992).

Volunteer breastfeeding helpers and LCs can serve one another. The volunteer may have seen a certain mother in her own home and thus may be able to alert the LC working in a hospital, doctor's office, or clinic to elements about the mother's home life which may bear on her lactation course. The LC may serve as a referral source for persons with complex problems. When the LC works in a medical center, where ongoing research is part of her role, she helps generate new knowledge. Both the volunteer and the paid LC can review written materials for the clients. The volunteer may be sensitive to ongoing issues that crop up after the mother has left the hospital or does not choose to mention to her health-care providers. The LC may be aware of aspects of the health-care system that influence breastfeeding. At St. Joseph's Medical Center in Wichita, Kansas, for example, the LC and the LLL Area Professional Liaison leader have an ongoing professional relationship, and they share information and resources.

Unfortunately, these relationships are not always compatible. Perhaps because their roles overlap, some LCs and some voluntary breastfeeding counselors view the other as competitors rather than as partners with the same goals (Frantz, 1988). Phillips (1990a) notes that the new lactation consultant often expects understanding and moral support from the volunteer counselors with whom she initially worked; instead, she may encounter overt or covert resentment of her decision to take on a paid professional role after having learned much of her craft in an unpaid capacity. Instead of identifying with one another as related sources of assistance for the breastfeeding mother, both the volunteer and the paid breastfeeding specialist may choose not to work with one another, erecting barriers that only contribute to additional misunderstanding (Auerbach, 1989). As Phillips (1990a) points out, each would do well to remember what other health-care providers also often forget: "No one *owns* breastfeeding; except, properly, the mother/baby dyad."

MARKETING

Kotler (1984) defines marketing as a "discipline used by business to convert people's needs into profitable company opportunities." Marketing is still poorly understood and appreciated by nurses and LCs; either they need to learn marketing techniques themselves or seek assistance from marketing experts. Some nurse/entrepreneurs call upon the assistance of small business centers at state universities, which help small business people at no cost. Also, there are marketing books available, as well as classes at various educational institutions.

Following are several basic marketing techniques that LCs might find useful:

- Collect data (demographics, attitudes) on potential clients; a marketing research example that the LC might use as a guide is one compiled by Shamansky and colleagues (1985) about attitudes of consumers towards services of nurse practitioners.
- Analyze strengths and weaknesses of competitors and focus on service needs not currently being met.
- Establish a small niche within the health-care market that is ignored by large health-care providers (Hirsch, 1987; Tinari, 1986).
- Promote the practice by advertising and public relations: brochures, newsletters, letterhead stationery, business cards, fact sheets, and radio and TV interviews all help to inform clients and other health workers about the LC's services (Gardner & Weinrauch, 1988).

The independent health practitioner has a much greater chance to survive if she markets her specific skills to compete with other health-care professionals who are covered by health insurance. Later in this chapter we discuss what LCs themselves have to say about effective methods of marketing their services.

NETWORKING

Networking is an established mechanism used by members of groups to exchange information, to assist others, and to get help in solving problems (Harter et al., 1987). Although most people think first of networking with physicians and others from whom referrals will be sought, LCs also develop a system with other lactation consultants and with volunteer breastfeeding counselors—a "good ole girl" network. Most LCs network with one or two to as many as 10 or more LCs on a regular basis. Generally, these networking contacts are with LCs who work in a similar setting such as a hospital or in a private practice—or with LCs who belong to affiliate groups of the International Lactation Consultant Association (ILCA).

Networking serves several purposes. First, it offers an opportunity to learn from one another. When a difficult case arises, many LCs feel much more comfortable if they can pick up the phone and work through the situation with another lactation consultant. Additional assessment of the problem and/or how to begin moving toward a solution might offer new insights or creative alternatives to the plan of ac-

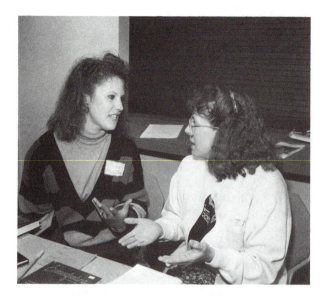

Figure 20–2 Making their "net" work for them, two LCs share experiences. (Courtesy of St. Joseph Medical Center, Wichita, KS.)

tion already considered. Networking also identifies job possibilities, colleagues who will cover for the LC when she is out of town, and referrals for clients needing equipment or specialized help. Networks may also be used to change systems and improve methods of providing care. Harter and colleagues (1987) describe how networking connected people with information and skills in a successful breastfeeding promotion project at Ohio State University.

REPORTING AND CHARTING

It is the responsibility of the lactation consultant, regardless of where she practices, to chart each contact with her clients and to provide complete reports to referring physicians and other health-care providers. Almost all record-keeping involves using a computer. Computer skills are rapidly becoming a necessity for health-care workers. As with other health providers, computers can be used to generate records, reports, and charts that:

- provide other health workers with valuable information
- reflect quality of care delivered (quality assurance and utilization review
- organize care

- highlight sometimes subtle observations or findings
- validate health services for insurance companies to determine reimbursement payment
- provide data that can be used for research
- serve as evidence in a legal dispute.

In the hospital, the mother's and infant's health record is a clinical record that contains information about the hospital stay and reports contact with everyone involved in their care. Because the mother and infant usually have separate charts, it is sometimes necessary to "double chart." At the same time, the care plans are geared to the mother, since it is she who is taught and the baby who is the recipient of her learning.

NURSING DIAGNOSIS

Nursing diagnosis is a way to identify and describe problems and concerns related to breastfeeding. Nursing diagnoses validate special skills and experience, pave the way for third-party reimbursement for client care, and enhance professional autonomy. Medical diagnoses are based upon disease groupings while nursing diagnoses are based upon how the problem affects the daily life of a person; thus, a nursing diagnosis is more appropriate to use for breastfeeding (Orlando, 1991).

The term *nursing diagnosis* began being used in the 1950s. The First National Conference on the Classification of Nursing Diagnosis was held in 1973; at that time a list of 34 diagnoses was developed. Since then, the concept has been tested, expanded, and refined. The definition of nursing diagnosis is "a clinical judgement about an individual, family, or community response to actual or potential problems or life processes that is derived through a systematic process of data collection and analysis, and provides the basis for prescription for definitive therapy for which the nurse is accountable" (Shoemaker, 1984).

The purposes of nursing diagnoses identified by the Organization for Obstetric, Gynecologic and Neonatal Nurses (NAACOG) are to clarify the focus of the care plan, define accountability, define the independent aspect of nursing practice, facilitate third-party reimbursement, and facilitate research (NAACOG, 1989).

In the late 1980s, The Department of Parent and Child Nursing at the University of Washington in Seattle, with a grant from Sigma Theta Tau, undertook the task of developing nursing diagnoses related to breastfeeding. The first breastfeeding diagnosis, Ineffective Breastfeeding, was accepted by the North American Nursing Diagnoses Association (NANDA) in 1987. Three years later in 1990, NANDA met in Orlando, Florida, and adopted the nursing diagnosis, Effective Breastfeeding (see Appendix C at the end of this book). Gorrie (1989) suggests other nursing diagnoses that may relate to breastfeeding/lactation:

- Alteration in comfort
- Alteration in nutrition (less than body requirements)
- Anxiety
- Disturbance in self-concept
- Knowledge deficit
- Potential for infection

METHODS OF CHARTING

The most commonly used methods of charting are narrative charting and problem-oriented charting. Flow sheets and standard care plans that are individualized are becoming more popular. They reduce paper work and save time (and money).

Narrative charting. Narrative documentation uses a diary or story format to document client-care events. It is a simple paragraph that describes the client's status and the care that was given. Narrative notes, sometimes called progress notes, are used less now with the advent of flow sheets and clinical care plans, which capture the routine aspects of care. Narrative notes can be easily combined with flow sheets or any other client record.

An example of a narrative note:

Date	Time	Progress note
6/11/91	0730	Alert, oriented, and in good spirits. Infant latches on breast effectively. Baby breastfed for 15 minutes until asleep.

Problem-oriented charting (POMA). Charting based on a problem uses a structured problem list and logical format for each entry in the medical record. The format used in problem-oriented charting is called the SOAP or SOAPIE method. Each letter stands for a different phase of the nursing process: Assessment (using subjective, objective data), plan,

---

PROBLEM-ORIENTED MEDICAL RECORD-KEEPING

S = Subjective data. What the mother herself tells you. *Example:* "My nipples feel sore." (Note: If the charting relates to only the infant, there will be no subjective data.)

O = Objective data. Concrete data you can observe. *Examples:* infant position at breast, temperature, infant weight.

A = Assessment and nursing diagnosis. An assessment of physical and psychosocial factors based upon subjective and objective data; what you think is going on. *Examples:* Infant not positioned well on the breast; breastfeeding at margin of nipple. **Nursing diagnosis:** Ineffective breastfeeding. An alternative is ineffective suckling.

P = Plan. Organized plan for care. Based upon the assessment, what you plan to do about the problem to help the breastfeeding mother and baby. *Example:* Will reposition infant on breast at next feeding.

I = Interventions. What you've done to/for the problem or what you plan to do. Includes teaching, referrals, finding the right pump. *Example:* Infant repositioned on mother's breast so that adequate breast tissue is being grasped by infant during suckling.

E = Evaluation. Review of outcomes. What happened? Was it effective? *Examples:* Infant appears to be suckling effectively at the breast. Baby breastfed four times during shift, three times following repositioning. Infant had bowel during feeding—appears well hydrated. In some cases in which a nursing care plan with diagnoses is used, evaluation may reflect only the presenting problem. Outcomes are then charted in the flow sheet.

---

interventions, and evaluation of care. (See the boxed list above which explains the codes.)

For the independent contractor, the completeness of reports also assists the referring health-care worker to understand the "how's" as well as the "why's" of a lactation consultant's practice and methods. Reporting provides a data base for all types of helpful information—for example, an increase in the number of referrals from a particular physician's practice. Early referrals might be for one or two common problems, while tracking over a time period may show that later referrals are for a wider variety of problems.

CLINICAL CARE PLANS

The purpose of a clinical care plan is to provide basic information about client assessment, diagnosis, and planned interventions. It also provides a guide for care, establishes a continuity of care, and provides a means of communication among all care-givers. There are two types of care plans: individual and standard. Individual care plans are developed "from scratch" for each client based on her specific needs.

A standard care plan is a preprinted plan of care* for a group of patients within the same DRG**or nursing diagnosis. Because each standard care plan must be tailored according to the needs of a particular client, they are designed to include space for adding information.

The Joint Commission on Accreditation of Healthcare Organizations (JCAHO) requires a care plan for each patient in the hospital as a requirement for accreditation; however, the plan of care can now be computer generated, preprinted, or appear in progress notes or standards of care (ANA, 1991a). Care plans are legal requirements of practice and may also serve as protocols and/or standards of care.

Traditionally, individual care plans are divided into three or four columns. The names of these columns change over the years to reflect new ideas in nursing, and some column labels are preferred over others. In this book, for instance, we have labeled

*Samples of clinical records that relate to lactation/breastfeeding are found in the *Lactation Consultant Series* (see especially Units 3 and 8), the *Journal of Human Lactation,* and lactation forms available from the Lactation Institute, 16161 Ventura Blvd., Suite 223, Encino, CA 91436.
**Diagnosis-related groups. See glossary in the accompanying study guide for other terminologies.

the clinical care plans with "assessment/interventions/rationale." Other commonly used labels are "problems/nursing goals/evaluation," "nursing diagnosis/patient outcomes/nursing action," or simply "intervention/evaluation." The critical care path is a new type of care plan used in hospitals. These "paths" are abbreviated care plans that focus on the client's length of stay in the hospital. A sample of one of these care plans is seen in Appendix K.

LEGAL CONSIDERATIONS

Whenever an LC offers advice or touches a mother or baby in the course of her evaluation of the breastfeeding course, she is risking a potential legal action. The kind of action that is most likely to be brought includes battery (when a client does not consent to be touched by another person); breach of warranty (meaning that a promise to provide a service—written or verbal—is not provided); or the infliction of emotional distress (usually through a reckless, intentional, or negligent act which results in a negative outcome, such as bodily harm of some kind) (Bornmann, 1986). People usually decide to sue health-care workers because they are angry at them; therefore, the most effective protection against such actions is establishing a mutually respectful relationship and rapport between client and helping professional. The LC's pattern of practice should include the following:

1. *Obtain permission—at least verbal, but preferably written—before touching the client or her infant.* Keep in mind that in different cultures, how one touches a baby may be important. For example, in Muslim cultures, use of the left hand to do a digital assessment of the baby's mouth is a highly offensive action and would be greatly resented by the mother. One way to avoid inadvertently offending a client is to ask if the baby may be touched—and to explain how the baby will be touched before doing so. In other settings, a female LC may easily obtain permission to touch another woman's breasts while assisting with breastfeeding.
2. *Make no promise or guarantee that will not be provided.* If the LC says she will make a home visit, such a visit should be provided. Generally, breach of warranty is raised as an actionable offense when one party guarantees a particular

outcome and that outcome is not forthcoming. The wise LC does not guarantee that the baby will be nursing fully on the breast, without needing other nutriment, within a specified number of breastfeeding episodes, hours, days, or weeks. Because each mother and baby is unique, as is their breastfeeding relationship, it is generally not possible to guarantee an outcome for one such couple based on the outcome of another pair. While similarities exist among mother-baby pairs, the LC should confine her comments to encouragement—without providing a guarantee, particularly one involving a specific time period or similar frame of reference.
3. *Avoid causing the mother, the baby, or any other member of the client's family emotional distress.* This might come about as a result of words said, reports written, or other actions that reflect the LC's relationship with the mother and baby. Judicious choice of words and actions is usually sufficient to avoid this problem.
4. *Maintain confidentiality about the mother, baby, and family.* To fail to do so is an invasion of privacy, a tort which involves confidential information that is revealed without permission to someone not entitled to know it.

A clearly written, detailed record of the health provider's actions, initial recommendations, and follow-up assistance (by phone and in person) is one of the most effective ways of avoiding legal action. Referrals increase following a well-written, complete report which was sent in a timely and professional manner. Client records are considered business records of the agency and are admissible as such under rules of evidence. Records will often prevent cases from going to court; lawsuits often are won and lost based on what is in the record. Although testimony is another form of evidence, the written health chart is viewed as more accurate and reliable.

LIABILITY COVERAGE
The LC who works in a doctor's office, clinic, or hospital is very apt to be part of the staff who are covered in an "umbrella" professional liability policy. The LC in private practice must determine for herself how much coverage she needs and what she can afford.

It is the rare LC in private practice who "goes bare" when she works in a country where litigation is a frequent occurrence. While legal action against an LC has not yet been reported, it can occur; therefore, every individual practitioner needs to consider how she will protect herself and her family against a judgment that could ruin her financially.

REIMBURSEMENTS

Physicians and hospitals are major providers recognized by third-party payers. Third party payers can be divided into three categories: private health insurance companies, such as Blue Cross/Blue Shield; government or public health insurance; and independent health plans, such as health maintenance organizations (HMOs). Reimbursement to the health-care provider can be either direct or indirect. Indirect payment involves billing by or through a health agency or physician. Major barriers to third-party reimbursement for nonphysician health-care workers are third-party payers who fear expansion of provider eligibility, state licensure laws, difficulties in procedures, and opposition by the medical profession (Caraher, 1988). More than 80% of Americans are covered by private insurance.

Insurance policies usually spell out by title who may be reimbursed. Payment to nurses and allied health workers is usually only by a physician's referral. Unfortunately, lactation consulting, as a profession, has not yet gained this official recognition. The possibility of coverage can be checked by calling the customer-service number of the client's insurance company. It is not necessary to have a special form to submit a claim for third-party reimbursement, as long as the insurance company has access to all the information. A special claim form, the so-called "lactation super-bill," developed at UCLA, may be helpful because it already lists procedure code numbers relating to breastfeeding; thus, it saves time and effort.*

In private practice, the easiest way to handle payment for services rendered or for equipment is to request payment from the client at the time of the service. The client, in turn, then requests reimbursement from her insurance company, providing the third-party payer with the needed information. If breastfeeding assistance is given as a part of routine home health care or as a postpartum visit, the employing agency usually requests the third-party reimbursement.

As of January, 1991, health services delivered by nurse practitioners and clinical nurse specialists (including certified nurse midwives) in rural areas can be directly reimbursed under the Medicare program. Rural areas are defined as nonmetropolitan statistical areas; this is the same definition used to distinguish rural hospitals for the Medicare program (ANA, 1991b).

PRIVATE PRACTICE

Inspired by the DRG revolution, nurses, LCs, and other health-care providers are developing private practices and home health-care alternatives to meet the demand of a population needing more care outside of the hospital setting (NAACOG, 1988; NAACOG, 1991; AJN, 1990). Many women and babies do not receive the extended care, perinatal education, and emotional support they need and deserve. Independent contracting helps fill this gap in health care. Nurses and LCs in private practices not only solve problems but also prevent problems; in at least one thriving nurse-run enterprise, a staff member makes a home visit the first full day the mother is home from the hospital (AJN, 1990).

Lactation consultants set up and operate practices in various ways. One of the authors of this chapter interviewed 13 lactation consultants who are in private practice in order to gain in-depth information about their experiences. These LCs serve the working classes as well as the affluent, and represent a variety of settings: rural, suburban, medium to large cities, and major metropolitan areas all across the United States—the Atlantic and Pacific coasts, the South, northern states and the Midwest. Some of the LCs have been in practice longer than 10 years; others for only a short time.

Nearly one-half of these LCs were La Leche League Leaders for five or more years, and nine were registered nurses. Three had educational backgrounds significantly removed from nursing or lactation; one has neither breastfed nor experienced motherhood. Almost all were IBCLC certified. Everyone with this credential reported that it has served them well in establishing their credibility as knowledgeable specialists in the field of lactation. One LC reported, "In the early

---

*"Lactation super-bills" may be ordered from UCLA Lactation Alumni, 2021 Grismer, #38, Burbank, CA 91504.

days, [other people] laughed. "Who needs credentials to help with *breastfeeding*?!' Now the local hospitals will only hire lactation consultants who are certified (IBCLC). It has become more important."

While all of these LCs began their practices with offices in their homes, two now maintain office space in commercial settings. Some of these women work as solo practitioners; others have one or more partners. Some of these partnerships serve the same client population; in other cases, the sharing is restricted to covering for a colleague when one of the partners is out of town.

In spite of differences in background and length of practice, the commonalities in their practices outweigh the differences. We describe their practices and concerns in order to assist those health-care workers who are weighing the decision to establish a private practice with a specialization in lactation.

WHY GO INTO PRIVATE PRACTICE?

The impetus for hanging up a shingle and going into private practice is recognizing that there is a need. One LC began her LC work by opening a breast pump rental depot. Another set up a private practice after receiving numerous calls from mothers who needed help with breastfeeding. This LC recognized a need for home health-care services that went beyond the limitations inherent in phone counseling and doctor visits. She said, "There was no need for [the mother] to go to a germ-ridden office and wait for an hour or more for the doctor to shrug his shoulders and say, 'I guess you could put the baby on formula,' in answer to her questions about breastfeeding." Several LCs who had been hospital nurses wanted to do more to help breastfeeding mothers than could be accomplished in the hospital and so decided to provide home health-care services. Some LCs in private practice see nearly all their clients in the mother's home rather than in an office. Still others found that a private practice in lactation consulting was a "natural" extension of their previous work as volunteer LLL leaders. Many of these women noted that phone assistance carried their clients only so far, and that a gap of services existed between hospital discharge and the first well-baby check-up. For one LC, the poor quality of the local hospital's breast pump rental service motivated her to set up a pump rental depot, out of which developed a full-service practice (see Fig. 20–3). More than one-half

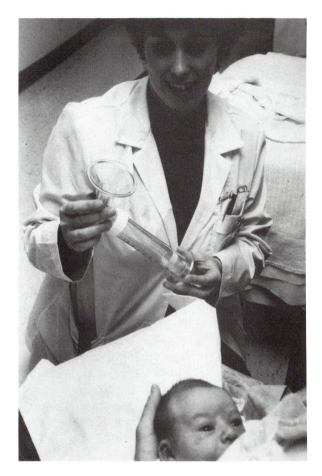

FIGURE 20–3 Lactation consulting sometimes requires knowing how to teach appropriate use of a breast pump.

of the LCs rent or sell breast pumps. The number of breast pumps carried ranges from three to more than 100. In some cases, breast pump rental income represents a substantial percentage of their income.

Many LCs mentioned the lack of correct information—or the existence of much *mis*information—as factors in their decision to offer what they considered an appropriate and needed service for the women in their communities. Finally, those women with growing children at home found that a lactation consultant practice—particularly when it was conducted out of the LC's home—offered an ideal alternative to the need for income and meeting family needs.

SETTING UP THE PRACTICE

Most of the LCs interviewed recommended that the practice should be located in a convenient place, such as her own home, if a room could be devoted exclusively to her practice. Such a space carries with it a minimum of overhead and financial outlay; however, the U.S. Internal Revenue Service *will not* allow a tax deduction on this space (including utilities, rent/mortgage, and cleaning fees) unless the room is used only for business. Seeing clients in the living room, storing files in the bedroom closet, and keeping breast pumps in the basement does not a home business make—at least in the eyes of the IRS.

If the lactation consultant is thinking of opening a practice in her home, she also needs to think about a private entrance. While most LCs in the survey group did not have a private entrance to their office, more than one LC recommended it. (Transforming an enclosed porch into an office with its own entrance might be a possibility.) The costs of such a transformation may, in some cases, represent nearly as large a financial investment as the rental of a commercial space for several months. If the LC plans to take out a business loan, the cost of renting commercial space needs to be a factor in determining the size of the loan. One LC who still dreams of a practice location outside her home said: "If I had to do it over again, I would bite the bullet and go for commercial property right from the beginning. I think it reflects on one's professionalism. I am still being confused with my La Leche League friends who offer free help out of their homes." Another LC, with an office in a commercial setting, noted that physicians and others viewed her as a professional much more than was the case when her office was in her home; her business has grown since she moved out of her home.

The best beginning location is space in a clinic, physician's office, or hospital where the LC receives referrals from the staff members of these organizations. A location that is easy to find and reach is another factor if clients are to frequent the LC in private practice. To prove this point, both of the LCs who maintain offices in commercial properties are located on a major traffic street with convenient parking. Inadequate road signs in suburban settings and/or in rural areas make maps on the backs of flyers and other advertisements a necessity.

"While there is something to be said for independence, there are pros and cons of private practice." Another LC echoed this sentiment: "A disadvantage is an uncertain income, whereas being an employee guarantees you a base salary. One aspect of the LC business is that it is never the same from day to day, to say nothing

---

ADVANTAGES AND DISADVANTAGES OF INCORPORATION

Advantages

- Life of the business is perpetual.
- Stockholders have a limited liability.
- Ownership transfer is easy.
- It is easy to raise capital and expand.
- Efficiency of management is maintained.
- The corporation is a legal entity.
- Possible tax advantages may be found.
- A corporation is adaptable to both small and large businesses.
- Other professionals may view the corporation as a sign that the business *is* a business rather than a "toy."

Disadvantages

- It is closely regulated; subject to many state and federal controls.
- It is more difficult and more expensive to organize.
- The corporate charter restricts the type of business activity one engages in.
- Extensive record-keeping is necessary.
- Double taxation may apply.

---

of from month to month. Some weeks, I'm starving; other weeks, I'm drowning in business!" The commitment of the clientele is another important consideration in job satisfaction. As one LC bluntly put it: "If you are working in private practice or with a physician's office, you will be working with patients who have already decided to breastfeed. This is much less likely in the hospital; there is something to be said for not having to beat your head against the wall every day working with mothers who say they will 'try' and then don't even do that."

THE BUSINESS OF DOING BUSINESS

One of the hardest lessons for a new LC to learn is that a private practice is a business; if she has no business experience, she must learn about it. Advertising is essential in establishing and/or maintaining a client pool. Generally, the best advertising is word-of-mouth referral from clients who are satisfied with the LC's services. Other successful advertising includes distributing flyers and sending personal letters to hospital staff, local physicians (pediatricians, family physicians, obstetricians), community women's groups, childbirth educators, and La Leche League leaders. Teaching a prenatal breastfeeding class is a form of advertising. At the same time, the LC has to be careful not to offer unlimited access to class members for later assistance and to make it clear that she charges for later visits.

Lactation consultants disagree about whether to advertise in local newspapers or on the radio. Several people said that such visibility "attracts the crazies." Others felt that regional newspapers, or those focused and distributed to a particular market— such as new parents—were an appropriate forum. However, most felt that advertising was far more costly than it was effective. One lactation consultant remarked that "newspaper articles, radio, or television interviews may provide name recognition, but they rarely result in generating clients."

The choice of words in advertisements or signs should be considered carefully. In one case, an LC posted a large sign with her name, but *not* the word 'breast' or 'lactation,' to alert passersby to her business. Said she: "The sign advertising your service must fit the place where you work. In my commu-

nity, it would not be wise for me to advertise my services using the word 'breast.' I chose the name of my practice very carefully with this in mind." Using 'family'- or 'mother'-related phrases works well in lieu of more obvious words. In other communities, inclusion of the words "breastfeeding" or "breast" may not be controversial.

More effective marketing techniques include meeting face-to-face with local physicians, their office staff, and hospital nurse managers, as well as attending professional meetings, such as hospital grand rounds or continuing education programs for nurses. See the boxed guidelines below for ways to generate referrals.

Incorporating the private practice should be considered only after carefully reviewing the advantages and disadvantages. (See the boxed checklist on p. 566.) A list of resources which apply to incorporation and other business considerations of private practice is included in the bibliography at the end of this chapter.

Lactation consultants—as do most women professionals—harbor a strong streak of idealism. While they may need to run their business *as a business,* all who were interviewed said that they have, on occasion, refrained from charging a client for their services when it was clear that the client could not pay. In every case, the LC provided the services in a spirit

---

Ways to Generate Referrals

Method	Target Audience
Teach a prenatal breastfeeding class	Mothers
One-on-one contacts	Physicians
	Hospital nurses
	Perinatal educators
	Postpartum/nursery managers
	Physicians' office nurses
A flyer describing the LC service	Anyone who is unfamiliar with what an LC does
Contacts with community groups geared to new, inexperienced mothers	Future referral sources
Informal relationships with physicians (or their spouses) who have had new babies and want to breastfeed	A satisfied customer is often the best advertisement
Providing pump rentals; use the free advertising often provided by the company	Such referrals may generate other nonpump business
Displays at baby fairs, community activities	The community unfamiliar with the services of an LC

of goodwill, either forgoing even writing a bill or writing it off after the client left. Some LCs have established an informal sliding scale to assist people for whom a total payment at the time of service is not possible. One LC noted that she has received payment as much as 18 months after the service was provided; others reported that only rarely are their bills not paid. Most people prefer to pay something rather than nothing; even when clients pay a very small amount for the care they receive, they are more inclined to follow through with the suggestions the LC has offered.

The amount of money LCs make varies around the country; it reflects the economy of each region and the location of the practice within that region. The average length of time LCs are in business before they are no longer putting their profits back into the practice is three years. In some cases, LCs make a profit within two years. The higher the overhead, the longer it takes before earnings exceed the costs of doing business. Another factor is "how hard you want to work." One LC noted that she would have been earning a profit sooner had she not limited the number of clients she sees: "My family's needs still come first with me. When the children are older, I will spend more time with my practice, and my income will reflect this."

Another aspect of doing business is setting fees. This issue seems to generate the greatest concern when lactation consultants first go into practice. Anxiety about how much to charge for their services may stem from having been a volunteer breastfeeding support person for many years and coming to value the helping relationships with the mothers— without thinking of charging for the service. This problem is not confined to LCs. Unlike men, women, in general, are reluctant to charge what their services are worth. This undervaluing of skills or services is part of a woman's socialization when she is growing up. In addition, lack of familiarity with running a business results in undervaluing the service provided.

The prospective private practice LC needs to set her fees based on having learned what other comparable professionals in her community are charging for similar services (e.g., other LCs in private practice, nurses who make home health visits, and pediatricians who make house calls). Other factors to consider in setting fees are the length of visits. Most LCs reported that while well-baby visits to a physician's office may last only 15 to 20 minutes, the usual first LC visit may run 60 to 90 minutes. Such a time differential needs to be taken into account. If the visits take place in the mother's home, travel time is included: one lactation consultant adds one hour to account for travel time to and from the client's home when she bills the visit.

Nearly all of the LCs surveyed have raised their fees since first going into business, which helps to keep the number of clients to a reasonable level. One sees clients on Saturdays at the same rate that she sees them during the rest of the week; however, a Sunday visit is charged at double the usual rate. This practice has resulted in a marked reduction in the number of clients seen on Sunday–not because the LC has refused to do so, but rather because clients choose not to spend the extra money.

While the lactation consultant should feel that she is being sufficiently reimbursed for her services, she must also feel comfortable that what she is charging is reasonable. She needs to assess what the market will bear. A rural community may require a lower fee schedule than an affluent bedroom community. The type of service may also vary. In some settings, exclusive home visiting may be the route to take in offering lactation services. In other places, a home office or an office setting elsewhere may be more acceptable to clients.

Phone consultations also need to be considered when establishing a fee structure. Some LCs provide "professional courtesy" for all other LCs and for volunteer breastfeeding helpers such as La Leche League leaders; they bill all other clients. LCs bill differently for phone consultations. Some bill for a specific amount of time within a set framework, such as up to one hour of calls within a week after the first visit. Others bill for each call separately. Still others provide free phone consultation for minor issues. For all other assistance, the client is asked to come in for an office visit or to consent to a home visit, for which the charge for that service is billed.

CONTACT WITH OTHER HEALTH-CARE WORKERS

LCs are most successful when they have an ongoing, comfortable relationship with physicians and nurses in the community who refer clients to them. The physicians may also act as mentors and are invaluable in helping the LC to understand the medical problems occurring in breastfeeding families.

Lactation consultants nearly always maintain informal arrangements with individual physicians or clinics. In some cases, the physicians' offices serve as a point of distribution for an LC's flyers or business cards. In other cases, office staff give this information to the physician's patients. Other referral sites are midwifery practices and obstetrics/gynecology offices—where LCs may teach prenatal breastfeeding classes. Relationships with physicians have established rules: one is that if a baby is thought to have a medical problem, before proceeding with lactation assistance, the LC refers the family to their baby's own pediatrician or family physician. One lactation consultant cautioned, "Never take responsibility that is beyond your expertise. Always counsel mothers to go back to their doctor to resolve a medical problem."

If the family does not have an attending physician, the lactation consultant has the responsibility of referring them to a reputable physician who is knowledgeable about breastfeeding. Some lactation consultants require that the baby be under a physician's care before they will offer their services. Such a plan of action assures that the case documentation has a place to go after the LC has seen the mother and baby—and that any medical problems are brought to the attention of the person most likely to provide medical care. It also offers a measure of legal protection for the LC against a charge that she is practicing medicine without a license. The referral is usually to a physician with whom the LC has a collaborative, trusting relationship. Said one LC: "I'm not a doctor and I'm not interested in being a doctor. I market myself as a breastfeeding management consultant, working with mother and baby and how they go together. Most problems I see aren't medical. I refer her back to her doctor or her baby's doctor if I spot something that is beyond my expertise to handle." Another LC reported that the next most frequent referral, after the pediatrician, is to a psychologist or psychiatrist who specializes in helping women with postpartum depression. She also encourages every private practice LC to know about local crisis hotlines in her community and to be prepared to refer women to them.

Essential to developing a professional reputation and high ethical standards is sending a written report to the referring physician and/or calling the physician after the patient has been seen. Referrals increase following a well-written, complete report that was sent in a timely and professional manner. Reported one lactation consultant: "Some physicians still think I'm one step above a witch doctor and on a par with a used-car salesman. My documentation of *every* mother and baby from their practice that I have seen has helped them to see that breastfeeding is more than slapping a baby on a breast and going on to the next case."

Being a professional requires that the lactation consultant present herself professionally—in her demeanor, the clothing she wears, the reports she writes, and the phone calls she makes. The professional LC knows her potential client population and how the professional system works in her area. "Don't go barging in there expecting to change things instantaneously," warned one LC. "Otherwise, you will speak to brick walls. When you offer services, do it professionally. Do what you do well; that establishes your reputation. The referrals will follow." Another lactation consultant urged:

> Be courteous; expect to learn something from them. Many people don't realize that what we do takes training and experience and that it is a profession. Approach them with the same respect you expect from them. While we can assume that they don't know as much as we do about lactation and breastfeeding, we can't let them know that we are assuming that!

HOSPITAL PRIVILEGES

The majority of the LCs interviewed did not have hospital privileges. This pattern appeared to be unrelated to whether they were licensed in some other health-care field, such as nursing. One LC did note that legal restrictions in her state mean that if she is asked to see a mother in the hospital by a referring physician, she can do so. However, she is limited to visiting and talking; she may not provide hands-on care. Of those who did have hospital privileges, one reported applying for them at one hospital in her community and being offered privileges in a competing hospital. She is classified, for purposes of seeing patients in the hospital, as an allied health professional. In another case, the LC has privileges that enable her to see patients who are part of the patient pool from a physicians' group practice with whom she is affiliated. This arrangement was not automatic, but required review by the hospital committees governing the issuance of hospital privileges.

Several LCs reported not wanting hospital privileges. While they recognized the value of very early teaching and intervention, the short length of stay minimizes most negative experiences in the hospital. They prefer to limit their work to their own office or to the mother's home.

PROBLEMS IN PRIVATE PRACTICE

A private lactation consulting practice is for pioneers, not for the faint of heart. There are a multitude of frustrations. The problem that is least likely to be solved in the short-term pertains to *misinformation and/or lack of education about the lactation process or breastfeeding behavior.* Both mothers and doctors were mentioned when these LCs were asked who was misinformed and lacked education. One LC remarked that until breastfeeding and bottle-feeding are no longer viewed as equivalent,

mothers are still going to think that breastmilk substitutes are adequate—"like mother's milk in a can; maybe not quite as good as the real thing, but almost as good." Additionally, she noted that most healthcare workers are not trained to know what kinds of questions to ask mothers; therefore, they are not in a position to provide appropriate help. One result is "16 different nurses giving 16 different suggestions. We need much more anticipatory guidance if mothers are to really get the kind of help they need before little problems become too big to handle without weaning." Still another LC noted that she is increasingly frustrated with poor advice from staff at physicians' practices in her community: "Even when mothers share what really worked—after the doctor's advice it suddenly didn't!—it's like the information goes in one ear and out the other. This is very frustrating."

Another difficulty is related to the timing of referrals:

SOLO PRACTICE VS. PARTNERSHIPS: ADVANTAGES AND DISADVANTAGES

Solo Practice

Advantages
- It is simple to organize.
- Start-up costs are low.
- Relative freedom from regulation.
- Owner is in direct control.
- Owner is free to make all decisions.
- Minimal working capital requirements.
- Legal restrictions.
- Tax advantages may apply to the small business owner.
- All profits go to the owner.
- The business is easy to dissolve.

Disadvantages
- Liability is unlimited.
- Must arrange for coverage when out-of-town.
- Skills are limited to those of the solo practitioner.
- It may be difficult to raise capital.

Partnerships

Advantages
- Easy to organize.
- Start-up costs may be low.
- Greater financial strength.
- Broader management base.
- Additional sources of venture capital.
- Provides combined managerial skills and judgments.
- A legally recognized business entity.
- Each partner has an interest in the business.
- Possible tax advantages.
- Limited outside regulation.
- Each partner can take time-off without closing the business.
- Networking is ongoing.

Disadvantages
- Unlimited liability.
- Lack of authority.
- Authority for decisions.
- Difficulty in raising additional capital.
- Finding a suitable partner may be difficult.
- Disagreements about work load, responsibility, income.
- Time-off activities must be coordinated.

Derived in part from Janet N. Repucci and Jacki R. Shina, Cofounders, Galatea Lactation Consultants, 1989.

"Most of the physicians in my area refer on the 11th hour of the 11th day. By the time I see the mother, I often end up picking up the pieces—if I'm able—or simply holding the mother's hand while she expresses regret about having 'failed.' She has not failed; we have failed her. There are times when I think you have to have the patience of Job to be an LC." Yet one LC cautioned: "Be careful of inadvertently sounding disgusted when the mother reports that the pediatrician gave some really bad or stupid advice."

Lack of time. Time management was a major problem: many LCs mentioned their frustration in attempting to juggle family and work needs; 'day' job and private practice demands; travel time between office and client; and scheduling each day as efficiently as possible. Related to this was the *paperwork* that such a business requires. Often, LCs mentioned that the time it took to generate referral letters seemed out of proportion to their effect on the referring physician's awareness of lactation issues. One LC uses a dictating service to get out from under the time constraints of such work. Others are considering such a service, having determined that the cost of the service will be more than made up in the time saved.

Lack of profits. This is related to the inconsistent nature of the LC business and to the fact that—especially in practices less than five years old—cash flow tends to move money out the door rather than into the cashbox! Sometimes low profits reflect a prevailing opinion that help for breastfeeding should be free. Several LCs suggested that this attitude stemmed from mothers' previous contact with volunteer breastfeeding support groups; others suggested that it reflects a prevailing belief that breastfeeding simply is not so important that advice pertaining to it should have a price tag.

Partnerships. Partnerships vary in how they are structured. In some cases, each partner sees all clients, and income that is generated is shared equally. In other practices, each partner maintains her own client group. Covering for a partner when the other's duties take precedence or the LC is out of town is automatic—as long as the partner is available. Going into a partnership requires that each LC be clear about what she wants from the arrangement at the outset. Complementary ways of working is a

plus; it is not necessary for each partner to be a "clone" of the other. However, when very different philosophies exist about how to provide client services, conflicts are more likely to arise that cannot be resolved. Like a marriage, a partnership has its high and low points, and several LCs reported that conflict between partners was particularly difficult: "Getting a partner doesn't always solve problems. Sometimes, partners can simply create a whole new set of problems." (See the boxed checklist on p. 566.)

Burnout. Failure to control an increase in demand for services can lead to burnout. While restructuring work can guard against burnout, the LC may need to sit down with someone who has a sympathetic and objective ear and make decisions about how many clients she can comfortably handle in a given space of time—and refuse to take on more. In some cases, LCs reported that changes in the needs of their own families often contributed to a sense of running in place even while the work piled up. Yet one LC noted: "But, children do grow up and things do get easier. Some doctors *have* changed; they refer earlier now. This has made my job easier: I have fewer situations where I'm 'picking up the pieces,' and more where I can help the mother work toward a more positive outcome."

Since advertising influences growth, one LC suggested limiting advertising in order to be able to handle the influx of patients that advertising generates: "Be realistic about the time you have to give and your other responsibilities and commitments. Don't expect too much; there is no way to know how quickly your practice will build."

Going slowly reduces burnout: "Don't feel like you are the breastfeeding 'goddess' of the community, the only one who can make or break a particular situation. Empower the mother and let her take over her experience. Burnout comes from trying to 'own' the situation." Advised another: "Lay the groundwork of your practice with an eye to the future. Try not to grow too quickly without realizing the implications, and complete the [paperwork] before you deposit the check."

One book to consider reading and then applying judiciously is *Office at Home* (Scott, 1987)—if that is the location of the LC's office. One LC advised: "Remember that the hours of an LC practice tend not to be limited to 9 to 5 Monday through Friday. How is this going to affect your personal life? You may be working on holidays, weekends, in the evening. And don't forget the need to provide coverage when you are going to be away." Another LC warned: "Be aware of the value of your service; don't give it away for free to those who can afford it."

Still other LCs have attempted to reduce the risk of burnout by going into partnership with one or more LCs or by limiting their practice to a specialized area. They refer some cases to nearby lactation consultants who, in turn, refer more complicated cases to the LC who has chosen to specialize.

Given the difficulties mentioned above, what do these lactation consultants advise others regarding pitfalls? Nearly all the LCs, in one way or another, urged tempering enthusiasm with an acceptance of reality and being willing to accept very slow change. One LC noted that after several years, her state now has a breastfeeding task force which meets regularly: "This snail is jogging. You have to be happy with tiny incremental improvements." Avoiding being thought of as radical was also mentioned. To illustrate her point, one LC said: "Don't use cabbage leaves to reduce engorgement on someone you've never seen before—even when you know it has worked for other mothers in similar circumstances."

THE BOTTOM LINE: WHY DO THEY DO IT?

Most of the LCs interviewed unequivocally stated that they loved their jobs, despite the problems and frustrations. "Would I do this again, knowing that I'm not going to make a lot of money? YES! It's something that goes beyond money. It's a field like none other," said one who has been in practice for six years. Another said that what she liked most about being a lactation consultant was empowering mothers: "I love being a change agent." An LC who has been in private practice for more than 10 years said: "I am delighted to get up in the morning and think about what my day will bring me. I'm lucky because I have a job that I enjoy. Most of my colleagues also love their work. How many people in other occupations can say that?"

Is a private practice something for every lactation consultant to consider? Clearly, no. However, of those who have done so and weathered the first five years, it can provide rewards that are rarely a part of another occupation. The independence, which is most frightening to persons who are used to a guaranteed salary and set working hours, also offers an opportunity to structure one's work in a way that may allow family involvement which simply is not possible otherwise.

DO'S AND DON'TS OF LACTATION CONSULTING

Following is a brief listing of do's and don'ts suggested by LCs in practice—either when establishing a private practice or when initiating an office-, clinic-, or hospital-based lactation consultant service.

DO . . .

- Network—with your LC colleagues, as well as other health-care workers with whom you come in contact.
- Avoid repeating problems other LCs have experienced by talking with them and learning from them. Follow ("shadow") them around for a while to see how they do things if you can arrange such mentoring.
- Begin by opening a breast pump rental depot in order to get a taste of what it is like to be in private practice (Rago, 1987).
- If you rent or sell equipment, know what you are doing, how the equipment works, and who should and shouldn't use it. Be aware that its availability from you may influence what you tell a client to do.
- Be aware of the marketing of artificial formula and what makes it attractive to mothers. Says one LC: "Don't let the medical folklore interfere with mothers' decisions to breastfeed; go armed with the facts."
- Learn how to use a computer, recommends another LC: "It can be a godsend, not just for working up practice notes, but also for maintaining the business end of things."
- Learn as much as possible about running a business. Get a competent business advisor for accounting, marketing, and taxes. Make sure those advisors understand exactly what you are trying to do.
- Bill the client directly for the service. The client then files a claim to her insurance company. Use a "lactation super-bill," standard forms for billing, and a letter that the client can use to seek insurance coverage.

- Develop a specialization within the field. Said one LC who has established induced lactation as her specialty area: "Get very good at what you do. This will help you build a reputation for good care."
- Always document what you have done and send the original to the primary care provider, whether or not this individual made the initial referral. Such documentation can help legitimize the service, particularly when repeated problems are resolved to the client's satisfaction and when references supporting care provided are shared with the primary care provider.

DON'T . . .

- "Don't make rounds at a hospital by announcing that you are the LC without having first obtained permission to see the client through the powers that be in that hospital."
- Don't get heavily involved in phone consultations, paid or unpaid, counsels another LC: "You are on shaky ground legally giving out such advice without having seen the mother and baby. Often the information may not be accurate." Plus, it's usually incomplete without an overall assessment.
- Don't give away your time without reimbursement.
- "Don't waste your money on a lot of expensive advertising. Advertise judiciously and be patient. Put everything you make back into the business for the first two years."
- "Don't give away free advice with breast pump or other equipment rentals; this sets a poor precedent for obtaining fees for other services."
- "Don't use someone else's opinion as a reason for doing something. Experiment; be creative. What works in one practice may not work in another one."
- Don't begin a private practice if you are working full-time elsewhere, warns one LC: "Your availability is so important; if you aren't available, your practice won't grow."
- Don't get too many partners at the beginning. Knowing how each partner works as an individual will not necessarily predict how each works as part of a group. The more partners one has the greater the number of problems that can arise. One LC posed the following rhetorical

question with a laugh: "Would you take on more than one husband at the same time?"
- Never forget that a happy mother and thriving baby are your best advertisements—and apt to generate more referrals than anything else.
- Don't forget to document what you have done with a mother; send the original form with this information on it to the primary care provider.

SUMMARY

The field of lactation is a health-care specialty that has grown rapidly in the last decade. The opportunity to work with healthy families and adorable babies—and to enhance early parenting and child health—has made it a popular, satisfying field. Although growth is welcomed, rapid growth causes growing pains. Some health professionals feel threatened by the emergence of new practitioners who expect to share their turf.

The experiences of the lactation consultant in this decade are similar to those of the childbirth educator in the 1960s and 1970s. Then, it was the childbirth educator who was the innovator and change agent who flew against the prevailing wind and traditional practices in birthing. These two disciplines share more than a common history: both have consistently acted as a health-related consumer advocate—for women and for families—during an age when technology and defensive medicine rule medical practice.

Those working with breastfeeding families cannot expect to become wealthy. However, they reap the reward of personal fulfillment as they assist other women in becoming empowered by their own breastfeeding experiences. This outcome has no price.

REFERENCES

American Journal of Nursing Company: Newborn RNs find niche: teaching how to parent (News), *AJN* 90:80–81, 1990.

American Nurses Association: Has JCAHO eliminated care plans? *Am Nurse,* June, 1991a, p. 6.

American Nurses Association: HCFA issues instructions for nurse reimbursement, *Am Nurse,* June 1991b, p. 39.

Anderson, E, and Geden, E: Nurses' knowledge of breastfeeding, *JOGNN* 20:58–64, 1991.

Auerbach, KG: A we/they dichotomy (editorial), *J Hum Lact* 5:121, 1989.

Auerbach, KG, and Walburn, J: Nebraska family practitioners' infant feeding recommendations, *Fam Pract Res J* 6:189–99, 1987a.

Auerbach, KG, and Walburn, J: Nebraska physicians' infant feeding recommendations, *Neb Med J* 72:168–74, 1987b.

Bachman, MC: The lactation consultant in a hospital setting, *J Hum Lact* 3:104–5, 1987.

Best, LJ: An option for LCs—adjunct staff member status, *J Hum Lact* 3:157–59, 1987.

Bornmann, PG: *Legal considerations and the lactation consultant—USA* (Unit 3), Lactation Consultant Series, Garden City Park, N.Y., 1986, Avery Publishing Group, Inc.

Brooten, D, et al.: A randomized clinical trial of early hospital discharge and home follow-up of very-low-weight infants, *N Engl J Med* 315:934–39, 1986.

Bull, P: Consent form to supplement newborns, *J Hum Lact* 2:27–28, 1986.

Caraher, MT: The importance of third-party reimbursement for NPs, *Nurse Pract* 13(4):50–54, 1988.

Clark, CC: Assertiveness issues for nursing administrators and managers. In Stone, S, et al.: *Management for nursing: a multidisciplinary approach,* St. Louis, 1984, The C. V. Mosby Company Co., pp. 74–75.

Cohen, SP: High tech-soft touch: breastfeeding issues, *Clin Perinatol* 4:187–96, 1987.

Davidson-Crews, E: Women working with women seminar, St. Joseph Medical Center, Wichita, Kansas, August 11, 1989.

Dodgson, J: Early identification of potential breastfeeding problems, *J Hum Lact* 5:80–81, 1989.

Dublin, P: Options for lactation consultants: the public health arena, *J Hum Lact* 5:19–20, 1989.

Eiger, MS: "For one brief shining moment . . . " (guest editorial), *J Hum Lact* 7:169–70, 1991.

Frantz, KB: Are there enough clients to go around? (editorial), *J Hum Lact* 4:99–100, 1988.

Gardiner, J, et al.: *Relationships and roles: the lactation consultant and lay breastfeeding groups* (Unit 7), Garden City Park, N.Y., 1986, Avery Publishing Group, Inc., pp. 6–8.

Gardner, KL, and Weinrauch, D: Marketing strategies for nurse entrepreneurs, *Nurse Pract* 13:46–49, 1988.

Gardner, SL: Mothering: the unconscious conflict between nurses and new mothers, *Keep Abreast J* 3:193–205, 1978.

Gerrard, JW: Breastfeeding: second thoughts, *Pediatrics* 54:757–64, 1974.

Gerrard, JW: Breast-feeding: should it be recommended? *CMAJ* 113:138–39, 1975.

Gilligan, C: *In a different voice,* Cambridge, 1982, Howard University Press.

Gorrie, TM: *A guide to the nursing of childbearing families,* Baltimore, 1989, The Williams & Wilkins Co.

Harter, C, et al.: Networking to implement effective health care, *MCN* 14:387–92, 1987.

Hill, LF: A salute to La Leche League International (letter), *J Pediatr* 73:161–62, 1968.

Jelliffe, DB, and Jelliffe, EFP: 'Breast is best': modern meanings, *N Engl J Med* 297:912–15, 1977.

Kantor, MB: *The change masters: innovation for productivity in the American corporation,* New York, 1983, Simon & Schuster, Inc., p. 409.

Kotler, P: *Marketing management: analysis, planning, and control* (5th ed.), Englewood Cliffs, N.J., 1984, Prentice–Hall.

Kutner, L: Nipple shield consent form: a teaching aid, *J Hum Lact* 2:25–27, 1986.

Marmet, C, and Shell, E: The role of the lactation consultant (Chapter 45). In Coates, MM, ed.: *The lactation consultant's topical review and bibliography of the literature on breastfeeding,* Franklin Park, Ill., 1990, La Leche League International, pp. 169–73.

Melia, J: *Breaking into the boardroom: what every woman needs to know,* New York, 1986, St. Martin's Press, Inc., pp. 13–33.

Mukasa, GK: A 12-month lactation clinic experience in Uganda, *J Trop Pediatr* 38:78–82, 1992.

NAACOG: NAACOG members offer home care, *NAACOG News* 18:7, 1991.

NAACOG: Nurses offer home health-care alternatives, Part 1, *NAACOG News* 15:3–4, 1988.

NAACOG: *Nursing diagnosis,* Washington, D.C., 1989, NAACOG, p. 2.

Orlando, R: *Breastfeeding care plans for the hospital-based lactation consultant,* La Leche League Conference, Miami Beach, Fla., July, 1991.

Phillips, V: Lactation consultants and voluntary breastfeeding counsellors: complementary roles or conflict? *Breastfeed Rev* 2:92–94, 1990a.

Phillips, V: The Nursing Mother's Association of Australia as a self-help organization. In Katz, AH, and Bender, EL: *Helping one another:* Self-help groups in a changing world, Oakland, Calif., 1990b, Third Party Publishing Co.

Rago, JL: Breast pump rental depot: a way to bridge the gap, *J Hum Lact* 3:156–57, 1987.

Riordan, J: A statistical overview of IBLCE certification exams, *J Hum Lact* 6:90–92, 1990.

Riordan, J, and Auerbach, KG: Lactation consultant certification candidates: the influence of background characteristics on test scores, *Birth* 14:196–98, 1987.

Scott, J: The importance of certification (Chapter 46). In Coates, MM, ed.: *The lactation consultant's topical review and bibliography of the literature on breastfeeding,* Franklin Park, Ill., 1990, La Leche League International, p. 175.

Scott, R: *Office at home,* New York, 1985, Charles Scribner's Sons; reviewed in *J Hum Lact* 3:168, 1987.

Shamansky, S, et al.: Determining the market for NP services: The New Haven experience, *Nurs Res* 34:242–47, 1985.

Shoemaker, JK: Essential features of a nursing diagnosis. In Kim, MJ, McFarlane, G, and McLane, A, eds.: *Classification of nursing diagnosis,* St. Louis, 1984, The C.V. Mosby Co., p. 109.

Shrago, LC: Product evaluation: nipple shields, *J Hum Lact* 4:169, 1988.

Sonstegard, L: A better way to market maternal-child care, *MCN* 13:395–402, 1988.

Tanis, AL, Coleman, AB, and Gross, L: I.B.C.L.C., *Pediatrics* 86:149, 1990.

Tinari, MA: Lactation consultant job proposal, *J Hum Lact* 2:114–15, 1986.

Williams, N: Creating a lactation consultant position, *J Hum Lact* 1:86–88, 1986.

Wilton, JM: Development of a hospital breastfeeding center, *J Hum Lact* 5:132–34, 1989.

Woolf, V: *A room of one's own,* New York, 1929, Harcourt, Brace and World.

SUGGESTED READINGS

Carnevali, D: *Nursing care planning: diagnosis and management,* 3rd ed., Philadelphia, 1983, J.B. Lippincott Co.

Carpenito, L: *Nursing diagnosis: application to practice,* 3rd ed., Philadelphia, 1989, J.B. Lippincott Co.

Clifford, D, and Warner, R: *The partnership book,* Berkeley, Calif., 1984, Nolo Press.

Doenges, M, Kenty, J, and Moorhouse, M: *Maternal newborn care plans: guidelines for client care,* Philadelphia, 1988, F.A. Davis Co.

Gulanick, M, Klapp, A, and Galanes, S: *Nursing care plans: nursing diagnosis and interventions,* St. Louis, 1986, The C.V. Mosby Co.

Iyer, PW, and Camp, NH: *Nursing documentation: a nursing process approach,* St. Louis, 1991, Mosby Year Book, The C.V. Mosby Co.

Scott, R: *Office at home,* New York, 1985, Charles Scribner's Sons.

The Small Business Association (SBA) has a variety of informational booklets appropriate to the entrepreneur interested in starting, managing, and incorporating a small business. Write for a listing of available offerings to the SBA, PO Box 30, Denver, CO 80201–0030.

Local members of the Senior Corps of Retired Executives (SCORE) provide counseling for persons interested in going into business. They are usually listed in local telephone directories. As with other business counselors, their helpfulness may be limited by their assumptions of what a lactation consulting business requires. Often, their members conduct SBA-sponsored workshops.

21

Research and Breastfeeding

ROBERTA J. HEWAT

Is intuition, gut reaction, or tradition the basis of breastfeeding practice and education? Or, is practice and education founded on a body of knowledge which is generated from data gathered and interpreted by systematic methods that practitioners continually question, study, and expand? Research is a process for developing a knowledge base for accountable and responsible practice that legitimizes professional care in today's society.

The intent of this chapter is to assist breastfeeding practitioners to develop an interest in—and understanding of—breastfeeding research, as well as to become what is known today as a research consumer. This entails reading articles to keep updated about current practices; understanding research methods to evaluate and determine whether study findings are relevant; incorporating appropriate findings into their practice; and consistently questioning practices to develop questions for further research.

APPROACHES TO RESEARCH METHODS

Qualitative and quantitative methodologies are two approaches for conducting research; both develop different kinds of knowledge. The research question—and whether knowledge is generated deductively or inductively—directs the approach used. Quantitative methods are traditional and have been most commonly used for breastfeeding research. However, since the mid-1980s, breastfeeding studies using qualitative methods are more evident in the literature. This trend is consistent with the gradual increase in use and recognition of qualitative methodologies in nursing research. The following section describes the characteristics of each approach.

THE QUALITATIVE APPROACH

Qualitative methodologies generate an understanding of the "meaning" that human values, beliefs, practices, or life experiences and events have for individuals. The aim is to discover new information or to gain a new perspective on a familiar topic. Therefore, all possible variables that influence individuals' perspectives are considered data; these data are broad and frequently complex. This humanistic approach is congruent with a holistic philosophy of providing health care.

The outcomes of qualitative studies are theory generation and/or rich descriptions of the meaning of experiences, events, or practices for individuals. Theory is generated by the process of inductive reasoning. Thus, from the study of a phenomenon such as an everyday life experience, variables and how they relate are identified. Further interpretation of the data can lead to conceptualization of the experience from which theoretical propositions are made.

Types of qualitative methods. The origins of qualitative methods are inherent in philosophy and the social sciences. Three major types of qualitative methods are phenomenology, ethnography, and grounded theory. Phenomenology and grounded-theory methods emanate from sociology; ethnographic methods are derived by anthropologists. Rigorous procedures for conducting research have been developed for each method.

"Phenomenology is . . . a distinctive philosophy, theory and method for studying the world of everyday life" (Anderson, 1991). The objective is to understand the meaning or essence of life experiences or events from the perspective of those living the experiences. Study findings provide greater understanding of clients' experiences, enabling practitioners to plan more relevant care.

A study addressing women's perceptions of the breastfeeding experience, conducted by Hewat and Ellis (1984), is an example of a phenomenological study. The impetus for this study was the result of unexpected findings from a quantitative study in which the breastfeeding period was not extended for women receiving additional information and support (Ellis & Hewat, 1984). Although some methodological issues may have contributed to the quantitative results, they compelled the investigators to explore the meaning of breastfeeding from women living the experience. Findings from the qualitative study describe similarities and differences of women who breastfeed for short and long duration (Hewat & Ellis, 1986) and discuss a conceptualization of the mother-infant breastfeeding relationship (Hewat & Ellis, 1984). These findings explain the complexity of the breastfeeding experience and provide direction for breastfeeding practitioners.

Ethnography is a method used to understand the beliefs, practices, and patterns of behavior from the perspective of individuals of a culture or subculture within the context of their environment. A "traditional" ethnography describes the many facets of an entire culture or subculture, whereas a "focused" ethnography portrays one aspect of a culture (Morse, 1991a). The purpose is to come to understand the cultural meanings people use to organize and interpret their experiences (Spradley, 1979).

A study by Neander and Morse (1989) is an example of a focused ethnography. The authors describe and compare infant feeding practices of the Northern Alberta Woodlands Cree when infants were born at home with practices followed after childbirth was relocated to the hospital. A decline in breastfeeding that occurred is associated with the mothers' loss of social support from native women and the lack of understanding by health professionals about Cree cultural beliefs and practices.

Grounded theory is a "field method that aims to generate theory which explains the action within the social context under study" (Stern, 1984). Using a rigorous and structured process (Strauss & Corbin, 1990), data based on individuals' realities are simultaneously collected and analyzed to develop theoretical constructs. The emerging theory represents reality because it is "grounded" in the data. From this new understanding, relevant interventions for clinical practice can evolve.

An example of breastfeeding research using the grounded-theory method is a study by Morse and Bottorff (1988) that examines mothers' attitudes toward breast expression. Study results report four major themes related to mothers' perceptions of breast expression. From the mothers' reported experiences, two models that illustrate the process were developed. One model portrays breast expression for mothers who feel they express successfully, and the other depicts the process for mothers who feel unsuccessful in breast expression. Implications for clinical practice suggest that health professionals remain sensitive to and explore women's feelings about breast expression in both the pre- and postnatal periods.

THE QUANTITATIVE APPROACH

Quantitative methodologies are traditional research methods advanced by the biological, physical, and social sciences. Key characteristics are objectivity, measurement, and control. Studies examine specific variables and control intervening variables. Data collection and analysis are conducted as objectively as possible to control prejudice on the part of the investigator and other sources of potential bias. Statistical procedures and principles of measurement determine relationships and/or examine cause and effect among variables.

Theories, principles, or conceptualizations are a common source of the variables or hypotheses for study. The process of studying components and their relationships deduced from a general premise is known as deductive reasoning.

The goal of quantitative studies is to determine relationships that are predictable and can be generalized to populations larger than the study sample. This may take many years of ongoing study by many independent investigators. The decades in which numerous studies were conducted before scientists declared that smoking is related to the development of lung cancer is an example.

Types of quantitative methods. The types of quantitative methods described represent three levels of inquiry identified by Brink and Wood (Brink & Wood, 1989; Roberts & Burke, 1989, p. 148; Wilson, 1989). They include methods for descriptive, correlational, and causal or experimental studies. The method chosen depends on the amount of knowledge known about the study topic and the purpose of the research.

Descriptive studies are appropriate when there is little knowledge about a topic of interest and specific information is desired. For example, the research question may address characteristics, influencing factors, or knowledge deficits related to a topic. Findings describe the studied phenomenon and may identify relationships among variables.

An example of a descriptive study is one conducted by Graef et al. (1988) on postpartum concerns of a group of 32 breastfeeding mothers during the first postpartum month. Graef and colleagues categorized the identified concerns as infant, maternal, and paternal/family issues, a modification of classifications previously developed. The percentage of mothers reporting each concern as well as a variance of concerns is described during the four-week postpartum period. The study findings are compared, and the similarities and differences with other studies are described and discussed. Findings of some descriptive studies may identify relationships between variables which form the basis for further study.

Correlational studies examine relationships between two or more variables and the type (negative or positive) and strength of the relationship(s). These studies require greater control than descriptive studies. Structuring the data that are collected is necessary in order to allow for numerical translation and correlational analysis to determine if the relationships between variables are statistically significant. In quantitative studies, the term significant is used only when a relationship is statistically significant.

Humenick's (1987) research regarding maturational rates of breastmilk is an example of a correlational study. The purpose of this study was to examine milk maturation rates of 98 mothers in relation to variables identified in the literature as possibly being associated with early milk maturation. Findings indicate significant and positive relationships between early milk maturation rates and the following variables: greater frequency of breastfeeding and longer feeding periods in the first 48 hours of life; increased infant weight gain at 28 days; and longer duration of breastfeeding. A significant relationship between lower milk maturation rates and higher transcutaneous bilimeter readings for infants at two and 14 days postpartum was also shown. In addition, findings indicate that in the first 48 hours postdelivery, the frequency and total number of feedings were significantly less for primiparas than for multiparas.

These study findings increase knowledge about milk maturation rates and provide direction for further investigations. For example, based on the finding that multiparas fed more frequently and for longer periods than primiparas in the first 48 hours, the following questions can be posed: Is milk maturation rate related to feeding practices or parity? Could a study in which primiparas are helped to increase breastfeeding frequency and duration show that practices are a cause which produces early milk maturation? Although not essential, evidence from correlational studies often supports the initiation of experimental research.

Experimental studies examine hypothesized relationships between variables in which the order of variable occurrence may suggest causation. Rigorous control is integral to conducting these studies. According to Nieswiadomy (1987), as well as Polit and Hungler (1991), criteria essential for a true experimental study include the following:

- the investigator controls (or manipulates) an experimental treatment (the independent variable)
- an experimental group of subjects receiving the treatment is compared to a control group
- a process of randomization assigns subjects to the study groups.

The study of human subjects, however, does not always permit such rigor. It is often not ethical, practical, or feasible to randomly assign individuals to groups and expose them to a specific treatment or experience. When the criteria of a true experimental study must be compromised, to take account of human subjects' rights or limitations, the research is *quasi-experimental.*

Lynch et al. (1986) used an experimental design to determine to what effect the services of a breastfeeding consultant (the treatment or independent variable) had on the duration of breastfeeding (the dependent or outcome variable). Two-hundred-and-seventy subjects were randomly assigned to experimental and control groups. Within a few days of hospital discharge all mothers were visited by a public-health nurse who provided information about breastfeeding concerns. In addition, mothers in the experimental group received a visit from a breast-feeding consultant within five days of hospital discharge. The consultant observed breastfeeding, provided assistance with positioning the infant at the breast, and discussed breastfeeding concerns. Weekly telephone calls were made to mothers during the first month, and monthly telephone calls were made during months two to six. Additional home visits and telephone calls were made to mothers with identified difficulties. The breastfeeding rate for all subjects was examined at one, three, six, and nine months. Study findings revealed no statistical differences between the control and experimental groups; therefore, Lynch et al. were unable to infer that a breastfeeding consultant prolonged breastfeeding duration.

The results of the Lynch et al. study may seem disappointing, but these findings are important for contributing knowledge about one method of providing breastfeeding support. These findings direct further questions for study that may produce different outcomes. Examples of questions include: What is the effect on breastfeeding duration of breastfeeding assistance from a lactation consultant during hospital stay and at home for four weeks following hospital discharge? What is the effect of breastfeeding assessment and information from a lactation consultant—during pregnancy, in hospital, and throughout the breastfeeding period—on patterns of infant feeding? Many additional studies are needed before the relationship between support and breastfeeding duration is understood. Research is an ongoing process; many experimental studies about a topic are necessary before conclusions are definitive.

QUANTITATIVE AND QUALITATIVE APPROACHES

In developing a scientific base for breastfeeding practice, both quantitative and qualitative approaches generate knowledge. Most studies use one approach; the choice depends on the research question addressed and whether theory is generated inductively or tested deductively. Some studies simultaneously use the two approaches (Field & Morse, 1985). This combined approach is known as *triangulation*. Triangulation may be used to enhance the comprehensiveness of quantitative data or to confirm or validate a data set. When using both approaches, researchers must be clear about the purpose of each and the separate strategies employed for collecting, analyzing, and interpreting data (Knafl & Breitmayer, 1991).

ELEMENTS OF RESEARCH

The elements of research are essential to writing proposals and reports, conducting research, and evaluating studies. The major elements are: the research problem and purpose; the review of literature; the protection of human subjects; the methodology; the analysis; and the results and discussion. Although the elements are similar for both qualitative and quantitative research approaches, the content and processes vary. The following section describes the elements and discusses the differences between qualitative and quantitative methods.

RESEARCH PROBLEM AND PURPOSE

The research problem is a critical component of a study. It identifies "what" is studied and with "whom." The purpose delineates "why" the study is conducted. There are many sources for generating research problems. Questioning clinical practice, observing clinical and societal patterns and trends, building on findings from previous studies, and examining theoretical propositions are ways of developing research questions.

A problem that is suitable for study should be important to the topic of breastfeeding and amenable to investigation by scientific inquiry. It should be meaningful to many individuals or have a distinct influence on a few. A descriptive survey conducted by Tanaka, Yeung, and Anderson (1989) regarding mothers' use of health professionals as sources of information on infant nutrition in metropolitan Toronto illustrates importance to many. Meier and Anderson's (1987) study of the responses of small, pre-term infants to bottle- and breastfeeding demonstrates impact on a few. Criteria that render a problem appropriate for scientific inquiry include:

- suitability of the research design for the research question
- accessibility of study participants
- feasibility of the study with regard to time, funding, and equipment
- potentiality of adhering to ethical requirements throughout all study phases.

Reviewing the literature about a study topic provides direction for asking a relevant question and selecting an appropriate method. A qualitative method is indicated when literature is limited about a phenomenon or when more in-depth knowledge is desired. However, when many studies about a topic have been undertaken, these study findings often provide a base and focus for further study, and a quantitative method is generally appropriate.

Research problems can be written as questions or declarative statements. Clearly identifying the topic, population, and variables for study is essential for quantitative methods. In qualitative studies less is known about the topic of interest; therefore, the research question is broader. The purpose is to discover variables relevant to a topic rather than examine variables previously identified. Examples of research questions that are applicable to specific research methods are shown in Table 21–1. All questions pertain to breastfeeding pre-term infants. For quantitative methods this has been further delineated to social network and breastfeeding pre-term infants, which is a topic and population studied by Kaufman and Hall (1989).

TABLE 21–1   EXAMPLES OF RESEARCH QUESTIONS AND RESEARCH METHODS

Qualitative Methods
Topic of Interest: Breastfeeding pre-term infants

Question	Research Method
What are mothers' perceptions of breastfeeding a pre-term infant?	Phenomenology
What are cultural influences on feeding patterns of preterm infants among Chinese women?	Ethnography
What is the experience of being a breastfeeding mother with a pre-term infant?	Grounded theory

Quantitative Methods

Topic: Social support and breastfeeding*
Population: Mothers of pre-term infants

Question	Research Method	Variables for Study
What kinds of social support are most useful to breastfeeding mothers of pre-term infants?	Descriptive	Social support
Is there a relationship between social network and choice of feeding method and duration of breastfeeding for mothers of pre-term infants? (Kaufman & Hall, 1989)	Correlational	Social network
		Choice of feeding method
		Breastfeeding duration
What is the effect on breastfeeding duration of scheduled visits by a lactation consultant to breastfeeding mothers of pre-term infants?	Experimental	Scheduled visits by a lactation consultant (independent variable)
		Breastfeeding duration (dependent variable)

*The topic and variables for study are usually more specifically identified in quantitative studies.

VARIABLES, HYPOTHESES, AND OPERATIONAL DEFINITIONS

Variables. Variables are defined as "attributes, properties, and/or characteristics of persons, events, or objects that are examined in a study" (Burns & Grove, 1987). Qualitative studies aim to discover variables that influence the study phenomenon, whereas quantitative studies identify specific variables for investigation. Experimental studies have at least one dependent and one independent variable. The *dependent* variable, also called the outcome variable, is what the investigator is most interested in understanding, explaining, or predicting. In the example of an experimental study cited in Table 21–1, the dependent variable is breastfeeding duration. The *independent* variable is thought to affect or change the dependent variable. It is the treatment or intervention that affects the outcome; in this example it is the scheduled visits by a lactation consultant.

Uncontrolled, confounding, or extraneous variables are those elements in quantitative studies that may affect the dependent or outcome variable. Sometimes such variables come between the occurrence of the treatment (independent variable) and the measurement of the outcome variable. For example, if mothers with pre-term infants view a television documentary on the advantages of breastmilk for pre-term infants, the television program—rather than the scheduled visits by the lactation consultant—may be the motivating factor for prolonging breastfeeding. To "control" the effect of these variables on experimental study outcomes, study participants are randomly assigned to an experimental group receiving visits by a lactation consultant or to a control group receiving existing care. The random placement of subjects in each group is expected to ensure that each group is similar in regard to background characteristics, practices, and opportunities. Therefore, if the participants of the experimental group breastfeed longer than those of the control group (as determined by statistical procedures), the increased breastfeeding duration is attributed to the visits by the lactation consultant that occurred in the experimental group.

Hypotheses. Hypotheses are "statements formulated to predict a relationship between two or more variables" (Seaman, 1987). Qualitative studies often generate hypotheses, whereas correlational and experimental studies examine and test relationships between identified variables.

Hypotheses for correlational studies focus on the association of variables. For the study by Kaufman and Hall (1989), an hypothesis may be written as follows: "For mothers of pre-term infants, there is a positive relationship between the mothers' perceptions of their social network and breastfeeding duration."

In experimental studies, an hypothesis represents a prediction of how an intervention or independent variable specifically influences an identified outcome or dependent variable. The written hypothesis includes these components as well as naming the study groups. For the experimental study in Table 21–1, a research hypothesis is written as follows: "Mothers of pre-term infants who have scheduled visits by a lactation consultant will breastfeed longer than mothers of pre-term infants who do not have scheduled visits by a lactation consultant." The experimental and control groups, the dependent and independent variables, and the predictor (longer breastfeeding duration) are identified.

For statistical purposes, some investigators prefer to write hypotheses in the null form. For example: "There will be *no* difference in the duration of breastfeeding between mothers of pre-term infants who receive scheduled visits by a lactation consultant and mothers of pre-term infants who do not receive scheduled visits by a lactation consultant." In using the null hypothesis, outcomes for the groups are considered the same until it is established that they are statistically different. When this occurs, the null hypothesis is rejected, and an inference is made that the visits by a lactation consultant are the reason for the different outcomes for the groups. The visits are then considered an effective intervention.

Operational definitions. Operational definitions are explicit descriptions of how the major variables are observed and measured—and how they are integral to correlational and experimental studies. In the Kaufman and Hall (1989) study, both major variables are defined so that numerical comparisons can be made. Breastfeeding duration is specified as "the number of postnatal days of any breast-feeding or expression," and social network is defined as a mother's perception of influence from social referents as measured by the Influence of Specific Referents (ISR) Scale.

In experimental studies, the independent variable must be clearly delineated. In the fictitious experimental study described in Table 21–1, a definition of the intervention regime—the scheduled visits by a lactation consultant—could be operationally defined in many ways. Examples include: a visit one to seven days prior to the infant's discharge from the special-care nursery; a visit twice a week for the duration of the infant's hospital stay; visits to the mother, two times per week, starting the week of delivery and ending when the infant is six weeks of age; or, a visit once a week from birth until four weeks after hospital discharge.

Operational definitions of breastfeeding are extensive. Table 21–2 illustrates differences in definitions used in studies. As the number of possible feeding categories increases, data regarding the variability of infant feeding patterns is more precise. The selection of definitions depends on the purpose of the study and can influence sample size. A large number of categories generally requires large samples.

How breastfeeding is operationally defined is of particular interest when evaluating and comparing study results because imprecise definitions of breastfeeding categories affect data analysis and study outcomes. Readers of research articles and reports must be cognizant of how breastfeeding is defined when determining the merits of a study. For example, infants who are only breastfed may be grouped with infants who are breastfed *once*. Likewise, exclusive or total breastfeeding may mean that the infant has ingested only breastmilk, or it may also include one formula feeding per week and/or supplements of water, glucose water, or juice. Auerbach, Renfrew, and Minchin (1991) illustrate, by providing reviews of breastfeeding definitions and outcomes of 43 studies, that "research purporting to compare breastfeeding with artificial feeding is seriously flawed." The authors outline guidelines for de-

TABLE 21–2 VARIANCE OF OPERATIONAL DEFINITIONS OF BREASTFEEDING

Study Title	Number of Categories	Definitions Distinguishing Breastfeeding Groups
Maternal characteristics associated with the duration of breastfeeding (Jones, West & Newcombe, 1986)	1	Breastfeeder: anyone who breastfed her baby at least once Nonbreastfeeder: all others
Factors predicting breastfeeding success (Hellings, 1984)	4	1 = total breastfeeding 2 = breastfeeding with less than 4 ounces of supplementation 3 = breastfeeding with more than 4 ounces of supplementation 4 = total formula-feeding
Evaluation of the efficacy of a breastfeeding clinic in prolonging the duration of breastfeeding (Ellis, Hewat & Livingstone, 1991)	6	Exclusive = total breastfeeding Primarily = breastfeeding or expressed breastmilk (EBM), plus a maximum of one alternate milk feeding per week Mainly = more than one breastfeeding or EBM feeding per day, plus more than one alternate milk feeding per week to a maximum of one alternate milk feeding per day Partial = more than one breastfeeding or EBM feeding per day, plus more than one alternate milk feeding per day Minimal = one or less breastfeeding or EBM feeding per day to one breastfeeding or EBM feeding per week Weaned = having stopped breastfeeding or EBM feeding for one week or more

fining feeding categories that should be considered by investigators when designing studies that compare different feeding groups. These include: detailed information about all types, combinations, volume, and frequency of any substance ingested by an infant; the method of feeding, e.g., gavage, bottle, or type of nipple used; and identification of the feeder, e.g., nurse or mother, if the infant is in a hospital or clinic.

In 1988 the Interagency Group for Action on Breastfeeding (IGAB), an international organization, started developing standard definitions for breastfeeding patterns that are internationally recommended for use (Armstrong, 1991). The definitions, published by Labbok and Krasovec (1990), include the following classifications: "full" breastfeeding, which is further delineated into subcategories of exclusive and almost exclusive breastfeeding; "partial" breastfeeding, with suggested (but not yet discretely differentiated) groupings of high, medium, and low; and "token" breastfeeding, which is described as minimal, occasional, and irregular breastfeeds. These definitions are a beginning; however, all subcategories of the classifications require further specification. This is a complex undertaking as the definitions must reflect cultural practices and meanings as well as satisfy the precision required for investigations. Further refining of the definitions is essential for more consistent and valid outcomes from breastfeeding research.

REVIEW OF LITERATURE

Reviewing literature on a study topic provides knowledge and understanding about the phenomenon. Findings from studies help to formulate the research problem and provide direction for research methods. The purpose of a review of literature can be different for qualitative and quantitative approaches. In qualitative studies, an initial review of literature is done primarily for investigator awareness of the studies conducted. Since the goal of qualitative methods is discovery, literature should not influence the mind set of the investigator during initial data collection. In the analysis stage, study findings reported in the literature are used to compare, contrast, and verify findings of the current study. Findings from a new study may even be combined with those of a previous study

to identify new insights and expand current knowledge about a phenomenon.

In quantitative studies, the existing literature will help to clarify the research problem and identify theories or concepts on which the study is based. Identification of key concepts and their relationships provides a conceptual framework or structure for the study. Literature is also useful in assisting with selection of a research design, providing strategies for data collection and analysis, and interpreting findings (Woods & Catanzaro, 1988).

PROTECTION OF THE RIGHTS OF HUMAN SUBJECTS

Most breastfeeding research involves human subjects. To protect the rights of study participants throughout the research process, investigators must adhere to ethical guidelines. International ethical standards, known as the Nuremberg Code, were first developed following World War II, when inhumane acts, described by the Nazis as scientific research, were revealed during the war crimes trials held in Nuremberg, Germany. This code is the basis of ethical standards developed by medicine and the behavioral science disciplines. The Declaration of Helsinki formulated by the World Medical Association (1964) provides further guidelines for physicians conducting clinical research. Ethical requirements for funded research are stipulated by governments and institutions, and individual codes have been developed by professional associations that represent researchers conducting human research. Specific ethical guidelines for nursing research have been adopted by the American Nurses' Association (ANA, 1985), the Canadian Nurses' Association (CNA, 1983), and the Royal College of Nursing of the United Kingdom (RCN, 1977).

Four basic rights of human subjects are recognized (Wilson, 1989). The first is freedom from risk or injury from physical, emotional, financial, or social harm. The second is full knowledge of the study purpose, procedures to be used, time commitments asked of the participants, and any other factors that may affect the subjects. The third is the assurance of the right to self-determination, which means that subjects may refuse to participate or withdraw from a study *at any time* without any effect on the care they receive. And the fourth is the affirmation of their privacy, anonymity, or confidentiality throughout all phases of the research.

Mechanisms, developed to ensure that research is ethically conducted, include the investigator's use of an informed-consent form and review of the proposed study by human subjects or ethical review boards. An informed-consent document describes the study, addresses how the rights of subjects will be maintained, and explains how the investigator may be contacted. It is presented to subjects when they are recruited. A subject's signature on the informed-consent document indicates an understanding of the study and willingness to participate. Ethical review boards—established by universities and many health-care agencies, school boards, or organizations which are resources for human subjects—review study proposals to ensure that the research process protects the rights of study participants.

METHODOLOGY

Each study method addresses setting, sample, data collection, and data analysis. An overview of these elements is presented, followed by examples of how they apply to studies using qualitative and quantitative research approaches.

Setting. A study setting is the locus of the study and/or source of participating subjects or sample. In all studies, the setting must be clearly described.

Population and sample. A population, which is often referred to as the target population, is the group of individuals in which the researcher is interested. For example, it could be all breastfeeding mothers, primiparas who breastfeed, mothers who work and breastfeed, or mothers of pre-term infants. Or, in some cases, an object, such as breastmilk, may be the phenomenon of interest rather than individuals. Because it is difficult to study an entire population, researchers generally study a subgroup of the larger population and this is the sample.

Sampling. Sampling is a process for selecting the sample from the population. Two basic types are probability and nonprobability sampling.

Probability sampling involves quantitative studies which aim to generalize findings from the sample studied to larger populations; therefore, it is important that the sample be representative of the target population. This is accomplished by the *random selection* of subjects from the population, a process

which requires that every individual in the population of interest has an equal and independent chance of being chosen. There are several methods of probability sampling.

Simple random sampling is achieved by numbering all members of the population and then selecting subjects by using a table of random numbers available in many quantitative research books. Other procedures include drawing subjects' names from a hat or flipping a coin.

Systematic sampling follows the procedure of choosing every "nth" (e.g., every eighth, 10th, or 100th) subject from a list of the population. To ensure that all possible subjects have an equal chance, the names on the list must not be grouped in any special way, such as alphabetical order or age of subjects. For example, in a study of the effect of hospital routines on early breastfeeding experience, selecting every nth case from the list of mothers admitted to a particular postpartum unit would be an appropriate sampling technique.

Stratified random sampling is a process of identifying subgroups of a population and selecting numbers of subjects that represent the distribution of the subgroups in the population. For example, if a researcher wishes to study a population of all mothers giving birth in a specific geographic location and learns that the population distribution is 40% primiparas and 60% multiparas, then the investigator will randomly select the numbers for each subgroup or "stratum" that reflects the population distribution.

In studies which involve human subjects, probability sampling is frequently not possible because all subjects in a population, for example all breastfeeding mothers, cannot be identified. Or, depending on the purpose of the study, random assignment of women to feeding groups may be unethical. Therefore, the majority of breastfeeding studies utilize nonprobability sampling.

Nonprobability sampling is the nonrandom selection of subjects for a study sample. There are several systematic methods for selecting the study participants.

Convenience sampling is a common method used for both qualitative and quantitative studies. The sample consists of consenting subjects from a readily available source—for example, all mothers giving birth at a hospital or attending a particular clinic.

Network, nominated, or snowball sampling is a

strategy that bases recruitment on asking current study participants to identify other individuals, similar to themselves, who may also consent to be study subjects. This method is useful in the study of an ethnic group or individuals with a specific condition for which a support group has been established, such as mothers with infants with Down syndrome.

Purposive sampling occurs when the investigator selects participants "according to the needs of the study" (Morse, 1991b). Participants are selected because they are thought to be "good informants" about the study topic. As the study progresses, additional participants are chosen to enrich the data and expand the developing theory.

Solicited or volunteer sampling is used when the investigator wishes to broaden the sample. Advertisements in newspapers and notices on bulletin boards regarding the research often entreat interested participants (Morse, 1991b).

Methods of data collection. Data are collected by asking questions, observing, and/or measuring key variables identified in the research question. The data collection method must be appropriate to the research methodology and the study population.

Self-report questionnaires are an effective and common way of obtaining specific information from a large sample. However, the construction of questionnaires which can be understood by all participants and are sufficiently broad in scope to reflect "true" meanings can be time-consuming and expensive to develop—and may be too long to result in a response rate sufficient to represent the potential whole of the population.

Interviews elicit more in-depth information; however, they are more time-consuming and expensive to administer. A skilled interviewer is required to ensure explicit and valid collection of data. When more than one interviewer is used, varying degrees of bias on the part of the interviewer must be considered as a potential limitation of the data.

Observations are useful for collecting data regarding patterns of behavior, activities, or interactions. Observations can be unstructured and recorded as field notes, or they can be structured for specific recording on checklists.

Biophysiological measurements, such as infant weight, length, head circumference, respirations, oxygen consumption, and heart rate, as well as the mother's temperature, prolactin levels, and milk composition, have been used in breastfeeding research. However, measurements are only as accurate as the equipment used and the investigator responsible for measuring and recording.

RELIABILITY AND VALIDITY

Reliability and validity are central issues concerned with error in research. Occurrence of error "anywhere during the research process compromises the outcomes of the study and limits the usability of the data" (Brink, 1991). *Reliability* refers to the accuracy, consistency, precision, and stability of measurement or data collection. *Validity* reflects truth, accuracy, and reality. To be valid, measures and methods of data collection must also be reliable.

DATA ANALYSIS

Data analysis is the process of examining, summarizing, and synthesizing the data collected to determine if study findings answer the research question. Strategies for data analysis are dependent on the research question, sample selection and size, and method and type of data collection.

APPLICATION OF METHODS TO QUALITATIVE APPROACHES

Specific methodological procedures for each qualitative method have been developed. Investigators should use the qualitative method and ascribed procedure that is most appropriate to the study problem. "Mixing" qualitative methods "violates assumptions of data collection techniques and methods of analysis of all the methods used" and may result in unreliable outcomes (Morse, 1991a).

SAMPLING

All nonprobability sampling methods are suitable for recruiting study participants, but a frequently used procedure is purposive or theoretical sampling. Purposive sampling permits the investigator to select participants thought to be the best informants for providing data about the population and the topic of interest. Sample size is determined through a process called *theoretical sampling*. This means that as data are simultaneously collected and analyzed from initial participants and descriptions of experiences are revealed, additional informants are recruited on the basis of expanding the developing knowledge base. Participants are recruited until no new information is disclosed and data are fully explored (Chenitz & Swanson, 1986). Sample sizes are generally small. Depending on the scope of the topic explored, sample size may range from five to 30 subjects (Roberts & Burke, 1989).

DATA COLLECTION

Methods of data collection include interviews, field observations, and review of documents. In-depth, unstructured interviews, which explore participants' perceptions and validate the investigator's subjective interpretation of the data, remain the most common method for the three qualitative methods described. The interviews are usually taped on audiocassette and then transcribed for detailed analysis. Participant observation, another common method, is particularly suitable for ethnographic research. For the circumstance under study, the investigator observes the activities, people, and physical aspects of the situation while engaging, either passively or actively, in the activities (Spradley, 1980). Recorded field notes of the observations are data for later analysis.

DATA ANALYSIS

Data analysis is ongoing throughout the period of data collection. Each piece of data, whether from transcriptions of interviews, detailed field notes, or documentation, is compared and contrasted with each other. As the study progresses, interpretations are made by the investigator and validated by study participants to ensure that findings represent true meanings.

In phenomenological studies, several processes of analysis have evolved (Giorgi, 1985; Spiegelberg, 1960; Van Kaam, 1969). An investigator should identify the procedure used in the study. An example of analytical steps developed by Giorgi include the following: compiling and examining descriptions about the meaning of a phenomenon; identifying common elements or units of meaning; delineating themes; naming abstract meanings; and generating what are called structural descriptions that embrace the meaning of the lived experience from the participants' perspectives. In ethnographic studies, data analysis comprises identifying domains and seman-

tic relationships, formulating larger taxonomies, and investigating multiple relationships for differences until cultural themes are revealed (Spradley, 1980). Grounded theory research follows a rigorous analytic process. Data are coded and categorized; a tentative conceptualization or theory is formulated and examined further until a core variable emerges that is the focus of the theory. Concept modification and integration continue through two processes called memoing and theoretical coding until a theory, substantiated by the data, is generated (Stern, 1984).

RELIABILITY AND VALIDITY

Ensuring reliability and validity requires ongoing examination by the investigator throughout the research process. Sources of error can occur in sampling, data collection, and analysis. Factors to evaluate include:

- the credibility of key informants providing accurate data
- the interviewer's skill in obtaining the participants' true perspectives
- the accuracy of field observations
- the generation of codes or units of analysis that represent data accurately within a social context
- the interpretations of the data to determine whether they represent true meanings.

The longitudinal nature of most qualitative studies can enhance reliability and validity of data because checks are often built into the process. Factors to consider include:

- the number of kinds of data collection used (because one method can validate another)
- the frequency with which data are collected from subjects using the same method
- the number of investigators collecting data
- the rigor in the process of analysis.

APPLICATION OF METHODS TO QUANTITATIVE APPROACHES

SAMPLING

Probability sampling methods, particularly for correlational and experimental studies, are preferred, so that the study findings can be generalized to a larger population. When probability sampling is used the optimal sample size can also be determined using statistical procedures. However, as previously discussed, many studies involving human subjects must employ nonprobability sampling methods, and an appropriate sample size is then more difficult to estimate. Factors to consider include: the study purpose, level of inquiry, design, and type of analysis. Generally, samples should be as large as possible, and sample size should increase as the number of variables for study increase (Burns & Grove, 1987). Following are general guidelines that may assist in determining the adequacy of sample size for levels of inquiry.

Descriptive studies that describe certain characteristics of a population may have smaller sample sizes because of the amount of data generated. In two studies describing postpartum concerns of breastfeeding mothers, sample sizes of 32 (Graef et al., 1988) and 50 (Chapman et al., 1985) are considered adequate.

Descriptive surveys and correlational studies that examine relationships among variables should have large numbers. Depending on the number of variables for investigation, a sample of 100 may be adequate. The correlational study previously described by Humenick (1987) had a sample size of 98 women. In a descriptive survey conducted by Tanaka, Yeung, and Anderson (1989), 404 mothers were interviewed to determine the kinds of infant nutrition information which were provided by a variety of health professionals throughout the pre-, intra-, and postpartum periods.

Another general guideline regarding sample size can be applied to quasi-experimental studies in which groups are compared. For each type of subject in a study, a minimum of 10 but preferably 20 to 30 subjects is recommended (Polit & Hungler, 1991). An example of numbers required for a study comparing breastfeeding with nonbreastfeeding mothers would be 60 (30 per group). If additional comparisons between primiparas and multiparas within each group is desired, then an additional 60 (another 30 per group) subjects would be added; the total sample then would be 120.

In these experimental or quasi-experimental studies, *random assignment* of subjects to experimental and control groups is advised. This has two purposes: all subjects have an equal and independent chance of receiving the treatment, and it increases the probability that each group is similar in regard to background characteristics. The latter serves as a control of extraneous variables that may influence effect of treatment. Random assignment should not be confused with random selection (previously discussed), which allows findings to be generalized to the population from which the sample was selected.

DATA COLLECTION

All methods of data collection previously described are applicable to quantitative studies if they are applied consistently and objectively. Descriptive studies gather data that are broader in scope or more subjective than correlational or experimental studies. However, questionnaires, interview schedules, and observation criteria must be structured so that the same data are collected in the same manner from all subjects. Measurement studies, such as correlational, quasi-experimental, and experimental studies, require data that can be reduced to numbers for applying statistical procedures. Reliable and valid questionnaires and observation checklists used for measuring variable relationships often take years to develop. Once established, they may be used in numerous studies.

An example of a breastfeeding questionnaire, named the "Infant Beastfeeding Assessment Tool" (IBFAT) (Matthews, 1988, 1991) is shown in Table 21–3. Using a Likert-type scale (see glossary at the end of this chapter), this measure rates a baby's feeding behaviors during a feeding. Because this questionnaire is specific to breastfeeding and has established interrater reliability and content validity, it has a great deal of potential for use. Further testing of reliability and validity of this measure with larger samples will make it invaluable for breastfeeding research and assessment in clinical practice.

RELIABILITY

Accuracy and consistency in the method of data collection, as well as the tools or instruments used, are essential in quantitative studies. Several types of reliability should be addressed.

Interrater reliability. This refers to the accuracy and consistency of data collection. When more than one individual observes phenomena, or when more than one instrument (such as a thermometer) is used for data collection, the probability of error be-

TABLE 21–3 INFANT BREASTFEEDING ASSESSMENT TOOL

Check the answer which *best* describes the baby's feeding behaviors at this feed.

1. When you picked baby up to feed was he/she?

(a) deeply asleep (eyes closed, no observable movements except breathing)	(b) drowsy	(c) quiet and alert	(d) crying
_____	_____	_____	_____

2. In order to get the baby to begin this feed, did you or the nurse have to?

(a) just place the baby on the breast as no effort was needed	(b) use mild stimulation such as unbundling, patting or burping	(c) unbundle baby; sit baby back and forward; rub baby's body or limbs vigorously at the beginning and during the feeding	(d) could not be aroused
3	2	1	0

3. Rooting (definition: at touch of nipple to cheek baby's head turns towards the nipple, the mouth opens and baby attempts to fix mouth on the nipple). When the baby was placed beside the breast, he/she?

(a) rooted effectively at once	(b) needed some coaxing, prompting, or encouragement to root	(c) rooted poorly even with coaxing	(d) did not try to root
3	2	1	0

4. How long from placing baby at the breast does it take for the baby to latch-on and start to suck?

(a) starts to feed at once (0–3 minutes)	(b) 3–10 minutes	(c) over 10 minutes	(d) did not feed
3	2	1	0

5. Which of the following phrases best describes the baby's feeding pattern at this feed?

(a) baby did not suck	(b) sucked poorly; weak sucking; some sucking efforts for short periods	(c) sucked fairly well (sucked off and on, but needed encouragement)	(d) sucked well throughout on one or both breasts
0	1	2	3

6. How do you feel about the way the baby fed at this feeding?

(a) very pleased	(b) pleased	(c) fairly pleased	(d) not pleased
_____	_____	_____	_____

Reprinted with permission. From Matthews, MK: Developing an instrument to assess infant breastfeeding behavior in the early neonatal period, *Midwifery* 4:154–65, 1988. See also Matthews, MK: Mothers' satisfaction with their neonates' breastfeeding behaviours, *JOGNN* 20:49–55, 1991.

tween the instruments or interviewers increases. To control this aspect, checks are made. Similar instruments should be calibrated until measurement is consistent. For individuals making similar observations, the degree of accuracy can be statistically de-termined and is reported as a coefficient. Generally, an interrater reliability of .85 between observers is considered suitable (Shelley, 1984). For the Infant Breastfeeding Assessment Tool shown above, inter-rater reliability was determined by comparing agreement of the mother's and the investigator's breastfeeding assessments. Overall, agreement was 91% accurate, although it was noted that infants who fed well or poorly were easier to assess than those who rated in the middle range and were classified as moderate feeders (Matthews, 1988, 1991).

Intrarater reliability. This refers to accuracy and consistency over time. When data are collected for more than six months, investigators may want to check the accuracy of the individual who is making the observations—and/or the instrument(s) used—every few months. An acceptable intrarater reliability coefficient reported for longitudinal observational studies is also in the range of .85.

Test-retest reliability. This indicates the stability of a measure, such as a questionnaire, over time. Results of two administrations to the same subjects, occurring approximately three weeks apart, are statistically compared. A coefficient reported as .80 or above is generally acceptable for measurement questionnaires which reflect attitudes or feelings that should be constant. However, for some events, such as postpartum adjustment, a low correlation coefficient (such as .40 or .50) may be desired since differences in individual scores over a period of time reflect inconsistency, which may indicate that the individual is changing or adjusting to a different lifestyle.

Internal consistency. This refers to the statistical agreement of several items on a questionnaire that reflect the meaning of a concept—for example, satisfaction with breastfeeding. Similarity in meaning or internal consistency of the items can be statistically determined. Cronbach's alpha is a reliability coefficient frequently computed to determine internal consistency. In the Kaufman and Hall (1989) study regarding influences of social network on choice and duration of breastfeeding pre-term infants, the authors report a Cronbach alpha coefficient for the Influence of Specific Referents Scale as .86. Since a coefficient of .70 to .80 is generally acceptable for a questionnaire measuring a construct (Nunnally, 1978), the data collected to measure this concept is considered reliable.

VALIDITY

Validity addresses the extent to which a questionnaire or measurement instrument reflects the mean-

ing of the concept that is being measured (Woods & Catanzaro, 1988). Types of validity referred to in quantitative studies are content, concurrent, and construct validity. Questionnaires and interview schedules used for descriptive studies should have *content* validity. This means that the questions reflect the study concepts. In developing questionnaires, investigators review the literature to include dimensions of the concept being studied and then submit the questionnaire to individuals who are considered experts on the research topic for review. This validation of content with literature and experts is known as content validity.

Questionnaires used to measure concepts should also be subjected to *concurrent* and *construct* validation. Both require psychometric testing or statistical validation of the meaning of concepts used in a specific context. Use of questionnaires shown to have either concurrent or construct validity enhances the validity of a study.

DATA ANALYSIS

Data analysis is the process of organizing, summarizing, examining, and synthesizing the data collected in order to reach conclusions about the research question. Numerical analysis of data is central to quantitative studies. The data collected is converted to numerical values in a variety of ways. Table 21–4 defines levels of measurement and provides examples. The level of measurement has implications for the statistical procedures applied.

Statistical procedures used for correlational and experimental or quasi-experimental studies can be classified as parametric or nonparametric. Parametric tests are more powerful and preferred because they permit inferences to be made from findings of the study sample to the larger population. Use of parametric procedures requires that the following assumptions be met: random selection of the sample; variables that are normally distributed among the study groups; and measurement of the dependent variable(s) at an interval level.

Nonparametric statistics are used in situations when the following characteristics are evident: small sample size; normal distribution of variables in the sample cannot be assumed; parameters of the population are unknown; and the level of measurement of variables is at a nominal or ordinal level.

The selection of an appropriate statistical proce-

TABLE 21–4   LEVELS OF MEASUREMENT

Type	Definitions	Examples
Nominal	Discreet categories of data that do not have any implied order	Gender: male/female Breastfed/not breastfed Marital status
Ordinal	Assigned categories of data that can be ranked in order, but intervals between categories are not equal	Most Likert-type scales Infant breastfeeding assessment scale (Matthews, 1991) Pain perception scale (Hewat & Ellis, 1986)
Interval/ratio	Categories of data that are ordered and are equal distances apart Ratio also has a known zero point	Body temperature Blood pressure Weight or length Duration of breastfeeding measured in specified days or weeks

dure is dependent on the type of study, sample size, sampling procedure, and type of data for analysis. Table 21–5 indicates commonly used procedures for study type and level of data. In experimental or quasi-experimental studies, the level of data of concern is the dependent variable. The purpose of the table is to assist research novices to recognize the appropriate use of statistics for reviewing studies. Extensive knowledge about statistical procedures is beyond the scope of this chapter.

There is controversy regarding the use of interval and ordinal data. Human feelings and perceptions do not fit the interval scale; most psychosocial variables can only be superimposed on an ordinal scale. Therefore, statistical procedures that traditionally require interval data are often used in human research with ordinal data.

Descriptive studies. Data collected to describe variables and their relationships are generally subjected to content analysis and descriptive statistics. Content analysis consists of examining the data, identifying similar content or meanings, and classifying those that are identified into mutually exclusive categories. These nominal data then can be used with the descriptive statistics identified in Table 21–5. Findings may be reported as frequency counts, percentages, or modes; they may be displayed in graphs, histograms, or contingency tables as shown in Table 21–6.

Contingency tables illustrate the relationships between variables and form the basis for determining the difference between groups using a statistical procedure known as chi-square.

Correlational studies. Correlational coefficients are statistical procedures for determining the relationship between two variables. The type of relationship is reported as positive (as one variable increases so does the other) or negative or inverse (as one variable increases the other decreases). The strength of the relationship is reported as a number between 1 and –1; stronger relationships are near 1 (positive) or –1 (negative), and 0 indicates no relationship. (See Table 21–5 for specific procedures.)

Experimental/quasi-experimental studies. The type of statistical procedure used to determine differences between groups depends on the number of groups and the level of measurement of the dependent variable, as shown in Table 21–5. Statistical differences are calculated using probability theory. Before analysis, the investigator decides on a level of significance—or a "p-value"—that will be used to accept that a statistically significant result indicates true differences between groups. The p-value reflects the possibility that the statistical result can occur by chance. In most breastfeeding research, a p-value of .05 is used. This indicates that the probability of a chance occurrence is 5 out of 100 (or 1 out of 20).

Multivariate analysis. Multivariate analysis is the concurrent analysis of three or more variables to

TABLE 21–5   USE OF APPROPRIATE STATISTICS FOR TYPE OF STUDY AND LEVEL OF DATA

Study Type	Statistical Procedure for Level of Data			
	Nonparametric	Data level	Parametric	Data level
Descriptive				
One variable	Frequency count	Nominal		
	Percentage	Ordinal		
	Mode	Nominal		
	Median	Ordinal		
	Mean	Interval		
	Standard deviation	Interval		
Two or more variables	Contingency table	Nominal		
	Cross tabulation	Nominal		
	Chi-square	Nominal		
Correlational	Spearman's Rho	Ordinal	Pearson-r	Interval
	Kendall's Tau	Ordinal		
Experimental/Quasi-Experimental				
Difference between two independent groups	Median test	Ordinal	t-test (independent sample)	Interval*
	Mann-Whitney U	Ordinal		
Difference between two dependent groups, e.g., pre-, posttests	Wilcoxon signed-rank	Ordinal	t-test (dependent sample)	Interval*
	McNemar chi-square	Nominal		
Difference among more than two groups	Chi-square	Nominal	ANOVA (F-test)	Interval*
	Kruskal-Wallis	Ordinal		
	Friedman test	Ordinal		

*Level of data of dependent variable

determine patterns of relationships between variables (Roberts & Burke, 1989). These advanced statistical procedures are suitable for studying complex phenomena, such as the various elements that can be associated with breastfeeding. As research of this topic increases in sophistication, the use of multivariate procedures is becoming more frequent. The procedures encountered include: multiple regression; path analysis; factor analysis; discriminant analysis; canonical correlation; and multivariate analysis of

TABLE 21–6   CONTINGENCY TABLE OF FEEDING MODE AND LABOR AND DELIVERY HIGH-RISK FACTORS AT THREE MONTHS POSTPARTUM*

High-risk factor present**	Feeding mode		
	Breast only	Not breast only	Total
Yes	13 (28)	33 (52)	46 (42)
No	33 (72)	31 (48)	64 (58)
Total	46 (42)	64 (58)	110 (100)

x^2 (1 df) = 5.96, $p < .05$
Note: Numbers in brackets are percentages.
*Data derived from a study conducted by Ellis and Hewat (1984).
**High-risk labor and delivery factors are: meconium staining, fetal heart aberrations, pre-eclampsia, infection, and malpresentation.

variance (MANOVA). Their use is appropriate for correlational and experimental studies of large numbers. Generally, interval level data are required.

RESULTS, DISCUSSION, AND CONCLUSIONS

Study results or findings should be clear, concise, and congruent with the research question(s) asked and the methodology used. The presentation of results varies for the type of study conducted. Qualitative studies are descriptive narratives which include participants' verbatim accounts that provide evidence of the researcher's data interpretations. The results may be rich descriptions of the study phenomenon, hypothetical propositions generated from the data, or a theory.

Quantitative studies frequently use tables and graphs to display results. Variables examined in descriptive studies should be precisely described, and responses should be numerically reported. Relationships of variables investigated in correlational studies and the procedures used to determine relationships must be clear. In studies that test hypotheses, the statistical procedures used, the results, and the decision for rejection or acceptance of the hypothesized relationships must be evident for each hypothesis stated. Significant, nonsignificant, and unexpected results must be reported. Findings in studies that are not what the investigator anticipates also contribute knowledge about the study topic; they can be an impetus for asking more relevant or more detailed research questions.

Interpreting study results is an intellectual process that gives meaning to the study (Burns & Grove, 1987). The investigator considers the study results with regard to the study process as well as findings from other studies that support or contradict current results. These can be addressed with the presentation of the results or separately in a section discussing the findings.

Limitations of a study are acknowledgements of factors that may affect study outcomes. Compromises are often necessary in the study process for pragmatic and ethical reasons. These can bring about weaknesses in design, sampling process, sample size, methods of data collection, or data analysis techniques. The extent to which study findings can be generalized to populations beyond the study sample should also be discussed. Stating limitations assists readers to evaluate the scientific merits of the study and enhances the credibility of the investigator.

Conclusions are concise statements that reflect the synthesis of the findings; they provide an overall account of the importance of the study and an understanding of the phenomenon in question. The conclusions must be pertinent to the findings and not expanded beyond the study parameters. Following the conclusions, implications of the findings for clinical practice are generally described, and suggestions for further research are identified.

EVALUATING RESEARCH REPORTS AND ARTICLES FOR USE IN PRACTICE

Evaluation is an analytical appraisal that makes judgments about the scientific merits of a study (Wilson, 1989). The analysis objectively addresses the study's strengths and weaknesses, poses questions about the research, and makes constructive recommendations. Purposes for evaluating studies include determining if study findings are useful for clinical decision-making, deciding if clinical practice should change, or concluding whether further study of a topic is indicated.

The process of evaluation starts with reading the research report or journal article several times to become familiar with the study. Analysis of the research elements can then proceed. Information in this chapter is a base for understanding the research process as well as expectations for research approaches and specific methodologies. A key issue in evaluation is that all components of the study are congruent with one another. This means that the following conditions are met: the design is consistent with the research question; sampling procedures and methods of data collection are compatible with the design; analysis is suitable for the type of data collected; and the findings answer the research question. Table 21–7 provides questions to ask when evaluating both qualitative and quantitative studies. Although not exhaustive, the guidelines will assist with the systematic review of studies.

Following examination of the research elements, the reviewer identifies the strengths and weaknesses of the study. All studies have flaws (Burns & Grove, 1987); therefore, weaknesses are considered in rela-

TABLE 21–7 GUIDELINES FOR EVALUATING QUANTITATIVE AND QUALITATIVE STUDIES

General Guidelines	Quantitative Studies	Qualitative Studies
1. Problem and purpose		
Clearly stated?	Provides direction for study?	Broadly stated?
Amenable to scientific investigation?		Exploratory?
Significant to breastfeeding?		
2. Review of literature		
Pertinent?	Includes recent and classic references?	Primary purpose is to acknowledge the existence of (or the lack thereof) literature on the topic?
Well organized?	Theoretical base or conceptual framework evident?	
3. Protection of human rights		
Subject's protection from harm ensured?		
Subjects suitably informed, e.g., by an informed-consent document?		
Study reviewed by ethics board or committee?		
Means for ensuring privacy, confidentiality, or anonymity are explained?		
4. Method		
Design congruent with research question?	Deductive approach?	Inductive approach?
Sampling procedure appropriate for research method?	Variables identified and defined?	Key informants are selected?
Method of data collection relevant for design?	Sample representative of population and adequate in size?	Theoretical sampling is addressed?
	Measuring tools suitable, reliable, and valid?	Data collection and analysis concurrent?
	Control of extraneous variables is evident?	Process for data collection and analysis described?
		Data saturated?
		Reliability and validity explained?
5. Results and discussion		
Analysis suitable for method and design?	Statistical procedures used suitable for data and sample size?	Examples of informants' accounts displayed?
Results clearly presented?	Tables clear and represent the data?	Rich descriptions or theory presented?
Interpretations clear and based on data?	Successful and unanticipated results reported?	Findings compared with literature?
Research question answered?		Theory logical and complete?
Limitations of study identified?		
Conclusions based on results?		
Implications for practice and research described?		

tion to how they affect outcomes and the overall meaning of the study. Judgments are made regarding the relevancy of knowledge generated and the usefulness of findings to clinical practice. Legitimate criticisms of a study should be presented with rational and constructive recommendations. Evaluation of studies is a skill that develops with practice, in-

creased knowledge and understanding of the research process, and awareness of studies related to a specific topic.

Research articles published in professional journals are the most common source of research reports. The limitations, particularly the length of the report, must be considered in the appraisal. Journal articles lack the detail of accounts of full research. Studies in refereed journals are subject to review before publication. Members of journal review boards, generally considered to be experts in the field, critique articles to judge them for their scientific merit and make recommendations regarding whether they are publishable. The beliefs that members of review boards have regarding the scientific value of qualitative research can influence publication of these kinds of studies. Recognition of qualitative research is recent, and publication of studies is gradually increasing, particularly in some of the nursing journals.

Breastfeeding encompasses many disciplines in the natural, social, and health sciences; therefore, breastfeeding practitioners must consult numerous and varied journals to keep current with new knowledge. Although a challenging task, it is essential for professional practice.

UTILIZATION OF RESEARCH IN CLINICAL PRACTICE

Implementing research findings into clinical practice is a challenge for researchers and practitioners. This will be accomplished more quickly by teamwork. Researchers can assist in the following ways:

- disseminating study findings directly to practitioners as soon as a study is completed
- encouraging practitioners to participate in research to develop interest and awareness
- listening to concerns about practice in order to generate problems for study that are relevant to a specific practice area
- assisting practitioners with evaluation of research articles.

The latter can enhance practitioners' knowledge about the research process and their confidence in judging research findings.

Practitioners have a responsibility to facilitate research. Accomplishing this includes:

- developing a questioning attitude and openness to change
- sharing concerns about practice with researchers to develop pertinent clinical studies
- critically reading and evaluating research arti-

cles and then utilizing relevant findings in practice
- telling other clinicians about study findings that assist practice.

Table 21–8 illustrates how findings from a qualitative, a quasi-experimental, and a correlational study can be applied to clinical practice.

Further research is indicated for all of the studies serving as examples in Table 21–8. However, utilizing the findings suggested will enhance care today. Scientific knowledge related to breastfeeding practice is in an early stage of development; the majority of published studies are descriptive, exploratory, and correlational. Few studies test interventions specific to clinical practice. Findings from many current studies are relevant, however, and can be applied to practice. It is important to try new methods and approaches, to question their effect, and to develop new studies. Through such an ongoing process knowledge will be expanded, and optimum practice will be facilitated. And mothers, infants, families, and society will all benefit.

SUMMARY

Research is a process for developing knowledge that is a base for accountable and responsible practice. Two approaches to conducting research are qualitative and quantitative methodologies. The research question asked—and whether knowledge is generated inductively or deductively—directs the approach used.

Qualitative methods generate an understanding of the "meaning" that reflect human values, beliefs, practices, and life experiences or events. Three types of qualitative methods are phenomenology, ethnography, and grounded theory. Characteristics of quantitative methods are objectivity, measurement, and control. Descriptive, correlational, experimental, and quasi-experimental studies use quantitative methods. Simultaneous use of qualitative and quantitative methods in one study is known as triangulation.

The major elements of research are the research problem and purpose, the review of literature, protection of human subjects, methodology, and results and discussion. The research problem identifies "what" is studied and with "whom," and the purpose

TABLE 21–8   APPLYING RESEARCH FINDINGS TO PRACTICE

Study Title	Sample	Major Findings	Application to Practice
The emotional experience of breast expression (Morse & Bottorff, 1988).	61 mothers, successful breastfeeders, well educated.	Breast expression is difficult and is a learned skill.	Hands-on assistance with breast expression is necessary. Information alone is not sufficient.
		Women have positive or negative feelings about breast expression.	Sensitivity to women's feelings about expression is essential. If negative, insisting she express may lead to feelings of failure and inadequacy. If positive, assistance is required.
A comparison of the effectiveness of two methods of nipple care (Hewat & Ellis, 1987).	23 breastfeeding women; own control; therefore, 46 breasts compared. Women followed for 10 days postpartum.	Women's perceptions of nipple pain and nipple trauma are the same when expressed breast milk (EBM) or lanolin is applied postfeeding.	For women who wish to apply a substance to nipples when breastfeeding, the effect of EBM and lanolin is similar.
		Positive *association* between nipple trauma and engorgement.	Prevention of engorgement is advised to decrease possibility of nipple trauma.
		75% of women did not have their breasts examined by a health professional during pregnancy.	Educate health professional to examine breasts/nipples during pregnancy. Advise women of results of assessment.
Infant feeding and childhood cancer (Davis, Savitz & Graubard, 1988).	201 children, 1.5–15 years, with cancer were compared with 181 controls.	An *association* between childhood cancer and infant feeding; those artificially fed and breastfed for short duration have increased risk of cancer compared with those breastfed for six months or more.	Awareness of this *potential* benefit of breastfeeding. Provide information to childbearing families and society of *possible* benefit.

delineates "why" the study is conducted. Research questions for quantitative methods are more specific than those of qualitative studies. In quantitative studies variables are delineated and operationally defined. How breastfeeding and the duration of breastfeeding are defined is of particular importance when conducting or evaluating studies.

Reviewing literature about a study topic assists in formulating the research problem and directs the research method. Qualitative methods are frequently used when little is known about a topic.

Research that involves human subjects must as-

sure the study participants of four basic rights. Mechanisms that assist in protecting subjects are use of an informed-consent form and evaluation of studies before they are conducted by ethical review boards or committees.

Study methods address setting, sample, data collection, and data analysis. The setting indicates the location of the study or the source of the participants. The sample is a subset of a larger population or group of individuals in whom the investigator is interested. Sampling is a process for selecting the sample from the population; two types are probability and nonprobability. Nonprobability sampling is used in all qualitative studies. Probability sampling is preferred in quantitative studies because findings can then be generalized from the study sample to the target population. This method requires random selection of subjects, which is not always possible; therefore, many quantitative studies involving human subjects also use nonprobability sampling.

Data are collected by the researcher asking questions, by making observations, and/or by measuring key variables identified in the research question. In-depth interviews and observations are the most common methods used for qualitative studies, and data collection and analysis occur simultaneously. Systematic and rigorous methods for collecting and analyzing data are developed for all qualitative methods. Methods for data collection in quantitative studies are highly structured and must be the same for every subject.

Reliability and validity are issues that must be addressed for all research. Reliability refers to accuracy, consistency, precision, and stability of data collected; validity reflects the true meaning of data. In qualitative studies, which are often longitudinal in nature, checks are built into the data collection and analysis process. In quantitative studies, reliability of measurement tools and investigators collecting data can be statistically estimated, as can the validity of the measurements used.

Data analysis is the process of organizing, summarizing, examining, and synthesizing the data collected to determine study findings. Qualitative studies generate rich descriptions and posit hypotheses and/or theory. Descriptive narratives of participants' verbatim accounts provide evidence of the investigator's interpretations. In quantitative studies, data are translated to numerical terms for statistical analysis. Depending on the type of study and the level of measurement of the data collected, a variety of statistical procedures can be employed. Results are displayed in tables and graphs.

Study results should be clear, concise, and congruent with the method used, as well as answer the research question(s). Significant, nonsignificant, and unexpected results are reported. Limitations of the study and the extent to which findings can be generalized to additional populations must also be addressed. The study conclusions reflect the study findings and do not expand beyond the parameters of the study.

Research reports or articles are evaluated to make judgments about their scientific merit and the usefulness of findings for clinical practice. A key issue in evaluation is that all study components are congruent.

Implementing research findings into clinical practice is a challenge for researchers and practitioners. This process can be expedited if both work together. Although findings from current studies are not generally definitive and further study is frequently recommended, utilization of relevant findings in practice often serve to question effects and generate new studies. Breastfeeding research is an ongoing process that expands knowledge and facilitates optimal practice for the benefit of mothers, infants, families, and society.

GLOSSARY

Applied research: Research that focuses on solving or finding an answer to a clinical or practical problem.

Basic research: Research that generates knowledge for the sake of knowledge.

Bias: Any factor, action, or influence that distorts the results of a study.

Bivariate: Statistics derived from the analysis of the relationship between two variables.

Chi-square: A statistical procedure that uses nominal level data and determines significant differences between observed frequencies in relation to the data and expected frequencies.

Concept: A word, idea, or phenomenon that generally has abstract meaning.

Conceptual framework: A structure of interrelated concepts that may be generated inductively by qualitative research or provide a base for a quantitative study.

Construct: A cluster of several concepts that has abstract meaning.

Correlation coefficient: A statistic that indicates the degree of relationship between two variables. The range in value is $+1.00$ to -1.00; 0.0 indicates no relationship, $+1.00$ is a perfect positive relationship and -1.00 is a perfect inverse relationship.

Deductive reasoning: The process of reasoning from a general premise to the concrete and specific.

Dependent variable: The variable the investigator measures in response to the independent or treatment variable; the outcome variable that is affected by the independent variable.

Design: The blueprint or plan for conducting a study.

External validity: The extent to which study findings can be generalized to samples different from those studied.

Extraneous variable: Variables that can affect the relationship of the independent and dependent variables, i.e., interfere with the effect of treatment. In experimental studies, strategies for controlling these variables are built into the research design.

Independent variable: The experimental or treatment variable that is manipulated by the investigator to influence the dependent variable.

Inductive reasoning: The process of reasoning from specific observations or abstractions to a general premise.

Internal validity: The extent to which manipulation of the independent variable really makes a significant difference on the dependent variable rather than on extraneous variables.

Likert scale: A scale that primarily measures attitudes by asking respondents their degree of agreement or disagreement for a number of statements.

Nonparametric statistics: Statistical procedures used when required assumptions for using parametric procedures are not met.

Operational definition: Explicit description of a concept or variable of interest in measurable terms.

Parametric statistics: Statistical procedures used when a sample is randomly selected, represents a normal distribution of the target population, and is considered sufficiently large in size and interval level data are collected.

Population: The total set of individuals that meet the study criteria from which the sample is drawn and about whom findings can be generalized.

Reliability: The degree to which collected data are accurate, consistent, precise, and stable over time.

Sample: A subset of the population selected for study.

Sampling: The procedure of selecting the sample from the population of interest.

Target population: The population that is of interest to the investigator and about which generalizations of study results are intended.

Univariate: Statistics derived from analysis of a single variable, e.g., frequencies.

Validity: The degree to which collected data are true and represent reality; the extent to which a measuring instrument reflects what it is intended to measure.

Variable: Attributes, properties, and/or characteristics of persons, events, or objects that are examined in a study.

REFERENCES

American Nurses' Association: *Human rights guidelines for nurses in clinical and other research*, Kansas City, Mo., 1985.

Anderson, J: The phenomenological perspective. In Morse, JM, ed.: *Qualitative nursing research: A contemporary dialogue*, London, 1991, Sage Publications Ltd., pp. 25–38.

Armstrong, HC: International recommendations for consistent breastfeeding definitions, *J Hum Lact* 7:51–54, 1991.

Auerbach, KG, Renfrew, MJ, and Minchin, MA: Infant feeding comparisons: A hazard to infant health? *J Hum Lact* 7:63–71, 1991.

Brink, PJ: Issues of reliability and validity. In Morse, JM, ed.: *Qualitative nursing research: A contemporary dialogue*, London, 1991, Sage Publications Ltd., pp. 164–86.

Brink, PJ, and Wood, MJ: *Advanced design in nursing research*, London, 1989, Sage Publications Ltd., p. 18.

Burns, N, and Grove, SK: *The practice of nursing research: Conduct, critique and utilization*, Philadelphia, 1987, W.B. Saunders Co.

Canadian Nurses' Association: *Ethical guidelines for nursing research involving human subjects*, Ottawa, 1983.

Chapman, JC, et al.: Concerns of breast-feeding mothers from birth to 4 months, *Nurs Res* 34:374–77, 1985.

Chenitz, WC, and Swanson, JM: *From practice to grounded theory*, Menlo Park, Calif., 1986, Addison-Wesley Publishing Co., Inc., pp. 96–98.

Davis, MK, Savitz, DA, and Graubard, BI: Infant feeding and childhood cancer, *Lancet* 2(8607):365–68, 1988.

Ellis, DJ, and Hewat, RJ: Factors related to breastfeeding duration, *Can Fam Phys* 30:1479–84, 1984.

Ellis, DJ, Hewat, RJ, and Livingstone, V: Evaluation of the efficacy of a breastfeeding clinic in prolonging the duration of breastfeeding (research in progress), University of British Columbia, School of Nursing and Department of Family Practice, Vancouver, B.C., 1991.

Giorgi, A: Sketch of a psychological phenomenological method. In Giorgi, A, ed.: *Phenomenology and psychological research*, Pittsburgh, 1985, Duquesne University Press, pp. 8–22.

Graef, P, et al.: Postpartum concerns of breastfeeding mothers, *J Nurs-Midwif*, 33:62–66, 1988.

Field, PA, and Morse, JM: *Nursing research: The application of qualitative approaches*, Rockville, Md., 1985, Aspen Publishers, Inc., p. 16.

Hellings, PJ: Factors predicting breastfeeding success, Ph.D. diss. University of Oregon, 1984.

Hewat, RJ, and Ellis, DJ: Breastfeeding as a maternal-child team effort: Women's perceptions, *Health Care Wom Int* 5:437–52, 1984.

Hewat, RJ, and Ellis, DJ: A comparison of the effectiveness of two methods of nipple care, Birth 14:41–45, 1987.

Hewat, RJ, and Ellis, DJ: Similarities and differences between women who breastfeed for short and long duration, *Midwifery* 2:1–7, 1986.

Humenick, SS: The clinical significance of breastmilk maturation rates, *Birth* 14:174–81, 1987.

Jones, DA, West RR, and Newcombe, RG: Maternal characteristics associated with the duration of breast-feeding, *Midwifery* 2:141–46, 1986.

Kaufman, KJ, and Hall, LA: Influences of the social network on choice and duration of breast-feeding in mothers of preterm infants, *Res Nurs Health* 12:149–59, 1989.

Knafl, KS, and Breitmayer, J: Triangulation in qualitative research: Issues of conceptual clarity and purpose. In Morse, JM, ed.: *Qualitative nursing research: A contemporary dialogue*, London, 1991, Sage Publications Ltd., pp. 226–39.

Labbok, M, and Krasovec, K: Toward consistency in

breastfeeding definitions, *Stud Fam Plann,* 21:226–30, 1990.

Lynch, SA, et al.: Evaluating the effect of a breastfeeding consultant on the duration of breastfeeding, *Can J Public Health* 77:190–95, 1986.

Matthews, MK: Developing an instrument to assess infant breastfeeding behaviour in the early neonatal period, *Midwifery* 4:154–65, 1988.

Matthews, MK: Mothers' satisfaction with their neonates' breastfeeding behaviours, *JOGNN* 20:49–55, 1991.

Meier, P, and Anderson, GC: Responses of small preterm infants to bottle- and breast-feeding, *MCN* 12:97–105, 1987.

Morse, JM: Qualitative nursing research: A free-for-all? In Morse, JM, ed.: *Qualitative nursing research: A contemporary dialogue,* London, 1991a, Sage Publications Ltd., pp. 14–22.

Morse, JM: Strategies for sampling. In Morse, JM, ed.: *Qualitative nursing research: A contemporary dialogue,* London, 1991b, Sage Publications Ltd., pp. 127–44.

Morse, JM, and Bottorff, JL: The emotional experience of breast expression, *J Nurs-Midwif* 33:165–70, 1988.

Neander, WL, and Morse, JM: Tradition and change in the northern Alberta Woodlands Cree: Implications for infant feeding practices, *Can J Public Health* 80:190–94, 1989.

Nieswiadomy, RM: *Foundations of nursing research,* Norwalk, Conn., 1987, Appleton & Lange, p. 130.

Nunnally, JC: *Introduction to psychological measurement,* Toronto, 1978, McGraw-Hill Book Co., p. 245.

Polit, DF, and Hungler, BP: *Nursing research: Principles and methods* (4th ed.), Philadelphia, 1991, J.B. Lippincott Co.

Roberts, CA, and Burke, SO: *Nursing research: A quantitative and qualitative approach,* Boston, 1989, Jones and Bartlett Publishers, Inc.

Royal College of Nursing of the United Kingdom: *Ethics related research in nursing,* London, 1977.

Seaman, CHC: *Research methods: Principles, practice and theory for nursing,* Norwalk, Conn., 1987, Appleton & Lange, p. 111.

Shelley, SI: *Research methods in nursing and health,* Boston, 1984, Little, Brown & Co., p. 340.

Spiegelberg, H: *The phenomenological movement,* The Hague, 1960, Martinus Nijhoff, pp. 658–701.

Spradley, JP: *The ethnographic interview,* New York, 1979, Holt, Rinehart and Winston, pp. 3–5.

Spradley, JP: *Participant observation,* New York, 1980, Holt, Rinehart and Winston.

Stern, PN: Qualitative research: The nurse as grounded theorist, *Health Care Wom Int* 5:371–85, 1984.

Strauss, A, and Corbin, J: *Basics of qualitative research: Grounded theory procedures and techniques,* Newbury Park, Calif., 1990, Sage Publications Inc., pp. 24–32.

Tanaka, PA, Yeung, DL, and Anderson, GH: Health professionals as sources of infant nutrition information for metropolitan Toronto mothers, *Can J Public Health* 80:200–204, 1989.

Van Kaam, A: *Existential foundation of psychology,* New York, 1969, Doubleday & Co., Inc., pp. 325–30.

Wilson, HS: *Research in nursing* (2nd ed), Redwood City, Calif., 1989, Addison-Wesley Publishing Co., Inc.

Woods, NF, and Catanzaro, M: *Nursing research: Theory and practice,* St. Louis, 1988, The C.V. Mosby Co.

World Medical Association: *Declaration of Helsinki: Recommendations guiding doctors in clinical research,* New York, 1964.

ADDITIONAL READINGS

Munhall, PL, and Oiler, CJ: *Nursing research: A qualitative perspective,* Norwalk, Conn., 1986, Appleton-Century-Crofts.

Waltz, CF, Strickland, OL, and Lenz, ER: *Measurement in nursing research* (2nd ed.), Philadelphia, 1991, F.A. Davis Co.

22

Issues in Human Milk Banking

LOIS D. W. ARNOLD

A small population of infants and children depend on banked human milk for health and even survival. Therefore, health professionals need to know about banked human milk: its availability, its safety, its standardization as a product, and its merits and limitations.

This chapter focuses on milk banking as it is practiced in the United States and Canada for two reasons. First, information about milk banking in other countries is difficult to obtain as there is no parent organization to which all milk banks belong, nor is there any central repository for data on existing milk banks—where they are located, whom to contact, and type of operation. Often there is little or no government support for or policy regarding milk banking. Many milk banks exist as a result of the commitment of a particular individual or group of individuals. Second, issues for milk banks in emerging nations are different, and the establishment of milk banks in these countries according to the standards of milk banks in industrialized countries presents a number of problems. For a more detailed discussion of these issues and guidelines based on practical experience, the reader is referred to Narayanan (1982) and Narayanan, Prakash, and Gujral (1982).

HISTORY OF HUMAN MILK BANKING

In ancient civilizations wet nurses (women who breastfed a biologically unrelated child) were essential to the survival of infants whose mothers died in childbirth or postpartum or whose mothers were unable to breastfeed them for numerous reasons. The quality of milk from the nonbiological mother was of concern from earliest times. Rules governing wet-nursing can be found in the Code of Hammurabi (1800 B.C.). Wet nurses were carefully chosen for both physical attributes and personality characteristics, since these were presumed to be transmitted through the milk to the nursing infant (Fildes, 1986; Lawrence, 1989).

In eighteenth century Europe, foundling hospitals with a policy of routine dry-nursing (i.e., hand or artificial feeding) their infants had much higher rates of mortality than those hospitals which either wet-nursed their infants in the hospital or sent them out to supervised wet nurses in the countryside (Fildes, 1988). During the late nineteenth and early twentieth centuries in Europe and the United States, studies showed, without exception, that infants breastfed by their own mothers or wet nurses had lower mortality rates than artificially fed infants (Cunningham, 1981). The clear benefits of breastfeeding for infant health and the difficulties of formulating artificial infant milk spurred the development of human milk banks.

In the United States during the early twentieth century wet nurses were difficult to find. Consequently, two Boston physicians, Denny and Talbot, developed the idea of stockpiling human milk. Both were aware of a 1911 study in Boston which showed that bottle-fed babies were six times more likely to die of diarrhea and enteritis during the first year of life than were breastfed babies (Davis, 1913). Both were medical directors of the Massachusetts Infant Asylum, which employed wet nurses to feed sick foundlings. Both were concerned about the quality of the stored product (Golden, 1988). Before milk was banked, donors were screened for tuberculosis, syphilis, and other contagious diseases (Arnold & Erickson, 1988; Talbot, 1911). Advances in dairy technology also benefitted early milk banks. Freezing, pasteurization, sterilization, and lyophilization (freeze-drying) were used, with varying success, to lengthen storage time so that an even supply of uncontaminated milk could be guaranteed (Arnold & Erickson, 1988; Emerson & Platt, 1933; Scheuer & Duncan, 1936; Smith, 1942; Smith & Emerson, 1924). In 1943, the American Academy of Pediatrics (AAP) published its first recommendations for operating human milk banks (AAP, 1943).

After World War II, milk banking fell out of favor in the United States, as the acceptance and use of formula increased. In the 1970s, with rapid advances in neonatal intensive care and recognition that human milk provided special properties that improved survival and decreased complications, milk banking once again became popular, and milk banks were established in many hospitals across the country. In the mid-to-late 1980s milk banking once again declined in North America because of concerns about viral transmission, particularly the human immunodeficiency viruses, and because of the development of special formulas for premature infants. In 1985, the Human Milk Banking Association of North America was formed to facilitate communications among North American milk banks, present a united front in matters of policy, public and professional education, and work with governmental regulatory agencies.

Milk banking is still a common practice in parts of Europe, where artificial formulas have never had the same acceptance and widespread use in the feeding of premature infants that they have had in the United States (Balmer & Wharton, 1992; Baum, 1989; Roy & Lescop, 1979; Siimes & Hallman, 1979). While milk banks dwindle in number in the United States, many emerging countries in Central America and the Caribbean are developing numerous milk banks as part of national campaigns to promote breastfeeding and the benefits of breastmilk. Help with funding for equipment has come from the United Nations Children's Fund (UNICEF) in many cases (Canahuati, personal communication, 1991; Jelliffe, personal communication, 1991).

The World Health Organization (WHO) and the United Nations Children's Fund (UNICEF), in a joint resolution issued in 1980, stated:

> Where it is not possible for the biological mother to breastfeed, the first alternative, if available, should be the use of human milk from other sources. Human milk banks should be made available in appropriate situations.

WHO/UNICEF Joint Statement: Meeting on infant and young child feeding, *J Nurs-Midwif* 25:31–38, p. 33, 1980.

CULTURAL ISSUES

Some cultures object to donated human milk. Narayanan et al. (1980) note that Muslim women object to their babies receiving milk from Hindu women, although Hindu mothers report no similar objections to donor milk from mothers practicing other religions. The Koran treats milk as altered blood; children suckled by the same woman become blood relations or milk siblings, and they are forbidden to marry each other. Therefore, donor milk should come from mothers of a baby who is the same sex as the recipient, in order to avoid the possibility of incest from a consanguineous marriage (Baumslag, 1987; Kocturk, 1989). In the United States certain religious groups such as Jehovah's Witnesses refuse blood transfusions. Donor milk may fall into a similar category if it is fresh-raw or fresh-frozen, because milk that is not heat-treated may contain live cells that can be transferred from donor to recipient.

CLINICAL USES

Occasional references appear in the literature about the theoretical potential for a graft vs. host (GVH) reaction to donor milk by the recipient when fresh breastmilk is used. Young animals fed breastmilk white cells from a different species exhibit this type of reaction (AAP, 1980). However, this has not been shown to occur in humans. In Toronto, fresh breastmilk was dispensed for many years within 24 hours of collection, without freezing or pasteurizing, and no ill effects were observed (Xanthou, 1987). The successful wet-nursing and cross-nursing that have gone on throughout history would also appear to negate the GVH theory. It is interesting to note that the possibility of a GVH reaction is raised when one mother's milk is provided for use by a baby of another mother of the same species. However, the same issue is not raised in considering crossing species lines, as when bovine milk is given to the human infant.

During 1986, between 1,000 and 1,500 babies received banked donor milk in the United States and Canada (Oxtoby, 1988). Over 260,000 ounces were dispensed; 72% went to infants in neonatal intensive-care nurseries (NICUs), 23% to infants at home, and 2% to patients in pediatric units of hospitals (Arnold, 1988). These numbers represent only milk from distributing milk banks. They do not include small, in-house hospital milk banks set up for their own NICU patients; most of the stored milk in these units is that of the biological mother for use by her own infant.

In some NICUs, banked milk is used routinely for the first feedings. British Columbia Children's Hospital (Vancouver), and the Medical Center of Delaware (Wilmington) use banked milk in their premature nurseries when mothers' milk is unavailable (Arnold, 1991).

Low-birth-weight (LBW) and very low-birth-weight (VLBW) infants have different nutritional requirements than full-term infants because of the nutrient malabsorption secondary to immaturity of their digestive systems. The composition of milk from preterm mothers differs for about the first two weeks postpartum from that of term mothers. Milk from term mothers is believed to have levels of protein, calcium, and phosphorus that are insufficient for the needs of the premature infant (AAP, 1985). There has also been a long-standing debate on whether VLBW and LBW infants can achieve proper growth on banked milk. Yet healthy VLBW infants can achieve intrauterine growth rates on banked human milk (Garza, 1990). There are several different ways to meet these nutrient requirements while feeding human milk. Enfamil Human Milk Fortifier (powder), Similac Natural Care (liquid), MCT oil (medium-chain triglycerides) and Polycose (carbohy-

drates in liquid form) can be added (Davis, 1990). These may be added directly to the human milk or, in the case of Similac Natural Care, fed alternately with human milk. In this way the infant continues to benefit from the immunological components of human milk. This extra fortification is usually discontinued once the infant reaches between 1800 and 2000 grams. In the United States, vitamins and minerals are also routinely added to feedings for premature infants (Brady et al., 1986).

However, commercial human milk fortifiers have a whey-to-casein ratio of 60:40, whereas human milk has a whey-to-casein ratio of approximately 80:20 (Brady et al., 1986). Moreover, these human milk fortifiers are derived from cow's milk, which always carries the risk of triggering an allergic response.

Health professionals attending the 1986 annual meeting of the Human Milk Banking Association of North America (HMBANA) observed that nurseries which routinely use human milk, either mother's own or that of donors, for initial feedings of premature infants have a lower incidence of necrotizing enterocolitis (NEC). Until recently the published data on NEC and the protective role of human milk feedings have been conflicting. Barlow and colleagues (1974), using the rat as a model, showed that fresh rat milk was protective against intestinal *Klebsiella* colonization and subsequent NEC in rat pups who were exposed daily to hypoxic conditions. However, one cannot automatically extrapolate these findings to humans. Many of the human studies were flawed with confounding variables, and a protective effect of breastmilk against NEC in humans was not proven conclusively (Bradley, 1986; Kliegman, Pittard & Fanaroff, 1979).

Lucas and Cole (1990) conducted a prospective multicenter study on 926 premature infants to look at the effect of early diet on the development of NEC. They found that NEC was 6 to 10 times more likely to develop in exclusively formula-fed infants than in those infants fed only breastmilk, and NEC was three times more common when the exclusively formula-fed infants were compared to those receiving both breastmilk and formula. Furthermore, pasteurized donor milk was as protective as unheated maternal milk. Eibl et al. (1988) found that giving oral immunoglobulin to formula-fed infants was prophylactic against NEC. Lucas and Cole believe that breastmilk may protect against NEC by providing IgA to the lumen of the intestine. Most IgA remains intact in donor milk during the heat treatment process, and banked milk would continue to be effective prophylaxis.

Another important finding of Lucas and Cole's study was that among formula-fed infants delay in starting feedings was associated with a significant reduction in the incidence of NEC. This was not the case with infants fed breastmilk. These infants could start enteral feedings much earlier without serious consequences. With the decrease in the use of breastmilk, both maternal and donor, in British neonatal units, Lucas and Cole estimate that exclusive formula-feeding could account for approximately 500 extra cases of NEC each year and 100 extra infant deaths per year in the United Kingdom.

Donor milk also has been used in the treatment of immunoglobulin-A (IgA) deficiencies (Marinkovich, 1988). As little as four ounces per day of fresh donor milk has supplied enough IgA to patients who are deficient in this immunoglobulin to combat allergic reactions. If milk is heat-treated, additional volume must be prescribed to compensate for the partial loss of IgA during heat treatment. Banked milk has also been used in patients with immunodepressed states related to bone marrow transplants or leukemia therapy (Asquith et al., 1987). Asquith also reports the use of banked milk in the treatment of such diseases as intractable diarrhea, gastroenteritis, ulcerative colitis, infantile botulism, sepsis, and pneumonia.

Banked milk is more commonly used for its nutritional properties and has been used in cases of malabsorption and several feeding intolerance conditions (Asquith et al., 1987). Malabsorption is a well-recognized complication of neonatal surgery. Banked milk is beneficial following surgery to repair NEC damage as well as following surgery for congenital anomalies of the gastrointestinal tract, such as gastroschisis, tracheoesophageal fistulas, intestinal atresia, intestinal obstruction, anorectal abnormalities, and diaphragmatic hernias (Rangecroft, de San Lazaro & Scott, 1978; Riddell, 1989).

Banked milk has been given to severely burned patients. The Central Massachusetts Regional Milk Bank supplied milk to an infant who was burned over 90% of his body. Although the infant died, the physician in charge of the case reported that the infant did very well on the banked milk (Erickson, personal communication, 1990). The benefits were both nutritional and immunological. Burn victims have an increased metabolism and thus greater energy requirements, but they do not metabolize glucose efficiently. They also have a high risk of sepsis and, therefore, need more immune factors. Finally, they lose nitrogen through their open wounds and need higher amounts of protein. Human milk provides lactose as a more easily metabolized energy source, in addition to providing protein, immunoglobulins, and bacteriostatic protection. Animal models show that complications from stress ulcers are fewer when elemental formulas (e.g., formulas that have fats, proteins, and carbohydrates broken down into their simplest elements) are added to the diet of burn victims (Young, Motil & Burke, 1981). Elemental formulas are formulated for adults (Brady et al., 1986), however, and are not meant for long-term pediatric use. Therefore, it would be better to use easily digestible human milk in pediatric burn cases, rather than risk stressing the child's intestinal tract with hyperosmolar elemental formulas.

Banked milk has also been used in cases of inborn errors of metabolism. In a rare case of molybdenum cofactor deficiency in Colorado, donor milk was the optimum feeding for this fatal condition because of its 1:1 ratio of methionine to cystine and the occurrence of these two amino acids in lesser amounts than in formula (Yannicelly, personal communication, 1991).

Other uses of human milk have been noted as well, e.g., as treatment for conjunctivitis and as food for the aged (Baumslag, 1987, 1991). The Centers for Disease Control (CDC) used breastmilk as a medical therapeutic in American Samoa during an outbreak of hemorrhagic conjunctivitis when they ran out of medicine (Baumslag, 1991). Human milk was also used in ancient India during eye and ear surgeries; it was used in eleventh-century Turkey for the treatment of ophthalmia.

CURRENT PRACTICE

The Human Milk Banking Association of North America (HMBANA), in consultation with the United States Food and Drug Administration (FDA), developed guidelines to standardize milk bank operations. These guidelines are presented in Appendix 22-1 and are being used as the basis for regulation of milk banking by the FDA. For comparison of North

American practices with those of two Scandinavian milk banks, see Tully (1991).

DONOR SELECTION AND SCREENING

In the early days of milk banking, mothers were paid for their milk by the ounce. They were also sometimes provided with transportation funds so that they could come to the milk bank to express their milk. In this way milk banks had control over the cleanliness of the mother and her expression technique and could ensure that the milk was not adulterated in any way (Chapin, 1923; Jones, 1928). The earliest guidelines (AAP, 1943; MacPherson & Talbot, 1939) include payment to mothers. MacPherson and Talbot's guidelines also include a test using a 0.25% aqueous solution of Nile blue sulfate to detect dilution or substitution of cow's milk by determining chloride content (Talbot, 1927; MacPherson & Talbot, 1939). Jones wrote that the Detroit milk bank checked the specific gravity of the milk to test for adulteration.

The current guidelines discourage payment of donors. Since the guidelines are patterned after blood-bank policies, most milk banks do not pay women for their milk, the exception being the Mothers' Milk Bank in Wilmington, Delaware. Established in 1947 when payment was a practice that was accepted in the AAP guidelines, the Wilmington milk bank continues to offer nominal payment, although most mothers will not accept it (Langerak & Arnold, 1991). For milk banks founded in the 1970s out of a strong sense of volunteerism, payment has never been an issue. Some countries in Europe continue to pay their "donors" (Tully, 1991). Williams et al. (1985) offer two reasons why mothers should not be paid: (1) to avoid the need for surveillance of milk for water dilution and/or addition of cow's milk; and (2) to assure that the mother's own infant is receiving adequate nutrition and not being deprived of milk in order that the mother earn more money. Concern about the health of the donor's infant has been in the literature since Talbot's time.

Donors are lactating mothers, usually of healthy term infants. Mothers of premature infants will often donate their excess pumped milk, although some milk banks do not use this milk until the donor's infant is either discharged or is nursing well. Occasionally, a mother whose baby has died will donate milk that she pumps as she is gradually decreasing lactation, at the same time working through the grieving process by helping another infant. One mother in Hawaii who had given her baby up for adoption also donated milk for a time. Donors are recruited from childbirth classes, breastfeeding support groups, and physicians' offices, as well as by newspaper articles publicizing a need for a specific infant and word of mouth from other donors.

FROM THE NEWS
BABIES DEPLETING HOSPITAL'S SUPPLY OF MOTHERS' MILK

Two-month-old Aaron Miki and other babies are guzzling the milk supply at the Hawaii Mother's Milk Bank at an alarming rate. Aaron is allergic to baby formula. His mother, Charlotte, is taking medication for an illness and cannot breastfeed. So they rely on the milk bank at Kapiolani Women's and Children's Medical Center. Since he was born, Aaron has consumed nearly 1500 ounces—$11\frac{1}{2}$ gallons—of milk from the bank, drastically reducing the supply there. Last month 1400 ounces of milk were doled out, said Lois Arnold, assistant administrator. That, plus the demand during the past two weeks, has left the milk bank with only 200 ounces. "We're supposed to maintain at least 500 ounces at all times," Arnold said. But because the bank depends on donations of milk from mothers who are breastfeeding their babies, it is not easy to keep an adequate supply on hand. Infants who need to use donor milk include those who are allergic to baby formula and whose mothers cannot breastfeed. Babies born prematurely may need a booster dose of banked milk because their mothers may not be able to supply an adequate amount.

Ambrose, J: Babies depleting hospital's supply of mothers' milk, *Honolulu Star-Bulletin*, August 14, 1984, p. A–3.

Definitions of Different Human Milk Preparations

Fresh-raw milk	Milk stored continuously at approximately 4°C for not longer than 72 hours following expression.
Fresh-frozen milk	Fresh-raw milk that has been frozen and held at approximately −20°C for less than 12 months.
Heat-treated milk	Fresh-raw and/or fresh-frozen milk which has been heated to not less than 56°C and held for 30 minutes—sometimes referred to as Holder Pasteurization.
Pooled milk	Milk from more than one donor.

All donors must be healthy and are screened for use of tobacco and alcohol, over-the-counter as well as prescription medications, and illegal drugs. Because the heterosexual population is increasingly at risk for HIV, it is critical that potential donors be serum-screened for HIV antibody (WHO, 1987). The issue of how often to serum-screen donors remains to be resolved because of the potentially long incubation period between exposure to the virus and the appearance of detectible antibodies in serum. Current recommendations are that long-term donors be rescreened every 6 months. Donors also must have negative serological tests for syphilis and hepatitis-B antigen. If a donor or member of her immediate family becomes ill, donations are temporarily halted at the discretion of the milk-bank coordinator.

Donors sign forms permitting the release of medical information from their physicians and forms releasing their milk to the milk bank. The latter allow the milk bank to dispense the donated milk to patients in need, or to release it for research purposes if the milk is unacceptable for human use.

HEAT TREATMENT

The FDA and the CDC recommend that all banked human milk be heat-treated. (See the following boxed list of definitions of human milk preparations.) Fresh-frozen milk is provided only for patients whose conditions necessitate milk which has not been heat-treated. An additional consent form which releases the milk bank from liability may be required of the recipient's family.

When a milk bank heat-treats milk, the frozen milk is first thawed and the contents of several containers

pooled. Most milk banks pool the milk of up to five donors to make up a batch. Pooling mixes milks of various fat concentrations to assure a more even concentration of fat from one batch to another (AAP, 1980). Banked milk can be sampled to determine the fat concentration by use of the creamatocrit. The test is simple, inexpensive, and accurate (Lemons, Schreiner & Gresham, 1980; Lucas et al., 1978).

Heat treatment destroys bacteria and viruses as well as some useful constituents of human milk. Finding the optimal temperature for heat-treating donor milk to assure destruction of harmful bacteria and viruses, while preserving as many of the properties of the milk as possible, was the goal of research commissioned by the FDA in 1989 and 1990. Human milk was spiked with various concentrations of either cell-free HIV or HIV-infected cells. Samples were heated for 30 minutes at 56°C or at 62.5°C, using the protocol in the HMBANA guidelines. Destruction of the virus was rapid at both temperatures, and no virus could be recovered through reculturing after processing at either temperature (McDougal, 1990). As new viruses are identified, it will be important to assess each virus individually for its viability in heat-treated banked milk.

Wallingford (1987) extensively reviewed studies of heat treatment methods; a summary of his findings on the effects of heat treatment at 62.5°C on antiinfective agents is presented in Table 22–1. At high temperatures, much of the bacteriostatic effect of human milk is destroyed, decreasing the benefit to the patient and making it more susceptible to later contamination (Bjorksten et al., 1980; Ford et al., 1977; Wills et al., 1982).

The effects of freezing, heating, and handling of

TABLE 22–1 EFFECTS OF HOLDER PASTEURIZATION* ON ANTIINFECTIVE AGENTS IN HUMAN MILK

Agent	Range of Survival (%)
Cells	None to 78% macrophages
Immunoglobulins	
Immunoglobulin A (IgA)	39–100
Immunoglobulin G (IgG)	66–86
Immunoglobulin M (IgM)	None to "substantial loss"
Enzymes	
Lactoperoxidase	53
Lipase	45
Protease	27
Lysozyme	61–105
Lactoferrin	27–44
Bile salt-stimulated lipase	None
Other	
Nonimmunoglobulin	Stable
Complement (C1–C9)	None
Lactobacillus bifidus growth factor	Stable
Thermostable lipid	Stable
Antiprotozoal activity	Some stability

*Milk held at 62.5°C for 30 minutes.
Derived from Wallingford, 1987.

human milk are cumulative. For example, Garza, Hopkinson, and Schanler (1986) report that freezing affects lipids in human milk by breaking down fat globule membranes, decreasing the size of the fat globules, and therefore increasing the surface available for lipase activity. This may lessen the digestibility and availability of fat to the patient. Heat treatment additionally alters other nutrients. Some immunological potency is lost during freezing, which destroys living cells in the milk. When previously frozen milk is heat-treated, further loss of immunoglobulins occurs. Even with this loss of bacteriostatic activity, some of the antiinfective properties remain intact, and the nutrients provided are still the most appropriate for the human infant.

Milk lipids have been shown to have antiviral activity against enveloped viruses, including HIV. McDougal (1990) noted this in spiked milk samples that sat on the counter as controls while other samples were being heat-treated. Isaacs and Thormar (1990) state that the appearance of this antiviral activity is lipoprotein-lipase dependent and occurs only in stored milk in which the lipase has had a chance to break lipids down into free fatty acids. The activity of the free fatty acids is cumulative (the more that are present, the more effective the antiviral activity), and viral killing is rapid when the free fatty acids come into contact with the envelope of the virus. In cases such as HIV infection, in which the virus may be found in the acellular fraction of the milk as well as the cellular fraction, these antiviral lipids may reduce the risk of viral transmission by destroying the free virus. The authors state that banked milk which has had the cellular portion lysed but retains its lipid antiviral potential may actually be less infectious than milk in which the cellular component remains intact.

Again using the HMBANA protocol for heat treatment, Eitenmiller (1990) looked at the effects of heat treatment on IgA, lactoferrin, lysozyme, and folic acid in samples of banked milk spiked with *Escherichia coli* and *Staphylococcus aureus* as bacterial markers. He found that enzymes and vitamins were much more stable than bacterial cells. His results are in general agreement with the results presented in Tables 22–1 and 22–2 (Wallingford, 1987). Eitenmiller found that the majority of vitamins are relatively stable at 56°C and 62.5°C; he also found that the loss rate is much more dependent on oxidation than on temperature. However, if milk is deaerated to preserve vitamins, more IgA and lactoferrin are lost. Since vitamin supplements are routinely given in intensive-care nurseries, opting for more lactoferrin and IgA would be the wiser choice.

Standard practice among milk banks has been Holder Pasteurization— rapidly heating the milk to 62.5°C and holding it at that temperature for 30 minutes. Based on the results of McDougal's and Eitenmiller's work, the HMBANA has amended its guidelines to make 56°C the lowest acceptable temperature for heat treatment. Some bacteriostatic properties will continue to be sacrificed in favor of being assured of viral and bacterial decontamination.

The use of lyophilization and irradiation to reduce bacterial and viral contamination has been explored. However, early reports indicate that both these methods also lower the concentration of immune substances (Liebhaber et al., 1977; Raptopoulou-Gigi,

TABLE 22–2 EFFECTS OF PASTEURIZATION* ON NUTRIENTS AND GROWTH FACTORS

Component	Range of Survival (%)
Vitamins	
Vitamin A	103
Vitamin D	103
Vitamin E	106
Thiamin	65–100
Riboflavin	94
Niacin	100
Biotin	99
Vitamin B_6	88–105
Folic acid	60–69
Vitamin C	65–90
Pantothenic acid	93
Epidermal growth factors	Stable
Lipids	67
Fatty acids	Stable
Nitrogen	No effect on retention

*Milk held at 62.5°C for 30 minutes.
Derived from Wallingford, 1987.

Marwick & McClelland, 1977). Oxtoby (1988) reports that they may not be effective in destroying HIV.

Some patients require milk which has not been heat-treated. For these patients there is serum-screening and verbal history-taking to ensure a quality product. One such patient is Lacie Smith (see the following case study).

PACKAGING FOR HEAT TREATMENT

Different milk banks use varying types of containers for heat-treating milk. The Breast Milk Service in Vancouver, British Columbia, uses an Oxford Human Milk Pasteurizer* and the bottles produced for use with that machine. Other milk banks use constant-temperature water baths and disposable four-ounce sterile glass bottles with new caps purchased for heat treatment. These caps may be ordered from

Anchor Hocking.** Milk is then refrozen in the same bottles for dispensing or in "volufeeds" in feeding-size portions.

COLLECTION, HANDLING, AND STORAGE

Donors are carefully instructed in methods for clean collection, handling, storage, and transportation of their milk. Milk banks supply donors with sterile glass or plastic containers for milk collection. These are often the two-ounce graduated containers used in the NICU, or four-ounce sterile water bottles. The Community Human Milk Bank (Georgetown University Hospital) in Washington, D. C., supplies its donors with polypropylene specimen cups. The Central Massachusetts Regional Milk Bank (Worcester) and the Denver Mothers' Milk Bank (Denver) occasionally accept milk collected in disposable plastic bottle liners ("baggies"), but the Massachusetts center uses this milk only for older infants who do not require as clean a product as a premature infant. Disposable plastic bottle liners are not generally recommended because they puncture and tear easily, thereby increasing the risk of contamination during processing.

The type of container used to collect milk can also have an effect on immune substances. Garza, Hopkinson, and Schanler (1986) reported loss of IgA when polyethylene bags were used. Paxson and Cress (1979) reported loss of leukocytes in fresh milk when glass containers were used, as the cells adhered to the surface. Later studies indicated that live cells detached from the walls of the containers after a period of time, and that cell count was more affected by the length of storage than by container type (Goldblum et al., 1981). Current recommendations are that glass containers are the best choice for storing milk (Hopkinson, Garza & Asquith 1990). There is no perfect container for human milk other than its original package. Donors are instructed to freeze their milk immediately after expressing it to preserve the immunological and nutritional elements.

---

*In order to obtain an Oxford Human Milk Pasteurizer, contact: Colgate Medical Ltd., 1 Fairacres Estate, Dedworth Rd., Windsor, Berkshire SL4 4LE U.K.

**Anchor Hocking Packaging Company, Metal Closures Division, 70 Sewell St., Glassboro, NJ 08028. When ordering, ask for Item # 68–2–1073. The description number is 040–0472–Infant Formula Item 2–1002. These caps must be ordered by the case. Each case contains 2,800 caps.

VITAL BREASTMILK SUPPLY FOR CHILD IS LOW

Doctors thought in the beginning that if Lacie Lynette Smith could live past her third birthday, she'd probably overcome her unique allergy to foods and be able to eat like other kids. Unfortunately, their prediction hasn't panned out.

Lacie, who is now eight-years-old, continues to survive on thousands of donated ounces of breastmilk. It's a precious staple which means the difference between life and death for her, and the supply is getting dangerously low.

"During the past nine months, we've been dipping into our reserves heavily," said Phyllis, Lacie's mother. "To amass the great quantity of mother's milk necessary to sustain Lacie, it has taken a team effort of thousands to make sure the shipments continue. There's a constant turnover as nursing mothers go back to work . . . "

Originally diagnosed when she was five-weeks-old with a rare intestinal disorder which rendered her unable to digest the sugars in her food, Lacie has undergone hundreds of tests as doctors have tried to find a workable treatment for the illness. Not until she was five-years-old did they determine that she actually had a rare condition called hypogammaglobulaanemia [sic].

"Lacie was born with immune factors which are produced to react against anything which isn't human tissue," Phyllis said. "The enzymes in her body are blocked and antigen, which rejects foreign substances to the body, is produced when she tries to eat. This causes major complications such as malabsorption and rapid transport, intestinal disorders which can be fatal."

In the last couple of years, Lacie has undergone food trials, but they have always caused major complications.

"Research drugs throughout the world have been used in conjunction with many more conventional drugs on an alternating basis," Phyllis said. "Under a restricted and regimented basis, Lacie can on occasion have small amounts of various basic foods, but to do this she must use approximately 36 drugs to help cut down on her body's reaction to the food."

"She is kind of like someone on chemotherapy when she's undergoing the food trial process," Phyllis said. "The repercussions from the process are difficult to handle. This last time, from January to March, Lacie was diagnosed with 27 major infections."

Lacie has been close to death many times. From the time Phyllis was forced to stop breastfeeding her five-week-old daughter because of the medications she herself was taking, to now, Lacie has tried to tolerate every foodstuff advised by the doctors. All have been unsuccessful, and all have done great internal damage.

"She was bombarded with 60 foods and formulas when she went off the breastmilk the day I went home from the hospital," said Phyllis. "The doctor thought she was just having a typical reaction to formula, and we began trying different ones. So many foods at once overloaded her immune system and made her allergic to all foods."

As a last resort, they decided to put Lacie back on mother's milk and that's when they discovered breastmilk, technically human tissue, was the only foodstuff she could tolerate.

Jacobs, R: Vital breast milk supply for child is low, *The Daily Ardmoreite*, Ardmore, Okla., August 20, 1989, pp. 1A, 3A.

Differences in collection methods can also affect the nutrient content, especially the amount of fat. Milk that is passively collected from one breast while the infant feeds at the other (drip milk) is basically skim milk; it lacks the fat content of milk from a breast that is "emptied" by nursing or pumping. Drip milk tends to be more contaminated (Lawrence, 1989). Milk banks in the United States and Canada try to minimize this problem by using only expressed milk.

The San Jose Mothers' Milk Bank (San Jose, California) requires that its donors hand express their milk, thereby avoiding extra equipment that might harbor bacteria. Other milk banks allow their donors to use pumps. The Community Human Milk Bank (Washington, D.C.) loans an electric pump to each of its donors. Donors are taught how to sterilize hand pumps and the parts for battery and electric pumps that come in contact with the milk. Rubber-bulb hand pumps, such as the bicycle horn pump and the old Evenflo pump that attaches directly to a bottle, are not allowed because of the high risk of contamination from the bulb. (See Chapter 11 for details on breast pumps.)

PACKAGING AND TRANSPORT

Milk is usually packed in ice and placed in a picnic cooler. Blue ice also works well in keeping milk frozen.

Locally, milk is transported by volunteers. The Central Massachusetts Regional Milk Bank (Worcester) has established depots in communities throughout the state where donors can leave their frozen milk. Volunteers then transport the milk from the depot to the milk bank. In Hawaii, volunteer collectors were on-call in different neighborhoods to pick up donor milk and take it to the milk bank. Some donors deliver their own milk to the milk bank.

Milk can be shipped over great distances by bus or airline. For long-distance shipping of milk, dry ice is used. Containers may be insulated boxes used to transport blood, styrofoam coolers, or the type of insulated box used by chemical companies for shipping frozen chemicals. Milk packed in dry ice can be successfully sent from one area of the country to another by overnight shipping companies—the same as other frozen medical supplies. Businesses are sometimes willing to donate their services to transport milk. For many years, Aloha Airlines shipped milk free of charge from neighbor-island donors to Oahu—and from Oahu to neighbor-island recipients for the Hawaii Mother's Milk Bank. Delta, Eastern, United, Federal Express, and Air Life Line airlines have also donated their services to transport milk. The American Red Cross has assisted many times with the transport of milk.

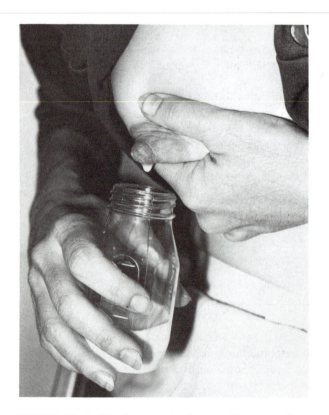

FIGURE 22–1. Hand expressing breastmilk into sterile container for the milk bank.

FUTURE TECHNOLOGICAL CHALLENGES

Recent advances in technology and new applications for established technology may have far reaching effects on the future of milk banking in the United States. Separating out constituents from cow's milk and adding them to human milk does not always give optimal results (Rumball, 1990). However, some researchers are applying the new process of lactoengineering to human milk with promising results. With lactoengineering, the components of human milk, such as protein, are fractionated and added to other human milks as fortifiers (Garza, Hopkinson & Schanler, 1986; Schanler, Garza & Nichols 1985). This technology may be important to patients in need of banked human milk.

The Hvidovre Milk Bank in Copenhagen, Denmark, has published results of a study using infrared analysis to measure protein, fat, and carbohydrate content of donor milk (Michaelsen et al., 1990). Individual milk donations can be analyzed and pooled to produce milks with the desired levels of proteins, fats, and carbohydrates to meet the requirements of premature infants.

Fat and fortifiers such as MCT oil can adhere to container walls and be lost (Mehta et al., 1988). This is an important issue when considering feeding methods, as fat adheres to the walls of the tubing used in gavage-feeding of premature infants (Stocks et al., 1985). (See Chapter 10 on high-risk infants.) Martinez and colleagues (1987) used ultrasonic homogenization of expressed milk to prevent fat from adhering to feeding tubes. Premature Brazilian infants with an average birthweight of 1400 grams were fed pasteurized, ultrasonically homogenized banked milk; they gained an average of five grams per day more than their counterparts receiving the same milk which had not been ultrasonically homogenized (Martinez, 1989). The group receiving the treated milk also had significantly greater gains in length, tricipital skinfold, and subscapular skinfold (Raiol et al., 1989). Furthermore, they achieved intrauterine growth rates, and hospital stays were shortened (Martinez, 1989).

Patients could derive great benefits from the improved nutrition that could be achieved as these techniques become a routine part of milk processing.

QUALITY ASSURANCE

Both donors and milk are screened to assure a safe product. The use of such tests as the creamatocrit or infrared analysis will help to assure a standard of nutritional quality of banked human milk appropriate for pre-term infants.

BACTERIAL SCREENING

In order to assure the safety of banked human milk, bacteria counts are done after heat treatment. Some milk banks also sample and do a bacterial count on each donor's milk prior to heat treatment or dispensing if the milk is to be used raw. This indicates whether the donor needs further education in clean collection techniques, including methods of pump sterilization. When more than one donor's milk is pooled, the sample of milk to be tested for bacteria is taken from the pool so that it represents what is actually being dispensed. Acceptable bacterial levels are given in Appendix 22–1. Milk samples are sent to either state or city health departments or to hospital laboratories for analysis.

The Health Sciences Centre in Winnipeg, Manitoba, studied bacteriological screening to determine whether it actually reduced the amount of bacteria

ingested by premature infants fed raw human milk (Law et al., 1989). It found that infants fed raw expressed milk were often exposed to large numbers of coagulase-negative staphylococci, but were less frequently exposed to *S. aureus* and gram-negative aerobic bacteria. The authors concluded that there was no clinical advantage to screening milk, since study infants fed raw milk showed no ill effects from it; in addition, the risk of sepsis from ingesting contaminated milk was probably very low. They felt that efforts to place upper limits on acceptable bacterial levels were misplaced and that the focus should be on what type of human milk to feed premature infants—e. g., fresh, frozen, or heat-treated milk. Narayanan (1982) also notes that in her experience dispensing fresh or fresh-frozen banked milk in India there were no instances in which the donor milk could be implicated in the transmission of a disease—even when that milk contained potentially pathogenic organisms. In fact, the occurrence of infection was significantly less in those infants receiving this milk than in artificially fed infants.

ENVIRONMENTAL POLLUTANTS

There is little information available to guide administrators of milk banks on what levels of environmental contaminants are acceptable. When contaminants are found in banked milk, each exposure has to be considered on a case-by-case basis and in consultation with experts from the FDA, the Environmental Protection Agency (EPA), and the AAP.

In Hawaii in 1981, cow's milk became contaminated with the pesticide heptachlor. Pregnant and/or lactating mothers were exposed through their consumption of cow's milk and local dairy products. It was necessary for Hawaii Mother's Milk, Inc., to test all donor milk for heptachlor before dispensing it to make sure that the pesticide content was within safe limits set by the EPA. Testing continued until banking operations ceased in 1988.

POLICIES AND PROCEDURES

Milk banks have written policies and procedures governing their operations. Milk banks operated by hospitals, such as the Community Human Milk Bank at Georgetown University Hospital (Washington, D.C.), have their policies reviewed and updated annually. Consent forms and release forms, as well as publicity and appeals for new donors, must also pass an institutional approval process. Milk banks establish advisory boards whose members are called upon for their expertise and advice in such areas as infection control, nutrition, and the law.

Milk banks that are part of a hospital or medical research facility are legally covered by the umbrella of that facility's insurance. In the past, a few free-standing milk banks existed. For example, Hawaii Mothers' Milk, Inc., was a separate, nonprofit entity housed in space donated by a hospital, but it was not part of the hospital's administrative structure. One of the reasons for its demise was its inability to get general liability insurance because of the risk involved in milk banking. So-called "kitchen" milk banks, operated out of a coordinator's home, have also been uninsurable— even when they have followed all the procedures and adopted all the policies for safe milk banking.

COST CONTAINMENT AND SURVIVAL

Milk banks would not exist were it not for the large body of volunteers who donate and transport the milk, help with fundraising, write newsletters, or act as file clerks, receptionists, and telephone operators. Sometimes the coordinators themselves are volunteers who receive no reimbursement for their efforts.

Financial solvency is a concern for all milk banks. In a few cases, a milk bank's budget is a part of the overall hospital budget. Such is the case at the Mother's Milk Bank at Central Baptist Hospital in Lexington, Kentucky. Financial shortages are covered by the hospital because of the positive community image the milk bank creates for the hospital. Other milk banks would not exist if they did not pay their own way. The Milk Bank at Georgetown University Hospital supports itself with income from pump rentals and lactation consulting, and it has actually made a profit over the last several years (Hughes, personal communication, 1990). The San Jose Milk Bank writes its own budget, including an overhead figure of 44%, which is paid to its parent institution, the California Institute for Medical Research (Asquith, personal communication, 1990).

All banks charge a processing fee for milk, usually between $2.00 and $2.50 an ounce. Recipients are not charged for the milk but rather for the labor, supplies, and equipment costs involved in collecting and processing the milk. Third-party reimbursement sometimes covers the processing fee. The WIC program in Hawaii has covered the fee, and currently it does so in Colorado and New Mexico. Medicaid covers the fee for eligible babies in Colorado, New York, and Massachusetts. Some private insurers pay reimbursement, but they are more likely to do so when the banked milk is used as part of in-hospital patient care.

MARKETING STRATEGIES

Milk banks offer many services, not all of which generate income (Arnold & Asquith, 1991). Hotlines with paging availability on off hours—or direct assistance to mothers by lactation consultants— may not require fees for service. Many milk banks publicize their services through brochures placed in hospitals and physicians' offices. Some milk banks actively publicize their services with public service announcements and participation in health fairs. Members of the staff of the milk bank may be part of a United Way speakers' bureau and give talks about milk bank services to community groups. Publicity of this nature, although not specifically for fund-raising, may generate income as well as new donors.

Processing fees do not begin to cover the actual expense involved in getting milk from a donor to a recipient. Methods of raising money to meet this shortfall include sales of pumps and supplies; pump rentals; fees for lactation consulting done by the staff of the milk bank; grant monies from charitable foundations, the United Way, and state and local governments; membership dues; individual bequests; and other fund-raisers, such as T-shirt and poster sales. Such fund-raising events are often handled creatively. The Hawaii milk bank, for example, held silent auctions in conjunction with wine-tasting parties. The milk banks in San Jose, California, and Lexington, Kentucky, organized "strollerthons" patterned after the March of Dimes Walkathon, in which mothers pushed decorated strollers. In 1990, this event netted more than $14,000 for the San Jose milk bank (Asquith, personal communication, 1990). Other events have included bake sales, garage sales, and sales of discount-coupon books.

SUMMARY

The availability of donor human milk is essential to a small but needy population. Without it, some patients would not survive. For others, banked donor milk—instead of artificial formulas—may help prevent long-term medical problems. While many experts agree on the efficacy of donor milk as therapy, much of the data is still in anecdotal form and not well documented. Too often breastmilk is tried as a last resort when damage is already severe. When the child dies, it is seen as a failure of the breastmilk, not as a failure of previous therapy that has placed the child in a condition from which recovery is unlikely. Katie from Massachusetts is one such example. Katie was born with short-gut syndrome and could not tolerate formula. Trials of every specialized formula failed. At four months of age, hyperalimentation seemed to be the only answer. At nine months of age, Katie developed total parenteral nutrition cholestasis (bile from the liver stopped being secreted), and hyperalimentation had to be discontinued with no viable alternative in sight. The case was presented at grand rounds in a well-known Boston hospital. A physician present, who had prescribed donor breastmilk for one of his own patients, suggested banked milk for Katie. It took three weeks to get the prescribed milk to the patient because of hospital red tape. The day the breastmilk arrived, Katie died. The autopsy revealed ruptured intestines (Erickson, 1987).

The challenge in North America now is to prevent further closings of human milk banks and to improve communication among existing milk banks so that any patient who needs banked human milk can have speedy access to it. Banked human milk needs to be considered more frequently by physicians in the treatment plan for certain infants and adults to prevent further trauma, disease, and suffering. While banked human milk as a therapeutic agent may not be the whole answer in all cases, in the absence of the biological mother's own milk it will "first do no harm."

ACKNOWLEDGMENTS

Appreciation is expressed to members of the Human Milk Banking Association of North America, Inc., for their assistance in reviewing this chapter. Portions of this chapter were completed in partial fulfillment of the requirements for a Masters in Public Health at the University of Hawaii, Honolulu, May 1990.

REFERENCES

Ambrose, J: Babies depleting hospital's supply of mothers' milk, *Honolulu Star-Bulletin,* August 14, 1984, p. A–3.

American Academy of Pediatrics, Committee on Mother's Milk: Recommended standards for the operation of mothers' milk bureaus, *J Pediatr* 23:112–28, 1943.

American Academy of Pediatrics, Committee on Nutrition: Human milk banking, *Pediatrics* 65:854–57, 1980.

American Academy of Pediatrics, Committee on Nutrition: Nutritional needs of low- birth-weight infants, *Pediatrics* 75:976–86, 1985.

Arnold, LDW: Milk bank survey—Preliminary report of findings and discussion, *HMBANA Newsl* 3:7–9, 1988.

Arnold, LDW: The statistical state of human milk banking and what's in the future, *J Hum Lact* 7:25–27, 1991.

Arnold, LDW, and Asquith, MT: The evolution of services in modern human milk banking, *J Hum Lact* 7:87–88, 1991.

Arnold, LDW, and Erickson, M: The early history of milk banking in the USA, *J Hum Lact* 4:112–13, 1988.

Asquith, MT, et al.: Clinical uses, collection, and banking of human milk, *Clin Perinatol* 14:173–85, 1987.

Balmer, SE, and Wharton, BA: Human milk banking at Sorrento Maternity Hospital, Birmingham, *Arch Dis Child* 67:556–59, 1992.

Barlow, B, et al.: An experimental study of acute neonatal enterocolitis—the importance of breast milk, *J Pediatr Surg* 9:587–95, 1974.

Baum, JD: *Milk banking in the UK;* Presentation at the annual meeting of the Human Milk Banking Association of North America, Vancouver, British Columbia, October 15, 1989.

Baumslag, N: Breastfeeding: Cultural practices and variations. In Jelliffe, DB, and Jelliffe, EFP, eds.: *Advances in international maternal and child health,* Vol. 7, Oxford, 1987, Oxford University Press, pp. 36–50.

Baumslag, N: *The mystery of the velvet bean;* Presentation at the Nineteenth Annual Seminar for Physicians, La Leche League International, Miami Beach, Fla., July 23, 1991.

Bjorksten, B, et al.: Collecting and banking human milk: To heat or not to heat? *Br Med J* 281:765–69, 1980.

Bradley, MW: Breastfeeding and necrotizing enterocolitis, *Indiana Med* 79:859–61, 1986.

Brady, MS, et al.: Specialized formulas and feedings for infants with malabsorption or formula intolerance, *J Am Diet Assoc* 86:191–200, 1986.

Chapin, HD: The operation of a breast milk dairy, *JAMA* 81:200–202, 1923.

Cunningham, AS: Breast-feeding and morbidity in industrialized countries: an update. In Jelliffe, DB, and Jelliffe, EFP, eds.: *Advances in international maternal and child health,* Oxford, 1981, Oxford University Press, pp. 128–68.

Davis, WH: Statistical comparison of the mortality of breast-fed and bottle-fed infants, *Am J Dis Child* 5:234–47, 1913.

Eibl, MM, et al.: Prevention of necrotizing enterocolitis in low-birth-weight infants by IgA-IgG feeding, *N Engl J Med* 319:1–7, 1988.

Eitenmiller, R: *An overview of human milk pasteurization;* Presentation at the annual meeting of the Human Milk Banking Association of North America, Lexington, Ky., October 15, 1990.

Emerson, PW, and Platt, W: The preservation of human milk. VI. A preliminary note on the freezing process, *J Pediatr* 2:472–77, 1933.

Erickson, M: Presidential address, annual meeting of the Human Milk Banking Association of North America, Raleigh, N.C., October 15, 1987.

Fildes, V: *Breasts, bottles and babies: A history of infant feeding,* Edinburgh, 1986, Edinburgh University Press.

Fildes, V: *Wet nursing: A history from antiquity to the present,* Oxford, 1988, Basil Blackwell, Ltd., pp. 144–89.

Ford, JE, et al.: Influence of the heat treatment of human milk on some of its protective constituents, *J Pediatr* 90:29–35, 1977.

Garza, C: Banked human milk for very low birth weight infants. In Atkinson, SA, Hanson, LA, and Chandra, RK, eds.: *Human Lactation 4: Breastfeeding, nutrition, infection and infant growth in developed and merging countries,* St. John's, Newfoundland, Canada, 1990, ARTS Biomedical Publisher, pp. 25–34.

Garza, C, Hopkinson, J, and Schanler, RJ: Human milk banking. In Howell, RR, Morriss, RH, and Pickering, LK, eds.: *Human milk in infant nutrition and health,* Springfield, Ill., 1986, Charles C Thomas, Publisher, pp. 225–55.

Goldblum, RM, et al.: Human milk banking. I. Effects of container upon immunologic factors in mature milk, *Nutr Res* 1:449–59, 1981.

Golden, J: From wet nurse directory to milk bank: The delivery of human milk in Boston, 1909–1927, *Bull Hist Med* 62:589–605, 1988.

Hopkinson, J, Garza, C, and Asquith, MT: Letter to the editor, *J Hum Lact* 6:104–5, 1990.

Isaacs, CE, and Thormar, H: Human milk lipids inactivate enveloped viruses. In Atkinson, SA, Hanson, LA, and Chandra, RK, eds.: *Human Lactation 4: Breastfeeding, nutrition, infection and infant growth in developed and emerging countries,* St. John's, Newfoundland, Canada, 1990, ARTS Biomedical Publisher, pp. 161–74.

Jacobs, R: Vital breast milk supply for child is low, *The Daily Ardmoreite,* Ardmore, Okla., August 20, 1989, pp. 1A, 3A.

Jones, K: The mothers milk bureau of Detroit, *Public Health Nurse,* pp. 142–43, March 1928.

Kliegman, RM, Pittard, WB, and Fanaroff, AA: Necrotizing enterocolitis in neonates fed human milk, *J Pediatr* 95:450–53, 1979.

Kocturk, T: Breast-feeding in Islam (letter), *Acta Paediatr Scand* 78:777–79, 1989.

Langerak, ER, and Arnold, LDW: The mothers' milk bank of Wilmington, Del.: History and highlights, *J Hum Lact* 7:197–98, 1991.

Law, BJ, et al.: Is ingestion of milk-associated bacteria by premature infants fed raw human milk controlled by routine bacteriologic screening? *J Clin Microbiol* 27:1560–66, 1989.

Lawrence, RA: *Breastfeeding: A guide for the medical profession,* St. Louis, 1989, The C.V. Mosby Co.

Lemons, JA, Schreiner, RL, and Gresham, EL: Simple method for determining the caloric and fat content of human milk, *Pediatrics* 66:626–28, 1980.

Liebhaber, M, et al.: Alterations of lymphocytes and of antibody content of human milk after processing, *J Pediatr* 91:897–900, 1977.

Lucas, A, and Cole, TJ: Breast milk and neonatal necrotising enterocolitis, *Lancet* 336:1519–23, 1990.

Lucas, A, et al.: Creamtocrit: Simple clinical technique for estimating fat concentration and energy value of human milk, *Br Med J* 1:1018–20, 1978.

MacPherson, CH, and Talbot, FB: Standards for directories for mother's milk, *J Pediatr* 15:461–68, 1939.

Marinkovich, V: *IgA deficiency and allergies;* Presentation at the annual meeting of the Human Milk Banking Association of North America, San Jose, Calif., September 30, 1988.

Martinez, FE: *Growth of premature neonates fed banked pasteurized human milk homogenized by ultrasonication;* Presentation at the annual meeting of the Human Milk Banking Association of North America, Vancouver, British Columbia, October 15, 1989.

Martinez, FE, et al.: Ultrasonic homogenization of expressed human milk to prevent fat loss during tube feeding, *J Pediatr Gastroenterol Nutr* 6:593–97, 1987.

McDougal, JS: *Pasteurization of human breast milk and its effect on HIV infectivity;* Presentation at the annual meeting of the Human Milk Banking Association of North America, Lexington, Ky., October 15, 1990.

Mehta, NR, et al.: Adherence of medium-chain fatty acids to feeding tubes during gavage feeding of human milk fortified with medium-chain triglycerides, *J Pediatr* 112:474–76, 1988.

Michaelsen, KM, et al.: Variation in macronutrients in human bank milk: Influencing factors and implications for human milk banking, *J Pediatr Gastroenterol Nutr* 11:229–39, 1990.

Narayanan, I: Human milk in the developing world: To bank or not to bank? *Ind Pediatr* 19:395–99, 1982.

Narayanan, I, Prakash, K, and Gujral, VV: Management of expressed human milk in a developing country—experiences and practical guidelines, *J Trop Pediatr* 28:25–28, 1982.

Narayanan, I, et al.: Partial supplementation with expressed breast-milk for prevention of infection in low-birth-weight infants, *Lancet,* September 13, 561–63, 1980.

Oxtoby, MJ: Human immunodeficiency virus and other viruses in human milk: Placing the issues in broader perspective, *Pediatr Infect Dis J* 7:825–35, 1988.

Paxson, CL, and Cress, CC: Survival of human milk leukocytes, *J Pediatr* 94:61–64, 1979.

Raiol, MRS, et al.: *Fat balance and growth of premature infants fed banked pasteurized human milk homogenized by ultrasound;* 14th International Congress of Nutrition, Seoul, Korea, August 20–25, 1989, Abstract F28–3, p. 429.

Rangecroft, L, de San Lazaro, C, and Scott, JES: A comparison of the feeding of the postoperative newborn with banked breast-milk or cow's-milk feeds, *J Pediatr Surg* 13:11–12, 1978.

Raptopoulou-Gigi, M, Marwick, K, and McClelland, DBL: Antimicrobial proteins in sterilized human milk, *Br Med J* 1:12–14, 1977.

Riddell, DG: *Use of banked human milk for feeding infants with abdominal wall defects;* Presentation at the annual meeting of the Human Milk Banking Association of North America, Vancouver, British Columbia, October 15, 1989.

Roy, CC, and Lescop, J: Human milk banking: High rate of interest for a still uncertain credit balance, *Am J Dis Child* 133:255–56, 1979.

Rumball, S: *Lactoengineering: An emerging science;* Presentation at International Lactation Consultant Association annual meeting, Scottsdale, Ariz., July, 1990.

Schanler, RJ, Garza, C, and Nichols, BL: Fortified mothers' milk for very low birth weight infants: Results of growth and nutrient balance studies, *J Pediatr* 107:437–45, 1985.

Scheuer, LA, and Duncan, JE: A method of preserving breast milk: A study of its clinical application, *Am J Dis Child* 51:249–54, 1936.

Siimes, MA, and Hallman, N: A perspective on human milk banking, 1978, *J Pediatr* 94:173–74, 1979.

Smith, CA: Human milk technology, *J Pediatr* 20:616–26, 1942.

Smith, LW, and Emerson, PW: Notes on the experimental production of dried breast milk, *Boston Med Surg J* 191:938–40, 1924.

Stocks, RJ, et al.: Loss of breast milk nutrients during tube feeding, *Arch Dis Child* 60:164–66, 1985.

Talbot, FB: A directory for wet-nurses: Its experiences for twelve months, *JAMA* 56:1715–17, 1911.

Talbot, FB: Directory for wetnurses, *Boston Med Surg J* 196:653–54, 1927.

Tully, MR: Human milk banking in Sweden and Denmark, *J Hum Lact* 7:145–46, 1991.

Wallingford, J: *Nutritional and anti-infective consequences of pasteurization of breast milk;* Presentation at the annual meeting of the Human Milk Banking Association of North America, Raleigh, N.C., October 15, 1987.

Williams, AF, et al.: Human milk banking, *J Trop Pediatr* 31:185–90, 1985.

Wills, ME, et al.: Short-time low-temperature pasteurization of human milk, *Early Hum Dev* 7:71–80, 1982.

World Health Organization: Breast-feeding/breast milk and human immunodeficiency virus (HIV), *Wkly Epidemiol Rec* 62:245–46, 1987.

World Health Organization/United Nations Children's Fund: Meeting on infant and young child feeding, *J Nurs-Midwif* 25:31–38, 1980.

Xanthou, M: Immunology of breast milk. In Stern, L, ed.: *Feeding the sick infant* (Nestlé Nutrition Workshop Series, Vol. 11), New York, 1987, Raven Press, pp. 101–17.

Young, VR, Motil, KJ, and Burke, JF: Energy and protein metabolism in relation to requirements of the burned pediatric patient. In Suskind, RM, ed.: *Textbook of pediatric nutrition,* New York, 1981, Raven Press, pp. 309–40.

Appendix 22–1

Guidelines for the Establishment and Operation of a Human Milk Bank*

PREFACE

This 1991 edition of *Guidelines for the Establishment and Operation of a Human Milk Bank* was accepted by member banks at the 1990 annual meeting and updated again by the Executive Committee. Lucas and Cole's recently published work confirming the long-held belief of many health-care professionals in milk banking and in neonatology—that banked human milk provides protection against necrotising enterocolitis—has been added to the bibliography (Lucas & Cole, 1990). Some of the procedures have been changed in light of research commissioned by the United States Food and Drug Administration which was reported at the annual meeting in Lexington, Kentucky.

Lois D. W. Arnold, M.P.H., I.B.C.L.C.
Mary Rose Tully, B.A., I.B.C.L.C.
Editors

PREFACE TO THE FIRST EDITION

This first edition of the *Guidelines for the Establishment and Operation of a Human Milk Bank* is the first recommendation on the practice of human milk banking drawn from the collective experience of operating milk banks in North America. It is being published to ensure that banked

human milk is a standard, high quality, safe, nutritious product. Efforts have been made to document the guidelines with current scientific data. Where no research information is available, the many years of collective experience of member milk banks of the Human Milk Banking Association of North America is used. Those areas where there is no research will be our priority for research.

As these guidelines were developed, they have undergone thorough and repeated scrutiny by professionals in the fields of milk banking, neonatology, pediatrics, nursing, infectious disease, immunology, pharmacology, nutrition, public health, and law. The input of these professionals has been invaluable. We are most grateful for their assistance.

It is the Association's hope that these guidelines will be useful to health-care providers in promoting and prescribing the use of banked human milk as a temporary form of therapy where appropriate. This is in keeping with the World Health Organization's policy statement that when it is not possible for the birth mother to breastfeed, the first alternative should be banked donor breast milk (WHO/UNICEF, 1980).

Lois D. W. Arnold, M.P.H., I.B.C.L.C. and
Mary Rose Tully, B.A., I.B.C.L.C.,
Editors

CONTRIBUTORS

Lois D. W. Arnold, M.P.H., I.B.C.L.C.
Hawaii Mother's Milk, Inc.
Honolulu, Hawaii

*Derived from Arnold, LDW, and Tully, MR: *Guidelines for the establishment and operation of a human milk bank* (1991 edition), West Hartford, Conn., 1991, HMBANA.

Maria Teresa Asquith
Susan Miksad
Mothers' Milk Bank
California Institute for Medical Research
San Jose, California

JoAnn Dalcin
Eastern Pennsylvania Milk Bank
Bethlehem, Pennsylvania

Nirmala Desai, M.D.
Human Milk Bank
University of Kentucky
Lexington, Kentucky

Miriam Erickson, B.S.
Central Massachusetts Regional Milk Bank
Medical Center of Central Massachusetts
Worcester, Massachusetts

Sandy Erickson, R.N.
Loraine Lockhart Borman, B.A.
Marianne Neifert, M.D.

Vergie Hughes, R.N., B.S.N., I.B.C.L.C.
Community Human Milk Bank
Georgetown University Hospital
Washington, District of Columbia

Elizabeth Langerak
Mothers' Milk Bank
Wilmington Hospital Medical Center of Delaware
Wilmington, Delaware

Judy Palsgraf, R.N., I.B.C.L.C.
Concepcion Sia, M.D.
Mother's Milk Bank
North Shore University Hospital
Manhasset, New York

Kate Y. Pierce, R.N., B.S.N., I.B.C.L.C.
Mother's Milk Bank
Central Baptist Hospital
Lexington, Kentucky

Agi Radcliffe, R.N., I.B.C.L.C.
A. G. F. Davidson, M.D.
Breast Milk Service
Children's Hospital
Vancouver, British Columbia

Joan Sechrist, R.D.
Karen Gibson, R.D.
Joy Seacat, C.H.A., M.S.
Mothers' Milk Bank
Women's & Children's Hospital, Presbyterian/St. Luke's
Medical Center
Denver, Colorado

Mary Rose Tully, B.A., I.B.C.L.C.
Piedmont Mother's Milk Bank
Wake Medical Center
Raleigh, North Carolina

Francie Vogel, R.N.
Fresh Breastmilk Program
Women's Hospital
Winnipeg, Manitoba

The HUMAN MILK BANKING ASSOCIATION OF NORTH AMERICA gratefully acknowledges the input of John Wallingford, Ph.D., of the Clinical Nutrition Branch, Center for Food Safety and Applied Nutrition, and James Weixel of the Consumer Safety Office, both of the Food and Drug Administration, Washington, D. C.; Edgar Marcuse, M.D., M.P.H., of the Committee on Infectious Diseases of the American Academy of Pediatrics; and J. D. Baum, M.D., of the Royal Hospital for Sick Children, University of Bristol, Bristol, England.

SECTION I. INTRODUCTION

In the early part of the 20th-century there was a growing recognition among physicians that infant mortality and morbidity were related to artificial feeding and formulae (Davis, 1913). To address this problem, the first human milk "bank" in the United States was founded in Boston, Massachusetts. The bank was a home for lactating women who were paid to wet-nurse infants in need while breastfeeding their own infants. The donors were all screened for TB and syphilis, and the bank was run under medical supervision (Talbot, 1911). In 1943, the American Academy of Pediatrics, Committee on Mothers' Milk, published standards for operation: collection, processing, storage, and dispensing of donated human milk. After World War II, interest in banked human milk declined simultaneously with a decrease in the incidence of breastfeeding in the United States.

In the 1970s there was a resurgence of interest in human milk banking because of both the increased interest in breastfeeding among new mothers and advances in neonatal intensive care, which has led to an increased survival rate for sick and very premature infants. Distributing milk banks were established in many communities in North America, either under the sponsorship of a medical facility or a volunteer organization of breastfeeding women. Frequently, hospitals established in-house milk banks to meet the needs of infants in their neonatal intensive care units whose mothers could not always provide their own breastmilk. The American Academy of Pediatrics published an updated policy statement on human milk banking in 1980 (AAP, 1980; Garza, Hopkinson & Schanler, 1986; Williams & Baum, 1984; Williamson et al., 1978).

Banked human milk has been shown to be efficacious in the treatment of both in-patients and out-patients ranging in age from premature infants to older at-risk children (Asquith et al., 1987; Narayanan et al., 1982; Rangecroft, de San Lazaro & Scott, 1978). Human milk has also been used effectively as therapy in the treatment of some adult conditions, such as stomach ulcers.

The HUMAN MILK BANKING ASSOCIATION OF NORTH AMERICA was established in 1985, drawing together representatives of milk banks and members of the medical community. The goals of the HMBANA are to:

1. provide a forum for networking among experts in the field on issues relating to human milk banking
2. provide information to the medical community on the benefits and appropriate uses of banked human milk
3. develop guidelines for milk banking practices in North America
4. communicate among member milk banks to assure adequate supplies for all patients
5. encourage research into the unique properties of human milk and its uses
6. act as a liaison between member institutions and governmental regulatory agencies.

SECTION II. DEFINITIONS

Human milk bank: A human milk bank is a service established for the purpose of collecting, screening, processing, storing, and distributing donated human milk to meet the specific needs of individuals for whom human milk is prescribed by physicians.
Donor milk: Donor milk is voluntarily given by women biologically unrelated to the recipient.
Preparations:

Fresh-raw milk—milk stored continuously at approximately 4°C for use not longer than 72 hours following expression.
Fresh-frozen milk—fresh-raw milk that has been frozen and held at approximately –20°C for less than 12 months.
Heat-processed milk—fresh-raw and/or fresh-frozen milk which has been heated to a minimum of 56°C for 30 minutes.
Pooled milk: Milk from more than one donor.

SECTION III. ORGANIZATION

Member milk banks are associated with a medical institution and maintain procedures and protocols which meet the minimum standards of the HMBANA.

GOVERNING STRUCTURE
The governing structure of a milk bank shall consist of a Medical Director and a Milk Bank Director, with the following functions and responsibilities:

Medical Director: The Medical Director shall be a licensed physician, and shall oversee the implementation of procedures and protocols, act as a liaison with the medical community, and be available for consultation with milk bank personnel.
Milk Bank Director: The Milk Bank Director shall have education, training, and experience as deemed suitable by the Medical Director. Duties shall include the planning, development, implementation, and evaluation of the administrative, medical, and educational services of the milk bank.

It is recommended that all milk banks develop a panel of consultants which may include, but not be limited to, specialists from the following areas: neonatology, pediatrics, nursing, immunology, microbiology, pharmacology, nutrition, public health, infectious diseases, obstetrics, pathology, food technology (i.e., milk processing), law, and consumer representation.

SECTION IV. DONOR SELECTION

DEFINITION OF A DONOR
1. Acceptable donors shall be healthy lactating women.
2. Potential donors shall be given educational materials informing them of the characteristics of the high-risk groups or activities which might put them at risk for blood-borne diseases. The standards of the American Association of Blood Banks for screening donors will be used (American Association of Blood Banks, 1989, Sections B1.260 to B1.264).

EXCLUSIONS
1. Potential donors shall be excluded on the basis of the following:
   a. history of receiving a blood transfusion or blood products within the last six months
   b. use of tobacco
   c. regular use of over-the-counter medications or systemic prescriptions, including birth-control pills (replacement hormones are acceptable)
   d. use of megadose vitamins and/or herbal preparations
   e. use of illegal drugs
2. A history of hepatitis B, systemic disorders of any kind, or chronic infections—for example, Human Immuno-

deficiency Virus (WHO, 1987)—will be sufficient to exclude donation of milk (see American Association of Blood Banks, 1989, Sections B1.260 to B1.264).

TEMPORARY DISQUALIFICATION

1. Active donors may be temporarily disqualified from donating milk under the following conditions:
   a. during an acute infection, including monilial and fungal infections, in the household (donors shall be instructed to report all such infections to the milk bank)
   b. during the four-week period following a case of rubella or the administration of an attenuated virus vaccine (e.g., measles, mumps, rubella)
   c. during a reactivation of latent infection with Herpes Simplex Virus (HSV) or Varicella zoster
   d. during episodes of clinical mastitis
   e. during the 12-hour period following consumption of alcohol (hard liquor, beer, or wine).
2. Any consumption of over-the-counter medication shall be reported to the milk bank.
3. Milk donation shall resume at the discretion of the milk bank director.

SEROLOGICAL TESTS

Each donor shall have had negative serological tests for HIV-1, hepatitis-B antigen, HTLV-1 and syphilis during the most recent pregnancy. In some geographic areas where certain diseases are endemic, additional screening tests may be warranted (e.g., TB, hepatitis C) (Oxtoby, 1988).

SECTION V. DONOR EDUCATION AND PROCEDURES

To ensure the highest quality of donated milk, donors shall be instructed in the appropriate methods for sanitary collection, handling, storage, and transportation of human milk.

WRITTEN INSTRUCTIONS

Donors shall be given written instructions covering:

1. clean techniques for milk collection including:
   a. washing and sterilizing breast pump parts
   b. hand washing and cleansing the breasts
   c. handling sterile containers
2. those times when donors should refrain from donating
3. labeling of donated milk, which shall include donor ID number and date of collection
4. frozen storage of milk

5. transportation of milk to the bank.

CONTAINERS

Donors shall store milk in sterile containers supplied and/or approved by the milk bank.

SECTION VI. MILK BANK PROCEDURES

The milk bank shall maintain a detailed procedures manual which is available to milk bank personnel at all times. The procedures manual shall be reviewed at least annually by the medical director and the milk bank director.

EQUIPMENT

1. Freezer temperatures shall be monitored by means of recording thermometers, or freezers shall be equipped with temperature-sensitive alarms.
2. Storage and processing equipment shall be calibrated annually.
3. All equipment manuals shall be available to milk bank personnel at all times.
4. No equipment intended for human milk banking—processing or storage—shall be used for, or be allowed to come into contact with biological, chemical, or other hazardous materials.

PROCESSING OF HUMAN MILK

Defrosting and Pooling

1. Frozen milk shall be defrosted completely by holding at 4°C over a 24-hour period.
2. Pooling of defrosted raw and fresh-raw milk shall be conducted under sanitary conditions.

Processing of Milk to be Used Raw

1. Each pool of milk shall have a sterile sample taken for bacteriological screening. Only milk from pools with $<10^4$ CFU/mL will be acceptable to dispense raw.
2. The presence of any pathogenic bacteria, gram-negative bacteria, *Staphylococcus aureus* (coagulase positive), or alpha or beta Streptococci is not acceptable.

Heat Processing

1. For milk banks using equipment specifically designed for human milk pasteurization, the procedures for use of the machine shall be followed, and containers specifically made for the unit shall be used.

2. For all other milk banks the procedure shall be as follows:
   a. Pooled milk shall be aliquoted into sterile containers of 120 ml or equivalent standard size. Original containers may be used as long as they have been maintained under sterile conditions.
   b. Containers shall be filled with not more than 105 ml of milk, leaving at least 20% void-volume in the container.
   c. All containers shall be capped sufficiently tightly to prevent contamination of milk during heat treatment.
   d. Aliquots of milk shall be processed by completely submerging the containers in a well-agitated or shaking water bath preheated to 56–58°C.
   e. At least one aliquot containing the same amount of milk as the most filled container in the batch shall be fitted with a calibrated thermometer to record milk temperature during heat processing.
   f. The thermometer shall be positioned such that approximately 25% of the milk volume is below the measuring point of the thermometer.
   g. The monitored aliquot shall be placed into the water bath after all other aliquots, and shall be positioned centrally among the treated aliquots.
   h. After the temperature of the monitored milk aliquot has reached 56°C, the heat treatment shall continue for 30 minutes.
   i. Milk temperature, bath temperature, and container leakage as indicated by released air bubbles shall be monitored at five-minute intervals.
   j. Leaky containers shall be discarded.

Chilling and Storage

1. Following heat processing, the milk is to be cooled by submersion in an ice slurry.
2. Containers shall be labeled with batch number and date.
3. An aliquot of processed milk shall be tested as described below.
4. Heat processed milk can be stored for up to 72 hours at 4°C or up to 12 months at approximately –20°C (based on customary and reasonable practice because of a lack of definitive research documentation).

BACTERIOLOGIC TESTING

1. Acceptable bacteriologic growth is no growth of non-pathogenic flora for heat-processed milk (based on customary and reasonable practice because of a lack of definitive research documentation).
2. The presence of any pathogenic bacteria (including gram- negative bacteria, *Staphylococcus aureus,* or alpha or beta Streptococci) is not acceptable.
3. Milk that does not meet acceptable bacteriologic standards may not be distributed to a recipient, but may be used for research.

SECTION VII. RECIPIENT SELECTION

All milk dispensed shall be heat treated unless the patient's condition indicates fresh-frozen milk, in which case the milk bank director shall consult with the medical director and advisory board to approve dispensing bacteriologically screened, fresh-frozen milk.

Banked human milk shall be dispensed only by prescription for the treatment of various medical conditions, including but not limited to:

1. prematurity
2. malabsorption
3. formula intolerance
4. immunologic deficiencies
5. congenital anomalies
6. postoperative nutrition.

If supplies of banked milk are sufficient, milk may also be dispensed by prescription in the following situations:

1. lactation failure
2. adoption
3. illness in the mother requiring temporary isolation
4. health risk to the infant from the milk of the biological mother
5. death of the mother who has been breastfeeding.

In the event that a milk bank is unable to supply the needs of its recipients, it will contact other milk banks for assistance in supplying milk. If unable to locate additional supplies of milk, it will dispense the milk available on a priority basis to the recipients in greatest need. The decision will be made by the milk bank director and medical director based on diagnosis, severity of illness, availability of alternative treatments, and history of previous milk use.

SECTION VIII. MILK BANK RECORDS

DONOR RECORDS

1. Donor records shall include:
   a. initial donor-screening form including medical history

b. confirmation of negative serology tests for HIV, hepatitis- B antigen, and syphilis
c. birthdate and gestational age of donor's infant
d. a log of each donation.
2. Each donor shall be assigned a unique ID number.
3. Donor records and ID numbers shall be treated as confidential.

ADMINISTRATIVE RECORDS

These shall include the following:

1. ID numbers of donors whose milk comprises each pool
2. batch information, including date of treatment, amount of milk treated, containers per batch, and heat treatment times and temperatures
3. bacteriologic test results by batch after pooling and/or pasteurization
4. freezer, refrigerator, and incubator temperatures
5. annual calibration records for all equipment
6. milk bank financial records.

RECIPIENT RECORDS

These shall include:

1. name of the ordering physician or hospital
2. batch numbers and amounts of all supplied milk
3. other pertinent information (such as diagnosis and medical outcome of patients).

REFERENCES

American Academy of Pediatrics, Committee on Nutrition: Human milk banking, *Pediatrics* 65:854–57, 1980.

American Academy of Pediatrics, Committee on Mothers' Milk: Recommended standards for the operation of mothers' milk bureaus, *J Pediatr* 23:1121–28, 1943.

American Association of Blood Banks: *Standards for blood banks and transfusion services,* Arlington, Va., 1989, American Association of Blood Banks.

Asquith, MT, et al.: Clinical uses, collection and banking of human milk, *Clin Perinatol* 14:173–85, 1987.

Canadian Paediatric Society: Statement on human milk banking, *CMAJ* 132:750–52, 1985.

Davis, WE: Statistical comparison of the mortality of breast-fed and bottle-fed infants, *Am J Dis Child* 5:234–47, 1913.

Garza, C, Hopkinson, J, and Schanler, RJ: Human milk banking. In Howell, RR, Morriss, FH, and Pickering, LK, eds.: *Human milk in infant nutrition and health,* Springfield, Ill., 1986, Charles C Thomas, Publisher, pp. 225–55.

Lucas, A, and Cole, TJ: Breast milk and neonatal necrotising enterocolitis, *Lancet* 336:1519–23, 1990.

Narayanan, I, et al.: A planned prospective evaluation of the anti-infective property of varying quantities of expressed human milk, *Acta Paediatr Scand* 71:441–45, 1982.

Oxtoby, MJ: Human immunodeficiency virus and other viruses in human milk: Placing the issues in broader perspective, *Pediatr Infect Dis J* 7:825–35, 1988.

Rangecroft, L, de San Lazaro, C, and Scott, JES: A comparison of the feeding of the postoperative newborn with banked breast-milk or cow's-milk feeds, *J Pediatr Surg* 13:11–12, 1978.

Talbot, FB: A directory for wet nurses: Its experiences for twelve months, *JAMA* 56:1715–17, 1911.

Williams, AF, and Baum, JD, eds.: *Human milk banking* (Nestlé Nutrition Series #5), New York, 1984, Raven Press.

Williamson, S, et al.: Organisation of bank of raw and pasteurised human milk for neonatal intensive care, *Br Med J* 1:393–96, 1978.

World Health Organization: Breast-feeding/breast milk and human immunodeficiency virus (HIV), *Wkly Epidemiol Rec,* 62:245–46, 1987.

World Health Organization/United Nations Children's Fund: Meeting on infant and young child feeding, *J Nurs-Midwif* 25:31–38, 1980.

Appendices

Appendix A (1)

ST. JOSEPH MEDICAL CENTER
THE FAMILY BIRTHPLACE

BREASTFEEDING POLICIES

DEFINITION AND PURPOSE

To promote a philosophy of maternal and infant care which advocates breastfeeding and supports the normal physiologic functions involved in this maternal-infant process. The goal is to assure that all families who elect to breastfeed their infants will have a successful and satisfying experience. These polices apply to the full term, normal newborn and may not apply to infants with certain clinical conditions, i.e., intra-uterine growth retardation (IUGR), prematurity, infant of diabetic mother.

I. GENERAL POLICIES

1. All pregnant women should receive information regarding the availability of classes on the benefits and management of breastfeeding.
2. Mothers who are undecided about feeding method will be encouraged to breastfeed.
3. Mothers expressing desire to breastfeed will have nipples examined for degree of eversion during admission procedures.
4. Educational pamphlets on breastfeeding shall be provided following birth, well before discharge.
5. Infants are to be put to breast as soon after birth as feasible for both mother and infant, with 20 minutes post-birth ideal and within the first 2 hours whenever possible.
6. Every mother is to be instructed in proper breastfeeding technique and re-evaluated before discharge. (See II: Functional Assessment of Infant at Breast.)

7. The infant is to be encouraged to nurse *at least* every 2 to 3 hours, for a minimum of 8 feedings per 24 hours.
8. Infants should feed from both breasts at all feedings, with a minimum of 6 minutes per breast. An infant may be returned to the first breast for continued suckling, if positioning is correct and nursing is comfortable.
9. If within the first 24–48 hours post-birth feedings at breast are incomplete or ineffective, the mother should be instructed to begin regular expression of her breasts, with continued assistance by an experienced staff member. The colostrum or milk obtained by expression should be given to the baby.
10. Supplementary water or formula is given for certain clinical conditions as ordered by the physician, but not on a routine basis. If prolonged supplementation is necessary, the physician will be contacted regarding formula choice and amount.
11. Mothers who wish to feed by both breast and bottle will be educated about breastfeeding and encouraged to breastfeed without supplement.
12. Pacifiers should not be used on a routine basis for the breastfeeding infant as a hunger satiety measure.
13. Breastfeeding mothers are to have their breasts examined for evidence of lactation or breastfeeding problems at least once every 24 hours.
14. Infants should remain at the mothers' bedside

621

both day and night. The nurse should plan with the mother and family for periods of rest/sleep both day and night. If the mother chooses to have the infant in the nursery, she will be encouraged to feed the baby on demand.

15. Commercial discharge packs containing water or formula are not to be given unless specifically ordered by the physician or requested by the mother.

16. At discharge, each mother is to be given a phone number to call for breastfeeding assistance.

17. Mothers who are separated from their infants will be instructed on the proper use of breast pumps as well as the storage and transportation of breast milk.

II. FUNCTIONAL ASSESSMENT OF THE INFANT AT BREAST (FAIB) POLICY*

A. Functional assessment of the infant at breast should be completed:
1. Within first 24 hours of life AND
2. Before discharge from birth setting.
3. Additional assessments should be performed anytime a breastfeeding problem is suspected (i.e., slow weight gain, persistent sore nipples, etc.).

B. Direct observation of breastfeeding is critical.

C. Assessment should be as nonobtrusive as possible.

D. Assessment is NOT necessary during the first breastfeeding experience. The first breastfeeding should be a "getting acquainted" session with lots of enthusiasm and little intervention from health care providers.

E. If the FAIB indicates difficulties with breastfeeding, the infant's physician will be notified prior to discharge.

Procedure

A. Four A's help guide assessment and documentation

1. Alignment

- Infant is in flexed position—relaxed, no muscular rigidity
- Infant's head is aligned with trunk

*Shrago, L, and Bocar, D: *JOGNN* 19:209–15, 1989.

- Infant's head is at breast level (no traction exerted on breast or nipple)
- Infant's head is straight on breast (not turned or hyperextended)
- Imaginary line drawn from ear to shoulder to iliac crest
- Mother is in comfortable position, supported with pillows

2. Areolar Grasp

- Mouth is opened widely, lips not pursed
- Lips are visible and flanged outward
- Tongue covers lower gum, curved (troughed) around areola
- Approximately 1/2 to 1 inch of areola is drawn SYMMETRICALLY into mouth
- Complete seal and strong vacuum is formed by infant's mouth
- No clicking or smacking sounds during feeding
- No drawing in or dimpling of cheek pads

3. Areolar Compression

- Mandible moves in a rhythmic motion
- Initially, approximately two sucks per second (non-nutritive sucking, "flutter" sucking); as milk/colostrum becomes available post Milk Ejection Reflex (M.E.R.), sucking slows to approximately one suck per second (nutritive sucking)
- Wavelike motion of tongue compresses lactiferous sinuses against hard palate (milk sprays from nipple pores)
- Confirmed by previous digital exam (exam not routinely performed at time of feeding)
- Tongue, jaw, lips move in single rhythmic unit

4. Audible Swallowing

- Quiet sound of swallowing is heard
- May be preceded by several sucking motions
- May increase in frequency and consistency after M.E.R.

B. Functional Assessment of Infant at Breast (FAIB) should be included in patient education to assure adequacy of breastfeeding upon discharge.

C. Document feedings on the newborn flow sheet

in the "Feeding" section utilizing the following abbreviations:

BO—Breastfeeding attempted

BAS—Breastfeed with audible swallowing

D. Document FAIB on mother's chart as a narrative notation:

"Mother and infant positioned correctly, unable to arouse sleepy baby, latch-on not accomplished."

"Infant accomplished latch-on with several bursts of 3–4 sucks."

"Audible swallowing at both breasts."

Above examples are more helpful than "breastfed well." Overemphasis on "number of minutes" of breastfeeding teaches clock watching rather than responding to infant behavior.

III. BREASTFEEDING ROUNDS POLICY:

In response to the Amercian Academy of Pediatrics, American College of Obstetricians and Gynecologists, and the World Health Organization's promotion of breastfeeding as the preferred method of infant feeding, and the Surgeon General's Health Promotion/Disease Prevention objective which states "by 2000, 75% of mothers will breastfeed when discharged and 35% will continue for the first 6 months," the Family Birthplace will provide "Breastfeeding Rounds"—an average length visit of 20 minutes is provided free of charge during the hospital stay. Women who have a short length of stay may not be seen by a consultant.

Procedure

A. A Certified Breastfeeding Educator or Certified Lactation Consultant who is a R.N. visits mothers who have chosen to breastfeed, in order to provide:

1. Information consistent with current research on practices relevant to successful lactation.

2. One-to-one patient education assisting mothers in identifying:
   - Infant's hunger cues and readiness to feed
   - Proper positioning and "latch-on" of the infant
   - Satiety cues of the infant, adequacy of milk supply
   - Problem signs indicating need for follow-up care

Breastfeeding rounds are charted on the "Breastfeeding Assessment" form, kept on clipboard with other mother/baby forms. Upon discharge, the original stays on mother's chart, copy to baby chart and copy to department.

3. When the Functional Assessment of the Infant at Breast (FAIB) indicates a dysfunction unrelated to maternal causes, a suck assessment will be performed. When a suck assessment reveals a dysfunction requiring intervention, the plan will be noted on the Care Plan and charted on the "Breastfeeding Assessment" form.

Procedure

a. Wash hands and don sterile glove or finger cot.

b. Perform digital oral motor exam.

c. Chart findings in "Breastfeeding Assessment" and discuss plan with physician and mother.

d. Add interventions to nursing care plan

4. Babies in NICU:

Mothers of babies in NICU will be visited by the Breastfeeding Educator/Lactation Consultant for the purpose of instructing the mother on the proper use of breast pumps as well as the storing and transporting of breast milk.

When the infant is deemed medically stable and able to be put to breast, the breastfeeding consultant will be available to perform one-time assessment of the infant at breast, if prior notification is received. The mother will be informed of the breastfeeding consultant's observations, and the session will be charted in the infant's record. Continued consultations must be noted as a physician's request in the infant's record and proper notification received.

5. Follow-up Phone Contact

The Breastfeeding Educator/Lactation Consultant will provide a one-time phone contact to breastfeeding mothers within 1 week of discharge. If the need for continued consultation/support or problems is identified, the physician will be contacted.

IV. USE OF BREASTFEEDING AIDS POLICY

A. Medela Nipple Shield

To be used only when the *cause* of the infant's

inability to achieve latch-on has been identified and documented. Nipple shields treat only the *symptom* of ineffective latch-on and *not the cause.*

Procedure

1. The shield will be initiated by the Breastfeeding Educator/Lactation Consultant.
2. The shield should be used as a tool for training an infant in developing an effective suckling pattern. Any patient discharged with a nipple shield must be referred to the Breastfeeding Educator/Lactation Consultant for follow-up care as shields have been shown to reduce milk volume by 22–58%.
3. Rubber bottle nipples over the mother's own nipple are not to be used.
4. Obtain the nipple shield from the supply cart, initiate appropriate charges, document use, obtain physician order for reimbursement as necessary.

B. Medela Breast Shells

Policy: Indications

1. Flat nipples causing difficult latch-on.
2. Inverted nipples.
3. Treatment of severely sore nipples after cause of soreness has been identified.

Procedure: Use to Erect Nipples

1. Obtain one package of breast shells (contains two shells) from supply cart.
2. Wash shells in soap-water before each use.
3. Instruct mother to wash her hands before handling shells.
4. Snap together dome and cone to form a shell.
5. Mother is to place shell inside her bra with the cone centered over nipple.
6. Shells are to be worn constantly between feedings when treatment is initiated after birth. Document use.
7. A physician order is necessary to obtain third party reimbursement.

Procedure: Use for Sore Nipples

1. Wash shells before each use.

2. Instruct mother to wash hands and snap together the dome and ring to form a shell.
3. Instruct mother to wear the shield inside bra between feedings, allowing nipples to dry and keeping clothing off sore nipple.
4. Bra pads may be necessary at lower border of shells if milk leakage is occurring.
5. Instruct mother to discard any milk that collects in the shells as this is not safe for the baby.

V. BREASTFEEDING CONSULTATION

Policy: To provide a mechanism for patients to receive consultation from a Breastfeeding Educator or Lactation Consultant.

1. Appropriate conditions for consultations include:
   a. Special situations (twins, premature infants, reluctant nursers, relactation).
   b. Patients at high risk for lactation failure (flat/inverted nipples, teenagers, uncommitted mothers, persistent sore nipples, use of nipple shield).
   c. Infants with a sucking disorder, slow weight gain, nipple confusion, anomalies.
   d. Breast/nipple problems (mastitis, abscess, clogged duct).

Procedure: Consult protocols approved by the Breastfeeding Committee; they will serve as guidelines for assessment and care and will be updated yearly and as needed.

1. Inpatient Visits
   a. Ideally, every breastfeeding mother is visited free of charge during her stay at the hospital (see Breastfeeding Rounds III.A). The average length of a visit is 20 minutes.
   b. Nursing staff identify mothers with questions or breastfeeding problems and make referrals to the Breastfeeding consultant.
   c. When problems exist, an order for a consultation is written by either the OB-GYN, family physician, or the baby's physician. Visits lasting more than 20 minutes are considered consults. Documentation of a diagnosis of "Infant Feeding Difficulties" in the medical record is helpful in obtaining third party reimbursement.

d. A breastfeeding consultation fee of $30.00 is initiated upon receiving the written order.

e. The Breastfeeding Assessment Record and/or progress notes are utilized for documentation of the consult.

2. Outpatient Visits. The breastfeeding consult does not take the place of routine pediatric health care visits; it is meant to assist the mother and infant in this special area only.

a. Routine appointments are made during regular working hours. Brief follow-up visits occur as needed. All patients need to check in at admissions either in the main lobby or the Emergency Room entrance.

b. During each visit both the mother and the nursing infant are evaluated. The infant is weighed, and a history is obtained to determine appropriate management. These routine appointments normally take one to two hours.

c. Documentation is made on the Clinical Progress Note. The original is sent to Medical Records along with physician orders, outpatient registration form and other documentation as needed. One copy of the Clinical Progress Note is sent to the referring physician and one copy for the department file.

d. An order for each consultation and a diagnosis of "Infant Feeding Difficulties" in the medical record are necessary for third party reimbursement.

e. A Breastfeeding Consultation fee of $30.00 is made for each routine appointment. If follow-up visits last longer than 20 minutes, the consult fee is initiated.

VI. EMPLOYEE BREASTFEEDING SUPPORT: "THE WHEY STATION"

Policy

1. To provide positive support for St. Joseph employees wishing to continue breastfeeding while coming back to work by providing a private area and an electric breast pump for their use.

Equipment and Supplies

1. Employees may use their own manual breast pump. All employees wishing to use the electric pump must first obtain their own accessory parts. These may be purchased at the PK Pharmacy located at 3305 East Harry or at any medical supply store.

2. If you deliver at SJMC, a Universal Pumping System can be obtained and charged to your inpatient account. The Universal System includes a manual breast pump, tubing and accessories to use for single and double pumping with the electric pump. Double pumping can be accomplished in about 10 minutes.

3. The employee will be responsible for cleaning her own manual breast pump and accessory breast pump parts.

Procedure

1. The breastfeeding pump room will be located on 4 North.

2. A sign-in book will be located in the room, in order to track frequency of usage.

3. Each employee will be responsible for spraying the breast pump and tubing with the hospital approved disinfectant after using the pump. Please wipe excess disinfectant off with clean washrags provided. Washrags may then be placed in laundry hamper. A bottle of dishwashing detergent will be provided to wash the breast pump parts.

4. Maintenance of the pump will be handled by the staff of The Family Birthplace or the Neonatal Intensive Care Unit. For problem solving please call 4 East, extension 5490 or NICU, extension 5475.

5. Employee is responsible for labeling and storing her own breastmilk. Containers for milk will not be provided. Infection Control has asked that any breastmilk being stored in a St. Joseph refrigerator be placed in a plastic bag. The plastic bags will be provided.

6. Assistance in choosing and using a pump, maintaining your milk supply or any breastfeeding concerns may be directed to the Breastfeeding Educator/Lactation Consultants by calling 689–5404 and leaving a message.

Appendix A (2)

WELLSTART
THE SAN DIEGO LACTATION PROGRAM

MODEL HOSPITAL BREASTFEEDING POLICIES

FOR FULL-TERM NORMAL NEWBORN INFANTS

DEFINITION AND PURPOSE

To promote a philosophy of maternal and infant care which advocates breastfeeding and supports the normal physiologic functions involved in this maternal-infant process. The goal is to assure that all families who elect to breastfeed their infants will have a successful and satisfying experience.

POLICY

1. Hospital administrative, medical, nursing and nutrition staff should establish a strategy which promotes and supports breastfeeding through the formation of an interdisciplinary team responsible for the implementation of hospital policies and provision of ongoing educational activities. [1,2,12,22]

2. All pregnant women should receive information regarding the benefits and management of breastfeeding prior to delivery. [1,2,10,13,14,15,21,22]

3. Infants are to be put to breast as soon after birth as feasible for both mother and infant. This is to be initiated in either the delivery room or recovery room. [7,10,13,15,19]

4. Every mother is to be instructed in proper breastfeeding technique and re-evaluated before discharge. [4,7,10,13,14,15]

5. Breastfeeding mother-infant couples are to room-in together on a 24 hour basis. [13,14,17]

6. The infant is to be encouraged to nurse *at least* every 2 to 3 hours, for a minimum of 8 feedings per 24 hours. Feeding may occur more frequently if needed. [6,10,13,15,19]

7. The time at the breast at each feeding should be approximately 10–15 minutes per side. Specific timing is not necessary. [6,10,11,13,14,20]

8. Infants should feed from both breasts at all feedings. [6,10,13,14,15,18]

9. If a feeding at the breast is incomplete or ineffective, the mother should be instructed to begin regular expression of her breasts in conjunction with continued assistance by an experienced staff member. The colostrum or milk obtained by expression should be given to the baby. [10,13,15]

10. No supplementary water or breast milk substitute is to be given to a breastfeeding infant unless specifically ordered by a physician or nurse practitioner. [3,5,10,16]

11. Pacifiers are not to be given to any breastfeeding infant unless specifically ordered by a physician or nurse practitioner. Bottles and nipples are to be used only when specifically ordered by a physician or nurse practitioner. [14,15]

12. Breastfeeding mothers are to have breasts examined for evidence of lactation or breastfeeding problems at least once every nursing staff shift. [10,15]

13. Discharge packs offered to breastfeeding mothers should contain only noncommercial materials which provide educational information and promote breastfeeding. [2,9,11,14,18,22]

14. All breastfeeding mothers are to be advised to arrange for their baby's first checkup within one week after discharge.[13,14]

15. If mothers and babies must be separated, policies 1, 2, 4, and 10 through 15 still apply.

16. Mothers who are separated from their babies are to be instructed in proper breast care and on how to maintain lactation.[8,13,14]

17. Mother's milk expressed during this period of separation is to be collected and made available to the infant as soon after expression as is feasible. If it cannot be offered to the infant, it is to be safely stored for use at a later time.

18. Separated infants should receive their own mother's expressed breastmilk unless alternate feeding orders have been written by the infant's physician or nurse practitioner.

19. At least 24 hours before discharge, mother and infant who have been separated should be brought together for an opportunity to reinstitute exclusive breastfeeding. The pair should be discharged only after breastfeeding is progressing normally.

20. In communities where telephones are available, at discharge each mother is to be given a phone number to call for breastfeeding assistance.[10,14]

Supporting References

1. American Academy of Pediatrics. The promotion of breast-feeding (Policy statement based on task force report). Pediatrics 1982; 69:654–661. (1,2)*

2. American Public Health Association. Breastfeeding. (Policy statement). Am J Public Health 1983; 73:347–348. (1, 2, 13)

3. Bergevin L, Dougherty C, and Kramer M. Do infant formula samples shorten the duration of breastfeeding? Lancet 1983; 1148–1151. (10)

4. Cohen S. High tech–soft touch: Breastfeeding issues. Clin Perinatol 1987; 14:187–196. (4)

5. de Carvalho M and Harvey D. Effects of water supplementation on physiological jaundice in breastfed babies. Arch Dis Child 1981; 56:568–569. (10)

6. de Carvalho M, Robertson S, Merkatz R, and Klaus M. Milk intake and frequency of feeding in breastfed infants. Early Hum Dev 1982; 7:155–163. (6, 7, 8)

7. de Carvalho M, Robertson S, Freidman A, and Klaus M. Effect of frequent breast-feeding on early milk pro-

duction and infant weight gain. Pediatrics 1983; 72:307–311. (3, 4)

8. Elander G and Lindberg T. Short mother-infant separation during first week of life influences the duration of breastfeeding. Acta Paediatr Scand 1984; 73:237–240. (16)

9. Frank D, Wirtz S, Sorenson J, and Heeren T. Commercial discharge packs and breast-feeding counseling: Effects on infant feeding practices in a randomized trial. Pediatrics 1987; 80:845–854. (13)

10. Lawrence R. The management of lactation as a physiologic process. Clin Perinatol 1987, 14:1–10. (3, 4, 6, 7, 8, 10, 12, 15)

11. L'Esperance C and Frantz K. Time limitation for early breastfeeding. JOGNN 1985; (Mar/Apr)114–118. (7)

12. Naylor A and Wester R. Providing professional lactation management consultation. Clin Perinatol 1987; 14:33–38. (1)

13. Neifert M and Seacat J. A guide to successful breast-feeding. Contemporary Pediatrics 1986, 3(Jul):26–45. (3, 4, 5, 6, 7, 8, 14, 16)

14. Neifert M and Seacat J. Medical management of successful breast-feeding. Pediatr Clin North Am 1986; 33:743–761. (4, 5, 7, 8, 11, 12, 14, 15, 16)

15. Neifert M and Seacat J. Contemporary breast-feeding management. Clin Perinatol 1985; 12:319–342. (3, 4, 6, 8, 11)

16. Nicoll A, Ginsburg R, and Tripp J. Supplementary feeding and jaundice in newborns. Acta Paediatr Scand 1982; 71:759–761. (10)

17. Procianoy R, Fernandex-Filho P, Lazaro L, Sartori N, and Drebes S. The influences of rooming-in on breastfeeding. J Trop Pediatr 1983; 29(Apr):112–114. (5)

18. Reiff M and Essock-Vitale S. Hospital influences on early infant-feeding practices. Pediatrics 1985; 76:872–879. (8)

19. Salariya E, Easton P, and Cater J. Duration of breastfeeding after early initiation and frequent feeding. Lancet 1978, 114–143. (3, 6)

20. Taylor P, Lamoni J, and Brown D. Early suckling and prolonged breast-feeding. Am J Dis Child 1986; 140 (Feb):151–154. (7)

21. Wiles L. The effect of prenatal breastfeeding education on breastfeeding success and maternal perception of the infant. JOGNN 1984; (Jul/Aug):253–257. (2)

22. Winikoff B, Myers D, Laukaran V, and Stone R. Overcoming obstacles to breastfeeding in a large municipal hospital: Applications of lessons learned. Pediatrics 1987; 80:423–433. (1, 2, 13)

*Numbers in parentheses refer to specific policies.

Appendix A (3)

ST. JOSEPH MEDICAL CENTER
THE FAMILY BIRTHPLACE

BREASTFEEDING EDUCATION PROTOCOL*

INTERVENTION/MANAGEMENT	RATIONALE	REFERENCES
POLICY #1: All pregnant women should receive information regarding the availability of classes on the benefits and management of breastfeeding.		
Mothers identified as choosing breastfeeding during prenatal contacts will be informed of the breastfeeding class in the childbirth education series. Childbirth education class schedules will be available on the labor-delivery-recovery-postpartum (LDRP) unit and at physicians' offices.	Breastfeeding success and performance is improved by specific knowledge and the support of significant others.	11, 13, 15, 18
POLICY #2: Mothers who are undecided about feeding method will be encouraged to breastfeed.		
Family Birthplace and perinatal education staff will inform mothers of the benefits of breastfeeding and human milk.	Demonstrates compliance with the American Academy of Pediatrics policy statement on breastfeeding and the Surgeon General's goal for the nation. Provides optimal nutritional composition for CNS development. Serves as standard for commercial infant formula.	1, 8, 9, 10, 11 11, 18

*Developed March 1991 by the Breastfeeding Committee: Gina Woodley, R.N., A.C.C.E., IBCLC; Rachel Lewis, R.N., C.B.E.; Pat Rierson, R.N.C., C.B.E.; Judy Angeron, R.N., IBCLC; Sharon Foster, R.N.C., M.N.; Jan Riordan, R.N., Ed.D.; Howard Whiteside, M.D.; Jean Broberg, R.N., M.N.

Adapted from: Arizona Healthy Mothers/Healthy Babies Wellstart-San Diego Lactation Program.

INTERVENTION/MANAGEMENT	RATIONALE	REFERENCES
	Decreases incidence of diarrhea, upper respiratory infections and some allergies; recent studies show decreased incidence in otitis media.	11, 18
	Promotes bonding and mother/infant closeness.	9, 11, 18
	Promotes uterine involution due to increased oxytocin secretion.	9, 10, 11, 14, 15, 20
	Economical and convenient.	
	Mother can always change her mind and discontinue breastfeeding.	

POLICY #3: Mothers expressing desire to breastfeed will have nipples examined for degree of eversion during admission procedures.

INTERVENTION/MANAGEMENT	RATIONALE	REFERENCES
Admitting nurse or resident will perform nipple palpation/pinch test during standard admissions procedures. Gently squeeze one inch behind the nipple base on the areola with thumb and forefinger. The nipple should protrude from the breast.	Identify mothers with non-protruding nipples prior to birth so the appropriate nursing care plan can be implemented.	8, 9, 10, 11, 18
	Infants may have difficulty latching on to non-protruding nipples. The pinch test can assist in determining how the nipple will react in the infant's mouth.	8, 9, 10, 11, 14, 15, 16

POLICY #4: Educational pamphlets on breastfeeding shall be provided following birth, well before discharge.

INTERVENTION/MANAGEMENT	RATIONALE	REFERENCES
Breastfeeding Educator or Primary Care Nurse provides appropriate pamphlet post-birth.	Literature can be used by breastfeeding educator and nursing staff for one-to-one patient education.	14, 15, 18, 26
	Provides consistency of information given by nursing staff and provides a frame of reference.	17, 18, 26
	Mother may refer to literature during hospital stay to reinforce learning.	

POLICY #5: Infants are to be put to breast as soon after birth as feasible for both mother and infant, with 20 minutes post-birth ideal and within the first 2 hours whenever possible.

INTERVENTION/MANAGEMENT	RATIONALE	REFERENCES
The baby will be given to the mother to nurse during the first two hours, and preferably within the first 20 minutes. This includes the alert, stable, post-cesarean birth, mother and baby.	Suck reflex is strongest 20–30 minutes post-birth; delaying gratification can make it difficult for infant to learn sucking process later on.	9, 10, 11, 18

INTERVENTION/MANAGEMENT	RATIONALE	REFERENCES
	Infant promptly receives immunologic benefits of colostrum and digestive peristalsis is stimulated.	11, 14, 15
	Suckling stimulates uterine involution and inhibits bleeding.	9, 10, 11, 14, 15, 18, 20
	Post-cesarean mothers may still be comfortable from epidural medications and interested in breastfeeding.	10, 14, 15, 18, 20
	Mothers should be permitted to engage in this normal, physiologic process regardless of birth method, as long as medically stable.	
Contraindications to immediate breastfeeding: 1. Heavily medicated mother. 2. Infant with Apgar <6. 3. Premature infant <36 weeks gestation.		

POLICY #6: Every mother is to be instructed in proper breastfeeding technique and re-evaluated before discharge.

INTERVENTION/MANAGEMENT	RATIONALE	REFERENCES
Nurse assists mother with breastfeeding and provides guidelines and support when indicated.	Assistance should support mother's efforts and be unobtrusive.	10, 18, 20
Nurse gives positive reinforcement of mother and baby's efforts and success. Pillows may be needed to support mother's arms and bring baby to breast level.	Nipple trauma can be prevented with proper attachment and nipple soreness minimized. Support and comfort of mother and baby prevent fatigue and facilitate proper positioning of the baby at breast. Pillow under baby prevents nipple trauma by raising baby to nipple height.	6, 8, 9, 10, 11, 12, 14, 15, 16, 18, 24
Functional assessment of infant at breast performed by nurse/breastfeeding educator within 24 hours of birth by utilizing the FAIB tool.	Provides for early identification of latch-on difficulties.	3, 20
	Direct observation of infant at breast assures adequacy of breastfeeding prior to discharge.	3, 20
	Provides opportunity for positive reinforcement of breastfeeding and assuring "baby getting something."	3, 20

INTERVENTION/MANAGEMENT	RATIONALE	REFERENCES
Infant's mouth should be at nipple level. Mother supports the breast using a "C" hold. The thumb is placed on top of the breast and the four fingers support the breast underneath. (All fingers should be well back from the areola.)	The "C" hold provides breast support and control and allows the infant to grasp the areola without interference.	9
Mother tickles the center of the infant's bottom lip with her nipple until the infant opens his mouth as wide as possible. The infant may take several minutes to do this.	Tickling the bottom lip causes the baby to open his mouth and assume a position wide enough to get well behind the nipple onto the areola.	
When infant's mouth is open very wide, mother should center her nipple quickly and draw the baby in close to her body.	Bringing baby in close to mother causes the jaws to bypass the centered nipple and come together on the areola.	
Infant's nose and chin should be touching the breast. There is no need to create an air space for most infants. Mother may be taught to lift baby's buttocks if needed.	Infant's nose touching the breast assures proper positioning and latch-on. Baby will not suffocate if close to the breast.	
Infant's mouth and lips should form a flanged seal around the breast tissue. The tongue should be curved around the breast, cupping it and extending over the gum line.	Negative pressure created by the flanged seal acts synergistically with positive pressure in the duct system to ensure transport of milk.	

POLICY #7: The infant is to be encouraged to nurse at least every 2 to 3 hours, for a minimum of 8 feedings/24 hours.

Breastfeeding shall be initiated as soon as possible post-birth.	Baby is more alert within the first 2 hours.	9, 10, 11, 14, 15, 18
Feeding every 2–3 hours will be supported by the nursing staff. Mothers will be assisted in identifying infant's hunger cues and readiness to feed, i.e., R.E.M., hand to mouth movement.	Breastmilk digests in 90 minutes. Eight feedings/24 hours has been associated with increased meconium passage and lower serum bilirubin levels of the infant.	4, 5, 9, 10, 11, 14, 15, 19, 27
Mother will be educated on the "supply and demand" principle of milk production.	Maternal prolactin levels fall after 3 hours. Every three hour feedings enhance milk production.	11, 14, 15, 18, 20
	Understanding of *basic* physiology enhances lactation success.	11, 18, 20

INTERVENTION/MANAGEMENT	RATIONALE	REFERENCES

POLICY #8: Infants should feed from both breasts at all feedings, with a minimum of 6 minutes per breast. An infant may be returned to the first breast for continued suckling, if positioning is correct and nursing is comfortable.

INTERVENTION/MANAGEMENT	RATIONALE	REFERENCES
Babies put to breast every 2–3 hours with at least 6 minutes active swallowing time/breast.	Feeding from both breasts provides regular breast stimulation and allows for greater volume of milk consumption. It often takes 2–3 minutes for milk to let down and may take as long as 6–10 minutes for oxytocin release with the onset of sucking.	9, 10, 11, 18
Mothers instructed on listening for quiet sounds of swallowing.	Audible swallowing is the most reliable indicator of intake.	10, 20
Mothers instructed to burp baby after first breast and put baby to second breast to complete feeding.	Limiting suckling time has not been shown to reduce nipple soreness. Breastfeeding is biphasic with larger volume of milk obtained when nursed from both breasts.	1, 6, 8, 9, 10, 11, 12, 14, 15, 16, 18, 24
Mothers will be instructed on observing baby's early cues for hunger (crying is a late hunger cue) and changes in suck/swallow patterns. Responding to infant's hunger cues takes priority over other events which may be delayed, i.e., infant "waiting" in nursery for lab work.	Restricting breastfeeding may increase degree of physiologic engorgement which occurs during transitional milk phase.	9, 10, 11, 14, 15, 18, 20

POLICY #9: If within the first 24–48 hours post-birth, feedings at the breast are incomplete or ineffective, the mother should be instructed to begin regular expression of her breasts, with continued assistance by an experienced staff member. The colostrum or milk obtained by expression should be given to the baby.

INTERVENTION/MANAGEMENT	RATIONALE	REFERENCES
The primary care nurse/breastfeeding educator will instruct the mother on pumping techniques using the electric breast pump, when infant consistently demonstrates inadequate suckling.	Piston electric pumps most closely imitate the suck cycle of the infant.	2, 11, 14, 18
	Electric system is time saving for the mother.	2, 9, 11, 14, 15, 18
	Breast stimulation and breast emptying are necessary to initiate and maintain lactation.	2, 9, 11, 14, 15, 18

INTERVENTION/MANAGEMENT	RATIONALE	REFERENCES
Expressed colostrum and breastmilk will be given to the infant in addition to any other supplement which may be indicated and prescribed by the physician.	Incomplete breast emptying may lead to insufficient milk due to pressure involution of glandular tissue.	14, 15
	Validates mother's pumping efforts as valuable and provides added benefits to baby.	3, 11, 18

POLICY #10: Supplementary water or formula is given for certain clinical conditions as ordered by the physician, but not on a routine basis. If prolonged supplementation is necessary, the physician will be contacted regarding formula choice and amount.

INTERVENTION/MANAGEMENT	RATIONALE	REFERENCES
Neonatal assessment completed as per nursing protocol.	Preterm or medically compromised infants may need additional nutritional support during the colostral phase of milk production.	10, 11, 14, 15, 18
Sterile water, glucose water or formula feedings are to be given only with specific written order of the attending physician.	Initial water feedings became standard for formula fed infants as formula and glucose water are irritating to the respiratory tree if aspirated. Colostrum is a physiologic substance and readily passes through the respiratory tree if aspirated.	10, 11, 19
	Colostrum and breastmilk will completely meet the newborn's nutritional and fluid needs (provides 17–20 cal./oz.).	9, 10, 11, 14, 15, 18
	Alteration of the flora of the baby's gut occurs with supplemental feedings.	11, 18
	Infants may be confused by a rubber nipple which requires a different tongue and jaw motion.	9, 10, 11, 14, 15, 16, 18 (22, 23)
	Water supplements have not been shown to prevent or cure hyperbilirubinemia in the neonatal period.	3, 4, 5, 10, 11, 14, 15, 18
	Higher protein levels in colostrum have a more stabilizing effect on blood glucose levels than glucose water.	10, 11, 18, 19
	Formula has a longer gut transit time than breastmilk and may decrease the infant's interest in nursing.	9, 10, 11, 14, 15, 18

INTERVENTION/MANAGEMENT	RATIONALE	REFERENCES
	Glucose water with 6 cal./oz. can give infant sense of fullness without providing adequate nutrition (colostrum and breastmilk provide 17–20 cal./oz.).	10, 11, 14, 15, 18, 19, 20
	Encouraging supplementation communicates that mother's milk is inadequate or inappropriate for her infant.	3, 17, 18

POLICY #11: Mothers who wish to feed by both breast and bottle will be educated about breastfeeding and encouraged to breastfeed without supplement.

INTERVENTION/MANAGEMENT	RATIONALE	REFERENCES
Primary care nurse/breastfeeding educator (PCN/BE) will educate mother on rationale for encouraging exclusive breastfeeding during the first weeks, and teach recommended time for introducing bottles.	Reduces mother's anxiety about "insufficient milk" by teaching how to establish and maintain adequate supply.	
	Exclusive breastfeeding during the first two weeks aids in the establishment of an adequate milk supply and appropriate breastfeeding technique.	9, 10, 11, 14, 15, 26
	Three to four weeks of age is the recommended age for introducing a bottle. Expressed breastmilk may be used for bottle feedings as well as infant formula.	9

POLICY #12: Pacifiers should not be used on a routine basis for the breastfeeding infant as a hunger satiety measure.

INTERVENTION/MANAGEMENT	RATIONALE	REFERENCES
Mothers shall be educated to respond to baby's cues for readiness to feed, and identify nutritive and non-nutritive sucking.	Pacifiers should be used for non-nutritive sucking needs.	
Pacifiers are not given to prolong length of time between breastfeedings in order to "get baby on a schedule."	Frequently needing a pacifier may be a sign of inadequate milk intake.	14, 15
	Infants with a weak or ineffective suck may be content to suck on a pacifier for both nutritive and non-nutritive sucking needs.	10, 11, 14, 15, 18

INTERVENTION/MANAGEMENT	RATIONALE	REFERENCES
POLICY #13: Breastfeeding mothers are to have breast examined for evidence of lactation or breastfeeding problems at least once every 24 hours.		
PCN examines breast during daily nursing assessments.	Provides appropriate maternity nursing care.	
BE/PCN examines nipples whenever concerns or complaints of sore nipples are expressed by mother.	Physiologic nipple tenderness occurs during the first few minutes of a feeding and eases up during the same feed. Pathologic nipple soreness is considered whenever mother complains of nipple pain throughout entire feeding or between feedings.	3, 9, 11, 14, 15, 18, 20
POLICY #14: Infants should remain at the mother's bedside both day and night. The nurse should plan with the mother and family for periods of rest/sleep both day and night. If the mother chooses to have the infant in the nursery, she will be encouraged to feed the baby on demand.		
Babies are cared for at the mothers' bedside as per Family Birthplace philosophy.	Infant's presence facilitates bonding and the attachment process. The infant's adaptation to extra-uterine life is aided by the mother's presence.	1, 3, 11, 18, 20
	Provides opportunity for individualized teaching. Aids mother in learning cues and behaviors of her baby.	26
The nurse shall plan with the mother for 1–2 hours of undisturbed rest twice daily.	Rest is an important physiologic and psychologic need for all post-partum mothers.	11, 18
	Adequate rest is essential to lactation.	11, 18
	With liberalized visiting hours, there is no time for mothers to rest unless naps are planned.	11
Infants will be cared for at night in the nursery at the request of the mother, but brought to the mother for demand feeding when exhibiting hunger cues or every 3 hours.	Prolactin levels are highest at night and may contribute to successful breastfeeding. Provides additional opportunities for mother and baby to establish effective nursing pattern prior to discharge.	1
POLICY #15: Commercial discharge packs containing water or formula are not to be given unless specifically ordered by the physician or requested by the mother.		
Mothers are not refused formula sample when requested.		

INTERVENTION/MANAGEMENT	RATIONALE	REFERENCES
Nurses who are concerned infant will not be adequately nourished at the breast due to poor latch-on shall inform the attending physician.	Assists in the development and implementation of a discharge plan which can meet both the infant's nutritional needs and the mother's breastfeeding goals.	
Discharge formula packs are not routinely given to breastfeeding mothers.	Endorses supplementation. Implies that breastmilk is inadequate to meet infant's needs.	17, 18, 19, 20

POLICY #16: At discharge, each mother is to be given a phone number to call for breastfeeding assistance.

Patients contacting physician office for mother/baby concerns reinforced and SJMC Lactation Program #689–5404 stamped on BF pamphlet; Ask-A-Nurse number 685–5700 for after-hours information.	Early discharge often occurs before lactation and breastfeeding well established.	10
	Reassurance can be given for transient breastfeeding difficulties (i.e., engorgement, sore nipples) and differentiated from situations requiring medical intervention.	14

POLICY #17: Mothers who are separated from their infant will be instructed on the proper use of breast pumps as well as the storing and transportation of breast milk.

When prolonged separation of mother and infant is expected (i.e., prematurity, ill infant), the mother will be provided the opportunity for pumping as soon after birth as medically feasible.	Involves mother in care for her infant. Allows her to make "unique" contribution.	3, 9, 11, 14, 15, 18
Pumping *may* need to be delayed if maternal cause for separation—i.e., pregnancy induced hypertension (P.I.H.).	Pumping may be regarded as additional stressor on already vulnerable patient. Certain medications used to treat P.I.H. and other medical conditions may be contraindicated.	11, 18
Breastfeeding Educator/PCN shall instruct the mother on use of the electric breast pump and pumping technique as per protocol.	Following protocol maintains consistency of information given.	11, 18, 20, 26
	Parents may need to have instructions repeated frequently.	11, 14, 15, 18
Breastfeeding Educator/PCN provides parents with written guidelines.	Parents want specific, concrete guidelines.	20
Discharge planning of the mother shall include pumping/expression options, with method decided upon noted in the record.	Emphasizes the importance of regular breast expression in maintaining lactation. Pumping sessions need to be part of daily routine. Pumping frequency and length guidelines are based on the method of expression.	11, 18

References

1. Anderson, G. C. (1989) Risk in mother-infant separation postbirth. *Image: Journal of Nursing Scholarship*, 21: 196–199.

2. Auerbach, K. (1990) Single or double pumping: Which method works best. *Rental Roundup*, 7: 1–4.

3. Cohen, S. P. (1987) High tech—soft touch: Breastfeeding issues. *Clin Perinatol*, 14: 187–195.

4. DeCarValho, M. et al. (1981) Effects of water supplementation on physiologic jaundice in breast-fed babies. *Arch Dis Child*, 56: 568–569.

5. DeCarValho, M., Klauss, M. & Merkatz, R. (1982) Frequency of breastfeeding and serum bilirubin concentration. *Am J Dis Child*, 136: 737–738.

6. DeCarValho, M., Robertson, S. & Klaus, M. (1984) Does the duration and frequency of early breastfeeding affect nipple pain? *Birth*, 11: 81–84.

7. Elander, G. & Lindberg, T. (1984) Short mother-infant separation during first week of life influences the duration of breastfeeding. *Acta Pediatr Scand*, 73: 237–240.

8. Frantz, K. B. (1980) Techniques for managing nipple problems and the reluctant nurser in the early postpartum period. In Freier, S. & Eidelman, A. I. eds. (1980) *Human Milk: Its biological and social value.* Excerptamedica, Amsterdam, pp. 314–317.

9. Huggins, K. (1990) *The Nursing Mother's Companion.* The Harvard Common Press, Boston.

10. Lawrence, R. A. (1987) The management of lactation as a physiologic process. *Clin Perinatol*, 14: 1–10.

11. Lawrence, R. A. (1989) *Breastfeeding: A Guide for the Medical Profession* (3rd edition). C. V. Mosby Co., St. Louis.

12. L'Esperance, C. & Frantz, K. (1985) Time limitation for early breastfeeding. *JOGNN*, 15: 114–118.

13. Naylor, A. & Weser, R. (1987) Providing professional lactation management consultation. *Clin Perinatol*, 14: 33–38.

14. Neifert, M. & Seacat, J. (1986) A guide to successful breastfeeding. *Contemp Pediatr*, 3: 26–45.

15. Neifert, M. & Seacat, J. (1985) Contemporary breastfeeding management. *Clin Perinatol*, 12: 319–341.

16. Newman, J. (1990) Breastfeeding problems associated with the early introduction of bottles and pacifiers. *J Hum Lact*, 6: 59–63.

17. Reiff, Michael & Essock-Vitale, S. (1985) Hospital influence on early infant feeding practices. *Pediatrics*, 76: 873–879.

18. Riordan, J. (1983) *A Practical Guide to Breastfeeding.* C. V. Mosby Co., St. Louis.

19. Shrago, L. (1981) Glucose water supplementation of the breastfed infant during the first three days of life. *J Hum Lact*, 3: 82–86.

20. Shrago, L. & Bucar, D. (1989) The infant's contribution to breastfeeding. *JOGNN*, 19:3 209–215.

21. Slaven, S. & Harvey, D. (1981) Unlimited suckling time improves breastfeeding. *Lancet*, (8216): 392–393.

22. Smith, W. et al. (1985) Physiology of sucking in the normal term infant using real-time US. *Radiology*, 156: 379–381.

23. Smith, W., Erenberg, A. & Nowak, A. (1988) Imaging evaluation of the human nipple during breastfeeding. *Am J Dis Child* 142: 76–78.

24. Walker, M. & Driscoll, J. (1989) Sore nipples: The new mother's nemesis. *MCN*, 14: 260–265.

25. Winikoff, B. et al. (1986) Dynamics of infant feeding: Mothers, professionals, and the institutional context in a large urban hospital. *Pediatrics*, 77: 357–365.

26. Winikoff, B. et al. (1987) Overcoming obstacles to breastfeeding in a large municipal hospital: Applications of lessons learned. *Pediatrics*, 80: 423–433.

27. Yamauchi, Y. & Yamanouchi, I. (1990) Breastfeeding frequency during the first 24 hours after birth in full-term neonates. *Pediatrics*, 86: 171–175.

Appendix B

Infant Assessment Form

Baby name _____ Dr. _____   Suck assessment performed _____ Yes _____ No

Birth date _____ Birth weight _____   Was baby able to latch on and nurse p̄ suck assessment?

              SGA   day 2 _____   (see suck assessment form)

Gestational Age _____ AGA   day 3 _____   _____ Yes _____ No

              LGA   day 4 _____   **Risk Factors:**

Phone # _____   Hx insufficient milk _____ Maternal employment _____

Insurance _____   Non-protruding nipples _____ Use of nipple shields _____

Date/time initial visit _____   Breast surgery _____ NICU _____

Questions/concerns of mother _____   Difficult latch on _____ Maternal illness _____

_____   Supplementation _____ Other _____

_____   Multiple birth _____ _____

Baby chart review: Last fed/time _____ how _____   **Physician notified:** _____

Supplementation _____ No _____ Yes   type and amount   _____

_____   Pamphlets given_____

Why given _____   **Nurses' Notes/recommendations: (date, time & signature upon entry)**

Function assessment of infant at breast performed _____ Yes

     _____ No   Results? _____

Position: ___ cradle ___ clutch ___sidelying _____ other

At this visit baby was: _____ deeply asleep

_____ drowsy _____ quiet/alert _____ crying

In order to get baby to nurse mother/nurse had to

_____ place baby at breast with no effort

_____ use mild stimulation

_____ use vigorous stimulation beginning and during feeding

_____ did not nurse

How long p̄ placing baby at breast did infant

latch on and suck?

_____ feeds immediately 0-3 min. _____ 3-10 min

_____ over 10 min. _____ does not feed

Baby's feeding pattern: _____sucks well

_____ sucks off and on, needs encouragement

_____ weak sucking, some effort for short periods

_____ baby did not suck

PATIENT IDENTIFICATION

ST. JOSEPH MEDICAL CENTER
WICHITA, KANSAS 67218
BREASTFEEDING ASSESSMENT RECORD
P1277 10/91

ORIGINAL: Mother's Chart / YELLOW COPY: Baby's Chart / PINK COPY: Department

Appendix C

Nursing Diagnosis Related to Breastfeeding

Approved diagnostic labels of the North American
Nursing Diagnosis Association (NANDA)

Effective Breastfeeding

Definition:
The state in which a mother-infant dyad/family exhibits adequate proficiency and satisfaction with breastfeeding process

Defining Characteristics
- Mother able to position infant at breast to promote a successful latch-on response
- Signs and/or symptoms of oxytocin release (let-down or milk ejection reflex)
- Adequate infant elimination patterns for age
- Eagerness of infant to nurse
- Maternal verbalization of satisfaction with the breastfeeding process

Related Factors
- Basic breastfeeding knowledge
- Normal breast structure
- Normal infant or structure

Ineffective Breastfeeding

Definition:
The state in which a mother or child experiences difficulty with the breastfeeding process

Defining Characteristics
- Mother unable to position infant at breast to promote a successful latch-on response
- Maternal reluctance to put infant at breast
- Inadequate infant elimination
- Maternal verbalization of dissatisfaction with breastfeeding
- Non-sustained suckling at the breast
- Infant does not receive nourishment at the breast for some or all of feedings
- Separation of mother and infant
- No signs or symptoms of oxytocin release (let-down)
- Nursing less than 7 in 24 hours (First month)

Related Factors
- Prematurity
- Maternal breast anomaly
- History of previous breastfeeding failure

Interrupted Breastfeeding

Definition:
A break in the continuity of the breastfeeding process as a result of inability or inadvisability to put baby to breast for feeding.

Defining Characteristics
- Infant does not receive nourishment at the breast for some or all of feedings
- Maternal desire to maintain lactation and provide (or eventually provide) her breastmilk for her infant's nutritional needs.
- Separation of mother and infant
- Lack of knowledge regarding expression and storage of breastmilk

Related Factors
- Maternal or infant illness
- Prematurity
- Maternal employment

- Infant gestation; age greater than 34 weeks
- Support source
- Maternal confidence

- Infant receiving supplemental feedings with artificial nipple
- Poor infant sucking reflex
- Non-supportive partner/family
- Knowledge deficit
- Maternal anxiety
- Delayed initiation of breast-feeding

- Contraindications to breastfeeding (e.g. drugs, true breastmilk jaundice)
- Need to abruptly wean infant

Appendix D

New York State Code in Support of Breastfeeding (Added 1984)*

(10(i) The hospital, with the advice of the maternity staff, shall formulate a program of instruction and provide assistance for each maternity patient(s) in the fundamentals of (normal) infant care including infant feeding choice and techniques, postpregnancy care and family planning.

(ii) The hospital shall provide instruction and assistance to each maternity patient who has chosen to breastfeed and shall provide information on the advantages and disadvantages of breastfeeding to women who are undecided as to the feeding method for their infants. As a minimum:

(a) the hospital shall designate at least one person who is thoroughly trained in breastfeeding physiology and management to be responsible for ensuring the implementation of an effective breastfeeding program; and

(b) policies and procedures shall be developed to assist the mother to breastfeed which shall include but not be limited to:

(1) prohibition of the application of standing orders for antilactation drugs;

(2) placement of the infant for breastfeeding immediately following delivery, unless contraindicated;

(3) restriction of the infant's supplemental feedings to those indicated by the medical condition of the infant or of the mother;

(4) provision for the infant to be fed on demand; and

(c) assurance that an educational program has been given as soon after admission as possible which shall include but not be limited to:

(1) the nutritional and physiological aspects of human milk;

(2) the normal process for establishing lactation, including care of breasts, common problems associated with breastfeeding and frequency of feeding;

(3) dietary requirements for breastfeeding;

(4) diseases and medication or other substances which may have an effect on breastfeeding;

(5) sanitary procedures to follow in collecting and storing human milk; and

(6) sources for advice and information available to the mother following discharge.

*Chapter V Subchapter A Article 2 Part 405 Hospitals—minimum standards (Statutory authority: Public health law § 2803) 405.8 Maternal, child health and newborn services

Appendix E

Prototype Lactation Consultant Job Proposal
or Description*

NOTE TO READER: In all cases, a job proposal or description should reflect those specific elements that are relevant to the setting and the individual offering to provide the service in question. This prototype job proposal/description is more inclusive than would be necessary in most settings.

QUALIFICATIONS NEEDED

1.0 Certification by the International Board of Lactation Consultant Examiners (I.B.L.C.E.)

2.0 Minimum five years experience working with childbearing families or maternal health nursing.

OBJECTIVES

1.0 Document the need for a lactation consultant.

1.1 Establish base-line data on the numbers and percentages within the institution's patient base of mothers who initiate breastfeeding and the length of time they continue to breastfeed after hospital discharge.

1.2. Collect and analyze data to determine when and what kind of support the breastfeeding mother would like to receive prior to her baby's birth, while she is in the hospital, and after she returns home.

1.3. Survey other health-care providers who staff the institution and/or who work in the community which the hospital serves regarding their perceived need for the assistance and resources that a lactation consultant could provide. [N.B.: In settings where the profession of lactation consultant is unknown,

this goal may need to be changed to determine the degree to which health providers—if given access to the resources of a lactation consultant—might choose to use such a service.]

2.0. Promote breastfeeding beyond the first few weeks of life and assist the mother to reach her own goals for breastfeeding.

2.1. Develop and implement guidelines and standards of care for assisting breastfeeding mothers in all areas of the institution where they might be served (emergency room, obstetrics/gynecology, family medicine, the midwifery service, employee health, women's health service, pediatrics, and internal medicine).

2.2. Clarify roles of and perceptions about breastfeeding support among all health providers in the hospital, paying particular attention to those care providers who are most likely to serve lactating women and their breastfeeding infants.

2.3. Develop a reference library of breastfeeding materials appropriate for both health-care providers and mothers interested in learning more about lactation. Particular attention should be paid to maintaining and regularly updating a file of journal articles and to obtaining reference works that include the latest information on lactation in a variety of contexts and circumstances.

2.4. Provide regular in-service education for all relevant medical, nursing, and ancillary staff. In some cases, hospital policies may determine the frequency with which such in-servicing must be offered and attended. In other cases, invitations may need to be secured from the administrative offices of the services in question.

*Derived in part from Tinari, MA: Lactation consultant job proposal, *J Hum Lact* 2:114–15, 1986.

2.5. Offer case conferences that highlight the particular needs of lactating mothers and/or their breastfeeding infants. Such case conferences may serve as a springboard for reexamining care routines and/or other aspects of the hospital experience of the mother-baby couple in question.

2.6. Set up a telephone warmline/hotline to provide continuing contact between the lactation consultant and the clients she has assisted in the hospital and others who may be referred to her for out-patient assistance.

2.7. Establish a regular follow-up system of continuing care for mothers first seen in the hospital. Such a system may be part of the hotline/warmline service, or it may consist of communication by postcard or letter, the incorporation of home visits by the hospital-based LC, or referral to a community-based breastfeeding counselor who makes home visits and reports back to the hospital LC. When such referral continues without reports, continuity of care is lost, although continued support for the breastfeeding mother may continue.

2.8. Provide an out-patient service for persons who were not initially seen in the hospital and/or who are not in the immediate postpartum period.

2.9. Offer regularly scheduled prenatal breastfeeding classes to inform prospective mothers of the services available in the institution that support the breastfeeding course and to provide them with sufficient information to make an informed choice about infant feeding.

2.10. Offer regularly scheduled postpartum breastfeeding classes to mothers who give birth in the institution prior to their return home.

2.11. Provide access to breastfeeding equipment and devices when their use is appropriate to the lactating mother and her breastfeeding infant. In most cases, such equipment will include breast pumps, breast shells, tube feeding devices, and the like. In some cases, such devices are available for purchase; in other cases, they are rented. In situations where the lactation consultant is unable or unwilling to provide such rental or purchase options, she needs to develop an ongoing relationship with those businesses in the community that do offer such a service, in order that she may assist the mother who needs such devices with a minimum of disruption to the lactation course.

3.0. Coordinate the services of the professional staff to the benefit of the lactating mother and her breastfeeding baby.

3.1. Document teaching and progress of the mother and baby on patient charts. In some cases, this may necessitate completing separate charts for the mother and the baby, a time-consuming duplication of effort. In other cases, lactation assessment charts have been developed whose copies can be appended to each patient's chart and/or sent to the physician seeing the mother and/or baby.

3.2. Confer regularly with the relevant obstetrician, pediatrician, mother-baby, and postpartum or nursery nursing staff member on each patient's progress, special needs, and continuity of care.

3.3. Develop and/or review all literature relating to infant feeding that is distributed to patients in the hospital and related to their discharge home.

3.4. Initiate and maintain contact with all relevant medical staff, particularly pediatric and obstetric/family medicine physicians regarding the policies and programs that affect their patients in order to effect a team approach to promoting successful breastfeeding.

3.5. Participate in a committee charged with evaluating relevant hospital policies that may influence the breastfeeding course of mothers and babies receiving care in the institution.

4.0. Participate in scholarly activities: research, publications, grants.

4.1. Maintain statistics on breastfeeding initiation and duration of all clients seen in the hospital or assisted in the out-patient clinic in order to periodically assess the effectiveness of the lactation consultant service within the institution.

4.2. Participate in the development, implementation, and dissemination of the results of research in which lactating mothers and/or their breastfeeding babies were subjects.

4.3. Write and submit articles for publication in the health-profession journals and maternal-child literature.

4.4. Apply for grants to support new clinical care procedures, research protocols evaluating some aspect of the maternal lactation course, and/or infant breastfeeding patterns.

5.0. Serve as a speaker/participant in public and professional forums providing programs relating to lactation and breastfeeding.

5.1. Participate in continuing education through seminars, workshops, conferences, and network with others in the field.

RESOURCES NEEDED

1. Office space and supplies, including lockable file cabinets in which to store client information forms and other records relating to the performance of the LC's duties.

2. Secretarial assistance in keeping with the needs of the LC or the LC practice.

3. Telephone with at least two lines. An answering machine and beeper system in order that the LC may be reached when she is not at her desk.

4. Small reference library.

5. Financial support for the LC to participate in regular continuing education at annual conferences and the purchase of books and other resource materials relevant to the practice of lactation consulting.

6. Computer with word processing and spreadsheet software**.

**"Rental Manager" spreadsheet software for reports and breast pump rental information is available from Medela, Inc., 4610 Prime Parkway, McHenry, IL 60050 USA; (815) 363–1166; or 1–800–435–8316; TELEX (815) 353–1246.

Appendix F

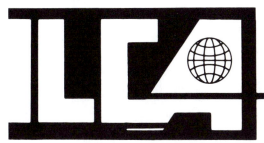

International Lactation Consultant Association

Recommendations and Competencies[1] for Lactation Consultant Practice[2]

Breastfeeding is a learned art and skill with proven benefits to the mother, baby, family and society. To maximize these benefits, lactation consultants function as members of the health care team, with their primary focus on breastfeeding. The overall goals of the lactation consultant are to enable mothers and families to make informed infant feeding choices, initiate and maintain lactation, overcome obstacles, prevent premature weaning and enhance maternal role satisfaction. Lactation consultants are linked to each other by the work they do, by the knowledge and skills they possess and by the way they use these skills to promote and protect the health of women and infants.

A profession's concern for the quality of its service constitutes the core of its responsibility to the public. Guidelines for practice promote unity in the lactation consultant profession by encouraging a common approach to practice. Lactation consultants have a variety of backgrounds and educational preparation, and they practice in diverse settings. A rational approach to providing guidelines within a framework of diversity is to identify competencies for practice rather than establishing rigid rules. A competency is a cognitive, affective or psychomotor skill.

This diversity in setting, personnel, style and delivery of lactation support in different cultural contexts requires that these guidelines allow for innovation and development of programs best suited to individual consumers and communities. They do not define a standard of care nor state exclusive rules for practice. This document presents general recognized recommendations intended as a foundation for specialty practice as a lactation consultant.

---

1. Adapted from *Competencies and Program Guidelines for Nurse Providers of Childbirth Education*, NAACOG, 1987.

2. Copyright, 1991 International Lactation Consultant Association. Not for reproduction without written permission. For more information about the International Lactation Consultant Association and to obtain additional copies of this Competency Statement for lactation consultants, contact ILCA, 201 Brown Avenue, Evanston, IL 60202-3601 USA; (708) 260-8874.

1.0 Breastfeeding Education and Advocacy

The lactation consultant will be able to:

1.1 Educate parents on all aspects of infant feeding for informed choice-making and supply listings of educational materials.

1.2 Review nutritional recommendations for lactation, provide written guidelines if necessary, and refer to a nutritionist or supplementary food program if needed.

1.3 Provide emotional support to parents through personal interaction and referral to resource personnel and support groups, if necessary.

1.4 Provide anticipatory guidance to reduce the occurrence of breastfeeding problems.

1.5 Discuss the effects of medications, recreational drugs, chemicals and home remedies on lactation and infant health.

1.6 Act as an advocate for breastfeeding in the community, work place and within the health care professions.

1.7 Act as an advocate for the breastfeeding family in the pursuit of optimal health care.

1.8 Educate the public and health workers on relevant aspects of lactation.

1.9 Develop the necessary understanding of cultural differences in the community as they relate to breastfeeding.

1.10 Teach breastfeeding classes for parents.

2.0 Clinical Management of Breastfeeding

2.1 Consent

2.1.1 Obtain informed consent from the mother after identification of need for lactation consultant services is made.
2.1.2 Obtain the mother's permission to conduct assessment.

2.2 History

2.2.1 Systematically obtain and update history of the mother and infant relative to lactation and breastfeeding, including: pregnancy, labor, delivery, previous breastfeeding experiences, current breastfeeding experience including feeding, elimination and sleep patterns, and current health of mother and baby.
2.2.2 Identify the possible conditions or problems based on history and assessment.
2.2.3 Evaluate the emotional status of the mother and the elements of her support system. Refer when indicated.

2.3 Assessment/Examination
2.3.1 Wash hands prior to examining mother or baby and maintain high standards of hygiene.
2.3.2 Examine the mother's breasts for:
2.3.2.1 Nipple protractility and breast elasticity.
2.3.2.2 Lumps, breast obstructions, inflammation, edema, engorgement, scars, and abnormal anatomy.
2.3.2.3 Alterations of breast and nipple skin integrity.
2.3.2.4 Breast, nipple and areolar size, appearance and symmetry.
2.3.3 Examine and/or observe the infant during non-feeding times for:
2.3.3.1 Level of alertness
2.3.3.2 Level of irritability
2.3.3.3 Body alignment and symmetry
2.3.3.4 Muscle tone and activity of body and mouth
2.3.3.5 Facial features and oral anatomy
2.3.3.6 Weight, weight for length ratio, length, head and chest circumference, and growth pattern since birth
2.3.3.7 Hydration status
2.3.3.8 Age appropriate reflexes and other developmental milestones
2.3.4 Observe mother and infant during a feeding.
2.3.4.1 Observe body position of mother and baby
2.3.4.2 Assess milk transfer
2.3.4.3 Observe and assess milk intake, noting:
• successful and proper attachment to the breast
• breathing pattern at the breast
• suckling pattern
• swallowing of milk

2.4 Analysis

2.4.1 Formulate and communicate a complete list of concerns, conditions and/or problems and verify with the mother.
2.4.2 Provide information to enable the mother to make decisions and to assume responsibility for her own health and her infant's health and feeding plan.
2.4.3 Initiate crisis intervention management when indicated.

2.5 Recommendations

2.5.1 Use accepted counseling techniques and communication skills with mothers and support persons.
2.5.2 Identify the need for consultation and referral to appropriate members of the health care team

or community support resources.

2.5.3 Develop with the mother a comprehensive feeding and care plan based on the history and assessment.

2.5.4 Evaluate with the mother possible goals and modify plans of care as needed.

2.5.5. Provide written instructions to the mother.

2.6 Reporting and Follow-up

2.6.1 Keep accurate and complete records on findings and care provided to mother and baby.

2.6.2 Regularly confer with and report progress, plans and evaluations to all primary health workers caring for the mother and baby.

2.6.3 Provide follow-up plans for each client contact.

3.0 Technical Knowledge

3.1 Demonstrate usual and special positioning techniques for mother and baby.

3.2 Select and explain assistance techniques based on history and assessment of the situation.

3.2.1 Increase or decrease infant milk intake.

3.2.2 Milk supply modification

3.2.3 Manual (hand) milk expression

3.2.4 Safe and effective collection and storage of breastmilk

3.2.5 Alternate massage

3.2.6 Maternal diet modification relative to sufficient intake, maternal or infant food intolerance, maternal or infant food allergies and their effect on the infant and lactation.

3.2.7 Finger-feeding with tubing, syringe, dropper

3.3 Discuss the risks and benefits of the use of the following items:

3.3.1 Breast pads

3.3.2 Nipple creams and oils

3.3.3 Nipple shields

3.3.4 Nursing bras

3.3.5 Slings and carriers

3.3.6 Nursing pillows

3.3.7 Special clothing

3.3.8 Pacifiers (dummies)

3.3.9 Mother's own milk, donor breastmilk and breast milk substitutes

3.4 Select and explain equipment based on history and assessment of the situation.

3.4.1 Breast pumps

3.4.2 Breast shells

3.4.3 Devices for dimpled nipples

3.4.4 Alternate feeding devices

    3.4.4.1 feeding tube devices

    3.4.4.2 cups

    3.4.4.3 bottles with artifical nipples/teats

    3.4.4.4 droppers

    3.4.4.5 syringes

    3.4.4.6 spoons

    3.4.4.7 bowls

4.0 Special Knowledge and Assistance

4.1 Develop special plans for the continuation of breastfeeding if any of the following conditions are present in the infant. Assist the mother in implementing those plans.

4.1.1 Hyperbilirubinemia

4.1.2 Problems with attachment ("latch-on")

4.1.3 Dysfunctional, disorganized or weak suck

4.1.4 "Nipple confusion" and nipple preference

4.1.5 Breast preference

4.1.6 Prematurity

4.1.7 Postmaturity

4.1.8 Low birth weight

4.1.9 Temporary mother-baby separation

4.1.10 Down Syndrome

4.1.11 Developmental disability

4.1.12 Physical challenges

4.1.13 Neurological impairment

4.1.14 Insufficient weight gain

4.1.15 Refusal to breastfeed

4.1.16 Cleft lip, cleft palate, other orofacial abnormalities

4.1.17 Digestive and metabolic disorders

4.1.18 Infectious and contagious diseases

4.1.19 Gastroenteritis

4.1.20 Other illness or conditions that may adversely affect breastfeeding

4.2 Develop and assist the mother in implementing special plans for the continuation of breastfeeding if any of the following conditions are present in the mother:

4.2.1 Breast engorgement

4.2.2 Nipple problems and anomalies

4.2.3 Breast pain

4.2.4 Milk ejection problems

4.2.5 Obstructed milk duct

4.2.6 Infectious and non-infectious mastitis

4.2.7 Breast abscess

4.2.8 Cystic breast disease

4.2.9 Variations in milk supply

4.2.10 Breast surgery

4.2.11 Cesarean birth

4.2.12 Induced lactation and relactation

4.2.13 Endocrine disorders

4.2.14 Enzyme deficiencies and other metabolic disorders

4.2.15 Seizure disorders

4.2.16 Affective disorders

4.2.17 Physical challenges

4.2.18 Adolescence

4.2.19 Infectious and contagious diseases

4.2.20 Acute or chronic medication use

4.2.21 Recreational drug use

4.2.22 Other illnesses or conditions that may adversely affect breastfeeding

4.3. Develop and assist the mother in the implementation of special plans for the following situations:
4.3.1 Separation from the infant
4.3.2 Relinquishing the infant for adoption
4.3.3 Death of the infant

5.0 Professional Responsibilities and Activities

5.1 Identify the need for consultation and collaboration with other members of the health care team. Make referrals as necessary to:
5.1.1 Peer or lay support groups
5.1.2 Other lactation consutlant with specific expertise
5.1.3 Physician, nurse practitioner, midwife, specialist, physical therapist, occupational therapist or other health care specialist

5.2 Coordinate services with other health workers.

5.2.1 Consult and confer with other lactation consultants as needed.
5.2.2 Inform client of consultations with other resources.

5.3 Make provisions for coverage outside of normal practice hours.

5.4 Pursue continuing education relevant to lactation consultant practice, including reading current professional journals, participation in workshops, seminars, in-service programs, conferences, accredited courses.

5.4.1 Present evidence of maintaining and expanding knowledge and skills through participation in any other professional development activities.

5.5 Support the development of relevant education and certification processes for the lactation consultant profession.

5.6 Assess equipment safety and effectiveness.

5.7 Observe guidelines for health workers in the International Code of Marketing of Breastmilk Substitutes.

5.8 Maintain professional credibility through membership in appropriate professional organizations.

5.9 Initiate, participate in, and report on research in the field of human lactation as opportunities arise.

5.10 Act as a resource to peer support groups.

5.11 Create peer support groups as indicated.

5.12 Create and staff breastfeeding hotline as needed.

5.13 Rent or sell breastfeeding equipment as desired.

5.14 When advertising the lactation consultant practice in any media, use the following guidelines, whether through telephone directory, periodicals, displays, newspapers, radio, television, written communications or other media:
5.14.1 Reflect support of the International Code of Marketing of Breastmilk Substitutes in all advertising.
5.14.2 Make no advertising claim which cannot be met in full without further qualification; provide accurate information regarding services and products.
5.14.3 Advertise in a manner which conforms to generally accepted standards of good taste; avoid practices, words, and illustrations that may be offensive.
5.14.4 Retain copy or recording of advertisement.

6.0 Business Practices/Legal Considerations

6.1 Maintain patient confidentiality.

6.2 Charge reasonable fees for services rendered, as determined by local community norms for comparable health care.

6.3 Make a clear statement to the mother regarding fees and billing prior to providing services.

6.4 Obtain written release when photographing a mother and/or baby.

6.5 Carry appropriate insurance coverage.

6.6 Follow local laws and codes.

6.7 Maintain patient records for an appropriate time period.

Appendix G

Breastfeeding Support Resources

ARGENTINA
Nunu (Asociación de Ayuda Materna)
Avda. San Martín 1450-Vte.
Vincente Lopez, 1636
Casilla Correo 69

AUSTRALIA
ACE (Andrea Robertson)
148 Hereford St.
Forest Lodge 2037
Tel.: 61–2–660 6149

Australian Lactation Consultants'
   Association
PO Box 1129
Carlton, Vic. 3053
Tel.: 61–3–398-3314/509–4929

CAPERS (Jan Cornfoot)
PO Box 567
Nundah, Qld. 4012
Tel.: 61–7–266–9573

Lactation Resource Centre
PO Box 231
Nunawading, Vic. 3131
Tel.: 61–3–877–7730

LLL Australia
c/o Cathy Rough
208 Payne Rd,
The Gap
Brisbane, Qld. 4061

N.M.A.A. (Nursing Mothers
   Association of Australia)
PO Box 231
Nunawading, Vic. 3131
Tel.: 61–3–877–5011

Parents' Centres Australia
32–4 Station St.
Harris Park, N.S.W. 2150
Tel.: 61–2–633–5899

Prahran College of TAFE
Childcare Studies Dept

High St.
Prahran, Vic. 3181
Tel.: 61–3–522–6700

BAHRAIN
LLL
c/o Laura Kyle
PO Box 14
Manama, Bahrain

BANGLADESH
Consumers Association of Bangladesh
House no. 320/2A
Road no. 8A (old-15)
West Dhanmondi, Dhaka

BARBADOS
LLL Cardon
Enterprise Coast Road
Christ Church

BELGIUM
Regionale Stillgruppe des
   deutschsprachingen Gebietes
   Belgiens
c/o J. Maes
Am. Neudorferberg 4
B–4730 Raeren, Belgium
Tel.: 32–87–86–6031

BELIZE
Breast is Best League
PO Box 1203
44 Gabourel Lane
Belize City

BRAZIL
Amigos do Peito
Av. Espitania Pessoa 1684/c 02
Ipanema
Rio de Janeiro

INAN
Sep/N Quadra 510
Conjunto A
70 750 Brasilia

Marina Rea
PO Box 8027
São Paulo SP, CEP 05403

Mothers' Group Sub-Program
Avenida General Guslo 274–40 Andar
Rio de Janeiro

CANADA
Alberta Social Services and
   Community Health
c/o Elva Pierdue
7th St. Plaza
10030–107 St
Edmonton, Alberta T5J 3E4

Canadian Lactation Consultant
   Association
c/o Eileen Shea
RR2 Mt. Hope
Ontario L0R 1W0
Tel.: 416–679–4939

Friends of Breastfeeding Society
Box 399
Mildmay, Ontario NOG 2J0

Health and Welfare Canada
Child and Family Health Programs
Health Promotion Directorate
4th Floor
Jeanne Mance Building
Tunneys Pasture
Ottawa, Ontario KIA IB4
Tel.: 613–996–1125

Ligue La Leche du Canada Francais
Case Postale 874
Ville St.
Laurent, Quebec

LLL Canada
2125 29 Ave. SW
Calgary, Alberta T2T 1N6

CHILE
Liga Chilena de la Lactancia Materna
Esmeralda–678–Piso
Santiago-Centro

COLOMBIA
LLL Area Co-ordinator for Central
   and South America
Apt. A 278
Zona B Envigado
Antioquia, Colombia

COSTA RICA
APOYO Centro Pro-Mujer
c/o Nancy Sabean
Apartado 470
San Pedro
Montes de Oca
San José 2070

CURAÇAO
Curaçao Breastfeeding Group
PO Box 2043
Willenstad, Curaçao
Netherlands Antilles

DENMARK
Ammelauget
c/o Ellyn Grubbe
Bregningevej 1
Gronnegade, Kettinge DK–4892
Tel.: 45–3–86–4533

Ammeradgviningen
c/o Susanne Heltzen
Figgardvej 5
Dommervy 7800 Skive
Foraeldre og Fodsel
Herlufsholmsallee 2
DK–4700 Naestved
Tel.: 45–1–15–7870

Foraeldre og Fodsel
Malmmosevej 71b
2830 Virum.
Tel.: 45–2–42–41–18

World Health Organisation
Regional Office for Europe
Dr. Elisabeth Helsing
8 Shcerfigvej
DK–2100 Copenhagen
Tel.: 45–1–29–01–11

ECUADOR
La Liga Ecuatoriana de la Lactancia
   Materna
Apartado 21–161
Eloy Alfaro
Quito

LLLI
c/o Ann Johnson
Casilla 6374 C.C.I.,
Quito
Tel.: 593–2–249–003

EGYPT
LLL Egypt
c/o Linda Zamora
PO Box 291
54 Rd. Maadi, Cairo

Society of Friends of Mothers' Milk
c/o Dr. Sayd Abd Allah
Damietta General Hospital
Maadi Medical Centre 21
ST. 105 Maadi, Cairo

EL SALVADOR
CALMA
Urbanización La Esperanza
Diagonal 2
Polígono L–226
San Salvador

FIJI
NM Association of Fiji
PO Box 4453
Samabula, Suva

FINLAND
Ensi-ja Turvakotien liito (BF
   Promotion Group)
Musseokatu 24A
00100 Helsinki
Ritva Kuusisto
Viidakkotie 6
SF–04260 Kerava

FRANCE
IFAM (professional group)
c/o Giselle Laviolle
65 Allée du Lac Inférieur
78110 le Vesinet

(Important for Francophone countries)
Info-Allaitement
c/o Dominique Couturier
Bayers 16460, Aunac

Lactarium
Institut de Puericulture
26, Blvd. Brune
F–75014 Paris

La Leche League
BP 18
L'Etang la Ville, France 78620
Tel.: 33–1–875–0289

Solidarilait
Centre Puercultrice
26, Blvd. Brune
F–75014 Paris

GERMANY
Arbeitsgemeinschaft Freier
   Stillgruppen,
Rheingaustr. 14
5429 Welterod Germany
Tel.: 37–6775–1368

LLL Deutschland e.V.
Postfach 96
D–8000 München 65, Germany

VELB (Verband Europäischer
   Laktationsberater/innen IBCLC)
Delpweg 14
3000 Hannover 91, Germany

GHANA
GINAN (Ghana Infant Nutrition
   Action Network
PO Box 6177
Accra North

GREECE
Maria Tsitsiloni-Lioulia
Salamionos 30
153 43 AG1A Paraskevi
Athens

GUATEMALA
National Commission for the
   Promotion of BF
PO Box 149
Guatemala City

HONDURAS
Proalma (Judy Canahuati)
PO Box 512
San Pedro Sula

HUNGARY
Dr. Eszter Bonta
1 Pagony St.
Budapest

ICELAND

Ahugafelag um brjostagof
c/o Anna Kristen Gunnarsdottir
Artun 19
550 Saudarkrokur
or Holavegur 13
550 Saudarkrokur
1124 Iceland

Nurses Association
c/o Edda Jona Jonasdottir
Lagmuli 7
108 Reykjavik

INDIA

Consumers' Guidance Society of
 India
c/o Dr. Raj Anand
55 Kavi Apts.
Worli, Bombay 400008
Tel.: 91–22–354699 (Office
 4 P.M.–6 P.M.)

Infant Nutrition Information Service
C–14 Community Centre
Safdarjung Development Area
New Delhi 110016

INDONESIA

Arif
Dr. Indra D. Elita
Jalan Liliroyor
Manado
Sulwesi Jtara

BK-PP-ASI
c/o Dept. Child Health
Gadjah Mada University
Jalan Pugeran 27
RS Pugeran 27
Yogyakarta

Breast Feeding Mothers Support
 Group
Jalan Senaya 16 Blok S1A
Kebayoran Baru
Jakarta Selatan

Department of Child Health
Contact: Dr. Sudaryat Suraatmaja
Udavana University
Denpasar, Bali

IRELAND

Association for Improvement in
 Maternity Services
48 Wyvern
Killiney Rd.

Dublin
Tel.: 353–1–85–6947

The Home Birth Centre
3 South Terrace
Inchicore, Dublin
Tel.: 353–8–71–7295

LLL Ireland
2 Rathdown Park
Greystones
Co. Wicklow
Tel.: 353–87–5368

Lactation Consultants of Ireland (LCI)
2 Kylemore Park
Taylor's Hill, Galway
Ireland

Well Woman Centre
63 Lr. Leeson St.
Dublin 2

ISRAEL

Israel Childbirth Education Centre
PO Box 3731
Haifa
Tel.: 972–4–313037 246 075

Israeli Lactation Consultant Associa-
 tion (ILCA)
PO Box 1172
Eilat

ITALY

Associazione per l'Allattamento
 Materno
c/o Anna Brennan
Colle Rasto I–00039

Zagarolo
Jenny Della Torre
via C. Goldoni 23
Milano 20129

IVORY COAST

Mlle Nicole Vial, Directrice
D'Inades-Documentation
Boite Postal 8
Abidjan 08

JAPAN

La Leche League (English)
c/o Diane Wiltshire
Kanagawa, 1–25–6
Minami Azabu
Minatuku 106
Tel.: 81–3–452–6027

La Leche League (Japanese)
c/o Reiko Yamamoto
6–18–12, Seijo
Satagaya Ku. 157

Tokyo Childbirth Education
 Association
c/o Diane Bond
2–5–17, Nakadai
Narita-shi
Tel.: 81–476–26–8954
Maya Shah, Tel.: 81–3–313–8665

KENYA

BIG (BF Information Group)
PO Box 59436
Nairobi

LIBERIA

Breastfeeding Advocacy Group
PO Box 1046
Monrovia
Tel.: 231–26–2610 26–1984

MALAYSIA

Consumers' Association of Penang
27 Jalan Kelawai
Penang

International Organisation of
 Consumer Unions Asia
PO Box 1045
Penang (04)
Tel.: 60–4–371–396
Fax: 60–4–366–506

Nursing Mothers Association of
 Penang
9 Jalan Chenghai
Tanjong Bungah Tolong
Penang

PPPI Malaysian Breastfeeding
 Advisory Association
25A Jalan Kampong Pandan
55100 Kuala Lumpur

MALTA

Marianne Theuma
5 Trafalgar Flats
Cardinal Street
Vittoriosa

MAURITIUS

MAPBIN
PO Box 1134
Port Louis

MEXICO
Breastfeeding Counsellors Project
Apartado Postal 82–109
Cuajimalpa 05000
Mexico

Produssep, A.C.
Patricio Sanz 449
Mexico D.F.

NETHERLANDS
La Leche League of Zoetermeer
Amalia Plaats 30
2713 B J Zoetermeer
Veriniging Borstvoeding Natuurlijk
Postbus 119
3960 BC Wijk bij Duurstede
2888884
Tel.: 31–1807–22430/31–2155–16026

NEW ZEALAND
CRY-SOS
c/o Dr. John Kirkland
Education Dept
Massey University
Palmerston North

LLL New Zealand
Box 13383
Johnsonville, Wellington
New Zealand Parents' Centres
    Federation
PO Box 11–310
Wellington

NICARAGUA
Génesis 11
Apartado 2829
Managua

NORWAY
AHIG (Ammehjelpen's International
    Group)
Postboks 110
Universitet
5027 Bergen

Ammehjelpen
Nordre Natlandsjellet 81
5030 Lnadaas
Tel.: 47–2–11–1470

PANAMA
Prolacma
Malvina Caballos
La Pulica A–20
Panama

PAPUA NEW GUINEA
Susu Mamas
Box 5857
Boroko

PERU
Perú-Mujer
Avda. Africa 755–B
Lima 18
Tel.: 51–14–46–5250
or Ford Foundation: 51–14–31–0111
Perú-Mujer, Avda. España 578, No.
    301
Lima 5

PHILIPPINES
BUNSO
6B K–6th St.
Kamias Rd.
Quezon City
Tel.: 63–2–922–8328
NMAP-KINI
c/o May Pascal
PO Box 883
Manila

POLAND
Ewa Nitecka
Lachmana 2/65
02–791 Warsaw

Institute of Mother and Child
c/o Krystyna Michiel-Kostyra
ul. Etiudy Rew, 42A
02–643 Warsaw

PUERTO RICO
Family Centred Education
Calle Rodeno 1565
El Paraíso
Río Piedras 00926
Tel.: Joanne Burris: 767–5083

SAMOA
Ms. Margaret Rhynd
Nutrition and Diet Unit
Apia, Western Samoa

SINGAPORE
Singapore BF Mothers' Support
    Group
c/o Trade Union House
Shenton Way 0106

SOLOMON ISLANDS
Lukaotem Picanini

c/o Box 390
Honiara

SOUTH AFRICA
Breastfeeding Association
3 Zwaanswyck Rd.
Stellenbosch 7600
Tel.: Noreen Wannacott: 27–751–388
June Francis: 27–651–071
LLL of South Africa
PO Box 4055
Old Oak, Bellville 7530

SWAZILAND
Nomajoni Ntombela
PO Box 1075
Mazini
Tel.: 268–44–326.
SINAN (Swaziland Infant Nutrition
    Action Newtork)
PO Box 1032
Mbabane

SWEDEN
Amningshjalpen
c/o Kvinnocentrum
Birger Jarlsgatum 22
S–114 34 Stockholm

Amningshjalpen
Box 20951
5–93102 Skelleftea
Tel.: 46–2–0910–19223

SWITZERLAND
Christian Medical Commission, WCC
150 route de Ferney
1211 Geneva

GP Femmes pour Allaitement
    Maternal
8 Rue des Bugrons
1217 Meyrin
Tel.: Tessa Osborne: 41–22–820054

Informationsdienst und Dritte Welt
Postfach 1686 (Monbijoustrasse 31)
    CH–3000 Berne
Tel.: 41–31–261232/3

LLLI Switzerland
Hinterbergweg 12
4153 Reinach

MCH Unit
Family Health Division
World Health Organisation
1211 Geneva 27

UNICEF
Palais de Nations
1211 Geneva 10

Verband Europaischer
    Laktationsberater/innen IBCLC
Postfach 94
C H–3000 Bern 25

World Health Organisation
1211 Geneva 27
Tel.: 41–22–91–21–11, x 3315

TAIWAN
Consumers Foundation ROC
28 sec 3
Jen-Ai Rd.
11F Taipei

THAILAND
Nursing Mothers Association of
    Thailand
c/o Dr. Kom Pongkham
66/1 M10, South Pattaya
Pattaya City, Chonburi 20260

TONGA
Nutrition Planning Co-ordinator
Central Planning Department
PO Box 827
Nuku'alofa 21–366

TRINIDAD
Housewives Association of Trinidad
    and Tobago
c/o Hazel Brown, Allison White
P.O. Box 410
Port of Spain
Tel.: 809–625–1796 (office)
809–632–2254 (home)

The Informationve Breastfeeding Service
c/o Marilyn Stollmeyer
16 Gray St.
St. Clair, Port of Spain
Tel.: 809–628–8234

UGANDA
Uganda Lactation Management
    Training Group
c/o Dr. Josephine Kasolo
PO Box 2395
Kampala

UNITED KINGDOM
AHRTAG
1 London Bridge St.

London SE 1 9SG
Tel.: 44–1–378–1403
FAX: 44–1–403–6003

Association of Breastfeeding Mothers
14 Pleasant Grove
or 131 Mayow Rd.
Sydenham
London SE26 4HZ
Tel.: 44–1–461–0022
44–1–659–5151
44–1–697–4585

Breastfeeding Promotion Group
The National Childbirth Trust
Alexandra House
Oldham Terrace, Acton
London W3 6NH
Tel.: 44–1–221–3833

HIFA (History of Infant Feeding
    Association)
2a Oxford St.
Gloucester GL1 3EQ

International Confederation of
    Midwives
57 Lower Belgrave Street
London, SW1W OLR

LLL Great Britain
BM 3424
London WCIV 6XX
Tel.: 44–1–404–5011

MIDIRS
Institute of Child Health
Royal Hospital for Sick Children
St. Michael's Hill
Bristol
BS28BJ
Tel.: 44–272–251–971

National Childbirth Trust Breast-
    Feeding Promotion Group
9 Queensborough Terrace
London W2 3 TB

Royal College of Midwives
15 Mansfield St.
London WIM OBE

TALC
PO Box 49
St. Albans
Herts ALI 4AX

Tropical Child Health Unit
Institute of Child Health
30 Guilford St.
London WC1 N 1EH

UNITED STATES
Boston Association for Childbirth
    Education
Nursing Mother's Council
PO Box 29
Newtonville, MA 01609
Tel.: 617–244–5102

Breastfeeding Connection
618 N. Wheaton Ave.
Wheaton, IL 60187
Tel.: 708–665–6848

Breastfeeding Infant Clinic
Pediatric Pavilion USC Clinic
1200 North State St.
Los Angeles, CA 90033
Tel.: 213–825–9305

Breastfeeding Support Consultants
164 Schoolhouse Rd.
Pottstown, PA 19464
Tel.: 215–326–9343

Center for Breastfeeding Information
PO Box 1209
Franklin Park, IL 60131–8209
Tel.: 708–455–7730

Child Survival Action News
1101 Connecticut Ave. NW
Suite 605
Washington, DC 20006

Clearinghouse on Infant Feeding and
    Maternal Nutrition
American Public Health Association
1015 Fifteenth St. NW
Washington, DC 20005
Tel.: 202–789–5600

Community Human Milk Bank
Georgetown University Hospital
3800 Reservoir Rd.
Washington, DC 20007

The Environmental Research Group
114 North First
Ann Arbor, MI 48104
Tel.: 313–662–3104

Family Health International
PO Box 13950
Research Triangle Park, NC 27709

FORMULA
PO Box 39051
Washington, DC 20016

Health Education Associates, Inc
8 Jan Sebastian Way
Sandwich, MA 02563
Tel.: 508–888–8044

International Board of Lactation
  Consultant Examiners (IBLCE)
2315 Wickersham Cove
Germantown, TN 38138
Tel.: 901–755–6233

International Childbirth Education
  Association (ICEA)
PO Box 20048
Minneapolis, MN 45420
Tel.: 612–854–8660

International Lactation Consultants
  Association (ILCA)
201 Brown Ave.
Evanston, IL 60202–3601
Tel.: 708–260–8874

Lactation Associates
254 Conant Rd.
Weston, MA 02193
Tel.: 617–893–3553

The Lactation Clinic, Inc.
401 South Green Rd.
Cleveland, OH 44121

Lactation Clinic and Childbearing
  Family Center
401 S. Green Rd.
Cleveland, OH 44121

Lactation Institute and Breastfeeding
  Clinic
16161 Ventura Blvd
Suite 215
Encino, CA 91436
Tel.: 818–995–1913

La Leche League International
9619 Minneapolis Ave.
Franklin Park, IL 60131
Tel.: 708–455–7730

LLL Around the World
Beryl Nielsen
46 Marina Vista Ave.
Larkspur CA 94939

Mothers' Milk Bank
Institute for Medical Research
751 South Bascom Ave
San Jose, CA 95128
Tel.: 408–998–4550/998–4554

NAPSAC
PO Box 267
Marble Hill, MO 63764
Tel.: 314–238–2010

Nursing Mothers Committee Family
  Centered Parents, Inc.
Box 142
Rockland, DE 19732

Nursing Mothers Council, Inc.
PO Box 50063
Palo Alto, CA 94303
Tel.: 408–272–1448

Nursing Mothers Services of Greater
  Philadelphia, Inc.
5 East Second Avenue
Conshohocken, PA 19428
Tel.: 215–828–0131

Pharmacy, Brigham and Women's
  Hospital
Boston, MA 02125
Tel.: 617–732–7166

Population Council
One Dag Hammarskjold Plaza
New York, NY 10017

San Diego Lactation Program
4062 1st Avenue
San Diego, CA 92103

UNICEF: Margaret Kyenkya-Isabirye
UNICEF H8F
3 UN Plaza
New York, NY 10017

Wellstart San Diego Lactation Program
4062 First Ave.
San Diego, CA 92103
Tel.: 619–295–5193

Women's International Public Health
  Network
7100 Oak Forest Lane
Bethesda, MD 20817
Tel.: 301–469–9211

VANUATU
Mama Bilong Vanuatu
PO Box 819
Port Vila

Vanuatu Nursing Mothers Group
National Planning Office
PO Box 741
Port Vila

VENEZUELA
Edificio Oriente
Avenida 5 de Julio
Puerto la Cruz

YEMEN
Technical Unit for Nutrition
PO Box 1330
Sana'a

YUGOSLAVIA
Maternal and Child Health

Dr. Stanka Kranjc-Simonetti
Zavod za zdravstveno varstvo
SR Slovenije
Trubarjeva 26100 Ljubljana

Mother and Child Health Institute
c/o Gordana Mrdjenovic
Str. Jurija Gagarina 196
11070 Belgrado

ZAMBIA
May Rea
PO Box 22415
Kitwe

National Breastfeeding
  Association
c/o National Food and Nutrition
  Committee
PO Box 32669
Lusaka

ZIMBABWE
Department of Nutrition
Ministry of Health
Government of Zimbabwe
Harare

LLL Zimbabwe
30 Alexander Rd.
Greendale, Harare

Zimbabwe Infant Nutrition Network
  (ZINN)
Box BE 7
Belvedere, Harare

**BREAST PUMPS AND BREASTFEED-
ING EQUIPMENT**
Ameda-Engell
764 Industrial Dr.
Cary, IL 60013 USA
Tel.: 800–323–8750

Lact-Aid, International
(Lact-Aid Nursing Trainer System)
PO Box 1066
Athens, TN 37303 USA

Medela, Inc.
4610 Prime Parkway
PO Box 660
McHenry, IL 60050 USA
Tel.: 800–435–8316

Nurse-Dri Breast Shield Co.
390 Corte Madera Ave.
Corte Madera, CA 94925 USA
Tel.: 415–927–1635

Nurse-Midwives' Assn. of Australia
(Supply Line)

PO Box 231
Nunawading, Vic. 3731
Australia

BOOKSTORES AND PUBLICA-
TIONS
Alma Seminars and Publications
PO Box 39
Wendouree, Vic. 3355

Australia
Tel.: 61–3–509–4929

Birth and Life Bookstore
PO Box 70625
Seattle, WA 98107 USA

Childbirth Graphics
PO Box 20540
Rochester, NY 14602–0540 USA
Tel.: 716–272–0300

ICEA Bookmarks
PO Box 200948
Minneapolis, MN 45420 USA
Tel.: 612–854–8660

La Leche League International
9619 Minneapolis Ave.
Franklin Park, IL 60131 USA
Tel.: 708–455–7730

Appendix H

Tables of Equivalencies and Methods of Conversion

METRIC

1 liter (L) = 10 deciliters (dl) = 1000 milliliters (ml) or 1000 cc

1 dl = 100 ml

1 ml = 0.001 L = 10^{-3} L = 1 cc = 1 gm (water)

1 kilogram (kg) = 1000 grams (gm)

1 gm = 100 milligrams (mg) = 0.001 kg

1 mg = 1000 micrograms (μg or mcg) = 0.001 gm = 10^{-3} gm

1 μg = 0.001 mg = 10^{-6} gm

1 nanogram (ng) = 0.001 μg = 10^{-9} gm

1 picogram (pg) = 0.001 ng = 10^{-12} gm

VOLUME

Household Measure	Fluid Ounces (Fl oz)	Metric Equivalent* (ml)	
1 cup (C)	8	240	1 C = 16 Tbsp
2 Tablespoons (Tbsp)	1	30	1 Tbsp = 3 tsp
1 Tbsp	not used	15	
1 teaspoon (tsp)	not used	5	
1 quart (qt)	32	960 ($\cong$ 1 L)	1 qt = 4 C = 2 pt
1 pint (pt)	16	480 ($\cong$ 500 ml)	1 pt = 2 C

WEIGHT

1 pound (1 lb or #) = 0.45 kg   1 oz = 28 gm $\cong$ 30 gm

1 kg = 2.2 lb

To convert lb to kg, divide lb by 2.2 *or* multiply lb times 0.45

To convert kg to lb, multiply kg times 2.2

LINEAR MEASURE

1 inch (in. or ″) = 2.54 centimeters (cm) ($\cong$ 2.5)

1 cm = 0.4 in.

To convert in. to cm, multiply in. times 2.5.

To convert cm to in., multiply cm times 0.4 *or* divide cm by 2.5.

TEMPERATURE

To convert Celsius (C) to Fahrenheit (F), $°C = \frac{5}{9}(°F - 32)$
(Subtract 32, then multiply times $\frac{5}{9}$)

To convert Fahrenheit to Celsius, $°F = \frac{5}{9} °C + 32$
(Multiply times $\frac{5}{9}$, then add 32)

*Equivalent is given to nearest multiple of five. Number given in parentheses may sometimes be used to simplify calculations.
$\cong$ means *approximately equals.*

Appendix I

Patient History

Name: _____ ☐ Boy Birthday: _____ Date of Visit: _____

Baby: _____ ☐ Girl Age of Baby: _____ Birthplace (Hosp.): _____

Mother: _____ Age: _____ Home Phone: _____

Father: _____ Age: _____

Obstetrician: _____ Phone: _____

Pediatrician: _____ Phone: _____

Mother's race/ethnicity (optional) _____ Mother's marital status _____

Reason for visit: | **For office use only**

MATERNAL HISTORY

1. Are you allergic to any medication? ☐ Yes ☐ No If yes, please list: _____

2. Have you ever had any of the following? Please check (✔) all that apply.
   - ☐ Abnormal pap smear
   - ☐ Allergy/asthma
   - ☐ Anemia
   - ☐ Cancer
   - ☐ Constipation/hemorrhoids
   - ☐ Depression/blues
   - ☐ Diabetes
   - ☐ Diarrhea (chronic)
   - ☐ Heart disease
   - ☐ High blood pressure
   - ☐ Infertility
   - ☐ Kidney disease/bladder infection
   - ☐ Liver disease/hepatitis
   - ☐ Thyroid disorders
   - ☐ Tuberculosis
   - ☐ Venereal disease
   - ☐ None known
   - ☐ Other: _____

3. Have you ever had any of the following problems or procedures related to your breasts? Please check (✔) all that apply.
   - ☐ Biopsy
   - ☐ Lumps
   - ☐ Nipple problems: _____
   - ☐ Surgery: _____
   - ☐ None

4. Are you taking the following medications? Please check (✔) all that apply.
   - ☐ Prenatal vitamin-mineral
   - ☐ Other vitamins
   - ☐ Iron
   - ☐ Other minerals
   - ☐ Diet pills
   - ☐ Antihistamines/cold remedies
   - ☐ Laxatives/antacids
   - ☐ Diuretics/water pills
   - ☐ Aspirin/pain pills
   - ☐ Birth control pills
   - ☐ Antibiotics
   - ☐ None of the above
   - ☐ Other drugs _____
   - _____

PERINATAL HISTORY List all pregnancies:

5.

Date Preg. Ended	Weeks Gesta-tion	Sex	Birth Weight	Complications of Pregnancy	Complications of Labor and Delivery	*Type of Anes-thesia	Type of Delivery		Breast-feeding Duration
							Vag.	C/S	

*Anesthesia: ① None ② Local ③ Epidural ④ Spinal ⑤ General (asleep)
⑥ Other _____

___/___/___/___/___

6. Did you have any of the following during this pregnancy? Please check (✔) all that apply.
   - ☐ Anemia (low iron level)
   - ☐ Fever
   - ☐ Gestational diabetes
   - ☐ High blood pressure
   - ☐ Nausea/vomiting (severe)
   - ☐ Premature labor
   - ☐ Urinary tract infection
   - ☐ Medication
   - ☐ None of the above
   - ☐ Other: _____

		For office use only

7. Did you have any of the following during this labor and delivery? Please check (✔) all that apply.
- ☐ Drugs to induce or speed labor: If yes, for how long during labor was this drug administered?
  _____hours
- ☐ Premature rupture of membranes
- ☐ Drugs to control high blood pressure
- ☐ Drugs to control pain
- ☐ Fever
- ☐ Antibiotics
- ☐ Hemorrhage
- ☐ None of the above
- ☐ Other:_____
  _____

8. With this labor and delivery, did you have any of the following? Please check (✔) all that apply.
- ☐ Total labor longer than 30 hours
- ☐ Pushing stage longer than 2 hours
- ☐ Episiotomy or vaginal tear
- ☐ Tear that involved the rectum (a "third or fourth degree" laceration)
- ☐ Breech presentation
- ☐ Forceps delivery
- ☐ Vacuum extraction
- ☐ None of the above

9. How would you rate your labor and delivery experience? Please check (✔) all that apply.
- ☐ Easy
- ☐ Difficult
- ☐ Painful
- ☐ Long
- ☐ Short
- ☐ Average length
- ☐ Just what I'd expected
- ☐ Not what I'd expected
- ☐ Other_____

10. Postpartum complications? Please check (✔) all that apply.
- ☐ Urinary/other infection
- ☐ Excessive bleeding (hemorrhage)
- ☐ High blood pressure
- ☐ Low blood pressure (shock)
- ☐ None of the above
- ☐ Other_____

11. Did the baby have any of the following shortly after birth? Please check (✔) all that apply.
- ☐ Breathing problems
- ☐ Fever
- ☐ High hematocrit
- ☐ Jaundice
- ☐ Low blood sugar
- ☐ Meconium aspiration
- ☐ None of the above

- ☐ Medications:_____
- ☐ Other:_____

12. How soon after delivery did you first put your baby to your breast? _____

13. Were you and your baby separated for more than 2 hours while in the hospital?   ☐ Yes   ☐ No

14. While in the hospital, how many times in 24 hours did you breastfeed your baby?
- ☐ Less than 8 times   ☐ 8-12 times (every 2-3 hours)   ☐ More than 12 times

15. While in the hospital, what was the longest time between breastfeeding?   Day:_____   Night:_____

16. Did you have any of the following problems with your breasts or with breastfeeding your baby while in the hospital? Please check (✔) all that apply.
- ☐ Attachment difficulties
- ☐ Engorgement
- ☐ None
- ☐ Sleepy baby
- ☐ Sore nipples
- ☐ Other:_____
- ☐ Preference for one breast
- ☐ Not enough milk

17. While in the hospital, was your baby given any supplements?   ☐ Yes   ☐ No
If yes, please check (✔) all that apply.
- ☐ Formula
- ☐ Water (plain)
- ☐ Sugar water
How were supplements given?   ☐ Bottle   ☐ Syringe   ☐ Dropper   ☐ Other:_____

18. While in the hospital, was your baby given a pacifier?   ☐ Yes   ☐ No

19. Did you and your baby go home at the same time?   ☐ Yes   ☐ No

20. How old was the baby at discharge? _____

21. Are you currently having vaginal bleeding?   ☐ Yes   ☐ No
Have your menstrual periods returned?   ☐ Yes   ☐ No   Date of last menstrual period:_____

22. Which of the following family planning methods are you using or do you plan to use?   ☐ None
- ☐ Birth control pills
- ☐ Other:_____

FEEDING HISTORY

23. How many times in 24 hours are you currently breastfeeding your baby?
- ☐ Less than 8 times   ☐ 8-12 times (every 2-3 hours)   ☐ More than 12 times

REV. 9/28/92

24. What is the longest time between breastfeedings? Day:_____   Night:_____

25. How long does your baby nurse on each breast? _____

26. While nursing, do you sense any of the following in your breasts?
☐ Filling   ☐ Burning   ☐ Milk dripping from other breast
☐ Tingling   ☐ Emptying   ☐ None of the above
☐ Other_____

27. Who decides when the feeding is over?   ☐ Mother   ☐ Baby

28. At home, has your baby received:
☐ Water   ☐ Formula   ☐ Liquids, other than formula   ☐ Any solids

29. How many times in 24 hours has your baby had: Wet diapers:_____   Bowel movements:_____

30. Does your baby spit up?   ☐ Never   ☐ Occasionally   ☐ Often

31. Is the baby content or sleeping between feedings?   ☐ Never   ☐ Occasionally   ☐ Often

32. Has your baby had any prolonged crying spells?   ☐ Never   ☐ Occasionally   ☐ Often

33. Is your baby given a pacifier?   ☐ Never   ☐ Occasionally   ☐ Often

34. Have you had any of the following problems with your breasts or with breastfeeding since coming home?
☐ Baby always hungry   ☐ Cracked/bleeding nipples   ☐ Painfully full breast(s)
☐ Baby prefers one breast   ☐ Nipple pain   ☐ Not enough milk
☐ Baby not interested   ☐ Breast pain   ☐ None of the above
☐ Other:_____

35. Have you used any of the following? Please check (✔) all that apply.
☐ Hand expression   ☐ Nursing bra (no underwire)   ☐ Breast or nipple shield
☐ Breast pump   ☐ Nursing bra (with underwire) ☐ None of the above
☐ Breast cream
☐ Other:_____

36. Your bra size: before pregnancy_____   now_____

FAMILY HISTORY

37. Does anyone on either side of the baby's family have any of the following?
☐ Allergy (food)   ☐ Allergy (hay fever)   ☐ Genetic disease
☐ Allergy (asthma)   ☐ Cancer (breast)   ☐ Thyroid disease
☐ Allergy (eczema)   ☐ Diabetes   ☐ None of the above
☐ Other:_____

38. How are members of your family adjusting to the new baby?
☐ Very well   ☐ Reasonably well   ☐ Poorly   ☐ Very poorly

39. Was your baby planned?   ☐ Yes   ☐ No

40. When did you decide to breastfeed this baby?
☐ Before pregnancy   ☐ During pregnancy   ☐ After delivery

41. How did you prepare for breastfeeding?
☐ Classes   ☐ Reading   ☐ Other:_____

42. Were you breastfed?   ☐ Yes   ☐ No   ☐ Not known

43. Was your baby's father breastfed?   ☐ Yes   ☐ No   ☐ Not known

44. How many previous babies have you breastfed?_____
How long? _____   Why did you stop? _____

45. Why do you wish to breastfeed your baby? _____

46. Is there anyone in your household/family who feels you should **not** breastfeed this baby?   ☐ Yes   ☐ No

47. For how long do you plan to breastfeed this baby?_____

48. Why do you think you will discontinue breastfeeding at that time?_____

For office use only

REV. 9/28/92

49. What was the highest grade or year of regular school you have completed?
   ☐ Less than 6 years   ☐ High school (12 years)   ☐ 4-year college (16 years)
   ☐ Elementary school (6 years)   ☐ 2-year college (14 years)   ☐ Graduate school (17+ years)
   ☐ Junior high school (9 years)

50. Usual occupation? Mother:_____ Father: _____
   When does mother plan to return to work? _____

NUTRITION

51. Did you see a nutritionist during your pregnancy?   ☐ Yes   ☐ No

52. Are there any foods that you avoid eating?   ☐ Yes   ☐ No   If yes, what: _____
   Why? _____

53. Are you now on any of these special diets?   ☐ Diabetic
   ☐ High protein   ☐ Low salt   ☐ No special diet
   ☐ Low fat   ☐ Weight loss   ☐ Other:_____
   If yes, who suggested the diet?_____

54. Are you trying to lose weight at this time?   ☐ Yes   ☐ No   If yes, how much?_____
   How?   ☐ Less food/more exercise   ☐ Program:_____   ☐ Other:_____

55. Are you a vegetarian?   ☐ Yes   ☐ No
   If yes, do you consume: ☐ Milk products (milk, cheese, yogurt)   ☐ Eggs?

56. How would you rate your appetite presently?   ☐ Good   ☐ Fair   ☐ Poor

57. How would you describe the type and amount of food in your household?
   ☐ Enough of the kind you want   ☐ Enough, but not always the kind you want
   ☐ Sometimes not enough   ☐ Often not enough

58. Are you receiving any of the following?
   ☐ Food stamps   ☐ Medi-Cal   ☐ Donated food/meals
   ☐ WIC   ☐ AFDC/welfare   ☐ None of the above
   ☐ Other:_____

59. Do you have someone to help you shop and prepare meals?   ☐ Yes   ☐ No

60. How many times a day do you eat meals:_____ and snacks:_____

61. How many cups (8 oz.) of the following liquids do you usually drink per day?
   _____ Water   _____ Sodas with sugar   _____ Coffee
   _____ Juice   _____ Diet soda, diet punch   _____ Tea
   _____ Milk   _____ Punch, Kool-Aid, Tang   _____ Other:_____

LIFESTYLE

62. How often are you now drinking beer, wine, hard liquor, or mixed drinks?
   ☐ Daily   ☐ Weekly   ☐ Monthly   ☐ Never
   When you drink, how many drinks do you have?   ☐ One   ☐ Two   ☐ Three   ☐ More

63. How many cigarettes do you smoke each day?
   ☐ Do not smoke   ☐ Fewer than 10 cigarettes   ☐ 11-20 cigarettes   ☐ More than 20 cigarettes

64. How often are you currently exercising (besides housework, child care)? _____
   What types of exercise do you do? _____

65. Do you feel you are getting adequate rest?   ☐ Never   ☐ Occasionally   ☐ Often

66. Having a new baby can be a stressful time for the family. What other stresses are present in your home?
   ☐ Relationship difficulties   ☐ Moving   ☐ Illness/death in the family
   ☐ Lack of help with home/child   ☐ Financial concerns   ☐ Other: _____
      care   ☐ Drug or alcohol use   ☐ None of the above

67. Who lives with you in your home? _____

68. Do you have any other concerns about yourself, your baby, or your family's health that you would like to discuss
   during your appointment?   ☐ Yes   ☐ No
   If yes, what?_____

For office use only

REV. 9/28/92

MATERNAL ANTHROPOMETRY

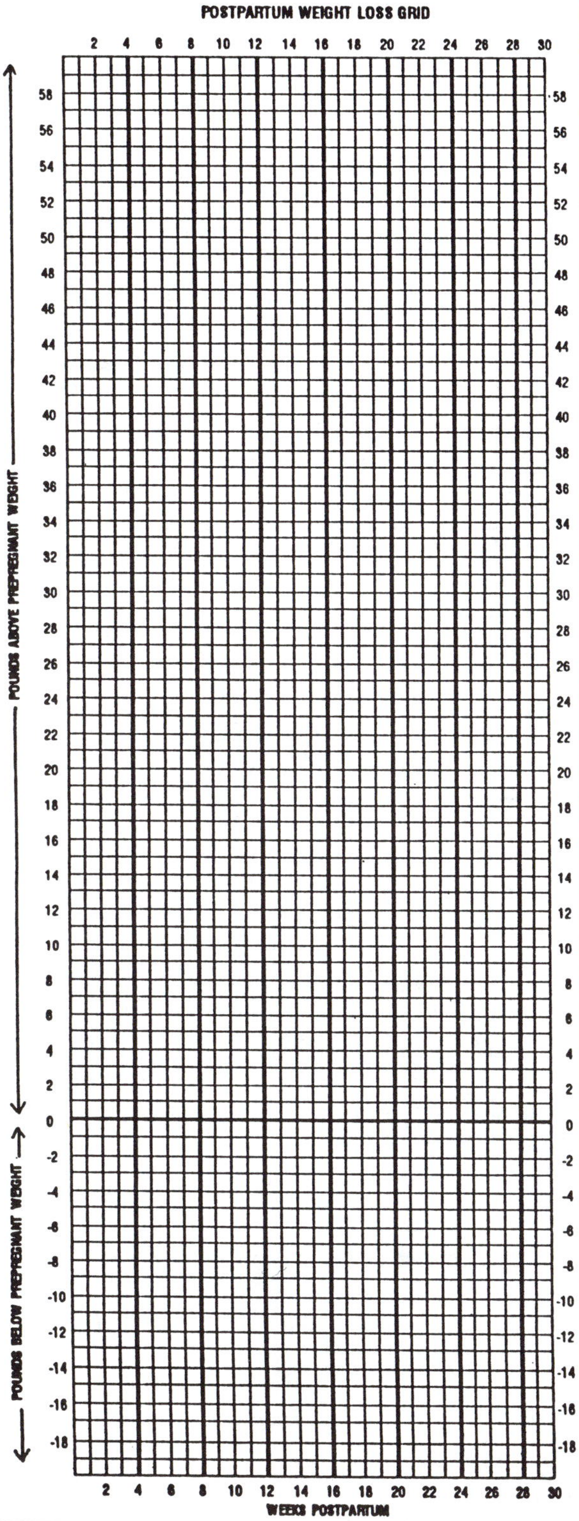

POSTPARTUM WEIGHT LOSS GRID

Grid chart with vertical axis labeled "POUNDS ABOVE PREPREGNANT WEIGHT" (upper) and "POUNDS BELOW PREPREGNANT WEIGHT" (lower), ranging from 58 down to -18. Horizontal axis labeled "WEEKS POSTPARTUM" ranging from 2 to 30.

Name_____

Age_____ Delivery date_____

Height_____ Desirable weight_____

Prepreg. weight_____ % Desir. wt._____BMI_____

Term weight_____ % Desir. wt._____BMI_____

Total preg. gain_____ Recomm. wt. gain_____

Date_____ Wks./mos. postpartum_____

Weight_____ % Desir. wt._____BMI_____

Date_____ Wks./mos. postpartum_____

Weight_____ % Desir. wt._____BMI_____

Date_____ Wks./mos. postpartum_____

Weight_____ % Desir. wt._____BMI_____

Date_____ Wks./mos. postpartum_____

Weight_____ % Desir. wt._____BMI_____

Date_____ Wks./mos. postpartum_____

Weight_____ % Desir. wt._____BMI_____

Date_____ Wks./mos. postpartum_____

Weight_____ % Desir. wt._____BMI_____

Date_____ Wks./mos. postpartum_____

Weight_____ % Desir. wt._____BMI_____

REV. 9/30/92

MOTHER'S PHYSICAL EXAM

Postpartum days/weeks	Height	Prepreg. wt.	Term wt.	Current wt.	Temperature	Blood Pressure
General Appearance			Thyroid			

BREASTS RIGHT	LEFT
AREOLA	
NIPPLES	
SECRETION	
OTHER	

INFANT'S PHYSICAL EXAM

DATE	AGE	WEIGHT (pounds)	(kg.)	HEIGHT (inches)	(cm.)	H.C. (inches)	(cm.)
	Birth						
Discharge:							
Today:							

GENERAL/BEHAVIOR	Temp.

Head		Heart	
Eyes		Pulses	
Ears		Abdomen	
Nose		Genitalia	
Mouth		Extremities	
Thorax		Neuro	
Lungs		Skin	

REV. 9/28/92

ORAL-MOTOR EXAMINATION/FUNCTION

MOUTH ☐ Normal ☐ Small ☐ Large

JAW ☐ Normal ☐ Receding ☐ Asymmetrical ☐ Thrusting ☐ Tight/poor opening

LIPS ☐ Normal ☐ Cleft ☐ Passively pulled in ☐ Pursed/tight

GUMS ☐ Normal ☐ Asymmetrical ☐ Excessive clenching/bite

TONGUE ☐ Normal resting position ☐ Flat ☐ Clicking ☐ Elevated ☐ Up in back
☐ Behind gum line ☐ Thrust/protruding ☐ Sucking

FRENULUM ☐ Normal ☐ Tight

PALATE ☐ Normal ☐ High arch ☐ Cleft

BREASTFEEDING OBSERVATION

Position used: ☐ Cradle ☐ Side-sitting ☐ Other:_____

Infant interest: ☐ Hungry, eager; goes easily to breast ☐ Willing, falls asleep quickly ☐ Awake, will not attach
☐ Willing but not insistent ☐ Sleepy, totally disinterested ☐ Awake, hungry, vigorously refuses
☐ Willing but distractable

Rooting: ☐ Normal ☐ Depressed/absent ☐ Tongue back/flat
☐ Frantic, disorganized

Attachment: ☐ Adequate ☐ Lips retracted ☐ Refuses
☐ Drops back ☐ Arches ☐ Other:_____
☐ Tongue malposition ☐ Cries _____

Milk ejection reflex: ☐ Prior to attachment ☐ After attachment, _____ sec / min ☐ Not apparent after _____ sec / min
☐ Hyperactive

Effectiveness: ☐ Good suck/rhythm ☐ Starts/stops repeatedly ☐ Excessive vertical movement
  suck:swallow _____:_____ ☐ Persistent flutter sucking only ☐ Clenching/biting
☐ Becomes ineffective ☐ Disorganized ☐ Other:_____
☐ Weak suction ☐ Cheeks dimple during suckling _____
☐ Attached, not suckling ☐ Tongue clicking _____

Swallow: ☐ Normal ☐ Uncoordinated

Comments:_____

Condition of nipple after nursing: (Right)
Color_____ Shape_____   Color_____ Shape_____

(Left)

Infant stress ⊢———⊣———⊣———⊣   **Maternal stress:** ⊢———⊣———⊣———⊣———⊣
Mellow,   Disturbed   Screaming,   At ease,   Anxious   Extremely
relaxed   slightly, not   resists   relaxed   tense
             screaming   positioning

Maternal interaction with infant: ☐ Hovering ☐ Attentive ☐ Harsh
☐ Over-stimulating ☐ Affectionate ☐ Detached

COMMENTS:

REV. 9/28/92

	ASSESSMENT	PLAN
MOTHER		
INFANT		
BREASTFEEDING		

COUNSELING	☐ Attachment ☐ Bras ☐ Burping ☐ Expression/storage ☐ Family adjustment ☐ Feeding frequency, duration	☐ Hand expression ☐ How to tell if baby is getting enough ☐ Hydration ☐ Maternal nutrition ☐ Nipple care	☐ Positioning ☐ Rapid growth period ☐ Waking ☐ Other_____ _____
HANDOUTS	☐ Blocked Duct ☐ Breastfeeding Record ☐ Calcium Rich Foods ☐ Candidiasis ☐ Daily Food Guide	☐ Engorgement ☐ Hand Expression ☐ How Much is Enough ☐ Is Baby Getting Enough ☐ Mastitis	☐ Mechanical Expression ☐ Increasing Milk Supply ☐ Milk Storage ☐ Nipple Trauma ☐ Other_____

Date	**Clinician**

Letter sent:_____

REV. 9/28/92

Appendix J

Conversion Tables

TABLE J–1   CONVERSION OF POUNDS TO KILOGRAMS FOR PEDIATRIC WEIGHTS

Pounds ⟶

	0	1	2	3	4	5	6	7	8	9
0	0.00	0.45	0.90	1.36	1.81	2.26	2.72	3.17	3.62	4.08
10	4.53	4.98	5.44	5.89	6.35	6.80	7.25	7.71	8.16	8.61
20	9.07	9.52	9.97	10.43	10.88	11.34	11.79	12.24	12.70	13.15
30	13.60	14.06	14.51	14.96	15.42	15.87	16.32	16.78	17.23	17.69
40	18.14	18.59	19.05	19.50	19.95	20.41	20.86	21.31	21.77	22.22
50	22.68	23.13	23.58	24.04	24.49	24.94	25.40	25.85	26.30	26.76
60	27.21	27.66	28.12	28.57	29.03	29.48	29.93	30.39	30.84	31.29
70	31.75	32.20	32.65	33.11	33.56	34.02	34.47	34.92	35.38	35.83
80	36.28	36.74	37.19	37.64	38.10	38.55	39.00	39.46	39.91	40.37
90	40.82	41.27	41.73	42.18	42.63	43.09	43.54	43.99	44.45	44.90
100	45.36	45.81	46.26	46.72	47.17	47.62	48.08	48.53	48.98	49.44
110	49.89	50.34	50.80	51.25	51.71	52.16	52.61	53.07	53.52	53.97
120	54.43	54.88	55.33	55.79	56.24	56.70	57.15	57.60	58.06	58.51
130	58.96	59.42	59.87	60.32	60.78	61.23	61.68	62.14	62.59	63.05
140	63.50	63.95	64.41	64.86	65.31	65.77	66.22	66.67	67.13	67.58
150	68.04	68.49	68.94	69.40	69.85	70.30	70.76	71.21	71.66	72.12
160	72.57	73.02	73.48	73.93	74.39	74.84	75.29	75.75	76.20	76.65
170	77.11	77.56	78.01	78.47	78.92	79.38	79.83	80.28	80.74	81.19
180	81.64	82.10	82.55	83.00	83.46	83.91	84.36	84.82	85.27	85.73
190	86.18	86.68	87.09	87.54	87.99	88.45	88.90	89.35	89.81	90.26
200	90.72	91.17	91.62	92.08	92.53	92.98	93.44	93.89	94.34	94.80

TABLE J–2   CONVERSION OF POUNDS AND OUNCES TO KILOGRAMS FOR PEDIATRIC WEIGHTS

Pounds	Kilograms	Ounces	Kilograms	Pounds	Kilograms	Ounces	Kilograms
1	0.454	1	0.028	9	4.082	9	0.255
2	0.907	2	0.057	10	4.536	10	0.283
3	1.361	3	0.085	11	4.990	11	0.312
4	1.814	4	0.113	12	5.443	12	0.340
5	2.268	5	0.142	13	5.897	13	0.369
6	2.722	6	0.170			14	0.397
7	3.175	7	0.198			15	0.425
8	3.629	8	0.227				

Appendix K

Critical Pathway

Critical Path for Postpartum Care of Breastfeeding Dyad; Vaginal Birth

Patient _____ Case # _____

DRG _____ Expected LOS _____

Date of Admission _____ Time _____ Date of Discharge _____

	LD/LDRP	First Shift	Second Shift	Third Shift	Day 2
Breastfeeding	First breastfeeding stat after delivery; arrange pillows; nipple/areola drawn into mouth	Observe latch-on, suckling Demonstrate optimal positioning	>3 feeds; teach feeding cues Assess positioning	Seen by LC; check hydration meconium	Baby latches on and suckles effectively; >6 feedings Teach different positions for feeding
Discharge planning				Assess support systems	Breastfeeding pamphlet/video Review/teach checklist Consults for community support

Glossary

Acinus Smallest division of a gland; a group of secretory cells arrayed around a central cavity. In the breast, an acinus secretes milk. Acini (pl). *See also*: Alveolus.

Aerobic Requiring air for metabolic processes, e.g., aerobic bacteria. Normal skin, including the breast, is colonized with aerobic bacteria.

Afferent Being conducted toward an organ or gland. Suckling produces afferent impulses that travel from the nipple to the pituitary gland, which then releases oxytocin causing milk to let down. The opposite of efferent.

Allergen Any substance causing an allergic response. Foods, drugs, or inhalants may be allergens. Cow's milk protein is a common allergen among infants.

Alphalactalbumin The principal protein found in the whey portion of human milk; it assists the synthesis of lactose. The dominant whey protein in cow's milk and most artificial infant milks, betalactoglobulin, is not found in human milk. *See also*: Non-casein protein.

Alveolar ridge The ridge on the hard palate immediately behind the upper gums. Movement of the infant's jaw during nursing compresses the areola between his tongue and alveolar ridge.

Alveolus In the mammary gland, a small sac at the terminus of a lobule in which milk is secreted and stored. Alveoli (pl). Groups of alveoli, organized in lobes, give the mammary gland the appearance of a "bunch of grapes." *See also*: Acinus.

Ampulla A normally dilated portion of a duct. Ampullae (pl). Ampullae in the lactiferous ducts underlie the areola near the base of the nipple. *See also*: Lactiferous sinus.

Anorectal abnormalities Anomalies of the rectum, the lower few inches of the large intestine, and the anus, the opening in the skin at the distal end of the rectum. An example is imperforate anus, in which the rectum ends in a blind pouch.

Antibody An immunoglobulin formed in response to an antigen, including bacteria and viruses. Antibodies then recognize and attack those bacteria or viruses, thus helping the body resist infection. Breastmilk contains antibodies to antigens to which either the mother or the infant have been exposed.

Antigen A substance which stimulates antibody production. It may be introduced into the body (as dust, food, or bacteria) or produced within it (as a by-product toxin).

Antigenemia The state of having an antigen of interest in the blood.

Areola Pigmented skin surrounding the nipple which overlies the ampullae or lactiferous sinuses. In order to suckle effectively, an infant should have his gums placed well back on the areola.

Artificial infant milk Any milk preparation, other than human milk, intended to be the sole nourishment of human infants.

Atopic eczema An inherited allergic tendency to rashes or inflammation of the skin. Exclusively breastfed infants are less likely to manifest this condition, as cow's milk protein is a common allergen.

Atresia, intestinal   Congenital blockage or closure of any part of the intestinal tract.

Axilla   The underarm area; in it lies the uppermost extent of the mammary ridge or milk line. Deep breast tissue (the axillary tail or "tail of Spence") extends towards and sometimes into the axilla. This tissue may engorge the axilla along with the rest of the breast in the early postpartum.

B-cell   A lymphocyte produced in bone marrow and peripheral lymphoid tissue which is found in breastmilk. It attacks antigens and is one type of cell which confers cell-mediated immunity.

Bactericidal   Capable of destroying bacteria. Breastmilk contains so many bactericidal cells that the bacteria count of expressed milk actually declines during the first 36 hours following expression.

Bacteriostatic   Capable of inhibiting the proliferation of bacterial colonies.

BALT/GALT/MALT   Bronchus/Gut/Mammary-Associated Immunocompetent Lymphoid Tissue. A lymphocyte pathway which causes IgA antibodies to be produced in the mammary gland after a lactating woman is exposed to an antigen on her intestinal or respiratory mucosa. These antibodies are then transferred through breastmilk to the breastfeeding infant, who thus may possess antibodies to antigens to which he has not been directly exposed.

Banked human milk   *See*: Donor milk.

Betalactoglobulin   The dominant protein present in the whey fraction of the milk of cows and other ruminants; it is absent from human milk.

Bioavailable   That portion of an ingested nutrient actually absorbed and used by the body. Because the nutrients in breastmilk are highly bioavailable, low concentrations may actually result in more nutrients being absorbed by the infant than do the higher, less bioavailable, concentrations in cow's milk or artificial infant milks.

Buccal pads   Fat pads sheathed by the masseter muscles in young infants' cheeks. The buccal pads touch and provide stability for the tongue, which enhances its ability to compress breast tissue during suckling. Breastfed infants typically have a plump-cheeked appearance because of well-developed buccal pads.

Candidiasis   A fungal infection caused by *Candida albicans* or "thrush." Common in the maternal vagina, it may inoculate the infant during delivery and be transferred from the infant's mouth to the mother's nipple. Candidiasis of the nipple and breast may produce intense nipple and breast pain. In the infant it may produce white spots on the oral mucosa and a bright red, painful rash ringing the anus. Formerly termed moniliasis.

Casein   The principal protein in milks of all mammals. Human milk has a ratio of soluble whey proteins to casein of about 65:35. Casein of human milk forms soft, easily digested curds in the infant stomach. The whey-to-casein ratio in cow's milk is 20:80; artificial infant milks have whey-to-casein ratios which vary from those of cow's milk to 40:60. Cow's milk casein forms firm curds which require a high expenditure of energy to digest.

Centers for Disease Control (CDC)   An agency of the United States Public Health Service established in 1973 to protect the public health of the nation by providing leadership and direction in the prevention and control of diseases and other preventable health conditions—and to respond to public health emergencies.

Certification   The process by which a nongovernmental professional association attests that an individual has met certain standards specified by the association for the practice of that profession.

Colostrum   The fluid in the breast at the end of pregnancy and in the early postpartum. It is thicker and yellower than mature milk, reflecting a higher content of proteins, many of which are immunoglobulins. It is also higher in fat-soluble vitamins (including A, E, and K) and some minerals (including sodium and zinc).

Congenital infection   An infection existing at birth which was acquired transplacentally. Infections which may be so acquired include HIV and TORCH organisms. *See also*: Human Immunodeficiency Virus; TORCH.

Conjunctivitis   Inflammation of the mucous membrane that lines the eyelid. In many traditional and some modern societies, fresh breastmilk is instilled into the eyes to alleviate this condition.

Contraception   Preventing conception. Breastfeeding provides significant contraceptive protection during the first few months postpartum—as long as the infant is fully breastfed, feeds during the night, and maternal menses have not resumed.

Cooper's ligaments Triangular, vertical ligaments in the breast which attach deeper layers of subcutaneous tissue to the skin.

Cord blood Blood remaining in the umbilical cord after birth.

Creamatocrit The proportion of cream in a milk sample determined by measuring the depth of the cream layer in a centrifuged sample. An indicator of caloric content of milk which must be used with care, the fat (and thus caloric) content of human milk varies between breasts, within a feed, diurnally, and over the entire course of lactation.

Cross nursing Occasional wet-nursing on an informal, short-term basis, usually in the context of child care.

Cytoprotective Any condition or factor which protects cells from inflammation or death.

Diagnostic-related grouping (DRG) A group of diagnoses for health conditions which result in similar intensity of hospital care and similar length of hospital stay for patients hospitalized with those conditions.

Disaccharide A carbohydrate composed of two monosaccharides. The principal sugar in human milk is lactose, a disaccharide; its constituent monosaccharides are glucose and galactose.

Donor milk Human milk voluntarily contributed to a human milk bank by women unrelated to the recipient.

Donor milk, fresh-frozen Fresh-raw milk that has been stored frozen at −20°C for less than 12 months.

Donor milk, fresh-raw Milk stored continuously at 4°C for not longer than 72 hours after collection.

Donor milk, heat-treated Fresh-raw milk or fresh-frozen milk which has been heated to a minimum of 56°C for 30 minutes.

Donor milk, pooled A batch of milk which contains milk from more than one donor.

Dopamine The "prolactin inhibiting factor" (PIF), or a mediator of the prolactin inhibiting factor, secreted in the hypothalamus. It blocks the release of prolactin into the bloodstream.

Drip milk Milk that leaks from a breast which is not being directly stimulated. Since its fat content is low, it should not be used regularly for infant feedings.

Ductules Small ducts in the mammary gland which drain milk from the alveoli into larger lactiferous ducts that terminate in the nipple.

Dyad A pair—e.g., the breastfeeding mother and her infant.

Eczema Skin inflammation or rash. *See also*: Atopic eczema.

Elemental formula Artificial infant milks containing fats, proteins, and carbohydrates in their simplest (most elemental) forms.

Eminences of the pars villosa Tiny swellings on the inner surfaces of an infant's lips which help the infant to retain a grasp on the breast during suckling.

Energy density The number of calories per unit volume; caloric density. Mature human milk averages 65 calories/100 ml, controlled largely by the fat content of the milk.

Envelope virus A virus which requires its coat (envelope) to infect other cells. If the envelope is destroyed—e.g., by heat or soap and water—the ability of the virus to produce infection is destroyed. Cytomegalovirus and Human Immunodeficiency Virus are two envelope viruses.

Epidemiology The study of the frequency and distribution of disease and the factors which cause that frequency and distribution.

Epiglottis Cartilaginous structure of the larynx. An infant's epiglottis lies just below the soft palate. It closes the larynx when the infant swallows, ensuring passage of milk to the esophagus.

Estrogen A hormone which causes growth of mammary tissue during part of each menstrual cycle, assists in the secretion of prolactin during pregnancy, and is one of the hormones whose concentration falls sharply at parturition.

Exogenous Derived from outside the body—e.g.,

iron supplements which provide the infant with exogenous iron.

Foremilk The milk obtained at the beginning of a breastfeed. Its higher water content keeps the infant hydrated and supplies water-soluble vitamins and proteins. Its fat content (1–2 gm/100 ml) is lower than that of hindmilk.

Frenulum Fold of mucous membrane, midline on the underside of the tongue, which helps to anchor the tongue to the floor of the mouth. A short or inelastic frenulum, or one attached close to the tip of the tongue, may restrict tongue extension enough to inhibit effective breastfeeding. The frenum.

Fructose A carbohydrate present in human milk in small quantities.

Galactorrhea Abnormal production of milk. It may occur under psychological influences or be a sign of pituitary tumor.

Galactose A monosaccharide present in small quantities in human milk. It is derived from lactose and in turn helps produce elements essential for the development of the human central nervous system.

Gastroenteritis Inflammation of the stomach and intestines resulting from bacterial or viral invasion. Breastfed infants are at less risk of this illness.

Gastroschisis An opening in the wall of the abdomen; a congenital malformation.

Gestational age An infant's age since conception, usually specified in weeks. Counted from the first day of the last normal menstrual period.

Hindmilk Milk released near the end of a breastfeed, after active let-down of milk. Fat content of hindmilk may rise to 6% or more, two or three times the concentration in foremilk.

Horizontal transmission Transmission of pathogens through direct contact. *See also*: Vertical transmission.

Human Immunodeficiency Virus (HIV) A retrovirus which disarms the body's immune system causing death from an opportunistic infection. First identified in 1981. The virus may be transmitted to unborn infants, and it is carried in the breastmilk, although not all breastfed infants born to HIV-positive mothers become ill themselves. The greatest risk to the infant is posed when a woman has her initial HIV-related illness while pregnant or breastfeeding.

Human milk Milk secreted in the human breast.

Human milk bank A service which collects, screens, processes, stores, and distributes donated human milk to meet the needs of those, usually infants, for whom human milk has been prescribed by a physician.

Human milk fortifiers Nutrients added to expressed human milk in order to enhance the growth and nutrient balances of very low-birth-weight infants. Added protein may be derived from protein components of donor human milk or from cow's-milk-based products. *See also*: Lactoengineering.

Hydration The water balance within a body. Adequate hydration is necessary to maintain normal body temperature and for most other metabolic functions. Breastmilk is 90% water. Therefore, even in hot or dry climates, a fully breastfed infant obtains all the water he requires through breastmilk.

Hyperalimentation The intravenous feeding of an infant, commonly a very premature infant, with a solution of amino acids, glucose, electrolytes, and vitamins.

Hyperosmolar A fluid that is of higher osmotic pressure than the reference fluid. Elemental formulas are hyperosmolar; breastmilk is iso-osmolar with human serum.

Hyper-prolactinemia Higher than normal prolactin levels, which may result in spontaneous breastmilk production and amenorrhea. Causes include pituitary tumors and some pharamaceuticals. *See also*: Prolactin.

Hypothalamus A gland which controls postpartum serum prolactin levels through release of dopamine. Inhibition of dopamine permits the release of prolactin, which controls the secretion of milk.

Immunity, active Immunity conferred by the production of antibodies by one's own immune system.

Immunity, passive Immunity conferred on an infant by antibodies manufactured by the mother and passed to the infant transplacentally or in breastmilk. Passive immunity is temporary but very important to the young infant.

Immunoassay Any method for the quantitative determination of chemical substances which uses the highly specific binding between antigen or hapten and homologous antibodies. E.g., radioimmunoassay, enzyme immunoassay, and fluoroimmunoassay.

Immunogen A substance which stimulates the body to form antibodies. *See also*: Antigen.

Immunoglobulin Proteins produced by plasma cells in response to an immunogen. The five types are IgG, IgA, IgM, IgE, and IgD. IgG is transferred in utero and provides passive immunity to infections to which the mother is immune; IgA is the principal immunoglobulin in colostrum and mature milk; IgM is produced by the neonate soon after birth and is also contained in breastmilk. *See also*: Non-casein protein.

Incubation period The period between exposure to infectious pathogens and the first signs of illness.

Infection control Practices—in hospitals formalized by protocols—which reduce the chance that infection will be spread between patients or between patients and staff. Handwashing and wearing of rubber gloves are two such practices.

International Code of Marketing of Breast-Milk Substitutes A set of resolutions which regulate the marketing and distribution of any fluid intended to replace breastmilk, certain devices used to feed such fluids, and the role of health-care workers who advise on infant feeding. Developed by members of a joint commission convened in 1979 by WHO and UNICEF, it was approved in 1981 by members of the World Health Organization (only the United States dissented). Intended as a voluntary model which could be incorporated into the legal code of individual nations in order to enhance national efforts to promote breastfeeding. Also referred to as the "WHO Code" or the "WHO/UNICEF Code."

Intracellular Occurring within cells. Viruses live within other cells during part of their reproductive lives. Although virus within cells may be passed to the infant in breastmilk, other cells in breastmilk enhance the destruction of these infected cells.

Intrauterine Within the uterus; in utero.

Intrauterine growth rate The normal rate of weight gain of a fetus. It is considered by many, but not all, physicians to be the ideal growth rate for premature infants.

Lactase Enzyme needed to convert lactose to simple sugars usable by the infant. Present from birth in the intestinal mucosa, its activity diminishes after weaning.

Lactase deficiency *See*: Lactose intolerance.

Lactiferous ducts Milk ducts. Fifteen to 24 tubes which collect milk from the smaller ductules and carry it to the nipple. They appear similar to stems on a bunch of grapes, the alveoli being the "grapes." The ducts open into nipple pores.

Lactiferous sinuses Dilations in the lactiferous ducts under the areola which act as small milk reservoirs. In order to nurse effectively, an infant must take enough breast into his mouth to be able to strip milk from these sinuses.

Lactobacillus bifidus Principal bacillus in the intestinal flora of breastfed infants. Low intestinal pH (5-6) of fully breastfed infants discourages the colonization of *Streptococcus faecalis*, *Bacteroides sp.* and *E. coli*, which are common in feces of infants fed cow's-milk-based infant milks.

Lactoengineering The process of fortifying human milk with nutrients derived from other batches of human milk, especially protein, calcium, and phosphorus, in order to meet the special nutritional needs of very low-birth-weight infants. *See also*: Human milk fortifiers.

Lactoferrin A protein which is an important immunological component of human milk. It binds iron in the intestinal tract, thus denying it to bacteria which require iron to survive. Exogenous iron may upset this balance. *See also*: Non-casein protein.

Lactogenesis The initiation of milk secretion. The initial synthesis of milk components which begins late in pregnancy may be termed lactogenesis I; the onset of copious milk production two or three days postpartum may be termed lactogenesis II.

Lactose The principal carbohydrate in human milk—about 4% of colostrum and 7% of mature milk. A disaccharide, it metabolizes readily to glucose, which is used for energy, and galactose, which assists lipids that are laid down in the brain. Lactose also enhances calcium absorption, thus helping prevent rickets in the breastfed infant, and it inhibits the growth of pathogens in the breastfed infant's intestine.

Lactose intolerance   The manifestation of lactase deficiency; the inability of the intestines to digest lactose, the principal carbohydrate in human milk. More common beyond early childhood because of diminished activity of intestinal lactase, especially in cultures which do not use milk or milk products as foods after early childhood.

Larynx   The region at the upper end of the trachea (windpipe) through which the voice is produced. In the infant, the larynx lies close to the base of the tongue; during swallowing it rises and is closed off by the epiglottis.

Lesion   Circumscribed area of injured or diseased skin.

Let-down   The milk-ejection reflex. Caused by contraction of myoepithelial cells surrounding the alveoli in which milk is secreted. It is under the control of oxytocin released during nipple stimulation and sometimes of psychological influences.

Leukocytes   Living cells, including macrophages and lymphocytes, which inhabit breastmilk and combat infection.

Licensure   The process whereby an agency of state government grants permission to an individual, who is accountable for the practice of a profession, to engage in that profession. The corollary of licensure is that unlicensed individuals are prohibited from legally practicing licensed professions. The purpose of licensure is to protect the public by ensuring professional competence.

Ligand   A small molecule that binds specifically to a larger molecule; e.g., the binding of an antigen to an antibody, or a hormone to a receptor.

Lipase   Enzyme which aids the digestion of milk fats by reducing them to a fine emulsion.

Low-birth-weight   Term applied to infants weighing less than 2500 gm at birth.

Lymphadenopathy   Abnormal swelling of lymph nodes.

Lymphocyte   A mature leukocyte; a lymph cell which is bactericidal.

Lyophilization   A process of rapid freeze drying of a fluid under a high vacuum. This process is used on human milk to obtain nutrient fractions used to fortify expressed human milk.

Lysozyme   Enzyme in breastmilk which is active against *E. coli* and *Salmonella*. *See also*: Non-casein protein.

Mammary bud   A clump of embryonic epithelial cells formed along the mammary ridge which extend into the underlying mesenchyme. It develops about 49 days postconception. From this bud sprout the precursors of the milk ducts.

Mammary ridge   Milk line. The linear thickening of epithelial cells to each side of the midline of the embryo. Develops during weeks five through eight. Later this ridge differentiates into breast and nipple tissue.

Mandible   The lower jaw. Strong, rhythmic closing of the mandible during breastfeeding drives the compression of the lacteriferous sinuses, one component of the infant's milking process.

Mature milk   Breastmilk commonly produced after about two weeks postpartum and containing no admixture of colostrum. It is higher in lactose, fat, and water-soluble vitamins. Its exact composition varies in response to infant needs.

Median   The middle number in a series of numbers; the number on either side of which exist an equal amount of numbers.

Mesenchyme   The embryonic mesoderm.

Mitosis   A type of cell division in which each daughter cell contains the same DNA as the parent cell.

Morbidity   The number of ill persons or instances of a disease in a specific population.

Mortality   The number of deaths in a specific population.

Mucocutaneous   Involving both mucous membranes and skin. Herpes blisters, for example, can form on both sites.

Multiparous   A woman who has carried two or more pregnancies to viability.

Myelination The process by which conducting nerve fibers develop a protective fatty sheath. The long-chain polyunsaturated fats which are important to myelination are abundant in human milk; they are much less abundant in cow's milk or cow's-milk-based infant milks. Loss of myelin is a characteristic of the disease multiple sclerosis.

Myoepithelial cells Contractile cells. In the breast these cells surround the milk-secreting alveoli; their contraction forces milk into the milk ducts. When many of these cells contract at the same time a "let-down" occurs. *See also*: Let-down.

Necrotizing enterocolitis Inflammation of the intestinal tract which may cause tissue to die. Premature infants not receiving human milk are at markedly greater risk for this serious complication of premature birth.

Neurotransmitter A chemical which is selectively released from a nerve terminal by an action potential and then interacts with a specific receptor on an adjacent structure to produce a specific physiologic response.

Nipple Cylindrical pigmented protuberance on the breast into which the lactiferous ducts open. The human nipple contains 15 to 20 nipple pores through which milk flows. The mammary papilla.

Nipple, inverted A nipple which is retracted into the breast both when at rest and when stimulated.

Non-casein protein The protein in the whey portion of milk. Non-casein proteins in human milk include alphalactalbumin, serum albumin, lactoferrin, immunoglobulins, and lysozyme.

Non-Governmental Organization (NGO) Title conferred by UNICEF on private organizations which command expertise valuable to UNICEF; such organizations are permitted to comment on and attempt to influence UNICEF activities. La Leche League International and the International Lactation Consultant Association are NGOs.

Nonprotein nitrogen (NPN) About one-fourth of the total nitrogen in human milk is derived from sources, such as urea, other than protein. NPN contains several free amino acids, including leucine, valine, and threonine, which are essential in the young infant's diet because he cannot yet manufacture them.

Nutriment Any nourishing substance.

Oligosaccharide Carbohydrate, comprised of a few monosaccharides, present in human milk. Some oligosaccharides promote the growth of *Lactobacillus bifidus*, thus increasing intestinal acidity, which discourages the growth of intestinal pathogens.

Oral rehydration therapy (ORT) The administration by mouth of a solution of water, salt, and sugar in order to replace body fluids lost during severe diarrhea. The proportions of elements in an oral rehydration solution are essentially the same as they are in breastmilk. Artificially fed infants are much more susceptible than those who are breastfed to the diarrhea which may lead to severe dehydration and the need for ORT.

Oxytocin A lactogenic hormone produced in the posterior pituitary gland. It is released during suckling (or other nipple stimulation) and causes ejection of milk as well as uterine contractions.

Palate, hard The hard, anterior roof of the mouth. A suckling infant uses his tongue to compress breast tissue against the hard palate.

Palate, soft The soft, posterior roof of the mouth, which lies between the hard palate and the throat. It rises during swallowing to close off nasal passages. The velum.

Parenchyma The functional parts of an organ. In the breast, the parenchyma include the mammary ducts, lobes, and alveoli.

Parenteral Introduction of fluids, nutrients, or drugs into the body by any avenue other than the digestive tract.

Pasteurization The heating of milk to destroy pathogens. Milk banks commonly heat donor milk to 56°C for 30 minutes.

Pathogen Substance or organism capable of producing illness.

Peristalsis Involuntary, rhythmic, wave-like action. Commonly thought of in relation to food and waste products moving along the gastrointestinal tract. In order to strip milk from the breast, an infant's tongue utilizes a peristaltic motion which begins at the tip of the tongue and progresses towards the back of the mouth.

Pharynx The muscular tube at the rear of the mouth, through which nasal air travels to the larynx and food from the mouth travels to the esophagus. During infant feeding, contraction of pharyngeal muscles moves a bolus of fluid into the esophagus.

Pituitary An endocrine gland at the base of the brain which secretes several hormones. Prolactin, which is essential for production of milk, is secreted by the anterior lobe; oxytocin, which is essential for milk let-down, is secreted by the posterior lobe.

Placenta The intrauterine organ which transfers nutrients from the mother to the fetus. The expulsion of the placenta at birth causes an abrupt drop in estrogen and progesterone, which in turn permits the secretion of milk.

Polymastia The presence of more than two breasts. These additional structures, which usually contain only a small amount of glandular tissue, may occur anywhere along the milk line from axilla to groin.

Premature infant One born before 37 weeks gestational age, regardless of birth weight.

Primary infection The first incidence of illness after exposure to a pathogen.

Primiparous A woman who has carried one pregnancy to viability.

Progesterone Hormone produced by the corpus luteum and placenta which maintains a pregnancy and helps develop the mammary alveoli.

Prolactin Hormone which is produced in the anterior pituitary gland. It stimulates development of the breast and controls milk synthesis. Normal concentrations are 10–25 ng/ml in a nonpregnant woman; 200–400 ng/ml at birth.

Prone Lying on one's stomach.

Respiratory syncytial virus (RSV) Organism causing a respiratory illness; breastfed infants are at less risk for this illness.

Rickets Abnormal calcification of the bones and changes in growth plates which lead to soft or weak bones. Rarely seen in breastfed children; exceptions include those not exposed to the sun.

Rotavirus A class of viruses which are a major cause of diarrheal illness leading to hospitalization of infants. Breastfed infants are at less risk for illness caused by this organism.

Rugae Corrugations on the hard palate behind the gum ridge which help the infant to retain a grasp on the breast during suckling.

Sebaceous glands Glands which secrete oil. Those on the areola are called tubercles of Montgomery. The oil they secrete is presumed to lubricate and provide bacteriostatic protection to the areola.

Secretory IgA An immunoglobulin abundant in human milk which is of immense value to the neonate. It is synthesized and stored in the breast; after ingestion by the infant it blocks adhesion of pathogens to the intestinal mucosa.

Secretory immune system The system which produces specific antibodies or thymus-influenced lymphocytes in response to specific antigens.

Sepsis The presence of bacteria in fluid or tissue.

Seroconvert For serum to show the presence of a factor which previously has been absent, or the reverse. When antibodies to an infecting agent such as cytomegalovirus become present, the person is said to have seroconverted.

Serological tests Tests performed on blood samples to ascertain the presence or absence of pathogens.

Seronegative Serum which does not demonstrate the presence of a factor tested for; "tests negative."

Seropositive Serum which demonstrates the presence of a factor tested for; "tests positive."

Serum Clear fluid portion of blood which remains after coagulation.

Serum albumin A protein in serum. *See also*: Noncasein protein.

Smooth muscle The type of muscle which provides the erectile tissue in the nipple and areola.

Somatic Pertaining to the body, especially nonreproductive tissue.

Spontaneous lactation Secretion and release of milk unrelated to a pregnancy or to nipple stimulation intended to stimulate milk production.

Suck, Suckle Used in this textbook interchangeably to mean the baby's milking action at the breast. In traditional usage, a baby at the breast "sucked," while a mother "suckled."

Sucking, non-nutritive Sucking not at the breast—e.g., as on a pacifier or on baby's own tongue. Or sucking at the breast characterized by alternating brief sucks and long rest periods during minimal milk flow. However, insofar as any milk is transferred, even this latter pattern of sucking may in fact be nutritive. *See also*: Sucking, nutritive.

Sucking, nutritive Steady rhythmic sucking during full, continuous milk flow. Insofar as any milk is transferred, other sucking patterns also may be nutritive. *See also*: Sucking, non-nutritive.

Symbiosis The intimate association of two different kinds of organisms. The breastfeeding dyad is considered by many to exemplify a mutually beneficial symbiosis.

Systemic immune system The nonspecific immune responses of the body.

T-cells Any of several kinds of thymic lymphoid cells or lymphocytes which help regulate cellular immune response. A subset of these cells (T4-cells) are preferentially attacked by Human Immunodeficiency Virus.

Teleological Describing the belief that all events are directed toward some ultimate purpose.

Thrombocytopenia Low levels of platelets in blood.

TORCH Acronym for organisms which can damage the fetus: Toxoplasmosis, Rubella, Cytomegalovirus, Herpes simplex.

Tracheoesophageal fistula (T-E fistula) An abnormal opening between the trachea and esophagus; this congenital malformation occurs in about 1:3000 births. T-E fistula may cause a neonate to aspirate fluids. Colostrum, a physiologic fluid, is much less irritating to the lungs than water, glucose water, or artificial infant milks.

Transcutaneous bilimeter A device which estimates bilirubin concentrations in the blood by measuring intensity of yellowish skin coloration.

Transitional milk Breast fluid of continuously varying composition produced in the first two-to-three weeks postpartum as colostrum decreases and milk production increases.

Transplacental Transferred from mother to fetus through the placenta. Nutrients and certain immunoglobulins are, and some infections may also be, transferred to the fetus transplacentally.

United Nations Childrens' Fund (UNICEF) Originally established in 1946 as the United Nations International Childrens' Emergency Fund. An agency of the United Nations charged with protecting the lives of children and enabling them to lead fuller lives. It assists member nations in providing health care, safe water, sanitation, nutrition, housing, education, and training to accomplish these goals.

Universal precautions Guidelines for infection control based on the assumption that every person receiving health care carries an infection which can be transmitted by blood, body fluids, or genital secretions.

Vaccine An infectious agent, or derivatives of one, given to a person so that his immune system will produce antibodies to that infection without a preceding illness.

Vertical transmission Transmission of infection from mother to child transplacentally or through breastmilk.

Very low-birth-weight Term applied to infants weighing less than 1500 gm at birth.

Virus Very small organisms which rely on material in invaded cells to reproduce. Viruses identified in breastmilk include cytomegalovirus, *Herpes zoster* and *Herpes simplex*, hepatitis, and rubella.

Water-soluble vitamins The B vitamins and vitamin C; pantothenic acid, biotin, and folate. These vitamins are present in serum; concentrations in breastmilk approximate those in serum. Concentrations reflect current maternal diet more directly than do fat-soluble vitamins (A, D, E, K).

Wet nurses   Women who breastfeed for pay infants who are not their own.

Whey   The liquid left after curds are separated from milk. Alphalactalbumin and lactoferrin are the principal whey proteins. Because human milk has a whey-to-casein ratio of about 65:35, it forms soft, easily digested curds in the infant stomach. *See also*: Casein; Non-casein protein.

Witch's milk   Colostrum, formed under the influ-ence of maternal hormones, which may be ex-pressed from temporarily enlarged mammary tissue in the neonate's breasts.

World Health Organization (WHO)   An agency of the United Nations charged with planning and coor-dinating global health care, as well as assisting mem-ber nations to combat disease and train health work-ers.

Xeropthalmia   Disease of the eyes caused by vita-min-A deficiency; it is endemic in parts of Africa. Human milk is a preventive.

Medical Abbreviations

>	greater than
<	less than
=	equal to
$\bar{a}$	before
ab	abortion
ABC	alternative birthing center
abd	abdomen
ABG	arterial blood gases
AIDS	Acquired Immunodeficiency Syndrome
BBT	basal body temperature
Bf	breastfed/breastfeeding
B/P	blood pressure
BPD	bronchopulmonary dysplasia
BSE	breast self-examination
BUN	blood urea nitrogen
C	centigrade
$\bar{c}$	with
CA	cancer
Ca	calcium
cal	calorie
CHD	congenital heart disease
CBC	complete blood count
cc	cubic centimeter
CMV	cytomegalovirus
CNS	central nervous system
CPAP	continuous positive airway pressure
C&S	culture and sensitivity
c/sec	cesarean birth
CNM	certified nurse-midwife

CSF	cerebral spinal fluid
CVA	cardiovascular accident
CVP	central venous pressure
D5W	5% dextrose in water
D&C	dilation and curettage
D/C	discharge
dc	discontinue
DR	delivery room
DRG	diagnostic related groups
dx	diagnosis
ECG	electrocardiogram
EDC	estimated date of confinement (due date)
EDD	estimated date of delivery
EEG	electroencephalogram
epis	episiotomy
EENT	eyes, ears, nose, throat
EFM	electronic fetal monitoring
ER	emergency room
ET	endotracheal tube
FAS	fetal alcohol syndrome
FBD	fibrocystic breast disease
FBS	fasting blood sugar
FLK	funny looking kid
FSH	follicular stimulating hormone
FTT	failure to thrive
FUO	fever of unknown origin
GDM	gestational diabetes mellitus
GI	gastrointestinal
gm	gram
gr	grain

grav	gravida (number of pregnancies)		p̄	after
GU	genitourinary		para	number of living children
GYN	gynecology		pc	after meals (refers to *post cibum*)
			PDA	patent ductus arteriosus
hct	hematocrit		peri	perineal
Hg	mercury		pH	degree of acidity/alkalinity
H&P	history and physical		PID	pelvic inflammatory disease
ht	height			
hx	history		PIH	pregnancy-induced hypertension
			PKU	phenylketonuria
IDDM	insulin-dependent diabetes mellitus		po	by mouth
IUGR	intrauterine growth retardation		prn	as needed
IM	intramuscular		PT	physical therapist
I&O	intake and output			
IUD	intrauterine device		q	every, each
IV	intravenous		qd	every day
			qid	4 times/day
JCAH	Joint Commission on the Accreditation of Hospitals		Ⓡ	right
			RBC	red blood cell
Kg	kilogram		RDA	recommended dietary allowances
			RDS	respiratory distress syndrome
L	liter		REM	rapid eye movement
Ⓛ	left		Rh	rhesus blood factor
lab	laboratory		R/O	rule out
LC	lactation consultant		Rx	medication/prescription
LGA	large for gestational age			
LMP	last menstrual period		s̄	without
			SGA	small for gestational age
Mcg	microgram		SIDS	sudden infant death syndrome
mec	meconium		SOAP	subjective data, objective data, analysis, plan
med	medication			
mg	milligram		staph	staphylococcus
ml	milliliter		STD	sexually transmitted disease
			strep	streptococcus
NANDA	North American Nursing Diagnosis Association			
			tid	3 times/day
NEC	necrotizing enterocolitis			
n/g	nasogastric		u/a	urinalysis
NPO	nothing by mouth		URI	upper respiratory infection
nsg	nursing (breastfeeding)		UTI	urinary tract infection
Ø	no, none		VBAC	vaginal birth after cesarean
OB	obstetrical			
OT	occupational therapy		WBC	white blood cell
OTC	over the counter		WIC	special supplemental food program for women, infants, and children
oz	ounce			

Index

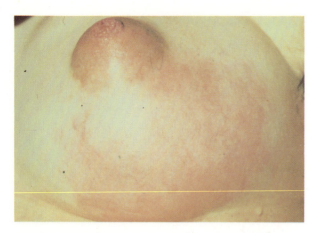

Mastitis. Involving the lower outer quadrant of the breast. The mother was placed on IV antibiotics in the hospital; lactation continued throughout the IV therapy. Her baby was housed with her during her hospitalization.

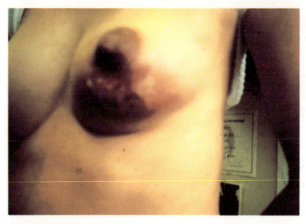

Breast Abscess. At the 4–8 o'clock position, following spontaneous rupture and drainage of purulent material. Breastfeeding continued throughout the period of healing of the abscess and for many months thereafter. (With permission from Beth Israel Medical Center, New York.)

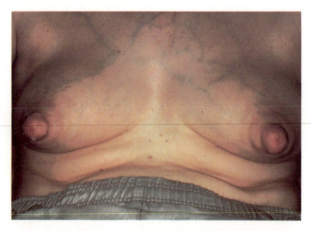

Veining of the breast. A lactating mother 26 weeks postpartum with prominent veining characteristic of lactation. (With permission from Chele Marmet.)

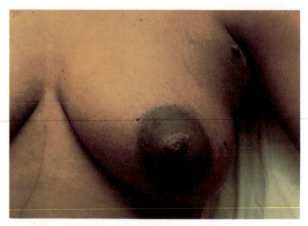

Auxiliary breast and nipple tissue. A common site for additional breast or nipple tissue. In the absence of stimulation, milk production and tissue swelling ceases.

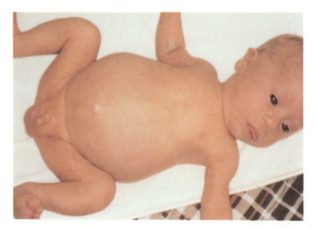

Baby with Down syndrome. Note the small genitalia characteristic of a child with Down syndrome. Poor head and neck control, weak jaw and other motor ability and a poor suck often require special assistance while the baby is learning how to suckle the breast. (With permission from Chele Marmet.)

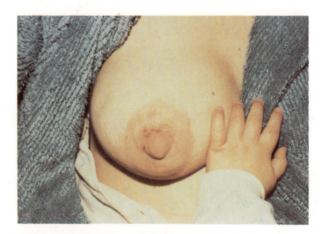

Herpes on the Areola. A 13-month-old nursing toddler contracted oral herpes by using a playmate's contaminated rattle. The mother then was infected. The breast lesion appeared soon after the baby's infection was identified. (With permission from Chele Marmet.)